ANTIBODIES

| Stimulation | Serology | | Comp. Binding | Immunoglobin Class | | Optimum Temperature | Clinical Significance | | Comments |
	Saline	AHG		IgM	IgG		HTR	HDN	
RBC	occ	yes	no	occ	yes	warm	yes	yes	Very rarely IgA anti-D may be produced; however, this is invariably with IgG.
RBC	occ	yes	no	occ	yes	warm	yes	yes	
RBC/NRBC	occ	yes	no	occ	yes	warm	yes	yes	Anti-E may often occur without obvious immune stimulation.
RBC	occ	yes	no	occ	yes	warm	yes	yes	
RBC	occ	yes	no	occ	yes	warm	yes	yes	Warm autoantibodies often appear to have anti-e-like specificity.
RBC	occ	yes	no	occ	yes	warm	yes	yes	
RBC	occ	yes	no	occ	yes	warm	yes	yes	
RBC/NRBC	occ	yes	no	occ	yes	warm	yes	yes	Anti-C^w may often occur without obvious immune stimulation.
RBC	occ	yes	no	occ	yes	warm	yes	yes	
RBC	occ	yes	no	occ	yes	warm	yes	yes	Antibodies to V and VS present problems only in the black population, where the antigen frequencies are in the order of 30 to 32.
RBC	occ	yes	no	occ	yes	warm	yes	yes	
RBC	occ	yes	some	occ	yes	warm	yes	yes	Some antibodies to Kell system have been reported to react poorly in low ionic media.
RBC	no	yes	no	rarely	yes	warm	yes	yes	
RBC	no	yes	no	no	yes	warm	yes	yes	Kell system antigens are destroyed by AET and by ZZAP.
RBC	rarely	yes	no	rarely	yes	warm	yes	yes	
RBC	rarely	yes	no	rarely	yes	warm	yes	yes	Anti-K1 has been reported to occur following bacterial infection.
RBC	no	yes	no	no	yes	warm	yes	yes	
RBC	no	yes	no	occ	yes	warm	yes	yes	The lack of Kx expression on RBCs and WBCs has been associated with the McLeod phenotype and CGD.
RBC	rare	yes	some	rare	yes	warm	yes	yes	Fy^a and Fy^b antigens are destroyed by enzymes. Fy (a–b–) cells are resistant to invasion by *P. vivax* merozoites, a malaria-causing parasite.
RBC	rare	yes	some	rare	yes	warm	yes	yes	
RBC	no	yes	rarely	no	yes	warm	yes	yes	FY3 and 5 are not destroyed by enzymes.
RBC	no	yes	?	no	yes	warm			FY5 may be formed by interaction of Rh and Duffy gene products. FY6 is a monoclonal antibody which reacts with most human red cells except Fy(a–b–) and is responsible for susceptibility of cells to penetration by *P. vivax*.

(Continued on inside back cover)

Modern Blood Banking & Transfusion Practices

SIXTH EDITION

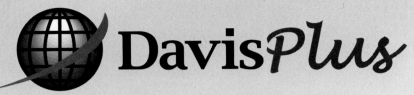
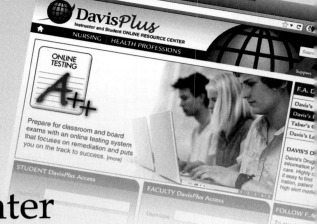
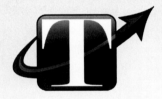

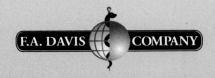

Modern Blood Banking & Transfusion Practices

SIXTH EDITION

Denise Harmening, PhD, MT(ASCP)
Director of the Online Masters in Clinical Laboratory Management
Adjunct Professor, Department of Medical Laboratory Science
College of Health Sciences
Rush University
Chicago, Illinois, USA

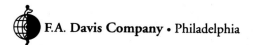 F.A. Davis Company • Philadelphia

F. A. Davis Company
1915 Arch Street
Philadelphia, PA 19103
www.fadavis.com

Copyright © 2012 by F. A. Davis Company

Printed in the United States of America

Last digit indicates print number: 10 9 8 7 6 5 4 3 2 1

Senior Acquisitions Editor: Christa Fratantoro
Manager of Content Development: George W. Lang
Developmental Editor: Nancy J. Peterson
Art and Design Manager: Carolyn O'Brien

As new scientific information becomes available through basic and clinical research, recommended treatments and drug therapies undergo changes. The author(s) and publisher have done everything possible to make this book accurate, up to date, and in accord with accepted standards at the time of publication. The author(s), editors, and publisher are not responsible for errors or omissions or for consequences from application of the book, and make no warranty, expressed or implied, in regard to the contents of the book. Any practice described in this book should be applied by the reader in accordance with professional standards of care used in regard to the unique circumstances that may apply in each situation. The reader is advised always to check product information (package inserts) for changes and new information regarding dose and contraindications before administering any drug. Caution is especially urged when using new or infrequently ordered drugs.

Library of Congress Cataloging-in-Publication Data

Modern blood banking & transfusion practices / [edited by] Denise Harmening.—6th ed.
    p. ; cm.
Modern blood banking and transfusion practices
Rev. ed. of: Modern blood banking and transfusion practices / [edited by] Denise M. Harmening. c2005.
Includes bibliographical references and index.
ISBN 978-0-8036-2682-9–ISBN 0-8036-2682-7
I. Harmening, Denise. II. Modern blood banking and transfusion practices. III. Title: Modern blood banking and transfusion practices.
[DNLM: 1. Blood Banks—methods. 2. Blood Grouping and Crossmatching. 3. Blood Transfusion—methods. WH 460]

615'.39—dc23

2011047863

*To all students—full-time, part-time, past, present,
and future—who have touched and will continue to
touch the lives of so many educators. . . .*

**It is to you this book is dedicated in the hope of
inspiring an unquenchable thirst for knowledge and
love of mankind.**

Foreword

Blood groups were discovered more than 100 years ago, but most of them have been recognized only in the past 50 years. Although transfusion therapy was used soon after the ABO blood groups were discovered, it was not until after World War II that blood transfusion science really started to become an important branch of medical science in its own right. In order to advance, transfusion science needs to be nurtured with a steady flow of new knowledge generated from research. This knowledge then must be applied at the bench.

To understand and best take advantage of the continual flow of new information generated by blood transfusion scientists and to apply it to everyday work in the blood bank, technologists and pathologists must have a solid understanding of basic immunology, genetics, biochemistry (particularly membrane chemistry), and the physiology and function of blood cells. High standards are always expected and strived for by technologists who work in blood banks and transfusion services. I strongly believe that technologists should understand the principles behind the tests they are performing, rather than performing tasks as a machine does.

Because of this, I do not think that "cookbook" technical manuals have much value in *teaching* technologists; they do have a place as reference books in the laboratory. During the years (too many to put in print) that I have been involved in teaching medical technologists, it has been very difficult to select one book that covers all of the information that technologists in training need to know about blood transfusion science without confusing them.

Dr. Denise Harmening has produced that single volume. She has been involved in teaching medical technologists for most of her career. After seeing how she has arranged this book, I would guess that her teaching philosophies are close to my own. She has gathered a group of experienced scientists and teachers who, along with herself, cover all of the important areas of blood transfusion science.

The chapters included in Part I, "Fundamental Concepts" (including a section on molecular phenotyping), provide a firm base on which the student can learn the practical and technical importance of the other chapters. The chapters in Part II, "Blood Groups and Serologic Testing," and Part III, "Transfusion Practice" (including a new chapter on cellular therapy), provide enough information for medical technologists without overwhelming them with esoteric and clinical details. Part IV covers leukocyte antigens and relationship (parentage) testing. The chapters in Part V, "Quality and Compliance Issues" (including new chapters on utilization management and tissue banking), complete the scope of transfusion science. Part VI: Future Trends describes tissue banking as a new role for the transfusion service.

Although this book is designed primarily for medical technologists, I believe it is admirably suited to pathology residents, hematology fellows, and others who want to review any aspect of modern blood banking and transfusion practices.

GEORGE GARRATTY, PhD, FIBMS, FRCPath
Scientific Director
American Red Cross Blood Services
Southern California Region
and
Clinical Professor of Pathology and Laboratory Medicine
University of California, Los Angeles

Preface

This book is designed to provide the medical technologist, blood bank specialist, and resident with a concise and thorough guide to transfusion practices and immunohematology. This text, a perfect "crossmatch" of theory and practice, provides the reader with a working knowledge of routine blood banking. Forty-four contributors from across the country have shared their knowledge and expertise in 28 comprehensive chapters. More than 500 illustrations and tables facilitate the comprehension of difficult concepts not routinely illustrated in other texts. In addition, color plates provide a means for standardizing the reading of agglutination reactions.

Several features of this textbook offer great appeal to students and educators, including chapter outlines and educational objectives at the beginning of each chapter; case studies, review questions, and summary charts at the end of each chapter; and an extensive and convenient glossary for easy access to definitions of blood bank terms.

A blood group Antigen-Antibody Characteristic Chart is provided on the inside cover of the book to aid in retention of the vast amount of information and serve as a review of the characteristics of the blood group systems. Original, comprehensive step-by-step illustrations of ABO forward and reverse grouping, not found in any other book, help the student to master this important testing, which represents the foundation of blood banking.

The sixth edition has been reorganized and divided into the following sections:

- Part I: Fundamental Concepts
- Part II: Blood Groups and Serologic Testing
- Part III: Transfusion Practice
- Part IV: Leukocyte Antigens and Relationship Testing
- Part V: Quality and Compliance Issues
- Part VI: Future Trends

In Part I, the introduction to the historical aspects of red blood cell and platelet preservation serves as a prelude to the basic concepts of genetics, blood group immunology, and molecular biology (including molecular phenotyping). Part II focuses on blood groups and routine blood bank practices and includes the chapters "Detection and Identification of Antibodies" and "Pretransfusion Testing." It also covers current technologies and automation.

Part III, "Transfusion Practice," includes a new chapter called "Cellular Therapy" and covers the more traditional topics of donor screening, component preparation, transfusion therapy, transfusion reactions, and apheresis. Certain clinical situations that are particularly relevant to blood banking are also discussed in detail in this section, including hemolytic disease of the fetus and newborn, autoimmune hemolytic anemias, and transfusion-transmitted diseases.

The human leukocyte antigens system and relationship testing are discussed in Part IV of the book. In Part V, quality and compliance issues are discussed, including a new chapter on utilization management. The chapters on quality management, transfusion safety and federal regulatory requirements, laboratory information systems, and legal and ethical considerations complete the scope of practice for transfusion services. Also included is the chapter "Tissue Banking: A New Role for the Transfusion Service," which introduces another responsibility already in place in several institutions.

This book is a culmination of the tremendous efforts of many dedicated professionals who participated in this project by donating their time and expertise because they care about the blood bank profession. The book's intention is to foster improved patient care by providing the reader with a basic understanding of modern blood banking and transfusion practices. The sixth edition is designed to generate an unquenchable thirst for knowledge in all medical technologists, blood bankers, and practitioners, whose education, knowledge, and skills provide the public with excellent health care.

DENISE M. HARMENING, PhD, MT(ASCP)

Contributors

Robert W. Allen, PhD
Director of Forensic Sciences
Center for Health Sciences
Oklahoma State University
Tulsa, Oklahoma, USA

Lucia M. Berte, MA, MT(ASCP)SBB, DLM; CQA(ASQ)CMQ/OE
President
Laboratories Made Better! P.C.
Broomfield, Colorado, USA

Maria P. Bettinotti, PhD
Director, HLA & Immunogenetics Department
Quest Diagnostics Nichols Institute
Chantilly, Virginia, USA

Cara Calvo, MS, MT(ASCP)SH
Medical Technology Program Director and Lecturer
Department of Laboratory Medicine
University of Washington
Seattle, Washington, USA

Lorraine Caruccio, PhD, MT(ASCP)SBB
National Institutes of Health
Rockville, Maryland, USA

Judy Ellen Ciaraldi, BS, MT(ASCP)SBB, CQA(ASQ)
Consumer Safety Officer
Division of Blood Applications
Office of Blood Research and Review
Center for Biologics Evaluation and Research
U.S. Food and Drug Administration
Rockville, Maryland, USA

Julie L. Cruz, MD
Associate Medical Director
Indiana Blood Center
Indianapolis, Indiana, USA

Paul James Eastvold, MD, MT(ASCP)
Chief Medical Officer
American Red Cross
Lewis and Clark Region
Salt Lake City, Utah, USA

Glenda A. Forneris, MHS, MT(ASCP)SBB
Program Director/Professor
Medical Laboratory Technology Program
Kankakee Community College
Kankakee, Illinois, USA

Ralph E. B. Green
Associate Professor
Discipline and Program Leader
Discipline of Laboratory Medicine
School of Medical Sciences
RMIT University
Melbourne, Australia

Steven F. Gregurek, MD
Assistant Professor
Clarian Health
Indianapolis, Indiana, USA

Denise Harmening, PhD, MT(ASCP)
Director of the Online Masters in Clinical Laboratory Management
Adjunct Professor, Department of Medical Laboratory Science
College of Health Sciences
Rush University
Chicago, Illinois, USA

Chantal Ricaud Harrison, MD
Professor of Pathology
University of Texas Health Sciences Center at San Antonio
San Antonio, Texas, USA

Elizabeth A. Hartwell, MD, MT(ASCP)SBB
Medical Director
Gulf Coast Regional Blood Center
Houston, Texas, USA

Darlene M. Homkes, MT(ASCP)
Senior Technologist for Transfusion Services
St. Joseph Hospital
Kokomo, Indiana, USA

Virginia C. Hughes, MS, MLS(ASCP)SBB
Director/Assistant Professor
Medical Laboratory Sciences
Dixie State College of Utah
St. George, Utah

Patsy C. Jarreau, MLS(ASCP)
Program Director and Associate Professor
Department of Clinical Laboratory Sciences
School of Allied Health Professions
Louisiana State University Health Sciences Center
New Orleans, Louisiana, USA

Susan T. Johnson, MSTM, MT(ASCP)SBB
Director: Department of Clinical Education and Specialist in Blood Banking (SBB) Program, Blood Center of Wisconsin
Director and Adjunct Associate Professor:
Marquette University Graduate School, Transfusion Medicine Program
Clinical Associate Professor: University of Wisconsin-Milwaukee, College of Health Sciences
Associate Director: Indian Immunohematology Initiative
Milwaukee, Wisconsin, USA

Melanie S. Kennedy, MD
Clinical Associate Professor Emeritus
Department of Pathology
College of Medicine
The Ohio State University
Columbus, Ohio, USA

Dwane A. Klostermann, MSTM, MT(ASCP)SBB
Clinical Laboratory Technician Instructor
Moraine Park Technical College
Fond du Lac, Wisconsin, USA

Barbara Kraj, MS, MLS(ASCP)CM
Assistant Professor
Georgia Health Sciences University
College of Allied Health Sciences
Department of Medical Laboratory, Imaging, and Radiologic Sciences
Augusta, Georgia, USA

Regina M. Leger, MSQA, MT(ASCP)SBB, CMQ/OE(ASQ)
Research Associate II
American Red Cross Blood Services
Southern California Region
Pomona, California, USA

Ileana Lopez-Plaza, MD
Division Head, Transfusion Medicine
Department of Pathology and Laboratory Medicine
Henry Ford Health System
Detroit, Michigan, USA

Holli Mason, MD
Director, Transfusion Medicine and Serology
Director, Pathology Residency Training Program
Harbor UCLA Medical Center
Associate Clinical Professor
David Geffen School of Medicine at UCLA
Torrance, California, USA

Gerald P. Morris, MD, PhD
Research Instructor
Department of Pathology and Immunology
Washington University School of Medicine
Saint Louis, Missouri, USA

Donna L. Phelan, BA, CHS(ASHI), MT(HEW)
Technical Supervisor
HLA Laboratory
Barnes-Jewish Hospital
St. Louis, Missouri, USA

Christine Pitocco, MS, MT(ASCP)BB
Clinical Assistant Professor
Clinical Laboratory Science Program
School of Health Technology and Management
Stony Brook University
Stony Brook, New York, USA

Valerie Polansky, MEd, MLS(ASCP)CM
Retired Program Director
Medical Laboratory Technology Program
St. Petersburg College
St. Petersburg, Florida, USA

Karen Rodberg, MBA, MT(ASCP)SBB
Director, Reference Services
American Red Cross Blood Services
Southern California Region
Pomona, California, USA

Susan Ruediger, MLT, CSMLS
Senior Medical Technologist
Henry Ford Cottage Hospital
Henry Ford Health System
Grosse Pointe Farms, Michigan, USA

Kathleen Sazama, MD, JD, MS, MT(ASCP)
Chief Medical Officer
LifeSouth Community Blood Centers, Inc.
Gainesville, Florida, USA

Scott Scrape, MD
Assistant Professor of Pathology
Director, Transfusion Medicine Service
The Ohio State University Medical Center
Columbus, Ohio, USA

Burlin Sherrick, MT(ASCP)SBB
Blood Bank Supervisor and Adjunct Clinical Instructor
Lima Memorial Hospital
Lima, Ohio

Ann Tiehen, MT(ASCP) SBB
Education Coordinator (f), Retired
North Shore University Health System
Evanston Hospital
Department of Pathology and Laboratory Medicine
Evanston, Illinois, USA

Kathleen S. Trudell, MLS(ASCP)CM SBBCM
Clinical Coordinator–Immunohematology
Clinical Laboratory Science Program
University of Nebraska Medical Center
Omaha, Nebraska, USA

Phyllis S. Walker, MS, MT(ASCP)SBB
Manager, Immunohematology Reference Laboratory, Retired
Blood Centers of the Pacific
San Francisco, California, USA

Merilyn Wiler, MA, MT(ASCP)SBB
Customer Regulatory Support Specialist
Terumo BCT
Lakewood, Colorado

Alan E. Williams, PhD
Associate Director for Regulatory Affairs
Office of Blood Research and Review
Center for Biologics Evaluation and Research
U.S. Food and Drug Administration
Silver Spring, Maryland, USA

Elizabeth F. Williams, MHS, MLS(ASCP)^{CM}, SBB
Associate Professor
Department of Clinical Laboratory Sciences
School of Allied Health Professions
LSU Health Sciences Center
New Orleans, Louisiana, USA

Scott Wise, MHA, MLS(ASCP), SBB
Assistant Professor and Translational Research Laboratory Manager
Medical College of Georgia
Department of Biomedical and Radiological Technologies
Augusta, Georgia, USA

Gregory Wright, MT(ASCP)SBB
Manager, Blood Banks
North Shore University Health System
Evanston, Illinois, USA

Patricia A. Wright, BA, MT(ASCP)SBB
Blood Bank Supervisor
Signature Healthcare-Brockton Hospital
Brockton, Massachusetts, USA

Michele B. Zitzmann, MHS, MLS(ASCP)
Associate Professor
Department of Clinical Laboratory Sciences
LSU Health Sciences Center
New Orleans, Louisiana, USA

William B. Zundel, MS, MLS(ASCP)^{CM}, SBB
Associate Teaching Professor
Clinical Laboratory Sciences Department
Associate Professor
Department. of Microbiology and Molecular Biology
Brigham Young University
Provo, Utah, USA

Reviewers

Terese M. Abreu, MA, MLS(ASCP)^{CM}
Director, Clinical Laboratory Science Program
College of Arts and Sciences
Heritage University
Toppenish, Washington, USA

Deborah Brock, MHS, MT(ASCP)SH
Instructor, Medical Laboratory Technology Program
Allied Health Department
Faculty Liaison for Professional Development
Academic Affairs Department
Tri-County Technical College
Pendleton, South Carolina, USA

Lynne Brodeur, MA, BS (CLS)
Lecturer
Department of Medical Laboratory Science
College of Arts & Sciences
University of Massachusetts–Dartmouth
North Dartmouth, Massachusetts, USA

Cynthia Callahan, MEd, MLS(ASCP)
Program Head, Medical Laboratory Technology
School of Health & Public Services
Stanly Community College
Locust, North Carolina, USA

Kay Doyle, PhD, MLS(ASCP)^{CM}
Professor and Program Director, Clinical Laboratory Sciences/Medical
Laboratory Science
Department of Clinical Laboratory and Nutritional Sciences
University of Massachusetts–Lowell
Lowell, Massachusetts, USA

Joyce C. Foreman, MS(CLS), MT(ASCP)SBB
Blood Bank Team Leader
Clinical Laboratory Department
Baptist Medical Center South
Montgomery, Alabama, USA

Michelle Lancaster Gagan, MSHS, MT(ASCP)
Instructor/Education Coordinator
Medical Laboratory Technology Program
Health and Human Services Department
York Technical College
Rock Hill, South Carolina, USA

Wyenona Hicks, MS, MT(ASCP)SBB
Assistant Professor, Program in Clinical Laboratory Sciences
College of Allied Health Sciences
University of Tennessee Health Science Center
Memphis, Tennessee, USA
Adjunct Faculty, Online Specialist in Blood Bank (SBB) Certificate Program
Rush University
Chicago, Illinois, USA

Shelly Hitchcox, RT (CSLT)
Medical Technologist
Blood Bank Department
Fletcher Allen Healthcare
Burlington, Vermont, USA

Judith A. Honsinger, MT(ASCP)
Associate Professor
Health & Human Services Department
River Valley Community College
Claremont, New Hampshire, USA

Fang Yao Stephen Hou, MB(ASCP)QCYM, PhD
Assistant Professor, Clinical Laboratory Science Department
College of Health Sciences
Marquette University
Milwaukee, Wisconsin, USA

Stephen M. Johnson, MS, MT(ASCP)
Program Director, School of Medical Technology
Saint Vincent Health Center
Erie, Pennsylvania, USA

Vanessa Jones Johnson, MBA, MA, MT(ASCP)
Program Director, Pathology & Laboratory Medicine Service
Overton Brooks VA Medical Center
Shreveport, Louisiana, USA

Douglas D Kikendall, MT(ASCP)
Blood Bank/Phlebotomy Supervisor
CLS Instructor, Blood Bank Department
Yakima Regional Hospital
Yakima, Washington, USA

Judith S. Levitt, MT(ASCP)SBB
Clinical Laboratory Manager
DeGowin Blood Center, Department of Pathology
University of Iowa Hospitals and Clinics
Iowa City, Iowa, USA

Beverly A. Marotto, MT(ASCP)SBB
Blood Bank Manager, Blood Bank Department
Lahey Clinic
Burlington, Massachusetts, USA

Tina McDaniel, MA, MT(ASCP)
Program Director, Medical Laboratory Technology
School of Health, Wellness, & Public Safety
Davidson County Community College
Thomasville, North Carolina, USA

Dora E. Meraz, MEd, MT(ASCP)
Laboratory Coordinator, Clinical Laboratory Sciences Program
College of Health Sciences
The University of Texas at El Paso
El Paso, Texas, USA

Gretchen L. Miller, MS, MT(ASCP)
MLT Program Director, Assistant Professor
Brevard Community College
Heath Science Institute
Cocoa, Florida, USA

Janis Nossaman, MT(ASCP)SBB
Manager, Donor Collections and Transfusion Services
Exempla St. Joseph Hospital
Denver, Colorado, USA

Karen P. O'Connor, MT(ASCP)SBB
Laboratory Instructor, Department of Medical Technology
College of Health Sciences
University of Delaware
Newark, Delaware, USA

Janet Oja, CLS (NCA)
Immunohematology Instructor
Department of Medical Laboratory Sciences
Weber State University
Ogden, Utah, USA

Susan H. Peacock, MSW, MT(ASCP)SBB, CQA(ASQ)
>Manager, Quality Assurance Department
>Gulf Coast Regional Blood Center
>Houston, Texas, USA

Emily A. Schmidt, MLS(ASCP)CM
>Clinical Instructor, School of Medical Technology
>Alverno Clinical Laboratory at St. Francis Hospital and Health Centers
>Beech Grove, Indiana, USA

Barbara J. Tubby, MSEd, BS, MT(ASCP)SBB
>Supervisor of Blood Bank
>Guthrie Health
>Sayre, Pennsylvania, USA

Amber G Tuten, MEd, MT(ASCP), DLM(ASCP)CM
>Assistant Professor, Clinical Laboratory Science Program
>Thomas University
>Thomasville, Georgia, USA

Meridee Van Draska, MLS(ASCP)
>Program Director, Medical Laboratory Science
>Department of Health Sciences
>Illinois State University
>Normal, Illinois, USA

Contents

Procedures Available on DavisPlus

The following procedures can be found on the textbook's companion website at DavisPlus.

Also available at DavisPlus (http://davisplus.fadavis.com/): Polyagglutination, by Phyllis S. Walker, MS, MT(ASCP)SBB.

Red Cell Antigen-
Serologic
Macroscopic

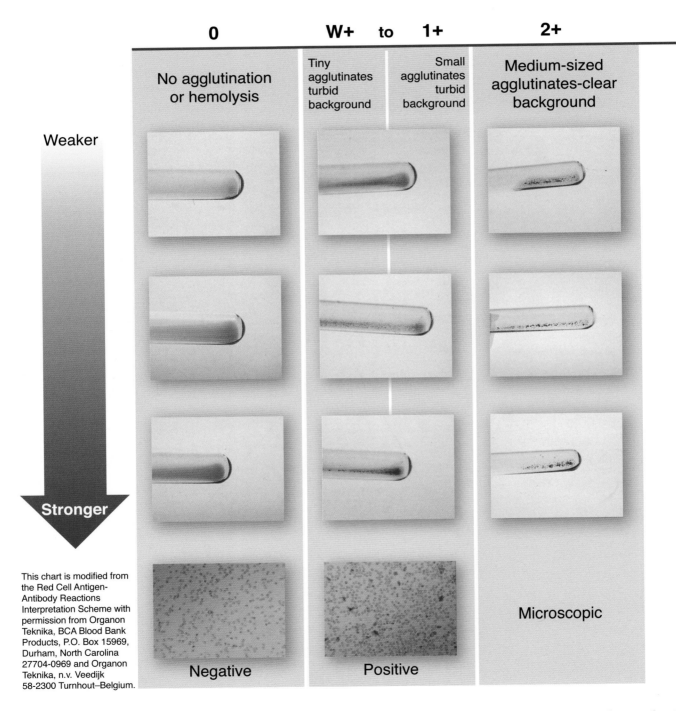

Plate 1. Red cell antigen-antibody reactions: serologic grading and macroscopic evaluation

Antibody Reactions
Grading
Evaluation

3+	4+
Several large agglutinates—clear background	One solid agglutinate

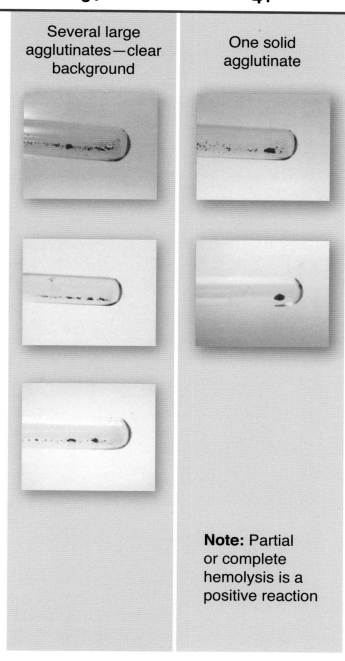

Note: Partial or complete hemolysis is a positive reaction

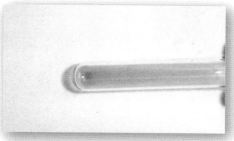

Negative: No aggregates

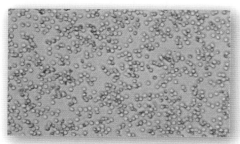

Negative: No aggregates (Microscopic)

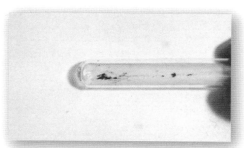

Pseudoagglutination or strong rouleaux (2+)

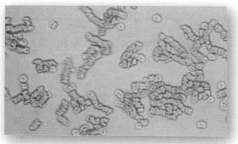

Rouleaux: Microscopic (original magnification x10; enlarged 240%)
Note: The "stack of coins" appearance of the agglutinates

Fundamental Concepts

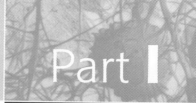

Part I

Chapter 1

Red Blood Cell and Platelet Preservation: Historical Perspectives and Current Trends

Denise M. Harmening, PhD, MT(ASCP) and Valerie Dietz Polansky, MEd, MLS(ASCP)CM

OBJECTIVES

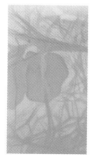

1. List the major developments in the history of transfusion medicine.

2. Describe several biological properties of red blood cells (RBC) that can affect post-transfusion survival.

3. Identify the metabolic pathways that are essential for normal RBC function and survival.

4. Define the hemoglobin-oxygen dissociation curve, including how it is related to the delivery of oxygen to tissues by transfused RBCs.

5. Explain how transfusion of stored blood can cause a shift to the left of the hemoglobin-oxygen dissociation curve.

6. State two FDA criteria that are used to evaluate new preservation solutions and storage containers.

7. State the temperature for storage of RBCs in the liquid state.

Continued

OBJECTIVES—cont'd

8. Define *storage lesion* and list the associated biochemical changes.

9. Explain the importance of 2,3-DPG levels in transfused blood, including what happens to levels post-transfusion and which factors are involved.

10. Name the approved anticoagulant preservative solutions, explain the function of each ingredient, and state the maximum storage time for RBCs collected in each.

11. Name the additive solutions licensed in the United States, list the common ingredients, and describe the function of each ingredient.

12. Explain how additive solutions are used and list their advantages.

13. Explain rejuvenation of RBCs.

14. List the name and composition of the FDA-approved rejuvenation solution and state the storage time following rejuvenation.

15. Define the platelet storage lesion.

16. Describe the indications for platelet transfusion and the importance of the corrected count increment (CCI).

17. Explain the storage requirements for platelets, including rationale.

18. Explain the swirling phenomenon and its significance.

19. List the two major reasons why platelet storage is limited to 5 days in the United States.

20. List the various ways that blood banks in the United States meet AABB Standard 5.1.5.1: "The blood bank or transfusion service shall have methods to limit and to detect or inactivate bacteria in all platelet components."

21. Explain the use and advantages of platelet additive solutions (PASs), and name one that is approved for use in the United States.

Introduction

People have always been fascinated by blood: Ancient Egyptians bathed in it, aristocrats drank it, authors and playwrights used it as themes, and modern humanity transfuses it. The road to an efficient, safe, and uncomplicated transfusion technique has been rather difficult, but great progress has been made. This chapter reviews the historical events leading to the current status of how blood is stored. A review of RBC biology serves as a building block for the discussion of red cell preservation, and a brief description of platelet metabolism sets the stage for reviewing the platelet storage lesion. Current trends in red cell and platelet preservation research are presented for the inquisitive reader.

Historical Overview

In 1492, blood was taken from three young men and given to the stricken Pope Innocent VII in the hope of curing him; unfortunately, all four died. Although the outcome of this event was unsatisfactory, it is the first time a blood transfusion was recorded in history. The path to successful transfusions that is so familiar today is marred by many reported failures, but our physical, spiritual, and emotional fascination with blood is primordial. Why did success elude experimenters for so long?

Clotting was the principal obstacle to overcome. Attempts to find a nontoxic anticoagulant began in 1869, when Braxton Hicks recommended sodium phosphate. This was perhaps the first example of blood preservation research. Karl Landsteiner in 1901 discovered the ABO blood groups and explained the serious reactions that occur in humans as a result of incompatible transfusions. His work early in the 20th century won a Nobel Prize.

Next came devices designed for performing the transfusions. Edward E. Lindemann was the first to succeed. He carried out vein-to-vein transfusion of blood by using multiple syringes and a special cannula for puncturing the vein through the skin. However, this time-consuming, complicated procedure required many skilled assistants. It was not until Unger designed his syringe-valve apparatus that transfusions from donor to patient by an unassisted physician became practical.

An unprecedented accomplishment in blood transfusion was achieved in 1914, when Hustin reported the use of sodium citrate as an anticoagulant solution for transfusions. Later, in 1915, Lewisohn determined the minimum amount of citrate needed for anticoagulation and demonstrated its nontoxicity in small amounts. Transfusions became more practical and safer for the patient.

The development of preservative solutions to enhance the metabolism of the RBC followed. Glucose was tried as early as 1916, when Rous and Turner introduced a citrate-dextrose solution for the preservation of blood. However, the function of glucose in RBC metabolism was not understood until the 1930s. Therefore, the common practice of using glucose in the preservative solution was delayed. World War II stimulated blood preservation research because the demand for blood and plasma increased. The pioneer work of Dr. Charles Drew during World War II on developing techniques in blood transfusion and blood preservation led to the establishment of a widespread system of blood banks. In February 1941, Dr. Drew was appointed director of the first American Red Cross blood bank at Presbyterian Hospital. The pilot program Dr. Drew established became the model for the national volunteer blood donor program of the American Red Cross.[1]

In 1943, Loutit and Mollison of England introduced the formula for the preservative acid-citrate-dextrose (ACD). Efforts in several countries resulted in the landmark publication of the July 1947 issue of the *Journal of Clinical Investigation*, which devoted nearly a dozen papers to blood preservation. Hospitals responded immediately, and in 1947, blood banks were established in many major cities of the United States; subsequently, transfusion became commonplace.

The daily occurrence of transfusions led to the discovery of numerous blood group systems. Antibody identification surged to the forefront as sophisticated techniques were developed. The interested student can review historic events during World War II in Kendrick's *Blood Program in World War II*, Historical Note.[2] In 1957, Gibson introduced an improved preservative solution called *citrate-phosphate-dextrose* (CPD), which was less acidic and eventually replaced ACD as the standard preservative used for blood storage.

Frequent transfusions and the massive use of blood soon resulted in new problems, such as circulatory overload. Component therapy has solved these problems. Before, a single unit of whole blood could serve only one patient. With component therapy, however, one unit may be used for multiple transfusions. Today, physicians can select the specific component for their patient's particular needs without risking the inherent hazards of whole blood transfusions. Physicians can transfuse only the required fraction in the concentrated form, without overloading the circulation. Appropriate blood component therapy now provides more effective treatment and more complete use of blood products (see Chapter 13, "Donor Screening and Component Preparation"). Extensive use of blood during this period, coupled with component separation, led to increased comprehension of erythrocyte metabolism and a new awareness of the problems associated with RBC storage.

Current Status

AABB, formerly the American Association of Blood Banks, estimates that there were 19 million volunteer donors in 2008.[3] Based on the 2009 National Blood Collection and Utilization Survey Report, about 17 million units of whole blood and RBCs were donated in 2008 in the United States.[3] Approximately 24 million blood components were transfused in 2008.[3] With an aging population and advances in medical treatments requiring transfusions, the demand for blood and blood components can be expected to continue to increase.[3] The New York Blood Center estimates that one in three people will need blood at some point in their lifetime.[4] These units are donated by fewer than 10% of healthy Americans who are eligible to donate each year, primarily through blood drives conducted at their place of work. Individuals can also donate at community blood centers (which collect approximately 88% of the nation's blood) or hospital-based donor centers (which collect approximately 12% of the nation's blood supply). Volunteer donors are not paid and provide nearly all of the blood used for transfusion in the United States.

Traditionally, the amount of whole blood in a unit has been 450 mL +/-10% of blood (1 pint). More recently, 500 mL +/-10% of blood are being collected. This has provided a small increase in the various components. Modified plastic collection systems are used when collecting 500 mL of blood, with the volume of anticoagulant-preservative solution being increased from 63 mL to 70 mL. For a 110-pound donor, a maximum volume of 525 mL can be collected, including samples drawn for processing.[5] The total blood volume of most adults is 10 to 12 pints, and donors can replenish the fluid lost from the 1-pint donation in 24 hours. The donor's red cells are replaced within 1 to 2 months after donation. A volunteer donor can donate whole blood every 8 weeks.

Units of the **whole blood** collected can be separated into three components: **packed RBCs**, **platelets**, and **plasma**. In recent years, less whole blood has been used to prepare platelets with the increased utilization of **apheresis** platelets. Hence, many units are converted only into RBCs and plasma. The plasma can be converted by **cryoprecipitation** to a clotting factor concentrate that is rich in **antihemophilic factor** (AHF, factor VIII; refer to Chapter 13). A unit of whole blood–prepared RBCs may be stored for 21 to 42 days, depending on the anticoagulant-preservative solution used when the whole blood unit was collected, and whether a preserving solution is added to the separated RBCs. Although most people assume that donated blood is free because most blood-collecting organizations are nonprofit, a fee is still charged for each unit to cover the costs associated with collecting, storing, testing, and transfusing blood.

The donation process consists of three steps or processes (Box 1–1):

1. Educational reading materials
2. The donor health history questionnaire
3. The abbreviated physical examination

BOX 1–1

The Donation Process

Step 1: Educational Materials

Educational material (such as the AABB pamphlet "An Important Message to All Blood Donors") that contains information on the risks of infectious diseases transmitted by blood transfusion, including the symptoms and sign of AIDS, is given to each prospective donor to read.

Step 2: The Donor Health History Questionnaire

A uniform donor history questionnaire, designed to ask questions that protect the health of both the donor and the recipient, is given to every donor. The health history questionnaire is used to identify donors who have been exposed to diseases that can be transmitted in blood (e.g., variant Creutzfeldt-Jakob, West Nile virus, malaria, babesiosis, or Chagas disease).

Step 3: The Abbreviated Physical Examination

The abbreviated physical examination for donors includes blood pressure, pulse, and temperature readings; hemoglobin or hematocrit level; and the inspection of the arms for skin lesions.

The donation process, especially steps 1 and 2, has been carefully modified over time to allow for the rejection of donors who may transmit transfusion-associated disease to recipients. For a more detailed description of donor screening and processing, refer to Chapter 13.

The nation's blood supply is safer than it has ever been because of the donation process and extensive laboratory screening (testing) of blood. Currently, 10 screening tests for infectious disease are performed on each unit of donated blood (Table 1–1). The current risk of transfusion-transmitted hepatitis C virus (**HCV**) is 1 in 1,390,000, and for hepatitis B virus (**HBV**), it is between 1 in 200,000 and 1 in 500,000, respectively.[6,7]

The use of **nucleic acid amplification testing** (NAT), licensed by the Food and Drug Administration (FDA) since 2002, is one reason for the increased safety of the blood supply. Refer to Chapter 18, "Transfusion-Transmitted Diseases" for a detailed discussion of transfusion-transmitted viruses.

RBC Biology and Preservation

Three areas of RBC biology are crucial for normal erythrocyte survival and function:

1. Normal chemical composition and structure of the RBC membrane
2. Hemoglobin structure and function
3. RBC metabolism

Defects in any or all of these areas will result in RBCs surviving less than the normal 120 days in circulation.

Table 1–1	**Current Donor Screening Tests for Infectious Diseases**
TEST	**DATE TEST REQUIRED**
Syphilis	1950s
Hepatitis B surface antigen (HBsAg)	1971
Hepatitis B core antibody (anti-HBc)	1986
Hepatitis C virus antibody (anti-HCV)	1990
Human immunodeficiency virus antibodies (anti-HIV-1/2)	1992[1]
Human T-cell lymphotropic virus antibody (anti-HTLV-I/II)	1997[2]
Human immunodeficiency virus (HIV-1)(NAT)*,**	1999
Hepatitis C virus (HCV) (NAT) **	1999
West Nile virus (NAT)	2004
Trypanosoma cruzi antibody (anti-T. cruzi)	2007

*NAT-nucleic acid amplification testing
**Initially under IND starting in 1999
[1] Anti-HIV-1 testing implemented in 1985
[2] Anti-HTLV testing implemented in 1988

RBC Membrane

Basic Concepts

The RBC membrane represents a semipermeable lipid bilayer supported by a meshlike protein cytoskeleton structure (Fig. 1–1).[8] Phospholipids, the main lipid components of the membrane, are arranged in a bilayer structure comprising the framework in which globular proteins traverse and move. Proteins that extend from the outer surface and span the entire membrane to the inner cytoplasmic side of the RBC are termed *integral* membrane proteins. Beneath the lipid bilayer, a second class of membrane proteins, called *peripheral* proteins, is located and limited to the cytoplasmic surface of the membrane forming the RBC cytoskeleton.[8]

Advanced Concepts

Both proteins and lipids are organized asymmetrically within the RBC membrane. Lipids are not equally distributed in the two layers of the membrane. The external layer is rich in glycolipids and choline phospholipids.[9] The internal cytoplasmic layer of the membrane is rich in amino phospholipids.[9] The biochemical composition of the RBC membrane is approximately 52% protein, 40% lipid, and 8% carbohydrate.[10]

As mentioned previously, the normal chemical composition and the structural arrangement and molecular interactions of the erythrocyte membrane are crucial to the normal length of RBC survival of 120 days in circulation. In addition, they maintain a critical role in two important RBC characteristics: deformability and permeability.

Deformability

To remain viable, normal RBCs must also remain flexible, deformable, and permeable. The loss of adenosine triphosphate (ATP) (energy) levels leads to a decrease in the phosphorylation of spectrin and, in turn, a loss of membrane deformability.[9] An accumulation or increase in deposition of membrane calcium also results, causing an increase in membrane rigidity and loss of pliability. These cells are at a marked disadvantage when they pass through the small (3 to 5 μm in diameter) sinusoidal orifices of the spleen, an organ that functions in extravascular sequestration and removal of aged, damaged, or less deformable RBCs or fragments of their membrane. The loss of RBC membrane is exemplified by the formation of "spherocytes" (cells with a reduced surface-to-volume ratio; Fig. 1–2) and "bite cells," in which the removal of a portion of membrane has left a permanent indentation in the remaining cell membrane (Fig. 1–3). The survival of these forms is also shortened.

Permeability

The permeability properties of the RBC membrane and the active RBC cation transport prevent colloid hemolysis and control the volume of the RBC. Any abnormality that increases permeability or alters cationic transport may decrease RBC survival. The RBC membrane is freely permeable to

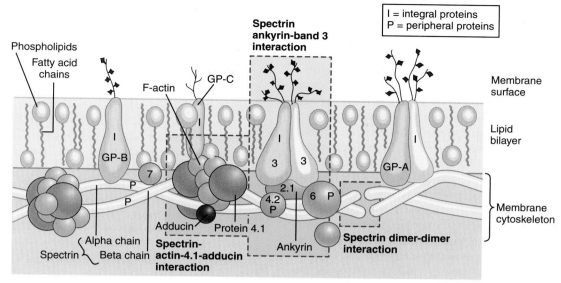

Figure 1–1. Schematic illustration of red blood cell membrane depicting the composition and arrangement of RBC membrane proteins. GP-A = glycophorin A; GP-B = glycophorin B; GP-C = glycophorin C; G = globin. Numbers refer to pattern of migration of SDS (sodium dodecyl sulfate) polyacrylamide gel pattern stained with Coomassie brilliant blue. Relations of protein to each other and to lipids are purely hypothetical; however, the positions of the proteins relative to the inside or outside of the lipid bilayer are accurate. (Note: Proteins are not drawn to scale and many minor proteins are omitted.) *(Reprinted with permission from Harmening, DH: Clinical Hematology and Fundamentals of Hemostasis, 5th ed., FA Davis, Philadelphia, 2009.)*

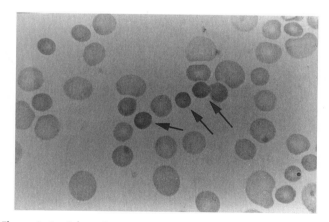

Figure 1–2. Spherocytes.

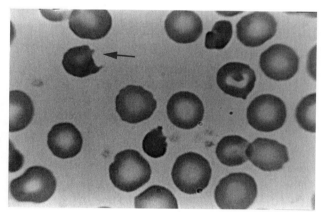

Figure 1–3. "Bite" cells.

water and anions. Chloride (Cl^-) and bicarbonate (HCO_3^-) can traverse the membrane in less than a second. It is speculated that this massive exchange of ions occurs through a large number of exchange channels located in the RBC membrane. The RBC membrane is relatively impermeable to cations such as sodium (Na^+) and potassium (K^+).

RBC volume and water homeostasis are maintained by controlling the intracellular concentrations of sodium and potassium. The erythrocyte intracellular-to-extracellular ratios for Na^+ and K^+ are 1:12 and 25:1, respectively. The 300 cationic pumps, which actively transport Na^+ out of the cell and K^+ into the cell, require energy in the form of ATP. Calcium (Ca^{2+}) is also actively pumped from the interior of the RBC through energy-dependent calcium-ATPase pumps. Calmodulin, a cytoplasmic calcium-binding protein, is speculated to control these pumps and to prevent excessive intracellular Ca^{2+} buildup, which changes the shape and makes it more rigid. When RBCs are ATP-depleted, Ca^{2+} and Na^+ are allowed to accumulate intracellularly, and K^+ and water are lost, resulting in a dehydrated rigid cell subsequently sequestered by the spleen, resulting in a decrease in RBC survival.

Metabolic Pathways

Basic Concepts

The RBC's metabolic pathways that produce ATP are mainly anaerobic, because the function of the RBC is to deliver oxygen, not to consume it. Because the mature erythrocyte has no nucleus and there is no mitochondrial apparatus for oxidative metabolism, energy must be generated almost exclusively through the breakdown of glucose.

Advanced Concepts

RBC metabolism may be divided into the anaerobic glycolytic pathway and three ancillary pathways that serve to maintain the structure and function of hemoglobin (Fig. 1–4): the pentose phosphate pathway, the methemoglobin reductase pathway, and the Luebering-Rapoport shunt. All of these processes are essential if the erythrocyte is to transport oxygen and to maintain critical physical characteristics for its survival. Glycolysis generates about 90% of the ATP needed by the RBC. Approximately 10% is provided by the pentose phosphate pathway. The methemoglobin reductase pathway is another important pathway of RBC metabolism, and a defect can affect RBC post-transfusion survival and function. Another pathway that is crucial to RBC function is the Luebering-Rapoport shunt. This pathway permits the accumulation of an important RBC organic phosphate, **2,3-diphosphoglycerate (2,3-DPG)**. The amount of 2,3-DPG found within RBCs has a significant effect on the affinity of hemoglobin for oxygen and therefore affects how well RBCs function post-transfusion.

Hemoglobin Oxygen Dissociation Curve

Hemoglobin's primary function is gas transport: oxygen delivery to the tissues and carbon dioxide (CO_2) excretion. One of the most important controls of hemoglobin affinity for oxygen is the RBC organic phosphate 2, 3-DPG. The unloading of oxygen by hemoglobin is accompanied by widening of a space between β chains and the binding of 2,3-DPG on a mole-for-mole basis, with the formation of anionic salt bridges between the chains. The resulting conformation of the deoxyhemoglobin molecule is known as the *tense (T) form*, which has a lower affinity for oxygen. When hemoglobin loads oxygen and becomes oxyhemoglobin, the established salt bridges are broken, and β chains are pulled together, expelling 2,3-DPG. This is the *relaxed (R) form* of the hemoglobin molecule, which has a higher affinity for oxygen. These **allosteric changes** that occur as the hemoglobin loads and unloads oxygen are referred to as the *respiratory movement*. The dissociation and binding of oxygen by hemoglobin are not directly proportional to the partial pressure of oxygen (pO_2) in its environment

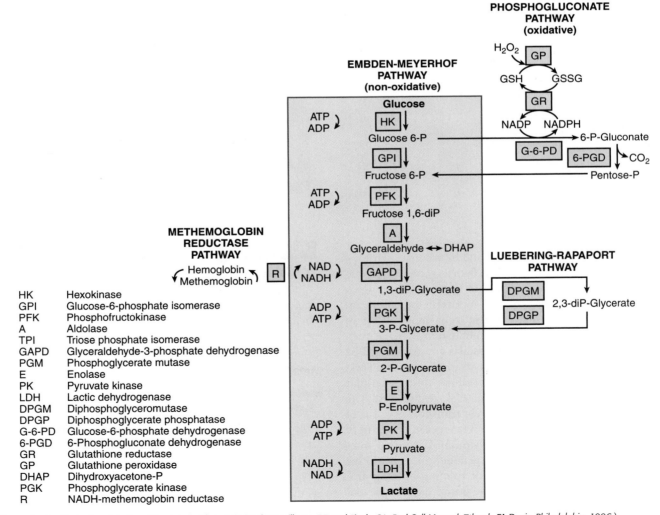

HK	Hexokinase
GPI	Glucose-6-phosphate isomerase
PFK	Phosphofructokinase
A	Aldolase
TPI	Triose phosphate isomerase
GAPD	Glyceraldehyde-3-phosphate dehydrogenase
PGM	Phosphoglycerate mutase
E	Enolase
PK	Pyruvate kinase
LDH	Lactic dehydrogenase
DPGM	Diphosphoglyceromutase
DPGP	Diphosphoglycerate phosphatase
G-6-PD	Glucose-6-phosphate dehydrogenase
6-PGD	6-Phosphogluconate dehydrogenase
GR	Glutathione reductase
GP	Glutathione peroxidase
DHAP	Dihydroxyacetone-P
PGK	Phosphoglycerate kinase
R	NADH-methemoglobin reductase

Figure 1–4.   Red cell metabolism. *(Reprinted with permission from Hillman, RF, and Finch, CA: Red Cell Manual, 7th ed., FA Davis, Philadelphia, 1996.)*

but instead exhibit a **sigmoid-curve** relationship, known as the *hemoglobin-oxygen dissociation curve* (Fig. 1–5).

The shape of this curve is very important physiologically because it permits a considerable amount of oxygen to be delivered to the tissues with a small drop in oxygen tension. For example, in the environment of the lungs, where the oxygen (pO_2) tension, measured in millimeters of mercury (mm Hg), is nearly 100 mm Hg, the hemoglobin molecule is almost 100% saturated with oxygen. As the RBCs travel to the tissues, where the (pO_2) drops to an average of 40 mm Hg (mean venous oxygen tension), the hemoglobin saturation drops to approximately 75% saturation, releasing about 25% of the oxygen to the tissues. This is the normal situation of oxygen delivery at a basal metabolic rate. The normal position of the oxygen dissociation curve depends on three different **ligands** normally found within the RBC: H^+ ions, CO_2, and organic phosphates. Of these three ligands, 2,3-DPG plays the most important physiological role. Normal hemoglobin function depends on adequate 2,3-DPG levels in the RBC. In situations such as hypoxia, a compensatory **shift to the right** of the hemoglobin-oxygen dissociation curve alleviates the tissue oxygen deficit. This rightward shift of the curve, mediated by increased levels of 2,3-DPG, decreases hemoglobin's affinity for the oxygen molecule and increases oxygen delivery to the tissues. A **shift to the left** of the hemoglobin-oxygen dissociation curve results, conversely, in an increase in hemoglobin-oxygen affinity and a decrease in oxygen delivery to the tissues. With such a dissociation curve, RBCs are much less efficient because only 12% of the oxygen can be released to the tissues. Multiple transfusions of 2,3-DPG–depleted stored blood can shift the oxygen dissociation curve to the left.[11]

RBC Preservation

Basic Concepts

The goal of blood preservation is to provide viable and functional blood components for patients requiring blood transfusion. RBC viability is a measure of **in vivo** RBC survival following transfusion. Because blood must be stored from the time of donation until the time of transfusion, the viability of RBCs must be maintained during the storage time as well. The FDA requires an average 24-hour post-transfusion RBC survival of more than 75%.[12] In addition, the FDA mandates that red cell integrity be maintained throughout the shelf-life of the stored RBCs. This is assessed as free hemoglobin less than 1% of total hemoglobin.[13] These two criteria are used to evaluate new preservation solutions and storage containers. To determine post-transfusion RBC survival, RBCs are taken from healthy subjects, stored, and then labeled with radioisotopes, reinfused to the original donor, and measured 24 hours after transfusion. Despite FDA requirements, the 24-hour post-transfusion RBC survival at outdate can be less than 75%;[12,14] and in critically ill patients is often less than 75%.[14,15]

To maintain optimum viability, blood is stored in the liquid state between 1°C and 6°C for a specific number of days, as determined by the preservative solution(s) used. The loss of RBC viability has been correlated with the **lesion of storage**, which is associated with various biochemical changes (Table 1–2).

Advanced Concepts

Because low 2,3-DPG levels profoundly influence the oxygen dissociation curve of hemoglobin,[16] DPG-depleted RBCs may have an impaired capacity to deliver oxygen to the tissues. As RBCs (in whole blood or RBC concentrates)

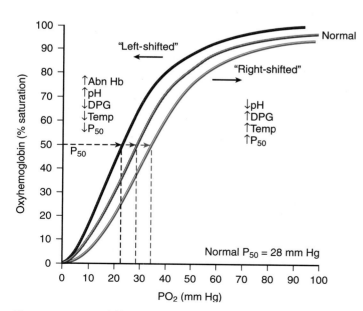

Figure 1–5. Hemoglobin-oxygen dissociation curve. *(Reprinted with permission from Harmening, DH: Clinical Hematology and Fundamentals of Hemostasis, 5th ed., FA Davis, Philadelphia, 2009.)*

Table 1–2	**RBC Storage Lesion**
CHARACTERISTIC	**CHANGE OBSERVED**
% Viable cells	Decreased
Glucose	Decreased
ATP	Decreased
Lactic acid	Increased
pH	Decreased
2,3-DPG	Decreased
Oxygen dissociation curve	Shift to the left (increase in hemoglobin and oxygen affinity; less oxygen delivered to tissues)
Plasma K^+	Increased
Plasma hemoglobin	Increased

are stored, 2,3-DPG levels decrease, with a shift to the left of the hemoglobin-oxygen dissociation curve, and less oxygen is delivered to the tissues. It is well accepted, however, that 2,3-DPG is re-formed in stored RBCs, after in vivo circulation, resulting in restored oxygen delivery. The rate of restoration of 2,3-DPG is influenced by the acid-base status of the recipient, the phosphorus metabolism, the degree of anemia, and the overall severity of the disorder.[11] It has been reported that within the first hour after transfusion, most RBC clearance occurs.[14] Approximately 220 to 250 mg of iron are contained in one RBC unit.[17] Therefore, rapid RBC clearance of even 25% of a single unit of blood delivers a massive load of hemoglobin iron to the monocyte and macrophage system, producing harmful effects.[13]

Anticoagulant Preservative Solutions

Basic Concepts

Table 1–3 lists the approved anticoagulant preservative solutions for whole blood and RBC storage at 1°C to 6°C. The addition of various chemicals, along with the approved anticoagulant-preservative CPD, was incorporated in an attempt to stimulate glycolysis so that ATP levels were better maintained.[18] One of the chemicals, adenine, incorporated into the CPD solution (CPDA-1) increases ADP levels, thereby driving glycolysis toward the synthesis of ATP. CPDA-1 contains 0.25 mM of adenine plus 25% more glucose than CPD. Adenine-supplemented blood can be stored at 1°C to 6°C for 35 days; the other anticoagulants are approved for 21 days. Table 1–4 lists the various chemicals used in anticoagulant solutions and their functions during the storage of red cells.

Advanced Concepts

It is interesting to note that blood stored in all CPD preservatives also becomes depleted of 2,3-DPG by the second week of storage. The reported pathophysiological effects of the transfusion of RBCs with low 2,3-DPG levels and increased affinity for oxygen include: an increase in cardiac output, a decrease in mixed venous (pO_2) tension, or a combination of these.[11] The physiological importance of these effects is not easily demonstrated. This is a complex mechanism with numerous variables involved that are beyond the scope of this text.

Stored RBCs do regain the ability to synthesize 2,3-DPG after transfusion, but levels necessary for optimal hemoglobin oxygen delivery are not reached immediately. Approximately 24 hours are required to restore normal levels of 2,3-DPG after transfusion.[19] The 2,3-DPG concentrations after transfusion have been reported to reach normal levels as early as 6 hours post-transfusion.[19] Most of these studies have been performed on normal, healthy individuals. However, evidence suggests that, in the transfused subject whose capacity is limited by an underlying physiological disturbance, even a brief period of altered oxygen hemoglobin affinity is of great significance.[14] It is quite clear now that 2,3-DPG levels in transfused blood are important in certain clinical conditions. Studies demonstrate that myocardial function improves following transfusion of blood with high 2,3-DPG levels during cardiovascular surgery.[11] Several investigators suggest that the patient in shock who is given 2,3-DPG–depleted erythrocytes in transfusion may have already strained the compensatory mechanisms to their limits.[11,20–22] Perhaps for this type of patient, the poor oxygen delivery capacity of 2,3-DPG–depleted cells makes a significant difference in recovery and survival.

It is apparent that many factors may limit the viability of transfused RBCs. One of these factors is the plastic material used for the storage container. The plastic must be sufficiently permeable to CO_2 in order to maintain higher pH levels during storage. Glass storage containers are a matter of history in the United States. Currently, the majority of blood is stored in polyvinyl chloride (PVC) plastic bags. One issue associated with PVC bags relates to the plasticizer di(ethylhexyl)-phthalate (DEHP), which is used in the manufacture of the bags. It has been found to leach from the plastic into the lipids of the plasma medium and RBC membranes of the blood during storage. However, its use or that of alternative plasticizers that leach are important because they have been shown to stabilize the RBC membrane and therefore reduce the extent of hemolysis during storage. Another issue with PVC is its tendency to break at low temperatures; therefore, components frozen in PVC bags must be handled with care. In addition to PVC, polyolefin containers, which do not contain DEHP, are available for some components, and latex-free plastic containers are available for recipients with latex allergies.[5]

Additive Solutions

Basic Concepts

Additive solutions (AS) are preserving solutions that are added to the RBCs after removal of the plasma with or

Table 1–3	**Approved Anticoagulant Preservative Solutions**	
NAME	**ABBREVIATION**	**STORAGE TIME (DAYS)**
Acid citrate-dextrose (formula A) *	ACD-A	21
Citrate-phosphate dextrose	CPD	21
Citrate-phosphate-double-dextrose	CP2D	21
Citrate-phosphate-dextrose-adenine	CPDA-1	35

* ACD-A is used for apheresis components.

Table 1–4   Chemicals in Anticoagulant Solutions

CHEMICAL	FUNCTION	PRESENT IN			
		ACD-A	CPD	CP2D	CPDA-1
Citrate (sodium citrate/citric acid)	Chelates calcium; prevents clotting	X	X	X	X
Monobasic sodium phosphate	Maintains pH during storage; necessary for maintenance of adequate levels of 2,3-DPG	X	X	X	X
Dextrose	Substrate for ATP production (cellular energy)	X	X	X	X
Adenine	Production of ATP (extends shelf-life from 21 to 35 days)				X

ACD-A = Acid citrate-dextrose (formula A); CPD = Citrate-phosphate dextrose; CP2D = Citrate phosphate double dextrose; CPDA-1 = Citrate phosphate dextrose adenine; 2,3-DPG = 2,3-diphosphoglycerate; ATP = adenosine triphosphate

without platelets. Additive solutions are now widely used. One of the reasons for their development is that removal of the plasma component during the preparation of RBC concentrates removed much of the nutrients needed to maintain RBCs during storage. This was dramatically observed when high-hematocrit RBCs were prepared. The influence of removing substantial amounts of adenine and glucose present originally in, for example, the CPDA-1 anticoagulant-preservative solution led to a decrease in viability, particularly in the last 2 weeks of storage.[14]

RBC concentrates prepared from whole blood units collected in primary anticoagulant-preservative solutions can be relatively void of plasma with high hematocrits, which causes the units to be more viscous and difficult to infuse, especially in emergency situations. Additive solutions (100 mL to the RBC concentrate prepared from a 450-mL blood collection) also overcome this problem. Additive solutions reduce hematocrits from around 70% to 85% to around 50% to 60%. The ability to pack RBCs to fairly high hematocrits before adding additive solution, also provides a means to harvest greater amounts of plasma with or without platelets. Box 1–2 summarizes the benefits of RBC additive solutions.

Currently, three additive solutions are licensed in the United States:

1. Adsol (AS-1; Baxter Healthcare)
2. Nutricel (AS-3; Pall Corporation)
3. Optisol (AS-5; Terumo Corporation)

The additive solution is contained in a **satellite bag** and is added to the RBCs after most of the plasma has been expressed. All three additives contain saline, adenine, and glucose. AS-1 and AS-5 also contain mannitol, which protects against storage-related hemolysis,[23] while AS-3 contains citrate and phosphate for the same purpose. All of the additive solutions are approved for 42 days of storage for packed RBCs. Table 1–5 lists the currently approved additive solutions.

Advanced Concepts

Table 1–6 shows the biochemical characteristics of RBCs stored in the three additive solutions after 42 days of storage.[4,24,25] Additive system RBCs are used in the same way

Table 1–5   Additive Solutions in Use in North America

NAME	ABBREVIATION	STORAGE TIME (DAYS)
Adsol (Baxter Healthcare)	AS-1	42
Nutricel (Pall Corporation)	AS-3	42
Optisol (Terumo Corporation)	AS-5	42

Table 1–6   Red Cell Additives: Biochemical Characteristics

	AS-1	AS-3	AS-5
Storage period (days)	42	42	42
pH (measured at 37°C)	6.6	6.5	6.5
24-hour survival*(%)	83	85.1	80
ATP (% initial)	68	67	68.5
2,3-DPG (% initial)	6	6	5
Hemolysis (%)	0.5	0.7	0.6

*Survival studies reported are from selected investigators and do not include an average of all reported survivals.

BOX 1–2

Benefits of RBC Additive Solutions

- Extends the shelf-life of RBCs to 42 days by adding nutrients
- Allows for the harvesting of more plasma and platelets from the unit
- Produces an RBC concentrate of lower viscosity that is easier to infuse

as traditional RBC transfusions. Blood stored in additive solutions is now routinely given to newborn infants and pediatric patients,[26] although some clinicians still prefer CPDA-1 RBCs because of their concerns about one or more of the constituents in the additive solutions.

None of the additive solutions maintain 2,3-DPG throughout the storage time. As with RBCs stored only with primary anticoagulant preservatives, 2,3-DPG is depleted by the second week of storage.

Freezing and Rejuvenation

RBC Freezing

Basic Concepts

RBC freezing is primarily used for autologous units and the storage of rare blood types. **Autologous transfusion** (*auto* meaning "self") allows individuals to donate blood for their own use in meeting their needs for blood transfusion (see Chapter 15, "Transfusion Therapy").

The procedure for freezing a unit of packed RBCs is not complicated. Basically, it involves the addition of a cryoprotective agent to RBCs that are less than 6 days old. Glycerol is used most commonly and is added to the RBCs slowly with vigorous shaking, thereby enabling the glycerol to permeate the RBCs. The cells are then rapidly frozen and stored in a freezer. The usual storage temperature is below –65°C, although storage (and freezing) temperature depends on the concentration of glycerol used.[16] Two concentrations of glycerol have been used to freeze RBCs: a high-concentration glycerol (40% weight in volume [w/v]) and a low-concentration glycerol (20% w/v) in the final concentration of the cryopreservative.[5] Most blood banks that freeze RBCs use the high-concentration glycerol technique.

Table 1–7 lists the advantages of the high-concentration glycerol technique in comparison with the low-concentration glycerol technique. See Chapter 13 for a detailed description of the RBC freezing procedure.

Currently, the FDA licenses frozen RBCs for a period of 10 years from the date of freezing; that is, frozen RBCs may be stored up to 10 years before thawing and transfusion. Once thawed, these RBCs demonstrate function and viability near those of fresh blood. Experience has shown that 10-year storage periods do not adversely affect viability and function.[27] Table 1–8 lists the advantages and disadvantages of RBC freezing.

Advanced Concepts

Transfusion of frozen cells must be preceded by a deglycerolization process; otherwise the thawed cells would be accompanied by hypertonic glycerol when infused, and RBC lysis would result. Removal of glycerol is achieved by systematically replacing the cryoprotectant with decreasing

Table 1–7	Advantages of High-Concentration Glycerol Technique Used by Most Blood Banks Over Low-Concentration Glycerol Technique	
ADVANTAGE	**HIGH GLYCEROL**	**LOW GLYCEROL**
1. Initial freezing temperature	–80°C	–196°C
2. Need to control freezing rate	No	Yes
3. Type of freezer	Mechanical	Liquid nitrogen
4. Maximum storage temperature	–65°C	–120°C
5. Shipping requirements	Dry ice	Liquid nitrogen
6. Effect of changes in storage temperature	Can be thawed and refrozen	Critical

concentrations of saline. The usual protocol involves washing with 12% saline, followed by 1.6% saline, with a final wash of 0.2% dextrose in normal saline.[5] A commercially available cell-washing system, such as one of those manufactured by several companies, has traditionally been used in the deglycerolizing process. Excessive hemolysis is monitored by noting the hemoglobin concentration of the wash supernatant. Osmolality of the unit should also be monitored to ensure adequate deglycerolization. Traditionally, because a unit of blood is processed in an **open system** (one in which sterility is broken) to add the glycerol (before freezing) or the saline solutions (for deglycerolization), the outdating period of thawed RBCs stored at 1°C to 6°C has been 24 hours. Generally, RBCs in CPD or CPDA-1 anticoagulant-preservatives or additive solutions are glycerolized and frozen within 6 days of whole blood collection. Red blood cells stored in additive solutions such as AS-1, AS-3, and AS-5 have been frozen up to 42 days after liquid

Table 1–8	Advantages and Disadvantages of RBC Freezing	
ADVANTAGES	**DISADVANTAGES**
Long-term storage (10 years)	A time-consuming process
Maintenance of RBC viability and function	Higher cost of equipment and materials
Low residual leukocytes and platelets	Storage requirements (–65°C)
Removal of significant amounts of plasma proteins	Higher cost of product

storage without **rejuvenation**. The need to transfuse RBCs within 24 hours of thawing has limited the use of frozen RBCs.

Recently, an instrument (ACP 215, Haemonetics) has been developed that allows the glycerolization and deglycerolization processes to be performed under **closed system** conditions.[28] This instrument utilizes a sterile connecting device for connections, in-line 0.22 micron filters to deliver solutions, and a disposable polycarbonate bowl with an external seal to deglycerolize the RBCs. RBCs prepared from 450-mL collections and frozen within 6 days of blood collection with CPDA-1 can be stored after thawing at 1°C to 6°C for up to 15 days when the processing is conducted with the ACP 215 instrument. The deglycerolized cells, prepared using salt solutions as in the traditional procedures, are suspended in the AS-3 additive solution as a final step, which is thought to stabilize the thawed RBCs. These storage conditions are based on the parameters used in a study by Valeri and others that showed that RBC properties were satisfactorily maintained during a 15-day period.[28] Further studies will broaden the conditions that can be used to prepare RBCs for subsequent freezing with closed system processing.

RBC Rejuvenation

Basic Concepts

Rejuvenation of RBCs is the process by which ATP and 2,3-DPG levels are restored or enhanced by metabolic alterations. Currently, Rejuvesol (enCyte Systems) is the only FDA-approved rejuvenation solution sold in the United States. It contains phosphate, inosine, pyruvate, and adenine. Rejuvesol is currently approved for use with CPD, CPDA-1, and CPD/AS-1 RBCs. RBCs stored in the liquid state can be rejuvenated at outdate or up to 3 days after outdate, depending on RBC preservative solutions used. Currently, only RBCs prepared from 450-mL collections can be rejuvenated.

Advanced Concepts

Rejuvenation is accomplished by incubating the RBC unit with 50 mL of the rejuvenating solution for 1 hour at 37°C. Following rejuvenation, the RBCs can be washed to remove the rejuvenation solution and transfused within 24 hours. More commonly, they are frozen, then washed in the post-freezing deglycerolization process. Because the process is currently accomplished with an open system, federal regulations require that rejuvenated or frozen RBCs are used within 24 hours of thawing.[28] It is possible that rejuvenated RBCs could be processed with the closed system ACP 215 instrument, thereby extending their shelf-life.

The rejuvenation process is expensive and time-consuming; therefore, it is not used often but is invaluable for preserving selected autologous and rare units of blood for later use.

Current Trends in RBC Preservation Research

Advanced Concepts

Research and development in RBC preparation and preservation is being pursued in five directions:

1. Development of improved additive solutions
2. Development of procedures to reduce and inactivate the level of pathogens that may be in RBC units
3. Development of procedures to convert A-, B-, and AB-type RBCs to O-type RBCs
4. Development of methods to produce RBCs through bio-engineering (blood pharming)
5. Development of RBC substitutes

Improved Additive Solutions

Research is being conducted to develop improved additive solutions for RBC preservation. One reason for this is because longer storage periods could improve the logistics of providing RBCs for clinical use, including increased benefits associated with the use of autologous blood/RBCs.

Procedures to Reduce and Inactivate Pathogens

Research is being conducted to develop procedures that would reduce the level of or inactivate residual viruses, bacteria, and parasites in RBC units. One objective is to develop robust procedures that could possibly inactivate unrecognized (unknown) pathogens that may be present, such as the viruses that have emerged in recent years. Although methods to inactivate pathogens in plasma have been used successfully for more than 20 years, **pathogen reduction** of cellular components has proven more challenging. Two methods that utilize alkylating agents that react with the nucleic acids of pathogens (S-303, Cerus/Baxter; Inactine, Vitex) have been evaluated in clinical trials in the United States. Work with Inactin (PEN110) has been discontinued, but clinical studies with S-303–treated RBCs are currently in progress at two U.S. blood centers. Clinical studies of riboflavin and UV light–treated RBCs are expected.[29] Areas of concern that must be addressed before pathogen-reduction and pathogen-inactivation technologies are approved for use in the U.S. are potential toxicity, immunogenicity, cellular function, and cost.

Formation of O-Type RBCs

The inadequate supply of O-type RBC units that is periodically encountered can hinder blood centers and hospital blood banks in providing RBCs for specific patients. Research over the last 20 years has been evaluating how the more available A and B type of RBCs can be converted to O-type RBCs. The use of enzymes that remove the carbohydrate moieties of the A and B antigens is the mechanism for forming O-type RBCs. The enzymes are removed by washing after completion of the reaction time. A clinical study sponsored by ZymeQuest, the company that is developing the technology, has shown that O-type RBCs manufactured from B-type RBCs were effective when transfused to O- and A-type patients in need of RBCs.[30]

Blood Pharming

Creating RBCs in the laboratory (**blood pharming**) is another area of research that has the potential to increase the amount of blood available for transfusion. In 2008, the Defense Advanced Research Projects Agency (DARPA) awarded a bioengineering company named Arteriocyte a contract to develop a system for producing O-negative RBCs on the battlefield. The company, which uses proprietary technology (NANEX) to turn hematopoietic stem cells (HSC) from umbilical cord into type-O, Rh-negative RBCs, sent its first shipment of the engineered blood to the FDA for evaluation in 2010.[31] FDA approval is required before human trials can begin. More recently, cultured RBCs generated from in vitro HSC has been reported that survive in circulation for several weeks.[32]

RBC Substitutes

Scientists have been searching for a substitute for blood for over 150 years.[33] After the discovery of blood groups in 1901, human-to-human blood transfusions became safer, but blood substitutes continued to be of interest because of their potential to alleviate shortages of donated blood. In the 1980s, safety concerns about **HIV** led to renewed interest in finding a substitute for human blood, and more recently, the need for blood on remote battlefields has heightened that interest. The U.S. military is one of the strongest advocates for the development of blood substitutes, which it supports through its own research and partnerships with private sector companies. Today the search continues for a safe and effective oxygen carrier that could eliminate many of the problems associated with blood transfusion, such as the need for refrigeration, limited shelf-life, compatibility, immunogenicity, transmission of infectious agents, and shortages. Box 1–3 lists the potential benefits of artificial oxygen carriers. Since RBC substitutes are drugs, they must go through extensive testing in order to obtain FDA approval. Safety and efficacy must be demonstrated through clinical trials. Table 1–9 outlines the different phases of testing.

Current research on blood substitutes is focused on two areas: **hemoglobin-based oxygen carriers** (HBOCs) and **perfluorocarbons** (PFCs).[34,35] Since the function of these products is to carry and transfer oxygen, just one of the many functions of blood, the term **RBC substitutes** is preferred to the original term *blood substitutes*. Recently the terms **oxygen therapeutics** and **artificial oxygen carriers** (AOC) have been used to describe the broad clinical applications envisioned for these products. Originally developed to be used in trauma situations such as accidents, combat, and surgery, RBC substitutes have, until now, fallen short of meeting requirements for these applications. Despite years of research, RBC substitutes are still not in routine use today. South Africa, Mexico, and Russia are the only countries where any AOCs

are approved for clinical use. None have received FDA approval for clinical use in the United States, although specific products have been given to individual patients under compassionate use guidelines.

Hemoglobin-Based Oxygen Carriers

By 1949, it was established that purified hemoglobin could restore blood volume and deliver oxygen; however, its transfusion resulted in serious side effects, such as **vasoconstriction** and renal failure. This toxicity was thought to be due to stromal remnants in the hemoglobin solutions.[36] **Ultrapurified stroma-free hemoglobin** (SFH) was developed, but it did not readily deliver oxygen to tissues. This was determined to be due to a loss of 2,3-DPG during processing, which caused a shift to the left of the oxygen dissociation

---

BOX 1–3

Potential Benefits of Artificial Oxygen Carriers

- Abundant supply
- Readily available for use in prehospital settings, battlefields, and remote locations
- Can be stockpiled for emergencies and warfare
- No need for typing and crossmatching
- Available for immediate infusion
- Extended shelf-life (1 to 3 years)
- Can be stored at room temperature
- Free of blood-borne pathogens
- At full oxygen capacity immediately
- Do not prime circulating neutrophils, reducing the incidence of multiorgan failure
- Can deliver oxygen to tissue that is inaccessible to RBCs
- Have been accepted by Jehovah's Witnesses
- Could eventually cost less than units of blood

Table 1–9	**Phases of Testing**
PHASE	**DESCRIPTION OF TESTING**
Preclinical	In vivo and animal testing
Phase I	Researchers test drug in a small group of people (20 to 80) for the first time to evaluate its safety, determine a safe dosage range, and identify side effects.
Phase II	The drug is given to a larger group of people (100 to 300) to see if it is effective and to further evaluate its safety.
Phase III	The drug is given to large groups of people (1,000 to 3,000) to confirm its effectiveness, monitor side effects, compare it to commonly used treatments, and collect information that will allow the drug to be used safely.
Phase IV	Post marketing studies to gather additional information about the drug's risks, benefits, and optimal use.

curve. Another problem was the product's short half-life, due to dissociation of the hemoglobin molecule into α and β dimers that were filtered by the kidneys and excreted in the urine.[32] Scientists began to look for ways to chemically modify the hemoglobin molecule to overcome these problems. **Cross-linking, polymerization,** and **pegylation** produced larger, more stable molecules. This reduced some, but not all, of the adverse effects.

To date, four generations of HBOCs have been developed.[33] HBOCs have been produced from human, bovine, and **recombinant hemoglobin. Bovine hemoglobin** has several advantages over human hemoglobin. It has a lower oxygen affinity and better oxygen uploading in ischemic tissues, and its availability is not dependent upon an adequate supply of outdated human RBCs. However, concerns about potential immunogenicity and transmission of prions have been raised.[37] Although several HBOCs have progressed to phase II and III clinical trials, currently none have been approved for clinical use in humans in the United States or Europe. Development of several products was terminated following clinical trials in which serious adverse side effects were discovered. Two HBOCs are still in clinical trials in the United States and Europe: Hemopure (OPK Biotech) and Hemospan (Sangart). Hemopure was approved for clinical use in South Africa in 2001 and a related product, Oxyglobin, has been used to treat canine anemia in the United States and Europe since 1998. An interesting side note is that a Spanish cyclist admitted to using Oxyglobin in the 2003 Tour de France. He crashed after experiencing nausea. Table 1–10 summarizes the history and status of several HBOCs.

A 2008 meta-analysis of 16 clinical trials involving 3,711 patients and five different HBOCs found a significantly increased risk of death and myocardial infarction associated with the use of HBOCs.[38] These findings make their widespread clinical use unlikely in the near future; however, some experts believe that HBOCs hold more promise than PFCs.[33,39] Table 1–11 lists the advantages and disadvantages of HBOCs.

Perfluorocarbons

Perfluorocarbons (PFCs) are synthetic hydrocarbon structures in which all the hydrogen atoms have been replaced with fluorine. They are chemically inert, are excellent gas solvents, and carry O_2 and CO_2 by dissolving them. Because of their small size (about 0.2 microns in diameter), they are able to pass through areas of vasoconstriction and deliver oxygen to tissues that are inaccessible to RBCs. PFCs have been under investigation as possible RBC substitutes since the 1970s. Fluosol (Green Cross Corp.) was approved by the FDA in 1989 but was removed from the market in 1994 due to clinical shortcomings and poor sales. Four other PFCs have proceeded to clinical trials. One, Perftoran (Perftoran), is in clinical use in Russia and Mexico. Two others are no longer under development, and one (Oxycyte, Oxygen Biotherapeutics) is currently being investigated as an oxygen therapeutic for treatment of wounds, decompression sickness, and traumatic brain injury.[40] Refer to Table 1–12 for further details, and review of PFCs. Table 1–13 for the advantages and disadvantages of Perfluorochemicals.

Table 1–10   Hemoglobin-Based Oxygen Carriers

PRODUCT	MANUFACTURER	CHEMISTRY/SOURCE	HISTORY/STATUS
HemAssist (DCLHb)	Baxter	Diaspirin cross-linked Hgb from outdated human RBCs	First HBOC to advance to phase III clinical trials in United States. Removed from production because of increased mortality rates.
PolyHeme (SFH-P)	Northfield Laboratories	Polymerized and pyridoxalated human Hgb	Underwent phase II/III clinical trials in United States. Did not obtain FDA approval. No longer produced.
Hemopure (HBOC-201)	Originally Biopure; currently OPK Biotech	Polymerized bovine Hgb	Still in phase II/III clinical trials in United States and Europe. Approved for use in S. Africa (2001).
Oxyglobin	Originally Biopure; now OPK Biotech	Polymerized bovine Hgb	Approved for veterinary use in United States and Europe.
Hemospan (MP4)	Sangart	Polyethylene glycol (PEG) attached to the surface of Hgb from human RBCs	In phase II trials in United States; phase III in Europe.
HemoLink	Hemosol	Purified human Hgb from outdated RBCs, cross-linked and polymerized	Abandoned due to cardiac toxicity.
HemoTech	HemoBioTech	Derived from bovine Hgb	Limited clinical trial outside of United States.
Oxy-0301	Oxygenix	Liposome-encapsulated hemoglobin	In experimental phase.

Table 1–11	Advantages and Disadvantages of Hemoglobin-Based Oxygen Carriers	
ADVANTAGES	**DISADVANTAGES**
Long shelf-life	Short intravascular half-life
Very stable	Possible toxicity
No antigenicity (unless bovine)	Increased O_2 affinity
No requirement for blood-typing procedures	Increased oncotic effect

Table 1–13	Advantages and Disadvantages of Perfluorochemicals	
ADVANTAGES	**DISADVANTAGES**
Biological inertness	Adverse clinical effects
Lack of immunogenicity	High O_2 affinity
Easily synthesized	Retention in tissues
	Requirement for O_2 administration when infused
	Deep-freeze storage temperatures

Platelet Preservation

Basic Concepts

Platelets are intimately involved in primary hemostasis, which is the interaction of platelets and the vascular endothelium in halting and preventing bleeding following vascular injury. Platelets are cellular fragments derived from the cytoplasm of megakaryocytes present in the bone marrow. They do not contain a nucleus, although the mitochondria contain DNA. Platelets are released and circulate approximately 9 to 12 days as small, disk-shaped cells with an average diameter of 2 to 4 µm. The normal platelet count ranges from 150,000 to 350,000 per µL. Approximately 30% of the platelets, that have been released from the bone marrow into the circulation, are sequestered in the microvasculature of the spleen as functional reserves.

Platelets have specific roles in the hemostatic process that are critically dependent on an adequate number in the circulation and on normal platelet function. Normal platelet function in vivo requires more than 100,000 platelets per microliter. Spontaneous hemorrhage may occur when the platelet count falls below 10,000. Assuming normal platelet function, a platelet count greater than 50,000/µL will minimize the chance of hemorrhage during surgery.[8] The role of platelets in hemostasis includes (1) initial arrest of bleeding by platelet plug formation and (2) stabilization of the hemostatic plug by contributing to the process of fibrin formation and (3) maintenance of vascular integrity. Platelet plug formation involves the adhesion of platelets to the subendothelium and subsequent aggregation, with thrombin being a key effector of these phenomena. Platelets, like other cells, require energy in the form of ATP for cellular movement, active transport of molecules across the membrane, biosynthetic purposes, and maintenance of a hemostatic steady state.

Advanced Concepts

The organelle region of the platelet is responsible for the metabolic activities in this cell. Like many other cells, platelets possess mitochondria and various cytoplasmic granules. Platelets, however, are anucleated and do not possess either a Golgi body or rough endoplasmic reticulum (RER). Generally, the most numerous organelles are the platelet granules. Platelets contain three morphologically distinct types of storage granules: dense granules, α granules, and lysosomes. The α granules are the most numerous (20 to 200 per platelet) and store a number of different substances, such as beta-thromboglobulin (β-TG), platelet factor 4 (PF4), platelet-derived growth factor (PDGF), thrombospondin, and factor V.

Table 1–12	Perfluorocarbons	
Fluosol-DA	Green Cross Corporation	The only oxygen therapeutic approved for human clinical use in the United States. Approved in 1989; discontinued in 1994 because of clinical shortcomings and poor sales.
Oxygent	Alliance Pharmaceutical Corporation	Phase III trial in Europe completed; phase III trial in United States terminated due to adverse effects. Development stopped due to lack of funding.
Oxyfluor	HemaGen	Early phase clinical trials completed. Development stopped due to loss of financial backing.
Oxycyte	Originally Synthetic Blood International; name changed to Oxygen Biotherapeutics in 2008	Shift in research from use as RBC substitute to other medical applications. Currently in phase II trials in Switzerland for treatment of traumatic brain injury.
Perftoran	Perftoran	Approved for use in Russia and Mexico.

Dense granules or bodies are smaller and fewer in number (2 to 10 per platelet) and appear as dense opaque granules in transmission electron microscopy (TEM) preparations.[8] Dense granules contain storage ADP, ATP, ionic calcium, serotonin, and phosphates. Platelet ADP and ATP are present in two cellular pools—a metabolic pool and a storage pool. The metabolic pool meets the platelet's ongoing metabolic needs, and the storage pool, which is located in the dense granules, is released when the platelet is stimulated.[19] Lysosomes contain microbicidal enzymes, neutral proteases, and acid hydrolases. Glycogen granules are also found within the organelle zone and function in platelet metabolism. The estimated 10 to 60 mitochondria present per platelet require glycogen as their source of energy for metabolism.[8] In the resting platelet, approximately 15% ATP (energy) production is generated by glycolysis and 85% by oxygen consumption through the tricarboxylic acid (TCA) cycle.[19] In the activated state, about half the ATP production in platelets occurs through the glycolytic pathway, increasing the rate of lactate production.[8] Platelets circulate in an inactivated state and require minimal stimulation for activation, ensuring their immediate availability for hemostasis.

The Platelet Storage Lesion

Basic Concepts

Platelet storage still presents one of the major challenges to the blood bank because of the limitations of storing platelets. In the United States, which has a storage limit of 5 days, approximately 30% of the platelet inventory is discarded either by the blood supplier or the hospital blood bank.[41] The two main reasons for the 5-day shelf-life for platelets is bacterial contamination at incubation of 22°C and the loss of platelet quality during storage (known as the **platelet storage lesion**). During storage, a varying degree of platelet activation occurs that results in release of some intracellular granules and a decline in ATP and ADP. This platelet activation often results in temporary aggregation of platelets into large sheets that must be allowed to rest for the aggregation to be reversed, especially when the **platelet concentrates (PCs)** are prepared with the **platelet-rich-plasma (PRP) method**.

The reduced oxygen tension (pO_2) in the plastic platelet storage container results in the platelets increasing the rate of glycolysis to compensate for the decrease in ATP regeneration from the oxidative (TCA) metabolism. This increases glucose consumption and causes an increase in lactic acid that must be buffered. This results in a fall in pH. During the storage of PCs in plasma, the principal buffer is bicarbonate. When the bicarbonate buffers are depleted during PC storage, the pH rapidly falls to less than 6.2, which is associated with a loss of platelet viability. In addition, when pH falls below 6.2, the platelets swell and there is a disk-to-sphere transformation in morphology that is associated with a loss of membrane integrity. The platelets then become irreversibly swollen, aggregate together, or lyse, and when infused, will not circulate or function. During storage of PCs, the pH will remain stable as long as the production of lactic acid does not exceed the buffering capacity of the plasma or other storage solution.

Advanced Concepts

The platelet storage lesion results in a loss of platelet quality and viability. When platelets deteriorate during storage, their membranes lose their ability to maintain normal lipid asymmetry and phosphatidylserine becomes expressed on the outer membrane surface.[41] The binding of annexin V, which has a high affinity for anionic phospholipids, can be used to measure this loss of membrane integrity using flow cytometry.[41] Flow cytometry is also used to measure the platelet degranulation process during storage by detecting the surface expression of CD62P or CD63.[41] Measurement of specific platelet α granules such as β-thromboglobulin and platelet factor 4 can also assess platelet degranulation during storage. Generally, the quality-control measurements required by various accreditation organizations for platelet concentrates include platelet concentrate volume, platelet count, pH of the unit, and residual leukocyte count if claims of leukoreduction are made.[42] In addition, immediately before distribution to hospitals, a visual inspection is made that often includes an assessment of **platelet swirl**.[41] The absence of platelet swirling is associated with the loss of membrane integrity during storage, resulting in the loss of discoid shape with irreversible sphering. Box 1–4 lists the in vitro platelet assays that have been correlated with in vivo survival.

Clinical Use of Platelets

Platelet components are effectively used to treat bleeding associated with thrombocytopenia, a marked decrease in platelet number. The efficacy of the transfused platelet concentrates is usually estimated from the **corrected count increment (CCI)** of platelets measured after transfusion. It should be noted that the CCI does not evaluate or assess function of the transfused platelets.[43]

Platelets are also transfused prophylactically to increase the circulating platelet count in hematology-oncology thrombocytopenic patients to prevent bleeding secondary

---

BOX 1–4

In Vitro Platelet Assays Correlated With In Vivo Survival

- pH
- Shape change
- Hypotonic shock response
- Lactate production
- pO_2

to drug and radiation therapy. Platelets are also utilized in some instances to treat other disorders in which platelets are qualitatively or quantitatively defective because of genetic reasons.

In the 1950s and 1960s, platelet transfusions were given as freshly drawn whole blood or platelet-rich plasma. Circulatory overload quickly developed as a major complication of this method of administering platelets. Since the 1970s, platelets have been prepared from whole blood as concentrates in which the volume per unit is near 50 mL in contrast to the 250- to 300-mL volume of platelet-rich plasma units. Today, platelets are prepared as concentrates from whole blood and increasingly by apheresis. The 2007 National Blood Collection and Utilization Survey found that only 17% of platelet doses in the United States were **whole blood derived** (WBD). Platelets still remain as the primary means of treating thrombocytopenia, even though therapeutic responsiveness varies according to patient conditions and undefined consequences of platelet storage conditions.[44,45] (See Chapter 13 for the methods for preparing platelet concentrates.)

Current Conditions for Platelet Preservation (Platelet Storage)

Basic Concepts

Platelet concentrates prepared from whole blood and apheresis components are routinely stored at 20°C to 24°C, with continuous agitation for up to 5 days. FDA standards define the expiration time as midnight of day 5. Primarily flatbed and circular agitators are in use. There are a number of containers in use for 5-day storage of WBD and apheresis platelets. In the United States, platelets are being stored in a 100% plasma medium, unless a platelet additive solution is used (see section on platelet additives on page 19). Although platelets can be stored at 1°C to 6°C for 48 hours,[46] it does not appear that this is a routine practice.

History of Platelet Storage: Rationale for Current Conditions

Advanced Concepts

The conditions utilized to store platelets have evolved since the 1960s as key parameters that influence the retention of platelet properties. Initially, platelets were stored at 1°C to 6°C, based on the successful storage of RBCs at this temperature range. A key study in 1969 by Murphy and Gardner showed that cold storage at 1°C to 6°C resulted in a marked reduction in platelet in vivo viability, manifested as a reduction in in vivo life span, after only 18 hours of storage.[47] This study also identified for the first time that 20°C to 24°C (room temperature) should be the preferred range, based on viability results.

The reduction in viability at 1°C to 6°C was associated with conversion of the normal discoid shape to a form that

is irreversibly spherical. This structural change is considered to be the factor responsible for the deleterious effects of cold storage. When stored even for several hours at 4°C, platelets do not return to their disk shape upon rewarming. This loss of shape is probably a result of microtubule disassembly. Based on many follow-up studies, platelets are currently stored at room temperature.

These studies provided an understanding of the factors that influenced the retention of platelet viability and the parameters that needed to be considered to optimize storage conditions. One factor identified as necessary was the need to agitate platelet components during storage, although initially the rationale for agitation was not understood.[48,49] Subsequently, agitation has been shown to facilitate oxygen transfer into the platelet bag and oxygen consumption by the platelets. The positive role for oxygen has been associated with the maintenance of platelet component pH.[50] Maintaining pH was determined to be a key parameter for retaining platelet viability in vivo when platelets were stored at 20°C to 24°C.

Although storage itself was associated with a small reduction in post-infusion platelet viability, an enhanced loss was observed when the pH was reduced from initial levels of near 7 to the range of 6.8 to 6.5, with a marked loss when the pH was reduced to levels below 6.[49] A pH of 6 was initially the standard for maintaining satisfactory viability. The standard was subsequently changed to 6.2 with the availability of additional data. As pH was reduced from 6.8 to 6.2, the platelets progressively changed shape from disks to spheres. This change is irreversible when the pH falls to less than 6.2.[19]

In the 1970s, when WBD platelets were initially stored as concentrates, a major problem was a marked reduction in pH in many concentrates. This limited the storage period to 3 days. The containers being used for storage were identified as being responsible for the fall in pH because of their limiting gas transfer properties for oxygen and carbon dioxide. Carbon dioxide buildup from aerobic respiration and as the end product of plasma bicarbonate depletion also influenced the fall in pH. The gas transport properties of a container are known to reflect the container material, the gas permeability of the wall of the plastic container, the surface area of the container available for gas exchange, and the thickness of the container. Insufficient agitation may also be a factor responsible for pH reduction because agitation facilitates gas transport into the containers.

Storage in Second-Generation Containers

Understanding the factors that led to the reduction in pH in first-generation platelet containers resulted in the development of **second-generation containers**, starting around 1982. The second-generation containers, with increased gas transport properties (allowing increased oxygen transport and carbon dioxide escape), are available and are being utilized for storing platelets for 5 days without pH substantially falling. Such containers are in use for WBD PCs and apheresis components.

Containers for platelet storage were originally constructed from polyvinyl chloride (PVC) plastic containing a phthalate plasticizer. The second-generation containers are constructed in some cases with PVC and in other cases with polyolefin plastic. For most PVC containers, alternative plasticizers (trimellitate and citrate based) have been used to increase gas transport. The nominal volumes of the containers are 300 to 400 mL and 1 to 1.5 L for WBD platelet concentrates and apheresis components, respectively. The size of the containers for apheresis components reflects the increased number of platelets that are being stored and hence the need for a larger surface area to provide adequate gas transport properties for maintaining pH levels near the initial level of 7 even after 5 days of storage. Box 1–5 lists factors that should be considered when using 5-day platelet storage containers.

Storing Platelets Without Agitation for Limited Times

Although platelet components should be stored with continuous agitation, there are data that suggest that platelet properties, based on in vitro studies, are retained when agitation is discontinued for up to 24 hours during a 5-day storage period.[51,52] This is probably related to the retention of satisfactory oxygen levels with the second-generation containers when agitation is discontinued, as occurs by necessity when platelets are shipped over long distances by, for example, overnight courier.

Measurement of Viability and Functional Properties of Stored Platelets

Viability indicates the capacity of platelets to circulate after infusion without premature removal or destruction. Platelets have a life span of 8 to 10 days after release from megakaryocytes. Storage causes a reduction in this parameter, even when pH is maintained. Platelet viability of stored platelets is determined by measuring pretransfusion and post-transfusion platelet counts (1 hour and/or 24 hours) and expressing the difference based on the number of platelets transfused (corrected count increment) or by determining the disappearance

rate of infused radiolabeled platelets to normal individuals whose donation provided the platelets.

The observation of the swirling phenomenon caused by discoid platelets when placed in front of a light source has been used to obtain a semiqualitative evaluation of the retention of platelet viability properties in stored units.[53] The extent of shape change and the hypotonic shock response in in vitro tests appears to provide some indication about the retention of platelet viability properties.[54] Function is defined as the ability of viable platelets to respond to vascular damage in promoting hemostasis. Clinical assessment of hemostasis is being increasingly used.

The maintenance of pH during storage at 20°C to 24°C has been associated with the retention of post-transfusion platelet viability and has been the key issue that has been addressed to improve conditions for storage at this temperature. There is also the issue of retaining platelet function during storage. Historically, room temperature storage has been thought to be associated with a reduction in platelet functional properties. However, the vast transfusion experience with room temperature platelets worldwide indicates that such platelets have satisfactory function. As has been suggested many times over the last 30 years, it is possible that room temperature–stored platelets undergo a rejuvenation of the processes that provide for satisfactory function upon introduction into the circulation.[55,56]

The better functionality of cold-stored platelets, based on some studies, especially ones conducted in the 1970s, may have reflected an undesirable activation of platelet processes as a result of storing platelets at a temperature range of 1°C to 6°C. Activation is a prerequisite for platelet function in hemostasis. During storage, it takes different forms. Even with storage at 20°C to 24°C, there is some activation, as judged by the release of granular proteins such as p-selectin (CD62) and platelet factor 4 and granular adenine nucleotides. There are some data that suggest that specific inhibitors of the activation processes may have a beneficial influence during storage.[57]

Table 1–14 summarizes platelet changes during storage (the platelet storage lesion). It should be noted that except for change in pH, the effect of in vitro changes on post-transfusion platelet survival and function is unknown, and some of the changes may be reversible upon transfusion.[58]

Platelet Storage and Bacterial Contamination

Basic Concepts

The major concern associated with storage of platelets at 20°C to 24°C is the potential for bacterial growth, if the prepared platelets contain bacteria because of contamination at the phlebotomy site or if the donor has an unrecognized bacterial infection.[59] Environmental contamination during processing and storage is another potential, though less common, source of bacteria. Room temperature storage and the presence of oxygen provide a good environment for bacterial proliferation. Sepsis due to contaminated

---

BOX 1–5

Factors to Be Considered When Using 5-Day Plastic Storage Bags

- Temperature control of 20°C to 24°C is critical during platelet preparation and storage.
- Careful handling of plastic bags during expression of platelet-poor plasma helps prevent the platelet button from being distributed and prevents removal of excess platelets with the platelet-poor plasma.
- Residual plasma volumes recommended for the storage of platelet concentrates from whole blood (45 to 65 mL).
- For apheresis platelets, the surface area of the storage bags needs to allow for the number of platelets that will be stored.

Table 1–14	**The Platelet Storage Lesion**
CHARACTERISTIC	**CHANGE OBSERVED**
Lactate	Increased
pH	Decreased
ATP	Decreased
Morphology scores change from discoid to spherical (loss of swirling effect)	Decreased
Degranulation (β-thromboglobulin, platelet factor 4)	Increased
Platelet activation markers (P-selectin [CD62P] or CD63)	Increased
Platelet aggregation	Drop in responses to some agonists

platelets is the most common infectious complication of transfusion.[60] A large-scale study at American Red Cross (ARC) regional blood centers from 2004 to 2006 detected bacteria in 186 out of 1,004,206 donations for a contamination rate of approximately 1 in 5,400.[61] Although the occurrence of patient **sepsis** is much lower, particularly troublesome is the fact that some septic episodes have led to patient deaths. An estimated 10% to 40% of patients transfused with a bacterially contaminated platelet unit develop life-threatening sepsis.[60] As a result, in 2002 the College of American Pathologists (CAP) added a requirement for laboratories to have a method to screen platelets for bacterial contamination, and AABB introduced a similar requirement in 2004.

Advanced Concepts

There are three commercial systems approved by the FDA for screening platelets for bacterial contamination: BacT/ALERT (bioMérieux), eBDS (Pall Corp.), and Scansystem (Hemosystem). BacT/ALERT and eBDS are culture-based systems. As the level of bacteria in the platelets at the time of collection can be low, samples are not taken until after at least 24 hours of storage. This provides time for any bacteria present to replicate to detectable levels. BacT/ALERT measures bacteria by detecting a change in carbon-dioxide levels associated with bacterial growth.[62] This system provides continuous monitoring of the platelet sample–containing culture bottles, which are held for the shelf-life of the platelet unit or until a positive reaction is detected. The eBDS system measures the oxygen content of the air within the sample pouch following incubation for 18 to 30 hours. A decrease in oxygen level indicates the presence of bacteria. BacT/ALERT and eBDS are the most widely used systems for screening platelets in the United States, and studies have documented good sensitivity and specificity;

however, false-negative test results have been documented. With both culture systems, the need to delay sampling and the requirement for incubation delay entry of the platelet products into inventory. Box 1–6 lists the disadvantages associated with the use of culture methods for the detection of bacterial contamination of platelets.

The third bacterial detection method approved by the FDA, Scansystem, is a laser-based, scanning cytometry method. In the United States, 100% of apheresis platelets are tested by the collection facility using culture-based assays.[63] Because screening individual units of WBD platelets by these methods is time-consuming, expensive, and uses a significant amount of the product, less sensitive methods, such as gram staining and dipstick tests for pH and glucose, were initially used for screening. Since these methods have a sensitivity of about only 50%, many transfusion services chose not to transfuse WBD platelets. This practice made it difficult for some blood banks to meet the demand for apheresis platelets, and WBD platelets became underutilized.

In November 2009, the FDA approved the first rapid test to detect bacteria in WBD platelets—the Pan Genera Detection (PGD) test (Verax Biomedical). The PDG test, which was previously approved by the FDA for testing leukocyte-reduced platelets as an adjunct to culture, is an immunoassay that detects lipoteichoic acids on gram-positive bacteria and lipopolysaccharides on gram-negative bacteria. Both aerobes and anaerobes are detected. The test can be performed on pools of up to 6 units of WBD platelets. A sample of only 500 µl is required. Following pretreatment, the sample is loaded into a disposable plastic cartridge with built-in controls that turn from yellow to blue-violet when the test is ready to be read, in approximately 20 minutes. A pink-colored bar in either the gram-positive or gram-negative test window indicates a positive result. The manufacturer states that the system has a specificity of 99.8% and can detect bacteria at 10^3 to 10^5 colony-forming units (CFU) per milliliter.[64] The PGD test can be performed by transfusion services just prior to release of platelet products. The optimum time for sampling is at least 72 hours after collection.

With the availability of this rapid and sensitive method for screening WBD platelets, AABB issued Interim Standard 5.1.5.1.1, which prohibits the use of the less-sensitive methods (microscopy, pH, glucose) after January 31, 2011.[65] Transfusion services must either obtain their platelets from a collection facility that performs an approved test for bacterial contamination, or they must perform an approved test themselves.[66] At this time, the approved tests are bacterial culture or the Verax PGD test.

The practice of screening platelets for bacterial contamination has reduced, but not eliminated, the transfusion of contaminated platelet products. False-negative cultures can occur when bacteria are present in low numbers and when the pathogen is a slow-growing organism. The American Red Cross received reports of 20 septic transfusion reactions from 2004 to 2006 following transfusion of culture-negative platelets. Eighty percent of the septic reactions were due to *Staphylococcus* spp., and 65% occurred with products transfused on day 5 after collection. Three of these reactions were fatal, for a fatality rate of 1 per 498,711 distributed products.[61]

Because current bacterial screening methods are not 100% sensitive, they must be supplemented by other precautions, such as the donor interview and proper donor arm disinfection. Another more recent precaution is the diversion of the first aliquot (about 20 to 30 mL) of collected blood into a separate but connected **diversion pouch**. This procedure minimizes the placement of skin plugs, the most common source of bacterial contamination, into the platelet products. The 2007 National Blood Collection and Utilization Survey found that 50.4% of blood collection facilities used diversion devices for collecting apheresis platelets, and one study found that diversion reduced bacterial contamination by 40% to 88%.[67]

In view of the ability to test for bacterial contamination and the use of diversion pouches and **sterile docking instruments**, there is now interest in being able to store pools of platelets up to the outdate of the individual concentrates. The retention of platelet properties during storage of pools has been shown in a number of studies. Traditionally, four to six WBD platelets are pooled into a single bag by the transfusion service just prior to issue. This facilitates transfusion but reduces the shelf-life of the platelets to 4 hours, because they are prepared in an open system.

In 2005, the FDA approved the use of **prestorage pooled platelets** prepared by Acrodose Systems (Pall Corp.). Acrodose platelets are pooled ABO-matched, leukoreduced WBD platelets that have been cultured and are ready for transfusion. Because they are produced in a closed system, they can be stored for 5 days from collection. They provide a therapeutic dose equivalent to apheresis platelets and at a lower cost,[68] but they do expose the recipient to multiple donors. A recent study comparing transfusion reactions from prestorage-pooled platelets, apheresis platelets, and poststorage-pooled WBD platelets found no difference in reaction rates among the different products.[69] Prestorage-pooled platelets may prove to be a useful adjunct to apheresis platelets, which are often in short supply, and may lead to improved utilization of WBD platelets.

Current Trends in Platelet Preservation Research

Advanced Concepts

Research and development in platelet preservation is being pursued in many directions, including the following:

1. Development of methods that would allow platelets to be stored for 7 days
2. Development of additive solutions, also termed *synthetic media*
3. Development of procedures to reduce and inactivate the level of pathogens that may be in platelet units
4. Development of platelet substitutes
5. New approaches for storage of platelets at 1°C to 6°C
6. The development of processes to cryopreserve platelets

Storage for 7 Days at 20°C to 24°C

In 1984, the FDA extended platelet storage from 5 to 7 days. Reports of septic transfusion reactions increased following this change, and in 1986 the storage time was changed back to 5 days. With the implementation of bacterial screening of platelets and its impact on their available shelf-life, there is renewed interest in being able to store platelets for 7 days. In 2005, the FDA approved a study called "Post Approval Surveillance Study of Platelet Outcomes, Release Tested" (PASSPORT) to collect data on the safety of apheresis platelets tested with an FDA-approved bacterial detection test and stored for 7 days. The study was suspended in 2008 because of safety concerns when interim data and published studies suggested that culture at 24 hours after collection may miss up to 50% of contaminated apheresis platelet units.[70] FDA and industry representatives discussed modifications to the study protocol that might increase the safety of 7-day platelets and allow resumption of the study—for example, increasing the size of the culture inoculum, performing anaerobic cultures in addition to aerobic cultures, and performing a second culture at 5 days of storage. Because consensus could not be reached, the PASSPORT study was not resumed.[70] Although work toward approval of safe and efficacious 7-day platelets is likely to continue, the shelf-life for platelets at this time remains 5 days.

Storage with Additive Solutions

Platelet additive solutions (PASs) were first developed in the 1980s[71] and have been used in Europe since 1995 to replace a large portion of the plasma in platelet suspensions prepared from whole blood by the **buffy coat method**. In 2010, the FDA approved the first PAS for use in the United States. This additive, called PAS-C, was approved for storage of apheresis platelets collected by the AMICUS Separator System (Fenwal/Baxter) for up to 5 days. Other PASs are under development and may gain FDA approval in the future.[72]

PASs are designed to support platelets during storage in reduced amounts of residual plasma. Historically, platelets have been stored in 100% plasma. With the addition of a PAS, residual plasma can be reduced to 30% to 40%[71] (35% with InterSol). One advantage is that this approach provides more plasma for fractionation. In addition, there are data indicating that optimal additive solutions may improve the quality of platelets during storage, reduce adverse effects associated with transfusion of plasma, and promote earlier detection of bacteria.[63,73,74] Box 1–7 lists the advantages of using a platelet additive solution for platelet storage.

Research is being conducted to improve the additive solutions in use. Gulliksson suggested that platelets could be stored for at least 18 to 20 days at 20°C to 24°C with an optimized additive medium based on considerations that indicate that storage could well inhibit platelet aging with the appropriate environments/medium.[75] Platelet additive solutions in use and those being developed contain varying quantities of citrate, phosphate, potassium, magnesium, and acetate. Citrate, magnesium, and potassium control platelet activation.[76] Acetate serves as a substrate for aerobic respiration (mitochondrial metabolism) while also providing a way to maintain pH levels as it reacts with hydrogen ions when it is first utilized. Some formulations also contain glucose, which seems to maintain pH better beyond day 5. This might give glucose-containing PASs an advantage over nonglucose PASs if extended storage of platelets becomes a reality.[77] Currently, glucose-containing PASs are not widely used because glucose caramelizes during the steam sterilization process that is used.[78] When nonglucose PASs are used, at least 20% to 35% of the plasma must be retained in order to provide the glucose the platelets need during storage.[78]

Procedures to Reduce and Inactivate Pathogens

Despite sensitive methods to detect bacteria in platelets, septic transfusion reactions still occur. As for RBCs, procedures are being developed to treat platelet components to reduce or inactivate any residual pathogens (bacteria, viruses, parasites) that may be present. The term *pathogen reduction* (PR) is preferred to *pathogen inactivation* (PI) because inactivation may not be complete.[79] PR/PI procedures could potentially add an additional level of safety by protecting against unknown and newly emerging pathogens.[79,80]

Two PR/PI methods, both using photochemical technologies to target nucleic acids, are approved for use in Europe but are approved only for clinical trials in the United States.[81] The targeting of nucleic acids is possible because platelets, like RBCs, do not contain functional nucleic acids. In the INTERCEPT system (Cerus Corp.), amotosalen is activated by ultraviolet (UV) light and binds to the nucleic acid base pairs of pathogens, preventing replication.[82] This system was approved for clinical use in Europe in 2002. The Mirasol PRT system (CaridianBCT Biotechnologies) uses riboflavin (vitamin B$_2$) and UV light to cause irreversible changes to the nucleic acids of pathogens.[83] Many studies suggest that PR of platelets is safe and effective; however, additional studies involving larger groups and pediatric patients are needed.[80] Some argue that since most patients who receive platelets also receive red cells, PR of platelets will be of limited value until there is an equivalent method for red cells.[79]

Development of Platelet Substitutes

In view of the short shelf-life of liquid-stored platelet products, there has been a long-standing interest to develop platelet substitute products that maintain hemostatic function. Platelet substitutes are in the early stages of development. It is understood that platelet substitutes may have use only in specific clinical situations because platelets have a complex biochemistry and physiology. Besides having a long shelf-life, platelet substitutes appear to have reduced potential to transmit pathogens as a result of the processing procedures. A number of different approaches have been utilized.[84] Apparently, one approach with the potential for providing clinically useful products is the use of lyophilization.

Two products prepared from human platelets are in preclinical testing. One preparation uses washed platelets treated with paraformaldehyde, with subsequent freezing in 5% albumin and lyophilization.[85] These platelets on rehydration have been reported to have hemostatic effectiveness in different animal models. A second method involves the freeze-drying of trehalose-loaded platelets.[86] Additional products that are apparently being developed include fibrinogen-coated albumin microcapsules and microspheres and modified RBCs with procoagulant properties as a result of fibrinogen binding. Fibrinogen is being used because in vivo this protein cross-links activated platelets to form platelet aggregates as part of the hemostatic process. Two other approaches include the development of platelet-derived microparticles that can stop bleeding and liposome-based hemostatic products.[84]

New Approaches for Storage of Platelets at 1°C to 6°C

Although storage of platelets at 1°C to 6°C was discontinued many years ago, there has been an interest in developing ways to overcome the storage lesion that occurs at 1°C to 6°C.[87] The rationale for the continuing effort reflects concerns about

---

BOX 1–7

Advantages of Using Platelet Additive Solutions

- Optimizes platelet storage in vitro
- Saves plasma for other purposes (e.g., transfusion or fractionation)
- Facilitates ABO-incompatible platelet transfusions
- Reduces plasma-associated transfusion side effects, such as febrile and allergic reactions, and may reduce risk of transfusion-related acute lung injury (TRALI)
- Improves effectiveness of photochemical pathogen reduction technologies
- Potentially improves bacterial detection

storing and shipping platelets at 20°C to 24°C, especially the chance for bacterial proliferation. Refrigeration would significantly reduce the risk of bacterial contamination, allowing for longer storage. Many approaches have been attempted without success, although early results showed some promise. The approaches primarily involve adding substances to inhibit cold-induced platelet activation, as this is thought to be the key storage lesion. Two reports concluded that platelets stored at 1°C to 6°C could conceivably have satisfactory in vivo viability and function if the surface of the platelets were modified to prevent the enhanced clearance (unsatisfactory viability) from circulation.[88,89]

Based on animal studies, it was suggested that cold-induced spherical platelets can remain in the circulation if abnormal clearance is prevented. Spherical platelets, manifested as a result of cold storage, have been assumed to be a trigger for low viability. The specific approach involves the enzymatic galactosylation of cold-stored platelets to modify specifically one type of membrane protein. The addition of uridine diphosphate galactose is the vehicle for the modificaiton.[89]

Frozen Platelets

Although considered a research technique and not licensed by the FDA, frozen platelets are used occasionally in the United States as autologous transfusions for patients who are refractory to allogeneic platelets. Platelets are collected by apheresis, the cryopreservative dimethyl sulfoxide (DMSO) is added, and the platelets are frozen at –80°C. The frozen platelets can be stored for up to 2 years. Prior to transfusion, the platelets are thawed and centrifuged to remove the DMSO. Although in vivo recovery after transfusion is only about 33%, the platelets seem to function effectively.[5]

SUMMARY CHART

- ✔ Each unit of whole blood collected contains approximately 450 mL of blood and 63 mL of anticoagulant-preservative solution or approximately 500 mL of blood and 70 mL of anticoagulant-preservative solution.

- ✔ A donor can give blood every 8 weeks.

- ✔ As of 2011, samples from donors of each unit of donated blood are tested by 10 screening tests for infectious diseases markers.

- ✔ Glycolysis generates approximately 90% of the ATP needed by RBCs, and 10% is provided by the pentose phosphate pathway.

- ✔ Seventy-five percent post-transfusion survival of RBCs is necessary for a successful transfusion.

- ✔ ACD, CPD, and CP2D are approved preservative solutions for storage of RBCs at 1°C to 6°C for 21 days, and CPDA-1 is approved for 35 days.

- ✔ Additive solutions (Adsol, Nutricel, Optisol) are approved in the United States for RBC storage for 42 days. Additive-solution RBCs have been shown to be appropriate for neonates and pediatric patients.

- ✔ RBCs have been traditionally glycerolized and frozen within 6 days of whole blood collection in CPD or CPDA-1 and can be stored for 10 years from the date of freezing.

- ✔ Rejuvesol is the only FDA-approved rejuvenation solution used in some blood centers to regenerate ATP and 2,3-DPG levels before RBC freezing.

- ✔ Rejuvenation is used primarily to salvage O-type and rare RBC units that are at outdate or with specific anticoagulant-preservative solution up to 3 days past outdate.

- ✔ Research is being conducted to improve on the current additive solutions.

- ✔ Research is being conducted to develop procedures to reduce or inactivate pathogens.

- ✔ RBC substitutes under investigation include hemoglobin-based oxygen carriers and perfluorocarbons.

- ✔ A platelet concentrate should contain a minimum of 5.5×10^{10} platelets (in 90% of the sampled units according to AABB standards) in a volume routinely between 45 and 65 mL that is sufficient to maintain a pH of 6.2 or greater at the conclusion of the 5-day storage period.

- ✔ When platelet concentrates (usually 4 to 6) are pooled using an open system, the storage time changes to 4 hours. A new method of pooling that uses a closed system allows the pool to be stored for 5 days from the date of collection.

- ✔ Apheresis components contain 4 to 6 times as many platelets as a PC prepared from whole blood. They should contain a minimum of 3.0×10^{11} platelets (in 90% of the sampled units).

- ✔ Platelet components are stored for up to 5 days at 20°C to 24°C with continuous agitation. When necessary, as during shipping, platelets can be stored without continuous agitation for up to 24 hours (at 20°C to 24°C) during a 5-day storage period. Platelets are rarely stored at 1°C to 6°C.

- ✔ If a platelet bag is broken or opened, the platelets must be transfused within 4 hours when stored at 20°C to 24°C.

Review Questions

1. What is the maximum volume of blood that can be collected from a 110-lb donor, including samples for processing?
   a. 450 mL
   b. 500 mL
   c. 525 mL
   d. 550 mL

2. How often can a blood donor donate whole blood?
   a. Every 24 hours
   b. Once a month
   c. Every 8 weeks
   d. Twice a year

3. When RBCs are stored, there is a "shift to the left." This means:
   a. Hemoglobin oxygen affinity increases, owing to an increase in 2,3-DPG.
   b. Hemoglobin oxygen affinity increases, owing to a decrease in 2,3-DPG.
   c. Hemoglobin oxygen affinity decreases, owing to a decrease in 2,3-DPG.
   d. Hemoglobin oxygen affinity decreases, owing to an increase in 2,3-DPG.

4. The majority of platelets transfused in the United States today are:
   a. Whole blood–derived platelets prepared by the platelet-rich plasma method.
   b. Whole blood–derived platelets prepared by the buffy coat method.
   c. Apheresis platelets.
   d. Prestorage pooled platelets.

5. Which of the following anticoagulant preservatives provides a storage time of 35 days at 1°C to 6°C for units of whole blood and prepared RBCs if an additive solution is not added?
   a. ACD-A
   b. CP2D
   c. CPD
   d. CPDA-1

6. What are the current storage time and storage temperature for platelet concentrates and apheresis platelet components?
   a. 5 days at 1°C to 6°C
   b. 5 days at 24°C to 27°C
   c. 5 days at 20°C to 24°C
   d. 7 days at 22°C to 24°C

7. What is the minimum number of platelets required in a platelet concentrate prepared from whole blood by centrifugation (90% of sampled units)?
   a. 5.5×10^{11}
   b. 3×10^{10}
   c. 3×10^{11}
   d. 5.5×10^{10}

8. RBCs can be frozen for:
   a. 12 months.
   b. 1 year.
   c. 5 years.
   d. 10 years.

9. What is the minimum number of platelets required in an apheresis component (90% of the sampled units)?
   a. 3×10^{11}
   b. 4×10^{11}
   c. 2×10^{11}
   d. 3.5×10^{11}

10. Whole blood and RBC units are stored at what temperature?
    a. 1°C to 6°C
    b. 20°C to 24°C
    c. 37°C
    d. 24°C to 27°C

11. Additive solutions are approved for storage of red blood cells for how many days?
    a. 21
    b. 42
    c. 35
    d. 7

12. One criterion used by the FDA for approval of new preservation solutions and storage containers is an average 24-hour post-transfusion RBC survival of more than:
    a. 50%.
    b. 60%.
    c. 65%.
    d. 75%.

13. What is the lowest allowable pH for a platelet component at outdate?
    a. 6
    b. 5.9
    c. 6.8
    d. 6.2

14. Frozen and thawed RBCs processed in an open system can be stored for how many days/hours?
    a. 3 days
    b. 6 hours
    c. 24 hours
    d. 15 days

15. What is the hemoglobin source for hemoglobin-based oxygen carriers in advanced clinical testing?

   a. Only bovine hemoglobin
   b. Only human hemoglobin
   c. Both bovine and human hemoglobins
   d. None of the above

16. Which of the following occurs during storage of red blood cells?

   a. pH decreases
   b. 2,3-DPG increases
   c. ATP increases
   d. plasma K^+ decreases

17. Nucleic acid amplification testing is used to test donor blood for which of the following infectious diseases?

   a. Hepatitis C virus
   b. Human immunodeficiency virus
   c. West Nile virus
   d. All of the above

18. Which of the following is NOT an FDA-approved test for quality control of platelets?

   a. BacT/ALERT
   b. eBDS
   c. Gram stain
   d. Pan Genera Detection (PGD) test

19. Prestorage pooled platelets can be stored for:

   a. 4 hours.
   b. 24 hours.
   c. 5 days.
   d. 7 days.

20. Which of the following is the most common cause of bacterial contamination of platelet products?

   a. Entry of skin plugs into the collection bag
   b. Environmental contamination during processing
   c. Bacteremia in the donor
   d. Incorrect storage temperature

References

1. Parks, D: Charles Richard Drew, MD 1904–1950. J Natl Med Assoc 71:893–895, 1979.
2. Kendrick, DB: Blood Program in World War II, Historical Note. Washington Office of Surgeon General, Department of Army, Washington, DC, 1964, pp 1–23.
3. United States Department of Health and Human Services: 2009 National Blood Collection and Utilization Survey Report. Retrieved August 2011 from http://www.hhs.gov/ash/bloodsafety/2009nbcus.pdf.
4. New York Blood Center. Blood Statistics. Retrieved August 30, 2011 from www.nybloodcenter.org/blood-statistics.do?sid0=85&page_id=202#bone.
5. Roback, J, Combs, M, Grossman, B, and Hillyer, C: Technical Manual, 16th ed. American Association of Blood Banks, Bethesda, MD, 2009.
6. Stramer, S: Current risks of transfusion-transmitted agents—a review. Arch Pathol Lab Med 131:702–707, 2007.
7. Zou, S, et al: Current incidence and residual risk of hepatitis B infection among blood donors in the United States. Transfusion 49:1609–1620, 2009.
8. Harmening, DM: Clinical Hematology and Fundamentals of Hemostasis, 5th ed. FA Davis, Philadelphia, 2009.
9. Mohandas, N, and Chasis, JA: Red blood cell deformability, membrane material properties and shape: Regulation of transmission, skeletal and cytosolic proteins and lipids. Semin Hematol 30:171–192, 1993.
10. Mohandas, N, and Evans, E: Mechanical properties of the genetic defects. Ann Rev Biophys Biomol Struct 23:787–818, 1994.
11. Koch, CG, Li, L, Sessler, DI, et al: Duration of red cell storage and complications after cardiac surgery. N Engl J Med 358(12):1229–1239, 2008.
12. Dumont, LJ, and AuBuchon, JP: Evaluation of proposed FDA criteria for the evaluation of radiolabeled red cell recovery trials. Transfusion 48(6):1053–1060, 2008.
13. Hod, EA, Zhang, N, Sokol, SA, et al: Transfusion of red blood cells after prolonged storage produces harmful effects that are mediated by iron and inflammation. Blood 115(21):4284–4292, 2010.
14. Luten, M, et al: Survival of red blood cells after transfusion: A comparison between red cells concentrates of different storage periods. Transfusion 48(7):1478–1485, 2008.
15. Zeiler, T, Muller, JT, and Kretschmer, V: Flow-cytometric determination of survival time and 24-hour recovery of transfused red blood cells. Transfus Med Hemother 30:14–19, 2003.
16. Valeri, CR: Preservation of frozen red blood cells. In Simon, TL, Dzik, WH, Snyder, EL, Stowell, CP, and Strauss, RG (eds): Rossi's Principles of Transfusion Medicine, 3rd ed. Williams & Wilkins, Baltimore, 2002.
17. Ozment, CP, and Turi, JL: Iron overload following red blood cell transfusion and its impact on disease severity. Biochim Biophys Acta 1790(7):694–701, 2009.
18. Beutler, E: Red cell metabolism and storage. In Anderson, KC, and Ness, PM (eds): Scientific Basis of Transfusion Medicine. WB Saunders, Philadelphia, 1994.
19. Simon, TL, Snyder, EL, Stowell, CP, et al (eds): Rossi's Principles of Transfusion Medicine, 4th ed. Wiley-Blackwell, Malden, MA, 2009.
20. Weinberg, JA, McGwin, G Jr, Marques, MB, et al: Transfusions in the less severely injured: Does age of transfused blood affect outcomes? J Trauma 65(4):794–798, 2008.
21. Offner, PJ, Moore, EE, Biffl, WL, Johnson, JL, and Silliman, CC: Increased rate of infection associated with transfusion of old blood after severe injury. Arch Surg 137(6):711–716, 2002.
22. Vandromme, MJ, et al: Transfusion and pneumonia in the trauma intensive care unit: An examination of the temporal relationship. J Trauma 67(1):97–101, 2009.
23. Högman, CF: Additive system approach in blood transfusion birth of the SAG and Sagman systems. Vox Sang 51:1986.
24. Högman, CF: Recent advances in the preparation and storage of red cells. Vox Sang 67:243–246, 1994.
25. Yasutake, M, and Takahashi, TA: Current advances of blood preservation—development and clinical application of additive solutions for preservation of red blood cells and platelets. Nippon Rinsho 55:2429–2433, 1997.
26. Jain, R, and Jarosz, C: Safety and efficacy as AS-1 red blood cell use in neonates. Transfus Apheresis Sci 24:111–115, 2001.
27. U.S. Department of Health and Human Services, Food and Drug Administration. Code of Federal Regulations, Title 21—Food and Drugs, Blood Products 600–680. U.S. Government Printing Office, Washington, DC, 2010.
28. Valeri, CR, et al: A multicenter study of in-vitro and in-vivo values in human RBCs frozen with 40% (wt/vol) glycerol and stored after deglycerolization for 15 days at 4°C in AS-3: assessment of RBC processing in the ACP 215. Transfusion 41:933–939, 2001.
29. Klein, HG, Glynn, SA, Ness, PM, and Blajchman, MA: Research opportunities for pathogen reduction/inactivation of blood components: Summary of an NHLBI workshop. Transfusion 49:1262–1268, 2009.

30. Kruskall, MS, et al: Transfusion to blood group A and O patients of group B RBCs that have been enzymatically converted to group O. Transfusion 40:1290–1298, 2000.

31. Arteriocyte: Cellular Therapies Medical Systems. Blood Pharming. www.arteriocyte.com. Retrieved August 30, 2011.

32. Giarratana, MC, et al: Proof of principle for transfusion of in vitro generated red blood cells. Published online before print. DOI:10.1182/blood-2011-06-362038; Blood September 1, 2011.

33. Chen, J, Scerbo, M, and Kramer, G: A review of blood substitutes: Examining the history, clinical trial results, and ethics of hemoglobin-based oxygen carriers. Clinics (Sao Paulo) <ONLINE> 64(8):803–813, 2009.

34. Reid, TJ: Hb-based oxygen carriers: Are we there yet? Transfusion 43:280–287, 2003.

35. Spahn, DR: Artificial oxygen carriers. Status 2002. Vox Sang 83:(Suppl 1):281–285, 2002.

36. Henkel-Hanke, T, and Oleck, M: Artificial oxygen carriers: a current review. AANA J 75(3):205–211, 2007.

37. Cohn, CS, and Cushing, MM: Oxygen therapeutics: Perfluorocarbons and blood substitute safety. Crit Care Clin 25:399–414, 2009.

38. Natanson, C, Kern, SJ, Lurie, P, Banks, SM, and Wolfe, SM: Cell-free hemoglobin-based blood substitutes and risk of myocardial infarction and death. JAMA 99(19):2304–2312, 2008.

39. Tappenden, J: Artificial blood substitutes. J R Army Med Corps 153(1):3–9, 2007.

40. Oxygen Biotherapeutics. www.oxybiomed.com. Retrieved August 31, 2011.

41. Devine, DV, and Serrano, K: The platelet storage lesion. Clin Lab Med 30: 475–487, 2010.

42. Keitel, S: Guide to the Preparation, Use, and Quality Assurance of Blood Components, 16th ed. Strasbourg (France), Council of Europe Publishing, 2011.

43. Horvath, M, Eichelberger, B, Koren, D, et al: Function of platelets in apheresis platelet concentrates and in patient blood after transfusion as assessed by Impact-R. Transfusion 50: 1036–1042, 2010.

44. Kelly, DL, et al: High-yield platelet concentrates attainable by continuous quality improvement reduce platelet transfusion cost and donor expense. Transfusion 37:482–486, 1997.

45. Van der Meer, PF, Pietersz, R, and Reesink, H: Leukoreduced platelet concentrates in additive solution: An evaluation of filters and storage containers. Vox Sang 81:102–107, 2001.

46. U.S. Department of Health and Human Services, Food and Drug Administration. Code of Federal Regulations, Title 21, Part 640.20 Subpart C–Platelets. U.S. Government Printing Office, Washington, DC, 2010.

47. Murphy, S, and Gardner, FH: Platelet preservation: Effect of storage temperature on maintenance of platelet viability—deleterious effect of refrigerated storage. N Engl J Med 280:1094–1098, 1969.

48. Slichter, SJ, and Harker, LA: Preparation and storage of platelet concentrates II: Storage variables influencing platelet viability and function. Br J Haematol 34:403–412, 1976.

49. Murphy, S: Platelet storage for transfusion. Semin Hematol 22:165–177, 1985.

50. Murphy, S, and Gardner, FH: Platelet storage at 22°C: Role of gas transport across plastic containers in maintenance of viability. Blood 46:209–218, 1975.

51. Moroff, G, and George, VM: The maintenance of platelet properties upon limited discontinuation of agitation during storage. Transfusion 30:427–430, 1990.

52. Hunter, S, Nixon, J, and Murphy, S: The effect of interruption of agitation on platelet quality during storage for transfusion. Transfusion 41:809–814, 2001.

53. Bertolini, F, and Murphy, S: A multicenter inspection of the swirling phenomenon in platelet concentrates prepared in routine practice. Transfusion 36:128–132, 1996.

54. Holme, S, Moroff, G, and Murphy, S: A multi-laboratory evaluation of in vitro platelet assays: The tests for extent of shape change and response to hypotonic shock. Transfusion 38:31–40, 1998.

55. Filip, DJ, and Aster, RH: Relative hemostatic effectiveness of human platelets stored at 4°C and 22°C. J Lab Clin Med 91:618–624, 1978.

56. Owens, M, et al: Post-transfusion recovery of function of 5-day stored platelet concentrates. Br J Haematol 80:539–544, 1992.

57. Holme, S, et al: Improved maintenance of platelet in vivo viability during storage when using a synthetic medium with inhibitors. J Lab Clin Med 119:144–150, 1992.

58. Kaufman, RM: Platelets: Testing, dosing and the storage lesion—recent advances. Hematology Am Soc Hematol Educ Program 492–496, 2006.

59. Brecher, ME, and Hay, SN: The role of bacterial testing of cellular blood products in light of new pathogen inactivation technologies. Blood Therapies Med 3:49–55, 2003.

60. Palavecino, EL, Yomtovian, RA, and Jacobs, MR: Detecting bacterial contamination in platelet products. Clin Lab 52:443–456, 2006.

61. Eder, AF, et al: Bacterial screening of apheresis platelets and the residual risk of septic transfusion reactions: The American Red Cross experience (2004–2006). Transfusion 47(7): 1134–1142, 2007.

62. Macauley, A, et al: Operational feasibility of routine bacterial monitoring of platelets. Transfusion Med 13:189–195, 2003.

63. Dumont, LJ, Wood, TA, Housman, M, et al: Bacterial growth kinetics in ACD-A apheresis platelets: Comparison of plasma and PAS III storage. Transfusion, 51(5): 1079-85, 2011.

64. FDA Clears the First Rapid Test to Detect Bacteria in Pooled Platelets. www.veraxbiomedical.com. Retrieved August 31, 2011.

65. AABB, Association Bulletin #10-05: Suggested options for transfusion services and blood collectors to facilitate implementation of BB/TS Interim Standard 5.1.5.1.1, August 19, 2010.

66. Rapp, H: Interim standard 5.1.5.1.1: What it means for facilities. AABB News, January 2011.

67. McDonald, CP: Bacterial risk reduction by improved donor arm disinfection, diversion and bacterial screening. Transfusion Medicine 16(6):381–396, 2006.

68. AcrodoseSM Platelet: Whole Blood Derived Platelets, Pooled. www.pall.com/medical_43849.asp. Retrieved August 31, 2011.

69. Tormey, CA, et al: Analysis of transfusion reactions associated with prestorage-pooled platelets. Transfusion 49(6):1242–1247, 2009.

70. Gambro BCT and Fenwal Suspend Passport Post-Market Surveillance Study for 7-Day Platelets. www.fenwalinc.com/En/Pages/GambroBCTandFenwalSuspendPassportPost-Market SurveillanceStudyfor7-DayPlatelets.aspx Retrieved January 30, 2011.

71. Wagner, SJ, et al: Calcium is a key constituent for maintaining the in vitro properties of platelets suspended in the bicarbonate-containing additive solution M-sol with low plasma levels. Transfusion 50:1028–1035, 2010.

72. AABB, Association Bulletin #10-06: Information concerning platelet additive solutions, October 4, 2010.

73. Yomtovian, R, and Jacobs, MR: A prospective bonus of platelet storage additive solutions: A reduction in biofilm formation and improved bacterial detection during platelet storage. Transfusion 50(11):2295–2300, 2010.

74. Greco, CA, et al: Effect of platelet additive solution on bacterial dynamics and their influence on platelet quality in stored platelet concentrates. Transfusion 50(11):2344–2352, 2010.

75. Gulliksson, H: Defining the optimal storage conditions for the long-term storage of platelets. Transfusion Med Rev 17:209–215, 2003.

76. Andreu, G, Vasse, J, Herve, F, Tardivel, R, and Semana, G: Introduction of platelet additive solutions in transfusion practice: Advantages, disadvantages, and benefit for patients. Transfus Clin Biol 14(1):100–106, 2007.

77. Sweeney, J: Additive solutions for platelets: Is it time for North American to go with the flow? Transfusion 49(2):199–201, 2009.

78. Vassallo, RR, et al: In vitro and in vivo evaluation of apheresis platelets stored for 5 days in 65% platelet additive solution/35% plasma. Transfusion 50(11):2376–2385, 2010.

79. Hervig, T, Seghatchian, J, and Apelseth, TO: Current debate on pathogen inactivation of platelet concentrates—to use or not to use? Transfus Apheresis Sci 43:411–414, 2010.

80. McClaskey, J, Xu, M, Snyder, EL, and Tormey, CA: Clinical trials for pathogen reduction in transfusion medicine: A review. Transfus Apheresis Sci 41:217–225, 2009.

81. Klein, HG, Glynn, SA, Ness, PM, and Blajchman, MA: Research opportunities for pathogen reduction/inactivation of blood components: Summary of an NHLBI workshop. Transfusion 49(6):1262–1268, 2009.

82. How INTERCEPT Works. Cerus Corporation, Concord, CA. www.cerus.com/index.cfm/ProductOverview. Retrieved August 31, 2011.

83. Mirasol Pathogen Reduction Technology. Caridian BCT Biotechnologies. www.caridianbct.com/location/north-america/Documents/306690227A-web.pdf. Retrieved August 31, 2011.

84. Blajchman, MA: Substitutes and alternatives to platelet transfusions in thrombocytopenic patients. J Thromb Haemostasis 1:1637–1641, 2003.

85. Fischer, TH, et al: Intracellular function in rehydrated lyophilized platelets. Brit J Haematol 111:167–174, 2000.

86. Crowe, JH, et al: Stabilization of membranes in human platelets freeze-dried with trehalose. Chem Phys Lipids 122:41–52, 2003.

87. Vostal, JG, and Mondoro, TH: Liquid cold storage of platelets: A revitalized possible alternative for limiting bacterial contamination of platelet products. Transfus Med Rev 11:286–295, 1997.

88. Hoffmeister, KM, et al: The clearance mechanism of chilled blood platelets. Cell 112:87–97, 2003.

89. Hoffmeister, KM, et al: Glycosylation restores survival of chilled blood platelets. Science 301:1531–1534, 2003.

Chapter 2

Basic Genetics

Lorraine Caruccio, PhD, MT(ASCP)SBB

OBJECTIVES

1. Explain Mendel's laws of independent segregation and random assortment, and describe how he developed them.
2. Correlate the concepts of dominant and recessive traits with examples of the inheritance of blood group antigens.
3. Explain the Hardy-Weinberg principle and how it applies to genetic traits.
4. Given the necessary information, solve Hardy-Weinberg problems for any blood group antigen.
5. Determine the inheritance pattern of a given trait by examining the pedigree analysis.
6. Describe the processes of mitosis and meiosis, and outline the differences between them.
7. Distinguish between X-linked and autosomal traits, and describe how each is inherited.
8. Describe in detail the processes of replication, transcription, and translation, including the basic mechanism of each.
9. List the various types of genetic mutations and describe how they can change the function of living cells and organisms.
10. Describe the cell's different mechanisms for correcting mutations.
11. Identify some of the ways in which genetics can be used in the modern transfusion laboratory, including the necessary background information for describing modern genetic testing techniques.
12. Describe in general the modern techniques used in the study of genetics.

Introduction

One of the most important areas of modern biology is the science of genetics. This chapter covers the basic concepts of genetics necessary to understand its role in modern blood banking. Knowledge of modern methods of analysis is also required to appreciate how problems in genetics are solved and explained. The more blood bank technologists become familiar with these techniques, the faster they can be applied to general use in blood bank laboratories and the faster they can be used to address questions and solve problems in transfusion medicine.

A solid understanding of classic genetics, including **Mendel's laws of inheritance** and **Hardy-Weinberg formulas**; cellular concepts that control chromosomes; cellular division such as mitosis and meiosis; and the biochemistry of the molecular structures of the nucleic acids and the proteins that are complexed with them is required to fully understand modern genetics. How these theories, concepts, and principles apply to transfusion medicine should be clearly understood, as genetics is a very dynamic science that has its greatest potential in direct applications. Many areas of transfusion medicine rely on an understanding of blood group genetics and on accurate and sensitive methods of pathogen testing to keep the blood supply safe. Most of the antigens in the various blood group systems (i.e., ABO, Rh, Kell, Kidd, etc.) generally follow straightforward inheritance patterns, usually of a **codominant** nature.

Historically, the major focus and role of genetics in blood banking has been more so in population genetics and inheritance patterns, but now cellular and molecular genetics are equally important. Increasingly, modern genetic techniques are playing a role in analyzing the profile of blood donors and recipients, which was once done only with serologic testing. Transfusion medicine physicians and technologists should still know classical genetics, such as interpretation of familial inheritance patterns. In addition, they must now master modern molecular methods that require a high level of training and skill, such as in **restriction mapping**, **sequencing**, **polymerase chain reaction (PCR)**, and **gene array** technology. (See Chapter 4, "Concepts in Molecular Biology.")

In this chapter, a general overview of genetics at three different levels (*population*, concerning genetic traits in large numbers of individuals; *cellular*, which pertains to the cellular organization of genetic material; and *molecular*, based on the biochemistry of genes and the structures that support them) is provided in some detail. It also gives a brief overview of modern molecular techniques. Chapter 4 explains in greater detail the modern testing methods of molecular biology, including recombinant DNA technology, Southern and Northern blotting, restriction fragment length polymorphism analysis, PCR techniques, and cloning and sequencing.

Classic Genetics

The science of genetics is one of the most important areas of modern biology. The understanding of the inheritance of blood group antigens and the testing for disease markers at the molecular level, both of which are vitally important in transfusion medicine, are based on the science of genetics. Modern genetics is based upon the understanding of the biochemical and biophysical nature of nucleic acids, including **deoxyribonucleic acid (DNA)**, **ribonucleic acid (RNA)**, and the various proteins that are part of the chromosomal architecture. In addition, genetics is concerned with population studies and epidemiology. The understanding of inheritance patterns in which genetic traits are followed and analyzed, as well as the biochemical reactions that result in gene mutations that can give rise to new alleles, are highly important in the study of genetics. New alleles can result in new blood groups and disease conditions that affect the health of blood donors and blood recipients.

All areas of transfusion medicine are influenced by genetics, including HLA typing, cell processing, parentage studies, viral testing, and blood services, and these would not be completely successful without a clear understanding of the principles of genetics and the laws of inheritance. The antigens present on all blood cells are expressed as a phenotype, but it is the genotype of the organism that controls what antigens may be expressed on the cell. For example, genotyping the donor or recipient DNA using leukocytes can determine which antigens may be present on the cells and therefore which antibodies can be made against them. This is especially true when a clear picture of the red cell antigens present on the red cells of a donor or recipient is not possible or if an antibody screening test gives ambiguous results. Using this simple example, we see that in modern blood banking, genetics has an important role.

Population Genetics

The major areas of population genetics of concern to blood banking include Mendel's laws of inheritance, the **Hardy-Weinberg principle**, and inheritance patterns.

Early Genetics and Mendel's Laws of Inheritance

The Swedish biologist Carolus Linnaeus started the first classification system of living things in the 17th century and used the unit of "species" as its principal definition. Determining factors that affected which classification group a species would be put into was based on physical traits and observations. There was no attempt made to understand the underlying reasons for one trait versus another trait occurring in one species or another. The amazing diversity of species and the processes that might contribute to it were not investigated further. In 1859, Charles Darwin published his epic book *On the Origin of Species* after many years of intense study of various and diverse life-forms. Darwin's ambition was to understand the diversity of life and how one organism could gain an advantage over another and better survive in a given environment, which is referred to as "natural selection." It created a revolution in the thinking of modern biology and is still controversial today.

The science of genetics found its modern development in the work of Gregor Mendel. Mendel was an Austrian monk and mathematician who used sweet pea plants growing in a monastery garden to study physical traits in organisms and how they are inherited. He determined the physical traits to be due to factors he called *elementen* within the cell. In modern genetics, we know the physical basis of these so-called elementen are genes within the nucleus of the cell. Mendel chose a good model organism for his observations. He studied the inheritance of several readily observable pea plant characteristics—notably flower color, seed color, and seed shape—and based his first law of inheritance, the law of independent or random segregation, on these results.

The first generation in the study, called the parental, pure, or P1 generation, consisted of all red or all white flowers that bred true for many generations. The plants were either homozygous for red flowers (RR, a dominant trait; dominant traits are usually written with uppercase letters) or homozygous for white flowers (rr, a recessive trait; recessive traits are usually written with lowercase letters). When these plants were crossbred, the second generation, called first-filial, or F1, had flowers that were all red. Thus the dominant trait was the only trait observed. When plants from the F1 generation were crossbred to each other, the second-filial, or F2, generation, of plants had flowers that were red and white in the ratio of 3:1 (Fig. 2–1). All the plants from the F1 generation are **heterozygous** (or hybrid) for flower color (Rr). The F2 generation has a ratio of three red-flowered plants to one white-flowered plant. This is because the plants that have the R gene, either RR **homozygous** or Rr heterozygous, will have red flowers because the red gene is dominant. Only when the red gene is absent and the white gene occurs in duplicate, as in the rr homozygous white-flowered plant, will the recessive white gene expression be visible as a phenotype. This illustrates Mendel's first law, the law of independent segregation. Therefore, each gene is passed on to the next generation on its own. Specifically, Mendel's first law shows that alleles of genes have no permanent effect on one another when present in the same plant but segregate unchanged by passing into different gametes.

An intermediate situation can also occur when alleles exhibit partial dominance. This is observed when the phenotype of a heterozygous organism is a mixture of both homozygous phenotypes seen in the P1 generation. An example of this is plants with red and white flowers that have offspring with pink flowers or flowers that have red and white sections. It is important to remember that although the phenotype does not show dominance or recessive traits, the F1 generation has the heterozygous genotype of Rr. It is essential to understand how a genotype can influence a

phenotype, and using flower color is a good basic model system to study this.

Unlike the flower color of many types of plants, most blood group genes are inherited in a codominant manner. In codominance, both **alleles** are expressed, and their gene products are seen at the phenotypic level. In this case, one gene is not dominant over its allele, and the protein products of both genes are seen at the phenotypic level. An example of this is seen in Figure 2–2 concerning the MNSs blood group system, in which a heterozygous MN individual would type as both M and N antigen positive. (See Chapter 8, "Blood Group Terminology and the Other Blood Groups.")

Mendel's second law is the law of independent assortment and states genes for different traits are inherited separately from each other. This allows for all possible combinations of genes to occur in the offspring. Specifically, if a homozygote that is dominant for two different characteristics is crossed with a homozygote that is recessive for both characteristics, the F1 generation consists of plants whose phenotype is the same as that of the dominant parent. However, when the F1 generation is crossed in the F2 generation, two general classes of offspring are found. One is the parental type; the other is a new phenotype called a *reciprocal type* and represents plants with the dominant feature of one plant and the recessive feature of another plant. Recombinant types occur in both possible combinations. Mendel formulated this law by doing studies with different types of seeds produced by peas and noted that they can be colored green or yellow and textured smooth or wrinkled in any combination. An illustration of independent assortment of Mendel's second law is given in Figure 2–3; his system of pea plant seed types are used as the example.

Mendel's laws apply to all sexually reproducing diploid organisms whether they are microorganisms, insects, plants, or animals, or people. However, there are exceptions to the Mendelian laws of inheritance. If the genes for separate traits are closely linked on a chromosome, they can be inherited as a single unit. The expected ratios of progeny in F1 matings may not be seen if the various traits being studied are linked.

Parental   RR   rr

Gametes   R   r

First-Filial   Rr

Second-Filial | R   r
                                  |
                         R | RR   Rr
                                  |
                         r | Rr   rr

Where R = red and r = White

Figure 2–1. A schematic illustration of Mendel's law of separation using flower color.

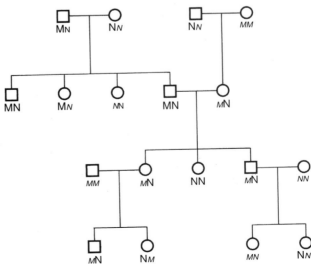

Figure 2–2. Independent segregation of the codominant genes of *M* and *N*.

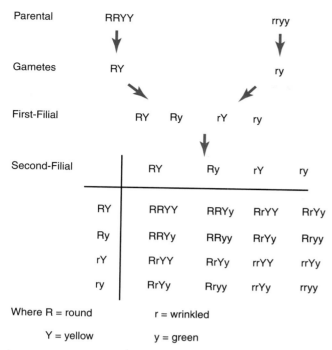

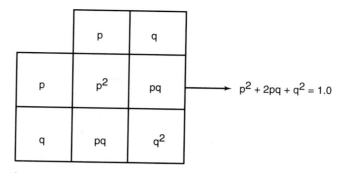

Figure 2–4.   Common inheritance patterns.

Where R = round   r = wrinkled

Y = yellow   y = green

Figure 2–3.   A schematic illustration of Mendel's law of independent assortment using seed types.

There can also be differences in the gene ratios of progeny of F1 matings, if recombination has occurred during the process of meiosis. An example of this in blood banking is the MNSs system, in which the MN alleles and the Ss alleles are physically close on the same chromosome and are therefore linked. Recombination happens when DNA strands are broken and there is exchange of chromosomal material followed by activation of DNA repair mechanisms. The exchange of chromosomal material results in new hybrid genotypes that may or may not be visible at the phenotypic level.

Mendel's laws of inheritance give us an appreciation of how diverse an organism can be through the variations in its genetic material. The more complex the genetic material of an organism, including the number of chromosomes and the number of genes on the chromosomes, the greater the potential uniqueness of any one organism from another organism of the same species. Also, the more complex the genetic material, the more complex and varied its responses to conditions in the environment. Therefore, as long as control is maintained during cell division and differentiation, organisms with greater genetic diversity and number can have an advantage over other organisms in a given setting.

Hardy-Weinberg Principle

G. H. Hardy, a mathematician, and W. Weinberg, a physician, developed a mathematical formula that allowed the study of Mendelian inheritance in great detail. The Hardy-Weinberg formula—$p + q = 1$, in which p equals the gene frequency of the dominant allele and q is the frequency of the recessive allele—can also be stated $p^2 + 2pq + q^2 = 1$ and specifically addresses questions about recessive traits and how they can be persistent in populations (Fig. 2–4). Like

many mathematical formulations, however, certain ideal situations and various conditions must be met to use the equations appropriately. These criteria are outlined in Box 2–1.

In any normal human population, it is almost impossible to meet these demanding criteria. Although large populations exist, collecting sample data from a significantly large enough segment of a population that correctly represents the members of the population is not always feasible. Also, mating is not always random, and there is mixing of populations on a global scale now that leads to "gene flow" on a constant basis. Recently, sequencing of the human genome has revealed that gene mutations occur much more commonly than originally thought. Some of these mutations affect the phenotype of an individual, such as loss of enzyme function, and some do not. Despite these drawbacks, Hardy-Weinberg is still one of the best tools for studying inheritance patterns in human populations and is a cornerstone of population genetics.

Most of the various genes controlling the inheritance of blood group antigens can be studied using the Hardy-Weinberg equations. A relevant example that shows how to use the Hardy-Weinberg formula is the frequency of the Rh antigen, D, in a given population. In this simple example, there are two alleles, D and d. To determine the frequency of each allele, we count the number of individuals who have the corresponding phenotype (remembering that both Dd and DD will appear as Rh-positive) and divide this number by the total number of alleles. This value is represented by p in the Hardy-Weinberg equation. Again, counting the alleles lets us determine the value of q. When p and q are added, they must equal 1. The ratio of homozygotes and heterozygotes is determined using the other form of the Hardy-Weinberg equation, $p^2 + 2pq + q^2 = 1$. If in our example we tested 1,000 random blood donors for the D antigen and found that

BOX 2–1

Criteria for Use of the Hardy-Weinberg Formula

- The population studied must be large.
- Mating among all individuals must be random.
- Mutations must not occur in parents or offspring.
- There must be no migration, differential fertility, or mortality of genotypes studied.

DD and Dd (Rh-positive) occurred in 84 percent of the population, and dd (Rh-negative) occurred in 16 percent, the gene frequency calculations would be performed as follows:

$$p = \text{gene frequency of D}$$
$$q = \text{gene frequency of d}$$
$$p^2 = DD, \; 2pq = Dd, \text{ which combined are 0.84}$$
$$q^2 = dd, \text{ which is 0.16}$$
$$q = \text{square root of 0.16, which is 0.4}$$
$$p + q = 1$$
$$p = 1 - q$$
$$p = 1 - 0.4$$
$$p = 0.6$$

This example is for a two-allele system only. A three-allele system would require use of the expanded binomial equation $p + q + r = 1$ or $p^2 + 2pq + 2pr + q^2 + 2qr + r^2 = 1$. More complex examples using this formula can be found in more advanced genetics textbooks.

Inheritance Patterns

The interpretation of **pedigree analysis** requires the understanding of various standard conventions in the representation of data figures. Males are always represented by squares and females by circles. A line joining a male and a female indicates a mating between the two, and offspring are indicated by a vertical line. A double line between a male and a female indicates a consanguineous mating. A stillbirth or abortion is indicated by a small black circle. Deceased family members have a line crossed through them. The propositus in the pedigree is indicated by an arrow pointing to it and indicates the most interesting or important member of the pedigree. Something unusual about the propositus is often the reason the pedigree analysis is undertaken.

Figure 2–5 shows examples of different types of inheritance patterns seen in pedigree analysis. Almost all pedigrees will follow one of these patterns or, rarely, a combination of them. The first example is a pedigree demonstrating autosomal-recessive inheritance. **Autosomal** refers to traits that are not carried on the sex chromosomes. A **recessive** trait is carried by either parent or both parents but is not generally seen at the phenotypic level unless both parents carry the trait. In some cases, a recessive trait can be genetically expressed in a heterozygous individual but may not be seen at the phenotypic level. When two heterozygous individuals mate, they can produce a child who inherits a recessive gene from each parent, and therefore the child is homozygous for that trait. An example from blood banking is when both parents are Rh-type Dd and have a child who is dd, which is Rh-negative.

In the second example, there is a case of a dominant X-linked trait. If the father carries the trait on his X chromosome, he has no sons with the trait, but all his daughters will have the trait. This is because a father always passes his Y chromosome to his sons and his X chromosome to his daughters. Women can be either homozygous or heterozygous for an X-linked trait; therefore, when mothers have an X-linked trait, their daughters inherit the trait in a manner identical to autosomal inheritance. The sons have a 50 percent

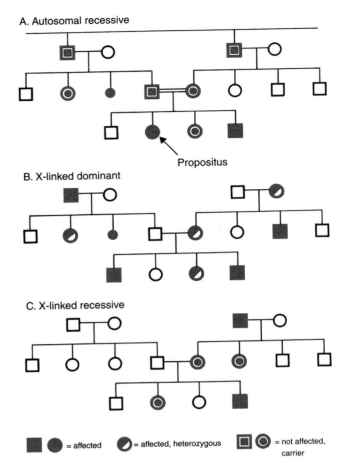

Figure 2–5. Schematic illustration of common inheritance patterns.

chance of inheriting the trait. Because the trait is dominant, the sons who inherit it will express it. The Xg^a blood group system is one of the few blood group systems that follow an X-linked inheritance pattern (refer to Chapter 8).

The third example illustrated is X-linked recessive inheritance. In this case, the father always expresses the trait but never passes it on to his sons. The father always passes the trait to all his daughters, who are then carriers of the trait. The female carriers will pass the trait on to half of their sons, who also will be carriers. In the homozygous state, X'Y, the males will express the trait, whereas only the rare homozygous females, X'X', will express it. In this situation, with an X-linked recessive trait, a disease-carrying gene can be passed from generation to generation, with many individuals not affected. A classic example of this is the inheritance of hemophilia A, which affected many of the royal houses of Europe.

In addition, there is autosomal-dominant, in which all the members of a family who carry the allele show the physical characteristic. Generally, each individual with the trait has at least one parent with the trait, and the gene is expressed if only one copy of the gene is present. Unlike X-linked traits, autosomal traits usually do not show a difference in the distribution between males and females, and this can be a helpful clue in their evaluation. Also, in autosomal and X-linked traits, if an individual does not have the trait, he or she can be a carrier and can pass it on to offspring. This is why recessive traits seem to skip generations, which is another helpful clue in determining inheritance patterns.

Autosomal-dominant traits are routinely encountered in the blood bank, as most blood group genes are codominant and are on autosomal chromosomes. They are passed on from one generation to the next and do not skip generations; therefore, they are usually present in every generation. Finally, unusually rare traits that occur in every generation and in much greater frequency than the general population are often the result of matings between related individuals. Table 2–1 provides examples of inheritance patterns in transfusion medicine.

Cellular Genetics

Organisms may be divided into two major categories: **prokaryotic**, without a defined nucleus, and **eukaryotic**, with a defined nucleus. Human beings and all other mammals are included in the eukaryotic group, as are birds, reptiles, amphibians, fish, and some fungus species. The nucleus of a cell contains most of the genetic material important for replication and is a highly organized complex structure. The nuclear material is organized into chromatin, consisting of nucleic acids and structural proteins, and is defined by staining patterns. **Heterochromatin** stains as dark bands, and **achromatin** stains as light bands and consists of highly condensed regions that are usually not transcriptionally active. **Euchromatin** is the swollen form of chromatin in cells, which is considered to be more active in the synthesis of RNA for **transcription**.

Most cellular nuclei contain these different types of chromatin. The chromatin material itself, which chiefly comprises long polymers of DNA and various basic proteins called **histones**, is compressed and coiled to form chromosomes during cell division. Each organism has a specific number of chromosomes, some as few as 4 and some as many as 50. In humans, there are 46 chromosomes. These 46 chromosomes are arranged into pairs, with one of each being inherited from each parent. Humans have 22 autosomes and one set of sex chromosomes, XX in the female and XY in the male. This comprises the 2N state of the cell, which is normal for all human cells except the gametes (sex cells). N refers to the number of pairs of chromosomes in a cell.

Table 2–1	Examples of Inheritance Patterns in Transfusion Medicine	
TYPE OF PATTERN	**EXAMPLE**
Autosomal-dominant	In (*Lu*) suppressor gene
Autosomal-recessive	*dd* genotype
X-linked dominant	*Xgᵃ* blood group system
X-linked recessive	Hemophilia A

Terminology

Remember that it takes two gametes to make a fertilized egg with the correct (2N) number of chromosomes in the nucleus of a cell. Therefore, each parent contributes only half (1N) of the inherited genetic information, or genes, to each child. In order to be completely healthy, each child must have the correct number of genes and chromosomes (2N), without major mutations affecting necessary biochemical systems.

The genetic material has a complex pattern of organization that has been evolving for millions of years to an amazing level of coordination and control. At the smallest level, genes are composed of discrete units of DNA arranged in a linear fashion, similar to a strand of pearls, with structural proteins wrapped around the DNA at specific intervals to pack it into tightly wound bundles. The DNA is organized at a higher level into chromosomes, with each chromosome being one incredibly long strand of duplex (double-stranded) DNA. A **gene** is a section, often very large, of DNA along the chromosome. The specific sequence of nucleotides and the location on the chromosome determines a gene. In addition, each gene has specific and general sequences that occur upstream (before the start site) and downstream (after the termination signals) that contribute to how the gene functions. The specific location of a gene on a chromosome is called a **locus** (plural = *loci*), and at each locus there may be only one or several different forms of the gene, which are called *alleles*.

It is important to keep in mind the distinction between **phenotype** and **genotype**. Genotype is the sequence of DNA that is inherited. The phenotype is anything that is produced by the genotype, including an enzyme to control a blood group antigen; the length of long bones of the skeleton; the curvature of the spine; the ratio of muscle fibers; the level of hormones produced; and such obvious traits as eye, skin, and hair color. Keep in mind that more than one gene can affect a particular trait (part of a phenotype), such as the height of an individual; all relevant genes can be considered as part of the genotype for that trait. Depending on the alleles inherited, an organism can be either homozygous or heterozygous for a specific trait. The presence of two identical alleles results in a homozygous genotype (i.e., AA), and the phenotype is group A blood. On the other hand, the inheritance of different alleles from each parent gives a heterozygous genotype.

Another important concept is that of the "silent" gene, or **amorph**, and the term **hemizygous**. An amorph is a gene that does not produce any obvious, easily detectable traits and is seen only at the phenotypic level when the individual is homozygous for the trait. *Hemizygous* refers to the condition when one chromosome has a copy of the gene and the other chromosome has that gene deleted or absent.

Mitosis

During cell division, the chromosomes are reproduced in such a way that all daughter cells are genetically identical to the parent cell. Without maintaining the same number and type of chromosomes, the daughter cells would not be viable. The process by which cells divide to create identical daughter cells is called **mitosis**. The chromosomes are duplicated, and one of each pair is passed to the daughter cells. During the process of mitosis, quantitatively and qualitatively identical DNA is delivered to daughter cells formed by cell division.

The complex process of mitosis is usually divided into a series of stages, characterized by the appearance and movement of the chromosomes. The stages are interphase, prophase, metaphase, anaphase, and telophase. The different phases of mitosis include **interphase** at the beginning, in which DNA is in the form of chromatin and is dispersed throughout the nucleus. This is the stage of the DNA when cells are not actively dividing. New DNA is synthesized by a process called *replication*. In the next stage, **prophase**, the chromatin condenses to form chromosomes. In prophase, the nuclear envelope starts to break down. In the next stage, **metaphase**, the chromosomes are lined up along the middle of the nucleus and paired with the corresponding chromosome. In this stage, chromosome preparations are made for chromosome analysis in cytogenetics. In **anaphase**, which occurs next, the cellular spindle apparatus is formed and the chromosomes are pulled to opposite ends of the cell. The cell becomes pinched in the middle, and cell division starts to take place. In the last stage, **telophase**, the cell is pulled apart, division is complete, and the chromosomes and cytoplasm are separated into two new daughter cells. The process of mitosis is illustrated in Figure 2–6 and outlined in Table 2–2.

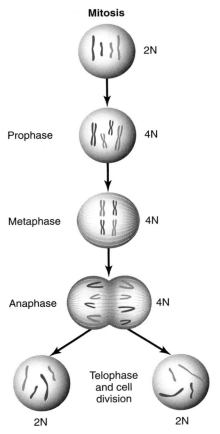

Figure 2–6. Mitosis leads to two daughter cells having the same number of chromosomes as the parent cell.

Table 2–2   Stages of Mitosis and Meiosis

MITOSIS

Stage	Description
1. Interphase (2N)	Resting stage between cell divisions; during this period, cells are synthesizing RNA and proteins, and chromatin is uncondensed.
2. Prophase (4N)	First stage of mitotic cell division. Chromosomes become visible and condense. Each chromosome has two chromatids from duplication of DNA, and chromatids are linked via the centromere.
3. Metaphase (4N)	Chromosomes move toward the equator of the cell and are held in place by microtubules attached at the mitotic spindle apparatus.
4. Anaphase (4N)	The two sister chromatids separate. Each one migrates to opposite poles of the cell, and the diameter of the cell decreases at equator.
5. Telophase (2N)	Chromosomes are at the poles of the cell, and the cell membrane divides between the two nuclei. The cell divides, and each cell contains a pair of chromosomes identical to the parent cell.

MEIOSIS

Stage	Description
1. Interphase (2N)	Resting stage between cell divisions; during this period, cells are synthesizing RNA and proteins, and chromatin is uncondensed.
2. Prophase I (4N)	First stage of meiotic division. Chromosomes condense. Homologous chromosomes pair to become bivalent. Chromosome crossing over occurs at this stage.
3. Metaphase I (4N)	Bivalent chromosomes align at cell equator. Bivalent chromosomes contain all four of the cell's copies of each chromosome.
4. Anaphase I (4N)	Homologous pairs move to opposite poles of the cell. The two sister chromatids separate.
5. Telophase I (2N)	The cell separates to become two daughter cells. The new cells are now 2N.
6. Metaphase II (2N)	Homologues line up at the equator.
7. Anaphase II (N)	Homologues move to opposite poles of the cell equator.
8. Telophase II (N)	Each cell separates into two new cells. There are now four (N) cells with a unique genetic constitution.

Meiosis

A different process is used to produce the gametes or sex cells. The process is called **meiosis** and results in four unique, rather than two identical, daughter cells. The uniqueness of the daughter cells generated with meiosis allows for great genetic diversity in organisms and controls the number of chromosomes within dividing cells. If cells with 2N chromosomes were paired, the resulting daughter cells would have 4N chromosomes, which would not be viable. Therefore, gametes carry a **haploid** number of chromosomes, 1N, so that when they combine, the resulting cell has a 2N configuration. Meiosis only occurs in the germinal tissues and is important for reproduction. Without the complicated process of meiosis, there would be no change from generation to generation, and evolution would not occur or happen too slowly for organisms to adapt to environmental changes.

The first stages of meiosis are nearly identical to those in mitosis, in which chromatin is condensed, homologous chromosomes are paired in prophase, and chromosomes are aligned along the center of the cell. However, there is no centromere division, and at anaphase and telophase, the cell divides and enters once again into interphase, in which there is no replication of DNA. This is followed by the second prophase, in which chromosomes are condensed, and then the second metaphase, with the centromeres dividing. Finally, in the second anaphase and telophase stages, the two cells divide, giving rise to four 1N daughter cells. In addition, during meiosis, crossing over and recombination can happen between maternal- and paternal-derived chromosomes. This allows for the creation of new DNA sequences that are different from the parent strains. Combined with random segregation, it is possible to have very large numbers of new DNA sequences. In humans with 23 pairs of chromosomes, the total possible number is several million. Meiosis is illustrated in Figure 2–7 and outlined in Table 2–2.

Cell Division

Cell division is also a complicated process and one that is important to understand. It also occurs with various specific stages. In eukaryotic cells such as human cells, the cell cycle is divided into four distinct stages and is represented by a clock or circular scheme indicating that it can repeat itself or can be stopped at any one point in the cycle. The first step or stage is the resting stage, or G_0, and is the state of cells not actively dividing. The prereplication stage is next and is called G_1. The step at which DNA is synthesized is the next stage, called the S stage. It is followed by the G_2 stage, or postreplication stage. Finally, there is the **M phase**, in which mitosis occurs.

Chromosomes are in the interphase stage of mitosis in the span from G_0 to the end of the G_2 phase. Cells that are completely mature and no longer need to divide to increase their numbers, such as nerve cells, can remain in the G_0 stage for a very long time. It is a hallmark of cancer cells, such as the transformed cells seen in the various leukemias and solid tumors, that they can go through the stages of cell division much faster than nontransformed, normal cells and therefore outgrow them. In this way, they take up the bulk of nutrients needed by the nontransformed cells and crowd them out of existence and potentially overgrow the adult organism in which they occur (Table 2–3).

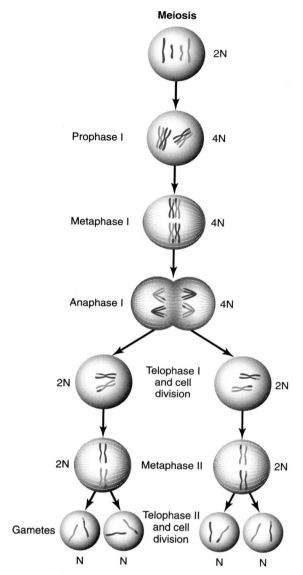

Figure 2–7. Meiosis produces four gametes having half the number of chromosomes present in the parent cell.

Table 2–3	**The Generative Cell Cycle**	
STAGE	**DESCRIPTION**	**CONFIGURATION**
G_0 (Gap 0)	Temporary resting period, no cell division	2N
G_1 (Gap 1)	Cells produce RNA and synthesize protein	2N
S (Synthesis)	DNA replication occurs	4N
G_2 (Gap 2)	During the gap between DNA synthesis and mitosis, the cell continues to synthesize RNA and produce new proteins	4N
M (Mitosis)	Cell division occurs	2N

Molecular Genetics

The study of genetics at the molecular level requires an understanding of the biochemistry of the molecules involved. This includes knowledge of the physical conformation of chromosomes as well as the biological and chemical nature of the polymers of the different nucleic acids and nuclear proteins.

Deoxyribonucleic Acid

Deoxyribonucleic acid (DNA) is a masterpiece of architectural evolution and the "backbone" of heredity. Chromatin is actually a type of polymer structure. Chromosomes are composed of long, linear strands of DNA tightly coiled around highly basic proteins called *histones* (Fig. 2–8). Each chromosome is a single, extremely long strand of duplex DNA. Remember that DNA is a nucleic *acid*, and therefore most of the proteins that interact with it have an overall *basic* pH. This helps to stabilize the overall complex structure. The complex of DNA and histone protein is referred to as a nucleosome. The DNA and protein complex is bound together so tightly and efficiently that extremely long stretches of DNA, several inches in length, can be packaged inside the nucleus of a cell on a microscopic level. The DNA and histones are held together by various proteins that keep the DNA in a very specific helical conformation. This conformation also protects the DNA from degradation when it is not being replicated or transcribed.

All DNA in human cells is in the form of a two-stranded duplex, with one strand in one direction and its complementary strand in the opposite direction (the strands are said to be **antiparallel**). DNA is composed of four nitrogenous bases, a 5-carbon sugar molecule called *deoxyribose* and a phosphate group. The sugar and phosphate moieties comprise the backbone of the DNA molecule, while the nitrogenous bases face in to each other and are stabilized by hydrogen bonding and Van der Waals forces. The backbone of a DNA molecule is joined by phosphodiester linkages. Unlike what is observed in proteins with an α-helical structure, there is little bonding forces between bases on the same strand, which allows DNA to be strong but flexible.

The four different bases are adenine (A), cytosine (C), guanine (G), and thymine (T). Adenine and guanine are **purines**, consisting of double-ring structures. Cytosine and thymine are **pyrimidines**, which are single-ring structures (Fig. 2–9). The hydrogen bonding in DNA is specific, in which A bonds only to T with two hydrogen bonds, thus forming the weaker pairing, and C bonds only with G with three hydrogen bonds, forming the stronger pairing. This is the classic Watson-Crick base pairing that occurs in the B-form, right-handed helical structure of DNA. It was first postulated by James Watson and Francis Crick, at Cambridge University in the early 1950s (Fig. 2–10).[1] Since then, it has been discovered that DNA can also occur in modified forms such as Z-DNA, which is a type of left-handed helix with a different three-dimensional conformation but that contains the same four nitrogenous bases.[2] In addition, there are some unusual forms of nitrogenous bases that can be incorporated into DNA templates.

The phosphates in the DNA backbone attach to the sugar at the third and fifth carbon atoms. Remember, all atoms in a molecular structure are numbered. The linkage of the purine or pyrimidine nitrogenous base to the sugar is at carbon 1. Therefore, the two DNA strands are antiparallel—that is, one strand is 5′ to 3′ (pronounced "5 prime to 3 prime") in one direction and the complementary strand is 5′ to 3′ in the other direction. During transcription, only one strand is copied, which is the complementary strand that gives the correct 5′ to 3′ sequence of messenger RNA (mRNA) that corresponds to the template, or coding strand, of the DNA molecule.

As there are only four different bases used to make up DNA templates and there are 20 different amino acids that are used to construct proteins, it is evident that any single nucleotide cannot code for any specific amino acid. What has been discovered is that triplets of nucleotides called a

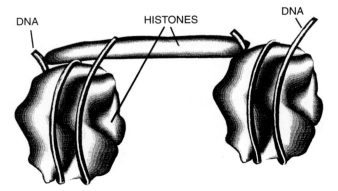

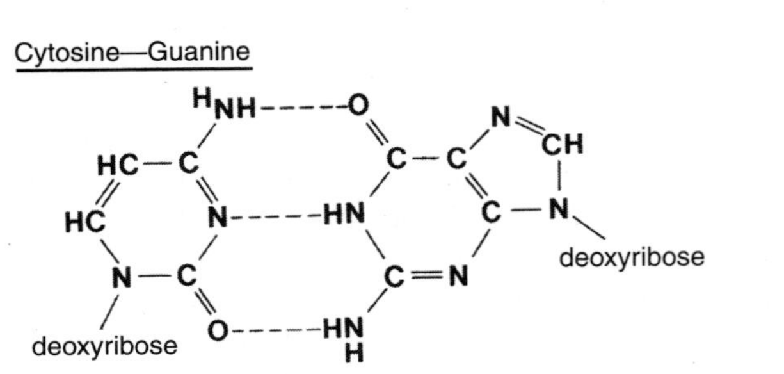

Figure 2–8. Nucleosomes consist of stretches of DNA wound around histone proteins.

Thymine—Adenine

Cytosine—Guanine

Dotted lines represent interatomic hydrogen bonds, which hold the base pairs together.

Figure 2–9. The pyrimidine and purine bases found in the DNA molecule.

The double helix has constant width

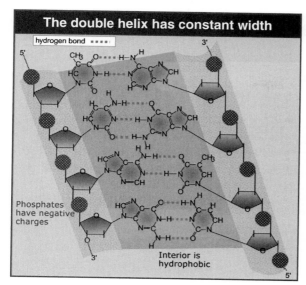

Figure 2–10. Base pairing in DNA and DNA structure. *(From Lewin B: Genes VIII. Prentice Hall/Pearson Education, New York, 2004, p 6. Reprinted with permission of the author.)*

The genetic code is triplet

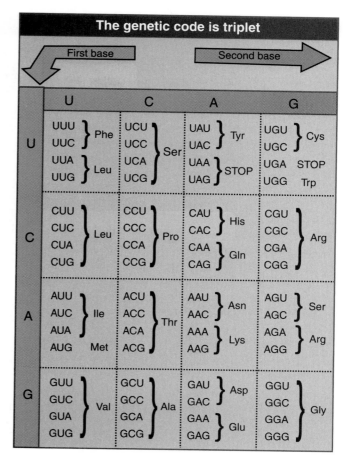

Figure 2–11. The genetic code. *(From Lewin B: Genes VIII. Prentice Hall/Pearson Education, New York, 2004, p 168. Reprinted with permission of the author.)*

codon, such as ATG, code for one specific amino acid. However, there is a redundancy to the genetic code in that some amino acids have more than one triplet, which codes for their addition to the peptide chain formed during translation. Generally, the more common the amino acid is in proteins, the greater the number of **codons** it has. There are four special codons, including the only codon specific for the initiation of transcription and translation, called the *start codon*, and three different codons that are used to stop the addition of amino acids in the process of peptide synthesis. Because these three codons cannot be charged with an amino acid, they are called **stop codons** and result in termination of the peptide being translated from mRNA. The genetic code is illustrated in Figure 2–11.

Replication

The **replication**, or copying, of DNA is a complex process involving numerous enzymes, nucleic acid primers, various small molecules, and the DNA helix molecule that serves as its own template for the replication process. DNA must be copied before mitosis can occur and must be copied in such a way that each daughter cell will have the same amount of DNA and the same sequence. Nearly all DNA replication is done in a bidirectional manner and is semiconservative in nature.[3] Specifically, as enzymes involved in the replication process open the double-stranded DNA helix, one strand of DNA is copied in a 5′ to 3′ manner, while the other strand is opened partially in sections and is copied 5′ to 3′ in sections as the double-stranded template continuously opens. In addition, each newly synthesized DNA strand will be paired with one of the parent strands. The replication process is shown in Figure 2–12.

In order for DNA to be replicated with the exact copying of the template and its sequence into a new double-stranded helix, many enzymes and proteins must participate in the process. DNA replication occurs in specific steps, and certain enzymes and other molecules are required at each step. First, sections of DNA must be uncoiled from its supercoiled (or double-twisted) nature, and the two strands must be separated and kept apart; this is done by the enzymes DNA gyrase (opens the supercoils) and DNA helicase (separates the two strands of duplex DNA). These enzymes, using energy derived from ATP hydrolysis, open the DNA molecules and keep the strands separate. In the next step, DNA polymerase III can synthesize a new strand in the 5′ to 3′ direction on the leading strand. Proteins called *single-stranded binding proteins* interact with the open strands of DNA to prevent hydrogen bonding when it is not needed during replication. DNA polymerase III also proofreads the addition of new bases to the growing DNA strands and can remove an incorrectly incorporated base, such as G paired to T.

In order for replication to take place on any piece of DNA, there must first be a short oligonucleotide (composed of RNA) piece that binds to the beginning of the region to be replicated. This "primes" the replication process; therefore, these short oligonucleotide sequences are called *primers*. All DNA is replicated in a 5′ to 3′ manner. Replication of the other parent strand, the lagging strand, is more complicated because of this restriction. As the helix is opened, RNA primer sequences are added to the area of the opening fork, and the RNA primers are extended in a 5′ to 3′ manner until

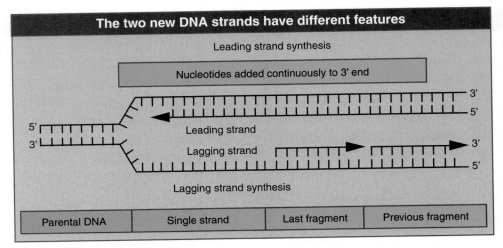

Figure 2–12.   DNA replication.

the polymerase reaches the previously synthesized end. Rather than being replicated in a continuous manner, these replication forks open up all along the lagging strand and are extended in this way. These small regions of newly replicated DNA are known as **Okazaki fragments**. The fragments must be joined together to make a complete and continuous strand. This is accomplished by the two enzymes DNA polymerase I and DNA ligase. The RNA primers are synthesized and added to the DNA strands by an enzyme called primase, which anneals to the parent strands. After replication of the leading and lagging strands is complete, DNA ligase joins the phosphodiester bonds of the DNA backbone to complete the intact molecule. Isomerase enzymes recoil the DNA; once this is completed and the DNA is proofread by proofreading enzymes, the cell can continue with mitosis and cell division.

Repair

DNA must be copied exactly or the information it contains will be altered, possibly resulting in a decrease in the organism's vitality. However, mistakes in the complex process of replication do occasionally occur, and a number of efficient mechanisms have evolved to correct these mistakes. The mechanisms can detect the mistakes, or changes, and correct the actual DNA sequence. One of the most important mechanisms for correcting DNA replication errors is the proofreading ability of DNA polymerases. The proofreading occurs in both the 5' to 3' and 3' to 5' directions and allows the polymerase to backtrack on a recently copied DNA strand and remove an incorrect nucleotide and insert the correct one in its place. In addition to the proofreading ability of DNA polymerase enzymes, there is a second type of editing called **mismatch repair**, where an incorrect nucleotide is removed and the correct one is inserted in its place.

In addition to errors in the primary nucleotide sequence of DNA molecules, there are other possible alterations that can affect the way the sequence information is processed. Many different chemicals and environmental factors can alter DNA by modifying it chemically or physically. These include alkylating agents, which react with guanine and result in

depurination. Some cancer treatments are often based on this principle that the faster-replicating DNA in cancer cells has greater damage and puts cancer cells at greater risk for cell death than normal cells. Ionizing radiation and strong oxidants such as peroxides can cause single-strand breaks. Ultraviolet (UV) radiation can alter thymine bases, resulting in thymine dimers. Certain drugs such as the antibiotic mitomycin C can form covalent linkages between bases on opposite strands; therefore, during replication, separation of the strands at that site will not occur correctly, and the resulting daughter strands will have mutations. Nearly all defects in DNA replication can be corrected by the various mechanisms used by the cell to maintain DNA integrity. However, if too many mistakes occur, the repair systems can be overwhelmed, and mistakes will not be corrected. The cell in which these mutations occur will have an altered DNA nucleotide sequence and may or may not be viable,

There are several major DNA repair systems. These include photoreactivation, excision repair (also referred to as *cut and patch repair*), recombinational repair, mismatch repair, and SOS repair (Box 2–2). DNA repair systems can recognize mismatched base pairs, missing nucleotides, and altered nucleotides in DNA sequences. For example, when thymine dimers are formed after exposure to UV light, the photoreactivation enzyme becomes active and enzymatically cleaves the thymine dimers. In addition to the photoreactivation system of DNA repair, thymine dimers can be removed by the rather complex process of excision repair, where the disrupted section of the DNA is removed. A cut is

---

BOX 2–2

DNA Repair Systems

- Photoreactivation
- Excision repair
- Recombinational repair
- Mismatch repair
- SOS repair

made on one side of the thymine dimer that bulges out from the rest of the duplex DNA. DNA polymerase I synthesizes a short replacement strand for the damaged DNA section. The old strand is removed by DNA polymerase I as it moves along the DNA. Finally, the old DNA strand is removed, and the newly formed DNA segment is ligated into place.

Recombinational repair uses the correct strand of DNA to fill in the strand where the error was deleted. Polymerase I and DNA ligase, then fill in the other strand. Mismatch repair is activated when base pairing is incorrect and a bulge occurs in the duplex DNA. Mismatch repair enzymes are able to remove the incorrect nucleotides and insert the correct ones. Methyl groups on adenines are used by the mismatch enzyme systems to determine which nucleotide is correct and which is a mistake. When DNA and cell damage occurs, SOS repair is induced. Damage can be caused by UV radiation, chemical mutagens, and excessive heat, and by such treatments as exposure to cross-linking agents. There are certain sections of highly conserved DNA that are activated when DNA is damaged, and the genes that are part of the SOS response system must work in a coordinated manner to repair the damaged DNA through recombination events that remove the damaged sections and replace them with the correct sequences. Repair systems exist and have been studied closely in both prokaryotes and eukaryotes. All of these systems are available to maintain the integrity of the DNA. The fact that so many repair systems exist in the cell proves how important the correct structure and sequence of DNA is to the cell. It also shows how complex the DNA molecule is in that many types of mutations can occur, and therefore many types of correction processes are present to repair them.

Mutations

Although many effective DNA proofreading and repair systems help to keep newly synthesized DNA from having mutations, none of the systems are foolproof and occasional mutations occur. Once a mutation is introduced into a DNA coding strand, the information in that strand is now altered. It may be altered at the protein level if the mutation encodes for a different amino acid or a change in reading frame. In general, a mutation is any change in the structure or sequence of DNA, whether it is physical or biochemical. An organism is referred to as a mutant if its DNA sequence is different from that of the parent organism. The original form of the DNA sequence, and the organism in which it occurs, is called the *wild type*. The various chemicals and conditions that can cause mutations are referred to as **mutagens**. Many mutagens are also carcinogens in that the cells in which they occur have an advantage in growth patterns that allows them to dominate the cells around them.

There are different types of mutations, and they may have very different consequences for the organisms in which they occur. Also, remember that mutations can be spontaneous. If they occur in the germinal tissue, they are passed on from one generation to the next. The simplest type of mutation is the point mutation, in which only one nucleotide in the DNA sequence is changed. Point mutations include substitutions, insertions, and deletions. Certain substitutions,

although they change the DNA sequence and the triplet codon(s), may not change the amino acid sequence in the corresponding protein because of redundancy in the genetic code. Recall that some of the amino acids have more than one codon that represents them. Therefore, if the new codon is for the same amino acid, the mutation will be silent, and the protein sequence will be the same. An example of this is the amino acid threonine, which has ACA, ACC, ACG, and ACU as possible codons. Therefore, a substitution of C, G, or U for A at the third position of the codon would still have a peptide with threonine at that position. A type of "silent mutation" also occurs when a mutation happens that causes a change in the peptide sequence, but that part of the peptide does not seem critical for its function; therefore, no mutation is seen at the phenotypic level, such as enzyme function or cell surface marker. A transition is a type of mutation in which one purine is substituted for another purine, or one pyrimidine is substituted for another pyrimidine. When a purine is substituted for a pyrimidine or a pyrimidine for a purine, it is called a **transversion**. Examples of DNA mutations are outlined in Table 2–4.[4]

Another type of mutation that can have a deleterious effect on the peptide sequence is called a **missense point mutation**. A missense mutation results in a change in a codon, which alters the amino acid in the corresponding peptide. These changes cannot be accommodated by the peptide while still maintaining its function. Typical examples of missense mutations include the alterations in the hemoglobin molecule at a single base pair, resulting in different types of inherited anemias.[5] A very specific type of serious mutation, called a *nonsense mutation*, results when a point change in one of the nucleotides of a DNA sequence causes one of the three possible stop codons to be formed. The three stop codons are amber (UAG), opal (UGA), and ochre (UAA), and these terminate the reading of the DNA sequence, so the resulting peptide is truncated at its 3′ end.

A more severe type of mutation happens when there is an insertion or deletion of one or more (but never multiplicities of three) nucleotides in the DNA sequence. The result of this

Table 2–4	**Examples of DNA Mutations in Blood Groups**	
TRANSITION		
	S antigen	s antigen
Amino acid	Methionine	Threonine
mRNA code	AUG	ACG
DNA code	TAC	TGC
TRANSVERSION		
	N antigen	He antigen
Amino acid	Leucine	Tryptophan
mRNA code	UUG	UGG
DNA code	AAC	ACC

type of mutation is a change in the triplet codon sequence and therefore an alteration in the frameshift reading so that a large change in the amino acid sequence occurs. Remember that the DNA sequence is read three nucleotides at a time, called codons, and each codon can be charged with a specific amino acid. In transfusion medicine, it has been shown that there is a single base pair deletion in the gene encoding for the transferase protein of the A blood group.[6] The **frameshift mutation** results in a nonfunctional transferase protein that is seen phenotypically as the O blood group.

Unusual genetic changes can also happen that cause gross mutations in the DNA sequence. Duplications, recombinations, and large deletions have a lower frequency rate than the mutations in the replication of DNA noted above. Duplications can occur quite frequently and give rise to **pseudogenes** and other so-called junk DNA that does not code for proteins. A large part of DNA consists of such junk DNA without apparent ill effects and may even be necessary to some extent for the structural integrity of DNA and chromosomes. Also, there are sequences "left over" from earlier evolution that are still present in human DNA, such as *Alu* sequences. In addition, there may be evolutionary pressures forcing duplications to occur. DNA contains short tandem repeats of various lengths throughout the entire DNA molecule.

In blood banking, there are two good examples of duplications. The first involves the *glycophorin A and B* genes; the second involves the genes *RHD* and *RHCE*. The Chido and Rodgers blood group antigens, carried on the complement components of the *C4A* and *C4B* genes, arose from duplications and mutations of the *C4* genes (refer to Chapter 8). In addition to these mutations, exchanges occasionally occur between chromosomes, such as the Philadelphia chromosome present in myelogenous leukemia. Mutations involving recombination or crossing over take place during the process of meiosis in the formation of gametes. It is very important to generate sex cells that are different from the parental cells. Recombination involves breaking both double-stranded DNA homologues, exchanging both strands of DNA, and then resolving the new DNA duplexes by reconnecting phosphodiester bonds. Crossing over can be single, double, or triple events (Fig. 2–13). An example of such an event resulting in a **hybrid formation** is seen in the MNSs blood group system. Crossover events have formed the genes for the Dantu and Mi V blood groups. One of the most important events in the immune system is the recombination of the *D, V,* and *J* genes, which gives rise to the vast array of immunoglobulin genes that are necessary to form the antibodies of the humoral system.

Deletion of large segments of DNA sequences covering hundreds and possibly even thousands of nucleotides is also possible. It is a type of mutation that is not capable of being corrected by any of the DNA repair systems due to the size and complexity of the mutation. Such mutations can result in complete loss of a peptide, a severely truncated peptide, or the formation of a nonfunctional peptide. An example of this type of mutation in transfusion medicine is the Rodgers negative phenotype, which results from a 30 kD deletion of both the complete *CD4* (Rodgers) and *21-hydroxylase* genes.[7]

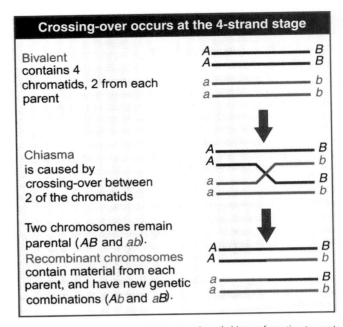

Figure 2–13. Crossing over of DNA strands and chiasma formation to create new sequences. *(From Lewin B: Genes VIII. Prentice Hall/Pearson Education, New York, 2004, p 20. Reprinted with permission of the author.)*

Isolation

The ability to successfully isolate DNA from cell cultures, blood, and other clinical specimens is fundamental to optimal performance of other molecular procedures described in Chapter 4. Common methods used for the isolation of nucleic acids use alkaline denaturation and precipitation with alcohol and high salt concentrations. They can be further purified from other unwanted cellular components, such as the cytoplasmic membrane, by use of specific columns or beads that will bind nucleic acids based on charge-charge interactions. Magnetic bead technology has become an efficient and popular way to isolate DNA and other molecules or even specific cell types, and it can be automated. Column chromatography has been in use for many years, and different materials are used to prepare columns, depending on the nature of the materials to be separated. In more traditional methods, DNA was isolated after treatment of cells with harsh mechanical or chemical agents often necessary to break open cell walls and disrupt proteins and fatty acids.

Sonication, phenol, and chloroform, or various chaotropic agents were used to disrupt cells, then followed by high-speed centrifugation on cesium chloride or sucrose gradients to isolate the nucleic acids. This was necessary to separate the high and low molecular weight DNA and RNA molecules within the cell. RNA requires greater care than DNA, as it is a single-stranded molecule and much more labile. Chemicals that will inactivate RNase enzymes must be used to obtain RNA that is not readily degraded and has its sequence intact. As mRNA is only a small part of the total RNA isolated, it can be purified by nature of its poly-A tail using a column that contains poly-T attached to resin bead molecules.

Methods such as complementary DNA (cDNA) synthesis, in which RNA is converted into a DNA copy in vitro, allows greater study of RNA sequences by making a more stable version of it. RNA isolation also requires greater disruption of the cellular material, usually with chaotropic agents such as guanidine thiocyanate, lithium salts, and mechanical means to disrupt cell membranes, such as douncing or shearing with a needle and syringe. Once DNA or RNA has been isolated, they can be stored in low salt buffers at the respective correct pH at –20°C or lower for DNA and RNA at –80°C for many months to many years. Storage in water is not recommended because the nucleic acids are polymers, hydrolysis reactions will degrade them, and water can contain contaminates that can degrade nucleic acids over time, even at low temperatures. Important is the pH of the buffer used in nucleic acid isolation and storage, as acidic pH can result in degradation of DNA and alkaline pH can degrade RNA.

Ribonucleic Acid

Ribonucleic acid (RNA) is similar to DNA in structure but has certain key differences. It has a very different role to play in the cell. One of the key structural differences is that unlike DNA, which is usually a double-stranded helix, RNA occurs most often as a single-stranded structure, although internal hydrogen bonding occurs frequently, probably to stabilize the RNA molecules. Both DNA and RNA are made up of nucleotides, but in place of thymine in DNA there is uracil in RNA. Uracil is very similar to thymine except that it lacks a methyl group. Another major difference is the substitution of the sugar ribose for deoxyribose in the backbone structure. The sugar in DNA, deoxyribose, lacks a hydroxyl group (-OH) at the 2′ carbon position (thus, the deoxyribonucleic acid, or DNA, name). Ribose in RNA has the hydroxyl group at this carbon position, whereas DNA has hydrogen.

In eukaryotes, RNA used to transmit genetic information (stored as DNA) from the nucleus to the cytoplasm is translated into peptides and proteins. DNA is copied into RNA by transcription, modified and transported out of the nucleus to the ribosomes, where it is translated into protein, which is then modified if necessary for its proper function. Therefore, RNA is the "go-between" of DNA, which stores genetic information and protein, which is the final product of the expression of that genetic information. It is worth mentioning that certain viruses can store genetic information as RNA, whereas others use DNA, either single- or double-stranded; some viruses use both during the different parts of their infectious cycles.

In eukaryotes there are four major types of RNA; each has a specific function as well as its own corresponding polymerase. The first class of RNA molecule is ribosomal RNA (rRNA), which makes up a large part of the ribosomal structure on the endoplasmic reticulum in the cytoplasm. It is here that RNA is translated into peptide. RNA polymerase I transcribes rRNA. It is the most abundant and consistent form of RNA in the cell. The second class of RNA is messenger RNA (mRNA); it is this form that is transcribed from DNA that encodes specific genes, such as those determining the various blood groups. RNA polymerase II transcribes mRNA. Unlike rRNA, mRNA molecules are very different from each other, depending on the gene they were transcribed from. In addition, mRNA undergoes postsynthesis processing before it can be transferred out of the nucleus and translated.

The third major class of RNA is transfer RNA (tRNA); it is involved in bringing amino acids to the mRNA bound on the ribosome. Each tRNA molecule can be charged with only one species of amino acid. However, as mentioned, the genetic code is redundant, and many amino acids have more than one type of tRNA that codes for them. In addition, tRNA has considerable internal hydrogen bonding to acquire its formal structure. This hydrogen bonding stabilizes tRNA as well.

The fourth major type of RNA includes small RNA molecules, which have other various functions within the cell. These RNA molecules, such as silencing RNA molecules, are necessary for proper gene expression and are altered in amount and type during cellular growth and differentiation.

Transcription

Transcription is the cellular process by which DNA is copied into RNA. Although mRNA accounts for only a small percent of the total RNA inside a eukaryotic cell, it has the extremely important role of being a "transportable" and disposable form of the genetic code. Messenger RNA allows for highly efficient processing of the genetic code into the proteins that play nearly all the functional roles within a cell. Transcription begins when the enzyme RNA polymerase II binds to the region upstream (to the left of the 5′ start site) of a gene. Certain DNA short sequences, called *consensus sequences*, such as the CAAT box and TATA box, are located at specific sections upstream of the gene to be transcribed; these are used to position RNA polymerase properly so transcription of a gene is started correctly. This region is referred to as the promoter and is important in how and when a gene is expressed.

Promoter regions also contain specific sequences that allow certain proteins, transcription factors, to bind to them preferentially. This allows for certain genes to be more or less active than other genes. Transcription factors are very critical to proper cell growth and differentiation. Upstream sequences are not part of the mRNA itself and are never transcribed; rather, they function to control transcription of mRNA. In addition to the promoter regions that can positively or negatively regulate various transcription factors and other transcription-specific protein effectors, there are regions of DNA sequence called enhancers that can affect transcription rates. Unlike promoters, these enhancer regions can have such effects without being close to the coding regions of the genes they influence. RNA is synthesized in a 5′ to 3′ direction; transcription starts at the 3′ end of the coding (or template) strand of the DNA duplex after it is opened to two single strands and proceeds to the 5′ end. In this way, a 5′ to 3′ coding strand is generated with U in place of T. The RNA transcript is complementary to the template strand and is equivalent to the coding strand of the DNA molecule. Transcription is illustrated in Figure 2–14.

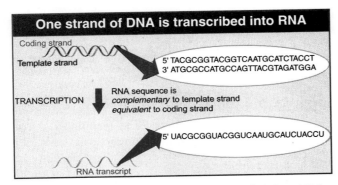

Figure 2–14.   Transcription of RNA from DNA. *(From Lewin B: Genes VIII. Prentice Hall/Pearson Education, New York, 2004, p 241. Reprinted with permission of the author.)*

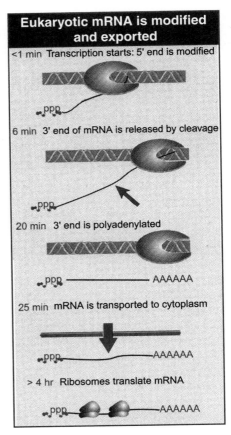

Figure 2–15.   Translation of RNA into protein. *(Lewin B: Genes VIII. Prentice Hall/Pearson Education, New York, 2004, p 122. Reprinted with permission of the author.)*

After RNA is transcribed, it is further processed before it is transported to the ribosome and translated into protein. One major modification to eukaryotic mRNA is the 5′ 7-methyl guanosyl cap that is added to protect the mRNA from degradation by nucleases. The 3′ end of mRNA is modified by the addition of a string of adenines that form a polyadenylation signal (poly-A tail), which can vary in length from about 20 to 200 nucleotides and is believed to increase mRNA stability. In addition to these steps, eukaryotic mRNA has intervening sequences called introns that do not code for protein or peptide and must be removed before translation can begin. The process by which introns are removed from mRNA is called *RNA splicing.* Specific nucleotide sequences at the beginning and end of each intron signal the necessary enzymes to remove the introns from the mRNA and degrade them. The remaining sequences, which contain only exons that code for peptides and proteins, are joined together by ligation to form a mature mRNA molecule. The mature mRNA is then transported out of the nucleus and to the ribosomes, where translation takes place.

Translation

Translation is the cellular process by which RNA transcripts are turned into proteins and peptides, the structural and functional molecules of the cell (Fig. 2–15). Like DNA and RNA, proteins have a direction, reading their sequences left to right from the amino (NH2-) terminal to the carboxy (-COOH) terminal. Peptides are composed of amino acids (aa) joined to make a linear chain. Peptides consist of one strand of amino acids, and polypeptides (proteins) consist of more than one strand. Many peptide strands have only primary and secondary structure. Proteins can also have more complicated tertiary and quaternary structure. The making of the peptide chain(s) in the correct sequence is complicated and requires multiple steps and many molecules to carry it out. Translation takes place on the rough endoplasmic reticulum (ER) in the cytoplasm. Also called the *rough ER,* it is the site of the ribosomes, which are organelles composed of proteins and ribosomal RNA (rRNA). In eukaryotic organisms, translation is monocistronic in that only one ribosome reads the mRNA transcript at any time as compared to polycistronic mRNA, which has coding regions representing more than one gene and is read differently.

Translation is a complicated process and involves three major steps: initiation, elongation, and termination. The first event of the initiation sequence is the attachment of a free methionine to a transfer RNA molecule called tRNAmet, which requires the presence of a high-energy molecule called *guanine triphosphate* (GTP) and a special protein called *initiation factor IF2.* When GTP, IF2, and factors IF1 and IF3 are present at the ribosome, tRNAmet is able to bind the small 40S subunit of the ribosome to form an initiation complex. The larger subunit of the ribosome, the 60S, also binds to the complex and hydrolyzes the GTP, and then the IFs are released. Translation is illustrated in Figures 2–16 and 2–17.

There are two sites present on the 60S ribosome unit—the A site and the P site. During translation, the charged tRNAmet must occupy the P site, and the A site next to the P site must have a charged tRNA with its correct matching amino acid in position. Peptide bond formation occurs by transferring the polypeptide attached to the tRNA in the P site to the aminoacyl-tRNA in the A site.

All tRNA molecules are long, single-stranded RNAs with a similar secondary structure with intramolecular hydrogen bonding. They are often described as having a cloverleaf-shaped conformation no matter which aa they are carrying to the translation machinery. There are two major functional areas of the tRNA molecule. The first is the anticodon; it consists of three nucleotides that hydrogen-bond to the corresponding correct site codon on the mRNA. It is this

Peptide bond synthesis involves transfer of polypeptide to aa-tRNA

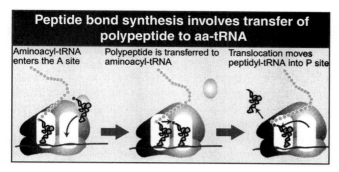

Aminoacyl-tRNA enters the A site

Polypeptide is transferred to aminoacyl-tRNA

Translocation moves peptidyl-tRNA into P site

Figure 2–16. Peptide bond synthesis in translation. *(Lewin B: Genes VIII. Prentice Hall/Pearson Education, New York, 2004, p 137. Reprinted with permission of the author.)*

hydrogen bonding that makes sure the correct aa is joined in the peptide chain by allowing only the correct tRNA molecule with the right anticodon to bond to the correct mRNA codon. The second part of the tRNA molecule is at the 3′ hydroxyl end and binds an amino acid. Only one aa can bind to one tRNA molecule; specificity is determined by the 3′ hydroxyl end. According to the recognition region, an aminoacyl synthase enzyme adds the specific aa to the correct tRNA molecule. Only when the tRNA is charged

with an amino acid can it transport it to the ribosome for translation.

During the elongation step of translation, the incoming tRNA binds to the A site in presence of the elongation factor called *E2F*. Again, GTP is hydrolyzed as the energy source to move the tRNA in the A site to the P site. As the tRNA in the A site is moved to the P site, the tRNA in the P site is released back to the cytoplasm to pick up another amino acid. In this way, tRNA molecules are conserved. The ribosomes move down the codons on the mRNA one at a time, adding a correct amino acid to the growing peptide chain. As the ribosome moves down the mRNA, it eventually comes to one of the three stop codons—UAA, UGA, or UAG—and translation of that mRNA is finished. Termination factors help the ribosome units to separate, and the peptide chain is further processed. Post-translational processing can consist of glycosylation, the addition of sugar groups, or the removal of leader peptide sequences that are used to traffic proteins to the cell membrane.

Processing can also consist of complicated folding schemes that ensure the protein is in its correct tertiary form, such as the formation of disulfide bonds via cysteine aa residues. A large family of proteins called **heat-shock proteins** assists new proteins to be folded correctly by binding to hydrophobic (water-avoiding) sections of the nascent protein chain. Hydrogen bonding, van der Waals forces, and hydrophilic (water-attracting) regions of proteins also help to give the new protein its correct three-dimensional conformation. After translation is complete, the mRNA is rapidly degraded by enzymes (a process that helps to control gene expression) or attaches to another ribosome, and the entire translation process starts all over again. See Figure 2–18.

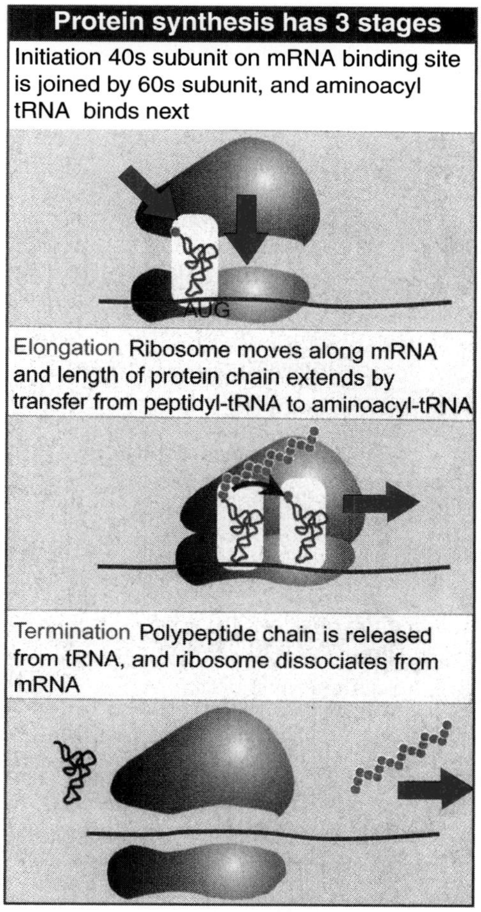

Protein synthesis has 3 stages

Initiation 40s subunit on mRNA binding site is joined by 60s subunit, and aminoacyl tRNA binds next

Elongation Ribosome moves along mRNA and length of protein chain extends by transfer from peptidyl-tRNA to aminoacyl-tRNA

Termination Polypeptide chain is released from tRNA, and ribosome dissociates from mRNA

Figure 2–17. Stages of protein synthesis in translation. *(Lewin B: Genes VIII. Prentice Hall/Pearson Education, New York, 2004, p 137. Reprinted with permission of the author.)*

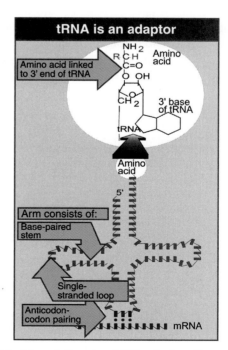

Figure 2–18 Schematic illustration of tRNA molecule and base pairing. *(Lewin B: Genes VIII. Prentice Hall/Pearson Education, New York, 2004, p 115. Reprinted with permission of the author.)*

Common Steps in Modern Genetics Techniques

Over the past three decades, the knowledge of genetics has advanced exponentially. Understanding the biochemical and biophysical nature of DNA, RNA, and peptides and proteins has allowed techniques to be developed to study these important molecules in great detail and to define the ways in which they interact in cells, groups of cells, complex multicellular organisms, and even in an entire human being. Most of the techniques used in molecular biology (the science of studying and manipulating genetic material) are based on the biochemical and biophysical properties of genes and chromosomes.

The following steps are common to most techniques used in molecular biology:

1. Any material that is to be studied must first be isolated intact without structural damage. This is often done with chemicals that interact with one part of the cellular material and not another. The methods to do this can be based on pH changes, salt gradients, detergent lysis, and enzyme activation.

2. There must be a way to visualize and locate the molecular species to be studied. This is often done with probes that act as signals or beacons that will bind specifically to the molecule being analyzed; for example, DNA, by interaction with parts of the molecule, such as hybridization with the hydrogen bonds of DNA. The probes can be synthesized with radiolabels, chemiluminescence molecules, fluorochromes, or nanoparticles.

3. A method to separate out different species and subspecies being studied, such as different sequences of DNA, must be available. An example of this involves running nucleic acids through gels, binding them to columns, hybridizing them to membranes, or binding them to other molecules.

4. A method to quantify the isolated and studied species has to be used to get differences in amount as exact as possible in the process studied. Changes in optical density when exposed to UV radiation, radioisotope emission levels, fluorescence energy detection, chemiluminescence emission that can be detected with optical imaging instruments can all be used to obtain data.

Several techniques used in molecular biology are reviewed in Chapter 4.

SUMMARY CHART

- ✔ *Genetics* is defined as the study of inheritance or the transmission of characteristics from parents to offspring. It is based on the biochemical structure of chromatin, which includes nucleic acids and the structural proteins that constitute the genetic material as well as various enzymes that assist in genetic processes such as replication.

- ✔ All living organisms have specific numbers of chromosomes. Humans have 22 pairs of autosomes and one set of sex chromosomes, females (XX) and males (XY), giving a total of 46 chromosomes in diploid cells.

- ✔ Mendel's law of independent assortment states that factors for different characteristics are inherited independent of each other if they reside on different chromosomes.

- ✔ Human chromosomes are composed of the genetic material chromatin, a complex of the nucleic acid polymer DNA wrapped around highly basic proteins called *histones*. The helical structure of DNA allows a lot of information to be packaged in a very small amount of space.

- ✔ Replication of DNA is semiconservative and is accomplished via the enzyme DNA polymerase, which produces a complementary duplicate strand of nucleic acid. Therefore, each strand of DNA can act as a template to be copied to make the opposite strand. DNA has a direction and is always read and written in the 5′ (left) to 3′ (right) direction unless specified differently for certain applications.

- ✔ *Mutation* refers to any structural alteration of DNA in an organism (mutant) that is caused by a physical or chemical agent (mutagen). Mutations can be beneficial or deleterious. Some mutations are lethal and therefore cannot be passed on to another generation. Some mutations are silent and have no consequence on the organism in which they occur and therefore have no selective pressure against them in the population.

- ✔ Transcription is an enzymatic process whereby genetic information in a DNA strand is copied into an mRNA complementary strand. Eukaryotic mRNA is modified after it is made by various processing steps, such as the removal of introns and addition of a poly-A tail to the 3′ end. These processing steps take place in the nucleus of the cell before the mRNA is exported to the cytoplasmic ribosomes for translation.

- ✔ Translation is the complex process by which mRNA, which contains a mobile version of the DNA template encoding the genes for an organism, is turned into proteins, which are the functional units of an organism and the cells that it consists of. Translation occurs on the ribosomes, and additional steps may be necessary to get a specific protein into its final correct form, such as proteins that require disulfide linkages and proteins that are positioned within the cell membrane. Proteins are made of strings of amino acids and are always read in an amino terminal (left) to carboxyl terminal (right) direction.

- ✔ The polymerase chain reaction (PCR) is an in vitro method for enzymatic synthesis and amplification of specific DNA sequences using a pair of primers, usually short nucleotide sequences, that hybridize to opposite DNA strands and flank the region of interest. Various modifications have made the PCR reaction more efficient and specific and allow more complex analysis.

Review Questions

1. Which of the following statements best describes mitosis?
   a. Genetic material is quadruplicated, equally divided between four daughter cells
   b. Genetic material is duplicated, equally divided between two daughter cells
   c. Genetic material is triplicated, equally divided between three daughter cells
   d. Genetic material is halved, doubled, then equally divided between two daughter cells

2. When a recessive trait is expressed, it means that:
   a. One gene carrying the trait was present.
   b. Two genes carrying the trait were present.
   c. No gene carrying the trait was present.
   d. The trait is present but difficult to observe.

3. In a pedigree, the "index case" is another name for:
   a. Stillbirth.
   b. Consanguineous mating.
   c. Propositus.
   d. Monozygotic twins.

4. Which of the following nitrogenous bases make up DNA?
   a. Adenine, leucine, guanine, thymine
   b. Alanine, cytosine, guanine, purine
   c. Isoleucine, lysine, uracil, leucine
   d. Adenine, cytosine, guanine, thymine

5. Proteins and peptides are composed of:
   a. Golgi bodies grouped together.
   b. Paired nitrogenous bases.
   c. Nuclear basic particles.
   d. Linear arrangements of amino acids.

6. Which phenotype(s) could not result from the mating of a Jk(a+b+) female and a Jk(a-b+) male?
   a. Jk(a+b–)
   b. Jk(a+b+)
   c. Jk(a–b+)
   d. Jk(a–b-)

7. *Exon* refers to:
   a. The part of a gene that contains nonsense mutations.
   b. The coding region of a gene.
   c. The noncoding region of a gene.
   d. The enzymes used to cut DNA into fragments.

8. PCR technology can be used to:
   a. Amplify small amounts of DNA.
   b. Isolate intact nuclear RNA.
   c. Digest genomic DNA into small fragments.
   d. Repair broken pieces of DNA.

9. *Transcription* can be defined as:
   a. Introduction of DNA into cultured cells.
   b. Reading of mRNA by the ribosome.
   c. Synthesis of RNA using DNA as a template.
   d. Removal of external sequences to form a mature RNA molecule.

10. When a male possesses a phenotypic trait that he passes to all his daughters and none of his sons, the trait is said to be:
    a. X-linked dominant.
    b. X-linked recessive.
    c. Autosomal dominant.
    d. Autosomal recessive.

11. When a female possesses a phenotypic trait that she passes to all of her sons and none of her daughters, the trait is said to be:
    a. X-linked dominant.
    b. X-linked recessive.
    c. Autosomal dominant.
    d. Autosomal recessive.

12. DNA is replicated:
    a. Semiconservatively from DNA.
    b. In a random manner from RNA.
    c. By copying protein sequences from RNA.
    d. By first copying RNA from protein.

13. RNA is processed:
    a. After RNA is copied from DNA template.
    b. After protein folding and unfolding on the ribosome.
    c. Before DNA is copied from DNA template.
    d. After RNA is copied from protein on ribosomes.

14. Translation of proteins from RNA takes place:
    a. On the ribosomes in the cytoplasm of the cell.
    b. On the nuclear membrane.
    c. Usually while attached to nuclear pores.
    d. Inside the nucleolus of the cell.

15. Meiosis is necessary to:
    a. Keep the N number of the cell consistent within populations.
    b. Prepare RNA for transcription.
    c. Generate new DNA sequences in daughter cells.
    d. Stabilize proteins being translated on the ribosome.

References

1. Watson, JD, and Crick, FHC: Molecular structure of nucleic acids: A structure for deoxyribose nucleic acid. Nature 171:737, 1953.
2. Garrett, RH, and Grisham, CM: Structure of nucleic acids. In Garret, RH, and Grisham, CM: Biochemistry, 4th ed. Brooks/Cole, Cengage Learning, Boston, 2010, pp 316–353.

3. Knippers, R, and Ruff, J: The initiation of eukaryotic DNA replication. In DNA Replication and the Cell Cycle. Springer-Verlag, New York, 1992, pp 2–10.
4. Antonarakis, SE, and Cooper, DN: Human gene mutation: mechanisms and consequences. In Speicher, MR, Antonarakis, SE, Motulsky, AG (eds): Vogel and Motulsky's Human Genetics: Problems and Approaches, 4th ed. Springer-Verlag, Berlin Heidelberg, 2010, pp 319–351.
5. Caskey, CT, et al: Triplet repeat mutations in human disease. Science 256:784–789, 1992.
6. Yamamoto, F, et al: Molecular genetic basis of the histo-blood group ABO system. Nature 345:229, 1990.
7. Le Van Kim, C, et al: Molecular cloning and primary structure of the human blood group RhD polypeptide. Proc Natl Acad Sci USA 89(22):10929, 1992.

Bibliography

Alberts, B, et al: Molecular Biology of the Cell, 4th ed. Garland Science, New York, 2002.

Calladine, CR, Drew, HR, Luise, BF, and Travers, AA: Understanding DNA, the Molecule and How it Works, 3rd ed. Elsevier, San Diego, CA, 2004.

Clark, DP, and Russell, LD: Molecular Biology Made Simple and Fun, 2nd ed. Cache River Press, St. Louis, MO, 2000.

Glick, BR, Pasternak, JJ, and Patten, CL: Molecular Biotechnology: Principles and Applications of Recombinant DNA, 4th ed. ASM Press, Washington, DC, 2009.

Harmening, DM: Modern Blood Banking and Transfusion Practices, 5th ed. FA Davis, Philadelphia, PA, 2005.

Hillyer, CD, Silberstein, LE, Ness, PM, Anderson, KC, and Roback, J: Blood Banking and Transfusion Medicine, Basic Principles and Practice. Churchill Livingstone, Philadelphia, PA, 2007.

Lewin, B: Genes VIII. Prentice Hall, New York, 2003.

Quinley, ED: Immunohematology: Principles and Practice, 3rd ed. Lippincott Williams & Wilkins, Philadelphia, PA, 2010.

Roback, J, Combs, M, Grossman, B, and Hillyer, C: Blood Group Genetics: Technical Manual, 16th ed. American Association of Blood Banks, Bethesda, MD, 2009.

Roback, J, Combs, M, Grossman, B, and Hillyer, C: Molecular Biology and Immunology in Transfusion Medicine: Technical Manual, 16th ed. American Association of Blood Banks Bethesda, MD, 2009.

Trent, RJ: Molecular Medicine, 3rd ed. Elsevier Academic Press, Burlington, MA, 2005.

Chapter 3

Fundamentals of Immunology

Lorraine Caruccio, PhD, MT(ASCP)SBB, and Scott Wise, MHA, MLS(ASCP)SBB

OBJECTIVES

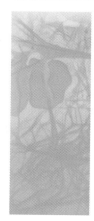

1. Outline the different components of the immune system and identify their functions.
2. Describe the characteristics of the major cells of the immune system and their functions.
3. List the major effector molecules and the roles they play in the immune response.
4. Outline the basic steps of hematopoiesis in the immune system.
5. Explain the function of the major histocompatibility complex (MHC) class I and II molecules.
6. Describe the physical characteristics of immunoglobulins in relation to structure and list the different subtypes.
7. Explain the activation sequences of the three major complement pathways and describe how they come to a common starting point.
8. List the methods used in the blood bank to detect antibodies and complement bound to red blood cells.
9. Describe the immune response, including antigen-antibody reactions, lymphocyte functions, and host factors that can activate and suppress the immune system.

Continued

10. List the traditional laboratory techniques used in blood bank testing.
11. Identify the various factors that affect agglutination reactions.
12. Describe some of the common diseases that can affect blood bank testing.

Introduction

The immune system (IS) is complicated, tightly controlled, and includes tissues, organs, cells, and biological mediators that coordinate to defend a host organism against intrusion by a foreign substance or abnormal cells of self-origin. **Immunity** refers to the process by which a host organism protects itself from attacks by external and internal agents. Immunity also confers protection from nonself and abnormal self-elements, which are controlled at different levels. The number of different types of nonself organisms includes unicellular and multicellular organisms, such as viroids, viruses, bacteria, mycoplasma, fungi, and parasites. Tumor cells, which are too old or misshapen to function, and cells destined for termination within the host must be recognized and eliminated.

The response and elimination of organisms and unwanted cells is accomplished through **cellular** and/or **humoral** mechanisms. The cellular defense mechanism is mediated by various cells of the IS, such as macrophages, T cells, and dendritic cells, which function to eliminate viruses, bacteria, cancer cells, and other cellular pathogens. In the humoral mechanism, specific antibodies and **complement** components are produced in plasma, saliva, and other bodily secretions. These antibodies bind to specific receptor sites on cells. Complement may also bind to **immunoglobulin** molecules that have specific complement receptor sites. The extent of activation and the amount of damage that occurs to red blood cells is dependent upon the complement pathway involved and on several other host factors.

Immunoglobulins, or antibodies, have special significance for transfusion medicine, because antigens present on transfused cells may cause reactions in the recipient and complicate therapy. The majority of blood bank testing is focused on the prevention, detection, and identification of blood group antibodies and on the typing of RBC antigens. Antigen characteristics, as well as host factors, have an impact on the immune response. Knowledge of these characteristics enables testing problems to be resolved. Understanding the IS and its responses is essential to understanding the factors that can affect agglutination reactions between RBCs and antibodies and various testing modifications.

Detection of **alloantibodies** or **autoantibodies** in routine blood bank testing procedures is of the utmost importance in providing compatible blood to patients. This detection is dependent upon several factors, including binding forces between antigens and antibodies, properties of the antibody itself, and individual host characteristics. Antigen-antibody reactions are influenced by a number of factors, including distance, antigen-antibody ratio, pH, temperature, and immunoglobulin type (Box 3–1).

> **BOX 3–1**
> ### Factors Affecting Antigen-Antibody Reactions
> - Distance
> - Antigen-antibody ratio
> - pH
> - Temperature
> - Immunoglobulin type

Both traditional and nontraditional laboratory testing methods are currently utilized in the transfusion service. These methods focus on either the detection of antigens or on the detection of antibodies. This chapter provides an introduction to the many areas of immunology and how they impact transfusion medicine. It will include a brief introduction to the biology and biochemistry of the immune system, and the application of testing procedures used in evaluating the immune response as related to blood transfusion. A brief description of immune-mediated diseases important to transfusion medicine is included at the end of the chapter.

Overview of the Immune System

Basic Concepts

All organisms at all levels of life are challenged constantly by various factors from their environment and must protect against them. The host organism is a rich source of nutrients and protection for an organism that is able to avoid the host's IS. One of the most fundamental concepts in immunology is the idea of **self** versus **nonself** and how the IS distinguishes between the two. The two terms have now been broadened in meaning. *Self* refers to anything that is derived from the host genome and the rearrangement of host genes. It includes cells, fluids, molecules, and more complex structures of a host organism. Anything put into the host body, even a close genetic match, can be regarded as nonself and therefore can be rejected by a response of the IS. *Nonself* refers to anything physically outside the host, whether a living organism (parasites, fungus) or nonliving toxin (poison ivy fluid, insect venom). When foreign objects or damaged host cells are detected by the IS, an immune response occurs. Immune responses occur at different levels and are either primary (natural, innate) or secondary (adaptive, acquired). The overall mechanisms and components of each are outlined in Table 3–1 and Table 3–2.

The **innate immune response** consists of physical barriers, biochemical effectors, and immune cells. The first step of

Table 3–1	**Comparison of the Major Mechanisms of the Immune System**
INNATE OR NATURAL IMMUNITY	**ACQUIRED OR ADAPTIVE IMMUNITY**
• Primary lines of defense	• Supplements protection provided by innate immunity
• Early evolutionary development	• Later evolutionary development–seen only in vertebrates
• Nonspecific	• Specific
◦ Natural–present at birth	◦ Specialized
◦ Immediately available	◦ Acquired by contact with a specific foreign substance
◦ May be physical, biochemical, mechanical, or a combination of defense mechanisms	◦ Initial contact with foreign substance triggers synthesis of specialized antibody proteins resulting in reactivity to that particular foreign substance
• Mechanism does not alter on repeated exposure to any specific antigen	• Memory
	◦ Response improves with each successive encounter with the same pathogen
	◦ Remembers the infectious agent and can prevent it from causing disease later
	◦ Immunity to withstand and resist subsequent exposure to the same foreign substance is acquired

Cellular and Humoral Immunity

The two major components of the vertebrate IS are cellular and humoral immunity. **Cellular immunity** is mediated by various IS cells, such as macrophages, T cells, and dendritic cells. Lymphokines are other effector molecules that play critical roles in the cellular system by activating and deactivating different cells, which allows cells to communicate throughout the host body. Lymphokines are powerful molecules that include cytokines and chemokines.

Humoral immunity consists of the fluid parts of the IS, such as antibodies and complement components found in plasma, saliva, and other secretions. One of the most important parts of humoral immunity is the antibody. **Antibodies** are also called *immunoglobulins*—**immune** because of their function, and **globulin** because they are a type of globular soluble protein. They are found in the gamma globulin portion of plasma or serum when it is separated by fractionation or electrophoresis. The function of the antibody is to bind to foreign molecules called *antigens*. Most antigens are found on the surface of foreign cells or on damaged internal cells.

A key feature of antigen-antibody reactions is their specificity. Only one antibody reacts with one antigen, or one part (an **epitope** or **antigenic determinant**) of a complex antigen. An immune reaction against an antigen stimulates the production of antibodies that will match the epitope of the antigen. The binding reaction of antigen and antibody has often been called a **lock and key** mechanism, referring to its specific conformation. Antigen-antibody complex formation inactivates the antigen and elicits a number of complicated effector mechanisms that will ultimately result in the destruction of the antigen and the cell to which it is bound. The laboratory study of antigen-antibody reactions is called **serology** and has been the basis of blood bank technology for many years. Antibody screening methods such as the indirect antibody test and crossmatching techniques rely on the detection of antigen-antibody complexes by screening for antibodies in the plasma or sera. The direct antiglobulin (**Coombs**) test relies on the detection of antibodies (and complement) bound to the surface of RBCs.

Innate and Acquired Immunity

One of the ways to characterize the immune system is by its cellular and humoral components. Another way is by the two major parts of the IS, which work to prevent infection and damaged cells from destroying the host; namely, innate and acquired immunity. The innate part of the system is less complicated and more primitive and does not function in a specific way; rather, it recognizes certain complex repeating patterns present on common invading organisms. The innate part can function immediately to stop host organisms from being infected.

The acquired immune response is more advanced and was developed after vertebrates had evolved. It relies on the formation of specific antigen-antibody complexes and specific cellular responses. Acquired immunity allows for a specific

innate defense is external, including skin and enzymes present on the skin's surface. The second line of innate defense is internal and can recognize common invaders with a **nonspecific** response, such as phagocytosis that does not have to be primed. The last line of defense is the acquired immune response that needs time and reorganization to mount an effective and **specific** reaction and that protects against a repeat attack by the same organism using immune memory. The IS's specificity also prevents the host from becoming attacked and damaged during an immune response. The localized nature of an immune reaction also prevents systemic damage throughout the host organism. The wide variety of potential organisms and substances that can invade the host requires a vast array of means to recognize and remove them. The acquired immune response must be capable of generating a near-infinite level of specific responses to all the different complex organisms and substances that the host can encounter over its lifetime.

Table 3–2 Cellular and Humoral Components of the Immune System

INNATE OR NATURAL IMMUNITY		ACQUIRED OR ADAPTIVE IMMUNITY
First Line of Defense	Second Line of Defense	Third Line of Defense
Internal Components	*Internal Components*	*Internal Components*
PHYSICAL	*CELLULAR*	*CELLULAR*
• Intact skin	• Phagocytic cells	• Lymphocytes
• Mucous membranes	○ Macrophages-Dendritic cells	○ T cells
• Cilia	○ Monocytes	○ T$_H$
• Cough reflex	○ PMNs: Large granular leukocytes	○ T$_C$
BIOCHEMICAL	○ NK cells	○ T memory cells
• Secretions	*HUMORAL (FLUID)/BIOCHEMICAL*	• B cells
○ Sweat	• Complement-alternate pathway	○ B memory cells
○ Tears	• Cytokines	○ Plasma cells
○ Saliva	○ Interferons	*HUMORAL*
○ Mucus	○ Interleukins	• Antibodies
• Very low pH of vagina and stomach	• Acute inflammatory reaction	• Complement-classic pathway
		• Cytokines

response, and IS memory allows resistance to a pathogen that was previously encountered. **Innate immunity** is the immediate line of immune defense.

There are two important features of innate immunity. First, the innate immune system is nonspecific. The same response is used against invading organisms, no matter what the source is, as long as the innate IS can recognize them as nonself. Innate immunity is present at birth and does not have to be learned or acquired. Second, it does not need modifications to function and is not altered with repeated exposure to the same antigen. Because innate immunity functions so well as a first line of defense, it was maintained in the IS of vertebrates during evolution.

Physical and biochemical barriers and various cells make up the innate IS. **Physical barriers** include intact skin, mucous membranes, cilia lining the mucous membranes, and cough reflexes. **Biochemical barriers** of the innate system include bactericidal enzymes such as lysozyme and RNases, fatty acids, sweat, digestive enzymes in saliva, stomach acid, and low pH. Innate immune cells include phagocytic leukocytes and natural killer (NK) cells. Phagocytic cells of different types are found in most tissues and organs of individuals, including the brain, liver, intestines, lungs, and kidneys. Phagocytes include circulating monocytes in the blood and peripheral macrophages (activated monocytes) that can move between vessel walls. Phagocytes recognize complex molecular structures on the surface of invading cells or in the secretions and fluids of the host body. They remove the

invading organisms by engulfing and digesting them with vesicle enzymes.

Two major cells that can use **phagocytosis** to remove pathogens are the polymorphonuclear cells (which include neutrophils, basophils, and eosinophils) and the mononuclear cells (which include the monocytes in plasma and the macrophages in tissues). Various molecules of the IS collaborate with the innate IS's cells. **Opsonins** are factors that include antibodies and complement components in plasma that coat pathogens and facilitate phagocytosis. When phagocytes ingest foreign cells and destroy them, they can become activated to release soluble polypeptide substances called cytokines that have various effects on other cells of the immune and vascular systems (Table 3–3 lists important cytokines). There are a large number of different cytokines; some have unique functions and others have overlapping functions. Some work together, and some oppose the functions of other cytokines. Many are secreted, and some are membrane receptors. Cytokines help to regulate the immune response in terms of specificity, intensity, and duration.

Another important component of the innate immune system is the **complement system**. Complement has three major roles in immunity: (1) the final lysis of abnormal and pathogenic cells via the binding of antibody, (2) **opsonization** and phagocytosis, and (3) mediation of inflammation. The proteins of the complement system are enzymes that are normally found in the plasma in a **proenzyme** inactive state. Three ways the complement proteins can be activated are the

Table 3–3   Cytokines and Their Functions

CYTOKINE	SOURCE	STIMULATORY FUNCTION
Interleukins		
IL-1	Mf, fibroblasts	Proliferation-activated B cells and T cells
IL-2		Induction PGE_2 and cytokines by Mf
IL-3		Induction neutrophil and T-cell adhesion molecules on endothelial cells
IL-4		Induction IL-6, IFN-b1, and GM-CSF
IL-5		Induction fever, acute phase proteins, bone resorption by osteoclasts
IL-6	T	Growth-activated T cells and B cells; activation NK cells
IL-7	T, MC	Growth and differentiation hematopoietic precursors
IL-8		Mast cell growth
IL-9	CD4, T, MC, BM stroma	Proliferation-activated B cells, T cells, mast cells, and hematopoietic precursor
IL-10		Induction MHC class II and Fc on B cells, p75 IL-2R on T cells
IL-11		Isotype switch to IgG1 and IgE
IL-12		Mf APC and cytotoxic function, Mf fusion (migration inhibition)
IL-13	CD4, T, MC	Proliferation-activated B cells; production IgM and IgA
		Proliferation eosinophils; expression p55 IL-2R
	CD4, T, Mf, MC, fibroblasts	Growth and differentiation B-cell and T-cell effectors and hemopoietic precursors
		Induction acute phase proteins
	BM stromal cells	Proliferation pre-B cells, CD4 cells, CD8 cells, and activated mature T cells
	Monocytes	Chemotaxis and activation neutrophils
		Chemotaxis T cells
		Inhibits IFN-g secretion
	T	Growth and proliferation T cells
	CD4, T, B, Mf	Inhibits mononuclear cell inflammation
	BM stromal cells	Induction acute phase proteins
	T	Activates NK cells
	T	Inhibits mononuclear phagocyte inflammation
Colony-Stimulating Factors		
GM-CSF	T, Mf, fibroblasts, MC, endothelium	Growth of granulocyte and Mf colonies
G-CSF	Fibroblasts, endothelium	Activated Mf, neutrophils, eosinophils
M-CSF	Fibroblasts, endothelium, epithelium	Growth of mature granulocytes
		Growth of macrophage colonies
Steel factor	BM stromal cells	Stem cell division (c-kit ligand)
Tumor Necrosis Factors		
TNF-a	Mf, T	
TNF-b	T	

Continued

Table 3–3 Cytokines and Their Functions—cont'd

CYTOKINE	SOURCE	STIMULATORY FUNCTION
Interferons		
IFN-a	Leukocytes	Antiviral; expression MHC I
IFN-b	Fibroblasts	
IFN-g	T	
Other		
TGF-b	T, B	
LIF	T	

Adapted from Delves, PJ, Martin, SJ, Burton, DR, Roitt, IM: Roitt's Essential Immunology, 8th ed. Wiley-Blackwell, Malden, 2011.
APC = antigen-presenting cells; BM = bone marrow; CSIF = cytokine synthesis inhibitory factor; Fc = immunoglobulin Fc receptor for IgE; G-CSF = granulocyte colony-stimulating factor; GM-CSF = granulocyte monocyte/macrophage colony-stimulating factor; IFN = interferon; IL = interleukin; LIF = leukocyte inhibitory factor; MC = mast cell; M-CSF = monocyte colony-stimulating factor; MHC = major histocompatibility complex; Mf = macrophage; NK = natural killer cells; PGE$_2$ = prostaglandin E$_2$; T = T lymphocyte; TGF = transforming growth factor; TNF = tumor necrosis factor.

classic, alternative, and lectin pathways; all have essentially the final result of cell lysis and inflammation. The classic pathway uses antigen-antibody binding and therefore is a specific activator of complement. The alternative pathway activates complement by recognizing polysaccharides and liposaccharides found on the surfaces of bacteria and tumor cells; therefore, it uses nonspecific methods of activation. The lectin pathway is activated by mannose binding proteins bound to macrophages.

Inflammation is also a critical component of the innate IS and is familiar to most people when they have a minor wound that has redness and warmth at the abrasion site. Inflammation is initiated by any type of tissue damage, whether it be to the skin or to an internal organ. Burns, infections, fractures, necrosis, and superficial wounds all elicit an inflammatory response that is characterized by an increase in blood flow to the wounded area, increased blood vessel permeability at the site to allow for greater flow of cells, a mobilization of phagocytic cells into the site, and a possible activation of acute phase and stress response proteins at the site of tissue damage. Eventually the wound is repaired, new tissue grows in place of the damaged tissue, and inflammation is stopped. Uncontrolled inflammation can result in unwanted damage to healthy tissues. The regulation of inflammation is tightly controlled and requires signals to effectively turn it on and off.

Acquired immunity is the other major arm of the host's IS and is the most highly evolved. It is also the most specific and allows the IS to have memory of pathogens it has encountered previously. The acquired system is present only in vertebrates. The term *acquired* refers to the fact that the immunity is acquired via specific contact with a pathogen or aberrant cell. The term *adaptive* refers to the ability to adapt to and destroy new complex pathogens, although it must first react to them through complex recognition processes. Acquired immunity is specific in recognition of new pathogens and has specific responses, depending on the type of pathogen it encounters.

The acquired IS uses antibodies as specific immune effectors. Antigen specificity and uniqueness determine the particular antibody that will bind to it. The antigen-antibody complex is a three-dimensional interaction that does not allow recognition of near misses. For example, antibodies against one blood group antigen do not react against another blood group antigen. An antigen that an antibody is made against is sometimes referred to as its **antithetical** antigen. The fact that acquired immunity has memory means medical histories of patients that require transfusions are absolutely critical. Antibodies do not always remain in plasma at levels observable with serologic testing, and if antigen-positive RBC units are transfused in a sensitized patient, the second antibody response against the transfused cell antigens can be more vigorous, resulting in intravascular RBC hemolysis.

Cells and Organs of the Immune System

The different types of immune system cells can be distinguished by the membrane markers they possess. These are referred to as **clusters of differentiation (CD)** markers and are detected by immunotyping methods. The immunization process requires many different types of cells and tissues, including phagocytic granulocytes of the innate system and monocytes and macrophages.

Lymphocytes are also important in acquired immunity. They are divided into two major types, the **T lymphocyte** (T cell) and the **B lymphocyte** (B cell). The T lymphocyte matures in the thymus gland and is responsible for making cytokines and destroying virally infected host cells. B lymphocytes mature in the bone marrow, and when stimulated by an antigen, evolve into **plasma cells** that secrete antibody. Natural killer cells are a type of lymphocyte that plays a role in immune protection against viruses. Dendritic cells are present throughout many systems of the body and are responsible for antigen processing. Macrophages can also process antigens. T and B cells communicate with each other and are both necessary for antibody production. B cells undergo gene rearrangement in order to have the correct antibody made that can react with the correct antigen.

T cells also have receptors that undergo gene rearrangement. The receptors on the cell membranes of T and B lymphocytes allow them to recognize foreign substances. Lymphocytes recognize only one specific antigen, which is determined by the genetic programming of that lymphocyte. Because there are so many different antigens that pathogens can carry, the IS has adapted to recognize millions of different antigens, with a specific antibody that will match only one particular antigen. Therefore, if a foreign antigen is present, only a small percentage of the host's antibodies and T-cell receptors will recognize it. In cases where an antigen is recognized by more than one antibody, a process of clonal selection happens, in which the different cells that recognize the different epitopes of the antigen are expanded. In transfusion medicine, this plays a role in selecting the best antibody reagents for testing, as not all epitopes of a complex antigen, including blood group antigens, will be equally reactive.

The maturation of B and T cells occurs after an antigen is encountered. Both B and T cells mature into what are called **effector cells**, which are the functional units of the IS. The final effect that B and T cells can cause is the elimination of pathogens and foreign cells. Immune memory is also acquired when lymphocytes mature into memory cells after antigenic stimulation; this allows the IS to recognize antigens from previous encounters. Once an infection is cleared, some of the cells that can recognize the antigen remain in circulation. The lymphocytes are permanently set to respond to the same antigen again by the process of memory. The second time this antigen is encountered, memory allows for a more effective and rapid immune response. Memory cells can persist for the lifetime of the host. It is one of the reasons that some immunizations with vaccines do not have to be repeated, except on a cautionary basis to keep the immunization active.

B Cells

Antibodies can be secreted or membrane-bound. Antibodies are secreted by mature B cells called *plasma cells* and bind to antigens in a specific manner. The antigens are usually in soluble form in the plasma. The receptor on the B cell that recognizes the antigen is a membrane-bound antibody. When the receptor antibody on the B cell reacts with a specific antigen and recognizes it, the B cell is activated to divide. The cells produced from this rapid division mature into plasma cells and memory B cells. Memory B cells have antibody on their surfaces that is of the same conformation as that of the B cell from which they were derived.

Plasma cells are antibody factories that make large amounts of one specific type of antibody in a soluble form

that remains in circulation in the plasma, body secretions, and lymphatics. Antibodies can neutralize toxic substances and antigens that are encountered by binding to them and therefore preventing them from interacting with the host. When the antigenic site is nonreactive because of antibody binding, it cannot interact with host cells to infect them or damage them. Also, binding of antigen by antibody brings about opsonization, which aids in the direct killing of pathogens by cell lysis. When complement is activated by an antigen-antibody complex, the pathogen can be destroyed. Pathogens can be destroyed intra- or extravascularly. Antibodies are one of the most important components of the IS and blood bank testing procedures.

T Cells

T cells are another very important component of the cellular part of acquired immunity. One of the major differences of cellular immunity compared to humoral immunity is that T cells recognize antigens that are internalized within a host cell. The antigens are then processed and presented on the host cell surface in small peptide fragments. T cell–mediated immunity is involved in the response against fungal and viral infections, intracellular parasites, tissue grafts, and tumors. T-cell receptors do not recognize foreign antigen on their own, as B cells do; they require help in the form of cell membrane proteins known as **major histocompatibility complex (MHC)** molecules. Therefore, there is a certain level of restriction placed on the acquired cellular branch of the IS, as determined by the inherited MHC molecules on host cells. The MHC genes determine the human leukocyte antigens (HLA) present on leukocytes and other cells; they have been known for many years to cause rejection of tissue grafts.

Advanced Concepts

There are two major classes of MHC genes and antigens: **MHC class I** and **MHC class II**. MHC class I antigens are found on most nucleated cells in the body, and MHC class II antigens are found on most antigen presenting cells. In humans, MHC class I genes code for the HLA-A, HLA-B, and HLA-C antigens; whereas MHC class II genes code for HLA-DR, HLA-DQ, and HLA-DC antigens. MHC classes I and II are important in the recognition of foreign substances and the immune reactions against them.

There are two major functions of T cells. The first major function is to produce immune mediating substances such as cytokines, which influence many immune functions throughout the body. The second major function is to kill cells that contain foreign antigen. When T cells are activated by antigen, they start to secrete cytokines and change their cellular interactions (see **Table 3–3**). T cells are also grouped into two major categories with two major functions: T helper (TH) cells and T cytotoxic (TC) cells. TH cells are also distinguished by the membrane marker CD4; TC cells are distinguished by the marker CD8. TH cells are further grouped into TH1 and TH2 and respond to different cytokines. T$_H$ cells have the ability to recognize antigen, along with MHC class II molecules, and provide help to B cells to evolve into plasma cells and make antibodies. T$_H$ cells therefore determine which antigens become IS targets, as well as which immune mechanisms will be used against them. T$_H$ cells aid in the proliferation of immune cells after they encounter antigen.

Antigen-Presenting Cells

There are several types of leukocytes that function as **antigen-presenting cells** (APCs), including macrophages, neutrophils, and some B cells. In addition to leukocytes, there are specialized immune cells capable of antigen presentation. These include the different types of dendritic cells present in the skin (Langerhans cells), nervous tissue (glial cells), lymph nodes, spleen, intestines, liver (Kupffer cells), bone (osteoclasts), and thymus. These APCs first phagocytize the foreign antigen, process it internally, and then with the help of MHC molecules, present short peptide sequences of the antigen on their cell membranes. T$_H$ cells can then recognize the antigen in the context of MHC presentation and respond to it by the appropriate immune reaction.

Immune System Organs

Basic Concepts

The organs of the IS are divided into primary and secondary systems. The primary lymphoid organs are the thymus and bone marrow, where immune cells differentiate and mature. The secondary lymphoid organs include the lymph nodes and spleen, in which immune cells interact with each other and process antigens (Table 3–4).

Immune Maturation

Because of the complexity and diversity of immune responses, a specific immediate immune response is not always possible. It usually takes days to months for all the aspects of an efficient immune response to happen from the moment an antigen is first encountered. The lag phase, until an appropriate immune response occurs, is called the **latency**, **preseroconversion**, or **window period**. It is during this time that antibody cannot be detected with serologic testing. During the latency period, however, T and B cells are very active in processing antigen and initiating the primary response to the antigen. The first antibodies made against the new antigen are different from the antibodies of the secondary response. The primary antibodies are the immunoglobulin M (IgM) subclass, whereas the antibodies of the secondary response are the immunoglobulin G (IgG) subclass and have a different structure. Figure 3–1 depicts the primary and secondary antibody responses.

After the antigen is cleared, memory cells are stored in immune organs of the host. When the same antigen is encountered again, the memory cells are activated and produce a stronger and more rapid response. IgG antibodies are formed during the secondary response and are made in great quantities, and although IgM is made during the primary response, there is a period when it overlaps with the production of IgG antibodies at the beginning of the secondary response. IgG secondary antibodies have a higher avidity for antigen and can be produced by much lower concentrations of antigen. Secondary antibodies can usually be measured within 1 to 2 days. For example, a primary antibody may require more than 100-fold excess of antigen to initiate the first response. Many of the antigens that stimulate the primary response have multiple repeating epitopes such as polysaccharides and therefore are good immune stimulators at lower concentrations.

Cell Lineages and Markers

Advanced Concepts

Nearly all cells of the host's body, especially the various leukocytes, have specific cell receptors that interact with other cells and receive signals from cellular messenger systems. Macrophages, NK cells, T and B cells, and APCs can interact directly with cell-to-cell communication or indirectly with soluble mediators through a complex system. These cell surface molecules are classified by complex in vitro testing using monoclonal antibodies. They specify cellular definitions and functions, including maturation levels and lineage specificity and are designated as CD markers. These markers on cells can change during the lifetime of the cell or in response to infection or activation. Currently, there are more than 200 different CD markers known. The first were identified on immune cells. CD markers are critical to identifying hematopoietic cell maturation stages and lineages.

All immune cells originate from pluripotent hematopoietic progenitors (or CD34-positive cells) through one of two pathways of lineage, the **myeloid** and the **lymphoid**. Various growth factors are responsible for differentiating

Table 3–4	**Lymphoid Organs Associated with the Acquired Immune System**	
PRIMARY LYMPHOID ORGANS	**SECONDARY LYMPHOID ORGANS**
• Thymus	• Lymph nodes
• Bone marrow	• Spleen
	• Mucosa-associated tissues
Site of maturation for T and B cells	Site of cell function for mature T and B cells
Lymphocytes differentiate from stem cells, then migrate to secondary lymphoid organs	Cells interact with each other and with accessory cells and antigens

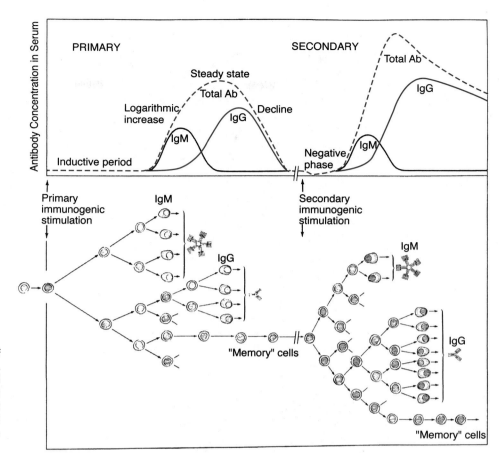

Figure 3–1. Schematic representation of primary and secondary antibody responses. Note the enhanced antibody production and expanded antibody-producing cell population during the secondary antibody response. *(From Herscowitz, HB: Immunophysiology. In Bellanti, JA [ed]: Immunology III. WB Saunders, Philadelphia, 1985, p 117, with permission.)*

and maturing stem cells into the many different cells of the IS. Growth factors also allow progenitor stem cells to reproduce and differentiate. The cells of the myeloid lineage consist of phagocytic cells such as the monocytes and macrophages, often referred to as the *mononuclear phagocytic system* (MPS); the granulocytes or polymorphonuclear cells (PMNs), the neutrophils, eosinophils, and the basophils; and the APCs such as the dendritic cells in the skin and liver. Erythrocytes and platelets originate from this system. The lymphoid lineage consists of the various subpopulations of lymphoid cells, the T cells, B cells, and NK cells.

The myeloid-monocyte precursors originate in the bone marrow and then differentiate into circulating blood monocytes. When monocytes encounter antigen, they can differentiate into tissue macrophages. Phagocytic cells process antigens for acquired immunity and can directly kill many pathogens such as bacteria and fungi as part of innate immunity. MPS cells present antigen to lymphocytes and interact with other immune cells via cell membrane receptors. The Fc part of the antibody receptor and the complement receptor CR1 are used by phagocytes during opsonization.[1] When these cells are functioning as APCs, they express the MHC class II molecules on their membranes and lack the Fc receptor. Granulocytes originate in the bone marrow. They are the predominant leukocyte in the circulation of the mature adult (60% to 70%).

Granulocytes all have granules in their cytoplasm and are of three types, distinguished by the hematologic staining of their granules. The neutrophils stain a faint purple or neutral color (neutral granules), the eosinophils a reddish orange color (acidic granules), and the basophils a bluish black color (basic granules). The main role of these cells is phagocytosis; they function primarily in acute inflammatory responses and have enzymes that allow them to destroy engulfed pathogens. All three types of granulocytes possess receptors for the Fc portion of IgG (CD16) and complement receptors C5a, CR1(CD35), and CR3(CD11b). Additionally, eosinophils possess low-affinity Fc receptors for IgE and therefore play a critical role in allergic reactions and inflammation in parasitic infections. Basophils and mast cells (a type of tissue basophil) possess high-affinity Fc immunoglobulin E (IgE) receptors, are powerful effectors of inflammation and allergic reactions, and can cause the release of localized histamine.

Lymphocytic cells are generated in the thymus or bone marrow and travel through the circulatory system to the lymph nodes and spleen, where they mature and differentiate. In a mature adult, the lymphocytes account for about 20% to 30% of the circulating leukocytes. In primary organs, these cells acquire receptors that enable them to interact with antigens and to differentiate between self and nonself antigens, a very critical part of lymphocyte maturation and the acquired IS in general.

In the secondary organs, immune cells are provided with a highly interactive environment in which immune responses are exchanged and made specific. Remember, there are two primary classifications of lymphocytes, T and B cells, and these similar-looking cells can be distinguished by the presence of specific cell markers by means of using sophisticated immunologic methods of testing, such as flow cytometry (discussed later in this chapter). Specific to the T cell is the T-cell receptor (TCR), which is in proximity to and usually identified with the CD3 complex on the T-cell membrane. It associates in cell-to-cell contacts and interacts with both antigenic determinants and MHC proteins. In addition to CD3 on T cells, there is the separate CD2 marker, which is involved in cell adhesion. It has the unique ability to bind with sheep erythrocytes in vitro.[2] Remember that T$_H$ cells have the CD4 marker and recognize antigen together with the MHC class II molecules, and T$_C$ cells possess CD8 markers and interact with MHC class I molecules.[3] The ratios of T cells with CD4 versus CD8-positive cells can be a marker for particular diseases. One of the defining features of AIDS is a reversal of the typical CD4 to CD8 ratio, which helped to explain some of the pathology of this illness.

There are also compounds referred to as **superantigens**, which can stimulate multiple T cells, causing them to release large amounts of cytokines. Certain bacteria toxins are superantigens and can lead to lethal reactions in the host if the immune system is overstimulated.

B cells are defined by the presence of immunoglobulin on their surface; however, they also possess MHC class II antigens (antigen presentation); the complement receptors CD35 and CD21; F$_C$ receptors for IgG; and CD19, CD20, and CD22 markers, which are the CD markers used to identify B cells. Membrane-bound immunoglobulin may act as an antigen receptor for binding simple structural antigens or antigens with multiple repeating determinants (referred to as *T cell–independent antigens*, meaning they do not require the intervention of T-cell help). When T cell–dependent antigens (structurally complex and unique substances) are encountered, B cells require the intervention of T cells to assist in the production of antibody. When B cells become activated, they mature and develop into plasma cells, which produce and secrete large quantities of soluble Ig into tissue or plasma.

The third major class of lymphocytes, the NK cells, are sometimes referred to as **third population cells** because they originate in the bone marrow from a developmental line distinct from those of T and B lymphocytes. They are also referred to as *large granular lymphocytes*. Unlike B cells, NK cells do not have surface Ig or secrete Ig, nor do they have antigen receptors like the TCR of T cells. NK cells have the CD56 and CD16 markers and do not require the presence of an MHC marker to respond to an antigen. They are thymus-independent and are able to lyse virally infected cells and tumor cells directly in a process known as **antibody-dependent cell-mediated cytotoxicity** (ADCC) by anchoring immunoglobulin to the cell surface membrane through an F$_C$ receptor.

Cytokines and Immunoregulatory Molecules

Cytokines are soluble protein or peptide molecules that function as powerful mediators of the immune response.

There are two main cytokine types: **lymphokines**, which are produced by lymphocytes, and **monokines**, which are produced by monocytes and macrophages. Cytokines function in a complex manner by regulating growth, mobility, and differentiation of leukocytes. One cytokine may act by itself or together with other cytokines. Other cytokines oppose the actions of one or more cytokines and function to quantitatively increase or decrease a particular immune reaction. Some cytokines are synergistic and need each other to have their full effect. The effects of cytokines can be in the immediate area of their release, or they can travel through the plasma to affect distant cells and tissues. There is often significant overlap in how cytokines function.

Major classes of cytokines include interleukins (IL), interferons (IFN), tumor necrosis factors (TNF), and colony-stimulating factors (CSF). Each class has several members (see **Table 3–3**). Cytokines act by binding to specific target cell receptors. When cytokines bind to their receptors on cells, the number of receptors is often increased as the cell is stimulated. Internal cellular signaling pathways become activated. The cell is no longer in a resting state and can have a new function. After cytokine binding, both the receptor and the cytokine become internalized, which induces the target cell to grow and **differentiate**. Differentiated cells have specialized functions such as secreting antibodies or producing enzymes. Immune cells and other host cells respond to cytokines and can react with chemoattraction, as well as antiviral, antiproliferation, and immunomodulation processes. Cytokines fine-tune the IS and also function as critical cell activators.

In addition to the cytokines, other mediator substances of the IS, including chemokines, immunoglobulins, complement proteins, kinins, clotting factors, acute phase proteins, stress-associated proteins, and the fibrinolytic system, are cellular products that can have powerful cellular effects. Cytokines typically communicate between cells through the plasma. Chemokines are attractant molecules that interact between cells, immunoglobulins, and complement proteins and are important in destroying pathogens. Acute phase proteins and fibrinolytic proteins play a role in inflammation, a process that recruits appropriate cells to an immune site and modifies the vascular system. In addition to inflammation and cell-to-cell communication, some cytokines are immunosuppressive. One of the important chemokine receptors in blood banking is the Duffy antigen group present on RBCs. The lack of these antigens can prevent certain types of malaria parasites from infecting the host. The Duffy antigen may also modulate immune response by acting as a sink for extra cytokines of the IL-8 family.

Immune System Genetics

Basic Concepts

Individuals have a unique immune response based on their genetic inheritance, and there are familial patterns of susceptibility and resistance. In blood banking this is important because not all transfusion recipients make antibodies to **alloantigens** on transfused RBCs. **Responders** are people who have a tendency based on their inheritance to make antibodies. The terms **high responders** and **low responders** describe individual responses to antigen challenges. When antigenic stimulation occurs, one B cell forms an antibody with a single specificity. During the lifetime of the cell, the cell can switch to make a different **isotypic** class of antibody that has the same antigen specificity. Isotype switching requires further DNA rearrangement in mature B cells. Class switching is dependent on antigenic stimulation and on the presence of cytokines released by T cells; this reflects the further adaptation of the immune response. Isotype switching is seen in blood banking when antibodies react at different temperatures and phases.

Advanced Concepts

The major histocompatibility complex (MHC) is the region of the genome that encodes the **human leukocyte antigen** (HLA) proteins. (Refer to Chapter 21, "The HLA System.") The MHC is critical in immune recognition and regulation of antigen presentation in cell-to-cell interactions, transplantation, paternity testing, and specific HLA patterns. It also correlates with susceptibility to certain diseases. HLA molecules are categorized into two classes: MHC classes I and II. Class I molecules are found on all nucleated cells except trophoblasts and sperm, and they play a key role in cytotoxic T-cell function. Class II molecules are found on antigen-presenting cells such as B lymphocytes, activated T cells, and the various dendritic cells. Class II molecules on APCs are essential for presenting processed antigen to CD4 T cells and are necessary for T-cell functions and B-cell help. In addition, there are class III molecules that encode complement components such as C2, C4, and factor B. The genes for MHC classes I through III molecules are located on the short arm of chromosome 6 and are highly **polymorphic** in nature with multiple alleles.

Characteristics of Immunoglobulins

Immunoglobulin (Ig), also called *antibody*, is a complex protein produced by plasma cells, with specificity to antigens (or immunogens), that stimulate their production. An Ig is a specific self protein produced by the host in response to a specific foreign, nonself protein, or other complex molecule not tolerated by the host. Immunoglobulins make up a high percentage of the total proteins in disseminated body fluids, about 20% in a normal individual. Antibodies bind antigen, fix complement, facilitate phagocytosis, and neutralize toxic substances in the circulation. Thus, antibodies have multiple functions, some more highly specialized and specific than others. Immunoglobulins are classified according to the molecular structure of their heavy chains. The five classifications are IgA (α [alpha] heavy chain), IgD (δ [delta] heavy chain), IgE (ε [epsilon] heavy chain), IgG (γ [gamma] heavy chain), and IgM (μ [mu] heavy chain).

Table 3–5 illustrates some of the various differences in the classes of immunoglobulins, such as molecular weight, percentage in serum, **valency** (number of antigen-binding sites), carbohydrate content, half-life in the blood, and whether they exist as monomers or multimers. IgG is the most concentrated in serum, comprising approximately 80% of the total serum Ig; next is IgA, at about 13% (although it is the major Ig found in body secretions); IgM is 6%; IgD is 1%; and IgE is the least common, present at less than 1%.[4]

Immunoglobulin Structure

All classes and subclasses of immunoglobulins (Igs) have a common biochemical structural configuration with similarities and are probably derived from a common evolutionary

Table 3–5 Characteristics of Serum Immunoglobulins

CHARACTERISTIC	IgA	IgD	IgE	IgG	IgM
Heavy chain type	Alpha	Delta	Epsilon	Gamma	Mu
Sedimentation coefficient(s)	7–15*	7	8	6.7	19
Molecular weight (kD)	160–500	180	196	150	900
Biologic half-life (d)	5.8	2.8	2.3	21	5.1
Carbohydrate content (%)	7.5–9	10–13	11–12	2.2–3.5	7–14
Placental transfer	No	No	No	Yes	No
Complement fixation (classical pathway)	No	No	No	+	+++
Agglutination in saline	+	0	0	±	++++
Heavy chain allotypes	A$_m$	None	None	G$_m$	None
Proportion of total immunoglobulin (%)	13	1	0.002	80	6

*May occur in monomeric or polymeric structural forms.

d = days; kD = kilodaltons; 0 = negative reactivity; ± = weak reactivity; + = slight reactivity; +++ = strong reactivity; ++++ = very strong reactivity.

molecular structure with well-defined function. In Figure 3–2, the basic Ig structural unit is composed of four polypeptide chains: two identical light chains (molecular weights of approximately 22,500 daltons) and two identical heavy chains (molecular weights from approximately 50,000 to 75,000 daltons). In Figure 3–3, covalent **disulfide bonding** holds the light and heavy chains together, and the covalent disulfide linkages in Ig molecules provide greater structural strength than do **hydrogen bonding** and **van der Waals forces**. However, they limit the flexibility of the Ig molecule. The heavy chains are also interconnected by disulfide linkages in the hinge region of the molecule. Although there are five types of heavy chains, there are only two types of light chains: κ (kappa) and λ (lambda). Both types are found in all classes of immunoglobulins, regardless of heavy chain classification.

Ig molecules are proteins and therefore have two terminal regions: the **amino** (-NH₂) terminal and the **carboxyl** (-COOH) terminal. The carboxyl region of all heavy chains has a relatively constant amino acid sequence and is named the *constant region*. Like the heavy chain, the light chain also has a constant region. Due to certain common Ig structures, enzyme treatment yields specific cleavage products of defined molecular weight and structure. The enzyme **papain** splits the antibody molecule at the hinge region to give three fragments: one crystallizable Fc fragment and two antigen-binding fragments, *Fab*. The Fc fragment encompasses that portion of the Ig molecule from the carboxyl region to the hinge region and is responsible for complement fixation and monocyte binding by Fc receptors on cells. The Fc fragment on IgG antibody only is also responsible for placental transfer. In contrast to the carboxyl terminal regions, the amino terminal regions of both light and heavy chains of immunoglobulins are known as the **variable** regions, because they are structured according to the great variation in antibody specificity. Structurally and functionally, the Fab fragments encompass the portions of the Ig from the hinge region to the amino terminal end and are the regions responsible for binding antigen (see **Fig. 3–2**).

The **domains** of immunoglobulins are the regions of the light and heavy chains that are folded into compact globular loop structures (see **Fig. 3–3**). The domains are held together by intrachain covalent disulfide bonds; the V region of the domain specifies the variable region, and the C is the constant region. The domains are also specified according to light and heavy chains. Looking at one half of an Ig molecule, one domain (V_L) is the variable region, one domain (C_L) is in the constant region of each light chain, and one variable domain (V_H) is on each heavy chain. The number of domains is determined by the isotype. There are three constant domains, C_H1 to C_H3, on the heavy chains of IgA, IgD, and IgG, and four constant domains, C_H1 to C_H4, on the heavy chains of IgE and IgM. The antigen-binding, or **idiotypic**, regions (which distinguish one V domain from all other V domains) are located within the three-dimensional structures formed by the V_L and V_H domains together. Certain heavy chain domains are associated with particular biological properties of immunoglobulins, especially those of IgG and IgM, and include complement fixation. They are identified with the C_H2 domain and the C_H3 domains, which serve as attachment sites for the Fc receptor of monocytes and macrophages.

Immunoglobulins Significant for Blood Banking

All immunoglobulins can be significant for transfusion medicine; however, IgG, IgM, and IgA have the most significance

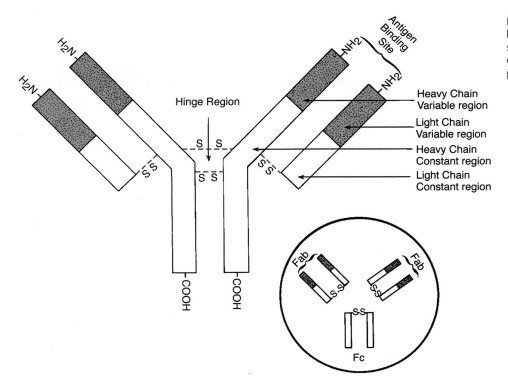

Figure 3–2. Schematic representation of basic immunoglobulin structure. The inset shows formation of Fab and Fc fragments after enzymatic cleavage of the IgG molecule by papain.

Heavy Chain Variable region
Light Chain Variable region
Heavy Chain Constant region
Light Chain Constant region

Hinge Region

Antigen Binding Site

H2N

COOH

Fab

Fc

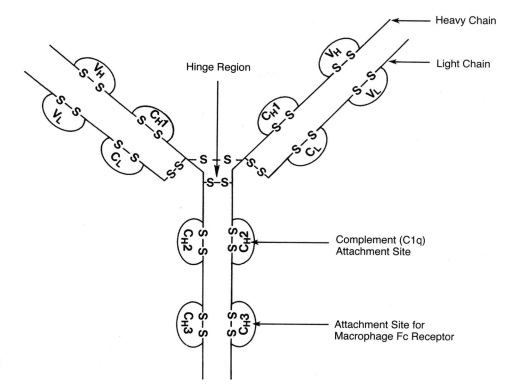

Figure 3-3. Schematic illustration of the domain structure within the IgG molecule.

for the blood bank. Most **clinically significant** antibodies that react at body temperature (37°C) are IgG isotype and are capable of destroying transfused antigen-positive RBCs, causing anemia and transfusion reactions of various severities. IgM antibodies are most commonly encountered as *naturally* occurring antibodies in the ABO system and are believed to be produced in response to commonly occurring antigens like intestinal flora and pollen grains. (Refer to Chapter 6, "The ABO Blood Group System.") Other blood groups such as Lewis, Ii, P, and MNS may also produce IgM antibodies, which usually react best at ambient temperature (22°C to 24°C). The primary testing problem encountered with IgM antibodies is that they can interfere with the detection of clinically significant IgG antibodies by masking their reactivity. Unlike IgG, IgM exists in both monomeric and polymeric forms (as pentamers) containing a J (joining) chain (Fig. 3–4).

Advanced Concepts

The pentameric form can be dissociated through cleavage of covalent bonds interconnecting the monomeric subunits and the J chain by chemical treatment with sulfhydryl reducing reagents such as β-2-mercaptoethanol (2-ME) or dithiothreitol (DTT). These reagents can distinguish a mixture of IgM and IgG antibodies, because only IgM is removed by the use of these compounds; therefore, the removal allows unexpected IgG antibodies to be detected. IgG antibodies are significant in transfusion medicine, because they are the class of immunoglobulins that are made in response to transfusion with nonself antigens on blood products. IgG antibodies are important in hemolytic

disease of the newborn (HDN), because antibodies can be formed in response against alloantigens on fetal RBCs that enter the mother's circulation, usually during delivery. HDN can be fatal. It is one area of medicine where immunohematology has provided prevention and treatment. Antibody screening, Rh typing, and passive anti-D antibody have prevented HDN from developing in D-negative mothers who give birth to D-positive babies.

IgG has the greatest number of subclasses: IgG_1, IgG_2, IgG_3, and IgG_4, and all four are easily separated by electrophoresis. The small differences in the chemical structure

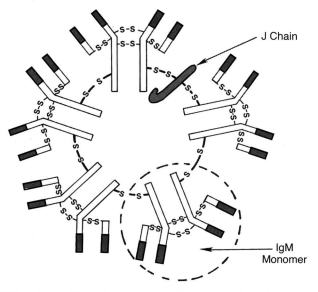

Figure 3-4. Schematic representation of the pentameric configuration of the IgM immunoglobulin.

within the constant regions of the gamma heavy chains designate the various subclasses, and the number of disulfide bonds between the two heavy chains in the hinge region of the molecule constitutes one of the main differences between subclasses. Functional differences between the subclasses include the ability to fix complement and cross the placenta (Table 3–6). IgG blood group antibodies of a single specificity are not necessarily one specific subclass; all four subclasses may be present, or one may predominate. For example, the antibodies to the Rh system antigens are mostly of the IgG_1 and IgG_3 subclasses, whereas anti-K (Kell), and anti-Fy (Duffy) antibodies are usually of the IgG_1 subclass. Anti-Jk (Kidd) antibodies are mainly IgG_3 and may account for the unusual nature of these different antibodies with regard to testing and clinical significance. The purpose for the existence of biological differences in subclass expression is still not completely understood. Especially important in blood banking, severe HDN has been most often associated with IgG_1 antibodies.[5]

Like IgM, IgA exists in two main forms—a monomer and polymer form—as dimers or trimers composed of two or three identical monomers, respectively, joined by a J chain. IgA is located in different parts of the IS, depending on subclass. Serum IgA is found in both monomeric and polymeric forms; however, secretory IgA is usually found in the mucosal tissues of the body. Its polymer form acquires a glycoprotein secretory component as it passes through epithelial cell walls of mucosal tissues and appears in nearly all body fluids. IgA is important in immunohematology, because about 30% of anti-A and anti-B antibodies are of the IgA class (the remaining percentages are IgM and IgG).[6] Also, anti-IgA antibodies can cause severe anaphylaxis if IgA are transfused in plasma products to patients who are deficient in IgA. Another reason for the importance of IgA is that it can increase the effect of IgG-induced RBC hemolysis.[7]

IgE is normally found only in monomeric form in trace concentrations in serum, about 0.004% of total immunoglobulins, and is important in allergic reactions. The Fc portion of the IgE molecule attaches to basophils and mast cells and facilitates histamine release when an allergen binds to the Fab portion of the molecule and cross-links with a second molecule on the cell surface. Histamine is critical for bringing about an allergic reaction. Although hemolytic transfusion reactions are not caused by IgE, urticaria may occur because of the presence of IgE antibodies. Because IgE causes transfusion reactions by release of histamines, patients who have several allergic reactions to blood products can be pretreated with antihistamines to counteract the response when receiving blood products.[2] IgD, present as less than 1% of serum immunoglobulins, appears to have functions that deal primarily with maturation of B cells into plasma cells. IgD is usually bound to the membrane of immature B cells. Therefore, IgD may be necessary for regulatory roles during B-cell differentiation and antibody production but is probably the least significant for blood banking.[8]

Immunoglobulin Variations

There are three main types of antibody-inherited variation: isotype, allotype, and idiotype. **Isotype variation** (or class variation) refers to variants present in all members of a species, including the different heavy and light chains and the different subclasses. All humans have the same Ig classes and subclasses. **Allotypic variation** is present primarily in the constant region; not all variants occur in all members of a species. **Idiotypic variation**, which determines the antigen-binding specificity (or **complementary determining regions**, [CDRs]) of antibodies and T-cell receptors, is found only in the variable (and **hypervariable**) regions and is specific for each antibody molecule.

The allotypes of a growing fetus may cause the maternal IS to become immunized to paternal allotypic determinants on fetal immunoglobulins.[4] Just as alloimmunization can occur during pregnancy, it can occur from transfusions, especially in patients who have received multiple transfusions of blood, plasma, or gamma globulin. Idiotypes can be seen as nonself because they are often present at concentrations too low to induce self-tolerance. Idiotypes are determined by the antigens that react with them and exist in a type of equilibrium with anti-idiotypic antibodies. The presence of antigen disrupts this equilibrium and may be important in controlling an immune response.

Table 3–6	**Biological Properties of IgG Subclasses**			
CHARACTERISTIC	**IgG_1**	**IgG_2**	**IgG_3**	**IgG_4**
Proportion of total serum IgG (%)	65–70	23–28	4–7	3–4
Complement fixation (classic pathway)	++	+	+++	0
Binding to macrophage Fc receptors	+++	++	+++	±
Ability to cross placenta	+	±	+	+
Dominant antibody activities:				
• Anti-Rh	++	0	+	±
• Anti-factor VII	0	0	0	+
• Anti-dextran	0	+	0	0
• Anti-Kell	+	0	0	0
• Anti-Duffy	+	0	0	0
• Anti-platelet	0	0	+	0
Biological half-life (days)	21	21	7–8	21

0 = negative reactivity; ± = weak (or unusual) reactivity; + = slight (or usual) reactivity; ++ = moderate (or more common) reactivity; +++ = strong reactivity.

Immunoglobulin Fc Receptors

Macrophages and monocytes have receptors for the attachment of IgG and can bind the C_H3 domain of the Fc portion.

Only the IgG$_1$ and IgG$_3$ subclasses are capable of attachment to phagocytic receptors. This is one way that incompatible RBCs coated with IgG antibody are removed by phagocytosis. The other phagocytic cells with Fc receptors include neutrophils, NK cells, and mature B cells.[4,9]

Complement System

Basic Concepts

The complement system, or complement, is a complex group of over 20 circulating and cell membrane proteins that have a multitude of functions within the immune response. Primary roles include direct lysis of cells, bacteria, and enveloped viruses as well as assisting with opsonization to facilitate phagocytosis. Another role is production of peptide fragment split products, which play roles in inflammatory responses such as increased vascular permeability, smooth muscle contraction, chemotaxis, migration, and adherence. Complement components circulate in inactive form as proenzymes, with the exception of factor D of the alternate pathway. The complement proteins are activated in a **cascade** of events through three main pathways: the classical, alternative, and lectin pathways. The three pathways converge at the activation of the component C3. The classical pathway is activated by the binding of an antigen with an IgM, IgG$_1$, or IgG$_3$ antibody. The alternative pathway is activated by high molecular weight molecules with repeating units found on the surfaces of target cells. The lectin pathway is activated by attachment of plasma mannose-binding lectin (MBL) to microbes. MBL in turn activates proteins of the classical pathway.

Advanced Concepts

Complement components are sequentially numbered C1 through C9, but this refers to their discovery date, not to their activation sequence. The four unique serum proteins of the alternative pathway are designated by letters: factor B, factor D, factor P (properdin), and IF (initiating factor). Some activation pathways require Ca^{2+} and Mg^{2+} cations as cofactors for certain components. In certain nomenclature, complement components that are active are designated by a short bar placed over the appropriate number or letter. The cleavage products of complement proteins are distinguished from parent molecules by suffixes such as C3a and C3b. The complement system is able to modulate its own reactions by inhibitory proteins such as C1 inhibitor (C1INH), factor H, factor I, C4-binding protein (C4BP), anaphylatoxin inactivator, anaphylatoxin inhibitor, membrane attack complex (MAC) inhibitor, and C3 nephritic factor (NF). This regulation of complement is important so that complement proteins do not destroy healthy host cells and inflammation is controlled. The evaluation of C3b and C3d complement components in transfusion medicine testing procedures is useful in the investigation of hemolytic transfusion reactions and autoimmune hemolytic anemias.

Classical Complement Pathway

The activation of the classical complement pathway is initiated when antibody binds to antigen. This allows the binding of the complement protein C1 to the Fc fragment of an IgM, IgG$_1$, or IgG$_3$ subclass antibody. Complement activation by IgG antibody depends on concentration of cell surface antigen and antigen clustering, in addition to antibody avidity and concentration. IgM is large and has Fc monomers close to each other on one immunoglobulin molecule; therefore, only one IgM molecule is necessary to activate complement. The C1 component is actually a complex composed of three C1 subunits, C1q, C1r, and C1s, which are stabilized by calcium ions. Without calcium present, there is no stabilization of the C1q, r, s complex, and complement is not activated.

In the C1 complex bound to antigen antibody, C1q is responsible for catalyzing the C1r to generate activated C1s. Activated C1s is a serine-type protease. The C1q, r, s complex (actually as a C1q[r, s]$_2$ unit) acts on C2 and C4 to form C4b2a. C4b2a uses component C3 as a natural substrate. By-products that result from the activation of the classical sequence include C3a; C4b, which binds to the cell surface; C4a, which stays in the medium and has modest anaphylatoxin activity; and C3b, which attaches to the microbial surface. Note that complement fragments that have the *b* type are usually bound to membranes, whereas the *a* fragments often have anaphylatoxic activity.

Human RBCs have CR1 receptors for C4d and C3b, and some of the cleavage products will attach to the RBC membrane. Eventually these fragments are further degraded to C4d and C3d through the action of C4BP, factor H (which binds C3b), and factor I (which degrades both C4b and C3b). Some of C3b binds to the C4b2a complex, and the resulting C4b2a3b complex functions as a C5 convertase. The C5 convertase then acts on C5 to produce C5a (a strong stimulator of anaphylatoxins) and C5b, which binds to the cell membrane and recruits C6, C7, C8, and C9 to the cell membrane. When C5b along with C6, C7, C8, and C9 are bound, the membrane attack complex forms; this causes cell lysis. Figure 3–5 shows the sequential activation of the complement system via the classical and alternative pathways. Figure 3–6 illustrates the mechanism of antibody-dependent cell-mediated cytotoxicity (ADCC).

Alternative Complement Pathway

The alternative pathway is older in evolution and allows complement to be activated without acquired immunity. The alternative pathway is activated by surface contacts with complex molecules and artificial surfaces such as dialysis membranes and dextran polymers. There are four important proteins in this pathway: factor D, factor B, properdin, and C3. In this pathway, complement component factor D is analogous to C1s in the classical pathway; factor B is analogous to C2; and the cleavage product C3b is analogous to C4. Also, factor C3bBbP is analogous to C4b2a, and C3b$_2$BbP is analogous to C4b2a3b in the classical pathway. Activation of the alternative pathway requires that a C3b molecule be bound to the surface of a target cell. Small

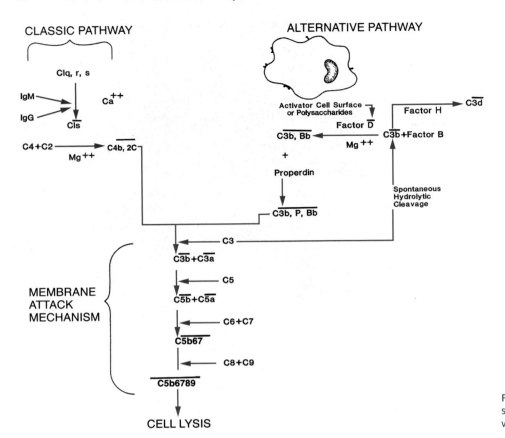

CLASSIC PATHWAY

ALTERNATIVE PATHWAY

MEMBRANE
ATTACK
MECHANISM

CELL LYSIS

Figure 3–5. Schematic diagram illustrating the sequential activation of the complement system via the classical and alternative pathways.

amounts of C3b are generated continuously, owing to the spontaneous hydrolytic cleavage of the C3 molecule. When C3b encounters normal cells, it is rapidly eliminated through the combined interactions of factors H and I. The accumulation of C3b on microbial cell surfaces is associated with attachment of C3b to factor B. The complex of C3b and factor B is then acted on by factor D. As a result of this action, factor B is cleaved, yielding a cleavage product known as Bb. The C3bBb complex is stabilized by the presence of properdin (P), yielding C3bBbP. This complex cleaves C3 into additional C3a and C3b. C3b, therefore, acts as a positive feedback mechanism for driving the alternative pathway. The $C3b_2BbP$ complex acts as a C5 convertase and initiates the later steps of complement activation (see **Fig. 3–5**).

Lectin Complement Pathway

The third pathway of activation, the lectin pathway, is activated by the attachment of MBL to microbes. The subsequent reactions are the same as those of the classical pathway. Remember that all three methods of activation lead to a final common pathway for complement activation and membrane attack complex (MAC) formation.

Membrane Attack Complex

The final step of complement activation is the formation of the MAC, which is composed of the terminal components of the complement sequence. There are two ways in which the MAC is initiated. In either classical or alternative pathways, the formation of C5 convertase is necessary. In the activation of the classical pathway, the MAC is initiated by the enzymatic activity of component C4b2a3b on C5. In the alternative pathway, it is $C3b_2Bb$ that has the ability to cleave C5. The next step in either pathway is the same. Component C5 is split into the fragments C5a (a potent anaphylatoxin) and C5b; the C5b fragment attaches to cell membranes and can continue the complement cascade by initiating the membrane attachment of C6, C7, and C8. After the attachment of C9

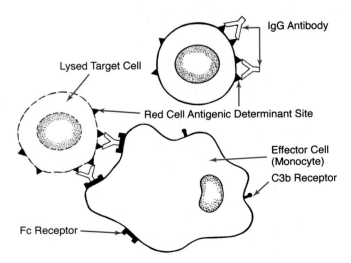

Figure 3–6. Schematic representation of the mechanism of antibody-dependent cell-mediated cytotoxicity (ADCC). Note the role of effector cell surface receptors for the Fc fragment of IgG.

to the C5b678 complex, a small transmembrane channel or pore is formed in the lipid bilayer of the cell membrane, and this allows for osmotic lysis and subsequent death of the cell.

Binding of Complement by RBC Antibodies

Basic Concepts

Disruption in the activation of either complement pathway can result in damage to the host's cells. Transfusion medicine specialists are concerned with the formation of antibodies with complement capacity that can bring about the destruction of RBCs. Recall that in order to initiate activation, C1 molecules bind with two adjacent Ig Fc regions. A pentameric IgM molecule provides two Fc regions side by side, thereby binding complement. A monomeric IgG molecule, on the other hand, binds C1q less efficiently, and two IgG molecules are needed in close proximity to bind complement. For example, as many as 800 IgG anti-A molecules may need to attach to one adult group A RBC to bind a single C1 molecule, so there is little complement activation by IgG anti-A immunoglobulins.[4]

Antibodies against the Rh antigens usually do not bind complement due to the low level of Rh antigens on RBC surfaces. Antibodies to the Lewis blood group system are generally IgM, and they can activate complement but rarely cause hemolytic transfusion reactions due to their low optimal reactivity temperature. Therefore, in blood banking, with the exception of the ABO system, only a few antibodies activate the complement sequence that leads to complement mediated intravascular hemolysis. However, extravascular hemolysis usually occurs as a result of antibody coating of RBCs, and the split products of complement activation can stimulate the reticuloendothelial system and cause anaphylatoxic effects.

Antibody-coated RBCs, either self or nonself, are removed by cells of the mononuclear phagocyte system and by the cells lining the hepatic and splenic sinusoids. These phagocytic cells are able to clear antibody-coated RBCs because they have cell surface receptors for complement CR1 (C3b) and Ig Fc receptors (see **Fig. 3–6**). IgM-coated RBCs are not eliminated through Fc receptor–mediated phagocytosis, but if erythrocytes are coated with IgG and complement, they will be cleared rapidly from circulation by monocytes and macrophages. If RBCs are coated with only C3b, they may not be cleared but only sequestered temporarily.

Characteristics of Antigens

The immune response is initiated by the presentation of an **antigen** (initiates formation of and reacts with an antibody) or **immunogen** (initiates an immune response). The term antigen is more commonly used in blood banking because the primary testing is the detection of antibodies to blood group antigens. The immune reaction to any immunogen, including antigens, is determined by the host response and

by several biochemical and physical characteristics of the immunogen. Properties such as size, complexity, conformation, charge, accessibility, solubility, digestibility, and biochemical composition influence the amount and type of immune response (Box 3–2).

Molecules that are too small cannot stimulate antibody production. Immunogens having a molecular weight (MW) less than 10,000 daltons (D), for example, are called **haptens** and usually do not elicit an immune response on their own; however, coupled with a carrier protein having a MW greater than 10,000 D, they can produce a reaction. Antibodies and cellular responses are very specific for an antigen's physical conformation as opposed to its linear sequence. Overall charge is important, as antibody response is also formed to the net charge of a molecule, whether it is positive, negative, or neutral. Obviously, an antigen must be seen by the IS, and so the accessibility of epitopes influences the immune response. Also, antigenic substances that are less soluble are less likely to elicit an immune response. The biochemical composition of the stimulus plays a role in immune stimulation. Remember that RBC antigens are very diverse in structure and composition and may be proteins (such as the Rh, M, and N blood group substances) or glycolipids (such as the ABH, Lewis, Ii, and P blood group substances). Human leukocyte antigens (HLAs) are glycoproteins. Because of these differences in structure, conformation, and molecular nature, not all blood group substances are equally immunogenic in vivo (Table 3–7).

Characteristics of Blood Group Antibodies

There are many different and important characteristics of blood group antibodies, such as whether they are polyclonal or monoclonal, naturally occurring or immune, and alloantibodies or autoantibodies.

Polyclonal and Monoclonal Antibodies

In laboratory testing, there are two types of antibody (reagent antibodies are called **antisera**) that are available for use; they are manufactured differently and have different properties. An antigen usually consists of numerous epitopes, and it is the epitopes and not the entire antigen that a B cell is

BOX 3–2

Characteristics of Antigens: Properties That Influence Immune Response

- Size
- Complexity
- Conformation
- Charge
- Accessibility
- Solubility
- Digestibility
- Chemical composition

Table 3–7	Relative Immunogenicity of Different Blood Group Antigens	
BLOOD GROUP ANTIGEN	**BLOOD GROUP SYSTEM**	**IMMUNO-GENICITY (%)***
D (Rh$_0$)	Rh	50
K	Kell	5
c (hr')	Rh	2.05
E (rh'')	Rh	1.69
k	Kell	1.50
e (hr'')	Rh	0.56
Fy^a	Duffy	0.23
C (rh')	Rh	0.11
Jk^a	Kidd	0.07
S	MNSs	0.04
Jk^b	Kidd	0.03
s	MNSs	0.03

Adapted from Kaushansky, K, et al: Williams Hematology, 8th ed. McGraw-Hill Professional, New York, 2010.
*Percentage of transfusion recipients lacking the blood group antigen (in the first column) who are likely to be sensitized to a single transfusion of red cells containing that antigen.

stimulated to produce antibody against. Therefore, these different epitopes on a single antigen induce the proliferation of a variety of B-cell clones, resulting in a heterogeneous population of serum antibodies. These antibodies are referred to as **polyclonal** or serum antibodies and are produced in response to a single antigen with more than one epitope.

In vivo, the polyclonal nature of antibodies improves the immune response with respect to quality and quantity. Antibodies against more than one epitope are needed to give immunity against an entire antigen, such as a pathogen. However, this diversity is not optimal in the laboratory, and in vitro reagents produced by animals or humans can give confusing test results. Consistency and reliability are needed in laboratory testing, and polyclonal sera can vary in antibody concentration from person to person and animal to animal. Sera from the same animal can also vary somewhat, depending on the animal's overall condition.

Individual sera also differ in the serologic properties of the antibody molecules they contain, the epitopes they recognize, and the presence of additional nonspecific or cross-reacting antibodies. One way to avoid this problem is to use monoclonal antibodies produced by isolating individual B cells from a polyclonal population and propagating them in cell culture with **hybridoma** technology. The supernatant from the cell culture contains antibody from a single type of B cell, clonally expanded, and therefore has the same variable region and a single epitope specificity. This results in a **monoclonal** antibody suspension. Monoclonal antibodies are preferred in testing because they are highly specific, well characterized, and uniformly reactive. Most reagents used

today are monoclonal in nature or are a blend of monoclonal antisera.

Naturally Occurring and Immune Antibodies

There are two types of antibodies that concern blood banking: one is **naturally occurring** and the other is **immune**. Both are produced in reaction to encountered antigens. RBC antibodies are considered naturally occurring when they are found in the serum of individuals who have never been previously exposed to RBC antigens by transfusion, injection, or pregnancy. These antibodies are probably produced in response to substances in the environment that resemble RBC antigens such as pollen grains and bacteria membranes.

The common occurrence of naturally occurring antibodies suggests that their antigens are widely found in nature and have a repetitive complex pattern. Most naturally occurring antibodies are IgM cold agglutinins, which react best at room temperature or lower, activate complement, and may be hemolytic when active at 37°C. In blood banking, the common naturally occurring antibodies react with antigens of the ABH, Hh, Ii, Lewis, MN, and P blood group systems. Some naturally occurring antibodies found in normal serum are manufactured without a known environmental stimulus.[10] In contrast to natural antibodies, RBC antibodies are considered immune when found in the serum of individuals who have been transfused or who are pregnant. These antigens have a molecular makeup that is unique to human RBCs. Most immune RBC antibodies are IgG antibodies that react best at 37°C and require the use of antihuman globulin sera (Coombs' sera) for detection. The most common immune antibodies encountered in testing include those that react with the Rh, Kell, Duffy, Kidd, and Ss blood group systems.[10]

Unexpected Antibodies

Naturally occurring anti-A and anti-B antibodies are routinely detected in human serum and depend on the blood type of the individual. Blood group A has anti-B; blood group B has anti-A; blood group O has both and anti-A, B. Blood group AB has neither antibody present in their serum. These naturally occurring antibodies, or **isoagglutinins**, are significant and useful in blood typing. They are easily detected by use of A and B reagent RBCs with a direct agglutination technique. In normal, healthy individuals, anti-A and anti-B are generally the only RBC antibodies expected to be found in a serum sample. People with an IS that does not function normally may not have the expected naturally occurring antibodies. All other antibodies directed against RBC antigens are considered unexpected and must be detected and identified before blood can be safely transfused, no matter their reaction strength or profile.

The reactivity of unexpected antibodies is highly varied and unpredictable, as they may be either isotype IgM or IgG; rarely, both may be present in the same sample. These antibodies may be able to hemolyze, agglutinate, or sensitize RBCs. Some antibodies require special reagents to enhance their reactivity and detection, especially if more than one antibody occurs in the sample. Due to the enormous polymorphism of the human population, a diversity of RBC alleles and antigens exist, requiring a variety of standardized immunologic techniques and reagents for their detection and identification.

The in vitro analysis of unexpected antibodies involves the use of antibody screening procedures to optimize antigen-antibody reactions. The majority of these procedures include reacting unknown serum from a donor or patient sample with known reagent cells at various amounts of time, temperature, and media. All routine blood bank testing requires the use of samples for both expected and unexpected antibodies.

Alloantibodies and Autoantibodies

Antibodies can be either alloreactive or autoreactive. Alloantibodies are produced after exposure to genetically different, or nonself, antigens, such as different RBC antigens after transfusion. Transfused components may elicit the formation of alloantibodies against antigens (red cell, white cell, and platelets) not present in the recipient. Autoantibodies are produced in response to self-antigens. They can cause reactions in the recipient if they have a specificity that is common to the transfused blood. Some autoantibodies do not have a detectable specificity.

Autoantibodies can react at different temperatures, and cold or warm autoantibodies may both be present. Patients with autoantibodies frequently have autoimmune diseases and may require considerable numbers of blood products and special techniques to find compatible units. A potentially serious problem for blood bankers is transfused patients who have alloantibodies that are no longer detectable in the patient's plasma or serum. If these individuals are transfused with the immunizing antigen again, they will make a stronger immune response against those RBC antigens, which can cause severe and possibly fatal transfusion reactions. These recipients will then have a positive autocontrol or **direct antiglobulin test** (DAT), which may also be referred to as the **direct Coombs' test**. This is why the previous history of any patient is a critical part of the testing. Autoantibodies can be removed from RBCs by special adsorption and elution techniques and then tested against reagent RBCs. Remember that in order to transfuse blood safely, the identity of antibodies should be determined and recorded.

Characteristics of Antigen-Antibody Reactions

There are many complex properties of antigen and antibody reactions that influence serologic and other testing methods involving antibodies. The antigen-binding site of the antibody molecule is uniquely designed to recognize a corresponding antigen; this antibody amino acid sequence cannot be changed without altering its specificity. The extent of the reciprocal relationship, also called the **fit** between the antigen and its binding site on the antibody, is often referred to as a lock and key mechanism. Factors influencing antigen-antibody reactions include intermolecular binding forces, antibody properties, host factors, and tolerance.

Intermolecular Binding Forces

Intermolecular binding forces such as hydrogen bonding, electrostatic forces, van der Waals forces, and hydrophobic bonds are all involved in antigen-antibody binding reactions. Stronger covalent bonds are not involved in this reaction, although they are important for the intramolecular conformation of the antibody molecule. Hydrogen bonds result from weak dipole forces between hydrogen atoms bonded to oxygen or nitrogen atoms in which there is incomplete transfer of the electronic energy to the more electronegative oxygen or nitrogen. When two atoms with dipoles come close to each other, there is a weak attraction between them. Although hydrogen bonds are singularly weak, many of them together can be strong. They are found in complex molecules throughout the human body.

Electrostatic forces result from weak charges on atoms in molecules that have either a positive or negative overall charge (like charges repel and unlike charges attract). This is seen in the formation of salt bridges. Van der Waals forces are a type of weak interaction between atoms in larger molecules. **Hydrophobic** (water-avoiding) bonds result from the overlap of hydrophobic amino acids in proteins. The hydrophobic amino acids bury themselves together to avoid water and salts in solution. The repulsion of these amino acids to prevent contact with water and aqueous solutions can be very strong collectively.

In addition, there are **hydrophilic** (water-loving) bonds that allow for the overlap of amino acids that are attracted to water. Hydrophobic and hydrophilic bonds repel each other, and these repulsive forces also play a role in the formation of the antigen-antibody bond. All of these bonds affect the total conformation and strength of antigen-antibody reactions and IS molecules.

Antibody Properties

There are many important terms that refer to the properties of antibody reactions. The first is antibody **affinity**; it is often defined as the strength of a single antigen-antibody bond produced by the summation of attractive and repulsive forces. The second term is **avidity**, which is used to express the binding strength of a multivalent antigen with antisera produced in an immunized individual. Avidity, therefore, is a measure of the **functional affinity** of an antiserum for the whole antigen and is sometimes referred to as a combination of affinities. Avidity can be important in blood banking because high-titer, low-avidity antibodies exhibit low antigen-binding capacity but still show reactivity at high serum dilutions.[11]

The **specificity** of an antiserum (or antibody) is one of its most important characteristics and is related to its relative avidity for antigen. Antibody specificity can be further classified as a specific reaction, cross-reaction, or no reaction (Fig. 3–7). A specific reaction implies reaction between similar epitopes. A cross-reaction results when certain epitopes of one antigen are shared by another antigen and the same antibody can react with both antigens. No reaction occurs when there are no shared epitopes.

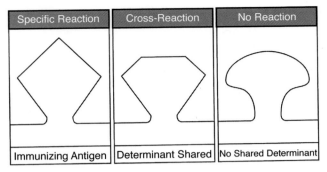

Specific Reaction	Cross-Reaction	No Reaction
Immunizing Antigen	Determinant Shared	No Shared Determinant

Figure 3–7.   Types of antigen-antibody reactions: specific reaction, cross-reaction, and no reaction.

In addition, there is the valency of an antibody, which is the number of antigen-binding sites on an antibody molecule or the number of antibody binding sites on an antigen. Antigens are usually multivalent, but antibodies are usually bivalent. IgM and IgA antibodies can have higher valences due to the multimeric nature of some of their structures. Because the biochemistry controlling the forces of antibody binding are well understood, the influence of these forces can be manipulated by using various reagents and methods to enhance the reactivity of certain RBC antigens with antibodies. When more than one antibody is present in a blood bank sample, it is often necessary to use special techniques to identify all the antibodies. These techniques and reagents were developed with an understanding of antibody reactivity.

Host Factors

Various host factors play a key role in an individual's immune response (Box 3–3). These factors are important in the host's overall immune response and in various specific immune reactions. Each individual's immune system is unique and determines how that individual is able to resist disease. Host factors include nutritional status, hormones, genetic inheritance, age, race, sex, physical activity level, environmental exposure, and the occurrence of disease or injury. It is also believed that immune function decreases as age increases; this may be one reason why so many diseases such as cancer and autoimmune conditions are seen at a later time in life. A decrease in antibody levels in older individuals may result in false-negative reactions, especially in reverse ABO blood typing.

BOX 3–3

Host Factors: Properties of the Host That Influence Immune Response

- Nutritional status
- Hormones
- Genetics
- Age
- Race
- Exercise level
- Disease
- Injury

In some instances, an individual's race may be a factor in susceptibility to certain diseases. A dramatic example of this is seen in malaria infection. The majority of African Americans who do not inherit the Duffy blood system antigens Fy^a or Fy^b are resistant to malarial invasion with *Plasmodium knowlesi* and *Plasmodium vivax*. The absence of these antigens may make these individuals ideal donors for those who have developed Duffy system antibodies. (Refer to Chapter 8, "Blood Group Terminology and the Other Blood Groups.") This illustrates once again the importance of the historical record of the patient or donor.

Tolerance

Advanced Concepts

Tolerance is defined as the lack of an immune response or an active immunosuppressive response. It has been observed post-transfusion for many years, but its mechanism is still unclear. Tolerance can be either naturally occurring or experimentally induced. Exposure to an antigen during fetal life usually produces tolerance to that antigen. An example of this type of tolerance is found in the **chimera**, an individual who receives an in utero cross-transfusion of ABO-incompatible blood from a dizygotic (fraternal) twin.[2] The chimera does not produce antibodies against the A and B antigen of the twin, and the ABO group of such an individual may appear as a testing discrepancy.

The induction of tolerance is used to prevent D-negative mothers from developing anti-D antibodies after delivering Rh-positive infants. When a D-negative woman gives birth to a D-positive infant, she is exposed to D-positive RBCs, most of which occurs during delivery. Approximately 50% to 70% of Rh-negative mothers develop anti-D antibodies on first exposure to D-positive cells. These antibodies can result in HDN upon later pregnancies with a D-positive fetus. Use of passive immunization to prevent the formation of these antibodies can prevent HDN. This is accomplished by administering IgG Rh-immune globulin (RHIG) within 48 to 72 hours after the birth of the infant. About 25% to 30% of D-negative individuals are nonresponders and do not produce anti-D antibodies, even when subjected to repeated exposure to D-positive cells. Because it is not known who will respond, it is recommended that all D-negative mothers who deliver D-positive newborns receive RHIG to prevent immunization.

Detection of RBC Antigen-Antibody Reactions

Basic Concepts

Various factors influence detection of RBC antigen-antibody reactions. These include having a correct sample and the proper reagents performing the correct test and understanding how the test should be done and interpreted.

Blood Samples Required for Testing

One of the most important steps in obtaining the correct and valid results of an analytical or diagnostic test is to have the correct sample. Different tests in the blood bank may require different samples. Some tests require the use of serum to ensure that adequate amounts of viable complement are available for fixation by blood group antibodies. Serum is obtained when no anticoagulant is used in the sample collection tube. The sample clots and is centrifuged to separate the clotted cells and the liquid serum fraction. An anticoagulated sample would not be conducive to complement activation studies, because anticoagulants bind divalent Ca^{2+} and Mg^{2+} ions and inhibit complement activity.

The commonly used anticoagulant ethylenediaminetetraacetic acid (EDTA) at a ratio of 2 mg to 1 mL of serum will totally inhibit complement activation by binding calcium and, to a lesser extent, magnesium. Another anticoagulant, sodium heparin, inhibits the cleavage of C4. These problems can be avoided by using serum instead of plasma for blood bank procedures that require fresh complement. Currently, however, plasma is used routinely in place of serum. Years of testing with both samples have shown that for most tests, plasma is comparable to serum. Plasma samples are preferred for DAT and elution studies because they lack fibrin strands, which can cause false-positives. Serum should be removed as soon as possible from a clotted blood sample. If testing cannot begin immediately, then serum should be removed and stored at 4°C for no longer than 48 hours. After this time, serum should be frozen at –50°C or lower to retain complement activity. The complement system may become activated during storage of preserved RBC products. For example, in citrate phosphate dextrose adenine (CPDA-1)–preserved RBCs, activation of the alternate pathway can be caused by contact of plasma C3 with plastic surfaces of blood bags. This may cause hemolysis that will become visible as the RBCs settle upon storage.[12]

Traditional Laboratory Testing Methods

The various complex immunologic responses that are important to blood banking have been studied by a number of immunologic methods. These in vitro testing methods were developed with an understanding of the biochemistry and biophysics of the IS. Many of the methods used today are modifications of previous blood bank techniques or more generalized immunologic testing methods that have been adapted to the needs of immunohematology laboratories. The routine methods used today have to be highly efficient to meet clinical laboratory requirements.

Advanced Concepts

Many different types of tests are available, and it is important to be familiar with the different purposes of each. In vitro testing for the detection of antigens or antibodies may be accomplished by commonly used techniques, including hemagglutination (a special type of agglutination), precipitation, agglutination inhibition, and hemolysis. Other techniques that quantify antigen or antibody with the use of a radioisotope, enzyme, or fluorescent label—such as radioimmunoassay (RIA), enzyme-linked immunosorbent assay (ELISA) or enzyme immunoassay (EIA), Western blotting (WB), and immunofluorescence (IF)—may be used in automated or semiautomated blood banking instrumentation.[2] These techniques are very important in testing for viral pathogens in donor units and patient samples. Recently, blood bank automated methods for the typing of whole blood units and patient samples have become more popular and may become routine in the near future.

In most transfusion laboratory testing, **hemagglutination** reactions are the major technique used. Hemagglutination methods for the analysis of blood group antigen-antibody responses and typing for ABO, Rh, and other blood group antigens is accomplished by **red cell agglutination** reactions. Agglutination is a straightforward process and can be shown to develop in two stages. In the first stage, *sensitization*, antigen binding to the antibody occurs. Epitopes on the surfaces of RBC membranes combine with the antigen-combining sites (Fab region) on the variable regions of the immunoglobulin heavy and light chains. Antigen and antibody are held together by various noncovalent bonds, and no visible agglutination is seen at this stage.

In the second stage, a **lattice**-type structure composed of multiple antigen-antibody bridges between RBC antigens and antibodies is formed. A network of these bridges forms, and visible agglutination is present during this stage. The development of an insoluble antigen-antibody complex, resulting from the mixing of equivalent amounts of soluble antigen and antibody, is known as a **precipitation reaction**.

Agglutination inhibition is a method in which a positive reaction is the opposite of what is normally observed in agglutination. Agglutination is inhibited when an antigen-antibody reaction has previously occurred in a test system. The antigen and antibody cannot bind because another substrate has been added to the reaction mixture and blocks the formation of the agglutinates. Inhibition reactions are used in **secretory studies** to determine whether soluble ABO substances are present in body fluids and secretions. The secreted substrate can combine with the antibody and block RBC antigen-antibody reactions. People who have blood group antibodies in their body fluids are called **secretors**.

Hemolysis represents a strong positive result and indicates that an antigen-antibody reaction has occurred in which complement has been fixed and RBC lysis occurs. The Lewis blood group antibodies anti-Le^a and anti-Le^b may be regarded as clinically significant if hemolysis occurs in their in vitro testing reactions.

RIA, ELISA (or EIA), WB, and IF techniques are immunologic methods based on detection and quantification of antigen or antibody by the use of a radioisotope, enzyme, or fluorescent labels. Either the antigen or the antibody can be labeled in these tests. These techniques measure the interaction of the binding of antigen with antibody and are extremely sensitive. Most of these techniques employ reagents that use either antigen or antibody, which is bound in a solid or liquid phase in a variety of reaction systems ranging from plastic tubes or plates to microscopic particles or beads. These methods use a separation system and washing steps to isolate bound and free fractions and a detection system to measure the amount of antigen-antibody interaction. The values of unknown samples are then calculated from the values of standards of known concentration.

Factors That Influence Agglutination Reactions

Basic Concepts

Various factors can influence reactivity of antigen-antibody RBC agglutination reactions. Typical of most biochemical reaction systems, agglutination reactions are influenced by the concentration of the reactants (antigen and antibody) and by factors such as pH, temperature, and ionic strength. The surface charge, antibody isotype, RBC antigen dosage, and the use of various enhancement media, antihuman globulin reagents, and enzymes are all important in antigen-antibody reactions. The most important factors are discussed in the following sections.

Centrifugation

Centrifugation is an effective way to enhance agglutination reactions because it decreases reaction time by increasing the gravitational forces on the reactants and bringing reactants closer together. High-speed centrifugation is one of the most efficient methods used in blood banking. Under the right centrifugation conditions, sensitized RBCs overcome their natural repulsive effect (zeta potential) for each other and agglutinate more efficiently. Having RBCs in closer physical proximity allows for an increase in antigen-antibody lattice formation, which results in enhanced agglutination.

Antigen-Antibody Ratio

Antigen and antibody have optimal concentrations; in ideal reactive conditions, an equivalent amount of antigen and antibody binds. Any deviation from this decreases the efficiency of the reaction and a loss of the **zone of equivalence** between antigen and antibody ratio that is necessary for agglutination reactions to occur. An excess of unbound immunoglobulin leads to a **prozone effect**, and a surplus of antigen leads to a **postzone effect** (Fig. 3–8). In either situation, the lattice formation and subsequent agglutination may not occur, which can give false-negative results. If this is suspected, simple steps can be taken to correct it. If the problem is excessive antibody, the plasma or serum may be diluted with the appropriate buffer. The problem of excessive antigen can be solved by increasing the serum-to-cell ratio, which tends to increase the number of antibodies available to bind with each RBC. Therefore, antigen-antibody test systems can be manipulated to overcome the effects of excessive antigen or antibody.

Another reason antigen amount may be altered is due to weak expression of antigen on RBCs (**dosage effect**). Weak expression occurs as a result of the inheritance of genotypes that give rise to heterozygous expression of RBC antigens and resultant weaker phenotypes. For example, M-positive RBCs from an individual having the genotype *MM* (homozygous) have more M antigen sites than M-positive cells from an individual having the *MN* (heterozygous) genotype. In the Kidd system, Jk^a homozygous inheritance has greater RBC antigen expression than Jk^a heterozygous. The same is true for Jk^b homozygous and heterozygous expression. In the Rh system, the C, c, E, and e antigens also show dosage

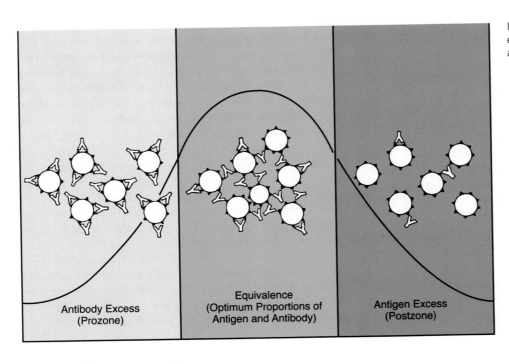

Figure 3–8. Schematic representation of the effects of varying concentrations of antigen and antibody on lattice formation.

Antibody Excess
(Prozone)

Equivalence
(Optimum Proportions of
Antigen and Antibody)

Antigen Excess
(Postzone)

effects. Dosage effect is sometimes used when preparing reagent RBCs for testing.

Effect of pH

The ideal pH of a test system for antigen-antibody reactions ranges between 6.5 and 7.5, which is similar to the pH of normal plasma or serum. Exceptions include some anti-M and some Pr(Sp₁) group antibodies that show stronger reactivity below pH 6.5.[13] Acidification of the test serum may aid in distinguishing anti-M and anti-Pr(Sp₁) antibodies from other antibodies.

Temperature

Different isotypes of antibodies may exhibit optimal reactivity at different temperatures. IgM antibodies usually react optimally at ambient temperatures or below 22°C at the **immediate spin (IS) phase** of testing, whereas IgG antibodies usually require 37°C incubation and react optimally at the **antihuman globulin (AHG) phase** of testing. Because clinically significant antibodies may be in both these temperature ranges, it is important to do testing with a range of temperatures (Fig. 3–9).

Immunoglobulin Type

Examples of IgM antibodies that have importance in blood banking include those against the ABH, Ii, MN, Lewis (Le^a, Le^b), Lutheran (Lu^a), and P blood group antigens. Important IgG antibodies are those directed against Ss, Kell (Kk, Js^a, Js^b, Kp^a, Kp^b), Rh (DCEce), Lutheran (Lu^b), Duffy (Fy^a, Fy^b), and Kidd (Jk^a, Jk^b) antigens (see **Fig. 3–8**). IgM antibodies are generally capable of agglutinating RBCs suspended in a 0.85% to 0.90% saline medium. The IgM antibody is 160 Å larger than an IgG molecule and approximately 750 times as efficient as IgG in agglutination reactions. This allows it to easily bridge the distance between two RBCs.[13]

Another factor that contributes to the difference in reactivity between the IgM and IgG molecules is the number of antigen-combining sites on each type of immunoglobulin. The IgM molecule has the potential to bind 10 separate antigen sites; however, an IgG molecule has only 2 binding sites per molecule, which implies that an IgG molecule would have to bind 2 RBCs with only 1 binding site on each cell.[13] IgM molecules rarely bind 10 sites, owing to the size and spacing of antigens in relation to the size and configuration of the IgM molecule. Typically, when the IgM molecule attaches to two RBCs, probably 2 or 3 antigen-combining sites attach to each RBC. Agglutination reactions involve more than one immunoglobulin molecule, and these conditions are multiplied many times in order to represent the agglutination reaction. Because of the basic differences in the nature of reactivity between IgM and IgG antibodies, different serologic systems must be used to optimally detect both classes of clinically significant antibodies. An overview of the serologic methods traditionally used for antibody detection in the blood bank laboratory is outlined in Table 3–8.

Enhancement Media

Agglutination reactions for IgM antibodies and their corresponding RBC antigens are easily accomplished in saline medium, as these antibodies usually do not need enhancement or modifications to react strongly with antigens. However, detection of IgM antibodies may not have the same clinical significance as the detection of most IgG antibodies, because IgG antibodies react best at 37°C and are generally responsible for hemolytic transfusion reactions and HDN. To discover the presence of IgG antibodies, there are many enhancement techniques or potentiators available (Table 3–9).

One of the key ways to enhance the detection of IgG antibodies is to increase their reactivity. Many of the commercially available enhancement media accomplish this by reducing the *zeta potential* of RBC membranes. The net negative charge surrounding RBCs (and most other human cells) in a cationic media is part of the force that repels RBCs from each other and is due to sialic acid molecules on the surface of RBCs. Most acids have a negative charge, and the large concentration of these molecules on RBCs creates a "zone" of negative charge around the RBC. This zone is protective and keeps RBCs from adhering to each other in the peripheral blood. A potential is created because of the ionic cloud of cations (positively charged ions) that are attracted to the zone of negative charges on the RBC membrane (Fig. 3–10).[13] This potential around the RBC is called the *zeta potential* and is an expression of the difference in electrostatic charges at the RBC surface and the surrounding cations. IgM and IgG antibodies have differences in how they react to the same zeta potential. Reducing the zeta potential allows the more positively charged antibodies to get closer to the negatively charged RBCs and therefore increases RBC agglutination by IgG molecules.

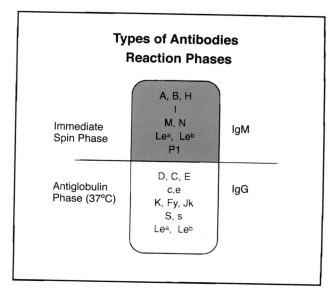

Figure 3–9. Types of antibodies and reaction phases. *(From Kutt, SM, Larison, PJ, and Kessler, LA: Solving Antibody Problems, Special Techniques. Ortho Diagnostic Systems, Raritan, NJ, 1992, p 10, with permission.)*

Table 3–8	**Serologic Systems Used in Traditional Laboratory Methods for Red Cell Antibody Detection**			
REACTION PHASE	**Ig CLASS COMMONLY DETECTED**	**PURPOSE AND MECHANISM OF REACTION**	**TESTS THAT USE SEROLOGIC SYSTEM**	**TYPE OF ANTIBODIES COMMONLY DETECTED**
Immediate spin	IgM	IgM antibodies react best at cold temperatures.	ABO reverse testing	Expected ABO alloantibodies
		IgM is an agglutinating antibody that has the ability to easily bridge the distance between red cells.	Cross-match	Unexpected cold-reacting alloantibodies or autoantibodies
37°C incubation	IgG	IgG antibodies react best at warm temperatures.	Antibody screening/identification	
			Autocontrol	
			Antibody screening/identification	
		No visible agglutination commonly seen.	Cross-match (if needed)	
		IgG is sensitizing antibody with fewer antigen binding sites than IgM and cannot undergo the second stage of agglutination, lattice formation.	Autocontrol	
		Complement may be bound during reactivity, which may or may not result in visible hemolysis.		
Antiglobulin test	IgG	Antihuman globulin (AHG) has specificity for the Fc portion of the heavy chain of the human IgG molecule or complement components.	Antibody screening/identification	Unexpected warm-reacting alloantibodies or autoantibodies
			Cross-match (if needed)	
			Autocontrol	
		AHG acts as a bridge cross-linking red cells sensitized with IgG antibody or complement.	Direct antiglobulin test (DAT)	

Protein Media

Colloidal substances, or **colloids**, are a type of clear solution that contains particles permanently suspended in solution. Colloidal particles are usually large moieties like proteins as compared with the more familiar **crystalloids**, which usually have small, highly soluble molecules, such as glucose, that are easily dialyzed. The colloidal solutes can be charged or neutral and go into solution because of their microscopic size. There are several colloidal solutions currently utilized in blood bank testing, and they are all used to enhance agglutination reactions. Colloids include albumin, polyethylene glycol (PEG), polybrene, polyvinylpyrrolidone (PVP), and protamine. These substances work by increasing the **dielectric constant** (a measure of electrical conductivity), which then reduces the zeta potential of the RBC.

Low Ionic Strength Solution Media

Low ionic strength solutions (LISS), or low salt media, generally contain 0.2% sodium chloride. They decrease the ionic strength of a reaction medium, which reduces the zeta potential and therefore allows antibodies to react more efficiently with RBC membrane antigens. LISS media are

Table 3–9	**Potentiators**		
REAGENT	**ACTION**	**PROCEDURE**	**TYPE OF ANTIBODY ID**
			Primarily IgM; IgG if incubated at 37°C
AHG	Cross-links sensitized cells, resulting in visible agglutination	1. DAT: AHG added directly to washed RBCs	1. Polyspecific; anti-IgG + anticomplement
		2. IAT: serum + screen cells; incubation at 37°C for time determined by additive used; cell washing before addition of AHG	2. IgG monospecific: anti-IgG only
22% albumin*	Causes agglutination by adjusting zeta potential between RBCs	Incubation at 37°C for 15–60 min; cell washing prior to indirect antiglobulin test (IAT)	IgG
LISS*	Low ionic strength environment causes RBCs to take up antibody more rapidly	Incubation at 37°C for 5–15 min; cell washing before IAT	IgG
PEG*	Increases test sensitivity;	Incubation at 37°C for 10–30 min; cell washing before IAT	IgG
	aggregates RBCs causing closer proximity of RBCs to one another, assisting in antibody cross-linking	NOTE: The test mixture cannot be centrifuged and examined reliably for direct agglutination after 37°C incubation.	
Enzymes	Reduces RBC surface charge; destroys or depresses some RBC antigens; enhances other RBC antigens	1. One step: enzymes added directly to serum/RBC mixture	Destroys Fy^a, Fy^b, MNS; enhances reactivity to Rh, Kidd, P_1, Lewis, and I antibodies
		2. Two step: RBC pretreated with enzymes before addition of serum	

*All additives should be added after the IS phase immediately before 37°C incubation
LISS = low ionic strength solutions; PEG = polyethylene glycol

often used because they result in an increased rate of antibody uptake during sensitization and a decreased reaction incubation time (from 30 to 60 minutes to 5 to 15 minutes as compared with protein potentiators such as albumin).[13,14] However, they can result in false-positive reactions and may require testing to be repeated with albumin.

Polyethylene Glycol and Polybrene

Advanced Concepts

PEG and **polybrene** are macromolecule additives used with LISS to bring sensitized RBCs closer to each other to facilitate antibody cross-linking and agglutination reactions. They are often used in place of albumin and have some advantages and possible drawbacks. Polybrene can detect ABO incompatibility and clinically significant IgG

alloantibodies, whereas PEG produces very specific reactions with reduction in false-positive or nonspecific reactions. PEG is considered to be more effective than albumin, LISS, or polybrene for detection of weak antibodies. These reagents have been used in automated and manual testing systems.

Proteolytic Enzymes

Enzymes are protein molecules that function by altering reaction conditions and bringing about changes in other molecules without being changed themselves. Only a small part of a large enzyme molecule reacts with a small part of another molecule, called its substrate. They are specific for the molecules they target and can modify proteins, nucleic acids, carbohydrates, or lipids. Proteolytic enzymes target protein molecules. Certain enzymes have been found to modify various blood group antigens and are useful in testing,

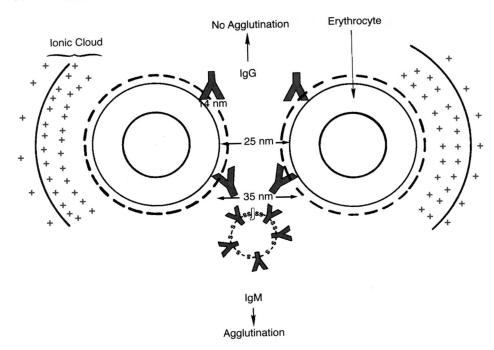

Figure 3–10. Schematic representation of the ionic cloud concept and its relevance to hemagglutination induced by IgM and IgG antibodies. Compare the size of the IgG antibody with that of the IgM molecule. The size of the IgG molecule is not large enough to span the distance between two adjacent RBCs.

especially in cases in which there are multiple antibodies present in a sample.

Enzymes used in the detection and identification of blood group antibodies include **ficin** (isolated from fig plants), papain (from papaya), **trypsin** (from pig stomach), and **bromelin** (from pineapple). It is thought that treating RBCs with enzymes results in the release of sialic acid from the membrane with a subsequent decrease in the negative charges and zeta potential of the RBCs. It has also been suggested that enzyme treatment removes hydrophilic glycoproteins from the membrane of RBCs, causing the membrane to become more hydrophobic, which would allow RBCs to come closer together. Also, because of the removal of glycoproteins from the membrane, antibody molecules may no longer be subject to steric hindrance from reacting with RBC antigens. The use of enzymes provides enhanced antibody reactivity to Rh, Kidd, P_1, Lewis, and I antigens and destroys or decreases reactivity to Fy^a, Fy^b, M, N, and S antigens.[14]

Antihuman Globulin Reagents

Basic Concepts

When RBCs become coated with antibody or complement or both but do not agglutinate in regular testing, special reagents are needed to produce agglutination. The direct antihuman globulin (AHG) test is designed to determine if RBCs are coated with antibody or complement or both. **Polyspecific AHG** can determine if RBCs have been sensitized with IgG antibody or complement (components C3b or C3d) or both. **Monospecific AHG** reagents react only with RBCs sensitized with IgG or complement.[14] Refer to Chapter 5, "The Antiglobulin Test."

Blood bank reagents can be either *polyclonal* or *monoclonal* in source. In the indirect antiglobulin test, the same AHG reagents are used to detect antibodies or complement that have attached to RBC membranes but with a prior incubation step with serum (or plasma). If the antibodies present in serum cannot cause RBC agglutination but only sensitize the RBCs, then the AHG reagents will allow for agglutination to occur by cross-linking the antibodies on the RBCs. The use of AHG reagents allows blood bank testing to be more sensitive. AHG is one of the most important reagents, and the development of AHG is one of the milestones in blood bank testing (see **Tables 3–8** and **3–9**).

Chemical Reduction of IgG and IgM Molecules

Advanced Concepts

There are special reagents available that can be used to help identify the different antibodies present in a mixture of alloantibodies or alloantibodies occurring with autoantibodies. The reagents generally act on covalent sulfhydryl bonds and facilitate antibody identification by removal of either IgG or IgM antibodies. Dithiothreitol (DTT) and β-2-mercaptoethanol (2-ME) are thiol-reducing agents that break the disulfide bonds of the J (joining) chain of the IgM molecule but leave the IgG molecule intact.[10] Another reagent, **ZZAP**, which consists of a thiol reagent plus a proteolytic enzyme, causes the dissociation of IgG molecules from the surface of sensitized RBCs and alters the surface antigens of the RBC.[2] Chemical reduction of the disulfide bond of the IgG molecule is also used to produce chemically modified reagents that react with RBCs in saline. Sulfhydryl compounds reduce the strong but less flexible covalent disulfide bonds in the hinge region of the IgG molecule, allowing the Fab portions more flexibility in facilitating agglutination reactions.[13]

Monoclonal Versus Polyclonal Reagents

Basic Concepts

Traditional polyclonal antisera reagents have been produced by immunizing donors with small amounts of RBCs positive for an antigen that they lack and then collecting the serum and isolating antibodies against that antigen. AHG reagents were originally made by injecting animals (usually rabbits) with human globulin components and then collecting the antihuman antibodies. One antigen can have a number of different epitopes, and polyclonal reagents are directed against multiple epitopes found on the original antigen used to stimulate antibody production. (Refer to Chapter 5.)

Monoclonal reagents are directed against specific epitopes and therefore are a potential solution. They are made by hybridoma technology with spleen lymphocytes from immunized mice that are fused with rapidly proliferating myeloma cells. The spleen lymphocytes have single epitope specificity; the myeloma cells (a type of immortalized, cultured cell) make vast amounts of antibody. After extensive screening and testing, these very efficient hybrid cells are selected and cultured to produce lines of immortal cell clones that make a lot of one type of antibody that reacts with one specific epitope. Monoclonal reagents do not use human donors and therefore do not use a human source for reagent purposes.

Monoclonal reagents have several important advantages over polyclonal reagents. Because monoclonal reagents are produced from immortal clones maintained in vitro, no batch variation exists, and nearly unlimited high titers of antibodies can be produced. Also, the immortal clones can be kept growing in in vitro culture for years without loss of production and are therefore cost-efficient. Monoclonal antibodies react very specifically and often have higher affinities. For these reasons, monoclonal reagents are not subject to cross-reactivity and interference from nonspecific reactions, and they can react strongly with the small quantities of antigen in some antigen subgroups; therefore, AHG phase testing may not be needed.

Unfortunately, there are some disadvantages of monoclonal antisera use, such as **overspecificity**. The fact that complement may not be fixed in the antigen-antibody reaction may cause false-negative results; problems with **oversensitivity** may cause false-positive results. Some of the disadvantages of monoclonal reagents may be overcome by using blends of different monoclonal reagents or by using polyclonal reagents and monoclonal reagents together.[2] Monoclonal antisera have generally replaced most of the polyclonal antisera and have been used for HLA typing, AHG testing, and RBC and lymphocyte phenotyping.

Nontraditional Laboratory Methods

Advanced Concepts

Sophisticated testing methods used in immunology research laboratories have become more commonplace in transfusion laboratories. These technologies are discussed in more detail in Chapter 12, "Other Technologies and Automation."

Flow Cytometry

Some of the most important techniques to study immunologic reactions and systems are fluorescence-assisted cell sorting (FACS) and flow cytometry. Flow cytometry makes use of antibodies that are tagged with a fluorescent dye. Fluorescence occurs when the compound absorbs light energy of one wavelength and emits light of a different wavelength. Cells that are coated with fluorescent-labeled antibody emit a brightly fluorescent color of a specific wavelength. Fluorescent dyes are used as markers in immunologic reactions, and a fluorochrome-labeled antibody can be visualized by an instrument that detects emitted light. There are many different fluorochromes available that have various colors, and they can be coupled to nearly any antibody with minimal problems with spectral overlap.

Flow cytometry can be used to obtain quantitative and qualitative data on cell populations and to sort different cell populations. There are direct and indirect procedures for labeling with fluorochromes. In a direct procedure, the specific antibody, called the *primary antibody*, is directly conjugated with a fluorescent dye and reacts with a specific antigen. Indirect procedures need a secondary antibody that is conjugated to a fluorochrome that reacts with an unlabeled specific primary antibody that has reacted with antigen. Indirect methods often require more complex analysis because these reactions have higher amounts of nonspecificity. The secondary antibody is usually made against the species of the primary antibody.

The principle of flow cytometry is based on the scattering of light as cells are bathed in a fluid stream through which a laser beam enters. The cells move into a chamber one at a time and absorb light from the laser. If labeled antibody is bound to the cell, then the light emitted is different from light emitted by cells without antibody. The flow cytometer instrument makes the distinction between different wavelengths of light. The light signal is amplified and analyzed. There are a number of components to the flow cytometry system that include: one or more lasers for cell illumination, photodetectors for signal detection, a possible cell sorting device, and a computer to manage the data.[15] Fluorescence is used in place of hemagglutination as the endpoint of the reaction. Immunofluorescent antibodies and flow cytometry have been used to quantify fetomaternal hemorrhage, identify transfused cells and follow their survival in recipients, measure low levels of cell-bound IgG, and distinguish homozygous from heterozygous expression of blood group antigens.[2]

Diseases Important in Blood Bank Serologic Testing

Advanced Concepts

A number of diseases that are immune-mediated are important in blood bank testing and merit a brief mention here. For further detail, please refer to the appropriate chapter in this textbook. However, some of these will be discussed within the context of this chapter to emphasize their importance in blood testing.

Immunodeficiency

Immunodeficiency diseases can result from various defects at many different levels of immune function and may be congenital or acquired. They can result from defects in either innate or adaptive immunity or both; the cause is often not known. Some of the more well-known immunodeficiencies are listed in Box 3–4.[16] Immunodeficiencies can influence blood bank test results and transfusion decisions, such as when there is a false-negative reverse grouping for ABO due to low immunoglobulin levels.

Hypersensitivity

Hypersensitivity (or allergy) is an inflammatory response to a foreign antigen and can be cell- or antibody-mediated or both. There are four different types of hypersensitive reactions, and the symptoms and treatment required for each are different. All four types can be caused by blood product transfusions and may be the first sign of a transfusion reaction. Type I reaction, also called *anaphylaxis* or *immediate* hypersensitivity, involves histamine release by mast cells or basophils with surface IgE antibody. It can occur in IgA-deficient individuals who receive plasma products containing IgA. *Urticarial* reactions (skin rashes) may also result from transfusion of certain food allergens or drugs in plasma products. A type II reaction can involve IgG or IgM antibody with complement, phagocytes, and proteolytic enzymes. HDN or transfusion reactions caused by blood group antibodies and autoimmune hemolytic reactions are all type II reactions.

Like type II reactions, type III reactions involve phagocytes and IgG and IgM and complement. Type III reactions result in tissue damage from the formation of immune complexes of antigen-antibody aggregates, complement, and phagocytes and are therefore very serious. Penicillin and

---

BOX 3–4

Classification of Immunodeficiency Disorders

Antibody (B Cell) Immunodeficiency Disorders

- X-linked hypogammaglobulinemia (congenital hypogammaglobulinemia)
- Transient hypogammaglobulinemia of infancy
- Common, variable, unclassifiable immunodeficiency (acquired by hypogammaglobulinemia)
- Immunodeficiency with hyper-IgM
- Selective IgA deficiency
- Selective IgM deficiency
- Selective deficiency of IgG subclasses
- Secondary B-cell immunodeficiency associated with drugs, protein-losing states
- X-linked lymphoproliferative disease

Cellular (T Cell) Immunodeficiency Disorders

- Congenital thymic aplasia (DiGeorge syndrome)
- Chronic mucocutaneous candidiasis (with or without endocrinopathy)
- T-cell deficiency associated with purine nucleoside phosphorylase deficiency
- T-cell deficiency associated with absent membrane glycoprotein
- T-cell deficiency associated with absent class I or II MHC antigens or both (base lymphocyte syndrome)

Combined Antibody-Mediated (B Cell) and Cell-Mediated (T Cell) Immunodeficiency Disorders

- Severe combined immunodeficiency disease (autosomal recessive, X-linked, sporadic)

- Cellular immunodeficiency with abnormal immunoglobulin synthesis (Nezelof syndrome)
- Immunodeficiency with ataxia-telangiectasia
- Immunodeficiency with eczema and thrombocytopenia (Wiskott-Aldrich syndrome)
- Immunodeficiency with thymoma
- Immunodeficiency with short-limbed dwarfism
- Immunodeficiency with adenosine deaminase deficiency
- Immunodeficiency with nucleoside phosphorylase deficiency
- Biotin-dependent multiple carboxylase deficiency
- Graft-versus-host disease
- Acquired immunodeficiency syndrome (AIDS)

Phagocytic Dysfunction

- Chronic granulomatous disease
- Glucose-6-phosphate dehydrogenase deficiency
- Myeloperoxidase deficiency
- Chediak-Higashi syndrome
- Job's syndrome
- Tuftsin deficiency
- Lazy leukocyte syndrome
- Elevated IgE, defective chemotaxis, and recurrent infections

other drug-induced antibodies can lead to hemolytic reactions through type III hypersensitivity. The type IV reaction involves only T cell–mediated responses and their cytokines and can be fatal if untreated. The most important type IV reaction is *graft-versus-host*, of which there is also more than one type. Immunocompromised and immunosuppressed patients must receive irradiated blood products so that T lymphocytes do not engraft and attack the host tissues. Type IV reactions are a problem for bone marrow transplant and stem cell transfusion recipients. (Refer to Chapter 16, "Adverse Effects of Blood Transfusion.")

Monoclonal and Polyclonal Gammopathies

Plasma cell neoplasms result in proliferation of abnormal immunoglobulin from either a single B-cell clone (monoclonal gammopathies) or multiple clones (in polyclonal gammopathies) and may be a specific isotype or only light or heavy chain molecules. Increased serum viscosity is a result of these diseases and can interfere with testing. The increased concentrations of serum proteins can cause nonspecific aggregation (as opposed to agglutination) of erythrocytes called **rouleaux**, which is seen as a stacking of RBCs. It often occurs in multiple-myeloma patients. If rouleaux is suspected, saline replacement technique may be needed to distinguish true cell agglutination from nonspecific aggregation. Roleaux primarily causes problems in the ABO reverse grouping, antibody screening, and compatibility testing procedures. However, excess immunoglobulin coating red cells can cause spontaneous aggregation to occur also.

Autoimmune Disease

Autoantibodies are produced against the host's own cells and tissues. It is unknown why this loss of tolerance to self-antigens occurs, but there are many possible explanations such as aberrant antigen presentation, failure to obtain clonal deletion, anti-idiotypic network breakdown, and cross-reactivity between self and nonself antigens. Autoimmune hemolytic anemias are an important problem in testing and transfusion. They may produce antibodies that cause RBC destruction and anemia and result in antibody- or complement-sensitized RBCs. The direct antiglobulin test should be done to detect sensitized RBCs and determine if the cells are coated with antibody or complement. Special procedures such as elution or chemical treatment to remove antibody from cells may be required to prepare RBCs for antigen typing. Serum autoantibodies may interfere with testing for clinically significant alloantibodies. Special reagents and procedures to denature immunoglobulins may be required to remove autoantibodies from serum so they do not interfere with the testing. (Refer to Chapter 20, "Autoimmune Hemolytic Anemias.")

Hemolytic Disease of the Newborn

Hemolytic disease of the fetus and newborn (HDFN) can result when the maternal IS produces an antibody directed at an antigen present on fetal cells but absent from maternal cells. The mother is exposed to fetal RBCs as a result of fetomaternal transfer of cells during pregnancy or childbirth. Maternal memory cells can cause a stronger response during a second pregnancy if the fetus is positive for the sensitizing antigens. IgG_1, IgG_3, and IgG_4 are capable of crossing the placenta and attaching to fetal RBCs, whereas IgG_2 and IgM are not. Severe HDFN is most often associated with IgG_1 antibodies and may require exchange transfusion. Antigens of the ABO, Rh, and other blood group systems such as Kell have been shown to cause HDFN. (Refer to Chapter 19, "Hemolytic Disease of the Fetus and Newborn [HDFN].")

Blood Product Transfusions and the Immune System

The immune system may undergo transient depression following the administration of blood and blood products. This is referred to as transfusion-related immunomodulation (TRIM). With a weakened immune system, there is an increased risk of an individual developing infections or cancer. The exact mechanism(s) causing TRIM are not known and have not been fully elucidated, but three major mechanisms seem to have emerged: clonal deletion, induction of anergy, and immune suppression. In clonal deletion, alloreactive lymphocytes are inactivated and removed, thus preventing a potential graft rejection (as in kidney organ). With induction of anergy, there is an unresponsiveness of the immune system most likely due to a failure of T cells to respond. In immune suppression, responding cells appear to be inhibited by some sort of cellular mechanism or cytokine.

Immune suppression can be due to a number of factors. Certain cytokines, including interleukins and some growth factors, can decrease immune responsiveness. Suppression of some IS components is critical at certain times, so the IS does not become overactivated and attack host cells. T and B cells that recognize host cells and might destroy them must be removed before they can develop into mature lymphocytes. Specific suppressor cells have recently been isolated. They have unique CD profiles and play a role in modulating lymphocyte function. Immune suppression can also occur when there is too little immunoglobulin made or when too many T and B cells are lost through severe infection, extreme immune stimulation, or IS organ failure.

It is believed that some constituents of cellular blood products may be responsible for TRIM. These constituents include allogeneic mononuclear cells, chemicals released by allogenic mononuclear cells as they age, and soluble HLA peptides I that circulate in plasma. Any decision to transfuse blood products must be approached with caution. Obviously, the best way to avoid TRIM is not to transfuse at all. If transfusion is required, the patient's immune status must be taken into consideration. The use of leukoreduction filters may help to reduce the risk for TRIM. (Refer to Chapter 15, "Transfusion Therapy.")

- ✔ The immune system interacts with other host systems and maintains the host equilibrium. The two major roles for the IS are:
  - Protection from pathogens and foreign substances
  - Removal of abnormal and damaged host cells
- ✔ The two major branches of the IS are:
  - Innate, or natural—the nonspecific primitive IS
  - Acquired, or adaptive—the specific, evolved IS
- ✔ The two major arms of the acquired IS are:
  - Humoral, mediated by B cells and antibody production
  - Cellular, mediated by T cells and lymphokines
- ✔ The basic mechanisms used by the IS are:
  - Recognition of self and nonself organisms, cells, and tissues
  - Removal of unwanted organisms, cells, and tissues (self or nonself)
  - Repair of damaged host tissues
- ✔ The acquired IS demonstrates diversity and uniqueness:
  - Individual B and T cells have vast arrays of unique membrane molecules that can have configurations to match nearly any antigen in the environment.
  - Each individual lymphocyte has one unique receptor per cell that recognizes one epitope.
  - Antibodies and T-cell receptors recognize and react only with the antigen that matches and fits their specific configuration.
  - Selected T and B cells can remain dormant and later respond more rigorously upon second exposure of a previously recognized antigen.
- ✔ The acquired IS demonstrates tolerance: this indicates that immune responses against the host are either removed or downregulated.
- ✔ There are three types of lymphocytes: T cells, B cells, and NK cells.
- ✔ T cells (or lymphocytes) have the TCR, which is usually associated with the CD3 complex, and T cells require APCs to respond to antigens.
- ✔ There are two well-characterized subpopulations of T cells distinguished by CD markers—T helper (T$_H$, CD4-positive) and T cytotoxic (Tc, CD8-positive) lymphocytes.
- ✔ T$_H$ lymphocytes have CD4 markers on their cell membranes, provide B-cell help to stimulate the immune response, release lymphokines when stimulated, and recognize antigens in association with MHC class II molecules.
- ✔ Tc lymphocytes have the CD8 marker on their membranes and can eliminate specific target cells without the help of antibody (cytotoxicity).
- ✔ B lymphocytes (or cells) make up about 5% to 15% of circulating lymphocytes and are characterized by their membrane-bound antibodies (or immunoglobulins)

- ✔ Membrane-bound antibodies are manufactured by B cells and inserted into their cell membranes, where they act as antigen receptors.
- ✔ Stimulated B cells differentiate into plasma cells to secrete humoral immunoglobulin; B cells receive T-cell help for antibody production and for immunologic memory; a single B cell clone manufactures Ig of a single specificity for a specific antigen for its entire cell lifetime.
- ✔ The primary, or original, immune response occurs after the first exposure to an antigen. The secondary, or anamnestic, immune response happens after a second exposure with the same specific antigen.
- ✔ Complement consists of a large group of different enzymatic proteins (convertases/esterases) that circulate in an inactive proenzyme form. Once the cascade is started, they activate each other in a sequence to form products that are involved in optimizing phagocytosis and cell lysis.
- ✔ Complement can be activated through three pathways:
  - The *classical* pathway is initiated by antigen-antibody complexes and requires C1q for activation to proceed.
  - The *alternative* pathway is activated by certain macromolecules on the cell walls of bacteria, fungi, parasites, and tumor cells and requires C3b, serum factors B, D, properdin, and initiating factor.
  - The *lectin* pathway is activated by binding of MBL to microbes.
- ✔ All three pathways meet at a common point in the cascade and result in the formation of the membrane attack complex to remove unwanted cells.
- ✔ There are five classes (or isotypes) of immunoglobulins, all of which have a basic four-chain protein structure consisting of two identical light chains and two identical heavy chains. Disulfide (covalent) bonds link each light chain to a heavy chain and link the two heavy chains to each other.
- ✔ Antibody molecules are isotypic (based on heavy chain subtype), allotypic (based on one heavy chain mutation), or idiotypic (based on hypervariable and variable regions of light and heavy chains) and are reflected in the Ig sequences.
- ✔ Blood group antibodies may be characterized by such factors as epitope and variable region diversity (monoclonal or polyclonal), mode of sensitization (naturally occurring or immune), expected or unexpected presence in routine serum samples, isotype class (IgM, IgG, or, rarely, IgA), activity (warm or cold reactive or both, agglutinating or sensitizing), clinical significance, alloantibody or autoantibody specificity, serum titer, and chemical reactivity (influence of enzymes, sensitivity to pH, DTT, or 2-ME reagents).

Review Questions

1. Which of the following is not involved in the acquired or adaptive immune response?
   a. Phagocytosis
   b. Production of antibody or complement
   c. Induction of immunologic memory
   d. Accelerated immune response upon subsequent exposure to antigen

2. Which cells are involved in the production of antibodies?
   a. Dendritic cells
   b. T lymphocytes
   c. B lymphocytes
   d. Macrophages

3. Which of the following cells is involved in antigen recognition following phagocytosis?
   a. B lymphocytes
   b. T lymphocytes
   c. Macrophages
   d. Granulocytes

4. The role of the macrophage during an antibody response is to:
   a. Make antibody
   b. Lyse virus-infected target cells
   c. Activate cytotoxic T cells
   d. Process antigen and present it

5. Which of the following immunoglobulins is produced in the primary immune response?
   a. IgA
   b. IgE
   c. IgG
   d. IgM

6. Which of the following immunoglobulins is produced in the secondary immune response?
   a. IgA
   b. IgE
   c. IgG
   d. IgM

7. Which of the following MHC classes are found on antigen presenting cells?
   a. Class I
   b. Class II
   c. Class III
   d. Class IV

8. Which of the following MHC classes encodes complement components?
   a. Class I
   b. Class II
   c. Class III
   d. Class IV

9. Which of the following immunoglobulins is most efficient at binding complement?
   a. IgA
   b. IgE
   c. IgG
   d. IgM

10. Which portion of the immunoglobulin molecules contains complement binding sites?
    a. Heavy chain variable region
    b. Light chain variable region
    c. Heavy chain constant region
    d. Light chain constant region

11. Which complement pathway is activated by the formation of antigen-antibody complexes?
    a. Classical
    b. Alternative
    c. Lectin
    d. Retro

12. Which of the following is known as the "recognition unit" in the classical complement pathway?
    a. C1q
    b. C3a
    c. C4
    d. C5

13. Which of the following is known as the "membrane attack complex" in the classical complement pathway?
    a. C1
    b. C3
    c. C4, C2, C3
    d. C5b, C6, C7, C8, C9

14. Which of the following immunoglobulin classes is capable of crossing the placenta and causing hemolytic disease of the newborn?
    a. IgA
    b. IgE
    c. IgG
    d. IgM

15. Which of the following refers to the effect of an excess amount of antigen present in a test system?
    a. Postzone
    b. Prozone
    c. Zone of equivalence
    d. Endzone

16. Which of the following refers to the presence of an excess amount of antibody present in a test system?
    a. Postzone
    b. Prozone
    c. Zone of equivalence
    d. Endzone

17. Which of the following refers to a state of equilibrium in antigen-antibody reactions?

   a. Postzone
   b. Prozone
   c. Zone of equivalence
   d. Endzone

18. Which one of the following properties of antibodies is NOT dependent on the structure of the heavy chain constant region?

   a. Ability to cross the placenta
   b. Isotype (class)
   c. Ability to fix complement
   d. Affinity for antigen

19. Molecules that promote the update of bacteria for phagocytosis are:

   a. Opsonins
   b. Cytokines
   c. Haptens
   d. Isotypes

20. Select the term that describes the unique confirmation of the antigen that allows recognition by a corresponding antibody:

   a. Immunogen
   b. Epitope
   c. Avidity
   d. Clone

21. Which of the following terms refers to the net negative charge surrounding red blood cells?

   a. Dielectric constant
   b. Van der Waals forces
   c. Hydrogen bonding
   d. Zeta potential

References

1. Waytes, AT, et al: Pre-ligation of CR1 enhances IgG-dependent phagocytosis by cultured human monocytes. J Immunol 146:2694, 1991.
2. Roback, J, Combs, M, Grossman, B, and Hillyer, C: Technical Manual, 16th ed. CD-ROM. American Association of Blood Banks, Bethesda, MD, 2009.
3. Sunshine, G, and Coico, R: Immunology: A Short Course, 6th ed. John Wiley & Sons, Hoboken, 2009.
4. Stites, DP, Parslow, TG, Imboden, JB, and Terr, AI (eds): Medical Immunology, 10th ed. McGraw-Hill, New York, 2001.
5. Nance, SJ, Arndt, PA, and Garratty, G: Correlation of IgG subclass with the severity of hemolytic disease of the newborn. Transfusion 30:381, 1990.
6. Rieben, R, et al: Antibodies to histo-blood group substances A and B: Agglutination titers, Ig class, and IgG subclasses in healthy persons of different age categories. Transfusion 31:607, 1991.
7. Sokol, RJ, et al: Red cell autoantibodies, multiple immunoglobulin classes, and autoimmune hemolysis. Transfusion 30:714, 1990.
8. Kerr, WG, Hendershot, LM, and Burrows, PD: Regulation of IgM and IgD expression in human B-lineage cells. J Immunol 146:3314, 1991.
9. Klein, HG, and Anstee, DJ (eds): Red cell antibodies against self-antigens, bound antigens and induced antigens. In Mollison's Blood Transfusion in Clinical Medicine, 11th ed. Wiley-Blackwell, Oxford, UK, 2007, pp 253–298.
10. Klein, HG, and Anstee, DJ (eds): ABO, Lewis and P groups and Ii antigens. In Mollison's Blood Transfusion in Clinical Medicine, 11th ed. Wiley-Blackwell, Oxford, UK, 2007, pp 114–162.
11. Turgeon, ML: Fundamentals of Immunohematology, 2nd ed. Lippincott Williams & Wilkins, Philadelphia, 2003.
12. Schleuning, M, et al: Complement activation during storage of blood under normal blood bank conditions: Effects of proteinase inhibitors and leukocyte depletion. Blood 79:3071, 1992.
13. Issitt, PD, and Anstee, DJ: Applied Blood Group Serology, 4th ed. Montgomery Scientific, Durham, NC, 1998, pp 34–35.
14. Kutt, SM, et al: Rh Blood Group System Antigens, Antibodies, Nomenclature, and Testing. Ortho Diagnostic Systems, Raritan, NJ, 1990, pp 13–14.
15. Stevens, CD: Clinical Immunology and Serology: A Laboratory Perspective, 3rd ed. FA Davis Company, Philadelphia, 2009.
16. Ammann, AJ: Mechanisms of immunodeficiency. In Stites, DP, Terr, AI, and Parslow, TG (eds): Basic and Clinical Immunology, 8th ed. Appleton & Lange, Norwalk, 1994.

Chapter 4

Concepts in Molecular Biology

Maria P. Bettinotti, PhD, dip. ABHI; Lorraine Caruccio, PhD, MT(ASCP)SBB; and Barbara Kraj, MS, MLS(ASCP)CM

OBJECTIVES

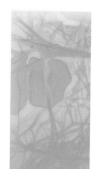

1. Refer to the contributions by Griffith, Avery, Hershey, and Chase, and explain how DNA was proven to be the carrier of genetic information.
2. Explain the significance of Chargaff's rules and x-ray diffraction studies by Wilkins and Franklin in Watson and Crick's discovery of the DNA double helix structure.
3. Describe DNA features fundamental in the design of molecular assays and define the applicable terms: *complementarity, hydrogen bonding, melting point, denaturation, annealing,* and *polarity*.
4. Explain what the central dogma of molecular biology is and how it expanded after the discovery of reverse transcriptase enzyme.
5. Explain what the recombinant DNA technology is and describe the tools used in molecular cloning: restriction endonucleases, vectors, and host cells.
6. Define *gene expression* and explain how it may be studied and used in manufacturing of recombinant proteins.
7. Summarize the procedures of plasmid DNA isolation and gel electrophoresis.
8. Explain the principles of the polymerase chain reaction as an in vitro molecular procedure mimicking the process of semiconservative DNA replication occurring in vivo.
9. Discuss the differences between classic PCR, reverse-transcriptase, and real-time PCR.
10. Describe the principle of transcription-mediated amplification.
11. Describe Sanger's sequencing dideoxy chain termination method.
12. Recognize the differences between immunoblotting and hybridization methods: Southern and Northern analysis, microarrays, and fluorescent in situ hybridization.
13. Explain major principles of methods used in studying gene polymorphisms: RFLP, VNTR, SSP, and SSOP.
14. Explain how nucleic acid testing (NAT) in donor blood improves the process of screening for infectious disease.
15. Describe the applications of RBC molecular antigen typing.

Introduction

Molecular biology is the science that studies the molecular interactions that take place in the living cell. For the molecular biologist, the master molecules are the nucleic acids: the deoxyribonucleic acid (**DNA**) and the ribonucleic acid (**RNA**). According to the original **central dogma** of molecular biology, the basic information of life flows from DNA through RNA to proteins.[1] By means of the **genetic code**, a sequence of nucleotides within a **gene** is transcribed and translated into a sequence of amino acids that form a peptide or protein. The processes of **transcription** and **translation** (reviewed in Chapter 2, "Basic Genetics") are referred to as **gene expression**. The key to the chemistry of life is the variety of gene expression products that are unique structural or functional protein molecules.

A protein may be shaped into a building component of a cell. For example, **spectrin** is a main structural protein of the red blood cell (RBC) skeleton. Defects in the spectrin gene lead to **hereditary spherocytosis** (HS), a condition characterized by fragile, spherical RBCs, which the spleen traps and destroys.

A protein may temporarily bind particular substrate molecules, enabling these molecules to chemically react with each other. Proteins that act as catalysts of these chemical reactions are called **enzymes**. A good example is the ABO blood group system. The *H* gene codes for protein fucosyl transferase, an enzyme that adds sugar L-fucose to a series of precursor structures. Once L-fucose has been added, the *A* and *B* gene–specified enzymes can add sugars to the chains that now carry the *H* residue. In other words, these genes determine a carbohydrate structure through the action of their encoded proteins acting as enzymes. (Refer to Chapter 6, "The ABO Blood Group System.") Some proteins may be shaped to bind to DNA at specific nucleotide sequences in the chromatin to influence gene expression. These proteins act as **transcription factors**. Through all these mechanisms, the genotype of a cell is translated into its phenotype.

Transfusion medicine is tied to three branches of molecular biology: (1) molecular genetics, because donor-recipient compatibility depends on the genetic transmission of polymorphic tissue markers, such as **blood groups** and **human leukocyte antigens** (HLA); (2) biotechnology, because of the production of recombinant proteins relevant to blood banking, such as growth factors, erythropoietin, and clotting factors; and (3) molecular diagnostics, because of the applications of molecular-based methods in the detection of transfusion-transmitted pathogens. Therefore, blood bankers must learn the basic principles of molecular biology.

Chapter 2 describes in detail the biochemistry of gene replication, transcription, and translation. In this chapter, some of the experiments and concepts that led to the discovery and understanding of the mechanisms underlying these phenomena are reviewed. These experiments are direct predecessors of modern benchtop molecular techniques relevant to immunohematology. This chapter provides a brief introduction to molecular biology and supplements the description of molecular applications presented in other sections of this book. **Blood group genotyping**, a relatively new and evolving application of molecular technology in transfusion medicine, is introduced at the end of this chapter.

DNA Is the Genetic Material

Living organisms can replicate and pass hereditary traits (genes) to successive generations; this is their most distinctive characteristic. Refer to Chapter 2 for an in-depth review of **Mendel's laws** and other concepts fundamental to heredity.

In 1928, the British microbiologist Frederick Griffith presented a model system that was key to demonstrating that DNA was the material that carried the genetic information responsible for the features of living organisms (Fig. 4–1). He used two naturally occurring strains of *Streptococcus pneumoniae* bacterium that differed in their infectivity of mice.[2] The virulent smooth (S) strain, which has a smooth polysaccharide capsule, kills mice through pneumonia. The nonvirulent rough (R) strain lacks the immunoprotective outer capsule and is nonlethal to mice because it is easily recognized and destroyed by the murine immune system. Injection of S-strain bacteria killed by heat does not cause any disease. However, simultaneous coinjection of the mixture of nonvirulent R strain with heat-killed S strain is lethal, and virulent S-strain bacteria can be recovered from mice infected with this mixture. Some heat-resistant component (a "transforming principle") from the heat-killed S strain is able to **transform** the living R strain from innocuous to virulent (S).

This experiment has been known as **Griffith's transformation**. It is still the basis for transfer of genetic material from one organism to another in the laboratory setting. Griffith

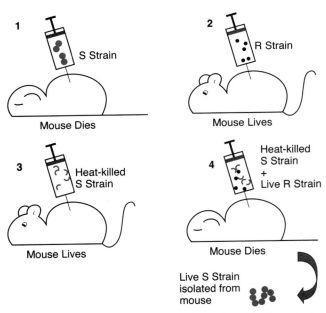

Figure 4–1. Griffith's transformation experiment. Bacterial cells can be transformed from nonpathogenic to virulent by heat-resistant component of the virulent strain: (1) Mice injected with encapsulated *Streptococcus pneumoniae* strain S die. The strain is virulent. (2) Mice injected with non-encapsulated *Streptococcus pneumoniae* strain R live. The strain is nonvirulent. (3) Mice injected with heat-killed S strain live. (4) Mice injected with a mixture of R live strain and heat-killed S strain die, and live S strain can be isolated from them.

was lucky choosing this particular species to demonstrate the transformation, because many cell types are very resistant to this process, which is now facilitated by harsh conditions like use of chemicals (detergents), electricity (electroporation), or liposomes.

But how do we know that this genetic transformation occurred due to transfer of DNA? Oswald T. Avery and his group at Rockefeller Institute were able to reproduce Griffith's transformation in vitro. In 1944, they reported that they had purified the "transforming principle."[3] By molecular composition and weight, it was mainly DNA. Moreover, treatment with RNA or protein hydrolytic enzymes did not degrade it, but treatment with DNase caused loss of activity. Avery's group's conclusion that DNA was responsible for the transformation was not accepted immediately. Some in the scientific community suspected that inadequately destroyed proteins that contaminated the isolated DNA caused the transformation.

In 1952, Alfred Hershey and Martha Chase reported an experiment that convinced the scientific community that genes are constituted by DNA (Fig. 4–2). They infected in parallel two bacterial cultures with phages (bacterial viruses), in which either the protein capsule was labeled with radioactive sulfur (^{35}S) or the DNA core was labeled with radioactive phosphorus (^{32}P). After dislodging the phage particles from the bacteria with a blender, they pelleted the bacteria by centrifugation. The phage particles were left in the supernatant. Following the centrifugation, ^{35}S (protein) was only in the supernatant and ^{32}P (DNA) was only in the pellet. From this pellet, a new generation of phages arose. The investigators concluded that the phage protein removed from the cells by stirring was the empty phage coat, whose mission was to transport the DNA from cell to cell. The DNA was the material of life, containing the phage genetic information necessary for the viral reproduction inside the bacteria.[4]

Features Relevant to Molecular Techniques

In 1950, Erwin Chargaff of Columbia University reported results of DNA quantitative analysis that became known as **Chargaff's rules**.[5] Later, Maurice Wilkins and Rosalind Franklin produced x-ray diffraction photographs of DNA that suggested a helical structure. Based on these clues, in 1953, James Watson and Francis Crick published a seminal in which they proposed that the DNA molecule was a double α helix.[6] DNA was a helical ladder, the rails of which were built from alternating units of deoxyribose and phosphate. Each rung of the ladder was composed of a pair of nitrogen-containing **nucleotides** (a base pair) held together by **hydrogen bonds**.

The double helix consisted of two strands of nucleotides that ran in opposite directions (they were antiparallel), designated by **polarity** (directionality) labels 3' and 5', which refer to the number assigned by convention to the deoxyribose carbon atom linked to either the hydroxyl or phosphate group (see Chapter 2 and **Fig. 2–10**). The **3' and 5' ends** determine the direction of DNA replication and transcription.

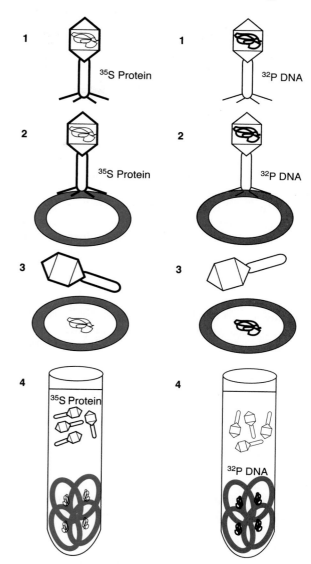

Figure 4–2. The Hershey-Chase phage experiment. DNA is the molecule that carries genetic information: (1) Bacteriophages were labeled with ^{35}S or with ^{32}P; ^{35}S was incorporated into proteins and ^{32}P into DNA. (2) Two *Escherichia coli* (*E. coli*) cultures were infected in parallel with the two different phages. (3) Phages were dislodged from bacteria by treatment with a blender. (4) After centrifugation, ^{35}S (proteins) were detected only in the supernatant of the first culture and ^{32}P (DNA) only in the pellet of the second culture. The phages remained in the supernatant and the bacteria in the pellet. From the bacterial pellet, a new generation of viruses could be raised.

Consistent with x-ray diffraction, about 10 base pairs were stacked on top of each other at each turn of a helix. Adenine always paired by two hydrogen bonds with thymine; guanine always paired by three hydrogen bonds with cytosine. Due to this **complementarity** resulting from formation of noncovalent hydrogen bonds, the nucleotide alphabet of one-half of the DNA helix determined the alphabet of the other half.

Chemistry and dynamics of hydrogen bonding is pivotal in understanding the fundamentals of molecular testing methods, as many procedures are based on the processes of DNA strands' separation (**denaturation**) and **annealing** (renaturation). These processes occur at different temperatures, depending on the total number of hydrogen bonds in the molecule, which determines the DNA **melting point (Tm)**. The value of Tm is necessary in calculations used to choose temperatures for **polymerase chain reaction** or other **hybridization**-based assays.[7] DNA melting point has nothing to do with the conversion of solid state into liquid, as the term could imply. Rather, it is the temperature at which half of all hydrogen bonds in the molecule are broken, while the other half are still intact. In other words, the Tm determines how much energy is needed to keep the strands of the helix apart. Temperatures above the Tm promote the separation of the strands, while temperatures below Tm keep the strands together.

The Watson-Crick model and the chemistry of hydrogen bonding reveal how DNA could replicate. During **replication**, the hydrogen bonds break, the strands separate, and each one functions as a template for the synthesis of another complementary half molecule. In this enzymatic process, two identical DNA molecules are generated, each containing the original strand and a new complementary strand. Because each daughter double helix contains an "old" strand and a newly synthesized strand, this model of replication is called **semiconservative**. The mechanism of DNA replication was studied using cellular components to reconstruct, in vitro, the biochemical reactions that occur within the cell. In this way, the whole process was dissected so that molecular testing procedures could be developed that mimicked the natural process that occurred in vivo. In eukaryotes, **DNA polymerase III** is able to form a new strand using **deoxyribonucleoside triphosphates** (dNTPs) as substrates, double-stranded DNA as template, and magnesium as an enzyme cofactor. This enzyme can add nucleotides onto the hydroxyl group (OH) at the 3' end of an existing nucleic acid fragment. Both strands are synthesized at the same time[8] (see Fig. 2–12).

The examples of techniques mimicking DNA replication are DNA sequencing and polymerase chain reaction (PCR), described later in this chapter.

Expression of Genetic Information

Genes act by determining the sequence of amino acids and therefore the structure of proteins. Knowledge of DNA structure revealed that the genetic information must be specified by the order of the four nitrogen-containing bases (A, C, G, and T). Proteins are polymers of 20 different amino acids, the sequence of which determines their structure and function. But how could the sequence of nucleotides determine the sequence of amino acids?

The discovery of the molecular basis of sickle cell anemia provided the first experimental evidence that the nucleotide sequence of a DNA molecule indeed determined the amino acid sequence of a protein. Sickle cell anemia is a genetic disease inherited according to an **autosomal-recessive pattern**. Patients with this disease have two copies of the mutated **beta globin chain** gene located on chromosome 11. Individuals with only one mutated copy of the gene show mild or no clinical manifestation and are called *carriers*. In 1949, Linus Pauling and Vernon Ingram showed that the hemoglobin

of individuals with and without sickle cell anemia had different mobility in an electric field (electrophoretic mobility).[9] This indicated that hemoglobin from the patients had a different electric charge; therefore, amino acid composition was different from normal hemoglobin. Carriers of the disease had both types of hemoglobin.

In 1957, Ingram identified that substituting valine for glutamic acid in the sixth amino acid position from the NH_2 end of the β-globin chain was the cause of the defective hemoglobin.[10] Thus, a direct link was established between a gene mutation and the structure of a protein. Concurrent research showed that proteins were synthesized in the cytoplasm in eukaryotic cells. These studies established that the microsomal fraction, which we now call **ribosomes**, was the major cellular component required for protein synthesis.[11]

Because DNA was in the nucleus, separated from the cytoplasm by the nuclear membrane, an intermediary molecule had to be responsible for conveying the genetic information from the nucleus to the cytoplasm. Ribonucleic acid (RNA) was a good candidate for this role. Its structure suggested that RNA could be produced based on a DNA template, and RNA was located mainly in the cytoplasm where protein synthesis occurred.

Experimental evidence supporting the role of RNA as the intermediary molecule came from the studies on bacterial viruses (**bacteriophages**). When bacteriophage T4 infects *E. coli*, the synthesis of bacterial RNA stops, and the only new RNA synthesized is transcribed from T4 DNA. Using radioactive labeling, Sidney Brenner, François Jacob, and Matthew Meselson showed that the newly synthesized T4 RNA associated with bacterial ribosomes, unlike ribosomal RNA.[12] These RNA molecules, which served as templates for protein synthesis, were given the name **messenger RNAs** (mRNAs).

But how could nucleotides direct the incorporation of an amino acid into a protein? The experimental answer to this question came again from studying cell-free extracts. In these experiments, a third type of RNA molecule, which we now call **transfer RNA** (tRNA), was isolated. These were short molecules, 70 to 80 nucleotides long, and some displayed the remarkable characteristic of having amino acids covalently attached to their 3' end. The enzymes responsible for attaching a specific amino acid to a specific tRNA were also isolated from cell-free extracts and were given the name **aminoacyl tRNA synthetases**. Sequencing of several tRNAs showed that they all had a common three-dimensional structure, but a unique three-nucleotide-long sequence was always present in a loop region. This sequence, which we now call **anticodon**, provided the specificity for each tRNA, carrying its specific amino acid, to align with the corresponding **codon** (triplet) in the mRNA.[8] (Refer to Chapter 2 and **Figs. 2–15 through 2–18** for more information on the process of translation.)

The next question was which triplet of nucleotides of the mRNA corresponded to which amino acid; in other words, it was time to decipher the genetic code. By 1966, Marshall Nirenberg and Har Gobind Khorana had cracked the code. Nirenberg used cell-free extracts containing ribosomes, amino acids, tRNAs, and aminoacyl tRNA synthetases, and added synthetic mRNA polymer containing only uracil (-UUUUUU-). He was able to produce in vitro a polymer peptide containing only the amino acid phenylalanine. In this way, he showed that UUU was the codon for phenylalanine.[13] During the next few years, all possible mRNA combinations were tried. The 61 different triplets were assigned to their corresponding amino acids, and 3 triplets were found to code for a stop signal (refer to **Fig. 2–11**). The genetic code is called **degenerate** because one amino acid may be encoded by more than one nucleotide triplet. This serves as a mechanism that protects the code from devastating effects of mutations occurring in the third or second base of the triplet. In most cases, the mutation results in amino acid change only when it affects the first base of the triplet.

The Central Dogma of Molecular Biology, Expanded

Deciphering the genetic code confirmed the central dogma of molecular biology. The genetic material is DNA. DNA is self-replicating and is transcribed into mRNA, which in turn serves as a template for the synthesis of proteins. Although the central dogma remains true, the knowledge acquired in the following years has refined and enlarged it, a process that continues now and into the future.

A different method of information flow in biological systems was discovered. A particular group of animal RNA viruses called tumor viruses can cause cancer in infected animals. In the early 1960s, Howard Temin discovered that replication of these viruses required DNA synthesis in the host cells. He formulated the hypothesis that RNA tumor viruses, subsequently called **retroviruses**, replicated via the synthesis of a DNA intermediate or **provirus**. In 1970, Temin and David Baltimore showed independently that these viruses contain an enzyme that catalyzes the synthesis of DNA using RNA as a template.[14,15]

The presence of viral DNA in replicating host cells was also demonstrated. The synthesis of DNA from RNA, now called **reverse transcription**, was thus definitely established as a mode of biological information transfer. In vitro reverse transcription is an important tool in molecular biology techniques. Natural or recombinant enzymes with **reverse transcriptase** activity can be used to generate DNA copies of any RNA molecule. Using reverse transcriptase mRNAs can be transcribed to its **complementary DNA** (cDNA) and studied by recombinant DNA techniques. For example, infectious disease screening assays designed to detect HIV in donors' blood and other specimens start with the process of reverse transcription, because HIV viruses are retroviruses and their genetic material consists of RNA. (Refer to Chapter 18, "Transfusion-Transmitted Diseases.") The cDNA synthesized during reverse transcription is subsequently amplified in polymerase chain reaction, which allows for creation of enough copies of genetic material to analyze (refer to "Reverse Transcriptase PCR" section in this chapter).

Scientists have added further disclaimers to the central dogma:

• Genes are not "fixed." Some of them do not have a designated chromosomal locus and function as transposable genetic elements in the eukaryotic genome. Another mechanism of physical rearrangement is in vivo DNA recombination. The examples are the immunoglobulin chain and T-cell receptor (TCR) gene rearrangements.

• DNA sequences and protein amino acid sequences do not exactly correspond to one another. In many organisms, including humans, coding sequences (exons) are interrupted by noncoding sequences (introns) that are excised from the immature RNA shortly after transcription. This introduces the possibility of alternative splicing to create different proteins from the same gene. Also, different reading frames can generate different mRNAs and therefore different proteins. Viruses frequently use this last mechanism. In vitro reverse transcription procedures will result in cDNA that corresponds only to sequences originally present within exons. Hence, cDNA derived from very long genes is a much shorter representation of the gene (Fig. 4–3). Scientists have discovered further roles for RNA. Some RNA molecules display catalytic activity; by **RNA interference**, small RNA molecules help to regulate gene expression.[16]

Figure 4–3. In eukaryotes, the coding sequences (exons) are interrupted by noncoding sequences (introns). Newly transcribed RNA (pre-mRNA) is considered heterogenous RNA (hnRNA) and loses the introns in the process of splicing. The mature mRNA is modified by polyadenylation of the 3′ end and addition of 7-methylguanine "cap" at the 5′ end, and it contains only the exons. In vitro reverse transcription procedures will result in cDNA that corresponds only to sequences originally present within exons. Hence, cDNA is a shorter representation of the gene. *(Modified from Buckingham, L, and Flaws, ML: Molecular Diagnostics. Fundamentals, Methods and Clinical Applications. F.A. Davis Company, Philadelphia, PA, 2007.)*

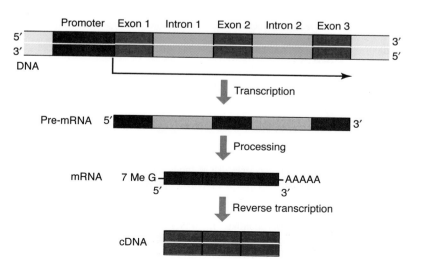

Recombinant DNA

The classic experiments in molecular biology, which we have described, used simple and rapidly replicating organisms (bacteria and viruses) as study models. However, the genomes of eukaryotes are much more complicated, and scientists had to explore new ways to isolate and study individual genes of these organisms. The big breakthrough came with the development of **recombinant DNA technology**. A fragment of DNA from one organism can be cut and pasted into a carrier DNA molecule or vector (e.g., a plasmid or bacteriophage). The new DNA molecule, which is a "recombinant" of the original DNA with the vector DNA, can be introduced using various techniques into another, usually simpler, host organism. Because the genetic code is almost universal, the host organism treats the gene as its own and replicates this "transgene" along with its own DNA. This technique is called **molecular cloning**. The ABO gene was cloned by Yamamoto's group in 1990[17] (Table 4–1).

Table 4–1   Major Events Leading to Establishment of Molecular Immunohematology

YEAR	MAJOR EVENT
1924	Bernstein, applying the Hardy-Weinberg principle, proposes that the ABO antigens are coded by one gene.
1944	Avery, MacLeod, and McCarty prove DNA as the carrier of inheritance (following Griffith's transformation in 1928).
1953	Watson and Crick decipher DNA structure based on Chargaff's rules (A + G = T + C and T = A and C = G) and x-ray studies by R. Franklin (Nobel '62 with Wilkins).
1970	Smith and Wilcox isolate the first restriction enzyme from *H. influenzae* (RFLP method developed in 1978). Temin and Baltimore discover enzyme reverse transcriptase.
1975	Maxam and Gilbert invent the first DNA sequencing method. Sanger improves it in 1977.
1977–78	First demonstration of a molecular basis for blood group polymorphisms: two aa differences in glycophorin A identified as the basis for M and N blood groups (several researchers).
1981	First demonstration of a molecular basis for rare blood group polymorphisms: basis for Mg and Mc rare blood group variants identified (H. Furthmayr and O. O. Blumenfeld groups).
1986	Kary Mullis publishes polymerase chain reaction (PCR) to amplify DNA fragments using thermostable Taq enzyme.
1986	Glycophorin A and glycophorin C are cloned.
1987	CD55 (DAF) responsible for the Cromer system and glycophorin B are cloned.
1990	F. Yamamoto and colleagues clone the ABO gene. R. D. Larsen and colleagues clone the FUT1 gene (H/h system).
1991	*RHD* and *RHAG* genes of the Rh system and KEL gene are cloned.
1992	Higuchi and others at Roche Molecular Systems and Chiron demonstrate real-time PCR (simultaneous amplification and detection).
1994	Genes responsible for the Lutheran system, Colton blood group antigens, and Kidd (JK) system are cloned.
1996	S. Iwamoto and colleagues identify promoter mutations as responsible for the Duffy a-b phenotype.
1999	The Blood Group Antigen Gene Mutation Database (BGMUT) is set up by O. Bloomenfeld and S. K. Patnaik. Moved in 2006 to National Center for Biotechnology Information site at www.ncbi.nlm.nih.gov/gv/mhc/xslcgi.cgi?cmd=bgmut/home.
2000	Complete sequence of the human genome is published.
2004	Consortium for Blood Group Antigens established with the purpose to "provide education for laboratories involved in DNA/RNA testing"; initiative by NYBC (M. Reid). First International Workshop of Molecular Blood Group Genotyping (ISBT initiative).
2005	Microarray-based blood group typing is described by multiple researchers (Transfusion, vol. 45).
2006	Ortho sponsors Rh molecular workshop in Heidelberg. FDA workshop Molecular Methods in Immunohematology (Transfusion, July 2007 suppl) www.fda.gov/downloads/BiologicsBloodVaccines/NewsEvents/WorkshopsMeetingsConferences/TranscriptsMinutes/UCM054428.pdf. AABB Annual Meeting—BioArray Solutions technology
2007	AABB News publishes "The Omics Revolution"

Modified from: dbRBC, Blood Group Antigen Gene Mutation Database.
Historical landmarks in the field of study of blood group systems. Available at www.ncbi.nlm.nih.gov/projects/gv/rbc/xslcgi.fcgi?cmd=bgmut/landmarks

Cloning is the reproduction of daughter cells from one single cell by fission or mitotic division, giving rise to a population of genetically identical clones. Successive divisions of the host cell create a population of clones containing the DNA fragment of interest. The gene or genes of interest can be studied using the techniques available for the host organism. These techniques have allowed detailed molecular studies of the structure and function of eukaryotic genes and genomes.[18]

The Coding Sequence of a Gene

In humans and most other eukaryotes, the coding part of a gene consists of **exons**, which in the genomic DNA alternate with noncoding **introns**. Newly transcribed RNA (**pre-mRNA**) is considered heterogenous RNA (**hnRNA**) and loses the introns in the process of **splicing**. The mature mRNA contains only the exons, the coding sequence of nucleotides that directs the process of translation into the amino acid sequence of the corresponding protein.[19]

Both the genomic DNA and the coding sequence of a gene can be cloned. First, the mRNA is reverse transcribed in vitro to its cDNA, using either synthetic or retroviral enzyme reverse transcriptase. Because eukaryotic mRNAs end with a **poly-A tail**, a short synthetic **oligo-dT** nucleotide can be used as a universal primer starting the cDNA synthesis (this process may also be achieved using the **random hexamers** or **sequence-specific primers**, depending on the application). The final product is a hybrid double strand of mRNA and cDNA. The mRNA is degraded, and a DNA strand complementary to the cDNA is synthesized using DNA polymerase. The cDNA, which has the information for the coding gene sequence, can be subjected to the same techniques as genomic DNA.[18]

Tools for DNA Cloning

The following sections describe the essential tools for molecular cloning: restriction endonucleases, gel electrophoresis, vectors, and host cells. An example of gene cloning follows.

Restriction Endonucleases

The first breakthrough in the production of recombinant DNA came with the discovery and isolation of **restriction endonucleases**. These enzymes cleave DNA at specific sequences and allow scientists to "cut" a DNA fragment in a controlled and predictable fashion and "paste" it into another fragment using other enzymes (**ligases**). Restriction endonucleases are isolated from bacteria. From the early 1950s, it was observed that certain strains of *E. coli* were resistant to infection by various bacteriophages. This form of primitive bacterial immunity was called *restriction* because the host was able to restrict the growth and replication of the virus. The resistant bacteria had enzymes that selectively recognized and destroyed foreign DNA molecules by cutting it into pieces (endonuclease activity). At the same time, these enzymes modified (by methylation) the host's chromosomal DNA, protecting it from self-destruction.

Numerous restriction endonucleases have been isolated from different bacteria. These enzymes have been classified as type I, II, and III according to their mechanism of action. Only the type II enzymes are relevant for our description of molecular cloning.

In 1970, Hamilton Smith and Kent Wilcox at Johns Hopkins University isolated the first type II restriction endonuclease. Type II restriction enzymes are extremely useful for the molecular biologist; they cut DNA at a precise position within its recognition sequence and have no modifying activity.[20] More than 200 restriction endonucleases, covering more than 100 different recognition sites, are available commercially. The name given to each enzyme reflects its origin. For example, Smith and Wilcox's endonuclease was called *HindII* because it was obtained from *Haemophilus influenzae* strain R_d. The number II indicates that it was the second endonuclease to be identified in these bacteria. Restriction endonucleases usually recognize sequences 4 to 8 nucleotides in length. The recognition sequences are **palindromic**; that is, they read the same in the 5' to 3' direction on both strands of the double helix. Some enzymes cut both strands in the middle of the target sequence, generating **blunt ends**. Some enzymes cut both strands off the center, generating staggered ends. For example enzyme *EcoRI*, isolated from *E. coli*, recognizes this sequence:

5'GAATTC3'
3'CTTAAG5'

EcoRI cuts after the first G in both strands, generating fragments with the following ends:

5'G AATTC3'
3'CTTAA G5'

The single-strand-overhanging ends are complementary to any end cut by the same enzyme. These **sticky**, or cohesive, ends are extremely useful for "cutting and pasting" DNA from different origins, thus creating recombinant DNA. Examples of other restriction endonucleases and corresponding recognition sequences are listed in Table 4–2.

Finding out the sequences in a given DNA recognized by these enzymes, and establishing the distance between such sites, is called **restriction enzyme mapping**. In case of short sequences (about a few thousand bp long), such as in plasmids, which are bacterial extrachromosomal DNA, the mapping is simple because there are only a few sites recognized by each enzyme. However, restriction maps of long eukaryotic genomes are quite complex. Restriction fragment sizes may be altered by changes in or between enzyme recognition sites. The restriction site may disappear upon various mutations, and a new enzyme recognition site may appear.

The discovery of these naturally and pathologically occurring changes contributed to the establishment of the **restriction fragment length polymorphism** (RFLP) method. The analysis of unique RFLP patterns of various loci proved useful in crime-victim identification and in kinship studies. Blood bank applications of this initially laborious method were expanded greatly after the discovery of polymerase

Table 4–2   Examples of Type II Restriction Endonucleases

ENZYME	RECOGNITION SEQUENCE
AluI	AG↓CT
AosI	TGC↓GCA
ApyI	CC↓(A,T)GG
AsuI	G↓GNCC
AsuII	TT↓CGAA
AvrII	C↓CTAGG
BalI	TGG↓CCA
BamHI	G↓GATCC
BclI	T↓GATCA
BglII	A↓GATCT
BstEII	G↓GTNACC
BstNI	CC↓(A,T)GG
BstXI	CCANNNNN↓NTGG
ClaI	AT↓CGAT
DdeI	C↓TNAG
EcoRI	G↓AATTC
EcoRII	↓CC(A,T)GG
Fnu4HI	GC↓NGC
FnuDII	CG↓CG
HaeI	(A,T)GG↓CC(T,A)
HaeII	PuGCGC↓Py
HaeIII	GG↓CC
HhaI	GCG↓C
HincII	GTPy↓PuAC
HindII	GTPy↓PuAC
HindIII	A↓AGCTT
HinfI	G↓ANTC
HpaI	GTT↓AAC
HpaII	C↓CGG
MboI	↓GATC
MstI	TGC↓GCA
NotI	GC↓GGCCGC
PstI	CTGCA↓G
RsaI	GT↓AC
SacI	GAGCT↓C
SacII	CCGC↓GG

chain reaction. For example, the PCR-RFLP method was used to discriminate between RHD+ and RHD genotypes, based on the different number of *Pst* I enzyme restriction sites in the region flanking the RHD gene (so called *Rhesus box*).[21]

Gel Electrophoresis

The restriction patterns mentioned in the previous section may be examined by gel electrophoresis (Fig. 4–4), another technique fundamental for DNA cloning. It allows not only for visual analysis of DNA fragments' length, but also for its isolation and purification for further applications.[18]

The word **electrophoresis** means "to carry with electricity." Agarose gel electrophoresis is a simple and rapid method of separating DNA fragments. The DNA sample is introduced into a well in a gel immersed in buffer and is exposed to electric current. The DNA molecules run at different speeds according to their size. After staining with a fluorescent dye, bands of DNA of specific length can be seen under ultraviolet (UV) light and isolated from the gel. In solution, at a neutral pH, DNA is negatively charged because of its phosphate backbone. When placed in an electric field, DNA molecules are attracted toward the positive pole (anode) and repelled from the negative pole (cathode).

To make a gel, molten **agarose** (a seaweed extract) is poured into a mold where a plastic comb is suspended. As it cools, the agarose hardens to form a porous gel slab with preformed wells. The gel has a consistency similar to gelatin and is placed in a tank full of buffer and with electrodes at opposing ends. The samples containing the DNA fragments are pipetted into the wells, after mixing them with a loading solution of high density, such as sucrose or glycerol. The dense solution helps the DNA sink when loaded into the wells and allows for monitoring of the progress of electrophoresis due to presence of **bromophenol blue** dye (a tracer). When electric current (80 to 120 V) is applied to electrodes on the tank, the DNA fragments migrate toward the anode. The porous gel matrix acts as a sieve through which larger molecules move with more difficulty than smaller ones. The distance run by a DNA fragment is inversely proportional to its molecular weight and therefore to its length or number of nucleotides.

DNA bands can be detected in the gel upon staining with a fluorescent dye, such as **ethidium bromide** (EB) or **SYBR Green**. The gel may be soaked in a diluted fluorescent dye solution, or, alternatively, the electrophoresis is run with a gel and buffer containing the dye. EB is a planar molecule, which intercalates between the stacked nucleotides of the DNA helix. This feature makes it a mutagenic factor, which calls for cautious handling of gels, equipment exposed to this agent, and waste.

SYBR Green dye isn't mutagenic, and many facilities have adopted this dye in their staining procedures to assure laboratory safety.[22] When the gel is exposed to ultraviolet light of 300 nm, the stained DNA fragments are seen as fluorescent orange (EB) or green (SYBR) bands and can be documented by photography. Each band of DNA is formed by millions of DNA molecules of equal length, which is established by comparison with standard bands of size marker reagents. Gel

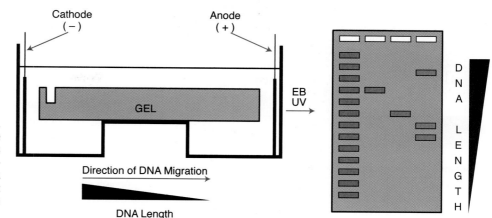

Figure 4–4. Agarose gel electrophoresis. Negatively charged DNA molecules migrate toward the positive pole. The agarose gel acts as a molecular sieve: The shorter the DNA molecule, the longer the distance of migration. DNA bands are detected by exposure to ultraviolet light (UV) after staining with the fluorescent dye ethidium bromide (EB) or SYBR Green.

electrophoresis, in **low melting point agarose**, is used in molecular cloning to isolate and purify the vector and insert, which will be used to form a recombinant DNA vector.

Vectors

A **vector** is a DNA molecule of known nucleotide sequence that is used to carry a foreign DNA fragment into a host organism. Vectors can be used to produce large quantities of a target DNA fragment. They can also be used to get a foreign gene expressed in a host cell to study the function of the gene or to manufacture large quantities of the encoded protein product.[18]

Plasmids. **Plasmids** are the simplest kind of vectors. They are bacterial, circular genetic elements that replicate independently from the chromosome. The plasmid vectors used in molecular cloning are "designer plasmids," modified to make perfect recombinant DNA carriers. A vast selection of plasmids are commercially available that are useful for different purposes, such as DNA sequencing, protein expression in bacteria, and protein expression in mammalian cells.

All plasmids contain an **origin of replication**. Plasmid vectors can be under "stringent" control of replication, in which case they replicate only once per cell division. By contrast, the "relaxed" plasmids replicate autonomously and can grow as hundreds of copies per cell. Relaxed plasmids are used to amplify large amounts of cloned DNA. Naturally occurring plasmids contribute significantly to bacterial genetic diversity by encoding functions, such as resistance to certain antibiotics, which provides the bacterium with a competitive advantage over antibiotic-sensitive strains. Plasmids used as vectors also contain genes that encode for antibiotic resistance. When bacteria grow in a culture medium with the given antibiotic, only host cells containing the plasmid will survive. Thus, a pure population of bacteria can be obtained. Examples of antibiotics used for bacterial cloning are listed in Box 4–1.

Cloning a DNA fragment requires inserting it into the plasmid vector. Plasmids are designed to contain one or more cloning sites, also called **polylinkers**, which are a series of recognition sequences for different restriction endonucleases. Most commonly, these are recognition sites for enzymes that cut both strands off the center, which generates cohesive

("sticky") ends. Otherwise, the procedure is called "blunt end cloning." The circular DNA of the plasmid is cut (or linearized) with a chosen restriction enzyme. The DNA fragment to be inserted is cut with the same enzyme. The sticky ends of the linearized plasmid can form hydrogen bonds with the complementary nucleotides in the overhang of the DNA fragment to be inserted (hence called an *insert*). Both fragments are run in a preparative, low-melting-point agarose gel. The bands corresponding to the expected size of the linearized plasmid and insert are cut out, and the purified DNA fragments are isolated. Both fragments are "pasted" together with DNA ligase, which forms phosphodiester bonds between adjacent nucleotides (Fig. 4–5).

Typical plasmid vectors consist of DNA 2 to 4 **kb** long and can accommodate inserts up to 15 kb long. Several other vectors are available for cloning fragments of DNA of different sizes.

Other Vectors. **Lambda (λ) vectors** contain the part of the bacteriophage's genome necessary for lytic replication in E. coli and one or more restriction endonuclease sites for insertion of the DNA fragment of interest. They can accommodate foreign DNA 5 to 14 kb long. The recombinant DNA is "packaged" into viral particles and used to infect E. coli.

Cosmids are vectors that can accept DNA 28 to 45 kb long. They are useful for producing large-insert genomic libraries. Cosmids have a small region of bacteriophage λ necessary for packaging viral DNA into λ particles. The linear genomic DNA fragment is inserted into the vector and packaged into bacteriophage particles. After infecting the E. coli cells, the

---

BOX 4–1

Antibiotics Used in Bacterial Cloning

- Ampicillin
- Carbenicillin
- Chloramphenicol
- Hydromycin B
- Kanamycin
- Tetracycline

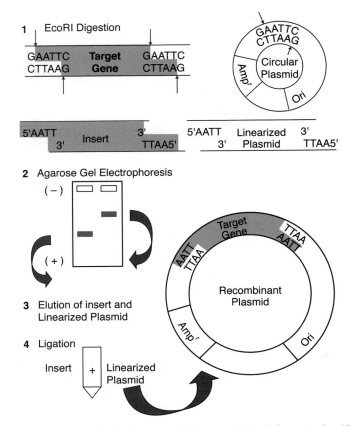

1 EcoRI Digestion

Figure 4–5. Gene cloning: part 1. (1) The target DNA and the vector plasmid are digested with *EcoRI*. (2) The insert and linearized plasmid are submitted to agarose gel electrophoresis. (3) The bands containing the insert and linearized plasmid are cut from the gel and the DNA fragments eluted. (4) Insert and linearized plasmid are ligated together and a recombinant plasmid containing the target gene is obtained.

vector circularizes into a large plasmid containing the DNA fragment of interest.

Bacterial artificial chromosomes (BACs) are circular DNA molecules that contain a unit of replication, or *replicon*, capable of carrying fragments as large as a quarter of the *E. coli* chromosome. BACs can maintain DNA inserts of up to 350 kb. A typical BAC library contains inserts of 120 kb.

Host Cells

The recombinant DNA molecule, which was produced in vitro, must then be introduced into a living cell to reveal if it is functional. The typical host organisms are various strains of *E. coli*. As we have previously described using the Griffith's experiment, the uptake and expression of foreign DNA by a cell is called *transformation*.[2] However, natural transformation that was observed due to DNA uptake by the rough (nonencapsulated) strain of *Streptococcus pneumoniae* is a rare event. The efficiency of the bacterial transformation can be increased by chemical or electrical (electroporation) methods that modify the cellular membrane.[18] The bacteria treated by these methods are called **competent**.

Because *E. coli* is a normal inhabitant of the human colon, it grows best in vitro at 37°C in a culture medium containing nutrients similar to those available in the human digestive

tract, including carbohydrates, amino acids, nucleotide phosphates, salts, and vitamins. To isolate individual colonies, cells are spread on the surface of agar plates containing an antibiotic used as a selectable marker. A suspension of the cells is diluted enough so that each cell will give rise to an individual colony. Plates are incubated at 37°C. After 12 to 24 hours (at the maximum rate, cells divide every 22 minutes), visible colonies of identical daughter cells appear. Individual colonies are picked and further propagated in liquid culture medium with antibiotic. The incubation proceeds with continuous shaking to maintain the cells in suspension and to promote aeration and production of cell mass that may be used for efficient isolation of vector DNA containing the insert.

Plasmid Isolation

Plasmids can be easily separated from the host's chromosomal DNA because of their small size and circular structure. A rapid method for making a small preparation of purified plasmid from 1 to 5 mL of culture is called **miniprep**. The overnight culture is centrifuged, and the pellet containing the bacteria is treated with a solution that includes sodium dodecyl sulfate (SDS) and sodium hydroxide. SDS is an ionic detergent that lyses the cell membrane, releasing the cell contents. Sodium hydroxide denatures DNA into single strands. Treating the solution with potassium acetate and acetic acid ("salting out"), causes an insoluble precipitate of detergent, phospholipids, and proteins and neutralizes the sodium hydroxide.

At neutral pH, the long strands of chromosomal DNA renature only partially and become trapped in the precipitate. The plasmid DNA renatures completely and remains in solution. After centrifugation, the pellet is discarded. Ethanol or isopropanol is added to the supernatant to precipitate the plasmid DNA out of the solution. After centrifugation, the DNA pellet is washed with 70% ethanol and dissolved in water or buffer. **RNase** is used to destroy the RNA that co-precipitates with the plasmid. A miniprep provides enough material for some downstream applications such as sequencing or subcloning into a different plasmid vector. However, it can be easily scaled up to a "midiprep" or "maxiprep" when more plasmid DNA is needed.

DNA Cloning: An Example

To summarize the process of DNA cloning, we will describe a hypothetical example in which a gene of interest, or target gene, is obtained from genomic DNA for sequencing purposes. In **Figure 4–5**, the target gene, flanked by two *EcoRI* restriction sites, is cut from genomic DNA and inserted into a plasmid vector. The plasmid contains an origin of replication (Ori) so it can be copied by the bacteria's DNA replication machinery. It also contains a gene that provides resistance to the antibiotic ampicillin (Amp^r); therefore, the bacteria that have the plasmid will be able to grow in culture medium with the antibiotic, whereas the bacteria that did not get the plasmid will die.

In **Figure 4–6**, competent *E. coli* are transformed with the plasmid and plated at a very low dilution in a Petri dish in solid LB medium with ampicillin. Only the bacteria containing

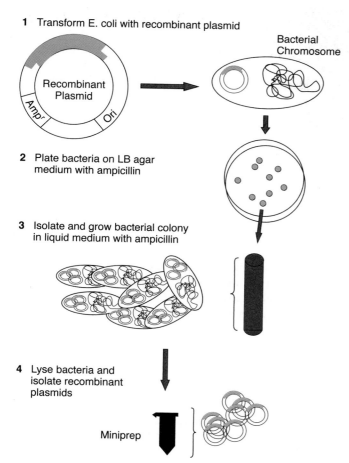

1 Transform E. coli with recombinant plasmid

Bacterial
Chromosome

Recombinant
Plasmid

Amp^r Ori

2 Plate bacteria on LB agar
medium with ampicillin

3 Isolate and grow bacterial colony
in liquid medium with ampicillin

4 Lyse bacteria and
isolate recombinant
plasmids

Miniprep

Figure 4–6. Gene cloning: part 2. (1) The recombinant plasmid is used to transform competent E. coli. (2) E. coli bacteria are plated onto solid agar medium containing ampicillin. Only bacteria containing the plasmid survive. Isolated colonies, each from a single cell, grow after overnight incubation at 37°C. (3) A colony is picked and cultured overnight in 1 to 5 mL of liquid LB medium containing ampicillin. (4) The recombinant plasmid is isolated from the bacterial culture ("miniprep").

the plasmid are able to grow and form colonies, which are visible after overnight incubation at 37°C. A colony is isolated and grown in liquid LB medium with ampicillin. The plasmid replicates independently from the bacterial chromosome, and several plasmids are formed inside each bacterium. From this cell suspension, the recombinant plasmid is isolated. The resulting miniprep contains abundant copies of the gene of interest (target gene) that can be used as a template for obtaining the sequence of the target gene. Currently, all genes coding for the 30 recognized human blood group systems have been cloned.[23]

Recombinant DNA Libraries

A way of isolating single genes is the production of recombinant DNA libraries. Instead of trying to fish one gene out of a mass of genomic DNA or cDNA, each gene is physically separated and introduced into a vector. The target gene is selected by screening each of the individual pieces with a specific probe. Recombinant **DNA libraries** are collections of clones that contain all genomic or mRNA sequences of a particular cell type. Clones containing a specific gene are identified by hybridization with a labeled

probe, such as a cDNA or genomic clone or a PCR product (see the "Detection of Nucleic Acids and Proteins" section).

As seen in the section on vectors, different vectors are useful for isolating DNA fragments of different sizes. For example, the Human Genome Project used BAC vectors to produce recombinant human genomic libraries. Genomic DNA was isolated from cells and partially digested with restriction enzymes, obtaining large fragments of around 100 to 200 kb. Inserts of these cloned BACs were subcloned as smaller fragments into phage or plasmid vectors, which were used for sequencing.[24] Complementary DNA libraries can be used to determine gene-coding sequences from which the amino acid sequence of the encoded protein can be deduced.

Oligonucleotides can be synthesized on the basis of partial amino acid sequence of the protein of interest and used to screen a recombinant cDNA library. The clones that contain the gene encoding the target protein are isolated and sequenced. The complete protein sequence can thus be obtained by translating the mRNA codons into amino acids. This approach was used in 1990 by Fumi-Chiro Yamamoto and his colleagues to isolate the gene that codes for the group A transferase.[17] Another approach for isolating a gene on the basis of the protein that it encodes is using antibodies specific against the target protein to screen **expression libraries**. In this case, the cDNA library is generated in an expression vector that drives protein synthesis in E. coli.

Expression of Cloned Genes: Recombinant Proteins in Clinical Use

The cost and effort necessary to isolate proteins with therapeutic functions from their original source make their use impractical. Also, the risk of viral contamination is a fundamental consideration in any therapeutic product that is purified from mammalian cells, in particular from human tissues. For these reasons, the use of engineered in vitro, **recombinant proteins** is a major improvement in the treatment of several diseases. Large amounts of recombinant proteins can be obtained for biochemical studies or for therapeutic use by molecular cloning of genes that code for them. The cloned gene is inserted into an expression vector, usually a plasmid, which directs the production of large amounts of the protein in either bacteria or eukaryotic cells. A great variety of expression vectors are available for recombinant protein expression in E. coli, yeast, insect cells, and mammalian cells.

The list of recombinant proteins used as therapeutic agents increases constantly. Interferon-α used to treat hairy cell leukemia and hepatitis C and B, recombinant hepatitis B vaccine, recombinant antihemophiliac factor, and recombinant coagulation factor IX are some examples of recombinant proteins useful for transfusion medicine. Granulocyte colony-stimulating factor (GCSF) is used to increase the production of hematopoietic stem cells (HSC) for HSC transplantation (HSCT). Epoetin alfa is used to treat anemia caused by chronic renal failure (Box 4–2).

Recombinant Proteins Used in Transfusion Medicine

- Factor VIII
- Factor IX
- Factor VII
- Factor XIII
- Thrombopoietin
- G-CSF
- GM-CSF
- Epoetin α
- Interferon-α

G-CSF = granulocyte colony stimulating factor; GM-CSF = granulocyte macrophage colony stimulating factor

Gene Therapy

Gene therapy is the introduction of new genetic material into the cells of an organism for therapeutic purposes. In the United States, only **somatic gene therapy** is allowed in humans—that is, the treated cells are somatic and not germline cells. The obvious clinical use of gene therapy is the treatment of inherited diseases. In the first clinical trial of that kind, the gene coding for **adenosine deaminase** was introduced into lymphocytes of children suffering from severe combined immunodeficiency disease.[25] However, several current clinical trials are focused on oncology. These treatments seek to enhance the host antitumor responses by overexpression of **cytokines** or by genetic alteration of the tumor cell.

One approach is the use of viral vectors, such as retroviruses, adenoviruses, herpesviruses, and lentiviruses. Most human clinical trials to date have used retroviral vectors. However, the use of these vectors carries serious potential risks that must be weighed against the severity of the underlying illness. The exogenous gene may cause disease if overexpressed or expressed in certain cell types. Contaminants may be introduced during vector manufacture. Also of concern is the potential for recombination of gene therapy vectors with human endogenous sequences. The search for better vectors is under way in animal models and holds promise for a safer and more effective gene therapy.

The Polymerase Chain Reaction

An alternative to cloning for isolating large amounts of a single DNA fragment or gene is the **polymerase chain reaction** (PCR), which was developed by Kary Mullis at Cetus Corporation in 1985.[26] As opposed to cloning, which is performed in a living cell, PCR is carried out completely in vitro. Provided that some sequence of the DNA molecule is known, PCR can be used to amplify a defined segment of DNA several million times.

In PCR, DNA (or cDNA) is replicated in the test tube or on a microtiter-like plate, replacing the steps that normally occur within a cell by adding synthetic or recombinant reagents and by cyclic changes in the reaction temperature. The role of the enzyme primase, which in vivo generates the primers to which DNA polymerase attaches the successive nucleotides, is replaced by synthetic oligonucleotides called **forward and reverse primers**. These primers are usually 15 to 20 nucleotides long and flank the target region to be amplified. In other words, the primers are designed to anneal to complementary DNA sequences at the 3' end of each strand of the DNA fragment (Fig. 4–7).

The product obtained (the **amplicon**) will have the sequence of the template bracketed by the primers. The two primers are mixed with a DNA sample containing the target sequence; thermostable DNA polymerase; the four deoxyribonucleoside triphosphates (dNTPs); and magnesium, which acts as enzyme cofactor. *Thermus aquaticus*, a bacterium that grew in hot springs, was the original source of heat-resistant polymerase, consequently named *Taq*.

Currently, numerous recombinant enzymes are on the market. The thermostability of the enzyme is of utmost importance because the first step of the PCR is heat *denaturation*. Applying high temperatures breaks the hydrogen bonds between the complementary nucleotides and plays the role of the helicases and gyrases that unwind the DNA so that the DNA polymerase complex can reach the template. At 94°C, the double helix is denatured into single strands. In the second step, annealing of the primers to the target sequences flanking the fragment of interest is achieved by cooling to a temperature of 50° to 60°C, which promotes renaturation (reestablishment of hydrogen bonds). The exact optimum temperature of annealing is determined by the number of G and C residues in the primers: The more GC, the more hydrogen bonds to break and the higher melting

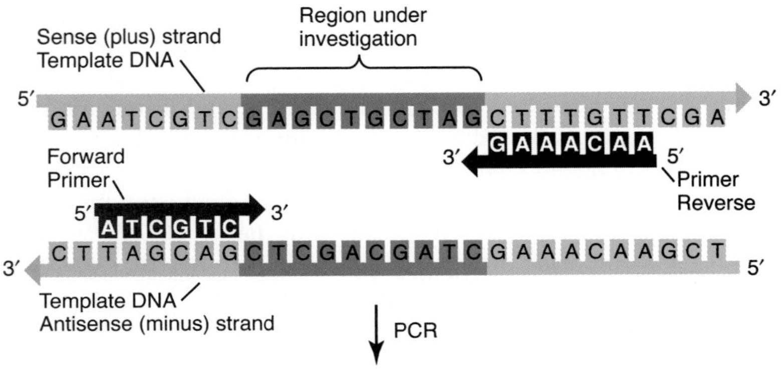

Figure 4–7. The FORWARD primer always anneals to the minus strand (also called *antisense strand*). It is complementary to the 3' end of the minus strand (and identical to the 5' end of the plus strand). The REVERSE primer always hybridizes with the plus strand (also called the *sense strand*). It is complementary to the 3' end of the plus strand and is identical to the 5' end of the minus strand. (*Modified from Buckingham, L, and Flaws, ML: Molecular Diagnostics. Fundamentals, Methods and Clinical Applications. F.A. Davis Company. Philadelphia, PA, 2007.*)

point Tm of the molecule. Typically, the optimum annealing temperature is 5 degrees Celsius below the Tm.

The third step, primer extension by DNA polymerase, is done at 72°C. This is the optimal temperature for the polymerase, which incorporates nucleotides to the 3' OH end of the primers using the target DNA as template. The cycles of DNA synthesis, which consist of denaturation, annealing, and extension, are repeated simply by repeating the cycle of temperatures. The reaction is carried out in a programmable heating and cooling machine called a **thermocycler**. The instrument contains a heating block built from materials characterized by high thermal conductivity (e.g., silver) that allow for rapid changes of temperatures and shortens time between the steps of each cycle. Figure 4–8 shows a schematic PCR reaction. In each cycle, an original template strand is copied to generate a complementary strand, which begins at the 5' end of the primer and ends wherever the Taq or other thermostable polymerase ceases to function. After the second cycle, DNA is synthesized, using the newly copied strands as templates. In this case, synthesis stops when it reaches the end of the molecule defined by the primer. By the end of the third cycle, a new blunt-ended double-stranded product is formed, with its 5' and 3' ends precisely coinciding with the primers.

These blunt-ended fragments accumulate exponentially during subsequent rounds of amplification, while the original DNA that was outside the region flanked by the primers isn't amplified. Thus, the majority of fragments in the later PCR cycles have both ends defined. A single DNA molecule amplified through 30 cycles of replication would theoretically yield 2^{30} (approximately 1 billion) progeny molecules. In reality, the exponential phase of product accumulation

during PCR is not indefinite; therefore, the theoretical number of product molecules is not reached. After a certain number of cycles, the accumulation of product reaches a plateau, the level of which depends on the initial number of target sequences, the quantity of reagents, and the efficiency of extension.

Aside from cloning, the PCR has numerous applications in immunohematology—for example, various modifications of this method have been used in the detection of infectious agents in donors' blood.[27,28] (Refer to Chapter 18.)

DNA Sequencing

Individual fragments of DNA can be obtained in sufficient amount for determining their nucleotide sequence either by molecular cloning or by PCR. Current methods of DNA sequencing are rapid and efficient. The easiest way of determining an amino acid sequence within a protein is the sequencing of a cloned gene, as the coding sequence of a gene can be unequivocally translated into the amino acid sequence of its encoded protein.

Modern sequencing is based on the **chain termination method** developed in 1977 by Fred Sanger at the Medical Research Council's Laboratory of Molecular Biology in Cambridge, England.[29] Just like the PCR, the Sanger sequencing method is a controlled in vitro process mimicking DNA synthesis. When a short synthetic primer (complementary to the beginning of the fragment to be sequenced) is hybridized to a single-stranded template in the presence of the four dNTPs, DNA polymerase can synthesize a new strand of DNA complementary to the template. The addition of an incoming nucleotide occurs via the 3' hydroxyl group in the deoxyribose

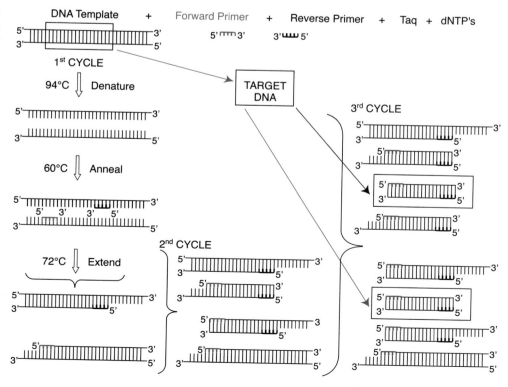

Figure 4–8. Polymerase chain reaction (PCR). Each cycle of PCR consists of denaturation of the double-stranded DNA by heating at 94°C, annealing of the forward and reverse primers to the template by cooling to 60°C, and extension at 72°C of the growing complementary strand catalyzed by the enzyme Taq polymerase. The target DNA sequence, bracketed by the forward and reverse primers, is indicated by a black box in the template DNA. In the third cycle, blunt-ended double-stranded products (also indicated by a black box) are formed with its 5' and 3' ends coinciding with the primers. These target DNA fragments continue to grow exponentially with each cycle.

necessary to form the phosphodiester linkage. The principle of Sanger method is based on including small amounts of modified dNTPs that are lacking that hydroxyl group into the reaction mix. These modified dNTPs are 2', 3'-**dideoxyribonucleoside triphosphates**. They are designated by a double *d* (ddNTPs). Upon incorporation into the newly synthesized DNA, they cause an immediate chain termination (hence the name of the method), as no new phosphodiester linkage with the following nucleotide is possible. Originally, Sanger sequencing required using radioisotopes and laborious casting of **polyacrylamide** electrophoretic gels in which the DNA fragments were separated by size in denaturing conditions created by the presence of urea.

Currently, most laboratories are using the automated fluorescent **cycle sequencing** method (Fig. 4–9). The reaction, which is carried out in a thermocycler, contains a DNA template, a primer, DNA polymerase, the four dNTPs, and four ddNTPs, each labeled with a different fluorescent dye. The reaction is heated to 94°C, which causes DNA denaturation to a single strand, followed by cooling to 65°C to allow annealing of the primer and its extension by enzymatic addition of nucleotides. Several cycles are repeated.

Working from the primer, the polymerase adds dNTPs or ddNTPs that are complementary to the DNA template. The ratio of dNTPs to ddNTPs is adjusted so that a ddNTP is incorporated into the elongating DNA chain, approximately once in every 100 nucleotides. Each time a ddNTP is incorporated, synthesis stops and a DNA fragment of a discrete size, labeled fluorescently according to its last nucleotide, is produced. At the end of 20 to 30 cycles of the reaction, millions of copies of the template DNA sequence are terminated at each nucleotide so a mixture of fragments is obtained, each longer by one nucleotide than the previous one. These fragments are separated by size by **capillary gel electrophoresis**. The fluorescent labels are detected as the terminated fragments pass a laser aimed at the capillary. When the fluorescent terminators are struck by the laser beam, each emits a colored light of a characteristic wavelength, which is collected by the detector and interpreted by the computer software as A (green), T (red), C (blue), or G (yellow). The final output is an electropherogram showing colored peaks corresponding to each nucleotide position.

Detection of Nucleic Acids and Proteins

The concepts of molecular cloning, creating expression DNA libraries and gene therapy, are fundamental in contemporary molecular research and development setting. Yet cloning may seem esoteric to a clinical laboratorian, presented with the task of identifying a specific mutation or confirming the presence of a pathogen. In the following paragraphs, some classical and newer methods for detecting specific nucleic acids and proteins will be described.

Nucleic Acid Hybridization

Base pairing between complementary strands of DNA or RNA allows the specific detection of nucleic acid sequences. Double-stranded nucleic acids denature at high temperature (90° to 100°C) and renature when cooled to form double-stranded molecules as dictated by complementary base pairing. This process of renaturation is called nucleic acid hybridization. Nucleic acid hybrids can be formed between two strands of DNA, two strands of RNA, or one strand of RNA and one of DNA. DNA or RNA sequences complementary to any purified DNA fragment can be detected by nucleic acid hybridization. The DNA fragment—for example, a cloned gene or a PCR product—is labeled using radioactive, fluorescent, or chemiluminescent tags. The labeled DNA is used as a probe for hybridization with any DNA or RNA complementary sequence. The resulting hybrid double strand will be labeled and can easily be detected by **autoradiography** or digital imaging.

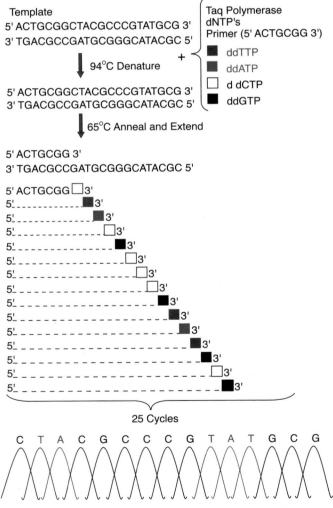

Figure 4–9. DNA sequencing: automated fluorescent cycle method. The double-stranded DNA template is denatured by heating at 94°C. Cooling to 65°C allows the annealing of the oligonucleotide primer. In the presence of the four dNTPs and the four fluorescently labeled ddNTPs, Taq polymerase incorporates nucleotides into the growing chain, following the template sequence in a 5' to 3' direction. Once in approximately 100 nucleotides, a ddNTP will be incorporated and synthesis will stop. A fragment of DNA is generated that contains a fluorescent tag in its last nucleotide. After capillary gel electrophoresis, the fluorescent labels are detected as the terminated fragments pass a laser aimed at the capillary. The final output is an electropherogram showing colored peaks corresponding to each nucleotide position.

Southern Blotting

In this technique developed by E. M. Southern, the DNA analyzed is digested with one or more restriction endonucleases, and the fragments are separated by agarose gel electrophoresis.[30] Due to an enormous number of some restriction enzyme recognition sites in genomic DNA, there may be hundreds of various-length fragments running on the gel within a short distance from one another, which upon staining is visible as a "smear" rather than well-distinguished bands. To capture only the fragments of interest, the gel is placed over a nitrocellulose or nylon membrane and overlaid with transfer buffer. The DNA fragments are transferred or "blotted," when vacuum is applied by the flow of a transfer buffer. The membrane-bound fragments have the same relative positions as the fragments separated by size on the gel. The filter is then incubated with a labeled probe under very specific temperature conditions. Upon hybridization, the fragments containing the sequence of interest are detected as labeled bands. The classical, laborious, and time-consuming **Southern blotting** is being replaced by PCR-based detection methods (Fig. 4–10).

Northern Blotting

This technique is a variation of Southern blotting and is used to detect RNA instead of DNA. Total cellular RNAs are extracted and fractioned by size through gel electrophoresis in the presence of substances, preventing RNA degradation by the ubiquitous RNases. The RNAs are then blotted onto a filter and detected by hybridization with a labeled probe. This technique is used for studying gene expression and is being replaced by quantitative reverse-transcriptase polymerase chain reaction (RT-qPCR).

DNA Microarrays

DNA **microarrays**, also called **gene chips**, allow tens of thousands of genes to be analyzed simultaneously.[31] A gene chip consists of a glass slide or a membrane filter onto which oligonucleotides or fragments of cDNA, which serve as multiple probes, are printed by a robot in small spots at high density. Because a chip can have more than 10,000 unique DNA sequences, scientists can produce DNA microarrays containing sequences representing all the genes in a cellular genome. A common application of this technique is the study of differential gene expression; for example, the comparison of the genes expressed by a normal cell as opposed to those of a tumor cell. Messenger RNA is extracted from both types of cells, and cDNA is obtained via reverse transcription. The two sets of cDNAs are labeled with different fluorescent dyes (typically red and green), and a mixture of the cDNAs is hybridized to the gene chip that contains many of the probes that represent genes already known in the human genome. The array is analyzed using a laser scanner. The ratio of red to green fluorescence at each specific spot on the array indicates the relative extent of transcription of the given gene in the tumor cells compared with the normal cells.

Another application of microarrays, especially desirable in contemporary immunohematology, is the analysis of the genome content rather than its expression. This represents a sophisticated form of genotyping (a process during which polymorphisms within multiple genes may be identified simultaneously). In 2007, a prototype BLOOD-1 Illumina BeadChip microarray-based system was developed in the United States and was used to screen for 18 **single nucleotide polymorphisms** (SNPs) within genes coding for RBC antigens in the Duffy, Colton, Lewis, Diego, and other blood groups.[32]

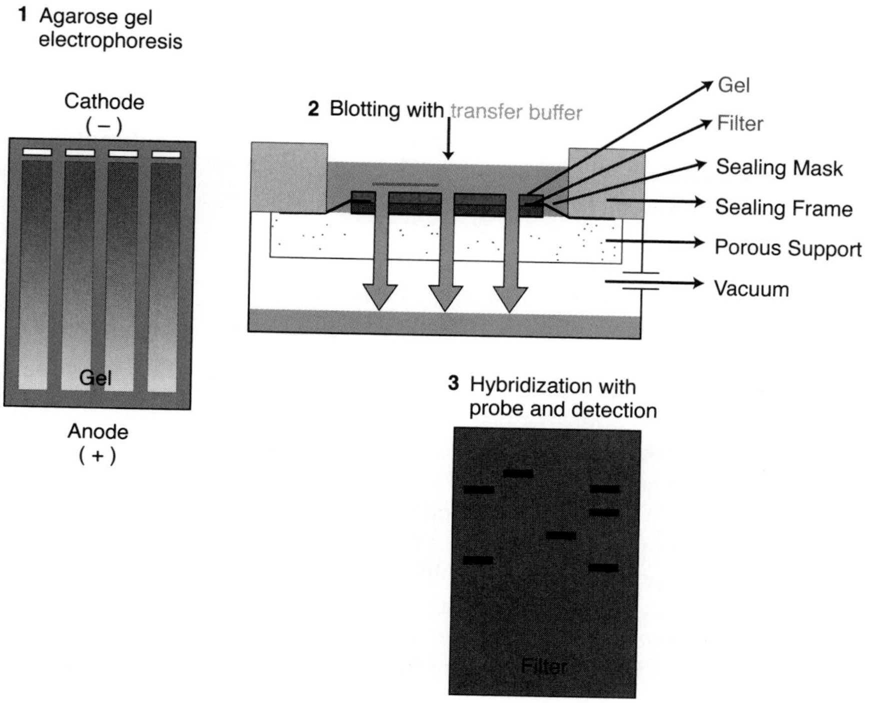

Figure 4–10. Southern blotting. (1) The DNA restriction digest is submitted to agarose gel electrophoresis. (2) The DNA fragments are transferred from the gel to a filter membrane by flow of buffer with negative pressure under vacuum. (3) The filter is hybridized with a labeled probe, and the labeled DNA bands are detected by digital imaging.

1 Agarose gel electrophoresis

Cathode
(–)

Gel

Anode
(+)

2 Blotting with transfer buffer

Gel
Filter
Sealing Mask
Sealing Frame
Porous Support
Vacuum

3 Hybridization with probe and detection

Filter

GenomeLab SNPStream by Beckman Coulter is another example of microarray technology that was customized for RBC antigen typing at the Genome Quebec Innovation Center, Canada.[33]

Fluorescent In Situ Hybridization

In this technique, scientists use fluorescent probes to detect homologous DNA or RNA sequences in chromosomes or intact cells. In this case, the hybridization of the probe to specific cells or subcellular structures is determined by direct microscopic examination. In 1995, this method was used to localize the ABO gene to chromosome 9.[34]

PCR-Based and Other Amplification Techniques

Amplification of DNA by PCR allows the detection of even single copies of DNA molecules. By contrast, Southern blotting has a detection limit of around 100,000 copies. The specificity of the PCR amplification depends on the primers that hybridize to complementary sequences of the template molecule spanning the target DNA fragment. With carefully chosen primers, PCR can be used to selectively amplify DNA molecules from complex mixtures, such as genomic DNA from cell extracts.

Real-Time PCR

In **real-time PCR**, conducted in a special type of thermocycler (**LightCycler**), the product formed during each cycle of amplification is detected by fluorescence at the same time that it is produced. In addition to primers, the real-time reaction mixture contains DNA probes that are complementary to the region between the primers (called **TaqMan** or **molecular beacons** or **FRET** probes), labeled with fluorophores that emit fluorescent light when binding to the newly synthesized amplicon. If the assay is used to detect polymorphism, a post-PCR monitoring of amplicon/probe separation upon slow increase of temperature is performed. This process is called **melting curve analysis** and allows for determination of homo- or heterozygosity. A classical example of melting curve analysis is the detection of factor V Leiden mutation in patients with this inherited coagulopathy.[35]

Real-time PCR allows the quantification of specific mRNAs in complex mixtures and is extremely useful in the study of gene expression when combined with reverse transcription.

Reverse Transcriptase PCR

Single copies of RNA can be detected by adding a step of cDNA synthesis by reverse transcription (RT), prior to the PCR amplification (RT-PCR). By RT-PCR, cDNA molecules can be specifically amplified from total RNA obtained from cell extracts, tissue sections, or plasma. The high sensitivity of PCR-based DNA and RNA detection techniques makes them valuable for early detection of transfusion-transmitted viruses, such as HIV and hepatitis B and C. The first RT-PCR assays developed by National Genetics Institute (UltraQual HIV-1) and by Roche (COBAS AmpliScreen HIV-1) were designed to detect these pathogens in donors' blood and were approved by the FDA in 2001 and 2003.[28,36] Real-time RT-PCR is employed in the **multiplex assay** for concurrent detection of HIV, HCV, and HBV (Roche Cobas TaqScreen MPX).[37]

Transcription Mediated Amplification

Other FDA approved tests for HIV, HCV, HBV, and West Nile virus in donors' blood are performed by means of another method developed by Gen-Probe: **transcription mediated amplification** (TMA). The starting material in this assay is RNA. The RNA serves as a template for a reverse transcriptase to synthesize a complementary DNA, which is bound to the RNA by hydrogen bonds to form a RNA/DNA hybrid. The DNA is never amplified in the assay. After enzymatic removal of the RNA from the hybrid, the DNA is transcribed to hundreds of RNA molecules. These multiple RNA molecules go through another reverse transcription process to produce more RNA/DNA hybrids, and the whole process is repeated many times. The detection of the pathogen (if its RNA is present in the sample) occurs via **hybridization protection assay** (HPA) technology. In this technology, ssDNA probes labeled with chemiluminescent molecules are added to form hybrids with the amplified RNA molecules produced during TMA. Light is emitted upon hybridization of the probes to the RNA and captured by a **luminometer**.

Nucleic acid testing (NAT) is rapidly becoming a standard method in blood banking. It allows the detection of pathogens before the appearance of a testable immune response, such as screening of antibodies. Narrowing the **preseroconversion** window (during which donors can be infected but do not yet test positive by serologic methods) helps to enhance the safety of blood products.[38,39] Since NAT implementation, the average seroconversion window for HIV has been shortened to 11 days (as compared to 22 days when using serologic testing and 16 days when performing the standard confirmatory p24 antigen testing). The average seroconversion window for HCV has been shortened to 10 days (as compared to the original 82 days when serologic testing is used). Consequently, the residual risk of HIV transmission decreased from 9.7 to 1.2 incidents per million donations, and the residual risk of HCV transmission decreased from 2 to 1 incident per million donations. A significant progress in testing for the transfusion-transmitted pathogens in donor units was the ability of the NAT assays to detect these pathogens concurrently. In 2008, the Gen-Probe assay, initially approved for detection of HIV-1 and HCV only, was also approved for the detection of HBV.[36]

Antibodies as Probes for Proteins

Gene expression at the protein level can be studied by using labeled antibodies as probes. In particular, monoclonal antibodies are widely used in the technique called **immunoblotting**.[40] This technique is also known as **Western blotting** by analogy to Southern and Northern blotting. Proteins in cell extracts are separated by polyacrylamide gel electrophoresis in the presence of the ionic detergent SDS. In **SDS-PAGE** electrophoresis, each protein binds many detergent molecules, which causes its denaturation and provides a negative charge. Proteins will migrate to the anode; the rate of migration depends on their size. The proteins are then transferred from the gel onto a filter membrane. The protein/antigen of interest is detected by incubation of the membrane with a specific labeled antibody. An example of Western blot is the HIV p24 confirmatory testing.

Techniques for Studying Gene Polymorphism

By recombinant DNA techniques, experimental analysis proceeds either from DNA into protein or from protein into DNA. An important consequence for transfusion medicine has been the introduction of techniques for typing molecular polymorphism, not only at the protein level but also at the genetic level. These techniques are usually grouped under the name of **DNA typing**.

Restriction Fragment Length Polymorphism

Restriction Fragment Length Polymorphism (RFLP) can be used to detect the glycosyl transferase gene in a person who is type AO or BO. The nucleotide deletion of the O allele results in the loss of a *BstEII* site (GGTGACC) and creation of a new *KpnI* site (GGTACC). RFLP can also be used to determine if an individual carries the mutation for sickle cell anemia. The gene that codes for hemoglobin S (HbS) has one nucleotide difference with the normal β-globin coding allele. The sixth codon of the defective gene is GTG (Val). The sixth codon of the normal gene is GAG (Glu). The restriction site for *MstII* (CCTGAGG) is lost in the mutated gene (CCTGTGG). RFLP is widely used in HLA typing for transplantation (Fig. 4–11), in paternity testing and in forensic science (refer to Chapter 22, "Relationship Testing").

PCR and Allele-Specific Probes

PCR can be used to amplify polymorphic genes from genomic DNA. The PCR products are blotted on a nylon filter and hybridized with specific probes that allow the distinction of the different known alleles. This method, usually called **dot blotting** or **sequence-specific oligonucleotide probe** (SSOP), is commonly used for HLA typing (Fig. 4–12).

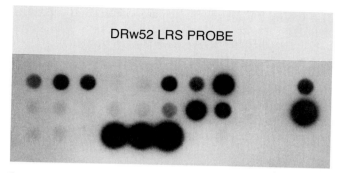

Figure 4–12.   Sequence-specific oligonucleotide probe (SSOP). Dot-blot of PCR products hybridized to an allelic-specific HLA probe.

A variation of this method is **sequence-specific PCR** (SSP), in which the alleles are distinguished by PCR amplification with primer pairs specific for one allele or a group of alleles. Genomic DNA is submitted to PCR amplification with a battery of primer pairs. The products of the different PCR reactions are run in an agarose gel and stained with EB or SYBR Green. The presence of fluorescent bands of a defined size in the gel indicates the presence of the allele for which the primer pair is specific (Fig. 4–13).

DNA Sequencing

Alleles of polymorphic genes can also be specifically amplified by PCR and sequenced after cloning into plasmid vectors. Alternatively, direct sequencing of PCR products can be done without previous cloning, if the product obtained is pure enough. This procedure is currently used in

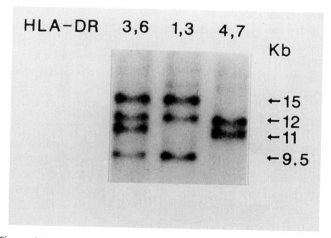

Figure 4–11.   Restriction fragment length polymorphisms (RFLPs). Southern blot analysis of genomic DNA to determine HLA-DR genotype.

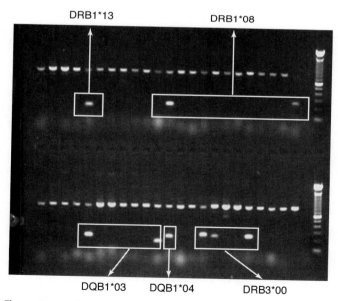

Figure 4–13.   Sequence-specific PCR (SSP). Genomic DNA was PCR amplified with primer pairs specific for different HLA class II alleles or group of alleles. Note the control band indicating successful PCR. (*Courtesy of HLA laboratory, Department of Transfusion Medicine, NIH.*)

HLA typing for allogeneic hematopoietic stem cell transplant (HSCT).

DNA Profiling or "Fingerprinting"

Minisatellites and **microsatellites** are regions of DNA interspersed in the human genome formed by **variable number of tandem repeats** (VNTRs) of short nucleotide sequences. The variability depends on the number of repeat units contained within each "satellite." Minisatellites or variable tandem repeats are composed of repeated units ranging in size from 9 to 80 bp. Microsatellites or **short tandem repeats** (STRs) contain repeat units of 2 to 5 nucleotides.

The polymorphism of these loci in the human population is so high that there is a very low probability that two individuals will have the same number of repeats. When several loci are analyzed simultaneously, the probability of finding two individuals in the human population with the same polymorphic pattern is extremely low. The independence of inheritance of the different loci tested is ensured by choosing loci on different chromosomes. The pattern of polymorphism (the differences in number of repeats or length) can be determined by RFLP or PCR analysis. In 1997, the Federal Bureau of Investigation recommended a panel of 13 STRs, plus an XY marker, for criminal investigations. With this number of independently inherited polymorphisms, the probability of even the most common combinations is less than 1 in 10 billion. Thus, modern DNA testing can uniquely identify each person, hence the name **DNA fingerprinting**. DNA profiling is used in forensic applications, paternity testing, and to follow chimerism after HSCT.

Systems Biology

The molecular techniques developed in recent years and older techniques, still valuable in the study of nucleic acids and the cellular processes they are involved in, keep improving and expanding. Many are being automated and miniaturized. While it is necessary to have the exact sequence of DNA that is of interest (e.g., if it is associated with an inherited disease), it is equally important to understand how that DNA is expressed inside of a living cell. As technology is developed, it will be interesting to see what new methods become available and occur in common use. Of particular interest to biotechnology is the development of nanotechnology and nanostring technology applications, high throughput DNA systems, and computational bioinformatics in which complex models of expression and regulation (such as proteasomes) are being assembled and analyzed.

Some of the most exciting recent advances in molecular biology have been the result of analyzing the complete nucleotide sequence of the human genome. A draft sequence of the human genome was published in 2001 by two independent teams of researchers.[24,41] The public effort was led by the International Human Genome Project, which used BAC libraries (briefly described in the "Tools for DNA Cloning" section). The other group, led by Craig Venter of Celera Genomics, used a "shotgun" approach in which small fragments of genomic DNA were cloned and sequenced.

Overlaps between the fragment sequences were used to assemble the whole genome. This draft encompassed about 90% of the euchromatin portion of the human genome. Continuing work by researchers around the world rendered a high-quality human genome sequence in 2003—50 years after the *Nature* paper in which Watson and Crick described the structure of DNA. This wealth of information, which is constantly updated, can be accessed through the National Center for Biotechnology Information (NCBI) website (www.ncbi.nlm.nih.gov).[42]

In its first 50 years, molecular biology has been primarily an analytical science, concerned mainly with reducing biological problems to the level of individual genes. This approach has been extraordinarily successful in finding the key genes involved in cellular replication and development and in identifying the genes involved in genetic disorders. The challenge for the next few decades is going to be understanding the synchronized activity of numerous genes during key biological events, such as development and memory, and understanding the multiple genes presumably involved in complex diseases such as cancer and diabetes. Another complication is the fact that several different proteins can be produced from a single gene by alternative RNA splicing and that additional forms are created by post-translational modifications.

To solve these complex issues, biologists are turning to more synthetic approaches that allow them to examine the coordinated expression of multiple genes. Experiments performed using DNA and protein chips are starting to show how hundreds or thousands of genes are expressed coordinately in response to different developmental and environmental stimuli. Analysis of these data is one of the applications of bioinformatics, a discipline that uses computer algorithms to manage and analyze large-scale experiments.

The functions of genes implicated in a specific pathway can be further explored by **reverse genetics**. Genes can be "knocked out" or "knocked in" as wild type or mutated into the germline of a mouse or other animal model.[43,44] The resulting **knockout transgenic animal** can be analyzed for metabolic or behavioral changes, which can give clues to the mechanism of function of the gene under study. A novel way of studying specific gene function is RNA interference, by which small synthetic RNA molecules can be used to silence a specific target gene.[16] This new biology that is emerging is called *systems biology*, and it requires integration of knowledge from experiments done in vitro, in vivo, and in silico (in a computer).

Red Cell Genotyping

Molecular RBC antigen typing could be of tremendous advantage in situations where serologic testing is impossible or inconclusive. Currently considered as supplemental rather than routine practice, it has the potential to revolutionize the way blood cell inventory may be searched for multiple antigen-negative units. The knowledge of theoretical principles and practical skills to perform red cell genotyping are becoming indispensable in contemporary blood banking.

Genetic Basis of Blood Groups

Early important events in the molecular biology of transfusion medicine includes the cloning and sequencing of the gene that codes for the MN polymorphism, *GYPA*, in 1986, followed by the *ABO* gene in 1990 (review Table 4–1). Now the genes for all the blood group systems have been identified and localized in specific chromosomal regions.[23] Also known are the alleles that code for the blood group polymorphisms, the structure of the gene products, and in many cases their function. This knowledge has allowed the development of red cell group typing at the DNA level. Molecular genotyping is being increasingly used in clinical blood banking, where it does not replace but complements traditional phenotyping. Molecular biology provides information to help make decisions in transfusion medicine, such as obtaining compatible blood in cases of massive transfusion or transplantation. The field of molecular biology is constantly changing and improving. Methods become more efficient and less expensive. As greater numbers of populations are analyzed, different alleles are discovered and added to databases that are updated frequently.

A committee of the International Society of Blood Transfusion (ISBT) is responsible for the nomenclature of red cell surface antigens. A monograph published in 2004 described the ISBT terminology for red cell surface antigens and genes and tabulated a complete classification.[45] Since then, two updates have been published.[46,47] The full current classification can be found at the ISBT/IBGRL website (http://ibgrl.blood.co.uk/).[48]

Most of the blood group systems are coded by variants of a single gene. There are four exceptions: Rh; Xg; Chido/Rodgers, which have two genes each; and MNS, which has three. As an example, the Rh system consists of two genes: *D* and *CE*. These genes have 97% homology, which can add difficulty in molecular methods for genotyping this system. Table 4–3 enumerates the blood group systems, their genes with the chromosomal location, and the corresponding antigens.

Molecular Basis of Blood Group Polymorphism

According to the Blood Group Antigen Gene Mutation Data base (dbRBC) as of July 7, 2010, there were 30 blood group systems, 39 genes, and 1,165 alleles known in the human population. The dbRBC contains a complete collection of genes and alleles and provides comprehensive information on blood groups antigens.[49] It is frequently updated and provides DNA sequences and alignments.

The systems ABO, P, Lewis, H, I, and MNS comprise antigens that are carbohydrates on glycoproteins or glycolipids. The genes that constitute these systems code for glycosyltransferases that catalyze oligosaccharide chain synthesis. For the rest of the blood group systems, the antigens are direct consequences of amino acid variation in the protein sequence. Most blood group variants are the result of one or more single nucleotide polymorphisms (SNPs) encoding amino acid substitutions in a glycosyltransferase or the extracellular domain of a membrane protein. Other mechanisms of polymorphism generation are gene deletion, single nucleotide deletion, insertion, and **intergenic recombination**. Clinically significant blood group systems are listed in **Table 4–3**.

Clinical Applications of Red Cell Genotyping

There are several important applications for red cell genotyping in use today.[50,51] These methods help to confirm serologic testing. In cases where serology is not possible or not sensitive enough or where discrepancies occur, genotyping provides results that can be used to obtain a blood type on a donor or patient. Applications of genotyping include fetal DNA typing, blood group typing of donors for alloimmunized patients, screening blood donors to locate rare blood group phenotypes, screening blood inventory for antigen-negative units, determining the frequency of blood group polymorphisms in a given population, determining zygosity for the fathers of fetuses at risk for hemolytic disease of the fetus and newborn (HDFN), and blood group typing of patients with autoimmune hemolytic anemia and other diseases.

Fetal DNA Typing

Initially, ABO and Rh typing should be done on a pregnant mother and should include an antibody screening. If the woman is D negative and has a negative antibody screen using IgG AHG techniques, she is a candidate for RhIG. If the antibody screening is positive, then the antibody specificity must be determined. If the father has the corresponding antigen, then his zygosity, either heterozygous or homozygous, should be established. If the father is heterozygous, then the genotype of the fetus can be determined using PCR testing of **amniocentesis** samples, **chorionic villus sampling**, or **cordocentesis** samples.

PCR has a very high sensitivity, approaching 100%, and a low false-negative rate, so it is an excellent method. DNA probes are known for most if not all genes playing a role in HDFN. As an alternate approach, the typing for the D antigen at the molecular level can be done on maternal samples as early as the second trimester. Fetal DNA in maternal samples is derived from **apoptotic syncytiotrophoblasts**; it increases in concentration throughout pregnancy and is cleared soon after delivery.

Maternal-only, sample DNA testing will likely become more routine in the near future, as it has many advantages. All DNA-based information allows earlier intervention in cases where HDFN is suspected.[52] (Refer to Chapter 19, "Hemolytic Disease of the Fetus and Newborn [HDFN].") In addition to HDFN, there is risk to the developing fetus in cases of platelet and neutrophil antigen incompatibility, resulting in **fetal and neonatal alloimmune thrombocytopenia** (FNAIT) and **neonatal alloimmune neutropenia** (NAN). Genotyping can help resolve these cases and determine if there is an associated risk due to maternal platelet and neutrophil antigens and HLA type.

Table 4–3 **Blood Group Systems with Number of Antigens, Coding Gene(s), and Chromosomal Location**

NO.	ISBT SYSTEM NAME	ISBT SYSTEM SYMBOL	GENE NAME(S)	CHROMOSOMAL LOCATION	NO. OF ALLELES
001	ABO	ABO	ABO	9q34.2	4
002	MNS	MNS	GYPA, GYPB, GYPE	4q31.21	46
003	P	P1	P1	22q11.2–qter	1
004	Rh	RH	RHD, RHCE	1p36.11	> 50
005	Lutheran	LU	LU	19q13.32	20
006	Kell	KEL	KEL	7q34	31
007	Lewis	LE	FUT3	19p13.3	6
008	Duffy	FY	DARC	1q23.2	6
009	Kidd	JK	SLC14A1	18q12.3	3
010	Diego	DI	SLC4A1	17q21.31	21
011	Yt	YT	ACHE	7q22.1	2
012	Xg	XG	XG, MIC2	Xp22.33	2
013	Scianna	SC	ERMAP	1p34.2	7
014	Dombrock	DO	ART4	12p12.3	6
015	Colton	CO	AQP1	7p14.3	3
016	Landsteiner-Wiener	LW	ICAM4	19p13.2	3
017	Chido/Rodgers	CH/RG	C4A, C4B	6p21.3	9
018	H	H	FUT1	19q13.33	1
019	Kx	XK	XK	Xp21.1	1
020	Gerbich	GE	GYPC	2q14.3	8
021	Cromer	CROM	CD55	1q32.2	15
022	Knops	KN	CR1	1q32.2	9
023	Indian	IN	CD44	11p13	4
024	Ok	OK	BSG	19p13.3	1
025	Raph	RAPH	CD151	11p15.5	1
026	John Milton Hagen	JMH	SEMA7A	15q24.1	5
027	I	I	GCNT2	6p24.2	1
028	Globoside	GLOB	B3GALT3	3q26.1	1
029	Gill	GIL	AQP3	9p13.3	1
030	Rh-associated glycoprotein	RHAG	RHAG	6p21-qter	3

Extensive Blood Group Typing of Donors for Alloimmunized Patients

Patients with multiple antibodies may require extensive testing to find compatible blood for transfusion. It is now possible to genotype potential donors and the patient to prevent further immunization and to characterize the donor at a more specific level.[53] DNA testing can be done in place of extensive family studies to determine the genotype. Sequencing of the entire gene of interest, often required to obtain sufficient information, may be labor-intensive. The amount of work may be lessened if exon sequencing is done first and if RFLPs can be done on certain areas of the gene at the beginning of the study. Focused sequencing with comparisons to antigenic profiles can also be used. Having extensive information on the patients' and the potential donors' genotypes allows transfusion to take place in a safer environment. Knowing the antigens that the patient does not have based on genotyping prevents further alloantibodies from being made from the transfusion of blood that is positive for these antigens. Because red cells have lost their nuclei, white cells can be used for genotyping and other normal adult diploid cells.

Screening of Blood Donors to Find Rare Blood Group Phenotypes

Using DNA-based methods to screen blood donors allows for a high-throughput system screening in comparison with serology-based methods. Blood group antisera often are not readily available for rare blood group phenotypes or are prohibitively expensive to use on a large scale. Genotyping with PCR techniques allows for the probes (or primers) to be synthesized at low cost and used in DNA-based methods, as long as information about the sequence of the gene is known. Different alleles can be tested at the same time in the multiplex PCR assays or on microarrays. Once known, the genotype information can be put into a database and does not require repeated testing, which saves considerable time and money. A rare donor profile can be generated, linking potential donors to potential recipients for better recruitment in cases of emergency. For patients requiring donor units with rare phenotypes, the costs and time involved in genotyping such donor units are acceptable.

Determining the Frequency of Blood Group Polymorphisms in a Population

Genotyping databases can be used to predict the possibility of finding a specific allele in a given population once a similar population has been analyzed at the genotype level. Because most blood group alleles are the result of a single nucleotide polymorphism, screening of blood samples for allele frequency can be relatively easy and done by simple DNA-based methods. Several different methods employed for this include RFLP and SSP-PCR (single or multiplex), real-time quantitative PCR, sequencing and microarray technology using DNA probes on chips.

Blood Group Typing of Patients With Autoimmune Hemolytic Anemia and Other Diseases

Patients with autoimmune hemolytic anemia and other conditions such as sickle cell anemia can have trouble obtaining compatible donor units. They are often sensitized to many antigens and have a rapid turnover of red cells, requiring frequent transfusion. Because they can have a complex population of red cells, with autologous cells mixed with transfused cells from more than one donor, genotyping methods are an excellent way to type these donors. A small amount of patient white cells or cheek cells can be used to determine the genotype using standard DNA-based methods, and the subsequent patient phenotype can be determined from the genotype.

Although crossmatching may not provide totally compatible results, especially with autoimmune diseases, at least alloantigens can be ruled out when transfusion is required, thereby preventing further alloimmunization in an already-difficult-to-transfuse patient. In addition to saving the time required for repeated adsorptions, elutions, and extensive phenotyping in these patients and in donor units, the information obtained by DNA-based methods is highly accurate and easy to obtain. It is a permanent record of the patient's genetic profile, and it is necessary information in cases where transplant may be considered. It is also a permanent record of the donor's profile when performed.

SUMMARY CHART

- ✔ The central dogma of molecular biology: DNA → RNA → protein.
- ✔ Proteins have structural, enzymatic, and gene-regulatory function. Through these mechanisms, the genotype of a cell is translated into its phenotype.
- ✔ DNA is the genetic material.
- ✔ DNA is a double helix, consisting of two antiparallel strands of stacked nucleotides paired through hydrogen bonds. Adenine (A) always pairs with thymine (T), and cytosine (C) always pairs with guanine (G).
- ✔ The structure of DNA determines its function. The sequence of nucleotides of one strand determines the sequence of its complementary strand, the basis for the semiconservative way of replication.
- ✔ A gene is transcribed into precursor RNA, and the spliced mRNA is translated into the amino acid sequence of the coded protein. The sequence of mRNA unequivocally determines the sequence of the protein.

Continued

SUMMARY CHART—cont'd

✔ Recombinant DNA is the DNA of one organism "cut and pasted" into a carrier vector. The foreign gene introduced in a host organism is functional because the genetic code is universal.

✔ By DNA cloning, recombinant genes of complex animals, such as humans, are introduced into simple organisms, such as bacteria, and other model organisms, such as mice, allowing structural and functional studies.

✔ Restriction endonucleases, bacterial enzymes that recognize and cut specific DNA sequences, are fundamental tools for DNA cloning.

✔ Gel electrophoresis separates nucleic acids by size.

✔ The most common host cell is the bacterium *E. coli*.

✔ Plasmids, the most commonly used vectors, are independently replicating circular DNA molecules modified to provide the host cell with resistance to antibiotics (selectable marker) and one or more restriction enzyme sites for inserting the recombinant gene.

✔ By reverse transcription, mRNA is transcribed into complementary DNA (cDNA).

✔ Automated fluorescent DNA sequencing based on the Sanger dideoxy, chain termination method is a standard laboratory procedure.

✔ DNA sequencing of a cloned cDNA corresponding to a given gene is the easiest way to determine the amino acid sequence of a protein.

✔ Genomic and cDNA libraries are collections of clones containing the genetic material of a cell.

✔ Base pairing between complementary strands of DNA or RNA (hybridization with a labeled probe) is used to detect specific nucleic acid sequences in complex mixtures.

✔ Southern blotting, Northern blotting, and dot blotting are hybridization-based techniques for nucleic acid sequence-specific recognition.

✔ The polymerase chain reaction (PCR) is an in vitro method for DNA amplification.

✔ Molecular polymorphism is studied at the genetic level by DNA typing. Methods for DNA typing relevant for transfusion medicine are restriction fragment length polymorphism, allele-specific oligonucleotide probe hybridization, allele-specific PCR amplification, DNA sequencing, and DNA profiling (DNA fingerprinting).

✔ PCR and TMA are used for the early detection of transfusion-transmitted pathogens.

✔ Other therapeutic uses of molecular biology are gene therapy and the clinical use of recombinant proteins, such as interferons, coagulation factors, and growth factors.

✔ Molecular RBC antigen typing is used to either confirm serologic testing or in cases where serology is not possible or is not sensitive enough or where discrepancies occur.

Review Questions

1. The central dogma of molecular biology states that:
   a. DNA is the genetic material
   b. RNA is the genetic material
   c. DNA is translated to mRNA
   d. Proteins are transcribed from mRNA

2. Recombinant-DNA technology is possible because:
   a. Restriction endonucleases cut RNA
   b. Restriction endonucleases cut proteins
   c. The genetic code is universal
   d. Bacteria are difficult to culture

3. Agarose gel electrophoresis is a technique used for:
   a. DNA synthesis
   b. RNA synthesis
   c. Separation of DNA molecules by size
   d. Oligonucleotide synthesis

4. Restriction fragment length polymorphism (RFLP) is based on the use of the enzymes:
   a. Reverse transcriptases
   b. Bacterial endonucleases
   c. DNA polymerases
   d. RNA polymerases

5. The polymerase chain reaction (PCR):
   a. Is carried out in vivo
   b. Is used for peptide synthesis
   c. Requires RNA polymerase
   d. Is used for the amplification of DNA

6. Plasmids are:
   a. Vectors used for molecular cloning
   b. Antibiotics
   c. Enzymes
   d. Part of chromosomes

7. Some model organisms:
   a. Simplify the study of human disease
   b. Are used to produce recombinant proteins
   c. Are prokaryotes and some are eukaryotes
   d. All of the above

8. DNA sequencing:
   a. Is more difficult than peptide sequencing
   b. Requires the use of RNA polymerase
   c. Can never be automated
   d. Is an enzymatic in vitro reaction

9. RFLP and SSP are techniques used for:
   a. Protein isolation
   b. RNA isolation
   c. DNA typing
   d. Protein typing

10. Recombinant DNA techniques:
   a. Are not used in a clinical setting
   b. Are useful research tools
   c. Are not used in blood banking
   d. Are useful only for research

11. Transcription mediated amplification:
   a. Requires thermostable DNA polymerase
   b. Is an isothermal procedure
   c. Is an obsolete method currently replaced by SSOP
   d. Utilizes probes labeled with fluorescent tags

12. Preseroconversion window:
   a. Is the time when donors can be infected but do not yet test positive by serologic methods
   b. May be narrowed by using molecular methods
   c. Refers mainly to viral pathogens
   d. All of the above

13. Red blood cell molecular antigen typing is useful in all listed situations except:
   a. In screening RBC inventory for antigen-negative units
   b. When reagent antibodies are weak or unavailable
   c. In quantitative gene expression analysis
   d. When resolving ABO discrepancies

References

1. Crick, F: Central dogma of molecular biology. Nature 227(5258):561–563, 1970.
2. Griffith, F: The significance of pneumococcal types. J Hyg (Lond) 27(2):113–159, 1928.
3. Avery, OT, MacLeod, CM, and McCarty M: Studies on the chemical nature of the substance inducing transformation of pneumococcal types. Induction of transformation by a desoxyribonucleic acid fraction isolated from *Pneumococcus* type III. J Exp Med 1;79(2):137–158, 1944.
4. Hershey, AD, and Chase, M: Independent functions of viral protein and nucleic acid in growth of bacteriophage. J Gen Physiol 36(1):39–56, 1952.
5. Chargraff, E, Magasanik, B, Visher, E, Green, C, Doniger, R, and Elson, D: Nucleotide composition of pentose nucleic acids from yeast and mammalian tissues. J Biol Chem 186(1):51–67, 1950.
6. Watson, JD, and Crick, FHC: Molecular structure of nucleic acids: A structure for deoxyribose nucleic acid. Nature 171:737–738, 1953.
7. Breslauer, KJ, et al: Predicting DNA duplex stability from the base sequence. Proc Natl Acad Sci USA 83(11):3746–3750, 1986.
8. Lewin, B: Genes VIII. Prentice Hall, New York, 2004, p 392.
9. Pauling, L, Itano, HA, et al: Sickle cell anemia a molecular disease. Science 110(2865):543–548, 1949.
10. Ingram, VM: Gene mutations in human hemoglobin: The chemical difference between normal and sickle cell hemoglobin. Nature 180:326–328, 1957.
11. Keller, EB, Zamecnik, PC, and Loftfield, RB: The role of microsomes in the incorporation of amino acids into proteins. J Histochem Cytochem 2(5):378–386, 1954.

12. Brenner, S, Jacob, F, and Meselson, M: An unstable intermediate carrying information from genes to ribosomes for protein synthesis. Nature 190:576–581, 1961.
13. Nirenberg, M, and Leder, P: RNA codewords and protein synthesis. Science 145:1399–1407, 1964.
14. Temin, HM, and Mizutani, S: RNA-dependent DNA polymerase in virions of Rous sarcoma virus. Nature 226:1211–1213, 1970.
15. Baltimore, D: RNA-dependent DNA polymerase in virions of RNA tumour viruses. Nature 226:1209–1211, 1970.
16. Sharp, PA: RNA interference—2001. Genes Dev 15:485–490, 2001.
17. Yamamoto, F, et al: Cloning and characterization of DNA complementary to human Histo-blood group A transferase mRNA. J Biol Chem 265:1146–1151, 1990.
18. Sambrook, J, and Russell, DW: Molecular Cloning: A Laboratory Manual, 3rd ed. Cold Spring Harbor Laboratory Press, Cold Spring Harbor, NY, 2001.
19. Alberts, B, et al: Molecular biology of the cell, 4th ed. Garland Publishing, New York, 2002.
20. Nathans, D, and Smith, HO: Restriction endonucleases in the analysis and restructuring of DNA molecules. Ann Rev Biochem 44:273–293, 1975.
21. Wagner FF, and Flegel, WA: *RHD* gene deletion occurred in the *Rhesus box*. Blood 95:3662–3668, 2000.
22. Kirsanov, KI, Lesovaya, EA, Yakubovskaya, MG, and Belitsky, GA: SYBR Gold and SYBR Green II are not mutagenic in the Ames test. Mutat Res 699(1-2):1–4, 2010.
23. Logdberg, L, Reid, M, and Zelinski, T: Human blood group genes 2010: Chromosomal locations and cloning strategies revisited. Transfus Med Rev 25(1):36–46, 2011.
24. International Human Genome Sequencing Consortium: Initial sequencing and analysis of the human genome. Nature 409:860–921, 2001.
25. Gaspar, HB: Bone marrow transplantation and alternatives for adenosine deaminase deficiency. Immunol Allergy Clin North Am 30(2):221–236, 2010.
26. Saiki, RK, Gelfand, DH, Stoffel, S, Scharf R, Higuchi, R, Horn, GT, et al: Primer-directed enzymatic amplification of DNA with a thermostable DNA polymerase. Science 239:487–491, 1988.
27. Busch, MP, and Kleinman, SH: Nucleic acid amplification testing of blood donors for transfusion-transmitted diseases. Report of the Interorganizational Task Force on nucleic acid amplification testing of blood donors. Transfusion 40:143–159, 2000.
28. Kraj, B, and Nadder, T: Blood donor screening process and infectious disease testing using molecular methods. Advance for Medical Laboratory Professionals, 17–20, October 8, 2007.
29. Sanger, F, Nicklen, S, and Coulson, AR: DNA sequencing with chain-terminating inhibitors. Proc Natl Acad Sci USA 74:5463–5467, 1977.
30. Southern, EM: Detection of specific sequences among DNA fragments separated by gel electrophoresis. J Mol Biol 98:503–517, 1975.
31. Brown, PO, and Botstein, D: Exploring the new world of the genome with DNA microarrays. Nat Genet 21:33–37, 1999.
32. Hashmi, G, et al: A flexible array format for large-scale, rapid blood group DNA typing. Transfusion 45(5):680–688, 2005.
33. Montpetit, A, et al: High-throughput molecular profiling of blood donors for minor red blood cell and platelet antigens. Transfusion 46(5):841–848, 2006.
34. Bennett, EP, et al: Genomic cloning of the human histo-blood group ABO locus. Biochem Biophys Res Commun 206(1):318–325, 1995.
35. Lyondagger, E, Millsondagger, A, Phan, T, and Wittwer, CT: Detection and Identification of base alterations within the region of factor V Leiden by fluorescent melting curves. Mol Diagn 3(4):203–209, 1998.

36. U.S. Food and Drug Administration: Complete list of donor screening assays for infectious agents and HIV diagnostic assays. Available at www.fda.gov/cber/products/testkits.htm.
37. Wiedmann, M, Kluwick, S, Walter, M, Fauchald, G, Howe, J, Bronold, M, et al: HIV-1, HCV and HBV seronegative window reduction by the new Roche cobas TaqScreen MPX test in seroconverting donors. J Clin Virol 39(4):282–287, 2007.
38. Glynn, SA, Kleinman, SH, Wright, DJ, and Busch, MP: International application of the incidence rate/window period model. Transfusion 42:966–972, 2002.
39. Dodd, RY, Notari, EP, Stramer, S: Current prevalence and incidence of infectious disease markers and estimated window period risk in the American Red Cross blood donor population Transfusion 42:975–979, 2002.
40. Kohler, G, and Milstein, C: Continuous cultures of fused cells secreting antibody of predefined specificity. Nature 256:495–497, 1975.
41. Venter, JC, et al: The sequence of the human genome. Science 291:1304–1351, 2001.
42. National Center for Biotechnology Information (NCBI) website: www.ncbi.nlm.nih.gov.
43. Capecchi, MR: Altering the genome by homologous recombination. Science 244:1288–1292, 1989.
44. Bronson, SK, and Smithies, O: Altering mice by homologous recombination using embryonic stem cells. J Biol Chem 269:27155–27158, 1995.
45. Daniels, GL, et al: Blood group terminology 2004: From the International Society of Blood Transfusion committee on terminology for red cell surface antigens. Vox Sanguinis 87:304–316, 2004.
46. Daniels, GL, et al. International Society of Blood Transfusion Committee on terminology for red cell surface antigens: Cape Town report. Vox Sanguinis 92:250–253, 2007.
47. Daniels GL, et al. International Society of Blood Transfusion Committee on terminology for red blood cell surface antigens: Macao report. Vox Sanguinis 96:153–156, 2009.
48. ISBT/IBGRL website: http://ibgrl.blood.co.uk/.
49. Blumenfeld, OO, and Patnaik, SK. Allelic genes of blood group antigens: A source of human mutations and cSNPs documented in the Blood Group Antigen Gene Mutation Database. Hum Mutat 23(1):8–16, 2004.
50. Reid, ME: Transfusion in the age of molecular diagnostics. Hematology 171–177, 2009.
51. Westhoff, CM: The potential of blood group genotyping for transfusion medicine practice. Immunohematology 24(4):190–195, 2008.
52. Finning, K, Martin, P, Summers, J, and Daniels, G: Fetal genotyping for the K (Kell) and Rh C, c, and E blood groups on cell-free fetal DNA in maternal plasma. Transfusion 47:2126–2133, 2007.
53. Anstee, DJ: Red cell genotyping and the future of pretransfusion testing. Blood 114:(2), 2009.
54. The dbRBC, Blood Group Antigen Gene Mutation Database. Historical landmarks in the field of study of blood group systems. Available at www.ncbi.nlm.nih.gov/projects/gv/rbc/xslcgi.fcgi?cmd=bgmut/landmarks.

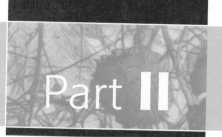

Chapter 5

The Antiglobulin Test

Ralph E. B. Green, BAppSc, FAIMLS, MACE and Dwane A. Klostermann, MSTM, MT(ASCP)SBB

OBJECTIVES

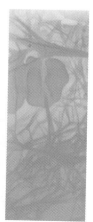

1. State the principle of the antiglobulin test.
2. Differentiate monoclonal from polyclonal and monospecific from polyspecific antihuman globulin (AHG) reagents.
3. Describe the preparation of monoclonal and polyclonal AHG reagents.
4. List the antibody requirements for AHG reagents.
5. Explain the use of polyspecific versus monospecific AHG in the indirect antiglobulin test (IAT).
6. List the advantages and disadvantages of anticomplement activity in polyspecific AHG.
7. Compare and contrast the IAT and the direct antiglobulin test (DAT).
8. Explain the principle and applications of red blood cell sensitization.
9. Explain the reasons for the procedural steps in the DAT and IAT.
10. Interpret the results of a DAT and IAT panel.
11. Identify the factors that affect the antiglobulin test.

Continued

Introduction

The **antihuman globulin test**, which is also referred to as the **Coombs' test**, is based on the principle that **antihuman globulins** (AHGs) obtained from immunized nonhuman species bind to human globulins such as **IgG** or **complement**, either free in serum or attached to antigens on red blood cells (RBCs). The antihuman globulin test (AGT) is an essential testing methodology when it comes to transfusion medicine; without its use, patients' well-being would be negatively impacted.

There are two major types of blood group antibodies: IgM and IgG. Because of their large pentamer structure, IgM antibodies bind to corresponding antigen and directly agglutinate RBCs suspended in saline. Some IgG antibodies are termed **nonagglutinating**, or **incomplete antibodies**, because their monomer structure is too small to directly agglutinate sensitized RBCs (refer back to the ionic cloud concept schematic found in Chapter 3, "Fundamentals of Immunology"). Adding AHG that contains anti-IgG to RBCs sensitized with IgG antibodies allows for hemagglutination of these sensitized cells. We use an anti-antibody to observe the formation of an Ag/Ab complex that would otherwise go undetected. Some blood group antibodies have the ability to bind complement to the RBC membrane. In such cases, an anticomplement component can be added to the AHG reagent, rendering it polyspecific. Antiglobulin tests detect IgG or complement-sensitized RBCs.

History of the Antiglobulin Test

Before the antiglobulin test was developed, only IgM antibodies were detected. The introduction of the AGT permitted the detection of nonagglutinating IgG antibodies and led to the discovery and characterization of many new blood group systems.

In 1945, Coombs and associates[1] described the use of the antiglobulin test for the detection of weak and nonagglutinating Rh antibodies in serum. In 1946, Coombs and coworkers[2] described the use of AHG to detect in vivo sensitization of the RBCs (later called the **direct antiglobulin test [DAT]**) of babies suffering from hemolytic disease of the newborn (HDN). Although the test was initially of great value in the investigation of Rh HDN, its versatility for detecting other IgG blood group antibodies soon became evident.

The first of the Kell blood group system antibodies[3] and the associated antigen were reported only weeks after Coombs had described the test. Although Coombs and associates[1] were instrumental in introducing the antiglobulin test

to blood group serology, the principle of the test had in fact been described by Moreschi[4] in 1908. Moreschi's studies used rabbit antigoat serum to agglutinate rabbit RBCs that were sensitized with low nonagglutinating doses of goat antirabbit RBC serum.

Coombs' procedure involved the injection of human serum into rabbits to produce **antihuman serum** (described in detail later in this chapter). After absorption to remove heterospecific antibodies and after dilution to avoid prozone, the AHG serum still retained sufficient antibody activity to permit cross-linking of adjacent RBCs sensitized with IgG antibodies. The cross-linking of sensitized RBCs by AHG produced hemagglutination, indicating that the RBCs had been sensitized by an antibody that had reacted with an antigen present on the cell surface.

Early AHG reagents were prepared using a crude globulin fraction as the **immunogen**. In 1947, Coombs and Mourant demonstrated that the antibody activity that detected Rh antibodies was associated with the anti–gamma globulin fraction in the reagent. In 1951, Dacie[5] presented the first indication that there might be another antibody activity present that influenced the final reaction. He observed that different reaction patterns were obtained when dilutions of AHG were used to test cells sensitized with warm as compared with cold antibodies. In 1957, Dacie and coworkers[6] published data showing that the reactivity of AHG to cells sensitized with warm antibodies resulted from anti–gamma globulin activity, whereas anti–nongamma globulin activity was responsible for the activity of cells sensitized by cold antibodies. The nongamma globulin component was shown to be beta globulin and had specificity for complement. Later studies[7,8] revealed that the complement activity was a result of C3 and C4.

The antiglobulin test can be used to detect RBCs sensitized with IgG alloantibodies, IgG autoantibodies, and complement components. **Sensitization** can occur either **in vivo** or **in vitro**. The use of AHG to detect in vitro sensitization of RBCs is a two-stage technique referred to as the **indirect antiglobulin test** (IAT). In vivo sensitization is detected by a one-stage procedure called the **direct antiglobulin test** (DAT). The IAT and DAT still remain the most common procedures performed in blood group serology.[9]

Antihuman Globulin Reagents

Several AHG reagents have been defined by the Food and Drug Administration (FDA) Center for Biologics Evaluation and Research (CBER). These are listed in Table 5–1 and are described in the following paragraphs. Antihuman globulin reagents can be polyspecific or monospecific.

Table 5–1   Antihuman Globulin Reagents

REAGENT	DEFINITION
Polyspecific	
1. Rabbit polyclonal	Contains anti-IgG and anti-C3d (may contain other anticomplement and other anti-immunoglobulin antibodies)
2. Rabbit/murine monoclonal blend	Contains a blend of rabbit polyclonal antihuman IgG and murine monoclonal anti-C3b and anti-C3d.
3. Murine monoclonal	Contains murine monoclonal anti-IgG, anti-C3b, and anti-C3d.
Monospecific Anti-IgG	
1. Rabbit polyclonal	Contains anti-IgG with no anticomplement activity (not necessarily gamma-chain specific)
2. IgG heavy-chain specific	Contains only antibodies reactive against human gamma chains
3. Monoclonal IgG	Contains murine monoclonal anti-IgG
Anticomplement	
Rabbit polyclonal	
1. Anti-C3d and anti-C3b	Contains only antibodies reactive against the designated complement
2. Anti-C3d, anti-C4b, anti-C4d	Component(s), with no anti-immunoglobulin activity
Murine Monoclonal	
1. Anti-C3d	Contains only antibodies reactive against the designated complement
2. Anti-C3b, anti-C3d	Component, with no anti-immunoglobulin activity

Data from Tyler, V (ed): Technical Manual, 12th ed. American Association of Blood Banks, Bethesda, MD, 1996.

Polyspecific AHG

Polyspecific AHG reagents contain antibody to human IgG and to the **C3d** component of human complement. Other anticomplement antibodies, such as anti-C3b, anti-C4b, and anti-C4d, may also be present. Therefore, its use can facilitate agglutination when RBCs have been sensitized with IgG or C3d or both. Commercially prepared polyspecific AHG contains little, if any, activity against IgA and IgM heavy chains. However, the polyspecific mixture may contain antibody activity to kappa and lambda light chains common to all immunoglobulin classes, thus reacting with IgA or IgM molecules.[10]

Monospecific AHG

Monospecific AHG reagents contain only one antibody specificity: either anti-IgG or antibody to specific complement components such as C3b or C3d (i.e., anticomplement). Licensed monospecific AHG reagents in common use are anti-IgG and anti-C3b-C3d.[10]

Anti-IgG

Reagents labeled anti-IgG contain no anticomplement activity. Anti-IgG reagents contain antibodies specific for the Fc fragment of the gamma heavy chain of the IgG molecule. If not labeled "gamma heavy chain–specific," anti-IgG may contain anti–light chain specificity and may therefore react with cells sensitized with IgM, IgA, and IgG.[10]

Anticomplement

Anticomplement reagents, such as anti-C3b, anti-C3d reagents, are reactive against only the designated complement components and contain no activity against human immunoglobulins.[10] Monospecific anticomplement reagents are often a blend of monoclonal anti-C3b and monoclonal anti-C3d (see the following sections for descriptions of monoclonal and polyclonal antibody production).

Preparation of AHG

The classic method of AHG production involves injecting human serum or purified globulin into laboratory animals such as rabbits. The human globulin behaves as foreign antigen, the rabbit's immune response is triggered, and an antibody to human globulin is produced. For example, human IgG injected into a rabbit results in anti-IgG production; human complement components injected into a rabbit result in anticomplement. This type of response produces a polyclonal antiglobulin serum. **Polyclonal antibodies** are a mixture of antibodies from different plasma cell clones. The resulting polyclonal antibodies recognize different antigenic determinants (epitopes), or the same portion of the antigen but with different affinities. Hybridoma technology can be used to produce monoclonal antiglobulin serum. **Monoclonal antibodies** are derived from one clone of plasma cells and recognize a single epitope.

Polyspecific AHG

Polyspecific AHG can be made using polyclonal or mono-clonal antibodies. The two types of antibody production processes are very different from one another, yielding two very different advantages and disadvantages in their usage.

Polyclonal AHG Production

Polyclonal AHG is usually prepared in rabbits, although when large volumes of antibody are required, sheep or goats may be used. In contrast with the early production methods, in which a crude globulin fraction of serum was used as the immunogen, modern production commences with the purifi-cation of the immunogen from a large pool of normal sera.

Conventional polyspecific antiglobulin reagents are pro-duced by immunizing one colony of rabbits with human immunoglobulin (IgG) antigen and another colony with human C3 antigen. Because of the heterogeneity of IgG mol-ecules, using serum from many donors to prepare the pooled IgG antigen to immunize the rabbits and the pooling of anti-IgG from many immunized rabbits is essential in producing polyclonal reagents for routine use that are capable of detecting the many different IgG antibodies. This is an advantage of using anti-IgG of polyclonal origin for antiglobulin serum.[11]

Both colonies of animals are hyperimmunized to produce high-titer, high-avidity IgG antibodies. Blood specimens are drawn from the immunized animals, and if the antibody potency and specificity meet predetermined specifications, the animals are bled for a production batch of reagent. Sep-arate blends of the anti-IgG and anticomplement antibodies are made, and each pool is then absorbed with A_1, B, and O cells to remove heterospecific antibodies. The preparation of polyclonal AHG is diagrammed in Figure 5–1. The total antibody content of each pool is determined, and the potency of the pools is analyzed to calculate the optimum antibody dilution for use. Block titrations for anti-IgG pools are performed by reacting dilutions of each antibody against cells sensitized with different amounts of IgG. This is a critical step in the manufacturing process because excess antibody, especially with anti-IgG, may lead to prozoning and, hence, false-negative test results.

Because it is not possible to coat cells with measured amounts of complement, the potency of anti-C3 pools is measured using at least two examples each of a C3b- and C3d-coated cell. Both anti-C3b (C3c) and anti-C3d are present in the polyclonal anti-C3 pool. The level of anti-C3d is critical in keeping false-positive tests to a minimum yet also detecting clinically significant amounts of RBC-bound C3d. Additionally, if the dilution of the anti-C3 pool is determined on the basis of the amount of anti-C3d present, the level of anti-C3b (C3c) varies. The inability to determine the potency of anti-C3b and anti-C3d individually is one of the difficulties with polyclonal reagents that can be avoided with monoclonal products.[11]

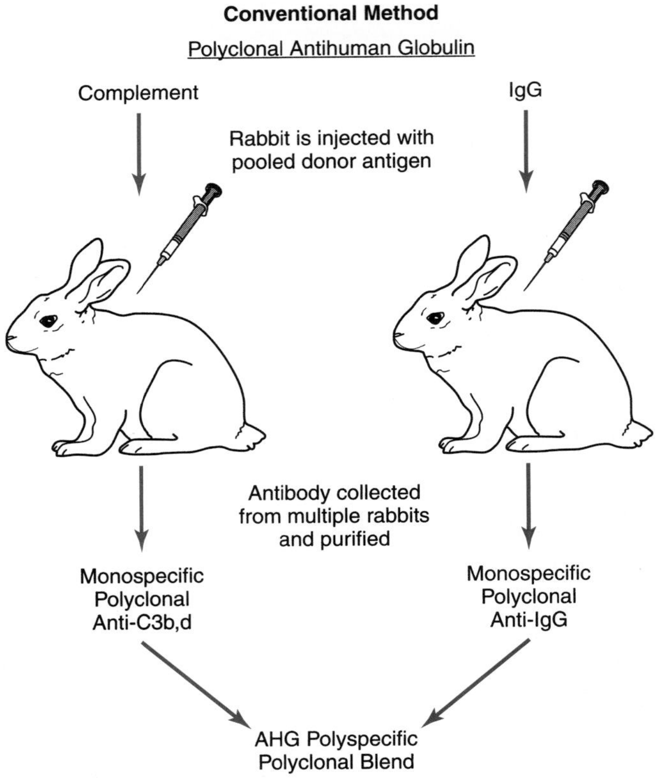

Monoclonal AHG Production

The monoclonal antibody technique devised by Kohler and Milstein[12] has been used to produce AHG and has proved particularly useful in producing high-titer antibodies with well-defined specificities to IgG and to the fragments of C3.[13–15]

Conventional Method

Polyclonal Antihuman Globulin

Figure 5–1. Preparation of polyclonal AHG reagents. Pooled donor antigen allows for a broader spectrum of reactivity, but the source of antibody is limited to the life span of the inoculated animal. Polyspecific antihuman globulin may be manufactured by combining polyclonal anti-IgG with either polyclonal or monoclonal anticomplement components.

Monoclonal antibody production begins with the immu-nization of laboratory animals, usually mice, with purified human globulin. After a suitable immune response, mouse spleen cells containing antibody-secreting lymphocytes are fused with myeloma cells. The resulting "hybridomas" are screened for antibodies with the required specificity and affinity. The antibody-secreting clones may then be propagated in tissue culture or by inoculation into mice, in which case the antibody is collected as ascites. Because the clonal line produces a single antibody, there is no need for absorption to remove heterospecific antibodies.

All antibody molecules produced by a clone of hybridoma cells are identical in terms of antibody structure and antigen specificity. This has advantages and disadvantages in AHG production. Once an antibody-secreting clone of cells has been established, antibody with the same specificity and reaction characteristics will be available indefinitely. This allows the production of a consistently pure and unconta-minated AHG reagent. The disadvantage is that all antibodies produced by a **clone** of cells recognize a single epitope pres-ent on an antigen. For antigens composed of multiple **epitopes** such as IgG, several different monoclonal anti-bodies reacting with different epitopes may need to be blended, or a monoclonal antibody specificity for an epitope on all variants of a particular antigen may need to be selected to ensure that all different expressions of the antigen are detected.

Monoclonal antibodies to human complement components anti-C3b and anti-C3d may be blended with polyclonal anti-IgG from rabbits to achieve potent reagents that give fewer false-positive reactions as a result of anticomplement. Immucor manufactures AHG reagents from an entirely monoclonal source. The anti-IgG component is produced by exposing mice to RBCs coated with IgG. The resulting monoclonal anti-IgG reacts with the C_H3 region of the gamma chain of IgG subclasses 1, 2, and 3. The antibody does not react with human antibodies of subclass IgG_4, but these are not considered to be clinically significant. Blending the monoclonal anti-IgG with a monoclonal anti-C3b and monoclonal anti-C3d results in a polyspecific AHG reagent. The preparation of monoclonal AHG is diagrammed in Figure 5–2.

Before the AHG is available for purchase, manufacturers must subject their reagents to an evaluation procedure, and the results must be submitted to the FDA for approval. Whether produced by the polyclonal or monoclonal technique, the final polyspecific product is one that contains both anti-IgG and anticomplement activity at the correct potency for immediate use. The reagent also contains buffers, stabilizers, and bacteriostatic agents and may be dyed green for identification.

Monospecific AHG

Monospecific AHG production process is similar to that described above for polyspecific AHG; however, it contains only one antibody specificity. Monospecific anti-IgG is produced as a monoclonal, polyclonal, or blended formula.

Antibodies Required in AHG

We have already discussed the need to use both polyspecific and monospecific AHG reagents. However, the reader should be aware of the specific requirements for the subclasses and components of IgG and complement required in the reagent.

Anti-IgG

AHG must contain antibody activity to nonagglutinating blood group antibodies. The majority of these antibodies are a mixture of IgG_1 and IgG_3 subclasses. Rarely, nonagglutinating IgM antibodies may be found; however, they have always been shown to fix complement and may be detected by anticomplement.[16] IgA antibodies with Rh specificity have been reported, but IgG antibody activity has always been present as well. The only RBC alloantibodies that have been reported as being solely IgA have been examples of anti-Pr,[17] and those antibodies were agglutinating. IgA autoantibodies have been reported, although very rarely.[18]

Figure 5–2.   Preparation of monoclonal AHG reagents. The production of antibody is longer lasting than the polyclonal source, as the hybridoma can live indefinitely. A monoclonal blend may be manufactured by blending monoclonal anti-C3b, monoclonal anti-C3d, and monoclonal anti-IgG. Monospecific antihuman globulin reagents can be manufactured by conventional or hybridoma technology.

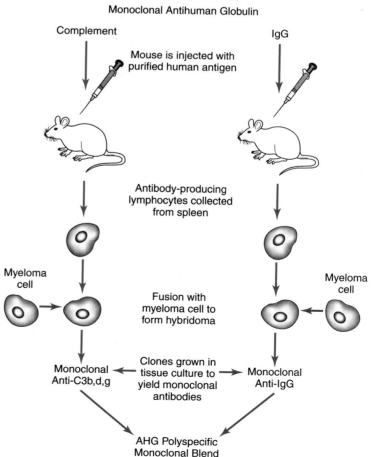

Therefore, anti-IgG activity must be present in the AHG reagent. Anti-IgM and anti-IgA activity may be present, but neither is essential. The presence of anti–light chain activity allows detection of all immunoglobulin classes.

Anticomplement

Some antibodies "fix" complement components to the RBC membrane after complexing of the antibody with its corresponding antigen. These antibodies are listed in Table 5–2 and are described in more detail in Chapters 6 through 9. The terms *most*, *some*, and *rare* in the table refer to antibodies that bind complement the vast majority of the time, that show variability in their ability to bind complement, and that rarely bind complement, respectively. These membrane-bound complement components can be detected by the anticomplement activity in AHG.

As a result of studies published during the 1960s[19–22] indicating the need for anticomplement activity in AHG to allow the IAT to detect antibodies, polyspecific reagent was introduced. Evidence was also presented showing that the presence of anticomplement activity would enhance the reactions of clinically significant antibodies (e.g., anti-Fy[a] and anti-K).[19]

During complement activation, C3 and C4 are split into two components. C3b and C4b bind to the RBC membrane, whereas C3a and C4a pass into the fluid phase. Further degradation of membrane-bound C3b and C4b occurs by removing C3c and C4c to leave C3d and C4d firmly attached to the RBC membrane.[23–25] The ISBT/ICSH Joint Working Party[26] considered anti-C3c to be the most important anticomplement component because of its limited capacity to cause nonspecific reactions. However, when RBCs are incubated with serum for

longer than 15 minutes, the number of C3c determinants falls rapidly because C3c is split off the C3bi molecule. This finding further supports the use of anti-C3d in international reference reagents by the Joint Working Party.

The final degradation step has been shown to occur in vivo[27] and is a common occurrence in both warm and cold autoimmune hemolytic anemias. Engelfriet and others[28] have also shown that degradation of C3b to C3d can occur in vitro, providing that the **incubation** period is greater than 1 hour. In 1976, Garratty and Petz[29] confirmed the need for anti-C3d activity in AHG for use in the DAT. They also confirmed Engelfriet's observation that, given sufficient time, cell-bound C3b could be degraded to C3d in vitro. Refer back to **Table 5–1** for a detailed listing of all AHG reagents' components.

Use of Polyspecific Versus Monospecific AHG in the IAT

As previously stated, polyspecific AHG contains both anti-IgG activity and anti-C3 activity. There is considerable debate among blood bankers over the use of monospecific anti-IgG versus polyspecific AHG for routine antibody detection and pretransfusion testing. Because most clinically significant antibodies detected during antibody screening are IgG, the most important function of polyspecific AHG is the detection of IgG antibodies.

There have been numerous reports of clinically significant RBC alloantibodies that were undetectable with monospecific anti-IgG but were detected with the anticomplement component of AHG.[30] Unfortunately, polyspecific AHG has also been associated with unwanted positive reactions that are not caused by clinically significant antibodies. To investigate these variables, Petz and coworkers[31] examined 39,436 sera comparing monospecific anti-IgG with polyspecific AHG. They also compared the albumin technique with **low ionic strength solutions** (LISS)-suspended RBCs. Four Jk[a] antibodies were detected only with polyspecific anti-IgG using albumin or LISS-suspended RBCs. An additional anti-Jk[a] was detected only with polyspecific AHG when using LISS but not with **albumin**. Also, five antibodies of anti-Kell, anti-Jk[a], and Fy[a] specificities were detected when using LISS, but not albumin, with both polyspecific AHG and anti-IgG. Their results concluded that some clinically significant antibodies are detected with the anticomplement component of AHG but not with anti-IgG. This is especially true for anti-Jk[a], a complement-binding IgG antibody often associated with delayed hemolytic transfusion reactions.

Petz and others[31] also determined the number of false-positive reactions obtained when using polyspecific AHG versus anti-IgG with LISS and albumin. False-positive reactions were defined as those caused by antibodies with no definable specificity or by antibodies considered to be clinically insignificant because of optimum reactivity at cold temperatures (anti-I, anti-H, anti-P$_1$, anti-M). Of the unwanted positive reactions, 93% were caused by C3 on the cells. The authors emphasize that, if the first step in evaluating a weakly positive AHG reaction is to repeat using the prewarmed technique, although not recommended, about 60% of the false-positive weak reactions become negative.

Table 5–2	**Antibodies Capable of Binding Complement**	
MOST	**SOME**	**RARE**
ABO	Xg^a	D
Le^a	LKE	P$_1$
Le^b	Lan	Lu^a
Jk^a		Lu^b
Jk^b		Kell
Sc1		Fy^a
Co3		Fy^b
Ge2		Co^a
Ge3		Co^b
li		Di^a
P		S
PP$_1$P^k		s
Vel		Yt^a

In a 3-year study, Howard and associates[32] found eight patients whose antibodies were detected primarily or solely by AHG containing anticomplement activity. Seven of these antibodies had anti-Jk^a or anti-Jk^b specificity. Some of them could be detected using homozygous Jk^a or Jk^b cells and an AHG containing only anti-IgG activity. Two of the anti-Jk^a antibodies were associated with delayed hemolytic transfusion reactions. The complement-only Kidd antibodies represented 23% of all Kidd antibodies detected during the study. The authors concluded that they would continue to use polyspecific AHG reagent for routine compatibility testing.

In summary, one must balance the advantage of detecting clinically significant complement-only antibodies with the disadvantages resulting from using antiglobulin serum containing anticomplement activity.[30] Deciding to use the AHG reagent for indirect tests is the prerogative of the individual blood bank. Many blood banks have begun using monospecific anti-IgG for routine pretransfusion testing, citing cost containment measures necessitated by the high number of repeats versus the rarity of complement-only detected antibodies such as anti-Jk^a. Milam[33] states that rare clinical transfusion intolerance, when using monospecific anti-IgG over polyspecific AHG reagents to screen for unexpected antibodies and to test for blood group compatibility, offers reliability without interference from common and clinically insignificant IgM-complement fixing antibodies.

Principles of the Antiglobulin Test

The antiglobulin test is based on the following simple principles:[10]

- Antibody molecules and complement components are globulins.
- Injecting an animal with human globulin stimulates the animal to produce antibody to the foreign protein (i.e., AHG). Serologic tests employ a variety of AHG reagents reactive with various human globulins, including anti-IgG antibody to the C3d component of human complement, and polyspecific reagents that contain both anti-IgG and anti-C3d activity.

AHG reacts with human globulin molecules, either bound to RBCs or free in serum. Washed RBCs coated with human globulin are agglutinated by AHG.

 The complete procedures for the direct and indirect antihuman globulin tests can be found in Procedures 5-1 and 5-2 on the textbook's companion website.

Figure 5–3 illustrates in vitro sensitization detected in the IAT and in vivo sensitization detected by the DAT.

Direct Antiglobulin Test

Described above are the overall principles of the antiglobulin test. **Figure 5–3** depicts two variations of the AGT, the DAT and the IAT. The following section details the DAT's principle, application, construct, and evaluation.

Principle and Application

The direct antiglobulin test (DAT) detects in vivo sensitization of RBCs with IgG or complement components. Clinical conditions that can result in in vivo coating of RBCs with antibody or complement are:

- Hemolytic disease of the newborn (HDN)
- Hemolytic transfusion reaction (HTR)
- Autoimmune and drug-induced hemolytic anemia (AIHA)

Table 5–3 lists the clinical application and in vivo sensitization detected for each situation.

The DAT is not a required test in routine pretransfusion protocols. Eder[34] tested the clinical utility of the DAT at a large tertiary care hospital in Philadelphia. A retrospective study was performed from 1999 to 2002. DATs with anti-IgG were performed on 15,662 pretransfusion patient samples; 15% were positive. Subsequent eluate testing revealed 76% were nonreactive, 9% were pan reactive, and 12% passively acquired ABO or D antibodies. Only one case demonstrated an RBC antibody in the eluate that was not detected in the serum, concluding that even in a tertiary care setting, the routine DAT is inefficient, yielding a positive predictive value of 0.16%. Judd and coworkers revealed similar findings on 65,049 blood samples in a 29-month period, where only 5.5% of samples resulted in a positive DAT.[35]

DAT Panel

Initial DATs include testing one drop of a 3% to 5% suspension of washed RBCs with polyspecific (anti-IgG, anti-C3d) reagent (please refer to the DAT procedure on DavisPlus website). Positive results are monitored by a DAT panel using monospecific anti-IgG and anti-C3d to determine the specific type of protein sensitizing the cell. In an effort to save valuable tech time, some institutions run polyspecific and monospecific reagents at one time as well as a saline control. The saline control serves to detect spontaneous agglutination of cells or reactions occurring without the addition of AHG reagents. In warm AIHA, including drug-induced hemolytic anemia, the RBCs may be coated with IgG or C3d, or both. Patterns of reactivity and the type of protein sensitization in AIHA are summarized in Table 5–4.

In a transfusion reaction workup, the DAT may demonstrate IgG or C3d, or both, depending on the nature and specificity of the recipient's antibody. In the investigation of HDN, testing for complement proteins is not necessary inasmuch as the protein sensitizing the newborn RBCs is

Table 5–3	**Direct Antiglobulin Test**
CLINICAL APPLICATION	**IN VIVO SENSITIZATION**
HDN	Maternal antibody coating fetal RBCs
HTR	Recipient antibody coating donor RBCs
AIHA	Autoantibody coating individual's RBCs

The Antihuman Globulin Test (AHG)

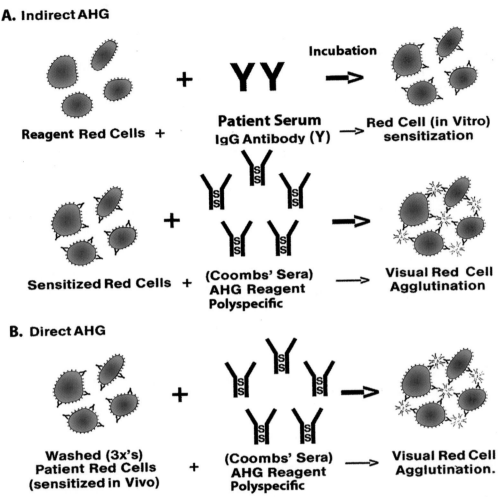

A. Indirect AHG

Reagent Red Cells + Patient Serum IgG Antibody (Y) → Incubation → Red Cell (in Vitro) sensitization

Sensitized Red Cells + (Coombs' Sera) AHG Reagent Polyspecific → Visual Red Cell Agglutination

B. Direct AHG

Washed (3x's) Patient Red Cells (sensitized in Vivo) + (Coombs' Sera) AHG Reagent Polyspecific → Visual Red Cell Agglutination.

Figure 5–3. The antihuman globulin (AHG) test. (A) Indirect AHG (IAT), with sensitization occurring in vitro, looking for unknown antibody in the patient's serum/plasma. (Note: If the IAT was identifying RBC antigens, the RBCs would be from the patient and the antibody would be the known reagent). (B) Direct AHG (DAT) with sensitization already occurring in vivo. (Note: The polyspecific AHG reagent is a mixture of anti-IgG and anti-C3d.)

presumed to be maternal IgG. Problems can arise in accurate D typing in the case of a newborn with a positive DAT. If the DAT is positive due to IgG and the immediate spin for D typing is negative, a test for weak D cannot be performed. The same is true for a patient with AIHA due to a warm IgG antibody coating the patient cells. The antibody must be removed from the RBCs for accurate phenotyping. Other techniques can be used to remove antibody from the patient's RBCs. These include chloroquine diphosphate, EDTA-glycine, and murine monoclonal antibodies.

Evaluation of a Positive DAT

Clinical consideration should dictate the extent to which a positive DAT is evaluated. Interpreting the significance of a positive DAT requires knowledge of the patient's diagnosis, drug therapy, and recent transfusion history. A

Table 5–4 DAT Panel: Patterns of Reactivity in Autoimmune Hemolytic Anemia*

ANTI-IgG	ANTI-C3d	TYPE OF AIHA
+	+	WAIHA
+	−	WAIHA
−	+	CAS; PCH, WAIHA
+	+	Mixed-type AIHA (cold and warm)

Data from Roback, JD, Combs, MR, Grossman, BJ, and Hillyer, CD (eds): Technical Manual, 16th ed. AABB, Bethesda, MD, 2008.

*The DAT with monospecific antiglobulin reagents is helpful in classifying AIHAs. Other procedures and studies are necessary to diagnose and characterize which form of autoimmune disease is present.

CAS = cold agglutinin syndrome; PCH = paroxysmal cold hemoglobinuria; WAIHA = warm autoimmune hemolytic anemia positive DAT may occur without clinical manifestations of immune-mediated hemolysis. Table 5–5 outlines the in vivo phenomena that may be associated with a positive DAT.

The AABB *Technical Manual* states that "a positive DAT alone is not diagnostic. The interpretation of the significance of this positive result requires knowledge of the patient's diagnosis; recent drug, pregnancy, and transfusion history; and information on the presence of acquired or unexplained hemolytic anemia."[36] Answering the following questions before investigating a positive DAT for patients other than neonates will help determine what further testing is appropriate:

- Is there evidence of in vivo hemolysis?
- Has the patient been transfused recently? If so, did the patient receive blood products or components containing ABO-incompatible plasma?
- Does the patient's serum contain unexpected antibodies?
- Is the patient receiving any drugs?
- Is the patient receiving antilymphocyte globulin or antithymocyte globulin?

- Is the patient receiving intravenous immune globulin (IVIG) or intravenous Rh immune globulin (IV RhIG)?
- Has the patient received a marrow or other organ transplant?

Indirect Antiglobulin Test

The IAT is performed to determine in vitro sensitization of RBCs and is used in the following situations:

- Detection of incomplete (nonagglutinating) antibodies to potential donor RBCs (compatibility testing) or to screening cells (antibody screen) in serum
- Determination of RBC phenotype using known antisera (e.g., Kell typing, weak D testing)
- Titration of incomplete antibodies

Table 5–6 lists the IATs and the in vitro sensitization detected for each application. For in vitro antigen-antibody reactions, the IAT tasks are listed and explained in Table 5–7.

Table 5–5   In Vivo Phenomena Associated With a Positive DAT

	CONDITION	CAUSE
Transfusion	1. Recipient alloantibody and donor antigen	Alloantibodies in the recipient of a recent transfusion that react with antigen on donor RBC
	2. Donor antibody and recipient antigen	Antibodies present in donor plasma that react with antigen on a transfusion recipient's RBCs
Drug induced	1. Type I (hapten-dependent Ab)	Drug binds covalently to membrane proteins and stimulates hapten-dependent Ab
	2. Type II (autoantibody)	Drug induces autoantibody specific for RBC membrane proteins through unknown mechanism; Ab reacts with normal RBCs in the absence of drug.
	3. Type III (drug-dependent Ab)	Drug induces Ab that binds to RBC only when drug is present in soluble form, unknown mech; Ab reacts with normal RBCs when soluble drug is present.
Autoimmune hemolytic anemia	1. WAIHA (IgG and/or C3)	Autoantibody reacts with patient's RBCs in vivo.
	2. CAS (C3)	Cold-reactive IgM autoagglutinin binds to RBCs in peripheral circulation (32°C). IgM binds complement as RBCs return to warmer parts of circulation; IgM dissociates, leaving RBCs coated only with complement.
	3. PCH (IgG)	The IgG autoantibody reacts with RBCs in colder parts of body, causes complement to be bound irreversibly to RBCs, and then elutes at warmer temperature.
Hemolytic disease of newborn	1. Maternal alloantibody crosses placenta (IgG)	Maternal (IgG) alloantibody, specific for fetal antigen, coats fetal RBCs. DAT is reactive with anti-IgG.
Miscellaneous	1. Absorbed proteins; administration of equine preparations of antilymphocyte globulin and antithymocyte globulin	Heterophile antibodies that are present in ALG or ATG coat recipient's RBCs. High levels of protein causing red cells to spontaneously agglutinate.
	2. Administration of high-dose IV gamma globulin and hypergammaglobulinemia	Non-antibody-mediated binding of immunoglobulin to RBCs in patients with hypergammaglobulinemia

Modified from Roback, JD, Combs, MR, Grossman, BJ, and Hillyer, CD (eds): Technical Manual, 16th ed. AABB, Bethesda, MD, 2008.
AIHA = autoimmune hemolytic anemia; CAS = cold agglutinin syndrome; PCH = paroxysmal cold hemoglobinuria.

Table 5–6   Indirect Antiglobulin Test

APPLICATION	TESTS	IN VITRO SENSITIZATION
Antibody detection	Compatibility testing	Recipient antibody reacting with donor cells
	Antibody screening	Antibody reacting with screening cells
Antibody identification	Antibody panel	Antibody reacting with panel cells
Antibody titration	Rh antibody titer	Antibody and selected Rh cells
RBC phenotype	RBC antigen detection (ex: weak D, K, Fy)	Specific antisera + RBCs to detect antigen

The DAT does not require the incubation phase because of the antigen-antibody complexes formed in vivo.

Factors Affecting the Antiglobulin Test

The DAT can detect a level of 100 to 500 IgG molecules per RBC and 400 to 1,100 molecules of C3d per RBC.[28]

For the IAT, there must be between 100 and 200 IgG or C3 molecules on the cell to obtain a positive reaction. The number of IgG molecules that sensitize an RBC and the rate at which sensitization occurs can be influenced by several factors, including:

- Ratio of serum to cells
- Reaction medium

Table 5–7   Tasks and Purposes of the Indirect Antiglobulin Test

TASK	PURPOSE
Incubate RBCs with antisera	Allows time for antibody molecule attachment to RBC antigen
Perform a minimum of three saline washes	Removes free globulin molecules
Add antiglobulin reagent	Forms RBC agglutinates (RBC Ag + Ab + anti-IgG)
Centrifuge	Accelerates agglutination by bringing cells closer together
Examine for agglutination	Interprets test as positive or negative
Grade agglutination reactions	Determines the strength of reaction
Add antibody-coated RBCs to negative reactions	Checks for neutralization of antisera by free globulin molecules (Coombs' control cells are D-positive RBCs coated with anti-D)

- Temperature
- Incubation time
- Washing of RBCs
- Saline for washing
- Addition of AHG
- Centrifugation for reading

Ratio of Serum to Cells

Increasing the ratio of serum to cells increases the sensitivity of the test system. Generally, a minimum ratio of 40:1 should be the target, and this can be achieved by using 2 drops of serum and 1 drop of a 5% volume of solute per volume of solution (v/v) suspension of cells.[34] When using cells suspended in saline, it is often advantageous to increase the ratio of serum to cells in an effort to detect weak antibodies (e.g., 4 drops of serum with 1 drop of a 3% [v/v] cell suspension will give a ratio of 133:1).

Reaction Medium

Reaction mediums include albumin, LISS, and polyethylene glycol.

Albumin

The macromolecules of albumin allow antibody-coated cells to come into closer contact with each other so that aggregation occurs. In 1965, Stroup and MacIlroy[37] reported on the creased sensitivity of the IAT if albumin was incorporated into the reaction medium. Their reaction mixture, consisting of 2 drops of serum, 2 drops of 22% (w/v) bovine albumin, and 1 drop of 3% to 5% (v/v) cells, was shown to provide the same sensitivity at 30 minutes of incubation as a 60-minute saline-only test. The use of albumin does not seem to provide any advantage over LISS techniques and adds to the cost of the test.[37] Petz and coworkers[31] also showed that an albumin technique may miss several clinically significant antibodies. Therefore, it is rarely, if ever, used as an IAT media for routine tests.

Low Ionic Strength Solutions

Low ionic strength solutions (LISS) enhance antibody uptake and allow incubation times to be decreased—from 30 to 60 minutes to 10 to 15 minutes—by reducing the zeta potential surrounding an RBC. Some LISS also contain macromolecular substances. The LISS technique, introduced by Low and Messeter,[38] has critical requirements with respect to the serum-to-cell ratio. Moore and Mollison[39] showed that optimum reaction conditions were obtained using 2 drops of serum and 2 drops of a 3% (v/v) suspension of cells in LISS. Increasing the serum-to-cell ratio increased the ionic strength of the reaction mixture, leading to a decrease in sensitivity and counteracting the shortened incubation time of the test. A LISS medium may be achieved by either suspending RBCs in LISS or using a LISS additive reagent, with the latter being more common practice.

Polyethylene Glycol

Polyethylene glycol (PEG) is a water-soluble linear polymer and is used as an additive to increase antibody uptake. Its action is to remove water molecules surrounding the RBC (the water of hydration theory), thereby effectively concentrating antibody. Anti-IgG is the AHG reagent of choice with PEG testing to avoid false-positive reactions.[10] Because PEG may cause aggregation of RBCs, reading for agglutination following 37°C incubation in the IAT is omitted. Several investigators[40] compared the performance of PEG as an enhancement media with that of LISS. Findings indicated that PEG increases the detection of clinically significant antibodies while decreasing detection of clinically insignificant antibodies. Barrett and associates[41] reported that as PEG has been used for pretransfusion antibody screening, 6,353 RBC components have been transfused without any reported acute or delayed HTRs.

Temperature

The rate of reaction for the majority of IgG antibodies is optimal at 37°C; therefore, this is the usual incubation temperature for the IAT. This is also the optimum temperature for complement activation.

Incubation Time

For cells suspended in saline, incubation times may vary between 30 and 120 minutes. The majority of clinically significant antibodies can be detected after 30 minutes of incubation, and extended incubation times are usually not necessary. If a LISS or PEG technique is being used,[38,39] incubation times may be shortened to 10 to 15 minutes. With these shortened times, it is essential that tubes be incubated at a temperature of 37°C. Extended incubation (i.e., up to 40 minutes) in the LISS technique has been shown to cause antibody to elute from the RBCs, decreasing the sensitivity of the test.[42] However, this could not be confirmed by Voak and coworkers.[43]

Washing of RBCs

When both the DAT and IAT are performed, RBCs must be saline-washed a minimum of three times before adding AHG reagent. Washing the RBCs removes free unbound serum globulins. Inadequate washing may result in a false-negative reaction because of neutralization of the AHG reagent by residual unbound serum globulins. The washing phase of a DAT and IAT becomes one of the most important steps in testing. The wash phase can be controlled using check cells, or group O cells sensitized with IgG.

Washing should be performed immediately after being removed from the incubator and in as short a time as possible to minimize the elution of low-affinity antibodies. The cell pellet should be completely resuspended before adding the next saline wash. All saline should be discarded after the final wash, because residual saline dilutes the AHG reagent and therefore decreases the sensitivity of the test. Centrifugation at each wash should be sufficient to provide a firm cell pellet and therefore minimize the possible loss of cells with each discard of saline.

Saline for Washing

Ideally, the saline used for washing should be fresh or buffered to a pH of 7.2 to 7.4. Saline stored for long periods in plastic containers has been shown to decrease in pH, which may increase the rate of antibody elution during the washing process, yielding a false-negative result.[44] One of the contributors (dk) has seen this phenomenon occur in working student labs when expiration dates are ignored to conserve resources. Changes in pH may have important implications when monoclonal AHG is used, inasmuch as monoclonal antibodies have been shown to have narrow pH ranges for optimum reactivity. Significant levels of bacterial contamination in saline have been reported;[45] this situation can contribute to false-positive results.

Addition of AHG

AHG should be added to the cells immediately after washing to minimize the chance of antibody eluting from the cell and subsequently neutralizing the AHG reagent. The volume of AHG added should be as indicated by the manufacturers. However, Voak and associates[46] have shown that adding two volumes of AHG may overcome washing problems when low levels of serum contamination remain. These authors indicated that the neutralization of AHG is a problem only with free IgG left in serum following inadequate saline washings and not with residual serum complement components. The complement fragments free in serum are not the same as the complement fragments bound to RBCs, and therefore residual serum does not contain C3b and C3d to neutralize the anti-C3b and anti-C3d in AHG reagent.

Centrifugation for Reading

Centrifugation of the cell pellet for reading of hemagglutination along with the method used for resuspending the cells is a crucial step in the technique. The CBER-recommended method for the evaluation of AHG uses 1,000 relative centrifugal forces (RCFs) for 20 seconds, although the technique described in this chapter suggests 500 RCFs for 15 to 20 seconds. The use of higher RCFs yields more sensitive results; however, depending on how the pellet is resuspended, it may give weak false-positive results because of inadequate resuspension or may give a negative result if resuspension is too vigorous. The optimum centrifugation conditions should be determined for each centrifuge.

Sources of Error

Some of the most common sources of error associated with the performance of the AHG test have been outlined in the previous section. Box 5–1 lists reasons for false-negative and false-positive AHG reactions. An anticoagulant such as EDTA should be used to collect blood samples for the DAT to avoid the in vitro complement attachment associated with refrigerated clotted specimens.[47]

All negative antiglobulin test reactions must be checked by the addition of IgG-sensitized cells. Adding IgG-coated

BOX 5–1

Sources of Error in Antihuman Globulin Testing

False-Positive Results

- Improper specimen (refrigerated, clotted) may cause in vitro complement attachment
- Overcentrifugation and overreading
- Centrifugation after the incubation phase when PEG or other positively charged polymers are used as an enhancement medium
- Bacterial contamination of cells or saline used in washing
- Dirty glassware
- Presence of fibrin in the test tube may mimic agglutination.
- Cells with a positive DAT will yield a positive IAT.
- Polyagglutinable cells
- Saline contaminated by heavy metals or colloidal silica
- Using a serum sample for a DAT (use EDTA, ACD, or CPD anticoagulated blood)
- Samples collected in gel separator tubes may have unauthentic complement attachment.
- Complement attachment when specimens are collected from infusion lines infusing dextrose solutions
- Preservative-dependent antibody directed against reagents

False-Negative Results

- Inadequate or improper washing of cells
- Failure to wash additional times when increased serum volumes are used
- Contamination of AHG by extraneous protein (i.e., glove, wrong dropper)
- High concentration of IgG paraproteins in test serum
- Early dissociation of bound IgG from RBCs due to interruption in testing
- Early dissociation of bound IgG from RBCs due to improper testing temperature (i.e., saline or AHG too cold or hot)
- AHG reagent nonreactive because of deterioration or neutralization (improper reagent storage)
- Excessive heat or repeated freezing and thawing of test serum
- Serum nonreactive because of deterioration of complement
- AHG reagent, test serum, or enhancement medium not added
- Undercentrifuged or overcentrifuged
- Cell suspension either too weak or too heavy
- Serum:cell ratios are not ideal
- Rare antibodies are present that are only detectable with polyspecific AHG and when active complement is present.
- Low pH of saline
- Inadequate incubation conditions in the IAT
- Poor reading technique

Modified from Roback, JD, Combs, MR, Grossman, BJ, and Hillyer, CD (eds): Technical Manual, 16th ed. AABB, Bethesda, MD, 2008.

RBCs to negative test reactions should demonstrate hemagglutination of these RBCs with the anti-IgG in the AHG reagent. If no hemagglutination follows the addition of IgG-coated RBCs, the test result is invalid and the test must be repeated. The most common technical errors that result in failure to demonstrate hemagglutination after the addition of IgG-coated RBCs are inadequate washing, nonreactive AHG reagent, and failure to add AHG reagent. While most blood banks do not check monospecific anti-C3d reactivity with the addition of C3d-coated RBCs to negative reactions, these cells are available and may also be produced in-house.[47]

Modified and Automated Antiglobulin Test Techniques

Modifications to the antiglobulin test technique (LISS, PEG, and albumin) have just been described; however, additional modifications may be used in special circumstances, including the low-iconic polybrene technique, enzyme-linked antiglobulin test, solid phase technology, and gel test.

Low Ionic Polybrene Technique

In 1980, Lalezari and Jiang[48] reported on the adaptation of the automated low ionic polybrene (LIP) technique for use as a manual procedure. The technique relies on low ionic conditions to rapidly sensitize cells with antibody. Polybrene, a potent rouleaux-forming reagent, is added to allow the sensitized cells to approach each other and permit cross-linking

by the attached antibody. A high ionic strength solution is then added to reverse the rouleaux; however, if agglutination is present, it will remain. The test can be carried through to an AHG technique if required. If this is performed, a monospecific anti-IgG reagent must be used, because the low ionic conditions cause considerable amounts of C4 and C3 to coat the cells and would give false-positive reactions if a polyspecific reagent were used.

The antiglobulin test has also been performed using microplates. Crawford and colleagues[49] used microplates for a number of different grouping procedures, including the IAT. Microplate technology is used increasingly in blood group serology, and many techniques are being adapted for it. Redman and associates[50] have adapted the LIP technique for use in microplates. Although their report does not include the use of an AHG phase, this additional step could easily be included.

It should also be mentioned that polybrene has a low sensitivity to detection of anti-Jk^a and –Jk^b and the Jk^a antigen.[51] Therefore, the potential exists for a clinically significant anti-Kidd antibody to be missed using the polybrene method of enhancement for IAT.

Enzyme-Linked Antiglobulin Test

In the enzyme-linked antiglobulin test (ELAT), an RBC suspension is added to a microtiter well and washed with saline. AHG, which has been labeled with an enzyme, is added. The enzyme-labeled AHG will bind to IgG-sensitized

RBCs. Excess antibody is removed, and enzyme substrate is added. The amount of color produced is measured spectrophotometrically and is proportional to the amount of antibody present. The optical density is usually measured at 405 nm. The number of IgG molecules per RBC can also be determined from this procedure.

Solid Phase Technology

Solid-phase technology may be used for performing antiglobulin tests. Several different techniques have been reported using either test tubes[51b] or microplates.[52,53] With the availability of microplate readers, this modification lends itself to the introduction of semiautomation. Direct and indirect tests can be performed using solid-phase methodology. In the former, antibody is attached to a microplate well, and RBCs are added. If antibody is specific for antigen on RBCs, the bottom of the well will be covered with suspension; if no such specificity occurs, RBCs will settle to the bottom of the well. In the latter, known RBCs are bound to a well that has been treated with glutaraldehyde or poly L-lysine. Test serum is added to RBC-coated wells, and if antibody in serum is specific for antigen on fixed RBCs, a positive reaction occurs as previously described. For a detailed description of this technology, see Chapter 12, "Other Technologies and Automation."

Gel Test

The **gel test** is a process that detects RBC antigen-antibody reactions by means of using a chamber filled with polyacrylamide gel. The gel acts as a trap; free unagglutinated RBCs form pellets in the bottom of the tube, whereas agglutinated RBCs are trapped in the tube for hours. Therefore, negative reactions appear as pellets in the bottom of the microtube, and positive reactions are fixed in the gel.

There are three different types of gel tests: neutral, specific, and antiglobulin. A neutral gel does not contain any specific reagent and acts only by its property of trapping agglutinates. The main applications of neutral gel tests are antibody screening and identification with enzyme-treated or untreated RBCs and reverse ABO typing. Specific gel tests use a specific reagent incorporated into the gel and are useful for antigen determination.

The gel low ionic antiglobulin test (GLIAT) is a valuable application of the gel test and may be used for the IAT or the DAT. AHG reagent is incorporated into the gel. For example, in an IAT gel, 50 µL of a 0.8% RBC suspension is pipetted onto a gel containing AHG, serum is added, and the tube is centrifuged after a period of incubation. At the beginning of centrifugation, the RBCs tend to pass through the gel, but the medium in which they are suspended remains above. This results in separation between the RBCs and the medium without a washing phase. RBCs come in contact with AHG in the upper part of the gel, and the positive and negative reactions are separated. The detection of unexpected antibodies by GLIAT compares favorably with conventional AHG methods and provides a safe, reliable, and easy-to-read AHG test.[54]

For the DAT, 50 µL of a 0.8% RBC suspension in LISS solution (ID-Diluent 2) is added to the top of each microtube of the LISS/Coombs ID cards. The cards are centrifuged at 910 rpm for 10 minutes.[55] In the case of a positive reaction, monospecific reagents (anti-IgG, anti-C3d) can be used in the gel test. For a detailed description of this technology, see Chapter 12.

Comparison of AHG Methodologies

Transfusion service departments typically work to detect all clinically significant antibodies, both DAT and IAT types, and none of the clinically insignificant antibodies such as warm and cold-reacting autoantibodies. A common question that arises in these departments is which detection method should be employed to reach such goals. This section briefly compares various AHG methods for DAT and IAT testing. Table 5–8 outlines some of the advantages and disadvantages in various AHG testing methodologies.

DAT Methods

There have been numerous studies comparing the tube and gel test when performing DATs. The main difference in the two techniques is that the former requires washing, and the latter omits a washing stage, resulting in discrepant results between the two methods. Multiple studies[56–60] concluded that a gel technique used for detecting in vivo sensitized RBCs was more sensitive than the conventional tube technique. However, a comparison study using solid-phase methodology for DAT has not been reported. The gel method, although more sensitive, isn't necessarily more sensitive only to clinically significant antibodies. Blood banks should be aware of the differences in the DAT when using the popular gel test over the tube technique. Additional comparative studies will add to the current body of knowledge.

IAT Methods

There has been a downward trend in conventional tube testing technique in AHG testing, with a gain in popularity for gel technology.[61] From a timing and sensitivity perspective, the conventional tube test using saline is the least preferred method.[61] The most popular tube medium is LISS followed by PEG.[62] Although the LISS and PEG methods are more sensitive than the saline tube method, they are the most labor-intense methods requiring the most skilled staff. One advantage they have over gel and solid phase is the lowered cost of required reagents. Bunker and colleagues[63] concluded in their study that the PEG IAT method was the most cost-effective pretransfusion antibody screening technique when compared to the solid red cell adherence assay.

Gel technology's introduction into the transfusion service department in the last decade has greatly benefitted the trend in laboratories to use generalist bench techs rather than department-focused techs. Gel technology is less labor-intensive than conventional tube testing and incorporates standardization both procedurally and in endpoint grading. This standardization cannot be duplicated using tube testing.

Table 5–8   Comparison of AHG Methodologies

TESTING METHODOLOGY	ADVANTAGES	DISADVANTAGES
Saline-CTT	• No additives • Reduced cost • Avoids reactivity with auto Abs • Ability to assess multiple phases of reactivity	• Long incubation • Least sensitive • Requires highly trained staff • Most procedural steps • Fewer method-dependent Abs detected
LISS-CTT	• Reduced cost • Avoids reactivity with auto Abs • Shortest incubation time • Increased Ab uptake • Most common tube method • Ability to assess multiple phases of reactivity	• Inability to be automated • Requires highly trained staff • Many procedural steps • Fewer method-dependent Abs detected
PEG-CTT	• Reduced cost • Decreased incubation time • Increased Ab uptake • Enhances most Abs • Ability to assess multiple phases of reactivity (not 37°C)	• Requires highly trained staff • Many procedural steps • Detects more unwanted Abs • Inability to be automated • Fewer method-dependent Abs detected
Gel	• More sensitive DAT method • No washing steps • No need for check cells • Stable endpoints • Small test volume • Enhanced anti-D detection • Ability to be automated	• Warm auto Abs enhanced • Mixed-cell agglutination with cold Abs • Increased costs • Increased need for additional instrumentation • Increased chances of detected unwanted Abs • Need to maintain backup method
Solid phase	• No need for check cells • Stable endpoints • Small test volume • Enhanced anti-D • Increased sensitivity for all Abs • Ability to be automated	• Increased sensitivity for all Abs • Detects unwanted Abs • Warm auto Abs enhanced • Increased costs • Increased need for additional instrumentation

Ab = antibody; CTT = conventional tube testing; LISS = low ionic strength saline; PEG = polyethylene glycol

Gel methods for IAT testing have been shown to be more sensitive than saline, LISS, and PEG at detecting passively acquired anti-D in postnatal patients.[64] Weisbach and associates[65] have also shown that labs using the gel method are more likely to detect weak antibody reactivity than the LISS tube method. An advantage to using the gel technology in a high-volume lab is its ability to operate as an automated system. A few disadvantages to using the gel method are the increased cost of instrumentation and reagents, the need to stay proficient with alternative methods for backup, and the increased likelihood of detecting unwanted autoantibodies.

Solid-phase technology can be incorporated as a manual or automated method for use in IAT. Like gel technology, solid-phase technology is more likely to detect weakly reactive antibodies than the LISS tube method.[65] However, with a higher sensitivity comes the detection of more nonspecific reactivity.[66,67] Thus, introducing additional costs required to investigate positive screening results. Garozzo and colleagues[68] showed that the solid-phase method is even more sensitive at detecting the anti-D than the gel method.

Over the coming years, the changes in blood bank technology, along with the changes in emphasis on the importance of crossmatching versus antibody screening, will probably further modify the role of the antiglobulin test. Method-dependent antibodies have been documented repeatedly in AHG method comparison studies. Some antibodies will be detectable using only one specific method of testing and will be negative in all others. However, AHG methods are comparable in regards to sensitivity and specificity.

When deciding which method to use in day-to-day operations, it is important to consider time, resources, facilities and staffing, and the cost of overall testing and how these factors will impact patient care. Current research is under way to utilize molecular diagnostic methods, particularly PCR, to identify RBC genotypes in place of the serologic phenotyping AHG methods. At present, however, serologic AHG testing methods remain the most important in the blood bank for detecting clinically significant antibodies to RBCs and RBC antigens and for detecting immune hemolysis.

CASE STUDIES

Case 5-1

You are working second shift at a Midwestern suburban hospital. Although you were trained in school using gel technology, your lab utilizes the conventional tube testing method using LISS as an enhancement medium, because the medical director refuses to adopt gel as the primary AHG methodology. About an hour before the end of your shift, the phlebotomist brings you a routine type and screen for a patient just admitted to the medical surgical floor. Because you are confident you can finish before your shift ends, you decide to proceed with testing. The patient types as an A-positive. The antibody screen results were negative in all phases of testing. Therefore, check cells were added to all tubes and the reactions after centrifuging were also negative.

1. Can the antibody screen be interpreted as negative?
2. What steps must be taken to resolve the problem?
3. What is the most likely cause for the discrepant results?
4. What are other causes for the results?

Case 5-2

A 34-year-old white male is admitted for an exploratory laparotomy. A type and screen is ordered prior to his scheduled surgery. ABO and Rh typing reveal the patient is O-positive, and the blood bank technologist performed an antibody screen using the patient serum and a two-cell screen using gel technology. One of the cells in the antibody screen is weakly reactive, so you proceed with an antibody identification using a ten-cell panel. However, only two cells are weakly reactive (1+) and show no pattern of reactivity. A second panel is run and yields similar results. You decide to run an antibody identification panel using the conventional tube testing method with LISS as your enhancement medium. All reactions are negative using LISS, including the cells that were previously positive.

1. Can the antibody screen be interpreted as negative?
2. Provide an explanation for the observed results.
3. Are there additional tests that should be conducted to complete testing on this patient? If so, which tests should be run?

SUMMARY CHART

- ✔ The antiglobulin test is used to detect RBCs sensitized by IgG alloantibodies, IgG autoantibodies, and complement components.
- ✔ AHG reagents containing anti-IgG are needed for the detection of IgG antibodies because the IgG monomeric structure is too small to directly agglutinate sensitized RBCs.
- ✔ Polyspecific AHG sera contain antibodies to human IgG and the C3d component of human complement.
- ✔ Monospecific AHG sera contain only one antibody specificity: either anti-IgG or antibody to anti–C3b-C3d.
- ✔ Classic AHG sera (polyclonal) are prepared by injecting human globulins into rabbits, and an immune stimulus triggers production of antibody to human serum.
- ✔ Hybridoma technology is used to produce monoclonal antiglobulin serum.
- ✔ The DAT detects in vivo sensitization of RBCs with IgG or complement components. Clinical conditions that can result in a positive DAT include HDN, HTR, and AIHA.

- ✔ The IAT detects in vitro sensitization of RBCs and can be applied to compatibility testing, antibody screen, antibody identification, RBC phenotyping, and titration studies.
- ✔ A positive DAT is followed by a DAT panel using monospecific anti-IgG and anti-C3d to determine the specific type of protein sensitizing the RBC.
- ✔ EDTA should be used to collect blood samples for the DAT to avoid in vitro complement attachment associated with refrigerated clotted specimens.
- ✔ There are multiple sources or error that can be introduced into the AHG procedure.
- ✔ LISS, PEG, polybrene, and albumin can all be used as enhancement media for AHG testing, with each having their own advantages and disadvantages.
- ✔ Conventional tube testing, gel technology, enzyme-linked technology, and solid-phase testing are available methods to use in AHG testing.
- ✔ Method-dependent antibodies do exist and should be evaluated on a case-by-case basis.

Review Questions

1. A principle of the antiglobulin test is:
   a. IgG and C3d are required for RBC sensitization.
   b. Human globulin is eluted from RBCs during saline washings.
   c. Injection of human globulin into an animal engenders passive immunity.
   d. AHG reacts with human globulin molecules bound to RBCs or free in serum.

2. Polyspecific AHG reagent contains:
   a. Anti-IgG.
   b. Anti-IgG and anti-IgM.
   c. Anti-IgG and anti-C3d.
   d. Anti-C3d.

3. Monoclonal anti-C3d is:
   a. Derived from one clone of plasma cells.
   b. Derived from multiple clones of plasma cells.
   c. Derived from immunization of rabbits.
   d. Reactive with C3b and C3d.

4. Which of the following is a clinically significant antibody whose detection has been reported in some instances to be dependent on anticomplement activity in polyspecific AHG?
   a. Anti-Jk^a
   b. Anti-Le^a
   c. Anti-P$_1$
   d. Anti-H

5. After the addition of IgG-coated RBCs (check cells) to a negative AHG reaction during an antibody screen, a negative result is observed. Which of the following is a correct interpretation?
   a. The antibody screen is negative.
   b. The antibody screen needs to be repeated.
   c. The saline washings were adequate.
   d. Reactive AHG reagent was added.

6. RBCs must be washed in saline at least three times before the addition of AHG reagent to:
   a. Wash away any hemolyzed cells
   b. Remove traces of free serum globulins
   c. Neutralize any excess AHG reagent
   d. Increase the antibody binding to antigen

7. An in vitro phenomenon associated with a positive IAT is:
   a. Maternal antibody coating fetal RBCs
   b. Patient antibody coating patient RBCs
   c. Recipient antibody coating transfused donor RBCs
   d. Identification of alloantibody specificity using a panel of reagent RBCs

8. False-positive DAT results are most often associated with:
   a. Use of refrigerated, clotted blood samples in which complement components coat RBCs in vitro.
   b. A recipient of a recent transfusion manifesting an immune response to recently transfused RBCs.
   c. Presence of heterophile antibodies from administration of globulin.
   d. A positive autocontrol caused by polyagglutination.

9. Polyethylene glycol enhances antigen-antibody reactions by:
   a. Decreasing zeta potential.
   b. Concentrating antibody by removing water.
   c. Increasing antibody affinity for antigen.
   d. Increasing antibody specificity for antigen.

10. Solid-phase antibody screening is based on:
    a. Adherence.
    b. Agglutination.
    c. Hemolysis.
    d. Precipitation.

11. A positive DAT may be found in which of the following situations?
    a. A weak D-positive patient
    b. A patient with anti-K
    c. HDN
    d. An incompatible crossmatch

12. What do Coombs' control cells consist of?
    a. Type A-positive cells coated with anti-D
    b. Type A-negative cells coated with anti-D
    c. Type O-positive cells coated with anti-D
    d. Type O-negative cells coated with anti-D

13. Which of the following methods requires the use of check cells?
    a. LISS
    b. Gel
    c. Solid-phase
    d. Enzyme-linked

14. Which factor can affect AHG testing, yet is uncontrollable in the lab?
    a. Temperature
    b. Antibody affinity
    c. Gravitational force in the centrifuge
    d. Incubation time

15. If you had the authority to decide which primary AHG methodology to utilize at your lab, which method would you choose based on the knowledge that the majority of the staff are generalists?
    a. LISS
    b. Polybrene
    c. Solid phase or gel
    d. Enzyme-linked

16. A 27-year-old group O mother has just given birth to a beautiful, group A baby girl. Since the mother has IgG anti-A in her plasma, it is likely that the baby is experiencing some in vivo red cell destruction. Which of the following methods and tests would be most effective at detecting the anti-A on the baby's RBCs?

   a. DAT using common tube technique
   b. DAT using gel
   c. IAT using common tube technique
   d. IAT using gel

References

1. Coombs, RRA, et al: A new test for the detection of weak and "incomplete" Rh agglutinins. Br J Exp Pathol 26:255, 1945.
2. Coombs, RRA, et al: In-vivo isosensitisation of red cells in babies with haemolytic disease. Lancet i:264, 1946.
3. Race, RR, and Sanger, R: Blood Groups in Man, 6th ed. Blackwell Scientific, Oxford, 1975, p 283.
4. Moreschi, C: Neue Tatsachen über die Blutkorperchen Agglutinationen. Zentralbl Bakteriol 46:49, 1908.
5. Dacie, JF: Differences in the behaviour of sensitized red cells to agglutination by antiglobulin sera. Lancet ii:954, 1951.
6. Dacie, JV, et al: "Incomplete" cold antibodies: Role of complement in sensitization to antiglobulin serum by potentially haemolytic antibodies. Br J Haematol 3:77, 1957.
7. Harboe, M, et al: Identification of the component of complement participating in the antiglobulin reaction. Immunology 6:412, 1963.
8. Jenkins, GC, et al: Role of C4 in the antiglobulin reaction. Nature 186:482, 1960.
9. Roback, J, Combs, M, Grossman, B, and Hillyer, C: Technical Manual, 16th ed. CD-ROM. American Association of Blood Banks, Bethesda, MD, 2009.
10. Brecher, ME (ed): Technical Manual, 14th ed. American Association of Blood Banks, Bethesda, MD, 2002.
11. Issitt, C: Monoclonal antiglobulin reagents. Dade International Online, 1997. Available at www.dadeinternational.com/hemo/papers/monoanti.htm.
12. Kohler, G, and Milstein, C: Continuous cultures of fused cells secreting antibody of predefined specificity. Nature 256:495, 1975.
13. Lachman, PJ, et al: Use of monoclonal antibodies to characterize the fragments of C3 that are found on erythrocytes. Vox Sang 45:367, 1983.
14. Holt, PDJ, et al: NBTS/BRIC 8: A monoclonal anti-C3d antibody. Transfusion 25:267, 1985.
15. Voak, D, et al: Monoclonal antibodies—C3 serology. Biotest Bull 1:339, 1983.
16. Mollison, PL: Blood Transfusion in Clinical Medicine, 7th ed. Blackwell Scientific, Oxford, 1983, p 502.
17. Garratty, G, et al: An IgA high titre cold agglutinin with an unusual blood group specificity within the Pr complex. Vox Sang 25:32, 1973.
18. Petz, LD, and Garratty, G: Acquired Immune Hemolytic Anemias. Churchill Livingstone, New York, 1980, p 193.
19. Polley, MJ, and Mollison, PL: The role of complement in the detection of blood group antibodies: Special reference to the antiglobulin test. Transfusion 1:9, 1961.
20. Polley, MJ, et al: The role of 19S gamma-globulin blood group antibodies in the antiglobulin reaction. Br J Haematol 8:149, 1962.
21. Stratton, F, et al: The preparation and uses of antiglobulin reagents with special reference to complement fixing blood group antibodies. Transfusion 2:135, 1962.
22. Stratton, F, et al: Value of gel fixation on Sephadex G-200 in the analysis of blood group antibodies. J Clin Pathol 21:708, 1968.
23. Lachman, PJ, and Muller-Eberhard, HJ: The demonstration in human serum of "conglutinogen-activating-factor" and its effect on the third component of complement. J Immunol 100:691, 1968.
24. Muller-Eberhard, HJ: Chemistry and reaction mechanisms of complement. Adv Immunol 8:1, 1968.
25. Cooper, NR: Isolation and analysis of mechanisms of action of an inactivator of C4b in normal human serum. J Exp Med 141:890, 1975.
26. Case, J, et al: International reference reagents: Antihuman globulin, an ISBT/ICSH Joint Working Party Report. Vox Sang 77:121, 1999.
27. Brown, DL, et al: The in vivo behaviour of complement-coated red cells: Studies in C6-deficient, Ce-depleted and normal rabbits. Clin Exp Immunol 7:401, 1970.
28. Engelfriet, CP, et al: Autoimmune haemolytic anemias: 111 preparation and examination of specific antisera against complement components and products, and their use in serological studies. Clin Exp Immunol 6:721, 1970.
29. Garratty, G, and Petz, LD: The significance of red cell bound complement components in development of standards and quality assurance for the anticomplement components of antiglobulin sera. Transfusion 16:297, 1976.
30. Petz, LD, et al: Clinical Practice of Transfusion Medicine, 3rd ed. Churchill Livingstone, New York, 1996, p 207.
31. Petz, LD, et al: Compatibility testing. Transfusion 21:633, 1981.
32. Howard, JE, et al: Clinical significance of the anticomplement component of antiglobulin antisera. Transfusion 22:269, 1982.
33. Milam JD: Laboratory medicine parameter: Utilizing monospecific antihuman globulin to test blood group compatibility. Am J Clin Pathol 104:122, 1995.
34. Eder, AF: Evaluation of routine pretransfusion direct antiglobulin test in a pediatric setting. Lab Med 24:680, 2003.
35. Judd, WJ, et al: The evaluation of a positive direct antiglobulin test in pretransfusion testing revisited. Transfusion 26:220, 1986.
36. Roback, JD, Combs, MR, Grossman, BJ, and Hillyer, CD (eds): Technical Manual, 16th ed. AABB, Bethesda, MD, 2008.
37. Stroup, M, and MacIlroy, M: Evaluation of the albumin antiglobulin technique in antibody detection. Transfusion 5:184, 1965.
38. Low, B, and Messeter, L: Antiglobulin test in low-ionic strength salt solution for rapid antibody screening and cross-matching. Vox Sang 26:53, 1974.
39. Moore, HC, and Mollison, PL: Use of a low-ionic strength medium in manual tests for antibody detection. Transfusion 16:291, 1976.
40. Shirley, R, et al: Polyethylene glycol versus low-ionic strength solution in pretransfusion testing: A blinded comparison study. Transfusion 34:5, 1994.
41. Barrett, V, et al: Analysis of the routine use of polyethylene glycol (PEG) as an enhancement medium. Immunohematology 11:1, 1995.
42. Jorgensen, J, et al: The influence of ionic strength, albumin and incubation time on the sensitivity of indirect Coombs' test. Vox Sang 36:186, 1980.
43. Voak, D, et al: Low-ionic strength media for rapid antibody detection: Optimum conditions and quality control. Med Lab Sci 37:107, 1980.
44. Bruce, M, et al: A serious source of error in antiglobulin testing. Transfusion 26:177, 1986.
45. Green, C, et al: Quality assurance of physiological saline used for blood grouping. Med Lab Sci 43:364, 1968.
46. Voak, D, et al: Antihuman globulin reagent specification: The European and ISBT/ICSH view. Biotest Bull 3:7, 1986.
47. Mallory, D, et al: Immunohematology Methods and Procedures. American National Red Cross, Washington, D.C., 1993, pp 40–41.

48. Lalezari, P, and Jiang, RF: The manual polybrene test: A simple and rapid procedure for detection of red cell antibodies. Transfusion 20:206, 1980.

49. Crawford, MN, et al: Microplate system for routine use in blood bank laboratories. Transfusion 10:258, 1970.

50. Redman, M, et al: Typing of red cells on microplates by low-ionic polybrene technique. Med Lab Sci 43:393, 1986.

51. Liu, JC, Wang, Y, Liu, FP, and He, YS: The manual polybrene test has limited sensitivities for detecting the Kidd blood group system. Scand J Clin Lab Investig 69:7, 797–800, 2009.

52. Moore, HH: Automated reading of red cell antibody identification tests by a solid phase antiglobulin technique. Transfusion 24:218, 1984.

53. Plapp, FV, et al: A solid phase antibody screen. Am J Clin Pathol 82:719, 1984.

54. Lapierre, Y, et al: The gel test: A new way to detect red cell antigen-antibody reactions. Transfusion 30:2, 1990.

55. Tissot, JD, et al: The direct antiglobulin test: Still a place for the tube technique? Vox Sang 77:223, 1999.

56. Chuansumrit, A, et al: The benefit of the direct antiglobulin test using gel technique in ABO hemolytic disease of the newborn. Southeast Asian J Trop Med Pub Health 28:428, 1997.

57. Lai, M, et al: Clinically significant autoimmune hemolytic anemia with a negative direct antiglobulin test by routine tube test and positive by column agglutination method. Immunohematology 18:109, 2002.

58. Mitek, JF, et al: The value of the gel test and ELAT in autoimmune haemolytic anaemia. Clin Lab Haem 17:311, 1995.

59. Das, SS, Chaudhary, R, and Khetan, D: A comparison of conventional tube test and gel technique in evaluation of direct antiglobulin test. Hematology 12(2):175–178, 2007.

60. Novaretti, MC, Jens, E, Pagliarini, T, Bonifacio, SL, Dorlhiac-Llacer, PE, and Chamone, DA: Comparison of conventional tube test technique and gel microcolumn assay for direct antiglobulin test: Large study. J Clin Lab Anal 18(5):255–258, 2004.

61. Casina, TS: In search of the Holy Grail: Comparison of antibody screening methods. Immunohematology 22(4):196–202, 2006.

62. Shulman, IA, Maffei, LM, and Downes, KA: North American pretransfusion testing practices, 2001–2004: Results from the College of American Pathologists Interlaboratory Comparison Program survey data, 2001–2004. Arch Pathol Lab Med 129(8):984–989, 2005.

63. Bunker, ML, Thomas, CL, and Geyer, SJ: Optimizing pretransfusion antibody detection and identification: A parallel, blinded comparison of tube PEG, solid-phase, and automated methods. Transfusion 41(5):621–626, 2001.

64. Klostermann, DA, Puca, KE, Scott, EA, and Johnson, ST: Comparison of methods for detection of antenatal anti-D. Transfusion 46(9S):148A, 2006.

65. Weisbach, V, et al: Comparison of the performance of microtube column systems and solid-phase systems and the tube low-ionic-strength solution additive indirect antiglobulin test in the detection of red cell alloantibodies. Transfusion Med 16(4):276–284, 2006.

66. Yamada, C, Serrano-Rahman, L, Vasovic, LV, Mohandas, K, and Uehlinger, J: Antibody identification using both automated solid-phase red cell adherence assay and a tube polyethylene glycol antiglobulin method. Transfusion 48(8):1693–1698, 2008.

67. Dwyre, DM, Erickson, Y, Heintz, M, Elbert, C, and Strauss, RG: Comparative sensitivity of solid phase versus PEG enhancement assays for detection and identification of RBC antibodies. Transfus Apher Sci 35(1):19–23, 2006.

68. Garozzo, G, et al: A comparison of two automated methods for the detection and identification of red blood cell alloantibodies. Blood Transfusion 5(1):33–40, 2007.

Chapter 6

The ABO Blood Group System

Denise M. Harmening, PhD, MT(ASCP), CLS (NCA); Glenda Forneris, MHS, MT(ASCP)SBB; Barbara J. Tubby MSEd, BS, MT(ASCP)SBB

OBJECTIVES

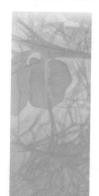

1. Describe the reciprocal relationships between ABO antigens and antibodies for blood types O, A, B, and AB.
2. Identify the frequencies of the four major blood types in the white, black, Hispanic, and Asian populations.
3. Explain the effect of age on the production of ABO isoagglutinins.
4. Describe the immunoglobulin classes of ABO antibodies in group O, A, and B individuals.
5. Predict the ABO phenotypes and genotypes of offspring from various ABO matings.
6. Explain the formation of H, A, and B antigens on the red blood cells (RBCs) from precursor substance to immunodominant sugars.
7. Describe the formation of H, A, and B soluble substances.
8. Explain the principle of the hemagglutination inhibition assay for the determination of secretor status.
9. Describe the qualitative and quantitative differences between the A_1 and A_2 phenotypes.
10. Describe the reactivity of *Ulex europaeus* with the various ABO groups.
11. Describe the characteristics of the weak subgroups of A (A_3, A_x, A_{end}, A_m, A_y, A_{el}).
12. Describe the characteristics of the Bombay phenotypes.
13. Explain the effects of disease on the expression of ABH antigens and antibodies.
14. Interpret the results from an ABO typing and resolve any discrepancies, if present.

Introduction

The ABO system is the most important of all blood groups in transfusion practice. It is the only blood group system in which individuals have antibodies in their serum to antigens that are absent from their RBCs. This occurs without any exposure to RBCs through transfusion or pregnancy. Due to the presence of these antibodies, transfusion of an incompatible ABO type may result in immediate **lysis** of donor RBCs. This produces a very severe, if not fatal, transfusion reaction in the patient. Testing to detect ABO incompatibility between a donor and potential transfusion recipient is the foundation on which all other pretransfusion testing is based.

Even today, transfusion of the wrong ABO group remains the leading cause of death in hemolytic transfusion reaction fatalities reported to the FDA; however, transfusion-related

Table 6–1 Transfusion-Related Fatalities by Complication, FY 2009

COMPLICATION	NUMBER	FY09
TRALI	13*	30%
HTR (non-ABO)	8	18%
HTR (ABO)	4	9%
Microbial infection	5	11%
TACO	12	27%
Anaphylaxis	1	2%
Other	1**	2%
TOTALS	44	100%

*In FY 2007, the review committee began using the Canadian Consensus Conference criteria[5,6] for evaluating TRALI cases; these numbers include both "TRALI" and "possible TRALI" cases.
**Other: Hypotensive Reaction[7] Key: HTR = hemolytic transfusion reaction; TACO = transfusion-associated circulatory overload; TRALI = transfusion-related acute lung injury
Data from 2009, F. R. (n.d.): Vaccines, Blood & Biologics; U.S. Food and Drug Administration. Fatalities Reported to FDA Following Blood Collection and Transfusion: Annual Summary for Fiscal Year 2009. Retrieved March 22, 2010, from www.fda.gov/BiologicsBloodVaccines/SafetyAvailability/ReportaProblem/TransfusionDonationFatalities/ucm204763.htm.

acute lung injury (TRALI) was the most frequent cause of death in fiscal year (FY) 2009[1] (Table 6–1). In FY 2009, there were four reports of fatal hemolytic transfusion reactions due to ABO incompatible blood transfusions (Box 6–1 lists the causes in each of these four cases).[1] This chapter presents the ABO blood group system and discusses the biochemistry, properties, and characteristics of ABO antigens and antibodies. In addition, weak subgroups and common discrepancies will be introduced to provide a working knowledge for routine ABO testing.

Historical Perspective and Routine ABO Testing

Karl Landsteiner truly opened the doors of blood banking with his discovery of the first human blood group system, ABO. This marked the beginning of the concept of individual uniqueness defined by the RBC antigens present on the RBC

BOX 6–1

Causes of Fatal Hemolytic Transfusion Reactions Due to ABO Incompatible Blood Transfusions in FY 2009

- Case 1: Recipient identification error at the time of transfusion (nursing error)
- Case 2: Patient sample labels switched (phlebotomist error)
- Case 3: Sample collected from incorrect patient (phlebotomist error)
- Case 4: Patient sample mistyped (lab error)

Data from 2009, F. R. (n.d.): Vaccines, Blood & Biologics; U.S. Food and Drug Administration. Fatalities Reported to FDA Following Blood Collection and Transfusion: Annual Summary for Fiscal Year 2009. Retrieved March 22, 2010, from www.fda.gov/BiologicsBloodVaccines/SafetyAvailability/ReportaProblem/TransfusionDonationFatalities/ucm204763.htm.

membrane. In 1901, Landsteiner drew blood from himself and five associates, separated the cells and serum, and then mixed each cell sample with each serum.[2] He was inadvertently the first individual to perform forward and reverse grouping. **Forward grouping** (front type) is defined as using known sources of commercial antisera (anti-A, anti-B) to detect antigens on an individual's RBCs. Figure 6–1 outlines the steps of performing the forward grouping for ABO (see color insert following page 128), and Table 6–2 lists the results of the forward grouping procedure.

Reverse grouping (back type) is defined as detecting ABO antibodies in the patient's serum by using known reagent RBCs, namely A_1 and B cells. Figure 6–2 outlines the steps of performing the reverse ABO grouping (see color insert following page 128), and Table 6–3 summarizes the results of the procedures. Table 6–4 lists the characteristics of the routine reagents used for ABO testing in the blood bank laboratory.

ABO forward and reverse grouping tests must be performed on all donors and patients.[3] ABO grouping is the

Table 6–2 ABO Forward Grouping: Principle—Detection of Antigens on Patient's RBCs With Known Commercial Antisera

PATIENT RBCS WITH ANTI-A	PATIENT RBCS WITH ANTI-B	INTERPRETATION OF BLOOD GROUP
0	0	O
4+	0	A
0	4+	B
4+	4+	AB

+ = visual agglutination
0 = negative
Note: Reaction gradings vary from patient to patient.

Table 6–3 ABO Reverse Grouping: Principle—Detection of ABO Antibodies (Isoagglutinins) in Serum of Patient With Known Commercial RBCs

PATIENT SERUM WITH REAGENT A_1 CELLS	PATIENT SERUM WITH REAGENT B CELLS	INTERPRETATION OF BLOOD GROUP
4+	4+	O
0	3+	A
3+	0	B
0	0	AB

+ = visual agglutination
0 = negative
Note: Reaction gradings vary from patient to patient.

Table 6–4   Characteristics of Routine Reagents Used for ABO Testing

Forward Grouping	ANTI-A REAGENT	ANTI-B REAGENT
	• Monoclonol antibody*	• Monoclonal antibody*
	• Highly specific	• Highly specific
	• IgM	• IgM
	• Clear blue colored reagent	• Clear yellow colored reagent (contains an acriflavine dye)
	• Expected 3+ to 4+ reaction	• Expected 3+ to 4+ reaction
	• Usually use 1–2 drops	• Usually use 1–2 drops

	REAGENT A₁ AND B CELLS
Reverse Grouping	• Human source • 4%–5% red cell suspension • Expected 2+ to 4+ reaction usually use one drop

*General rule: Always drop clear solutions first and RBCs second to make sure you have added both a source of antibody and antigen.

most frequently performed test in the blood bank. There is always an inverse reciprocal relationship between the forward and reverse type; thus, one serves as a check on the other. For example, if the individual has A antigens only on their red cells, there will be an "expected" naturally occurring anti-B antibody in their serum since they lack the B antigen.

It has been postulated that bacteria, pollen particles, and other substances present in nature are chemically similar to A and B antigens. Bacteria are widespread in the environment, which constantly exposes individuals to A-like and B-like antigens. This exposure serves as a source of stimulation of anti-A and anti-B. All other defined blood group systems do *not* regularly have in their serum expected "**naturally occurring**" antibodies to antigens they lack on their RBCs. Antibody production in most other blood group systems requires the introduction of foreign RBCs by transfusion or pregnancy, although some individuals can occasionally have antibodies present that are not related to the introduction of foreign RBCs. (These antibodies are usually of the IgM type and are not consistently present or expected in everyone's serum.) Therefore, performance of serum

grouping is unique to the ABO blood group system. The regular occurrence of anti-A and/or anti-B in persons lacking the corresponding antigen(s) serves as a confirmation of results in ABO grouping. Table 6–5 summarizes the forward and reverse grouping for the common ABO blood groups.

The frequency of these blood groups in the white and black populations is outlined in Table 6–6.[4] Group O and A are the most common blood types, and blood group AB is the rarest. However, frequencies of ABO groups differ in a few selected populations and ethnic groups (Table 6–7).[4] For example, group B is found twice as frequently in blacks and Asians as in whites. In addition, there is a significant decrease in the distribution of group A in these two ethnic populations in comparison to whites. It has been reported that subgroup A₂ is rarely found in Asians.[5]

ABO Antibodies

Individuals normally produce antibodies directed against the A and/or B antigen(s) absent from their RBCs. These antibodies have been described as *naturally occurring* because they are

Table 6–5   Summary of Forward and Reverse Groupings

BLOOD GROUP	Forward Group Patient's Cells With Reagents			Reverse Group Patient's Serum With Reagents		
	ANTI-A	ANTI-B	ANTIGEN(S) ON RBCS	A₁ CELLS	B CELLS	ANTIBODY(IES) IN SERUM
O	0	0	No A or B antigen	4+	4+	A and B
A	4+	0	A	0	2+	B
B	0	4+	B	3+	0	A
AB	3+	3+	A and B	0	0	No A or B antibodies

0 = negative (no agglutination)
+ = visual agglutination
Note: Reaction gradings vary from patient to patient.

Table 6–6	**Frequency of ABO Blood Groups in the United States***

	RACE	
Blood Group	**Whites**	**Blacks**
O	45%	50%
A	40%	26%
B	11%	20%
AB	4%	4%

*Percentages rounded to the nearest whole number
Data from Garratty, G, Glynn, SA, and McEntire, R: ABO and Rh (D) phenotype frequencies of different racial/ethnic groups in the United States. Transfusion 44:703–706, 2004.

produced without any exposure to RBCs. The ABO antibodies are predominantly IgM, and they activate complement and react at room temperature or colder.[5] ABO antibodies produce strong direct **agglutination** reactions during ABO testing. The production of ABO antibodies is initiated at birth, but **titers** are generally too low for detection until the individual is 3 to 6 months of age.[6] Therefore, most antibodies found in cord blood serum are of maternal origin. Results of serum ABO testing before 3 to 6 months of age cannot be considered valid because some or all of the antibodies present may be IgG maternal antibodies that have crossed the placenta. As a result, it is logical to perform only forward grouping on cord blood from newborn infants.

Antibody production peaks when an individual is between 5 and 10 years of age and declines later in life.[6] Elderly people usually have lower levels of anti-A and anti-B; therefore, antibodies may be undetectable in the reverse grouping (see the "ABO Discrepancies" section later in this chapter). ABO antibodies can cause rapid intravascular **hemolysis** if the wrong ABO group is transfused; this can result in the patient dying.[1]

Although anti-A (from a group B individual) and anti-B (from a group A individual) contains predominantly IgM antibody, there may be small quantities of IgG present.[5] Serum

Table 6–7	**ABO Phenotype Frequencies of Ethnic Groups in the United States**

U.S. FREQUENCIES (%) (ROUNDED TO THE NEAREST WHOLE NUMBER)

Phenotype	**Whites**	**Blacks**	**Hispanic***	**Asian****
O	45	50	56	40
A	40	26	31	28
B	11	20	10	25
AB	4	4	3	7

*Hispanic includes Mexican, Puerto Rican, Cuban, and other Hispanics.
**Asian includes Chinese, Filipino, Indian, Japanese, Korean, and Vietnamese.
Data from Garratty, G, Glynn, SA, and McEntire, R: ABO and Rh (D) phenotype frequencies of different racial/ethnic groups in the United States. Transfusion 44:703–706, 2004.

from group O individuals contains not only anti-A and anti-B but also anti-A,B, which reacts with A and B cells. Anti-A,B antibody activity, originally thought to be just a mixture of anti-A and anti-B, cannot be separated into a pure specificity when adsorbed with either A or B cells.[7] For example, if group O serum is adsorbed with A or B cells, the antibody eluted will react with both A and B cells.[7] Anti-A,B antibody is *not* a combination of anti-A and anti-B but is a separate "cross-reacting" antibody that is usually IgG in nature.[7] Knowing the amount of IgG anti-A, anti-B, or anti-A,B in a woman's serum sometimes allows prediction or diagnosis of hemolytic disease of the fetus and newborn (HDFN) caused by ABO incompatibility.[8] Often cord blood samples from babies of group O mothers are examined for possible ABO HDFN (see Chapter 19, "Hemolytic Disease of the Fetus and Newborn [HDFN]"). Both immunoglobulin classes of ABO antibodies react preferentially at room temperature (20°C to 24°C) or below and efficiently activate complement at 37°C.[9]

Testing RBCs with reagent anti-A,B is not required as a routine part of ABO testing.[10] However, some believe that anti-A,B is more effective at detecting weakly expressed A and B antigens than reagent anti-A or anti-B. However, the production and use of **monoclonal antisera** have made anti-A and anti-B reagents much more sensitive, to the point where weak A and B antigens can be detected routinely. Therefore, anti-A,B reagent is not usually used in routine ABO red cell testing on patient samples. It is still routinely used when performing ABO confirmation of blood donors, because it is more economical to use one reagent (anti-A,B) than to use two reagents (anti-A and anti-B) to verify group O donor units.[3] Reagent anti-A,B can be prepared using blended monoclonal anti-A and anti-B; **polyclonal** human anti-A,B; or a blend of monoclonal anti-A, anti-B, and anti-A,B.[3] Consult the manufacturer's package insert to determine if a reagent anti-A,B reacts with a specific weak A phenotype.

Inheritance of the ABO Blood Groups

The theory for the inheritance of the ABO blood groups was first described by Bernstein in 1924. He demonstrated that an individual inherits one *ABO* gene from each parent and that these two genes determine which ABO antigens are present on the RBC membrane. The inheritance of *ABO* genes, therefore, follows simple **Mendelian genetics**. ABO, like most other blood group systems, is codominant in expression.[9] (For a review of genetics, see Chapter 2, "Basic Genetics.") One position, or **locus**, on each chromosome 9 is occupied by an *A*, *B*, or *O* gene.[11,12] The *O* gene is considered an **amorph**, as no detectable antigen is produced in response to the inheritance of this gene. Therefore, the group O phenotype is an **autosomal** recessive trait with the inheritance of two *O* genes that are nonfunctional.

The designations group A and B refer to phenotypes, whereas *AA*, *BO*, and *OO* denote genotypes. In the case of an O individual, both phenotype and genotype are the same, because that individual would have to be **homozygous** for the *O* gene. An individual who has the phenotype A (or B) can have the genotype *AA* or *AO* (or *BB* or *BO*). Box 6–2 lists

BOX 6–2

ABO Genotypes and Phenotypes

Genotype	Phenotype
A_1A_1	A_1
A_1A_2	A_1
A_1O	A_1
A_2A_2	A_2
A_2O	A_2
A_1B	A_1B
A_2B	A_2B
OO	O
BB	B
BO	B

the ABO genotypes and phenotypes. **Serologically**, it is not possible to determine the genotype from the phenotype of an A or B individual. Family studies or molecular assays would have to be performed to determine the exact genotype. The phenotype and genotype are the same in an AB individual because of the inheritance of both the *A* and *B* gene. Table 6–8 lists possible ABO phenotypes and genotypes from various matings.

Formation of A, B, and H Red Cell Antigens

The formation of ABH antigens results from the interaction of genes at three separate loci (ABO, Hh, and Se). These genes do not actually code for the production of antigens but rather produce specific **glycosyltransferases** that add sugars to a basic precursor substance (Table 6–9). A, B, and H antigens are formed from the same basic precursor material (called a **paragloboside** or **glycan**) to which sugars are attached in response to specific enzyme transferases elicited by an inherited gene.[11–13]

The **H antigen** is actually the precursor structure on which A and B antigens are made. Inheritance of the *H* gene results in the formation of the H antigen. The *H* and *Se* genes are closely linked and located on chromosome 19, in contrast to *ABO* genes, which are located on chromosome 9. The *H* and *Se* genes are not part of the ABO system; however, their inheritance does influence A and B antigen expression. The *H* gene must be inherited to form the ABO antigens on the RBCs, and the *Se* gene must be inherited to form the ABO antigens in secretions. The precursor substance on erythrocytes is referred to as type 2. This means that the terminal galactose on the precursor substance is attached to the N-acetylglucosamine in a beta $1 \rightarrow 4$ linkage (Fig. 6–3). A type 1 precursor substance refers to a beta $1 \rightarrow 3$ linkage between galactose and N-acetylglucosamine, which will be described below. ABH antigens on the RBC are constructed on oligosaccharide chains of a type 2 precursor substance.[14]

The ABH antigens develop early in fetal life but do not increase much in strength during the gestational period. The RBCs of the newborn have been estimated to carry anywhere from 25% to 50% of the number of antigenic sites found on the adult RBC.[10] As a result, reactions of newborn RBCs with ABO reagent antisera are frequently weaker than reactions

Table 6–8   ABO Groups of Offspring from Various Possible ABO Matings

OFFSPRING POSSIBLE PHENOTYPES	MATING GENOTYPES	MATING PHENOTYPES (AND GENOTYPES)
A × A	AA × AA	A (AA)
	AA × AO	A (AA or AO)
	AO × AO	A (AA or AO) or O(OO)
B × B	BB × BB	B (BB)
	BB × BO	B (BB or BO)
	BO × BO	B (BB or BO) or O (OO)
AB × AB	AB × AB	AB (AB) or A (AA) or B(BB)
O × O	OO × OO	O (OO)
A × B	AA × BB	AB (AB)
	AO × BB	AB (AB) or B (BO)
	AA × BO	AB (AB) or A (AO)
	AO × BO	AB (AB) or A (AO) or B (BO) or O (OO)
A × O	AA × OO	A (AO)
	AO × OO	A (AO) or O (OO)
A × AB	AA × AB	AB (AB) or A (AA)
	AO × AB	AB (AB) or A (AA or AO) or B (BO)
B × O	BB × OO	B (BO)
	BO × OO	B (BO) or O (OO)
B × AB	BB × AB	AB (AB) or B (BB)
	BO × AB	AB (AB) or B (BB or BO) or A (AO)
AB × O	AB × OO	A (AO) or B (BO)

with adult cells. The expression of A and B antigens on the RBCs is fully developed by 2 to 4 years of age and remains constant throughout life.[8] In addition to age, the phenotypic expression of ABH antigens may vary with race, genetic interaction, and disease states.[15]

Interaction of *Hh* and *ABO* Genes

Individuals who are blood group O inherit at least one *H* gene (genotype *HH* or *Hh*) and two *O* genes. The *H* gene elicits the production of an enzyme called α-2-L-fucosyltransferase, which transfers the sugar L-fucose to an **oligosaccharide chain** on the **terminal galactose** of **type 2 chains**.[13] The sugars that occupy the terminal positions of this precursor chain and confer blood group specificity are called the **immunodominant sugars**. Therefore, L-fucose is

Table 6–9	**Glycosyltransferases and Immunodominant Sugars Responsible for H, A, and B Antigen Specificities**		
GENE	**GLYCOSYLTRANSFERASE**	**IMMUNODOMINANT SUGAR**	**ANTIGEN**
H	α-2-L-fucosyltransferase	L-fucose	H
A	α-3-N-acetylgalactosaminyltransferase	N-acetyl-D-galactosamine	A
B	α-3-D-galactosyltransferase	D-galactose	B

the sugar responsible for H specificity (blood group O; Fig. 6–4). The *O* gene at the ABO locus, which is sometimes referred to as an amorph, does not elicit the production of a catalytically active polypeptide transferase; therefore, the H substance remains unmodified.[13] Consequently, the O blood group has the highest concentration of H antigen. The H substance (L-fucose) must be formed for the other sugars to be attached in response to an inherited *A* and/or *B* gene.

The *H* gene is present in more than 99.99% of the random population. Its allele, "h," is quite rare, and the genotype *hh* is extremely rare. The term **Bombay** has been used to refer to the phenotype that lacks normal expression of the ABH antigens because of the inheritance of the *hh* genotype. The *hh* genotype does not elicit the production of α-2-L-fucosyltransferase. Therefore, L-fucose is not added to the type 2 chain, and H substance is not expressed on the RBC. Even though Bombay (*hh*) individuals may inherit *ABO* genes, normal expression, as reflected in the formation of A, B, or H antigens, does not occur. (See "The Bombay Phenotypes" section.)

In the formation of blood group A, the *A* gene (*AA* or *AO*) codes for the production of **α-3-N-acetylgalactosaminyltransferase**, which transfers an **N-acetyl-D-galactosamine(GalNAc) sugar** to the H substance. This sugar is responsible for A specificity (blood group A; Fig. 6–5). The A-specific immunodominant sugar is linked to a type 2 precursor substance that now contains H substance through the action of the *H* gene.

The *A* gene tends to elicit higher concentrations of transferase than the *B* gene. This leads to the conversion of practically all of the H antigen on the RBC to A antigen sites. As many as 810,000 to 1,170,000 antigen sites exist on an A$_1$ adult RBC in response to inherited genes.[5] Individuals who are blood group B inherit a *B* gene (*BB* or *BO*) that codes for the production of α-3-D-galactosyltransferase, which attaches D-galactose (Gal) sugar to the H substance previously placed on the type 2 precursor substance through the action of the *H* gene.[14] This sugar is responsible for B specificity (blood group B; Fig. 6–6). Anywhere from 610,000 to

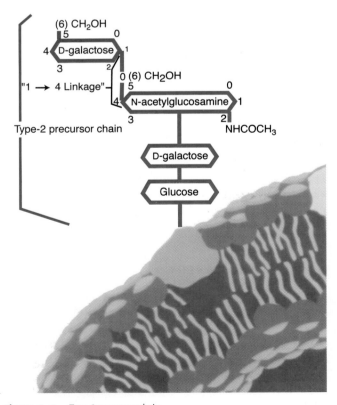

Figure 6–3. Type 2 precursor chain.

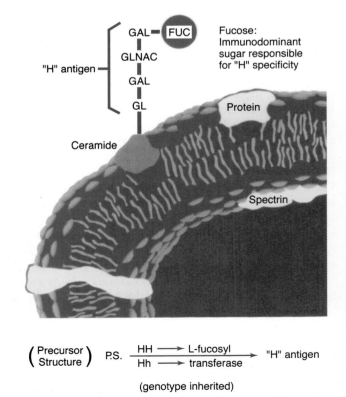

Figure 6–4. Formation of the H antigen.

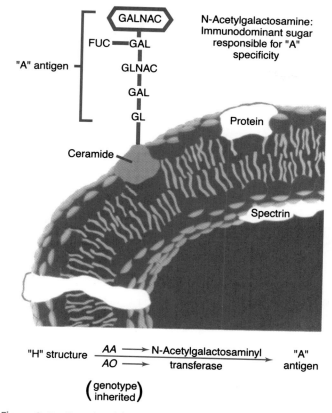

"A" antigen

GALNAC

N-Acetylgalactosamine: Immunodominant sugar responsible for "A" specificity

FUC — GAL
GLNAC
GAL
GL

Protein

Ceramide

Spectrin

| "H" structure | $\dfrac{AA \longrightarrow}{AO \longrightarrow}$ | N-Acetylgalactosaminyl transferase | $\longrightarrow$ | "A" antigen |

$\binom{\text{genotype}}{\text{inherited}}$

Figure 6–5.   Formation of the A antigen.

D-Galactose: Immunodominant sugar responsible for "B" specificity

GAL

FUC — GAL
GLNAC
GAL
GL

"B" antigen

Ceramide

Protein

Spectrin

| "H" structure | $\dfrac{BB \longrightarrow}{BO \longrightarrow}$ | Galactosyl transferase | $\longrightarrow$ | "B" antigen |

$\binom{\text{genotype}}{\text{inherited}}$

Figure 6–6.   Formation of the B antigen.

830,000 B antigen sites exist on a B adult RBC in response to the conversion of the H antigen by the α-3-D-galactosyltransferase produced by the *B* gene.[5]

When both *A* and *B* genes are inherited, the B enzyme (α-3-D-galactosyltransferase) seems to compete more efficiently for the H substance than the A enzyme (α-3-N-acetylgalactosaminyltransferase). Therefore, the average number of A antigens on an AB adult cell is approximately 600,000 sites, compared with an average of 720,000 B antigen sites.[5] Interaction of the *Hh* and *ABO* genes is reviewed in Figure 6–7.

Molecular Genetics of *ABO*

Advanced Concepts

Since the cloning in 1990 of the complementary DNA corresponding to messenger RNA transcribed at the blood group *ABO* locus,[13] more than 200 ABO **alleles** have been identified by molecular investigation.[14,15] The *ABO* gene is located on chromosome 9 and consists of seven **exons**.[16,17] The last two exons (6 and 7) encode for the catalytic domain of the ABO glycosyltransferases, with most of the coding sequence lying in exon 7. Exons 6 and 7 constitute 77% of the gene.[16,17]

Amino acid substitutions, resulting primarily from mutations within these two exons of the coding DNA of variant ABO glycosyltransferases, are responsible for transferring the immunodominant sugar to H substance, resulting in ABO phenotypes.[18] The seven common *ABO* alleles include A_1, A_1variant (A_1v), A_2, B_1, O_1, O_1variant(O_1v), and O_2.[19,20]

All ABO antigens arise from mutations in the single *ABO* gene; however, only three specific mutations, which show a high frequency in the population, indirectly lead to changes in the **epitope structures** resulting in A, B, or O specificities. Two of the mutations (substitutions) change the specificity of the enzyme from an α-N-acetylgalactosaminyltransferase (the A enzyme) to an α-3-D-galactosyltransferase (the B enzyme).[20] These glycosyltransferases, in turn, introduce an α 1,3 N-acetylgalactosamine (A) or an α 1,3 galactose (B) carbohydrate at the ends of **type H oligosaccharide (glycan) chains**. The third mutation is a deletion within the 5' region of the catalytic domain that results in a frameshift and inactivates the enzyme altogether, leaving the H glycan unmodified.[21] These different glycans define the A, B, or O antigens or epitopes.

ABO genotyping is complicated by the remarkable diversity at the **ABO locus**. **Recombination** or gene conversion between common alleles may lead to hybrids that result in unexpected ABO phenotypes. Furthermore, numerous mutations associated with weak subgroups, **nondeletional null (O) alleles**, and hybrids resulting from recombinational crossing-over between exons 6 and 7 of chromosome 9, have been described.[21] These amino acid substitutions, resulting from deletions, mutations, or gene recombination within these two exons of the coding DNA of variant ABO

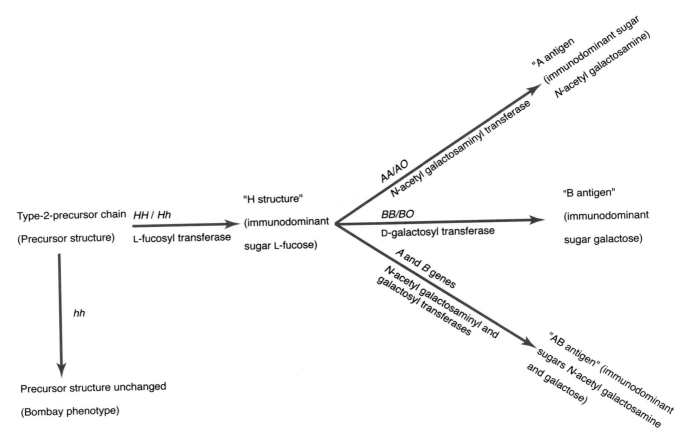

Figure 6–7.   Interaction of the *Hh* and *ABO* genes.

glycosyltransferases, are responsible for the less efficient transfer of the immunodominant sugar to H substance. This results in weak serologic reactions observed in ABO subgroups.[17,18]

Formation of A, B, and H Soluble Antigens

ABH antigens are integral parts of the membranes of RBCs, endothelial cells, platelets, lymphocytes, and epithelial cells.[8] ABH-soluble antigens can also be found in all body secretions. Their presence is dependent on the *ABO* genes inherited and on the inheritance of another set of genes called *Sese* (secretor genes) that regulate their formation. Eighty percent of the random U.S. population are known as secretors because they have inherited a secretor gene (*SeSe* or *Sese*). The inheritance of an *Se* gene codes for the production of a transferase (α-2-L-fucosyltransferase) that modifies the type 1 precursor substance in secretions to form H substance.[22] This H substance can then be modified to express A and B substance (if the corresponding gene is present) in secretions such as saliva. For example, a group A individual who is a secretor (*SeSe* or *Sese*) will secrete **glycoproteins** carrying A and H antigens. However, the *Se* gene does not affect the formation of A, B, or H antigens on the RBC. It is the presence of the *Se* gene–specified α-2-L-fucosyltransferase that determines whether ABH-soluble substances will be secreted (Fig. 6–8).[22] People who inherit the *sese* genotype are termed **nonsecretors.**

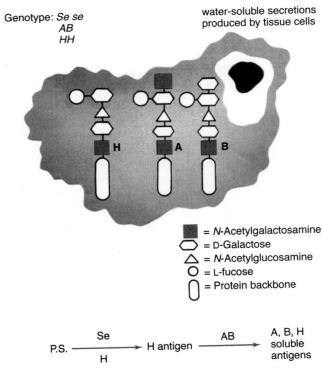

Genotype: *Se se*
       AB
      HH

water-soluble secretions produced by tissue cells

■ = *N*-Acetylgalactosamine
⬡ = D-Galactose
△ = *N*-Acetylglucosamine
○ = L-fucose
∪ = Protein backbone

P.S. $\xrightarrow[\text{H}]{\text{Se}}$ H antigen $\xrightarrow{\text{AB}}$ A, B, H soluble antigens

Figure 6–8.   Secretor ABH glycoprotein substances.

Comparison of A, B, and H Antigens on RBCs with A, B, and H Soluble Substances

The formation of soluble A, B, and H substances is the same as that described for the formation of A, B, and H antigens on the RBCs, except for a few minor distinctions that are compared in Table 6–10.

In the past, tests for ABH secretion have been used to establish the true ABO group of an individual whose RBC antigens are poorly developed. The demonstration of A, B, and H substances in saliva is evidence for the inheritance of an *A* gene, *B* gene, *H* gene, and *Se* gene. The term **secretor** refers only to secretion of A, B, and H soluble antigens in body fluids. The **glycoprotein-soluble substances** (or antigens) normally found in the saliva of secretors are listed in Table 6–11. Both ABH red cell antigens and ABH soluble substances are formed due to the attachment of an immunodominant sugar to an oligosaccharide chain. Although several types of oligosaccharide chains exist, types 1 and 3 are primarily associated with body secretions, while types 2 and 4 are associated with the red cell membrane.[22] It is interesting to note that types 1 and 2 are more abundant, and they differ only in the linkage position of **galactose** (Gal) to **N-acetylglucosamine** (GlcNAc); namely type 1 has a beta 1→3 linkage and type 2 has a beta 1→4 linkage.[22] Adding specific immunodominant sugars to the type 2 and 4 chains leads to formation of A, B, and H antigens on the red cell membrane, with the majority being present on type 2 chains.

Table 6–10	Comparison of ABH Antigens on RBCs with A, B, and H Soluble Substances	
ABH ANTIGENS ON RBCs	**A, B, AND H SOLUBLE SUBSTANCES**
RBC antigens can be glycolipids, glycoproteins, or glycosphingolipids.	Secreted substances are glycoproteins.
RBC antigens are synthesized only on type 2 precursor chains.	Secreted substances are primarily synthesized on type 1 precursor chains.[12]
Type 2 chain refers to a beta 1→4 linkage in which the number one carbon of the galactose is attached to the number four carbon of the N-acetylglucosamine sugar of the precursor substance.	Type 1 chain refers to a beta-1→3 linkage in which the number one carbon of the galactose is attached to the number three carbon of the N-acetylglucosamine sugar of the precursor substance.
The enzyme produced by the H gene (α-2-L-fucosyltransferase) acts primarily on type 2 chains, which are prevalent on the RBC membrane.	The enzyme produced by the *Se* gene (α-2-L-fucosyltransferase) preferentially acts on type 1 chains in secretory tissues.

Table 6–11	ABH Substance in the Saliva of Secretors (*SeSe* or *Sese*)*		
	SUBSTANCES IN SALIVA		
ABO Group	**A**	**B**	**H**
O	None	None	↑↑
A	↑↑	None	↑
B	None	↑↑	↑
AB	↑↑	↑↑	↑

* Nonsecretors (*sese*) have no ABH substances in saliva.
↑↑ and ↑, respectively, represent the concentration of ABH substances in saliva.

Adding the same immunodominant sugars to the type 1 and 3 chains in the body secretions allow for A, B, and H soluble substances to be made in body secretions. Box 6–3 summarizes the body fluids in which ABH-soluble substances can be found.

The procedure for determining the secretor status (saliva studies) can be found as Procedure 6-1 on the textbook's companion website.

ABO Subgroups

The original reports of most ABO subgroups were made before the availability of the monoclonal typing reagents currently used in routine ABO grouping. ABO subgroups represent phenotypes that show weaker variable serologic reactivity with the commonly used human polyclonal anti-A, anti-B, and anti-A,B reagents.

A Subgroups

Basic Concepts

In 1911, von Dungern described two different A antigens based on reactions between group A RBCs and anti-A and anti-A[1].[23] Group A RBCs that react with both anti-A and anti-A[1] are classified as A[1], whereas those that react with anti-A and not anti-A[1] are classified as A[2] (Table 6–12 and Figs. 6–9 and 6–10). RBCs from A[1] and A[2] individuals react

BOX 6–3
Fluids in Which A, B, and H Substances can be Detected in Secretors

- Saliva
- Tears
- Urine
- Digestive juices
- Bile
- Milk
- Amniotic fluid
- Pathological fluids: pleural, peritoneal, pericardial, ovarian cyst

Table 6-12   A₁ Versus A₂ Phenotypes

REACTIONS OF PATIENT'S RBCS WITH

Blood Group	Anti-A Reagent (anti-A plus anti-A₁)	Anti-A₁ Lectin Reagent
A₁	+	+
A₂	+	0

+ = positive (agglutination)
0 = negative (no agglutination)

equally strong with current reagent monoclonal anti-A in ABO forward typing tests.[2]

The A subgroups are generally more common than B subgroups. The weaker serologic reactivity of ABO subgroups is attributed to the decreased number of A and B antigen sites on their red cells. Classification into A₁ and A₂ phenotypes accounts for 99% of all group A individuals. The cells of approximately 80% of all group A (or AB) individuals are A₁ (or A₁B), and the remaining 20% are A₂ (or A₂B) or weaker subgroups. The differences between A₁ and A₂ are both quantitative and qualitative (Table 6-13).

The production of both types of antigens is a result of an inherited gene at the ABO locus. Inheritance of an A₁

gene elicits production of high concentrations of the enzyme α-3-N-acetylgalactosaminyltransferase, which converts almost all of the H precursor structure to A₁ antigens on the RBCs. The very potent gene A₁ creates from 810,000 to 1,170,000 antigen sites on the adult RBC; whereas inheriting an A₂ gene, results in the production of only 240,000 to 290,000 antigen sites on the adult A₂ RBC.[10] The immunodominant sugar on both A₁ and A₂ RBCs is **N-acetyl-ᴅ-galactosamine**.

Qualitative differences also exist, since 1% to 8% of A₂ individuals produce anti-A₁ in their serum, and 22% to 35% of A₂B individuals produce anti-A₁.[8] This antibody can cause discrepancies between forward and reverse ABO testing and incompatibilities in crossmatches with A₁ or A₁B cells. Because anti-A₁ is a naturally occurring IgM cold-reacting antibody, it is unlikely to cause a transfusion reaction because it usually reacts only at temperatures well below 37°C. It is considered clinically significant if it is reactive at 37°C.

It is now known through ABO genotyping that **polymorphism** at the ABO locus results in subgroup alleles such as the A₂ allele, which is characterized by a single-base substitution at nucleotide 467 and a single-base substitution at nucleotide 1059. These substitutions alter the active site of the coding region and subsequently change the specificity of the A glycosyltransferase.[24] It should be noted that in routine forward grouping, the reagent anti-A strongly agglutinates

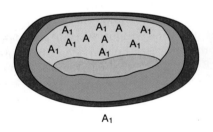
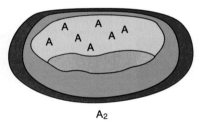

Figure 6-9. A₁ versus A₂ phenotypes.

Reactions of Patients' Red Cells with

Blood Group	Antigen Present	Anti-A (Anti-A plus Anti-A₁)	Anti-A₁ lectin
A₁	A₁ A	+	+
A₂	A	+	0

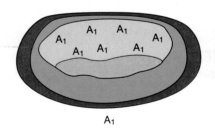
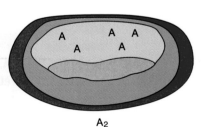

Figure 6-10. A₁ versus A₂ phenotypes (alternative conceptual presentation).

Reactions of Patients' Red Cells with

Blood Group	Antigen Present	Anti-A (Anti-A plus Anti-A₁)	Anti-A₁ lectin
A₁	A₁	+	+
A₂	A	+	0

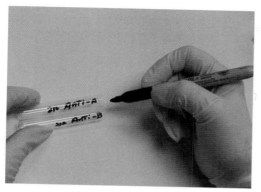

Step 1: Label test tubes.

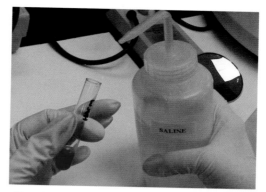

Step 2: Make a 2–5% patient red cell suspension.

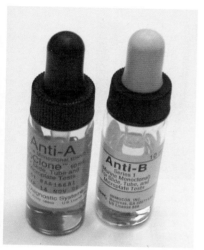

Step 3: Add reagent antisera*
(approximately 1 drop).

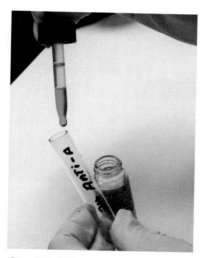

Step 3A: Add reagent Anti-A antisera*
(approximately 1 drop).

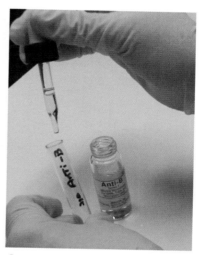

Step 3B: Add Anti-B reagent antisera*
(approximately 1 drop).

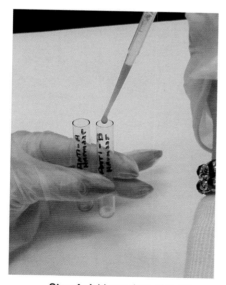

Step 4: Add one drop of 2–5%
suspension of patient red cells to
each tube.

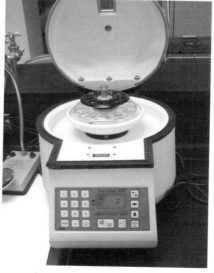

Step 5: Mix and centrifuge
(approximately 20 seconds).

* Consult manufacturer's package insert for specifics.

ure 6–1. Procedure for forward grouping. Principle: Detection of antigens on the patient's RBCs with known commercial antisera (continued on following page).

Step 6: Read and record agglutination reactions.

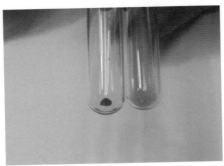

Group B
4+ Agglutination with Anti-B
0 Agglutination with Anti-A

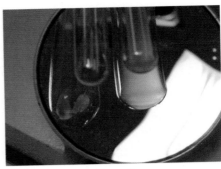

Group B
4+ Agglutination with Anti-B
0 Agglutination with Anti-A

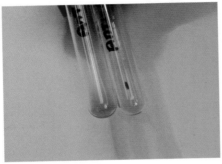

Group A
4+ Agglutination with Anti-A
0 Agglutination with Anti-B

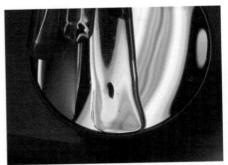

Group A
4+ Agglutination with Anti-A
0 Agglutination with Anti-B

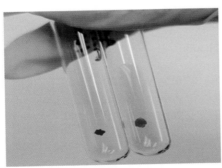

Group AB
4+ Agglutination with Anti-A and Anti-B

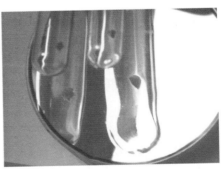

Group AB
4+ Agglutination with Anti-A and Anti-B

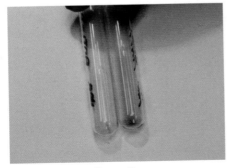

Group O
No Agglutination with Anti-A or Anti-B

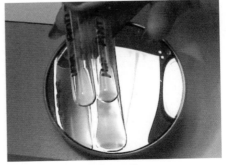

Group O
No Agglutination with Anti-A and Anti-B

Figure 6–1.—cont'd

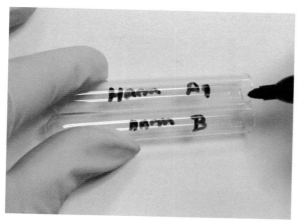

Step 1: Label test tubes.

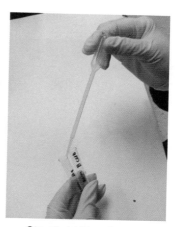

Step 2: Add two drops of patient serum to each tube.

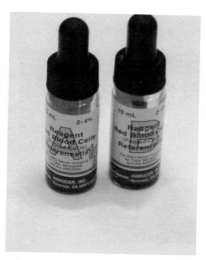

Step 3: Add one drop of reagent cells* to each test tube.

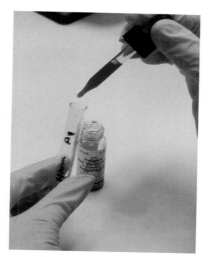

Step 3A: Add one drop of reagent A₁ cells.

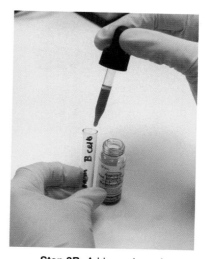

Step 3B: Add one drop of reagent B cells.

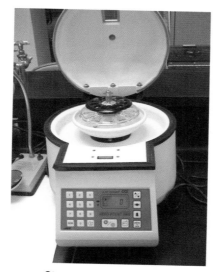

Step 4: Mix and centrifuge (approximately 20 seconds).

* Consult manufacturer's package insert for specifics.

Figure 6–2. Procedure for reverse grouping. Principle: Detection of antibodies in the patient's serum with known commercial antisera (continued on following page).

Step 5: Resuspend cells button; interpret and record results.

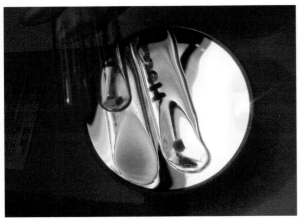

Group A
4+ Agglutination with B Cells
0 Agglutination with A_1 Cells

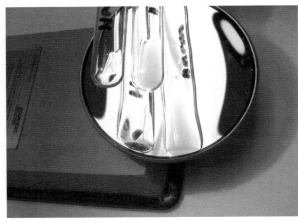

Group B
4+ Agglutination with A_1 Cells
0 Agglutination with B Cells

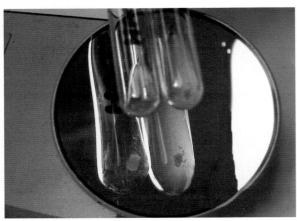

Group O
4+ Agglutination with A_1 Cells
3+ Agglutination with B Cells

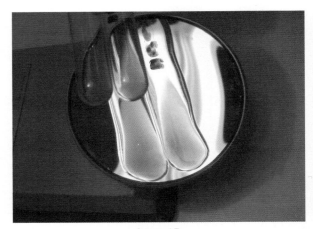

Group AB
0 Agglutination with A_1 Cells
No Agglutination with A_1 and B Cells

Figure 6–2.—cont'd

Table 6–13 Quantitative and Qualitative Differences of Subgroups A₁ and A₂

QUANTITATIVE	QUALITATIVE
• ↓ Number of antigen sites	• Differences in the precursor oligosaccharide chains
• ↓ Amount of transferase enzyme	• Subtle differences in transferase enzymes
• ↓ Amount of branching	• Formation of anti-A1, in a percentage of some subgroups

both A₁ and A₂ phenotypes. Differentiation of A₁ and A₂ phenotypes can be determined by using a reagent made from the seeds of the plant *Dolichos biflorus*, which serves as a source of anti-A₁. This reagent is known as anti-A₁ lectin.

Lectins are seed extracts that agglutinate human cells with some degree of specificity. This reagent agglutinates A₁ (or A₁B) cells but does not agglutinate A₂ (or A₂B cells). Box 6–4 lists the lectins used in blood banking. The characteristics of the A₁ and A₂ phenotypes are presented in Table 6–14. Because the A₂ glycosyltransferase activity is weaker in adding the immunodominant sugar to the H antigen precursor, A₂ red cells will show increased reactivity in comparison to A₁ red cells with the reagent anti-H lectin.

H antigen is found in greatest concentration on the RBCs of group O individuals. H antigen may not be detectable in group A₁ individuals, because in the presence of the A₁ gene, almost all of the H antigen is converted to A₁ antigen by placing the large N-acetyl-D-galactosamine sugar on the H substance. Because of the presence of so many A₁ antigens, the H antigen on A₁ and A₁B RBCs may be hidden and therefore may not be available to react with anti-H antisera. In the presence of an A₂ gene, only some of the H antigen is converted to A antigens, and the remaining H antigen is detectable on the cell.

Weak subgroups of the A antigen will often have an inverse reciprocal relationship between the amount of H antigen on the RBC and the amount of A antigens formed (i.e., the more A antigen formed, the less H antigen expressed on the RBC). The H antigen on the RBCs of A₁ and A₁B individuals is so well hidden by N-acetyl-D-galactosamine that anti-H is occasionally found in the serum. This anti-H is a naturally occurring IgM cold agglutinin that reacts best below room temperature. As can be expected, this antibody is formed in response to a natural substance and reacts most strongly with cells of group O individuals (which have the greatest amount of H substance on their RBCs).

Anti-H reacts weakly with the RBCs of A₁B individuals (which contain small amounts of H substance). It is an insignificant antibody in terms of transfusion purposes, because it has no reactivity at body temperature (37°C). However, high-titered anti-H may react at room temperature and present a problem in antibody screening procedures, because reagent screening cells are group O (see Chapter 9, "Detection and Identification of Antibodies"). This high-titered anti-H may also present a problem with compatibility testing (see Chapter 10, "Pretransfusion Testing"). Anti-H lectin from the extract of the plant *Ulex europaeus* closely parallels the reactions of human anti-H. Both antisera agglutinate RBCs of group O and A₂ and react very weakly or not at all with groups A₁ and A₁B.[10] Group B cells give reactions of variable strength (Fig. 6–11).

Advanced Concepts

The discussion thus far has presented a basic overview of the two major ABO subgroups, A₁ and A₂. A more plausible, yet more detailed, theory of ABO subgroups has been proposed by the identification of four different forms of H antigens, two of which are **unbranched straight chains (H₁, H₂)** and two of which are **complex branched chains (H₃, H₄;** Fig. 6–12).[22,25] The antigens H₁ through H₄ correspond to

BOX 6–4

Lectins Used in Blood Banking

- *Dolichos biflorus*—agglutinates A₁ or A₁B
- *Bandeiraea simplicifolia*—agglutinates B cells
- *Ulex europaeus*—agglutinates O cells (H specificity) and other ABO blood groups depending on the amount of H antigen available.

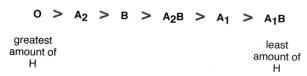

$$O > A_2 > B > A_2B > A_1 > A_1B$$

greatest amount of H   least amount of H

Figure 6-11. Reactivity of anti-H antisera or anti-H lectin with ABO blood groups.

Table 6–14 Characteristics of A₁ and A₂ Phenotypes

	REAGENTS				ANTIBODIES IN SERUM		OTHER	
Phenotypes	Anti-A	Anti-B	Anti-A,B	Anti-A₁	Common	Unexpected	Substances Present in Saliva of Secretors	Number of Antigen Sites RBC × 10³
A₁	4+	0	4+	4+	Anti-B	None	A, H	810–1,170
A₂	4+	0	4+	0	Anti-B	Anti-A₁ (1%–8% of cases)	A, H	240–290

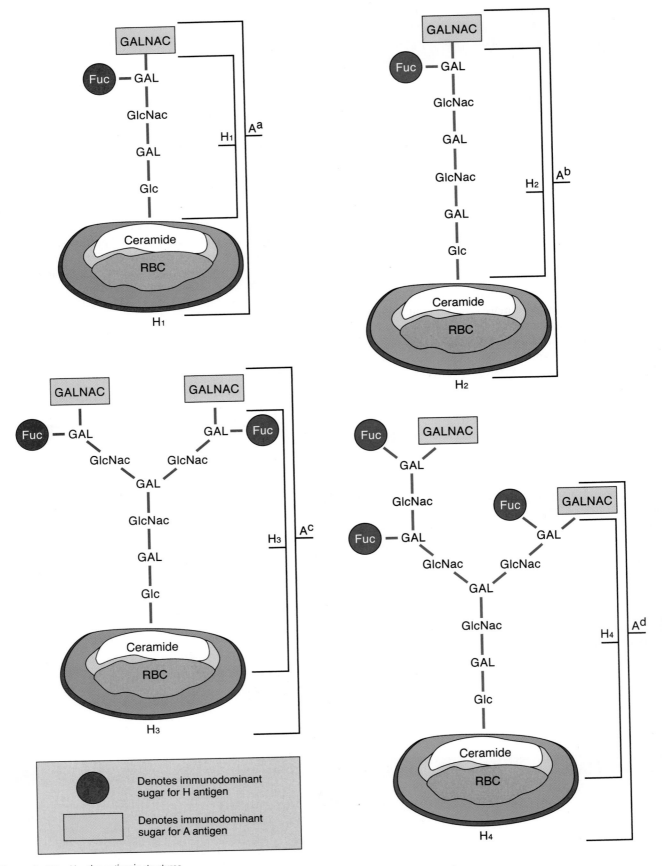

Figure 6–12.   H-active antigenic structures.

the precursor structures on which the A enzyme can act to convert H antigen to blood group A active glycolipids. Although the chains differ in length and complexity of branching, the terminal sugars giving rise to their antigenic specificity are identical. Studies on the chemical and physical characteristics of the A_1 and A_2 enzyme transferases have demonstrated that these two enzymes are different qualitatively.[13,14] Straight chain H_1 and H_2 glycolipids can be converted to A^a and A^b antigens, respectively, by both A_1 and A_2 enzymes, with the A_2 enzyme being less efficient. The more complex branched H_3 and H_4 structures can be converted to A^c and A^d antigens by A_1 enzyme and only very poorly by A_2 enzyme.[25] As a result, more unconverted H antigens (specifically H_3 and H_4) are available on group A_2 RBCs, and only A^a and A^b determinants are formed from H_1 and H_2 structures.[25]

On the RBCs of some A_2 individuals, A^c is extremely low and A^d is completely lacking (Box 6–5). These are the individuals in whom one would likely find anti-A_1 in the serum. This anti-A_1 antibody could really be an antibody to A^c and A^d determinants, which these A_2 individuals lack. Also, in 22% to 35% of A_2B individuals, anti-A_1 can be found in the serum. Since the B enzyme transferase is usually more efficient than the A enzyme in converting H structures to the appropriate antigen, A_2 enzymes would probably fail completely when paired with a B enzyme. As a result, A_2B individuals would be far more likely to lack A^c and A^d components with subsequent production of anti-A^c and anti-A^d (anti-A_1).

As stated previously, most group A infants appear to be A_2 at birth, with subsequent development to A_1 a few months later. Newborns have a deficiency of the branched H_3 and H_4 antigens and therefore the A^c and A^d antigens as well, possibly accounting for the A_2 phenotype. Adult cells contain a higher concentration of branched H_3 and H_4 structures and therefore A^c and A^d determinants of the A antigen in A_1 individuals.[26]

Weak A Subgroups

Basic Concepts

Subgroups weaker than A_2 occur infrequently and are most often recognized through an ABO discrepancy (unexpected reactions in the forward and reverse grouping). These subgroups of A make up 1% of those encountered in the laboratory and therefore are mainly of academic interest.[27] Characteristics of weak A subgroups include:

- Decreased number of A antigen sites per RBC (resulting in weak or no agglutination with human polyclonal anti-A)
- Varying degrees of agglutination by human anti-A,B[8]
- Increased variability in the detectability of H antigen, resulting in strong reactions with anti-H
- Presence or absence of anti-A_1 in the serum

Secretor studies, adsorption-elution tests, and molecular testing can be utilized to subdivide A individuals into A_3, A_x, A_{end}, etc.[28] (Table 6–15).

Occasionally, weak subgroups of A may present practical problems; for example, if an A_x donor was mistyped as a group O and was transfused to a group O patient. This is potentially dangerous because the group O patient possesses anti-A,B, which agglutinates and lyses A_x RBCs, causing rapid intravascular hemolysis.

BOX 6–5

Structural Characteristics of A_1 and A_2 RBCs

- A_2 RBCs: Predominantly A^a and A^b and unconverted H_3 and H_4 antigen sites
- A_1 red cells: A^a, A^b, A^c, and A^d determinants and no unconverted H_3 and H_4 antigen sites

---

Table 6–15 Characteristics of Weak ABO Phenotypes

	REAGENTS				ANTIBODIES IN SERUM			OTHER		
Phenotypes	Anti-A	Anti-B	Anti-A,B	Anti-H	Anti-A	Anti-B	Anti-A_1	Substances present in saliva of secretors	Presence of A transferase in serum	Number of antigen sites RBC $\times 10^3$
A_3	++mf	0	++mf	3+	no	Yes	Sometimes	A, H	Sometimes	35
A_x	wk/0	0	2+	4+	o/wk	Yes	Almost always	H	Rarely	5
A_{end}	wk mf	0	wk mf	4+	no	Yes	Sometimes	H	No	3.5
A_m*	0/wk	0	0/+	4+	no	Yes	No	A, H	Yes	1
A_y*	0	0	0	4+	no	Yes	No	A, H	Trace	1
A_{el}*	0	0	0	4+	some	Yes	Yes	H	No	.7

*A specificity demonstrated only by absorption/elution procedures
0 = negative; mf = mixed-field agglutination; wk = weak

Advanced Concepts

Weak A phenotypes can be serologically differentiated using the following techniques:

- Forward grouping of A and H antigens with anti-A, anti-A,B, and anti-H
- Reverse grouping of ABO isoagglutinins and the presence of anti-A_1
- Adsorption-elution tests with anti-A
- Saliva studies to detect the presence of A and H substances
- Additional special procedures such as molecular testing for mutations or serum glycosyltransferase studies for detecting the A enzyme can be performed for differentiation of weak subgroups.[27,28]

Absence of a disease process should be confirmed before subgroup investigation, because ABH antigens are altered in various malignancies and other hematologic disorders. (Refer to the "ABH Antigens and Antibodies in Disease" and "ABO Discrepancies" sections).

Weak A subgroups can be distinguished as A_3, A_x, A_{end}, A_m, A_y, and A_{el}, using the serologic techniques mentioned previously (see **Table 6–15**). The characteristics of each weak A subgroup are presented in the following paragraphs.

A_3 RBCs characteristically demonstrate a mixed-field pattern of agglutination with anti-A and most anti-A,B reagents.[6] **Mixed-field** can be defined as small agglutinates within predominantly unagglutinated red cells. The estimated number of A antigen sites is approximately 35,000 per RBC.[6] Weak α-3-N-acetylgalactosaminyltransferase activity is detectable in the serum. However, there appears to be molecular **heterogeneity** in the A_3 glycosyltransferases isolated from various A_3 phenotypes. A_3 enzyme is a product of an allele at the ABO locus inherited in a dominant manner; however, the A_3 blood group has been reported to be very heterogeneous at the molecular level.[29–32] Anti-A_1 may be present in serum of A_3 individuals, and A substance is detected in the saliva of A_3 secretors.

A_x RBCs characteristically are not agglutinated by anti-A reagent but do agglutinate with most examples of anti-A,B.[6] The estimated number of A antigen sites is approximately 4,000 per RBC.[33] Anti-A can be adsorbed and then eluted from A_x cells without difficulty. A transferase is not usually detectable in the serum or in the RBC membranes of A_x individuals. The molecular genetics of A_x reflects the considerable heterogeneity of the serologic phenotypes.[33] A_x individuals almost always produce anti-A_1 in their serum. Routine secretor studies detect the presence of only H substance in A_x secretors. However, A_x secretors contain A substance detectable only by agglutination/inhibition studies using A_x RBCs as indicators.[25] Caution should be used in interpreting results of secretor studies using A_x indicator cells and anti-A, because not all A_x cells are agglutinated by anti-A.

A_{end} RBCs characteristically demonstrate mixed-field agglutination with anti-A and anti-A,B, but only a very small percentage of the RBCs (10% or less) agglutinate.[34] The estimated number of A antigen sites on the few agglutinable RBCs is approximately 3,500 per RBC, whereas no detectable A antigens are demonstrated on RBCs that do not agglutinate.[34] No A glycosyltransferase is detectable in the serum or in the RBC membranes of A_{end} individuals. A_{end} is inherited as an allele at the ABO locus.[34] Secretor studies detect the presence of only H substance in the saliva of A_{end} secretors. Anti-A_1 is found in some A_{end} sera.[35] The phenotypes of A_{finn} and A_{bantu} are considered by some investigators to represent variants of the A_{end} subgroup.[36]

A_m RBCs are characteristically not agglutinated, or are agglutinated only weakly, by anti-A or anti-A,B.[37] A strongly positive adsorption or elution of anti-A confirms the presence of A antigen sites. The estimated number of A antigen sites varies from 200 to 1,900 per RBC in A_m individuals.[37] An A enzyme of either the A_1 or A_2 type previously described is detectable in the serum of A_m subgroups.[37] A_m is inherited as a rare allele at the ABO locus.[38] These individuals usually do not produce anti-A_1 in their sera. Normal quantities of A and H substance are found in the saliva of A_m secretors.[38]

A_y RBCs are not agglutinated by anti-A or anti-A,B. Adsorption and elution of anti-A is the method used to confirm the presence of A antigens. Activity of **eluates** from A_y RBCs is characteristically weaker than that of eluates from A_m RBCs. Trace amounts of A glycosyltransferase is detectable in the serum of A_y individuals, and saliva secretor studies demonstrate H and A substance, with A substance present in below-normal quantities.[37] A_y individuals usually do not produce anti-A_1. The A_y phenotype can be observed in siblings, implicating a recessive mode of inheritance. This phenotype does not represent expression of an alternate allele at the ABO locus but rather as a **germline mutation** of an A gene within a family.[4]

A_{el} RBCs typically are unagglutinated by anti-A or anti-A,B; however, adsorption and elution can be used to demonstrate the presence of the A antigen. No detectable A enzyme activity can be demonstrated in the serum or in the RBC membranes of A_{el} individuals by glycosyltransferase studies.[39] The A_{el} phenotype is inherited as a rare gene at the ABO locus.[39,40] A_{el} individuals usually produce an anti-A_1 that is reactive with A_1 cells and sometimes produce anti-A, which agglutinates A_2 RBCs.[39] Secretor studies demonstrate the presence of only H substance in the saliva of A_{el} secretors.

It should be noted that there are still some reported A variants that do not fit into any of the weak subgroups described, alluding to the existence of new alternate alleles or regulation by modifier genes.[41,42]

A general flowchart for the process of elimination and identification of various subgroups is presented in Figure 6–13. It is assumed that the patient's medical history, such as recent transfusion, pregnancy history, disease states, and medications, has been investigated and excluded as a source of the discrepancy.

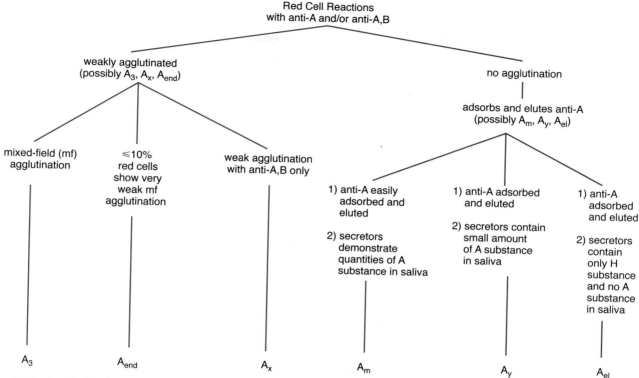

Figure 6–13.   Investigation of weak A subgroups.

Weak B Subgroups

Basic Concepts

Subgroups of B are very rare and much less frequent than A subgroups. Subgroups of B are usually recognized by variations in the strength of the reaction using anti-B and anti-A,B. Inheritance of B subgroups, similar to that of the majority of A subgroups, is considered to be a result of alternate alleles at the B locus. Criteria used for differentiation of weak B phenotypes include the following serologic techniques:

• Strength and type of agglutination with anti-B, anti-A,B, and anti-H
• Presence or absence of ABO isoagglutinins in the serum
• Adsorption-elution studies with anti-B
• Presence of B substance in saliva
• Molecular testing

Advanced Concepts

RBCs demonstrating serologic activity that is weaker than normal are designated weak B phenotypes or B subgroups and include B_3, B_x, B_m, and B_{el} phenotypes[43] (Table 6–16). There are no B subgroups reported that are equivalent to A_{end} or A_y. A classification system similar to A subgroups has been used because of common serologic characteristics. Subgroups of B are usually recognized by variations in the strength of the reaction using anti-B and anti-A,B.

Serologic techniques can be used to characterize B subgroups in the following categories: B_3, B_x, B_m, and B_{el}. The **B_3** phenotype generally results from the inheritance of a rare gene at the ABO locus and is characterized by a mixed-field pattern of agglutination with anti-B and anti-A,B.[44] B glycosyltransferase is present in the serum but not in the RBC membranes of these individuals. Anti-B is absent in the serum of B_3 phenotypes, but B substance is present in normal amounts in the saliva of secretors. The B_3 subgroup is the most frequent weak B phenotype.[44,45]

B_x RBCs typically demonstrate weak agglutination with anti-B and anti-A,B antisera. B glycosyltransferase has not been detected in the serum or in the RBC membranes of B_x phenotypes, but a weakly reactive anti-B usually is produced.[46] B_x RBCs readily adsorb and elute anti-B. Secretor studies demonstrate large amounts of H substance and some B substance that often can only be detected by inhibiting agglutination of B_x cells with anti-B. Family studies suggest that B_x is a rare allele at the ABO locus.[47]

B_m RBCs are characteristically unagglutinated by anti-B or anti-A,B. The B_m RBCs easily adsorb and elute anti-B. B glycosyltransferase is present in the serum of B_m phenotypes but is usually lower in activity and varies from individual to individual.[29] Only very small amounts of B transferase activity is demonstrated in B_m RBC membranes. Reduced activity of B enzyme in hematopoietic tissue is clearly the defect causing the formation of the B_m subgroup, since normal B plasma incubated with B_m RBCs and uracil diphosphate (UDP)-galactose transforms this subgroup into a normal group B phenotype. Anti-B is not

Table 6–16	**Characteristics of B Phenotypes**							
	REAGENTS				**ANTIBODIES IN SERUM**		**OTHER**	
Phenotypes	**Anti-A**	**Anti-B**	**Anti-A,B**	**Anti-H**	**Common**	**Unexpected**	**Substances Present in Saliva of Secretors**	**Presence of a B Transferase in Serum**
B	0	4+	4+	2+	Anti-A	None	B,H	Yes
B_3	0	++mf	++mf	3+	Anti-A	None	B,H	Yes (wk pos)
B_x	0	wk	wk	3+	Anti-A	Weak anti-B	H	No
B_m*	0	0/wk	0/wk	3+	Anti-A	None	B,H	Yes (wk pos)
B_{el}*	0	0	0	3+	Anti-A	Sometimes a weak anti-B	H	No

*B specificity demonstrated only by adsorption/elution procedures.

0 = negative; mf = mixed-field; wk = weak

characteristically present in the serum of B_m individuals. Normal quantities of H and B substance are found in the saliva of B_m secretors.

The B_m phenotype is usually the result of inheritance of a rare allele at the ABO locus, although the subgroup B_m may be the product of an interacting modifying gene linked closely to the ABO locus.[48] This modifier gene may depress expression of the *B* gene, resulting in decreased B enzyme activity.[49] The B_m subgroup is reported to be more frequent in Japan.[49]

B_{el} RBCs are unagglutinated by anti-B or anti-A,B. This extremely rare phenotype must be determined by adsorption and elution of anti-B. No B glycosyltransferase has been identified in the serum or RBC membrane of B_{el} individuals. B_{el} is inherited as a unique mutation in exon 7 of the *B* gene at the ABO locus.[50] A weak anti-B may be present in the serum of this subgroup. Only H substance is demonstrated in saliva of B_{el} secretors.

Other weak B phenotypes have been reported that do not possess the appropriate characteristics for classification into one of the groups previously discussed.[51] These may represent new classifications and new representations of ABO polymorphism.

The Bombay Phenotypes (O_h)

Basic Concepts

The Bombay phenotype was first reported by Bhende in 1952 in Bombay, India.[52] It represents the inheritance of a double dose of the *h* gene, producing the very rare genotype hh. As a result, the *ABO* genes cannot be expressed, and ABH antigens cannot be formed, since there is no H antigen made in the Bombay phenotype (Box 6–6).

More than 130 Bombay phenotypes have been reported in various parts of the world.[53] These RBCs are devoid of normal ABH antigens and, therefore, fail to react with anti-A, anti-B, and anti-H. In RBC testing using anti-A and anti-B, the Bombay would phenotype as an O blood group.

However, the RBCs of the Bombay phenotype (O_h) do not react with the anti-H lectin (*Ulex europaeus*), unlike

BOX 6–6

The Bombay Phenotype (O_h)

- *hh* genotype
- No H antigens formed; therefore, no A or B antigens formed
- Phenotypes as blood group O
- Anti-A, anti-B, anti-A,B, and anti-H present in the serum
- Can only be transfused with blood from another Bombay (O_h)

those of the normal group O individual, which react strongly with anti-H lectin.[53] Bombay serum contains anti-A, anti-B, anti-A,B, and anti-H. Unlike the anti-H found occasionally in the serum of A_1 and A_1B individuals, the Bombay anti-H can often be potent and reacts strongly at 37°C. It is an IgM antibody that can bind complement and cause RBC lysis. Transfusing normal group O blood (with the highest concentration of H antigen) to a Bombay recipient (anti-H in the serum) would cause immediate cell lysis. Therefore, only blood from another Bombay individual will be compatible and can be transfused to a Bombay recipient.

ABH substance is also absent in saliva.[53] The (O_h) Bombay phenotype is inherited as an autosomal recessive trait. The underlying molecular defect is most commonly a mutation in the gene *FUT1* (*H* gene), which produces a **silenced gene** that is incapable of coding for the enzyme, $\alpha(1,2)$fucosyltransferase (H transferase).[53] This enzyme catalyzes the transfer of fucose in an α-1,2 linkage to the terminal galactose of the precursor molecule on RBCs forming the H antigen. This mutation underlying the Bombay phenotype is also associated with a silenced *FUT2* gene (*Se* gene), which normally encodes a very similar $\alpha(1,2)$fucosyltransferase and normally transfers a fucose to form H antigens in **secretions** when active.[53] Box 6–7 summarizes the general characteristics of the Bombay phenotype. When family studies demonstrate which *ABO* genes are inherited in the Bombay phenotype, the genes are written as superscripts (Oh^A, Oh^B, Oh^{AB}).[54]

BOX 6–7

General Characteristics of Bombay O_h (H_{null}) Phenotypes

- Absence of H, A, and B, antigens; no agglutination with anti-A, anti-B, or anti-H lectin
- Presence of anti-A, anti-B, anti-A,B, and a potent wide thermal range of anti-H in the serum
- A, B, H nonsecretor (no A, B, or H substances present in saliva)
- Absence of α-2-L-fucosyltransferase (H-enzyme) in serum and H antigen on red cells
- Presence of A or B enzymes in serum (depending on ABO genotype)
- A recessive mode of inheritance (identical phenotypes in children but not in parents)
- RBCs of the Bombay phenotype (O_h) will not react with the anti-H lectin (Ulex europaeus)
- RBCs of the Bombay phenotype (O_h) are compatible only with the serum from another Bombay individual

The Para-Bombay Phenotypes

Advanced Concepts

The para-Bombay phenotypes are those rare phenotypes in which the RBCs are completely devoid of H antigens or have small amounts of H antigen present.[54] RBCs of these individuals express weak forms of A and B antigens, which are primarily detected by adsorption and elution studies. If a person is genetically A or B, the respective enzymes can be detected, but no H enzyme is detectable, even though it has been shown that there is limited production of H antigen on the RBC.[55] The notations A_h and B_h, respectively, have been used to describe these individuals. AB_h individuals have also been reported. A_h, B_h, and AB_h have been reported mainly in individuals of European origin.[54] No H, A, or B antigen is present in the saliva, and anti-H is present in the serum. The serum of A_h individuals contains anti-B and no anti-A, although anti-A_1 is usually present.[54]

In B_h serum, anti-A is always present, and anti-B may be detected.[54] It is postulated that homozygous inheritance of a mutant H (FUT1) gene codes for the production of low levels of H transferase activity. The small amount of H substance on the RBC is completely used by the A or B transferase present. This results in small quantities of A or B antigen being present on the RBC with no detectable H antigen. The anti-H present in the serum is weaker in reactivity than the anti-H found in the Bombay phenotype, although it may be reactive at 37°C.[55] The genetic basis for the para-Bombays is a mutated FUT1 (H gene) with or without an active FUT2 (Se gene) or a silenced FUT1 gene with an active FUT2 gene.[56]

In the case of the mutated FUT1 gene para-Bombay, the encoded α(1,2)fucosyltransferase enzyme activity is greatly reduced, so very low amounts of H, A, and B antigens are produced. These antigens are serologically undetectable in routine ABO testing. Remember, these very weakly expressed antigens are detectable using only adsorption and elution techniques with the appropriate reagents. In the silenced FUT1 gene with the active FUT2 gene para-Bombays, the α(1,2)fucosyltransferase enzyme associated with the FUT2 gene (α2FucT2) produces H, A, B, type 1 antigens in secretions, including plasma. These type 1 antigens in plasma may adsorb onto the RBC membrane, yielding very weakly expressed H, A, and B antigens, which can be detected only by adsorption and elution techniques. H-deficient secretors have been found in a variety of ethnic groups and nationalities.[56]

RBCs have little or no A, B, and H antigens. RBCs of O_h secretors are not agglutinated by most examples of anti-H but may be agglutinated by strong anti-H reagents. Adsorption and elution of anti-H may reveal the presence of some H antigen on the RBC.[56] Cells are not usually agglutinated by anti-A and anti-B; however, some $O_h{}^A$ RBCs can mimic the behavior of A_x cells and can be agglutinated by anti-A,B and potent examples of anti-A. The same reactions with anti-A,B and potent examples of anti-B can be seen with $O_h{}^B$ RBCs.[4] A weak H-like antibody, called anti-IH, that is reactive at low temperature is almost always present in the serum (see Chapter 8, "Blood Group Terminology and the Other Blood Groups"). This antibody is nonreactive with cord cells and is not inhibited by secretor saliva. Because of their secretor status, normal levels of H substances are present in the saliva.[55] A and B substances are present in the secretions when A and B genes are present.[55]

ABH Antigens and Antibodies in Disease

Associations between ABH antigens and practically any disorder known to man can be found throughout medical literature. Even more profound are the associations of blood group specificity with such things as a more pronounced "hangover" in A blood groups, "criminality" in group B blood groups, and "good teeth" in group O individuals. There are also several papers correlating blood groups with personality traits. It is no surprise that many scientists refer to these associations as a part of blood group mythology. However, more relevant associations between blood groups and disease are important to the blood banker in terms of blood group serology.

Various disease states seem to alter red cell antigens and result in progressively weaker reactions or additional acquired pseudoantigens, which can be seen during forward grouping. Leukemia, chromosome 9 translocations, and any hemolytic disease that induces stress hematopoiesis (e.g., thalassemia)[29] have been shown to depress antigen strength. Often the cells will appear to show a mixed-field agglutination (tiny agglutinates in a sea of unagglutinated cells). Hodgkin's disease also has been reported to weaken or depress ABH red cell antigens, resulting in variable reactions during forward grouping similar to those found in leukemia. The weakening of the antigen tends to follow the course of the disease. The antigen strength will increase again as the patient enters remission.

The isoagglutinins (anti-A, anti-B, or anti-A,B) also may be weak or absent in those leukemias demonstrating **hypogammaglobulinemia**, such as chronic lymphocytic leukemia (CLL). Various lymphomas, such as the malignant (non-Hodgkin's) variety, may yield weak isoagglutinins, owing to moderate decreases in the **gamma globulin fraction**. Also, immunodeficiency diseases, such as congenital agammaglobulinemia, will also yield weak or absent isoagglutinins. If this problem is suspected, a simple serum protein electrophoresis will confirm or rule out this condition. Individuals with intestinal obstruction, carcinoma of the colon or rectum, or other disorders of the lower intestinal tract may have increased permeability of the intestinal wall, which allows passage of the bacterial polysaccharides from *Escherichia coli* serotype O_{86} into the patient's circulation. This results in the **acquired B** phenomenon in group A_1 individuals. The patient's group A red cells absorb the B-like polysaccharide, which reacts with human-source anti-B.

A lack of detectable ABO antigens can occur in patients with carcinoma of the stomach or pancreas. The patient's red cell antigens have not been changed, but the serum contains excessive amounts of blood group–specific soluble substances (BGSS) that may neutralize the antisera utilized in the forward grouping. All these disease states previously mentioned may result in discrepancies between the forward and reverse groupings, indicating that the patient's red cell group is not what it seems. All ABO discrepancies must be resolved before blood for transfusion is released for that patient. In some cases, secretor or molecular studies may help confirm the patient's true ABO group.

ABO Discrepancies

ABO discrepancies occur when unexpected reactions occur in the forward and reverse grouping. These can be due to problems with the patient's serum (reverse grouping), problems with the patient's red cells (forward grouping), or problems with both the serum and cells. The unexpected reaction can be due to an extra positive reaction or a weak or missing reaction in the forward and reverse grouping. All ABO discrepancies must be resolved prior to reporting a patient or donor ABO group.

Technical Errors

Technical errors can also cause ABO discrepancies. This includes errors in labeling the blood sample at the patient's bedside or in the laboratory; therefore, patient and sample identification are essential! Other errors include the failure to add reagents or the addition of incorrect reagents or sample. Therefore, it is recommended that serum and antiserum be added first, then the patient or reagent red cells. It is also recommended that results be recorded immediately to avoid transcription errors. In addition, contaminated reagents can cause errors in testing. Therefore, looking at all the reagent vials when performing ABO testing and during quality control testing is extremely important. Some of the common causes of technical errors leading to ABO discrepancies in the forward and reverse groupings are listed in Box 6–8.

BOX 6–8

Common Sources of Technical Errors Resulting in ABO Discrepancies

- Incorrect or inadequate identification of blood specimens, test tubes, or slides
- Cell suspension either too heavy or too light
- Clerical errors or incorrect recording of results
- A mix-up in samples
- Missed observation of hemolysis
- Failure to add reagents
- Failure to add sample
- Failure to follow manufacturer's instructions
- Uncalibrated centrifuge
- Overcentrifugation or undercentrifugation
- Contaminated reagents
- Warming during centrifugation

Resolution

If the initial test was performed using RBCs suspended in serum or plasma, repeat testing the same sample using a saline suspension of RBCs can usually resolve the ABO discrepancy. It is important to make sure that any and all technical factors that may have given rise to the ABO discrepancy are reviewed and corrected. It is also essential to acquire information regarding the patient's age, diagnosis, transfusion history, medications, and history of pregnancy. If the discrepancy persists and appears to be due to an error in specimen collection or identification, a new sample should be drawn from the patient and the RBC and serum testing repeated.

When a discrepancy is encountered, results must be recorded, but interpretation of the ABO type must be delayed until the discrepancy is resolved. If blood is from a potential transfusion recipient, it may be necessary to administer group O–compatible RBCs before the discrepancy is resolved. In general, when investigating ABO discrepancies, it should be noted that RBC and serum grouping reactions are very strong (3+ to 4+); therefore, the weaker reactions usually represent the discrepancy. Figure 6–14 shows an algorithm for resolving ABO discrepancies.

Categories of ABO Discrepancies

ABO discrepancies may be arbitrarily divided into four major categories: group I, group II, group III, and group IV discrepancies.

Group I Discrepancies

Group I discrepancies are associated with unexpected reactions in the reverse grouping due to weakly reacting or missing antibodies. These discrepancies are more common than those in the other groups listed. When a reaction in the serum grouping is weak or missing, a group I discrepancy should be suspected, because, normally, RBC and serum grouping reactions are very strong (4+). One of the reasons for the missing or weak isoagglutinins is that the patient has depressed anti-

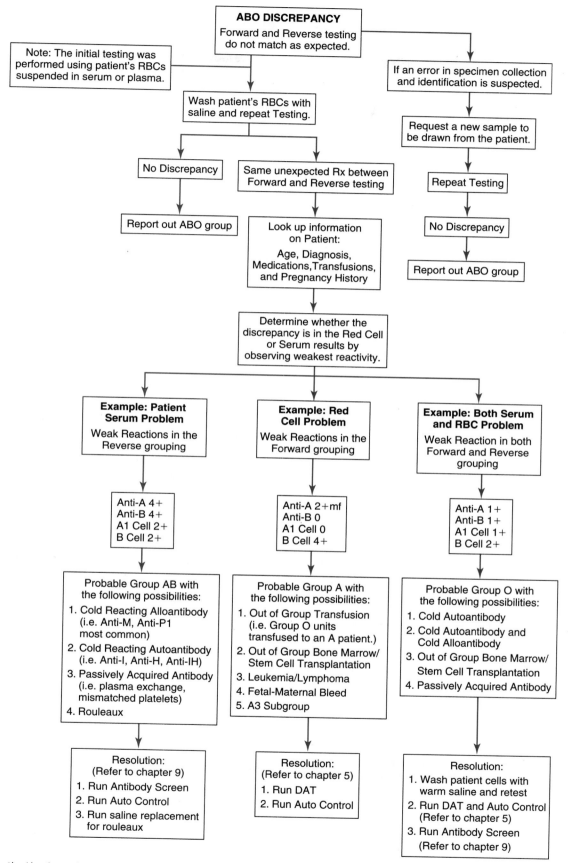

Figure 6–14. Algorithm for resolving ABO discrepancies.

body production or cannot produce the ABO antibodies. Common populations with discrepancies in this group are:

- Newborns (the production of ABO antibodies is not detectable until 4 to 6 months of age)
- Elderly patients (the production of ABO antibodies is depressed)
- Patients with a leukemia (e.g., chronic lymphocytic leukemia) or lymphoma (e.g., malignant lymphoma) demonstrating hypogammaglobulinemia
- Patients using immunosuppressive drugs that yield hypogammaglobulinemia
- Patients with congenital or acquired agammaglobulinemia or immunodeficiency diseases
- Patients with bone marrow or stem cell transplantations (patients develop hypogammaglobulinemia from therapy and start producing a different RBC population from that of the transplanted bone marrow)
- Patients whose existing ABO antibodies may have been diluted by plasma transfusion or exchange transfusion
- ABO subgroups

Resolution of Common Group I Discrepancies

Obtaining the patient's history may resolve this type of discrepancy, such as a newborn sample that would not have ABO antibodies in the serum until the child was 4 to 6 months of age. If the history indicates an elderly individual, or the diagnosis indicates hypogammaglobulinemia, then the best way to resolve this discrepancy is to enhance the weak or missing reaction in the serum. This is usually performed by incubating the patient serum with reagent A_1 and B cells at room temperature for approximately 15 to 30 minutes or by adding one or two drops more plasma or serum to the test. If there is still no reaction after centrifugation, the serum-cell mixtures can be incubated at 4°C for 15 minutes. An **auto control** and O **cell control** must always be tested concurrently with the reverse typing when trying to solve the discrepancy, since the lower temperature of testing will most likely enhance the reactivity of other commonly occurring cold agglutinins (such as anti-I) that react with all adult RBCs (see Chapter 8). Table 6–17 shows a type of discrepancy that may be seen with weak or missing antibodies.

The red cell results present a group O individual and the serum results present an AB individual. Since serum problems are more common, it is more likely that the serum immunoglobulins are decreased.

Group II Discrepancies

Group II discrepancies are associated with unexpected reactions in the forward grouping due to weakly reacting or missing antigens. This group of discrepancies is probably the least frequently encountered. Some of the causes of discrepancies in this group include:

- Subgroups of A (or B) may be present (see the "ABO Subgroups" section)
- Leukemias may yield weakened A or B antigens (Table 6–18), and Hodgkin's disease has been reported in some cases to mimic the depression of antigens found in leukemia.
- The "acquired B" phenomenon will show weak reactions with anti-B antisera and is most often associated with diseases of the digestive tract (e.g., cancer of the colon). Table 6–19 shows the ABO testing results of an acquired B phenomenon.

Resolution of Common Group II Discrepancies

The agglutination of weakly reactive antigens with the reagent antisera can be enhanced by incubating the test mix-

---

Table 6–17   Example of ABO Discrepancy Seen With Weak or Missing Antibodies

	FORWARD GROUPING REACTION OF PATIENT'S CELLS WITH		REVERSE GROUPING REACTION OF PATIENT'S SERUM WITH	
	Anti-A	Anti-B	A_1 Cells	B Cells
Patient	0	0	0	0
		Patient's probable group: O (elderly patient or newborn)		

Note: The absence of agglutination with reagent cells in the reverse type is because the production of ABO antibodies can be weak or absent in the elderly.
Resolution: (1) Check age of the patient. (2) Increase incubation time to 30 minutes (not appropriate for newborn sample). (3) Lower the temperature to 4°C for 15 minutes (include O cells and an autocontrol).

Table 6–18   Serologic Reactions Typical of Leukemia

	FORWARD GROUPING REACTION OF PATIENT CELLS WITH		REVERSE GROUPING REACTION OF PATIENT SERUM WITH	
Patient Phenotype	Anti-A	Anti-B	A_1 Cells	B Cells
A	+mf	0	0	3+
B	0	±/+	4+	0

Note: Weak reactivity with anti-A and anti-B is because the disease, leukemia, has resulted in the weakened expression of the corresponding antigen.

Table 6–19   Example of ABO Discrepancy Caused by an Acquired B Antigen

	FORWARD GROUPING REACTION OF PATIENT'S CELLS WITH		REVERSE GROUPING REACTION OF PATIENT'S SERUM WITH	
	Anti-A	Anti-B	A₁ Cells	B Cells
Patient	4+	2+	0	4+

Patient's probable group: A

Note: Patient RBCs have acquired a B-like antigen that reacts with reagent anti-B and is associated with cancer of the colon or other diseases of the digestive tract.
Resolution: (1) Acidify Anti-B reagent to a pH of 6. (2) Run DAT (refer to Chapter 5, "The Antiglobulin Test"). (3) Run autocontrol.

ture at room temperature for up to 30 minutes, which will increase the association of the antibody with the RBC antigen. If it is still negative, incubate the text mixture at 4°C for 15 to 30 minutes. Include group O and autologous cells as controls. RBCs can also be pretreated with enzymes and retested with reagent antisera.

The acquired B antigen arises when bacterial enzymes modify the immunodominant blood group A sugar (N-acetyl-D-galactosamine) into D-galactosamine, which is sufficiently similar to the group B sugar (D-galactose) and cross-reacts with anti-B antisera. This **pseudo-B antigen** is formed at the expense of the A₁ antigen and disappears after recovery.[39] The reaction of the appropriate antiserum with these acquired antigens demonstrates a weak reaction, often yielding a mixed-field appearance (see **Table 6–19**).

Blood group reagents of a monoclonal anti-B clone (ES4) strongly agglutinate cells with the acquired B antigen. The pH of reagents containing ES4 has been lowered; consequently, only those cells with the strongest examples of acquired B antigen react with the antisera. Testing the patient's serum or plasma against autologous RBCs gives a negative reaction, because the anti-B in the serum does not agglutinate the patient's RBCs with the acquired B antigen. The acquired B antigen is also not agglutinated when reacted with anti-B that has a pH greater than 8.5 or less than 6.[40] Secretor studies can be performed when trying to characterize the acquired B phenomenon. If the patient is in fact a secretor, only the A substance is secreted in the acquired B phenomenon. Treating RBCs with acetic anhydride reacetylates the surface molecules, then markedly decreases the reactivity of the cells tested with anti-B. The reactivity of normal B cells is not affected by treatment with acetic anhydride.[24]

Rare Group II Discrepancies

Advanced Concepts

Weakly reactive or missing reactions in RBC grouping may be due to excess amounts of blood group–specific soluble (BGSS) substances present in the plasma, which sometimes occurs with certain diseases, such as carcinoma of the stomach and pancreas. Excess amounts of BGSS substances will neutralize the reagent anti-A or anti-B, leaving no unbound antibody to react with the patient cells. This yields a false-negative or weak reaction in the forward grouping. Washing the patient cells free of the BGSS substances with saline should alleviate the problem, resulting in correlating forward and reverse groupings.

Antibodies to low-incidence antigens in reagent anti-A or anti-B may also result in weakly reactive or missing reactions in RBC grouping (Table 6–20). It is impossible for manufacturers to screen reagent antisera against all known RBC antigens. It has been reported (although rarely) that this additional antibody in the reagent antisera has reacted with the corresponding low-incidence antigen present on the patient's RBCs. This gives an unexpected reaction of the patient's cells with anti-A or anti-B, or both, mimicking the presence of a weak antigen. The best way to resolve this discrepancy is by repeating the forward type, using antisera with a different lot number. If the cause of the discrepancy is a low-incidence antibody in the reagent antisera reacting with a low-incidence antigen on the patient's cells, the antibody probably will not be present in a different lot number of reagent. This is only seen when human source antiserum is used. Most ABO reagents in use today are monoclonal antibodies, and these reagents are free of contaminating antibodies to low-incidence antigens.

Chimerism is defined as the presence of two cell populations in a single individual (Table 6–21). It was discovered

Table 6–20   Example of ABO Discrepancy Caused by Low-Incidence Antibodies in the Reagent Antisera

	FORWARD GROUPING REACTION OF PATIENT CELLS WITH		REVERSE GROUPING REACTION OF PATIENT SERUM WITH	
	Anti-A	Anti-B	A₁ Cells	B Cells
Patient	0	1+	4+	4+

Patient's probable group: O

Note: Reaction with anti-B in the forward type is due to agglutination between a low-incidence antibody in reagent anti-B and the corresponding antigen on the patient's cells.
Resolution: Use a different lot number for reagent Anti-B

Table 6–21   ABO Grouping in Chimera Twins

PATIENT	ANTI-A	ANTI-B	ANTI-A,B	A₁ CELLS	B CELLS	RBC %
Twin 1	0	2+mf	2+mf	4+	0	70% **B**; 30% **O**
Twin 2	0	+wk	+wk	4+	0	30% **B**; 70% **O**

0 = negative; mf = mixed field; wk = weak

in twins (born to a group O mother and group B father) who had a mixture of both B and O cells instead of the expected group of either B or O. Detecting a separate cell population may be easy or difficult, depending on what percentage of cells of the minor population are present. Reactions from chimerism are typically mixed field.

True chimerism, which occurs in twins, is rarely found, and the two cell populations will exist throughout the lives of the individuals. In utero exchange of blood occurs because of vascular **anastomosis**. As a result, two cell populations emerge, both of which are recognized as self, and the individuals do not make anti-A or anti-B. Therefore, expected isoagglutinins are not present in the reverse grouping, depending on the percentage of the population of red cells that exist in each twin. If the patient or donor has no history of a twin, then the chimera may be due to **dispermy** (two sperm fertilizing one egg) and indicates **mosaicism**. More commonly, artificial chimeras occur, which yield mixed cell populations as a result of:

- Blood transfusions (e.g., group O cells given to an A or B patient)
- Transplanted bone marrows or peripheral blood stem cells of a different ABO type
- Exchange transfusions
- Fetal-maternal bleeding

Group III Discrepancies

These discrepancies between forward and reverse groupings are caused by protein or plasma abnormalities and result in rouleaux formation or pseudoagglutination, attributable to:

- Elevated levels of globulin from certain disease states, such as multiple myeloma, Waldenström's macroglobulinemia, other plasma cell dyscrasias, and certain moderately advanced cases of Hodgkin's lymphomas
- Elevated levels of fibrinogen

- Plasma expanders, such as dextran and polyvinylpyrrolidone
- Wharton's jelly in cord blood samples
- Table 6–22 shows an example of ABO discrepancy caused by rouleaux formation.

Resolution of Common Group III Discrepancies

Rouleaux is a stacking of erythrocytes that adhere in a coin-like fashion, giving the appearance of agglutination. It can be observed on microscopic examination (Fig. 6–15). Cell grouping can usually be accomplished by washing the patient's RBCs several times with saline. Performing a saline replacement technique will free the cells in the case of rouleaux formation in the reverse type. In this procedure, serum is removed and replaced by an equal volume of saline. In true agglutination, RBC clumping will still remain after the addition of saline. Rouleaux can be a nuisance in the laboratory, since it is an in vitro problem observed during laboratory

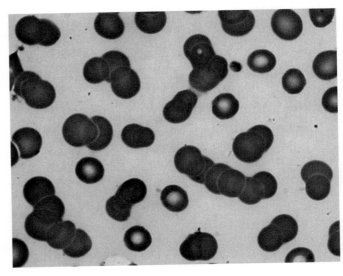

Figure 6–15.   Rouleaux.

Table 6–22   Example of ABO Discrepancy Caused by Rouleaux Formation

	FORWARD GROUPING REACTION OF PATIENT CELLS WITH		REVERSE GROUPING REACTION OF PATIENT SERUM WITH	
	Anti-A	Anti-B	A₁ Cells	B Cells
Patient	4+	4+	2+	2+
Patient's probable group: AB				

Note: Agglutination with A₁ and B cells in reverse type is due to rouleaux formation as a result of increased serum protein or plasma abnormalities.
Resolution: (1) Microscopic examination (2) Saline replacement technique (3) Wash cells with saline three times (4) Run antibody screen (refer to Chapter 9)

testing. It is not an in vivo problem for the patient. (Refer to companion website for the saline replacement procedure.)

Cord blood samples received in the laboratory can also pose a problem in ABO testing, since cord cells may be contaminated with a substance called Wharton's jelly, which may cause the red cells to aggregate. Washing cord cells six to eight times with saline should alleviate spontaneous rouleaux due to Wharton's jelly. This substance is a viscous mucopolysaccharide material present on cord blood cells, and thorough washing should result in an accurate ABO grouping. However, because testing is usually not performed on cord serum (because the antibodies detected are usually of maternal origin), reverse grouping may still not correlate with the RBC forward grouping.

Group IV Discrepancies

These discrepancies between forward and reverse groupings are due to miscellaneous problems and have the following causes:

- Cold reactive autoantibodies in which RBCs are so heavily coated with antibody that they spontaneously agglutinate, independent of the specificity of the reagent antibody (Fig. 6–16 and Table 6–23).
- Patient has circulating RBCs of more than one ABO group due to RBC transfusion or marrow/stem cell transplant

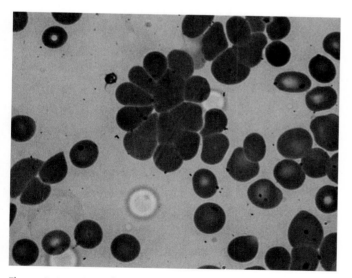

Figure 6–16.   Autoagglutination in a patient with cold agglutinin disease.

- Unexpected ABO isoagglutinins
- Unexpected non-ABO alloantibodies

Resolution of Common Group IV Discrepancies

Potent cold autoantibodies can cause spontaneous agglutination of the patient's cells. These cells often yield a positive direct **Coombs'** or antiglobulin test (see Chapter 20, "Autoimmune Hemolytic Anemias"). If the antibody in the serum reacts with all adult cells—for example, anti-I—the reagent A_1 and B cells used in the reverse grouping also agglutinate.

To resolve this discrepancy, the patient's RBCs could be incubated at 37°C for a short period, then washed with saline at 37°C three times and retyped. If this is not successful in resolving the forward type, the patient's RBCs can be treated with 0.01 M dithiothreitol (DTT) to disperse IgM-related agglutination. As for the serum, the reagent RBCs and serum can be warmed to 37°C, then mixed, tested, and read at 37°C. The test can be converted to the antihuman globulin phase if necessary. Weakly reactive anti-A or anti-B may not react at 37°C, which is outside their optimum thermal range. If the reverse typing is still negative (and a positive result was expected), a cold autoabsorption (patient cells with patient serum) could be performed to remove the cold autoantibody from the serum. The absorbed serum can then be used to repeat the serum typing at room temperature. (Refer to Chapter 9 for cold autoadsorption and alloadsorption with rabbit erythrocyte stroma [REST] for the removal of cold autoantibodies.)

Unexpected ABO isoagglutinins in the patient's serum react at room temperature with the corresponding antigen present on the reagent cells (Table 6–24). Examples of this type of ABO discrepancy include A_2 and A_2B individuals, who can produce naturally occurring anti-A_1, or A_1 and A_1B, individuals who may produce naturally occurring anti-H. (Refer to the previous sections on ABO subgroups.) Serum grouping can be repeated using at least three examples of A_1, A_2, B cells; O cells; and an autologous control (patient's serum mixed with patient's RBCs).[3] The specificity of the antibody can be determined by examining the pattern of reactivity (e.g., if the antibody agglutinates only A_1 cells, it can most likely be identified as anti-A_1). The patient's RBCs can be tested with *Dolichos biflorus* to confirm the presence of the ABO subgroup. *Dolichos biflorus* will agglutinate cells of the A_1 but not the A_2 phenotype.

Unexpected alloantibodies in the patient's serum other than ABO isoagglutinins (e.g., anti-M) may cause a discrepancy in the reverse grouping (Table 6–25). Reverse grouping

---

Table 6–23   Example of ABO Discrepancy Caused by Cold Autoantibodies

	FORWARD GROUPING REACTION OF PATIENT CELLS WITH		REVERSE GROUPING REACTION OF PATIENT SERUM WITH	
	Anti-A	Anti-B	A_1 Cells	B Cells
Patient	2+	4+	4+	2+
Patient's probable group: B				

Note: Reaction with anti-A in forward type is due to spontaneous agglutination of antibody coated cells; reaction with B cells in reverse type is due to cold autoantibody (e.g., anti-I) reacting with I antigen on B cells.

Resolution: (1) Wash patient cells with warm saline and retest; (2) Run DAT and autocontrol; (3) Run antibody screen (refer to Chapter 9)

Table 6–24   Example of ABO Discrepancy Caused by an Unexpected ABO Isoagglutinin

	FORWARD GROUPING REACTION OF PATIENT CELLS WITH		REVERSE GROUPING REACTION OF PATIENT SERUM WITH	
	Anti-A	Anti-B	A_1 Cells	B Cells
Patient	4+	4+	1+	0
	Patient's probable group: A_2B			

Note: Reactions with patient serum are due to anti-A_1 agglutinating A_1 reagent red cells.
Resolution: (1) Test cells with anti-A_1 lectin; (2) Test serum with A_1, A_2, and O cells; (3) Run an autocontrol

Table 6–25   Example of ABO Discrepancy Caused by an Unexpected Non-ABO Alloantibody

	FORWARD GROUPING REACTION OF PATIENT CELLS WITH		REVERSE GROUPING REACTION OF PATIENT SERUM WITH	
	Anti-A	Anti-B	A_1 Cells	B Cells
Patient	4+	4+	1+	1+
	Patient's probable group: AB			

Note: Reactions with patient serum are due to non-ABO alloantibody agglutinating an antigen other than A_1 and B on reagent red cells.
Resolution: (1) Run an antibody screen and panel (refer to Chapter 9)

cells possess other antigens in addition to A_1 and B, and it is possible that other unexpected antibodies present in the patient's serum will react with these cells. In this situation, an antibody identification panel should be performed with the patient's serum. Once the unexpected alloantibodies are identified, reagent A_1 and B cells negative for the corresponding antigen can be used in the reverse grouping.

Rare Group IV Discrepancies

Advanced Concepts

Antibodies other than anti-A and anti-B may react to form antigen-antibody complexes that may then adsorb onto patient's RBCs. One example is an individual who has an antibody against acriflavine, the yellow dye used in some commercial anti-B reagents. The acriflavine-antiacriflavine complex attaches to the patient's RBCs, causing agglutination in the forward type. Washing the patient's cells three times with saline and then retyping them should resolve this discrepancy.

Cis-AB refers to the inheritance of both AB genes from one parent carried on one chromosome and an O gene inherited from the other parent. This results in the offspring inheriting three ABO genes instead of two (Fig. 6–17). The designation cis-AB is used to distinguish this mode of inheritance from the more usual AB phenotype in which the alleles are located on different chromosomes. The cis-AB phenotype was first discovered in 1964, when a Polish family was described in which the father was group O, and the mother was group AB and gave birth to children who were all group AB. It was resolved by the fact that the A and B genes were inherited together and were both on the same, or cis, chromosome; thus the term *cis-AB*.

RBCs with the cis-AB phenotype (a rare occurrence) express a weakly reactive A antigen (analogous to A_2 cells) and a weak B antigen.[4] The B antigen usually yields a weaker reaction with the anti-B from random donors, with mixed-field agglutination typical of subgroup B_3

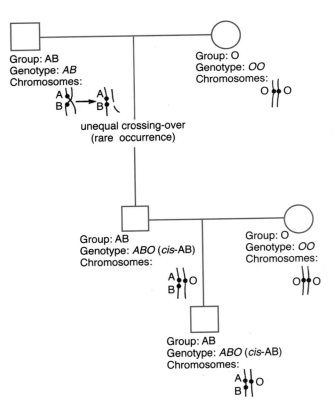

Figure 6–17. Example of cis-AB inheritance to unequal crossing-over. O = male; □ = female.

reported in several cases. Weak anti-B (present in the serum of most cis-AB individuals) leads to an ABO discrepancy in the reverse grouping. The serum of most cis-AB individuals contains a weak anti-B, which reacts with all ordinary B RBCs, yet not with cis-AB RBCs. A and B transferase levels are lower than those found in ordinary group AB sera.[4]

Various hypotheses have been offered to explain the cis-AB phenotype. Many favor an unequal crossing over between the *A* and *B* gene with gene fusion and the formation of a new gene. However, the banding pattern of the distal end of the long arm of chromosome 9 representing the ABO locus is normal. There have been other examples of cis-ABs that do not fit the above scenario. In these examples, there was a point mutation at the ABO locus, and an enzyme was produced that was capable of transferring both A-specific and B-specific sugars to the precursor molecule.[41] Many families have been reported in other parts of the world, with a high incidence of cis-AB being found in Japan.

Table 6–26 provides some examples of serologic reactions involving ABO discrepancies, with possible causes and resolution steps. Figure 6–18 provides a simplified summary of ABO discrepancies.

Table 6–26   ABO Discrepancies Between Forward and Reverse Grouping

Patient	FORWARD GROUPING		REVERSE GROUPING				Possible Cause	Resolution Steps
	Anti-A	Anti-B	A₁ Cells	B Cells	O Cells	Auto-Control		
1	0	0	0	0	0	0	Group O newborn or elderly patient; patient may have hypogammaglobulinemia or agammaglobulinemia, or may be taking immunosuppressive drugs	Check age and diagnosis of patient and immunoglobulin levels if possible; incubate at RT for 30 min or at 4°C for 15 min; include group O and autologous cells at 4°C
2	4+	0	1+	4+	0	0	Subgroup of A: probable A₂ with anti-A₁	React patient cells with anti-A₁ lectin, test serum against additional A₁, A₂, and O cells; run auto control.
3	4+	4+	2+	2+	2+	2+	(1) Rouleaux (multiple myeloma patient; any patient with reversed albumin-to-globulin ratio or patients given plasma expanders) (2) Cold autoantibody (probable group AB with an auto anti-I) (3) Cold autoantibody with underlying cold or RT reacting alloantibody (probable group AB with an auto anti-I and a high-frequency cold antibody [e.g., anti-P₁, anti-M, anti-Leᵇ])	(1) Wash RBCs; use saline dilution or saline replacement technique (2) Perform cold panel and autoabsorb or rabbit erythrocyte stroma (REST) absorb (see Chapter 9) or reverse type at 37°C (3) Perform cold panel autoabsorb or REST, and run panel on absorbed serum; select reverse cells lacking antigen for identified alloantibody; repeat reverse group on absorbed serum to determine true ABO group or at 37°C

Continued

Table 6–26   ABO Discrepancies Between Forward and Reverse Grouping—cont'd

Patient	FORWARD GROUPING		REVERSE GROUPING				Possible Cause	Resolution Steps
	Anti-A	Anti-B	A$_1$ Cells	B Cells	O Cells	Auto-Control		
4	4+	4+	1+	0	0	0	Subgroup of AB; probabe A$_2$B with anti-A$_1$	Use anti-A$_1$ lectin, test serum against additional A$_1$, A$_2$, and O cells
5	4+	0	0	4+	3+	0	A$_1$ with potent anti-H	Confirm A$_1$ group with anti-A$_1$ lection; test additional A$_2$, O, and A$_1$ cells and an O$_h$ if available
6	0	0	4+	4+	4+	0	O$_h$ Bombay	Test with anti-H lection; test O$_h$ cells if available; send to reference laboratory for confirmation
7	0	0	2+	4+	0	0	Subgroup of A; probable A$_x$ with anti-A$_1$	Perform saliva studies or absorption/elution
8	4+	2+	0	4+	0	0	Group A with an acquired B antigen	Check history of patient for lower gastrointestinal problem or septicemia; acidify anti-B typing reagent to pH 6.0 by adding 1 or 2 drops of 1N HCl to 1 mL of anti-B anti-sera, and measure with a pH meter (this acidified anti-B antisera would agglutinate only true B antigens *not* acquired B antigens), test serum against autologous cells
9	4+	4+	2+	0	2+	0	Group AB with alloantibody	Perform antibody screen and panel, identify room temperature antibody, repeat serum type with antigen negative *reagent* cells or perform serum type at 37°C
10	0	4+	4+	1+	1+	1+	Group B with cold autoantibody	Enzyme-treat RBCs and perform autoabsorption at 4°C or perform prewarmed testing

*AutoAbsorption should not be performed on patient's cells that have been transfused within the last 3 months.
RT = room temperature

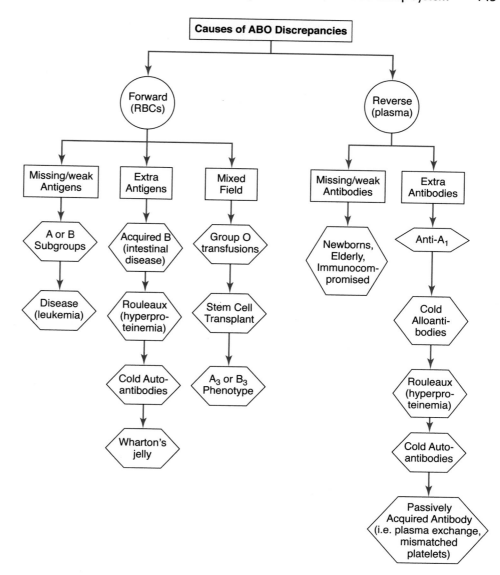

Figure 6–18. Simplified Summary of ABO Discrepancies

CASE STUDY

Case 6-1

A 45-year-old woman, who has given birth to three children and has a history of five cases of dilation and curettage, is scheduled for a partial hysterectomy at a community hospital. Preoperation laboratory tests include a type and screen. There is no history of transfusions.

Part 1
ABO and Rh Typing

Anti-A	Anti-B	Anti-A,B	A₁Cells	B Cells	Anti-D
3+	0	3+	2+	4+	3+

Antibody Screen

	37°C	AHG	CC
SCI	0	0	√
SCII	0	0	√
SCIII	0	0	√

1. Where is the discrepancy?
2. What testing would you perform next to resolve the discrepancy?

Part 2

The patient's serum was then tested with A_2 cells and O cells and the patient's red cells with Anti-A_1 lectin.

	A_2 Cells	O Cells	Anti-A_1 Lectin
Patient serum	0	0	Patient RBCs 0

3. How would you interpret these results?
4. Why were O+ RBCs chosen for transfusion?

SUMMARY CHART

✔ ABO frequencies: group O, 45%; group A, 40%; group B, 11%; group AB, 4%.

✔ ABO blood group system has naturally occurring antibodies that are primarily IgM.

✔ *ABO* genes, like those of most other blood groups, are inherited in a codominant manner.

✔ ABH-soluble antigens are secreted by tissue cells and are found in all body secretions. The antigens secreted depend on the person's ABO group.

✔ ABO reverse grouping is omitted from cord blood testing on newborns, because their antibody titer levels are generally too low for detection.

✔ ABO RBC antigens can be glycolipids, glycoproteins, or glycosphingolipids; ABO-secreted substances are glycoproteins.

✔ L-fucose is the immunodominant sugar responsible for H specificity.

✔ *N*-acetylgalactosamine is the immunodominant sugar responsible for A specificity.

✔ D-galactose is the immunodominant sugar responsible for B specificity.

✔ The *hh* genotype is known as the Bombay phenotype, or O_h, and lacks normal expression of the ABH antigens.

✔ Group O persons have the greatest amount of H substance; group A_1B persons contain the least amount of H substance.

✔ Approximately 80% of the individuals inherit the A gene phenotype as A_1; the remaining 20% phenotype as A_2 or weaker subgroups.

✔ Approximately 1% to 8% of A_2 persons produce anti-A_1 in their serum.

✔ Glycoproteins in secretions are formed on type 1 precursor chains.

✔ The ABH antigens on RBCs are formed on type 2 precursor chains.

✔ Forward and reverse grouping normally yield strong (3+ to 4+) reactions.

✔ Group A persons have anti-B in their serum; group B persons have anti-A in their serum; group AB persons have neither anti-A nor anti-B in their serum; group O persons contain both anti-A and anti-B in their serum.

✔ Approximately 78% of the random population inherit the *Se* gene and are termed *secretors*; the remaining 22% inherit the *se* gene and are termed *nonsecretors*.

✔ The *Se* gene codes for the production of L-fucosyltransferase.

Review Questions

1. An ABO type on a patient gives the following reactions:

Patient Cells With		Patient Serum With	
Anti-A	Anti-B	A_1 cells	B cells
4+	4+	Neg	Neg

What is the patient's blood type?
   a. O
   b. A
   c. B
   d. AB

2. The major immunoglobulin class(es) of anti-B in a group A individual is (are):
   a. IgM
   b. IgG
   c. IgM and IgG
   d. IgM and IgA

3. What are the possible ABO phenotypes of the offspring from the mating of a group A to a group B individual?
   a. O, A, B
   b. A, B
   c. A, B, AB
   d. O, A, B, AB

4. The immunodominant sugar responsible for blood group A specificity is:
   a. L-fucose
   b. *N*-acetyl-D-galactosamine
   c. D-galactose
   d. Uridine diphosphate-*N*-acetyl-D-galactose

5. What ABH substance(s) would be found in the saliva of a group B secretor?
   a. H
   b. H and A
   c. H and B
   d. H, A, and B

6. An ABO type on a patient gives the following reactions:

Patient Cells With			Patient Serum With	
Anti-A	Anti-B	Anti-A_1	A_1 cells	B cells
4+	4+	Neg	2+	Neg

The reactions above may be seen in a patient who is:
   a. A_1 with acquired B
   b. A_2B with anti-A_1
   c. AB with increased concentrations of protein in the serum
   d. AB with an autoantibody

7. Which of the following ABO blood groups contains the least amount of H substance?

   a. A_1B

   b. A_2

   c. B

   d. O

8. You are working on a specimen in the laboratory that you believe to be a Bombay phenotype. Which of the following reactions would you expect to see?

   a. Patient's cells + *Ulex europaeus* = no agglutination

   b. Patient's cells + *Ulex europaeus* = agglutination

   c. Patient's serum + group O donor RBCs = no agglutination

   d. Patient's serum + A_1 and B cells = no agglutination

9. An example of a technical error that can result in an ABO discrepancy is:

   a. Acquired B phenomenon.

   b. Missing isoagglutinins.

   c. Cell suspension that is too heavy.

   d. Acriflavine antibodies.

10. An ABO type on a patient gives the following reactions:

Patient Cells With		Patient Serum With			
Anti-A	Anti-B	A_1 cells	B cells	O cells	Autocontrol
4+	Neg	2+	4+	2+	Neg

These results are most likely due to:

   a. ABO alloantibody.

   b. Non-ABO alloantibody.

   c. Rouleaux.

   d. Cold autoantibody.

References

1. 2009, F. R. (n.d.): *Vaccines, Blood & Biologics; U.S. Food and Drug Administration.* Fatalities reported to FDA following blood collection and transfusion: Annual summary for fiscal year 2009. Retrieved March 22, 2010, from www.fda.gov/BiologicsBloodVaccines/SafetyAvailability/ReportaProblem/TransfusionDonationFatalities/ucm204763.htm.

2. Landsteiner, K: Uber agglutinationserscheinungen normalen menschlichen blutes. Wien Klin Wschr 14:1132–1134, 1901.

3. Roback, D, Combs, MR, Grossman, BJ, and Hillyer, CD: Technical Manual, 16th ed. American Association of Blood Banks, Bethesda, MD, 2008.

4. Garratty, G, Glynn, SA, and McEntire, R: ABO and Rh (D) phenotype frequencies of different racial/ethnic groups in the United States. Transfusion 44:703–706, 2004.

5. Daniels, G, and Bromilow, I: Essential Guide to Blood Groups. Blackwell Publishing, Malden, MA, 2007.

6. Simon, TL, Snyder, EL, Stowell, CP, Strauss, RG, Solheim, BG, and Petrides, M (eds): Rossi's Principles of Transfusion Medicine, 4th ed. Wiley-Blackwell, Malden, MA, 2009.

7. Dumont, LJ, AuBuchon, JP, Herschel, L, Roger, J, White, T, and Stassinopoulos, A: Random healthy donor sera show varying effectiveness in hemolyzing ABO Incompatible red blood cells. Blood (ASH Annual Meeting Abstracts) 108(11):958, 2006.

8. Murphy, MF, and Pamphilon, DH: Practical Transfusion Medicine, 3rd ed. Wiley-Blackwell, Hoboken, NJ, 2009.

9. Klein, HG, and Anstee, DJ: Mollison's Blood Transfusion in Clinical Medicine, 11th ed. Blackwell Publishing, Malden, MA, 2005.

10. American Association of Blood Bank Standards, 26th ed. American Association of Blood Banks, Bethesda, MD, 2009.

11. Olsson, ML, and Chester, MA: Polymorphism and recombination events at the ABO locus: A major challenge for genomic ABO blood grouping strategies. Transfus Med 11:295–313, 2001.

12. Chester, MA, and Olsson, ML: The ABO blood group gene: A locus of considerable genetic diversity. Transfus Med Rev 15:177–200, 2001.

13. Yamamoto, F, Clausen, H, White, T, Marken, J, and Hakamori S: Molecular genetic basis of histo-blood group ABO system. Nature 345:229–233, 1990.

14. Cohen, M, Hurtado-Ziola, N, and Varki, A: ABO blood group glycans modulate sialic acid recognition on erythrocytes. Blood 114:3668–3676, 2009.

15. Donghaile, DO, Jenkins, VP, McGrath, R, et al: Defining the molecular mechanisms responsible for the ABO high expresser phenotype. Blood (ASH Annual Meeting Abstracts) 114:2119, 2009.

16. Yamamoto, F: Cloning and regulation of the ABO genes. Transfus Med 11:281–294, 2001.

17. Seltsam, A, et al: Systematic analysis of ABO gene diversity within exons 6 and 7 by PCR screening reveals new ABO alleles. Transfusion 43:428–439, 2003.

18. Olsson, ML, Irshaid, NM, Hosseini-Maaf, B, et al: Genomic analysis of clinical samples with serologic ABO blood grouping discrepancies: Identification of 15 novel A and B subgroup alleles. Blood 98:1585–1593, 2001.

19. Seltsam, A, Hallensleben, M, Kollmann, A, and Blaszyk, R: The nature of diversity and diversification at the ABO locus. Blood 102:3035–3042, 2003.

20. Hosseini-Maaf, B, Hellberg, A, Chester, MA, and Olsson, ML: An extensive polymerase chain reaction-allele-specific polymorphism strategy for clinical ABO blood group genotyping that avoids potential errors caused by null, subgroup, and hybrid alleles. Transfusion 47(11):2110–2125, 2007.

21. Blumenfeld, OO: The ABO gene—more variation! Blood 102:2715, 2003.

22. Svensson, L, Pettersson, A, and Henry, SM: Secretor genotyping for A385T, G428A, C571T, 685delTGG, G849A, and other mutations from a single PCR. Transfusion 40:856–860, 2000.

23. Watkins, WM: The ABO blood group system: Historical background. Transfus Med 11:243–265, 2001.

24. Yan, L, Zhu, F, Liu, Y, Xu, X, and Hong, X: Sequences variations in 5'-flanking region of ABO gene and correlation with ABO alleles in the indigenous Chinese. Vox Sang 94(3):227–233, 2008.

25. Fujitani, N, et al: Expression of H type 1 antigen of ABO histio–blood group in normal colon and aberrant expressions of H type 2 and H type 3/4 antigens in colon cancer. Glycoconj J 17:331–338, 2000.

26. Hosoi, E, Hirose, M, and Hamano, S: Expression levels of H-type alpha (1,2)-fucosyltransferase gene and histo-blood group ABO gene corresponding to hematopoietic cell differentiation. Transfusion 43:65–71, 2003.

27. Mizuno, N, Ohmori, T, Sekiguchi, K, et al: Alleles responsible for ABO phenotype-genotype discrepancy and alleles in individuals with a weak expression of A or B antigens. J Forensic Sci 49(1):21–28, 2004.

28. Seltsam, A, and Blaszyk, R: Missense mutations outside the catalytic domain of the ABO glycosyltransferase can cause weak blood group A and B phenotypes. Transfusion 45(10):1663–1669, 2005.

29. Novaretti, MCZ, Domingues, AE, Pares, MMNS, et al: Rapid detection of 871G>A mutation by sequence specific PCR in ABO*A301 blood donors. Blood (ASH Annual Meeting Abstracts) 104:4098, 2004.

30. Barjas-Castro, ML, et al: Molecular heterogeneity of the A3 group. Clin Lab Haematol 22:73–78, 2000.

31. Domingues, AE, Novaretti, MCZ, Dorlhiac-Llacer, PE, and Chamone, DAF: Systematic analysis of ABO gene in A3 and A3B individuals reveals new ABO variants. Blood (ASH Annual Meeting Abstracts) 110:2898, 2007.

32. Olsson, ML, Irshaid, NM, Hosseini-Maaf, B, et al: Genomic analysis of clinical samples with serologic ABO blood grouping discrepancies: Identification of 15 novel A and B subgroup alleles. Blood 98:1585–1593, 2001.

33. Deng, ZH, Yu, Q, Wu, GG, et al: Molecular genetic analysis for Ax phenotype of the ABO blood group system in Chinese. Vox Sang 89(4):251–256, 2005.

34. Nishimukai, H, Fukumori, Y, Tsujimura, R, et al: Rare alleles of the ABO blood group system in two European populations. Leg Med (Tokyo): 11(Suppl 1):S479–S481, 2009.

35. Hillyer, CD (ed): Blood Banking and Transfusion Medicine, 2nd ed. Churchill Livingston Elsevier, Philadelphia, PA, 2007.

36. Hosseini-Maaf, B, Smart, E, Chester, MA, and Olsson ML: The Abantu phenotype in the ABO blood group system is due to a splice-site mutation in a hybrid between a new O1-like allelic lineage and the A2 allele. Vox Sang 88(4):256–264, 2005.

37. Catron, JP, et al: Assay of alpha-N-acetylgalactosaminyltransferase in human sera: Further evidence for several types of Am individuals. Vox Sang 28:347–365, 1975.

38. Asamura, H, et al: Molecular genetic analysis of the Am phenotype of the ABO blood group system. Vox Sang 83:263–267, 2002.

39. Yu, Q, Wu, GG, Liang, YL, Deng, ZH, Su, YQ, and Wang, DM: Study on molecular genetic structure of Ael blood subgroup. Zhonghua Yi Xue Yi Chuan Xue Za Zhi 23(2):173–176, 2006.

40. Sun, CF, Chen, DP, Tseng, CP, Wang, WT, and Liu, JP: Identification of a novel A1v-O1v hybrid allele with G829A mutation in a chimeric individual of AelBel phenotype. Transfusion 46(5):780–789, 2006.

41. Yazer, MH, Hosseini-Maaf, B, and Olsson, ML: Blood grouping discrepancies between ABO genotype and phenotype caused by O alleles. Curr Opin Hematol15(6):618–624, 2008.

42. Zhu, F, Tao, S, Xu, X, et al: Distribution of ABO blood group allele and identification of three novel alleles in the Chinese Han population. Vox Sang 98(4):554–559, 2010.

43. Cai, XH, Jin, S, Liu, X, et al: Molecular genetic analysis for the B subgroup revealing two novel alleles in the ABO gene. Transfusion 48(11):2442–2447, 2008.

44. Cho, D, Yazer, MH, Shin, M, et al: Dispermic chimerism in a blood donor with apparent B3 blood group and mosaic 47, XYY Syndrome. *Blood (ASH Annual Meeting Abstracts)*. 2005;106(11):1896.

45. Xu, XG, Hong, XZ, Liu, Y, Zhu, FM, Lv, HJ, and Yan, LX: A novel M142T mutation in the B glycosyltransferase gene associated with B3 variant in Chinese. Zhonghua Yi Xue Yi Chuan Xue Za Zhi 26(3):254–257, 2009.

46. Hosseini-Maaf, B, Letts, JA, Persson, M, et al: Structural basis for red cell phenotypic changes in newly identified, naturally occurring subgroup mutants of the human blood group B glycosyltransferase. Transfusion 47(5):864–875, 2007.

47. Seltsam, A, Wagner, FF, Gruger, D, Gupta, CD, Bade-Doeding, C, and Blasczyk, R: Weak blood group B phenotypes may be caused by variations in the CCAAT-binding factor/NF-Y enhancer region of the ABO gene. Transfusion 47(12):2330–2335, 2007.

48. Seltsam, A, Gruger, D, Just, B, et al: Aberrant intracellular trafficking of a variant B glycosyltransferase. Transfusion 48(9):1898–1905, 2008.

49. Koscielak, J, Pacuszka, T, and Dzierkowa-Borodej, W: Activity of B-gene-specified galactosyltransferase in individuals with Bm phenotypes. Vox Sang 30:58–67, 1976.

50. Lin, PH, et al: A unique 502C>T mutation in exon 7 of ABO gene associated with the Bel phenotype in Taiwan. Transfusion 43:1254–1259, 2003.

51. Hosseini-Maaf, B, Hellberg, A, Rodrigues, MJ, Chester, MA, and Olsson, ML: ABO exon and intron analysis in individuals with the A weak B phenotype reveals a novel O1v-A2 hybrid allele that causes four missense mutations in the A transferase. BMC Genet 4:17, 2003.

52. Bhende, YM, Deshpande, CK, Bhatia, HM, et al: A "new" blood group characteristic related to the ABO system. Lancet 1:9034, 1952.

53. Storry, et al: Identification of six new alleles at the FUT1 and FUT2 loci in ethnically diverse individuals with Bombay and para-Bombay phenotypes. Transfusion 46(12):2149–2155, 2006.

54. Salmon, C, et al: H-deficient phenotypes: A proposed practical classification of Bombay Ah, H2, Hm. Blood Transfus Immunohaematol 23:233–248, 1980.

55. Yan, L, Zhu, F, Xu, X, Hong, X, and Lv, Q: Molecular basis for para-Bombay phenotypes in Chinese persons, including a novel nonfunctional FUT1allele. Transfusion 45:725–730, 2005.

56. Storry, JR, and Olsson, ML: The ABO blood group system revisited: a review and update. Immunohematology, vol 25(2):48–59, 2009.

Chapter 7

The Rh Blood Group System

Susan T. Johnson, MSTM, MT(ASCP)SBB and Merilyn Wiler, MA, MT(ASCP)SBB

OBJECTIVES

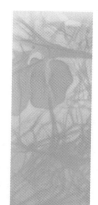

Explain the derivation of the term *Rh*.

1. Differentiate Rh from LW blood group systems.

2. Compare and contrast the Fisher-Race and Wiener theories of Rh inheritance.

3. Translate the five major Rh antigens, haplotypes, and predicted haplotypes, from one nomenclature to another, including Fisher-Race, Wiener, Rosenfield, and ISBT.

4. Define the basic biochemical structure of Rh.

5. Compare and contrast the genetic pathways for the regulator type of Rh_{null} and the amorphic Rh_{null}.

6. Describe and differentiate five mechanisms that result in weakened expression of D on red blood cells.

7. List one instance in which the weak-D status of an individual must be determined.

8. List and differentiate four types of Rh typing reagents, and provide two advantages of each type.

9. Define three characteristics of Rh antibodies.

10. Describe three symptoms associated with an Rh hemolytic transfusion reaction.

11. Compare and contrast Rh_{null} and Rh_{mod} and describe the role of RhAG in Rh antigen expression.

12. List four Rh antigens (excluding DCcEe), and give two classic characteristics of each antigen.

13. Determine the most probable genotype of an individual when given the individual's red blood cell typing results, haplotype frequencies, and ethnicity.

Introduction

This chapter describes in detail the Rh blood group system. It is imperative to have a basic understanding of Rh, as RhD typing is a critical component of pretransfusion testing. In addition, clinically important Rh antibodies are relatively common in pregnancy and in patients requiring blood transfusion.

The term Rh refers to a specific red blood cell (RBC) antigen (D) and to a complex blood group system currently composed of over 50 different antigenic specificities. Although Rh antibodies were among the first to be described, scientists have spent years unraveling the complexities of the Rh blood group system from its serology to its mode of inheritance, genetic control, and the biochemical structure of the Rh antigens. Rh-specific antigens reside on proteins versus the carbohydrate antigens ABO and Hh.

Rh is the second most important blood group system in terms of transfusion, as the Rh system antigens are very **immunogenic**. Unlike ABO antibodies that are typically found in individuals who lack the corresponding antigen, Rh antibodies are produced only after exposure to foreign red blood cells. Once present, they can produce significant **hemolytic disease of the fetus and newborn** (HDFN) as well as hemolytic transfusion reactions.

The terms Rh-positive or positive and Rh-negative or negative are routinely used by the public and by experts in the field when referring to blood type—for example, A-positive or A-negative. **Rh-positive** indicates that an individual's red blood cells possess one particular Rh antigen, the D antigen, on their red blood cells. **Rh-negative** indicates that the red blood cells lack the D antigen.

History

Before 1939, the only significant blood group antigens recognized were those of the ABO system. Transfusion medicine was thus based on matching ABO groups. Despite ABO matching, blood transfusions continued to result in morbidity and mortality. As the 1930s ended, two significant discoveries were made that would further the safety of blood transfusion and eventually define the most extensive blood group system known. It began when Levine and Stetson[1] described a hemolytic transfusion reaction in an obstetrical patient. After delivering a stillborn infant, this woman required transfusions. Her husband, who had the same ABO type, was selected as her donor. After transfusion, the recipient demonstrated classic symptoms of an **acute hemolytic transfusion reaction** (AHTR). Subsequently, an antibody was isolated from the mother's serum that reacted both at 37°C and at 20°C with the father's RBCs. It was postulated that the fetus and the father possessed a common factor the mother lacked. While the mother carried the fetus, she was exposed to this factor and subsequently produced an antibody that showed positive reactivity when tested against the transfused RBCs from the father.

One year later, Landsteiner and Wiener[2] reported on an antibody made by guinea pigs and rabbits when they were transfused with Rhesus macaque monkey RBCs. This antibody,

which agglutinated 85% of human RBCs, was named Rh after the Rhesus monkey. Another investigation by Levine and coworkers[3] demonstrated that the agglutinin (antibody causing direct agglutination of RBCs) causing the hemolytic transfusion reaction and the antibody described by Landsteiner and Wiener appeared to define the same blood group. Many years later it was recognized that the two antibodies were different. However, the name Rh was retained for the human-produced antibody, and **anti-Rhesus** formed by the animals was renamed **anti-LW** in honor of those first reporting it (Landsteiner and Wiener).

Further research resulted in defining Rh as a primary cause of hemolytic disease of the fetus and newborn (HDFN, also called **erythroblastosis fetalis**) and a significant cause of hemolytic transfusion reactions. Continued investigation[4-7] showed additional blood group factors were associated with the original agglutinin. By the mid-1940s, five antigens made up the Rh system. Today the Rh blood group system contains over 57 different specificities and continues to grow in number as new genetic mutations are discovered.

Terminology

Terminologies used to describe the Rh system are derived from four sets of investigators. Two terminologies are based on postulated genetic theories of Rh inheritance. The third common terminology used describes only the presence or absence of a given antigen. The fourth is the result of the combined efforts of the International Society of Blood Transfusion (ISBT) Committee on Terminology for Red Cell Surface Antigens. The molecular basis of the Rh blood group system as we know it today is described in detail in the "Molecular Genetics" section after the discussion of nomenclature to provide context to the terminology used.

Fisher-Race: DCE Terminology

In the 1940s, Fisher and Race[8] were investigating antigens found on human RBCs, including the newly defined Rh antigen. They postulated that the antigens of the system were produced by three closely linked sets of **alleles** (Fig. 7–1). Each gene was responsible for producing a product (or antigen) on the RBC surface. Each antigen and corresponding gene were given the same letter designation (when referring to the gene, the letter is italicized).

Fisher and Race named the antigens of the system D, d, C, c, and E, e. Now it is known that "d" represents the

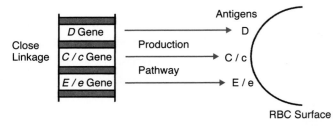

Figure 7–1. Fisher-Race concept of Rh (simplified). Each gene produces one product.

Table 7–1	Frequency of Common Rh Antigens in Caucasians	
ANTIGEN	**GENE FREQUENCY (%)**	
D	85	
No D (absence of D)	15	
C	70	
E	30	
c	80	
e	98	

absence of D antigen; however, the term continues to be utilized with Fisher-Race terminology as a placeholder. The **phenotype** (antigens expressed on the RBC detected by typing) of a given RBC is defined by the presence of D, C, c, E, and e expression. The gene frequency in the Caucasian population for each Rh antigen is given in Table 7–1, and the Rh **haplotype** (the complement of genes inherited from either parent) frequencies are given in Table 7–2. Notice how the frequencies vary with ethnic background.

According to the Fisher-Race theory, each person inherits a set of *Rh* genes from each parent (i.e., one *D* or *d,* one *C* or *c,* and one *E* or *e*) (see **Fig. 7–1**). Because *Rh* genes were thought to be **codominant**, each inherited gene expresses its corresponding antigen on the RBC. The combination of maternal and paternal haplotypes determines one's **genotype** (the *Rh* genes inherited from each parent) and dictates one's phenotype. An individual's Rh phenotype is reported as DCE rather than CDE because Fisher postulated that the *C/c* locus lies between the *D/d* and *E/e* loci. This information is based on frequencies of the various gene combinations.

Table 7–2	Fisher-Race Haplotypes of the Rh System		
	PREVALENCE (%)		
Haplotype	**White**	**Black**	**Asian**
DCe	42	17	70
dce	37	26	3
DcE	14	11	21
Dce	4	44	3
dCe	2	2	2
dcE	1	< 0.01	< 0.01
DCE	< 0.01	< 0.01	1
dCE	< 0.01	< 0.01	< 0.01

Modified from Roback, JD, Combs, MR, Grossman, B, Hillyer, C (eds): Technical Manual, 16th ed. AABB, Bethesda, MD, 2008.

It is essential to remember that d does not represent an antigen but simply represents the absence of D antigen. C, c, E, and e represent actual antigens recognized by specific antibodies. There has never been an antibody that recognizes d antigen, supporting the fact that d antigen does not exist. Further discussion on the absence of D follows later in the chapter. For many students and working laboratory scientists, the Fisher-Race terminology represents the easiest way to think about the five major Rh system antigens, but it has shortcomings. Many antigens assigned to the Rh blood group system were given names using a variety of terminologies. In addition, as the number of Rh antigens continues to grow, the original Fisher-Race terminology is becoming too limiting.

In very rare instances, an individual may fail to express any allelic antigen at one or both Rh loci; that is, a person may lack E and e, or all CcEe antigens. The probable genotype for the Rh (D)-positive person exhibiting a deletion phenotype such as these is written *DC-* or *Dc-*, or *D–*. A deletion of Cc with Ee has not been reported. The person expressing no Rh antigens on the RBC is said to be **Rh$_{null}$**, and the phenotype may be written as —/—. Weakened expression of all Rh antigens of an individual has also been reported. These individuals are said to have the **Rh$_{mod}$** **phenotype**. Placing parenthesis around (D), (C), and (e) indicates weakened antigen expression.

Wiener: Rh-Hr Terminology

In his early work defining the Rh antigens, Wiener[9] believed there was one gene responsible for defining Rh that produced an agglutinogen containing a series of blood factors. According to Weiner, this *Rh* gene produced at least three factors within an **agglutinogen** (Fig. 7–2). The agglutinogen may be considered the phenotypic expression of the haplotype. Each factor is an antigen recognized by an antibody. Antibodies can recognize single or multiple factors (antigens).

Table 7–3 lists the major agglutinogens and their respective factors, along with the shorthand term that has come to represent each agglutinogen. Wiener's terminology is complex and unwieldy; nevertheless, many blood bankers use modified Wiener terminology interchangeably with other nomenclatures. This terminology allows one to convey Rh antigens inherited on one chromosome or haplotype and makes it easier to discuss a genotype. A medical laboratory scientist conveying a probable genotype to a coworker would have to say DcE/DcE. However, R$_2$R$_2$ is much easier to verbally communicate.

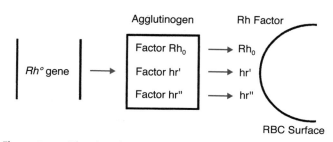

Figure 7–2. Wiener's agglutinogen theory. Antibody will recognize each factor within the agglutinogen.

Table 7–3   Rh-Hr Terminology of Wiener

GENE	AGGLUTINOGEN	BLOOD FACTORS	SHORTHAND DESIGNATION	FISHER-RACE ANTIGENS
Rh^0	Rh_0	$Rh_0hr'hr''$	R_0	Dce
Rh^1	Rh_1	$Rh_0rh'hr''$	R_1	DCe
Rh^2	Rh_2	$Rh_0hr'rh''$	R_2	DcE
Rh^z	Rh_z	$Rh_0rh'rh''$	R_z	DCE
rh	rh	$hr'hr''$	r	ce
rh'	rh'	$rh'hr''$	r'	Ce
rh''	rh''	$hr'rh''$	r''	cE
rh^y	rh_y	$rh'rh''$	r^y	CE

Fisher-Race nomenclature may be converted to Wiener nomenclature and vice versa. It is important to remember that an agglutinogen in Wiener nomenclature actually represents the presence of a single haplotype expressing three different antigens (see **Table 7–3**). When describing an agglutinogen, the uppercase R denotes the presence of the original factor, the D antigen. The lowercase r indicates the absence of D antigen. The presence of uppercase C is indicated by a 1 or a single prime ('). Lowercase c is implied when there is no 1 or ' indicated. (It is assumed that the third antigen is e). That is, R_1 is the same as DCe; r' denotes Ce; and R_0 is equivalent to Dce. The presence of E is indicated by the Arabic number 2 or double prime ("). Lowercase e is implied when there is no 2 or " indicated—that is, R_2 is the same as DcE; r'' denotes cE, and r is equivalent to ce. (Again, it is assumed that a c antigen is present.) When both C and E are uppercase, the letter z or y is used. R_z denotes DCE, whereas r^y represents CE. See Table 7–4 for a summary of this shorthand nomenclature.

Italics or superscripts are used when describing *Rh* genes in the Wiener nomenclature (i.e., R_1 *or* R_2, R^1 or R^2).

Standard type is used to describe the gene product or agglutinogen. Subscripts are used with the uppercase R and superscripts with the lowercase r (i.e., R_1 or R_2 or r'). Phenotypes of Rh_{null} and Rh_{mod} are written as stated. The genotype for the Rh_{null} that arises from an amorphic gene at both Rh loci is written as $\overline{\overline{rr}}$ and pronounced "little r double bar."

When referring to the Rh antigens (or blood factors) in Wiener nomenclature, the single prime (') refers to either C or c and the double prime (") to either E or e. If the r precedes the h (i.e., rh' or rh''), this refers to the C or E antigens, respectively. When the h precedes the r, this refers to either the c (hr') or e (hr'') antigen. Rh_0 is equivalent to D. In the Wiener nomenclature, there is no designation for the absence of D antigen. By using these designations, the laboratorian should be able to recognize immediately which antigens are present on the RBCs described. However, it is difficult to use the Wiener nomenclature to adequately describe additional alleles within an agglutinogen. Because of this, many of the more recently described antigens of the Rh system have not been given Rh-Hr designations.

Table 7–4   Weiner Haplotype Terminology

	SYMBOL	D	C	E	c*	e*	SHORTHAND DESIGNATION
R	1	+	+	0	*0*	+	**R_1**
r	'	0	+	0	*0*	+	**r'**
R	2	+	0	+	+	*0*	**R_2**
r	''	0	0	+	+	*0*	**r''**
R	z	+	+	+	*0*	*0*	**R_z**
r	y	0	+	+	*0*	*0*	**r^y**
R	0	+	0	0	+	+	**R_0**
r	None	0	0	0	+	+	**r**

*c and e typings are assumed based on symbols used to indicate phenotype.

Rosenfield and Coworkers: Alphanumeric Terminology

As the Rh blood group system expanded, it became more difficult to assign names to new antigens using existing terminologies. In the early 1960s, Rosenfield and associates[10] proposed a system that assigns a number to each antigen of the Rh system in order of its discovery or recognized relationship to the Rh system (Table 7–5). This system has no genetic basis, nor was it proposed based on a theory of Rh inheritance, but it simply demonstrates the presence or absence of the antigen on the RBC. A minus sign preceding a number designates the absence of the antigen. If an antigen has not been typed, its number will not appear in the sequence. An advantage of this nomenclature is that the RBC phenotype is thus succinctly described.

For the five major antigens, D is assigned Rh1, C is Rh2, E is Rh3, c is Rh4, and e is Rh5. For RBCs that type D + C + E + c negative, e negative, the Rosenfield designation is Rh: 1, 2, 3, –4, –5. If the sample was not tested for e, the designation would be Rh: 1, 2, 3, –4. All Rh system antigens have been assigned a number.

The numeric system is well suited to electronic data processing. Its use expedites data entry and retrieval. Its primary limiting factor is that there is a similar nomenclature for numerous other blood groups such as Kell, Duffy, Kidd, Lutheran, Scianna, and more. K:1,2 refers to the K and k antigens of the Kell blood group system. Therefore, when using the Rosenfield nomenclature on the computer, one must use both the alpha (Rh:, K:) and the numeric (1, 2, –3, etc.) to denote a phenotype.

International Society of Blood Transfusion Committee: Updated Numeric Terminology

As the world of blood transfusion began to cooperate and share data, it became apparent there was a need for a universal language. The International Society of Blood Transfusion (ISBT) formed the Committee on Terminology for Red Cell Surface Antigens. Its mandate was to establish a uniform nomenclature that is both eye- and machine-readable and is in keeping with the genetic basis of blood groups.[11] The ISBT adopted a six-digit number for each authenticated antigen belonging to a blood group system. The first three numbers represent the system and the remaining three the antigenic specificity. Number 004 was assigned to the Rh blood group system, and then each antigen assigned to the Rh system was given a unique number to complete the six-digit computer number. Table 7–6 provides a listing of these numbers.

When referring to individual antigens, an alphanumeric designation similar to the Rosenfield nomenclature may be used. The alphabetic names formerly used were left unchanged but were converted to all uppercase letters (e.g., Rh, Kell became RH, KELL). Therefore, D is RH1, C is RH2, and so forth. (Note: There is no space between the RH and the assigned number.)

The phenotype designation includes the alphabetical symbol that denotes the blood group, followed by a colon and then the specificity numbers of the antigens defined. A minus sign preceding the number indicates that the antigen was tested for but was not present. The phenotype D + C – E + c + e + or DcE/ce or R_2r would be written RH:1, –2, 3, 4, 5.

Table 7–5 Common Rh Types by Three Nomenclatures

	WIENER	FISHER-RACE	ROSENFIELD PHENOTYPE	PHENOTYPE FREQUENCY (%) (APPROX., CAUCASIAN)
Common genotypes	R^1r	DCe/dce	Rh:1, 2, –3, 4, 5	34.9
	R^1R^1	DCe/DCe	Rh:1, 2, –3, –4, 5	18.5
	rr	dce/dce	Rh: –1, –2, –3, 4, 5	15.1
	R^1R^2	DCe/DcE	Rh:1, 2, 3, 4, 5	13.3
	R^2r	DcE/dce	Rh:1, –2, 3, 4, 5	11.8
	R^2R^2	DcE/DcE	Rh:1, –2, 3, 4, –5	2.3
Rarer genotypes	r'r	dCe/dce	Rh: –1, 2, –3, 4, 5	0.8
	r'r'	dCe/dCe	Rh: –1, 2, –3, –4, 5	Rare
	r''r	dcE/dce	Rh: –1, –2, 3, 4, 5	0.9
	r''r''	dcE/dcE	Rh: –1, –2, 3, 4, –5	Rare
	R^0r (R^0R^0)	Dce/dce(Dce/Dce)	Rh:1, –2, –3, 4, 5	2.1
	r'r'' (r^yr)	dCe/dcE(dCE/dce)	Rh: –1, 2, 3, 4, 5	0.05

Table 7–6   Antigens of the Rh Blood Group System in Four Nomenclatures

NUMERIC	FISHER-RACE	WEINER	ISBT NUMBER	OTHER NAMES OR COMMENT
Rh1	D	Rh_0	004001	
Rh2	C	rh'	004002	
Rh3	E	rh''	004003	
Rh4	c	hr'	004004	
Rh5	e	hr''	004005	
Rh6	ce	hr	004006	f
Rh7	Ce	rh_i	004007	
Rh8	C^w	rh^{w1}	004008	
Rh9	C^x	rh^x	004009	
Rh10	V	hr^v	004010	ce^s
Rh11	E^w	rh^{w2}	004011	
Rh12	G	rh^G	004012	
Rh13[†]		Rh^A	004013	
Rh14[†]		Rh^B	004014	
Rh15[†]		Rh^C	004015	
Rh16[†]		Rh^D	004016	
Rh17		Hr_0	004017	
Rh18		Hr	004018	Hr^S (High prevalence)
Rh19		hr^s	004019	
Rh20	VS	e^s	004020	
Rh21	C^G		004021	
Rh22	CE	Rh	004022	Jarvis
Rh23	D^w		004023	Wiel
Rh24[†]	E^T		004024	
Rh25*/[†]			004025	
Rh26	c-like		004026	Deal
Rh27	cE	rh_{ii}	004027	
Rh28		hr^H	004028	Hernandez
Rh29			004029	Total Rh
Rh30	D^{cor}		004030	Go^a (low prevalence) DIVa
Rh31		hr^B	004031	
Rh32		$\bar{\bar{R}}^N$	004032	Troll (low prevalence)
Rh33		R_0^{Har}	004033	D^{HAR} (low prevalence)
Rh34		Hr^B	004034	Bastiaan
Rh35			004035	(low prevalence)
Rh36			004036	Be^a (Berrens; low prevalence)

Table 7–6   Antigens of the Rh Blood Group System in Four Nomenclatures—cont'd

NUMERIC	FISHER-RACE	WEINER	ISBT NUMBER	OTHER NAMES OR COMMENT
Rh37			004037	Evans (low prevalence)
Rh38†				Formerly Duclos
Rh39	C-like		004039	
Rh40	Tar		004040	Targett (low prevalence)
Rh41	Ce-like		004041	
Rh42	Ce^S, Cce^S	rh_i^s	004042	Thornton
Rh43			004043	Crawford (low prevalence)
Rh44			004044	Nou (high prevalence)
Rh45			004045	Riv
Rh46			004046	Sec (high prevalence)
Rh47	"Allelic"	to $\bar{\bar{R}}^N$	004047	Dav (high prevalence)
Rh48			004048	JAL (low prevalence)
Rh49			004049	Stem
Rh50			004050	FPTT (low prevalence)
Rh51			004051	MAR (high prevalence)
Rh52			004052	BARC (low prevalence)
Rh53			004053	JAHK (low prevalence)
Rh54			004054	DAK (low prevalence)
Rh55			004055	LOCR (low prevalence)
Rh56			004056	CENR (low prevalence)
Rh57			004057	CEST

*Rh25 was formerly assigned to the LW antigen. LW is now known as LWᵃ and is no longer considered a member of the Rh system.
†Obsolete names: Rh13, Rh14, Rh15, Rh16 former classification of partial D types, Rh 24, Rh25 formerly LW, Rh38 formerly Duclos.

When referring to a gene, an allele, or a haplotype, the symbols are italicized. A haplotype is followed by a space or an asterisk, and then the numbers of the specificities are separated by commas. The R^1 haplotype or DCe would be RH 1,2,5 or RH*1,2,5.

Overview of Rh Terminologies

Blood bankers must be familiar with Fisher-Race, Wiener, Rosenfield, and ISBT nomenclatures and must be able to translate among them when reading about, writing about, or discussing the Rh blood group system.

Tables 7–4, 7–5, and **7–6** summarize the data presented in this section. These tables also include probable genotypes based on the antigens found in selected RBC populations. Table 7–7 correlates Rh phenotypes with the most probable or predicted genotype in a designated population. Results of typing do not define genotype, only phenotype. Other possible genotypes that can occur with the given test results are also listed, but they are not commonly seen.

Determining probable or predicted genotypes was useful for parentage studies, also known as *relationship testing*, and for population studies. Other molecular methods are proving more powerful today. Probable genotypes are useful in predicting the potential for HDFN in offspring of Rh-negative women with anti-D; however, molecular testing, commonly referred to as **zygosity testing,** can be performed to confirm whether the father possesses one or two copies of the *RHD* gene.

There are substantial differences in phenotypes and predicted genotypes of various populations. For example, the phenotype D+C-E-c+e+ is most commonly seen in the black population but is considered relatively rare in whites (see Tables 7–5 and 7–7). These differences must be remembered when trying to locate compatible blood for recipients with unusual or multiple Rh antibodies.

Table 7–7   Eighteen Possible Reaction Patterns With Five Antisera*

D	C	E	c	e	WHITES (%)	BLACKS (%)	WHITES	BLACKS	OTHER POSSIBILITIES (BOTH GROUPS)
+	+	−	+	+	34.9	15 9	DCe/dce	DCe/Dce or DCe/dce	dCe/Dce
+	+	−	−	+	18.5	3	DCe/DCe	DCe/DCe	DCe/dCe
+	+	+	+	+	13.3	4	DCe/DcE	DCe/DcE	DCe/dcE, dCe/DcE, DCE/dce, DCE/Dce, or dCE/Dce
+	−	+	+	+	11.8	10 6	DcE/dce	DcE/Dce or DcE/dce	dcE/Dce
+	−	+	+	−	2.3	1	DcE/DcE	DcE/DcE	DcE/dcE
+	−	−	+	+	2.1	19 23	Dce/dce	Dce/Dce, or Dce/dce	−
−	−	−	+	+	15.1	7	dce/dce	dce/dce	−
−	+	−	+	+	0.8	1	dCe/dce	dCe/dce	−
−	−	+	+	+	0.8	rare	dcE/dce	dcE/dce	−
−	+	+	+	+	0.05%	rare	dCe/dcE		dCE/dce
−	+	−	−	+	rare	rare	dCe/dCe		−
−	−	+	+	−	rare	rare	dcE/dcE		−
+	+	+	−	+	0.2%	rare	DCE/DCe		DCE/dCe
+	+	+	+	−	0.1%	rare	DCE/DcE		DCE/dcE
+	+	+	−	−	0.1%	rare	DCE/DCE		DCE/dCE
−	+	+	−	+	rare	rare	dCE/dCe		−
−	+	+	+	−	rare	rare	dCE/dcE		−
−	+	+	−	−	rare	rare	dCE/dCE		−

*Percentages are rounded off.

To further emphasize the interchangeable use of the terminologies for the basic antigens, see **Table 7–5**, which defines common genotypes using the Fisher-Race, Wiener, and Rosenfield nomenclatures. Frequencies listed are for those found in the Caucasian population.

Finally, as the genetics and biochemistry of the Rh blood group system have been unraveled, the terminology has continued to change. For consistency of use, *RHD* and *RHCE*, all uppercase and in italics, will be used from this point forward in the text to indicate genes. RhD, RhCe, RhcE, Rhce, and RhCE will be used to designate proteins on which the Rh antigens reside.

Molecular Genetics

Several theories have been described to explain genetically the results of serologic and biochemical studies in the Rh system. Two theories of Rh genetic control were initially postulated. Wiener hypothesized that a single gene produces a single product that contains separately recognizable factors (see **Fig 7–2**). In contrast, Fisher and Race proposed that the Rh locus contains three distinct genes that control production of their respective antigens (see **Fig 7–1**). Later, Tippett correctly proposed two *RH* genes, *RHD* and *RHCE*, that control expression of Rh antigens.[12]

RH Genes

It is now known that only two closely linked genes located on chromosome 1 control expression of Rh proteins—namely, *RHD* and *RHCE*.[13–15] The gene *RHD* codes for the presence or absence of the RhD protein, and the second gene *RHCE* codes for either RhCe, RhcE, Rhce, or RhCE proteins (Fig. 7–3). *RHD* and *RHCE* genes each have 10 exons and are 97% identical.

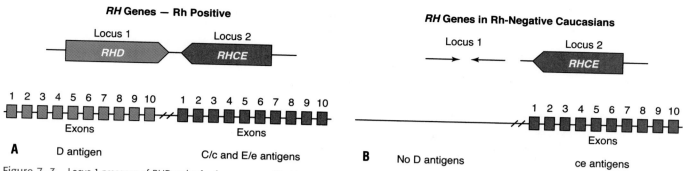

Figure 7–3.   Locus 1 presence of *RHD* codes for the presence of D (A) or no D (B). Locus 2 codes for Ce, CE, cE, ce. Each gene consists of 10 coding exons.

Another gene important to Rh antigen expression is *RHAG*, and it resides on chromosome 6.[16] The product of this gene is **Rh-associated glycoprotein** (RhAG). This polypeptide is very similar in structure to the Rh proteins, with the difference being it is glycosylated (carbohydrates attached). Within the RBC membrane, it forms complexes with the Rh proteins. RhAG is termed a *coexpressor* and must be present for successful expression of the Rh antigens. However, by itself, this glycoprotein does not express any Rh antigens. When mutations in the *RHAG* gene occur, it can result in missing or significantly altered RhD and RhCE proteins, affecting antigen expression. In rare instances, individuals express no Rh antigens on their RBCs. These individuals are said to have the Rh$_{null}$ phenotype and are discussed in more detail later in this chapter. RHAG has been assigned as a blood group system and is discussed in further detail in Chapter 8, "Blood Group Terminology and the Other Blood Groups."

Rh-Positive Phenotypes

As predicted, *RH* genes are inherited as codominant alleles. Rh-positive individuals inherit one or two *RHD* genes, which result in expression of RhD antigen and are typed Rh-positive. In addition to the *RHD* gene(s), two *RHCE* genes are inherited, one from each parent. Figure 7–4 is an example of a normal Rh inheritance pattern.

Numerous mutations in the *RHD* gene have been discovered that cause weakened expression of the RhD antigen detected in routine testing. This is generally termed weak D or weak expression of D and will be discussed in more detail later in the chapter.

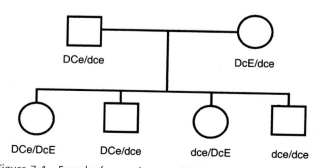

Figure 7-4.   Example of a normal pattern of Rh inheritance.

Rh-Negative Phenotypes

Rh-negative individuals can arise from at least three different mutations. These mutations are most often found in individuals falling into three different ethnic backgrounds: European, African, and Asian.

European Ethnicity

Common Rh-negative white individuals have a deletion of the *RHD* gene—that is, they possess no *RHD* gene but have inherited two *RHCE* genes.[17]

Advanced Concepts

African Ethnicity

An unusual form of the *RHD* gene occurs in 66% of individuals of African ethnicity termed *RHD* pseudogene or *RHDψ*. This gene is an *RHD*-negative allele whose sequence is identical to the *RHD* gene except for missense mutations in exon 5 and exon 6, a nonsense mutation in exon 6, and a 37-bp insertion at the intron 3/exon 4 boundary.[18] Individuals with this gene do not produce RhD protein.

Asian Ethnicity

Another mutation has been described in Asians that alters the *RHD* gene, causing an individual to type as D-negative.[19] This is termed D$_{el}$ and will be discussed further in the section on weak D phenotypes.

Numerous mutations have been described in the *RH* genes. Greater than 150 alleles have been determined in the *RHD* gene, and greater than 60 alleles have been found in the *RHCE* allele and the number continues to grow.[20] Fortunately for the medical laboratory scientist, these mutations rarely change the serology observed in day-to-day testing.

Biochemistry

Basic Concepts

The product of *RH* genes are nonglycosylated proteins. This means no carbohydrates are attached to the protein. Rh antigens reside on **transmembrane proteins** and are an integral part of the RBC membrane.[21] The gene products of *RHD* and *RHCE* are remarkably similar in that both encode for proteins composed of 416 amino acids that traverse the cell membrane 12 times. Their proteins differ by only 32 to 35 amino acids.[22] Amino acid position 103 is important in determining C or c expression and position 226 differentiates E from e (Fig. 7–5). Only small loops of Rh proteins are exposed on the surface of the RBC and provide the conformational requirements for many serologic differences between the Rh blood types.

Advanced Concepts

In researching the biochemistry of Rh antigens, investigations have been performed to determine the quantity of antigen sites on RBCs of various Rh phenotypes. In comparison with ABO and Kell (K) blood groups, A_1 cells possess approximately 1×10^6 A antigens, whereas RBCs possessing a double-dose expression of the K antigen have 6,000 K sites. Hughes-Jones and coworkers measured the number of D antigen sites on a variety of Rh phenotypes.[23] The results are summarized in Table 7–8. The greatest number of D antigen sites are on cells of the rare Rh phenotype D (refer to the "Deletions" section). However, of the commonly encountered Rh genotypes, R^2R^2 cells possess the largest number of D antigen sites.

Rh Function

RhD and RhCE proteins and RhAG are exclusively on red blood cells. As they are transmembranes, it is not surprising they play a role in maintaining the structural integrity of red cells. Based on their structure, it appears they may also be transporters. Westhoff and colleagues showed they may have a role in transporting ammonia.[24] An alternative hypothesis is that they may be CO_2 transporters.[25]

Weak D: Variations of D Antigen Expression

When Rh-positive RBC samples are typed for the D antigen, they are expected to show strong positive reactivity with anti-D reagents. However, some individuals have RBCs that

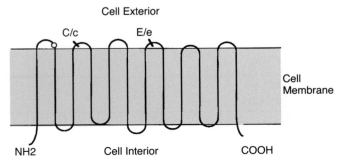

Figure 7–5. Model of Rh polypeptide; "o" denotes where the sequence of D diverges from C/c or E/e. The C/c and E/e, respectively, denote the region responsible for the serologic difference between C/c and E/e.

Table 7–8	Number of D Antigen Sites of Cells with Various Phenotypes

Rh PHENOTYPE	NUMBER OF D ANTIGEN SITES
R_1r	9,900–14,600
R_0r	12,000–20,000
R_2r	14,000–16,600
R_1R_1	14,500–19,300
R_1R_2	23,000–31,000
R_2R_2	15,800–33,300
D--	110,000–202,000

possess D antigen that requires an indirect antiglobulin test to detect the presence of D antigen. RBCs carrying weaker D antigen have historically been referred to as having the D^u type based on the original description of what the investigators thought was a new antigen.[26] It was later proven that this was not a new antigen since individuals did not produce anti-D^u; they produced anti-D.

For many years, all individuals with altered D antigen were referred to as having weak D because their RhD antigen was altered. Now these individuals with altered D antigen are categorized into different phenotypes defined as weakened D due to C in *trans* to *RHD*, weak D, partial D, and D_{el}. It has been shown that 1% to 2% of individuals with European ancestry possess some altered form of D antigen.[27] Altered D antigen occurs more often in individuals of African descent, but the exact prevalence is not known. Finally, to further complicate matters, there are rare individuals who possess D epitopes on their RhCE protein.[28,29]

C in *Trans* to *RHD*

The first mechanism that may result in weakened expression of D antigen was originally described as a position effect or gene interaction effect.[30] The allele carrying *RHD* is *trans* (or in the opposite haplotype) to the allele carrying *C*; for example, *Dce/dCe*. The Rh antigen on the RBC is normal, but the steric arrangement of the C antigen in relationship to the D antigen appears to interfere with the expression of D antigen. This interference with D expression does not occur when the *C* gene is inherited in the *cis* position to *RHD*, such as *DCe/dce*. It is not possible to serologically distinguish genetic weak D from the position effect weak D. Molecular studies would differentiate the two types. Practically speaking, this is unnecessary because the D antigen is structurally complete. These individuals can receive D-positive RBCs with no adverse effects.

Weak D

The second mechanism results from inheritance of *RHD* genes that code for a weakened expression of the D antigen.[31]

The D antigens expressed appear to be complete but fewer in number. On a molecular level, mutations in the *RHD* gene occur, causing changes in amino acids present in the transmembrane or intracellular region of the RhD protein, thus causing conformational changes in the protein. Mutations for weak D type 1 and 2 are indicated on Figure 7–6. When these changes occur, normal RhD antigen expression is altered. Individuals with weak D phenotype rarely make anti-D, since changes in their RhD protein occur "inside" the red cell. Mutations in the *RHD* gene causing this altered expression have been categorized into types 1 through 53 and counting. Type 1 through 3 are the most common mutations found in individuals of European ancestory.[25]

Partial D

The third mechanism in which D antigen expression can be weakened is when one or more D epitopes within the entire D protein is either missing or altered, termed *partial D*.[32] Some individuals have red cells with **partial-D** antigen that may type weaker than expected or that may not react at all when routine procedures are used with most commercial anti-D reagents. Others have partial-D types that may show normal typing with reagent anti-D.

In the early 1950s, several reports[33,34] described individuals who were typed D-positive but who produced an anti-D that reacted with all D-positive samples except their own. The formation of alloanti-D by D-positive individuals required explanation.

Wiener and Unger[35] postulated that the D antigen is made of antigenic subparts, genetically determined, that could be absent in rare instances. If an individual lacked one (or more) pieces, or epitopes, of the total D antigen, alloantibody can be made to the missing epitope(s) if exposed to RBCs that possess the complete D antigen. This theory has become well accepted.

Tippett and Sanger[36] worked with RBCs and sera of partial-D individuals to classify these antigens. Their work was based on testing anti-D sera from D-positive people, with RBCs from other D-positive people who also made anti-D. This led to a method of categorizing partial D. Seven categories were recognized, designated by Roman numerals I through VII. Category I is now obsolete, and a few of the categories have been further subdivided.

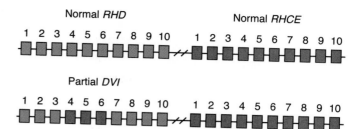

Figure 7–7. One type of partial DVI gene where three exons of *RHCE* gene are inserted into *RHD* gene.

Today, partial-D antigens can be classified on a molecular level and are attributed to hybrid genes resulting from portions of the *RHD* gene being replaced by portions of the *RHCE* gene, as shown in Figure 7–7. The resulting protein contains a portion of RhD and RhCE in various combinations, depending on the hybrid gene's makeup. These protein changes occur external to the red cell membrane. If an individual with a hybrid RhD-RhCe-RhD protein is exposed to red blood cells possessing normal RhD protein, they will make antibody to the portion of the RhD protein they are missing.[37]

Anti-D made by individuals expressing partial D can cause hemolytic disease of the fetus and newborn (HDFN) or transfusion reactions, or both. Once anti-D is identified, Rh-negative blood should be used for transfusion. The identification of a person with a partial-D routinely occurs after the person begins producing anti-D unless there are discrepant Rh (D) typings. This discovery should prompt collection of additional samples to be sent to an immunohematology reference laboratory for further RhD classification.

Advanced Concepts

With the advent of monoclonal antibodies and the depletion and deterioration of the available anti-D made by persons with partial-D phenotypes, Tippett and coworkers[38] pursued the classification of partial-D antigens using monoclonal anti-D (MAb-D). Table 7–9 presents a summary of the partial-D categories known at the time of the study. Today, a commercial monoclonal anti-D panel is available. Although helpful, it does not define all partial D and weak D types clearly. A combination of serologic typing and molecular analysis are often required to accurately categorize partial-D types.

D$_{el}$

D$_{el}$ is a phenotype occurring in individuals whose red blood cells possess an extremely low number of D antigen sites that most reagent anti-D are unable to detect. Adsorbing and eluting anti-D from the individual's red cells is often the only way to detect the D antigen. This procedure requires incubating anti-D with the RBCs in question at 37°C followed by eluting the anti-D off the adsorbed red cells. The 37°C incubation provides time for the anti-D to bind to the few D antigen sites present on these red cells. Molecular studies can detect a mutant *RHD*

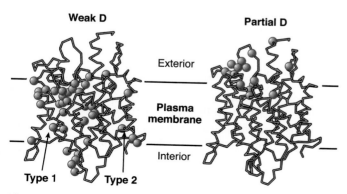

Weak D   **Partial D**

Exterior

Plasma membrane

Interior

Type 1   **Type 2**

Figure 7–6. Three-dimensional illustrations of weak and partial D. From: Chou ST, Westhoff CM. The Rh System. In: Roback JD, Grossman BJ, Harris T, Hillyer CD, eds. *Technical Manual.* 17th edition. AABB, Bethesda, MD, pp. 389–410, 2011.

Table 7–9   Epitope Profiles of Partial D Antigens

	REACTIONS WITH MONOCLONAL ANTI-D ANTIBODIES							
Cells	**epD1**	**epD2**	**epD3**	**epD4**	**epD5**	**epD6/7**	**epD8**	**epD9**
I	+	±	+	0	+	+	+	0
IIIa	+	+	+	+	+	+	+	+
IIIb	+	+	+	+	+	+	+	+
IIIc	+	+	+	+	+	+	+	+
IVa	0	0	0	+	+	+	+	0
IVb	0	0	0	0	+	+	+	0
Va	0	+	+	+	0	+	+	+
VI	0	0	+	+	0	0	0	+
VII	+	+	+	+	+	+	0	+
DFR	±	±	+	+	±	±	0	+
DBT	0	0	0	0	0	±	+	0
R_0Har	0	0	0	0	±	±	0	0

+ = positive reaction; 0 = negative reaction; ± = positive with some antibodies and negative with other antibodies.

gene that alters expression of the RhD protein. This phenotype is relatively common in individuals of Asian ethnicity, occurring in 10% to 30% of that population.[19] It is rare in whites.

D Epitopes on RhCE Protein

Like RhD proteins that can express some RhCE protein, resulting in the partial-D phenotypes, RhCE protein can express RhD epitopes detected by some monoclonal anti-D. This can cause discrepant RhD type results with historical information on a patient or donor. There are rare individuals who possess these unusual proteins and when typed with anti-D will show positive reactivity even though the D epitope is on the RhCE protein. Examples of these unusual phenotypes include D^{HAR} and ceCF (Crawford).

$R_0{}^{Har}$, also known as D^{HAR}, results from a **hybrid gene** RHCE-RHD-RHCE where only a small portion of RHD is inserted into the RHCE gene (Fig. 7–8).[28] If this hybrid gene is paired with a normal RHD gene, the individual will type Rh-positive. However, if paired with a D-deletion, they may type D-positive, depending on the anti-D reagent being used. These individuals should be classified as RhD-negative since they essentially lack the RhD protein.

The Crawford (ceCF) phenotype is found in individuals of African descent. It results from a specific amino acid change in the RHce gene, resulting in an RhD epitope on the Rhce protein.[29]

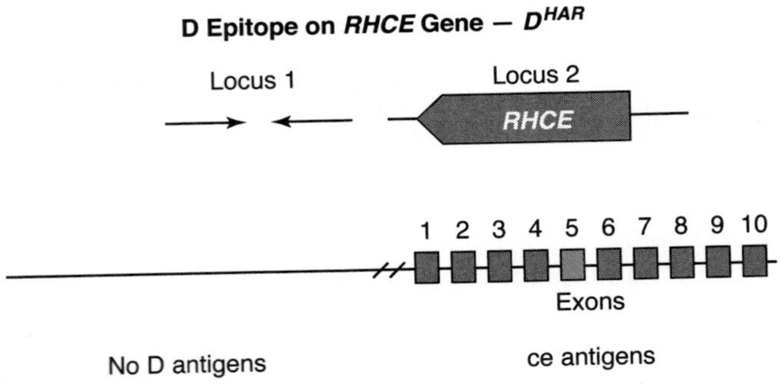

Detection of Rh Antibodies and Antigens

Basic Concepts

Rh antibodies are fairly straightforward to detect and identify as compared to understanding the molecular genetics and biochemistry of the Rh blood group system. Further discussion on detecting antibodies made by individuals to Rh antigens follows.

D Epitope on RHCE Gene — D^{HAR}

Figure 7–8.   D^{HAR} results from one RHD exon inserted into the RHCE gene.

Rh Antibodies

Although the Rh system was first recognized by saline tests used to detect IgM antibodies, most Rh antibodies are IgG immunoglobulins and react optimally at 37°C or after antiglobulin testing in any method used for antibody detection. Rh antibodies are usually produced following exposure of the individual's immune system to foreign RBCs, through either transfusion or pregnancy. Rh antibodies may show dosage, reacting preferentially with RBCs possessing double-dose Rh antigen. For example, anti-E may show 3+ positive reactivity with E+e- RBCs versus 2+ positive reactivity with E+e+ RBCs. In addition, Rh antibodies are enhanced when testing with enzyme-treated RBCs.

Rh antigens are highly immunogenic; the D antigen is the most potent.[39] This is not surprising given that most Rh-negative individuals lack the entire RhD protein, resulting in a difference of 32 to 35 amino acids.[22] Exposure to less than 0.1 mL of Rh-positive RBCs can stimulate antibody production in an Rh-negative person. While the D antigen is most immunogenic, c antigen is the next most likely Rh antigen to elicit an immune response, followed by E, C, and e. It is not uncommon to see several Rh antibodies in a patient; for example, anti-D and anti-C or anti-c and anti-E (see Case Study 7-2 and Figure 7-9).

IgG_1, IgG_2, IgG_3, and IgG_4 subclasses of Rh antibodies have been reported. IgG_1 and IgG_3 are of the greatest clinical significance because the reticuloendothelial system rapidly clears RBCs coated with IgG_1 and IgG_3 from the circulation. IgA Rh antibodies have also been reported but are not routinely tested for in the blood bank.[35]

As with most blood group antibodies, IgM Rh antibodies are formed initially, followed by a transition to IgG. Rh antibodies often persist in the circulation for years. An individual with low-titer Rh antibody may experience an anamnestic (secondary) antibody response if exposed to the same sensitizing antigen. Therefore, in the clinical setting, accuracy of D typing is essential, as is the careful checking of patient history to determine whether an Rh antibody has been identified previously. Most commonly found Rh antibodies are considered clinically significant. Therefore, antigen-negative blood must be provided to any patient with a history of Rh-antibody sensitization, whether the antibody is currently demonstrable or not.

Rh antibodies do not bind **complement**. For complement to be fixed (or the complement cascade activated), two IgG immunoglobulins must attach to an RBC antigen in close proximity to each other. Rh antigens (to which the antibody would attach) are not situated on the RBC surface this closely. Therefore, when an Rh antibody coats the RBCs, intravascular, complement-mediated hemolysis does not occur. RBC destruction resulting from Rh antibodies is primarily extravascular. However, a few rare examples of complement binding Rh antibodies have been reported.

Because Rh antibodies are primarily IgG and can traverse the placenta and because Rh antigens are well developed early in fetal life, Rh antibodies formed by Rh-negative pregnant women cross the placenta and may coat fetal RBCs that carry the corresponding antigen. This results in the fetal cells having a positive **direct antiglobulin test**; in HDFN, the coated fetal cells are removed prematurely from the fetal circulation (see Chapter 19, "Hemolytic Disease of the Fetus and Newborn [HDFN]"). Until the discovery of Rh immune globulin, anti-D was the most frequent cause of HDFN.

D　>　c　>　E　>　C　>　e

Figure 7–9.　Immunogenicity of common Rh antigens.

Rh Typing Reagents

Reagents used to type for D and for the other Rh antigens may be derived from a variety of sources. The reagents may be high-protein-based or low-protein-based, saline-based, chemically modified, monoclonal, or blends of monoclonals. The goal is to use a reagent anti-D that will allow for typing individuals' RBCs as quickly and accurately as typing for ABO.

Saline reactive reagents, which contain IgM immunoglobulin, were the first typing reagents available to test for the D antigen. **Saline anti-D** has the advantage of being low-protein-based and can be used to test cells that are already coated with IgG antibody, as in patients who have warm autoantibodies binding to their RBCs. If a high-protein-based reagent was used when typing these antibody-coated RBCs, a false-positive reaction would be obtained because the RBCs would agglutinate on their own without the addition of anti-D. The primary disadvantages of saline typing reagents are their limited availability, cost of production, and lengthy incubation time. Because saline anti-D is an IgM immunoglobulin, it cannot be used for weak-D typing.

In the 1940s, **high-protein anti-D** reagents were developed that consisted primarily of IgG anti-D. Human plasma containing high-titer D-specific antibody was used as the raw material. Potentiators of bovine albumin and macromolecular additives such as dextran or polyvinylpyrrolidone were added to the source material to optimize reactivity in the standard slide and rapid tube tests to allow for direct agglutination of red cells using an IgG anti-D.[40] In essence, this media causes RBCs to be in closer proximity to each other and allows IgG anti-D to crosslink and cause direct agglutination. These reagents are commonly referred to as high-protein reagents.

However, the presence of potentiators and the higher protein concentration increase the likelihood of false-positive reactions. To assess the validity of the high-protein Rh typing results, a control reagent was manufactured and had to be tested in parallel with each Rh test. If the control reacted, the test result was invalid and had to be repeated using a different technique or reagent anti-D. The major advantages of high-protein anti-D reagents are reduced incubation time and the ability to perform weak-D testing and slide typing with the same reagent. This type of anti-D reagent is also polyspecific. More than one clone of anti-D is produced by immunized human donors and is therefore able to recognize multiple epitopes on the RhD protein.

In the late 1970s, scientists chemically modified the IgG anti-D molecule by breaking the disulfide bonds that maintain the antibody's rigid shape.[41] This allows the antibody to relax and to span the distance between RBCs in a low-protein medium. The chemically modified reagents can be used for both slide and tube testing and do not require a separate, manufactured Rh control as long as the samples type as A, B, or O. When samples test AB Rh-positive or when the Rh test is performed by itself, a separate saline control or 6% to 8% albumin control must be used to ensure the observed reactions are true agglutination and not a result of spontaneous agglutination. Fewer false-positive test reactions are obtained because of the lower-protein suspending medium. Because of its lower-protein base and ready availability, the chemically modified anti-D replaced the need for saline (IgM) anti-D reagents.

As monoclonal antibody production became available, Rh monoclonal antibodies were produced. These reagents are derived from single clones of antibody-producing cells. The antibody-producing cells are hybridized with myeloma cells to increase their reproduction rate, thereby maximizing their antibody-producing capabilities. Because the D antigen is composed of many epitopes and the monoclonal Rh antibodies have a narrow specificity, monoclonal anti-D reagents are usually a combination of monoclonal anti-D reagents from several different clones to ensure reactivity with a broad spectrum of Rh-positive RBCs. Some companies also blend IgM and IgG anti-D to maximize visualization of reactions at immediate spin testing and to allow indirect antiglobulin testing for weak D antigen with the same reagent.[42] Monoclonal blends can be used for slide, tube, microwell, and most automated Rh testing. Because these reagents are not human-derived, they lack all potential for transmitting infectious disease.

As with all commercial typing reagents, Rh antigen typing must be performed with strict adherence to manufacturer's directions, use of proper controls, and accurate interpretation of test and control results. Table 7–10 summarizes several common causes of false Rh typing results and suggests corrective actions that may be taken to obtain an accurate Rh type.

Clinical Considerations

Determining an individual's RhD type and testing to identify antibodies to Rh antigens has been reviewed. When Rh antibodies are identified it is important to understand the clinical implications when Rh incompatibility exists.

Transfusion Reactions

Rh antigens are highly immunogenic. The D antigen is the most immunogenic antigen outside the ABO system. When anti-D is detected, a careful medical history will reveal RBC exposure through pregnancy or transfusion of products containing RBCs. Circulating antibody appears within 120 days of a primary exposure and within 2 to 7 days after a secondary exposure.

Rh-mediated hemolytic transfusion reactions, whether caused by primary sensitization or secondary immunization, usually result in extravascular destruction of immunoglobulin-coated RBCs. The transfusion recipient may have an unexplained fever, a mild bilirubin elevation, and a decrease in hemoglobin and haptoglobin. The direct antiglobulin test

Table 7–10   False Reactions With Rh Typing Reagents

FALSE-POSITIVES		FALSE-NEGATIVES	
Likely Cause	Corrective Action	Likely Cause	Corrective Action
1. Cell suspension too heavy	1. Adjust suspension, retype	1. Immunoglobulin-coated cells (in vivo)	1. Use saline-active typing reagent
2. Cold agglutinins	2. Wash with warm saline, retype	2. Saline-suspended cells (slide)	2. Use unwashed cells
3. Test incubated too long or drying (slide)	3. Follow manufacturer's instructions precisely	3. Failure to follow manufacturer's directions precisely	3. Review directions; repeat test
4. Rouleaux	4. Use saline-washed cells, retype	4. Omission of reagent manufacturer's directions	4. Always add reagent first and check before adding cells
5. Fibrin interference	5. Use saline-washed cells, retype	5. Resuspension too vigorous	5. Resuspend all tube tests gently
6. Contaminating low-incidence antibody in reagent	6. Try another manufacturer's reagent or use a known serum antibody	6. Incorrect reagent selected	6. Read vial label carefully; repeat
7. Polyagglutination	7. See chapter on polyagglutination	7. Variant antigen	7. Refer sample for further investigation
8. Bacterial contamination of reagent vial	8. Open new vial of reagent, retype	8. Reagent deterioration	8. Open new vial
9. Incorrect reagent selected	9. Repeat test; read vial label carefully		
10. Centrifugation too long	10. Repeat test using shorter centrifugation time	10. Centrifugation too short	10. Repeat test using longer centrifugation time
11. rpm too high	11. Repeat test using lower rpm	11. rpm too low	11. Repeat testing using higher rpm

is usually positive, and the antibody screen may or may not demonstrate circulating antibody. When the direct antiglobulin test indicates that the recipient's RBCs are coated with IgG, elution studies may be helpful in defining the offending antibody specificity. If antibody is detected in either the serum or eluate, subsequent transfusions should lack the implicated antigen. It is not unusual for a person with a single Rh antibody to produce additional Rh antibodies if further stimulated.[39]

Hemolytic Disease of the Fetus and Newborn

Hemolytic disease of the fetus and newborn (HDFN) is briefly described here because of the historic significance of the discovery of the Rh system in elucidating its cause; it is covered in more detail in Chapter 19. As stated previously, anti-D was discovered in a woman after delivery of a stillborn fetus. The mother required transfusion. The baby's father donated blood for the transfusion, and the mother subsequently experienced a severe hemolytic transfusion reaction. Levine and Stetson[1] postulated that the antibody causing the transfusion reaction also crossed the placenta and destroyed the RBCs of the fetus, causing its death. The offending antibody was subsequently identified as anti-D.[3]

HDFN caused by Rh antibodies is often severe because the Rh antigens are well developed on fetal cells, and Rh antibodies are primarily IgG, which readily cross the placenta.

After years of research, a method was developed to prevent susceptible (D-negative) mothers from forming anti-D, thus preventing RhD HDFN. Rh-immune globulin, a purified preparation of IgG anti-D, is given to D-negative woman during pregnancy and following delivery of a D-positive fetus.[43] Rh-immune globulin is effective only in preventing RhD HDFN. No effort has been made to develop immune globulin products for other Rh antigens (e.g., C, c, E, e). When present, Rh HDFN may be severe and may require aggressive treatment. Refer to Chapter 19 for a more detailed discussion of HDFN—its etiology, serology, and treatment.

Rh Deficiency Syndrome: Rh$_{null}$ and Rh$_{mod}$

Rare individuals have Rh deficiency or Rh$_{null}$ syndrome and fail to express any Rh antigens on the RBC surface. This syndrome is inherited in one of two ways—amorphic and regulator. Other rare individuals exhibit a severely reduced expression of all Rh antigens, a phenotype called Rh$_{mod}$.

Individuals who lack all Rh antigens on their RBCs are said to have Rh$_{null}$ syndrome, which can be produced by two different genetic mechanisms.[37] In the regulator-type Rh$_{null}$ syndrome, a mutation occurs in the *RHAG* gene. This results in no RhAG protein expression and subsequently no RhD or RhCE protein expression on the RBCs, even though these individuals usually have a normal complement of *RHD* and *RHCE* genes. These individuals can pass normal *RHD* and *RHCE* genes to their children.

In the second type of Rh$_{null}$ syndrome (the amorphic type), there is a mutation in each of the *RHCE* genes inherited from each parent and the common deletion of the *RHD* gene found in most D-negative individuals. The *RHAG* gene is normal.

It should be noted that Rh$_{null}$ individuals of either regulator or amorphic type are negative for the **high prevalence antigen** LW and for FY5, an antigen in the Duffy blood group system. S, s, and U antigens found on glycophorin B may be depressed.[44]

Individuals with Rh$_{null}$ syndrome demonstrate a mild compensated hemolytic anemia,[45] reticulocytosis, stomatocytosis, a slight-to-moderate decrease in hemoglobin and hematocrit levels, an increase in hemoglobin F, a decrease in serum haptoglobin, and possibly an elevated bilirubin level. The severity of the syndrome is highly variable from individual to individual, even within one family. When transfusion of individuals with Rh$_{null}$ syndrome is necessary, only Rh$_{null}$ blood can be given.

Individuals of the Rh$_{mod}$ phenotype have a partial suppression of *RH* gene expression caused by mutations in the *RHAG* gene. When the resultant RhAG protein is altered, normal Rh antigens are also altered, often causing weakened expression of the normal Rh and LW antigens. Rh$_{mod}$ RBCs exhibit other blood group antigens; however, like Rh$_{null}$, S, s, and U antigen expression may be depressed.[45] Rh$_{mod}$ individuals exhibit features similar to those with the Rh$_{null}$ syndrome; however, clinical symptoms are usually less severe and rarely clinically remarkable.[46]

Unusual Phenotypes and Rare Alleles

Several of the less frequently encountered Rh antigens are described briefly in the following paragraphs. Refer to other textbooks for in-depth discussions.[28,47–49]

C^w

C^w was originally considered an allele at the *C/c* locus.[50] Later studies showed that it can be expressed in combination with both *C* and *c* and in the absence of either allele. It is now known that the relationship between C/c and C^w is only phenotypic and that C^w is antithetical to the high-prevalence antigen MAR.[51] C^w results in a single amino acid change most often found on the *RhCe* protein. C^w is found in about 2% of whites and is very rare in blacks.

Anti-C^w has been identified in individuals without known exposure to foreign RBCs and after transfusion or pregnancy. Anti-C^w may show dosage (i.e., reacting more strongly with cells from individuals who are homozygous for *C^w*). Because of the low prevalence of C^w, C^w antigen–negative blood is readily available.

f (ce)

The f antigen is expressed on the RBC when both *c* and *e* are present on the same haplotype; it has been called a compound antigen.[52] However, f is likely a single entity resulting from conformational changes in the Rhce protein.[53] The antigen f was included in a series of these compound antigens, which were previously referred to as *cis*-products to indicate that the antigens were on the same haplotype. It is now known they are expressed on the Rhce protein. Phenotypically, the following samples appear the same when tested with the five major Rh antisera: D+C+E+c+e+, resulting in the predicted genotypes of *DCE/dce* or *DcE/DCe*. However, when tested with anti-f, only the *DCE/dce* shows positive reactivity, confirming the former genotype.

Anti-f is generally a weakly reactive antibody often found with other antibodies. It has been reported to cause HDFN and transfusion reactions. In case of transfusion, f-negative blood should be provided. Anti-f is not available as a reagent; however c-negative or e-negative blood may be provided since all c-negative or e-negative individuals are f-negative.

rh$_i$ (Ce)

Similar to f, rh$_i$ was considered a compound antigen present when *C* and *e* are on the RhCe protein.[52] A sample with the phenotype D +C +E +c +e + can be either *DcE/DCe* or *DCE/dce*. Anti-rh$_i$ shows positive reactivity only with *DCe/dce* RBCs.

Antigens cE and CE or Rh22 also exist, but antibodies produced to these antigens are not commonly seen.

G

G is an antigen present on most D-positive and all C-positive RBCs. The antigen results from the amino acid serine at position 103 on the RhD, RhCe, and RhCE protein. In antibody identification testing, anti-G reacts as though it were a combination of anti-C plus anti-D because all C-positive and D-positive cells are G+.[54] G was originally described in an rr person who received D+C−E−c+e+ RBCs. Subsequently, the recipient produced an antibody that appeared to be anti-D plus anti-C, which should be impossible because the C antigen was not on the transfused RBCs. Further investigation showed the antibody was directed toward D + G, not anti-C. This also explains situations in which an Rh-negative individual who has received Rh-negative blood will look like they made anti-D. The Rh-negative blood the patient received was C-positive, thus G-positive and the antibody produced is actually anti-G, not anti-D and anti-C.

Anti-G versus anti-D and anti-C is important when evaluating obstetric patients. If the patient has produced anti-G and *not* anti-D, they are considered a candidate for RhIg. Elaborate adsorption and elution studies, usually performed in an immunohematology reference laboratory, are valuable in these situations to discriminate anti-D from anti-C from anti-G.

For transfusion purposes, it is not necessary to discriminate anti-D and anti-C from anti-G, as the patient would receive D-C blood regardless if the antibody is –D, –C or –G.

Rh13, Rh14, Rh15, and Rh16

> ### Advanced Concepts
>
> Rh13, Rh14, Rh15, and Rh16 define four different parts of the D mosaic, as it was originally described.[55] Although these parts are included in the partial-D categories II to VII as defined by Tippett and Sanger,[36] they are not directly comparable. These antigens are now obsolete.

Rh17 (Hr$_0$)

Rh17, also known as Hr$_0$, is an antigen present on all RBCs with the "common" Rh phenotypes (e.g., R$_1$R$_1$, R$_2$R$_2$, rr).[56] In essence, this antibody is directed to the entire protein resulting from the *RHCE* genes. When RBCs phenotype as D−, the most potent antibody they make is often one directed against Rh17 (Hr$_0$).

Rh23, Rh30, and Rh40

Rh23, Rh30, and Rh40 are all low-prevalence antigens associated with a specific category of partial-D. These low-prevalence antigens result from the formation of the hybrid proteins seen in individuals with partial-D phenotypes. Rh23 (also known as Wiel and D^w) is an antigenic marker for category Va partial-D.[57] Rh30 (also known as Go^a or D^{cor}) is a marker for partial DIVa.[58] Rh40 (also known as Tar or Targett) is a marker for partial DVII.[59] Rh52 or BARC is associated with some partial-DVI types.[36]

Rh33 (Har)

The low-prevalence antigen Rh33 is most often found in whites and is associated with the rare variant haplotype called R$_0$^{Har}.[60] R$_0$^{Har} gene codes for normal amounts of c, reduced amounts of e, reduced f, reduced Hr$_0$, and reduced amounts of D antigen written as (D)c(e). The D reactions are frequently so weak that the cells are often typed as Rh-negative. As previously discussed, R$_0$^{Har} or D^{HAR} results from a hybrid gene *RHCE-RHD-RHCE* in which only a small portion of *RHD* is inserted into the *RHCE* gene.

Rh32

Rh:32 is a low-prevalence antigen associated with a variant of the $R^1[D(C)(e)]$ haplotype called $\overline{\overline{R}}^N$.[61] The C antigen and e antigen are expressed weakly. The D antigen expression is exaggerated or exalted. This gene has been found primarily in blacks.

Rh43 (Crawford)

Rh43, also known as the Crawford antigen, is a low-prevalence antigen on a variant Rhce protein.[29] The Crawford (ceCF) antigen is of very low prevalence found in individuals of African descent.

e Variants

Like the variant D antigen seen in individuals possessing a hybrid or mutated *RHD* gene, some individuals of African or mixed ethnic backgrounds possess e antigen that exhibits similar qualities as those described for partial-D phenotypes—that is, an individual may phenotype e-positive but produce antibodies behaving as anti-e.[62] These variant types result from multiple mutations in the *RHCE* gene.[63] Individuals who possess two altered *RHCE* genes may phenotype e-positive but produce antibodies behaving as anti-e.

The Rh antigens hr[B] and hr[S] are rarely considered in routine blood banking. They are normally present in individuals who possess normal RhCe or Rhce protein but are lacking in individuals with normal RhcE or RhCE proteins (i.e., e-negative). Several antigens, most notably hr[B] and hr[S], are lacking on the resulting Rhce proteins encoded by some variant *RHCE* genes. If individuals with these variant genes who are hr[B]-negative or hr[S]-negative are immunized, they may produce anti-hr[B] or anti-hr[S]. In routine antibody identification, these antibodies are generally nonreactive with e-negative red cells (and therefore are also hr[B]-negative and hr[S]-negative), appearing to have anti-e-like specificity.

To further complicate this, the variant *RHCE* gene associated with the hr[B]-negative phenotype is usually found with a variant *RHD-CE-D* hybrid gene. The *RHCE* is inserted in the middle of the *RHDIIIa* gene. The resulting protein lacks D antigen but possesses an unusual form of the C antigen. The hybrid gene occurs in 22% of individuals of African decent.[18,64] This haplotype that includes the *RHDIIIa-RHCE-DIIIa* hybrid gene and variant *RHCE* genes is referred to as r's[(C)ce[s]].

V and VS

V and VS are antigens of low prevalence in the Caucasian population but are more prevalent among African Americans. These antigens can be used as predictors of an individual's ethnic background because of this difference in prevalence.

The V antigen, also historically referred to as ce[S],[65] is found in about 30% of randomly selected African Americans. It is most often found in individuals with Gly263 amino acid change in Rhce; several other mutations also occur in this gene.

The VS antigen, also known as e[S], occurs in 32% in blacks.[66] It results from a single amino acid change that occurs at position Val245 in the Rhce protein. Most hr[B]- individuals with r's genotype are VS+. The Val245 mutation in this haplotype is found in the hybrid *RHDIIIa-RHCE-RHDIIIa* gene described previously.[67] Most V+ individuals are also VS+.

Deletions

There are very uncommon phenotypes that demonstrate no Cc and/or Ee reactivity. Many examples lacking all *Cc* or *Ee* often have an unusually strong D antigen expression, frequently called *exalted D*. The deletion phenotype is indicated by the use of a dash (–), as in the following example: D–. This phenotype results from individuals possessing normal *RHD* gene(s) and hybrid *RHCE-RHD-RHCE* in which the Rhce protein is replaced with RhD. This helps explain the exalted D, as there are extra D antigens recognized on the resulting hybrid protein. The antibody made by D–/D– people is called anti-Rh17 or anti-Hr$_0$.[49]

A variation has been recognized within the deletion D–, called D••. The D antigen in the D•• is stronger than that in DC–, or Dc– samples but weaker than that of D– samples. A low-prevalence antigen called Evans (Rh:37) accompanies the Rh structure of D•• cells.[68]

Some deletion phenotypes are missing E/e only and are indicated as Dc- or DC-. To date, a deletion of only C/c has not been reported.

Transfusion of individuals with a D– or D•• phenotype is difficult, as blood of a similar phenotype or even the rarer Rh$_{null}$ blood, all lacking Rh17, would be required.

Landsteiner Weiner Blood Group System

Basic Concepts

A discussion of the Landsteiner Weiner (LW) antigen begins with the time when Rh antigens were first recognized. The antibody produced by injecting rhesus monkey RBCs into guinea pigs and rabbits was identified as having the same specificity as the antibody Levine and Stetson[1] described earlier. The antibody was given the name anti-Rh, for *anti-rhesus*, and the blood group system was established. Many years later, it was recognized that the two antibodies were not identical; the anti-rhesus described by Landsteiner and Wiener[2] was renamed anti-LW in their honor.

Phenotypically, there is a similarity between the Rh and LW systems. Anti-LW reacts strongly with most D-positive RBCs, weakly with Rh-negative RBCs (and sometimes not at all), and never with Rh$_{null}$ cells. Anti-LW usually shows stronger positive reactivity with D-positive RBCs than with D-negative adult RBCs. A weak anti-LW may be positive only with D-positive RBCs, and enhancement techniques may be required to demonstrate its reactivity with D-negative cells. Anti-LW shows equal reactivity with cord cells regardless of their D type.[69] This is an important characteristic to remember when trying to differentiate anti-LW from anti-D. Also, anti-LW more frequently appears as an autoantibody, which does not present clinical problems. Further discussion can be found in Chapter 8, "Blood Group Terminology and the Other Blood Groups."

Because of the complexity of the Rh blood group system, a tremendous amount of literature exists. The inquisitive reader can continue to piece together the puzzle by consulting the sources included in the references.

CASE STUDIES

Case 7-1

Two units of blood are ordered for an 89-year-old woman with myelodysplastic syndrome. She had been transfused 3 years ago and has six children. Routine pretransfusion testing follows.

Anti-A	Anti-B	Anti-D	A₁ Cells	B Cells	Interpretation
0	0	0	4+	4+	

1. What is the patient's ABO, Rh type?

	Rh						MNS				LU		P	Lewis		Kell		Duffy		Kidd		GEL
	D	C	E	c	E	f	M	N	S	s	Luᵃ	Luᵇ	P₁	Leᵃ	Leᵇ	K	k	Fyᵃ	Fyᵇ	Jkᵃ	Jkᵇ	IAT
1	+	+	0	0	+	0	+	+	+	+	0	+	+	+	0	+	+	+	0	0	+	2+
2	+	0	+	+	0	0	+	0	+	0	0	+	+	0	+	0	+	+	+	+	0	2+

2. How would you interpret the results of the antibody detection test/screen?
3. What information can you obtain from your evaluation of the antibody detection test/screen?
4. What additional testing should be performed?

Gel Antibody Identification Panel

	Rh						MNS				Lu		Pl	Lewis		Kell		Duffy		Kidd		IAT
	D	C	E	c	e	f	M	N	S	s	Luᵃ	Luᵇ	P₁	Leᵃ	Leᵇ	K	k	Fyᵃ	Fyᵇ	Jkᵃ	Jkᵇ	
1	+	+	0	0	+	0	+	+	+	+	0	+	0	+	0	0	+	0	+	0	+	2+
2	0	0	0	+	+	+	+	0	+	0	0	+	+	0	+	+	0	+	+	+	0	0
3	0	0	+	+	0	0	0	+	0	+	0	+	+	0	+	+	+	+	0	0	+	0
4	+	+	0	0	+	0	+	0	+	+	0	+	0	0	0	0	+	+	+	+	+	2+
5	0	0	+	+	+	+	+	+	0	+	0	+	0	0	+	0	+	0	+	0	+	0
6	0	+	0	0	+	0	+	+	0	+	0	+	+	0	+	+	+	+	+	+	+	0
7	+	0	+	+	0	0	0	+	0	+	0	+	0	0	+	0	+	0	+	+	0	2+
8	0	0	0	+	+	+	+	0	+	0	0	+	+	0	+	0	+	+	0	0	+	0
9	+	+	0	+	+	+	+	+	0	+	0	+	+	+	0	0	+	0	+	+	0	2+
10	+	0	+	+	0	0	0	+	+	+	0	+	+	+	0	0	+	+	0	+	0	2+
11	+	0	0	+	+	+	0	+	0	0	0	+	+	0	+	0	+	0	+	+	+	2+
AC																						0

NOTE: In this case study, antibodies are excluded only if the patient's serum does not react with panel cells that possess a double-dose expression of the antigen (from a donor with homozygous expression).

5. What antibody(ies) is(are) present in the patient's plasma?

Case 7-2

A 25-year-old woman, pregnant with her second child, had routine orders for a "type and screen," with the following results:

Anti-A	Anti-B	Anti-D	A₁ Cells	B Cells	Interpretation
0	0	3+	4+	4+	

1. How would you interpret the results of the ABO, Rh type and antibody detection test (screen)?

	Rh						MNS				LU		P	Lewis		Kell		Duffy		Kidd		IS	37C	PEG
	D	C	E	c	E	f	M	N	S	s	Luᵃ	Luᵇ	P₁	Leᵃ	Leᵇ	K	k	Fyᵃ	Fyᵇ	Jkᵃ	Jkᵇ			
1	+	+	0	0	+	0	+	+	+	+	0	+	+	+	0	+	+	+	0	0	+	0	NH	IAT
2	+	0	+	+	0	0	+	0	+	0	0	+	+	0	+	0	+	+	+	+	0	0	NH	3+

NH = No hemolysis observed

An antibody identification panel is set up and results follow.

	Rh						MNS				Lu		Pl	Lewis		Kell		Duffy		Kidd			PEG	
	D	C	E	c	e	f	M	N	S	s	Lua	Lub	P1	Lea	Leb	K	k	Fya	Fyb	Jka	Jkb	IS	37C	IAT
1	+	+	0	0	+	0	+	+	+	+	0	+	0	+	0	0	+	0	+	0	+	0	NH	0
2	0	0	0	+	+	+	+	0	+	0	0	+	+	0	+	+	0	+	+	+	0	0	NH	0
3	0	0	+	+	0	0	0	+	0	+	0	+	+	0	+	+	0	+	+	+	0	0	NH	3+
4	+	+	0	0	+	0	+	0	+	0	0	+	+	0	+	+	0	+	0	0	+	0	NH	3+
5	0	0	+	+	+	+	+	+	0	+	0	+	0	0	0	0	+	+	+	+	+	0	NH	0
6	0	+	0	0	+	0	0	+	0	+	0	+	0	0	+	0	+	0	+	0	+	0	NH	3+
7	+	0	+	+	0	0	0	+	0	+	0	+	0	0	+	+	+	+	0	+	0	0	NH	0
8	0	0	0	+	+	+	+	0	+	0	0	+	+	0	+	0	+	+	0	0	+	0	NH	3+
9	+	+	0	+	+	+	+	+	0	+	0	+	+	+	0	0	+	0	+	+	0	0	NH	3+
10	+	0	+	+	0	0	0	+	+	+	0	+	+	+	0	0	+	+	0	+	0	0	NH	3+
11	+	0	0	+	+	+	0	+	0	0	0	+	+	+	0	0	+	+	0	+	0	0	NH	3+
AC											+	0	+	+	0	0	+	0	0	+	+	0	NH	0

NOTE: In this case study, antibodies are excluded only if the patient's serum does not react with panel cells that possess a double-dose expression of the antigen (from a donor with homozygous expression).

2. What antibody(ies) cannot be ruled out based on the panel results?
3. What additional testing should be performed?

The patient was phenotyped for the following antigens:

	Anti-C	Anti-E	Anti-c	Anti-e	Anti-K
Patient	4+	0	0	4+	4+

4. Using Fisher-Race and Weiner nomenclature, what are the possible Rh phenotypes?
5. Using Fisher-Race and Weiner nomenclature, what is the most probable genotype?
6. Does the patient's antigen type confirm or conflict with your antibody identification?
7. Which Rh antibodies are difficult to rule out on a double-dose (homozygous) antigen-positive cell in this case? Explain why.

Case 7-3 (Advanced)

A 29-year-old female, pregnant for the first time, presented to her OB physician in her early first trimester for initial prenatal care. She had no known prior transfusions.

Forward			Reverse		
Anti-A	Anti-B	Anti-D	A1	B	Interpretation
4+	0	0	0	4+	

1. What is the patient's ABO, Rh type?

	Rh						MNS				LU		P	Lewis		Kell		Duffy		Kidd		GEL
	D	C	E	c	E	F	M	N	S	s	Lua	Lub	P1	Lea	Leb	K	k	Fya	Fyb	Jka	Jkb	IAT
1	+	+	0	0	+	0	+	+	+	+	0	+	+	+	0	+	+	+	0	0	+	0
2	+	0	+	+	0	0	+	0	+	0	0	+	+	0	+	0	+	+	+	+	0	0

Approximately 1 month later, the Transfusion Service received a call from the OB physician, stating the patient had been previously typed as "A-positive" at another facility and her donor card states "A-positive." A sample is sent to the laboratory for repeat ABO, Rh typing.

The patient's repeat ABO, Rh type showed the same results: A Rh-negative. Because of the reported discrepancy, the patient's Rh (D) typing was performed using several different anti-D reagents.

Results with various anti-D reagents are as follows:

Anti-D Reagent	IS	IAT	Control IAT
G-clone (monoclonal)	0	4+	0
O-clone (monoclonal)	0	3+	0
Gel IgG (polyspecific—human)		0	0
Polyspecific—human	0	3+	0

Typing with different anti-D reagents showed variability. All required a weak D test or indirect antiglobulin test to detect the weakened D antigen.

The Rh typing was reported as follows: A-negative—for transfusion purposes and candidacy for RhIG at the testing facility, patient is considered "Rh(D)-negative" (patient to receive Rh[D]-negative blood products and RhIG prophylaxis recommended).

Further testing was performed to determine if the patient possessed a partial-D antigen. The Rh phenotype results follow:

	Anti-C	Anti-E	Anti-c	Anti-e
Patient	3+	0	4+	4+
Positive control	4+	4+	4+	4+
Negative control	0	0	0	0

2. Using Fisher-Race and Weiner nomenclature, what are the possible Rh phenotypes?
3. Using Fisher-Race and Weiner nomenclature, what is the most probable genotype?

The sample was sent to an immunohematology reference laboratory for further characterization. A commercial monoclonal anti-D panel was available for testing to aid in differentiating weak D from partial D. The patient's RBCs were typed with this kit.

Anti-D Cell Line	Weak D type 1 and 2	DII and DNU	DIII	DIV	DV	DCS	DVI	DVII	DOL	DFR	DMH	DAR	DAR-E	DHK and DAU-4	DBT	Ro^Har	POS Cont	Neg Cont	Pt
LHM 76/58	+	+	+	+	+/0	+	0	+	+	+	+	+	0	0	0	(+)/0	4	0	0
LHM 76/59	+	+	+	0	+	+	+	+	+	+	+	+	+	+	0	0	4	0	3+
LHM 174/102	(+)/0	+	+	0	0	+	0	+	0	0	+	0	0	0	0	0	4	0	0
LHM 50/28	+	+	+	+	+	+	0	+	+	+	+	+	+	0	0	4	0	0
LHM 169/81	+	+	+	0	0	+	0	+	+	+	+	0	0	0	0	0	4	0	0
ESDI	+	+	+	0	+	+	+	+	+	+	+	+	+	0	0	4	0	4+
LHM 76/55	+	+	+	0	+	+	+	+	+	+	+	+	+	0	0	4	0	3+
LHM 77/64	+	0	+	0	+	+	+	+	+	+	+	+	+	+/0	0	0	4	0	3+
LHM 70/45	(+)/0	+	+	0	0	0	0	+	0	0	0	0	0	0	0	0	4	0	0
LHM 59/19	+	+	+	+	+	+	0	0	0	0	0	0	(+)	+	+	0	4	0	0
LHM 169/80	+	+	+	+	+	+	0	+	+	+	+	+	+	0	0	0	4	0	0
LHM 57/17	+	+	+	+	+	0	0	+	+	0	+	+	+	0	+	0	4	0	0

The results are consistent with a partial DVI. Discrepancies in RhD typing are dependent on reagents and methods used to detect RhD antigen.

SUMMARY CHART

- ✔ The Rh antibody was so named on the basis of antibody production by guinea pigs and rabbits when transfused with rhesus monkey RBCs.
- ✔ Historically, Rh was a primary cause of HDFN, erythroblastosis fetalis, and a significant cause of hemolytic transfusion reactions.
- ✔ Fisher-Race DCE terminology is based on the theory that antigens of the system are produced by three closely linked sets of alleles and that each gene is responsible for producing a product (or antigen) on the RBC surface.
- ✔ A person who expresses no Rh antigens on the RBC is said to be Rh_{null}, and the phenotype may be written as ——/——.
- ✔ In the Wiener Rh-Hr nomenclature, it is postulated that the gene responsible for defining Rh actually produces an agglutinogen that contains a series of blood factors in which each factor is an antigen recognized by an antibody.
- ✔ It is currently accepted that two closely linked genes control the expression of Rh; one gene (*RHD*) codes for the presence of RhD, and a second gene (*RHCE*) codes for the expression of CcEe antigens.
- ✔ In the Rosenfield alpha/numeric terminology, a number is assigned to each antigen of the Rh system in order of its discovery (Rh1 = D, Rh2 = C, Rh3 = E, Rh4 = c, Rh5 = e).
- ✔ Rh antigens are characterized as nonglycosylated proteins in the RBC membrane.
- ✔ The most common phenotype in whites is R_1r (31%); the most common phenotype in blacks is R_0r (23%), followed by R_0R_0 at 19%.
- ✔ The Rh antigens are inherited as codominant alleles.
- ✔ A partial-D individual is characterized as lacking one or more pieces or epitopes of the total D antigen and may produce alloantibody to the missing fraction if exposed to RBCs with the complete D antigen.
- ✔ Blood donor units for transfusion are considered Rh-positive if either the D or weak-D test is positive; if both the D and weak-D tests are negative, blood for transfusion is considered Rh-negative.
- ✔ Most Rh antibodies are IgG immunoglobulin and react optimally at 37°C or following antiglobulin testing; exposure to less than 0.1 mL of Rh-positive RBCs can stimulate antibody production in an Rh-negative person.
- ✔ Rh-mediated hemolytic transfusion reactions usually result in extravascular hemolysis.
- ✔ Rh antibodies are IgG and can cross the placenta to coat fetal (Rh-positive) RBCs.

Review Questions

1. The Rh system was first recognized in a case report of:
   a. A hemolytic transfusion reaction.
   b. Hemolytic disease of the fetus and newborn.
   c. Circulatory overload.
   d. Autoimmune hemolytic anemia.

2. What antigen is found in 85% of the white population and is always significant for transfusion purposes?
   a. d
   b. c
   c. D
   d. E

3. How are weaker-than-expected reactions with anti-D typing reagents categorized?
   a. Rh_{mod}
   b. Weak D
   c. DAT positive
   d. D^w

4. Cells carrying a weak-D antigen require the use of what test to demonstrate its presence?
   a. Indirect antiglobulin test
   b. Direct antiglobulin test
   c. Microplate test
   d. Warm autoadsorption test

5. How are Rh antigens inherited?
   a. Autosomal recessive alleles
   b. Sex-linked genes
   c. Codominant alleles
   d. X-linked

6. Biochemically speaking, what type of molecules are Rh antigens?
   a. Glycophorins
   b. Simple sugars
   c. Proteins
   d. Lipids

7. Rh antibodies react best at what temperature (°C)?
   a. 22
   b. 18
   c. 15
   d. 37

8. Rh antibodies are primarily of which immunoglobulin class?
   a. IgA
   b. IgM
   c. IgG
   d. IgD

9. Rh antibodies have been associated with which of the following clinical conditions?
   a. Erythroblastosis fetalis
   b. Thrombocytopenia
   c. Hemophilia A
   d. Stomatocytosis

10. What do Rh_{null} cells lack?
    a. Lewis antigens
    b. Normal oxygen-carrying capacity
    c. Rh antigens
    d. MNSs antigens

11. What antigen system is closely associated phenotypically with Rh?
    a. McCoy
    b. Lutheran
    c. Duffy
    d. LW

12. Anti-LW will not react with which of the following?
    a. Rh-positive RBCs
    b. Rh-negative RBCs
    c. Rh_{null} RBCs
    d. Rh:33 RBCs

13. Convert the following genotypes from Wiener nomenclature to Fisher-Race and Rosenfield nomenclatures, and list the antigens present in each haplotype.
    a. R_1r
    b. R_2R_0
    c. R_zR_1
    d. r^yr

14. Which Rh phenotype has the strongest expression of D?
    a. R_1r
    b. R_1R_1
    c. R_2R_2
    d. D–

15. Which of the following most commonly causes an individual to type RhD positive yet possess anti-D?
    a. Genetic weak D
    b. Partial D
    c. C in *trans* to *RHD*
    d. D epitopes on RhCE protein

16. An individual has the following Rh phenotype: D+C+E+c+e+. Using Fisher-Race terminology, what is their most likely Rh genotype?
    a. DCE/Dce
    b. DCE/dce
    c. DCe/dcE
    d. DCe/DcE

17. Which of the following is the most common Rh phenotype in African Americans?
    a. Dce/dce
    b. DcE/dce
    c. DCe/dce
    d. Dce/dCe

References

1. Levine, P, and Stetson, RE: An unusual case of intragroup agglutination. JAMA 113:126, 1939.
2. Landsteiner, K, and Wiener, AS: An agglutinable factor in human blood recognized by immune sera for rhesus blood. Proc Soc Exp Biol (NY) 43:223, 1940.
3. Levine, P, et al: The role of isoimmunization in the pathogenesis of erythroblastosis fetalis. Am J Obstet Gynecol 42:925, 1941.
4. Race, RR, et al: Recognition of a further common Rh genotype in man. Nature 153:52, 1944.
5. Mourant, AE: A new rhesus antibody. Nature 155:542, 1945.
6. Stratton, F: A new Rh allelomorph. Nature 158:25, 1946.
7. Levine, P: On Hr factor and Rh genetic theory. Science 102:1, 1945.
8. Race, RR: The Rh genotypes and Fisher's theory. Blood 3 (Suppl 2):27, 1948.
9. Wiener, AS: Genetic theory of the Rh blood types. Proc Soc Exp Biol (NY) 54:316, 1943.
10. Rosenfield, RE, et al: A review of Rh serology and presentation of a new terminology. Transfusion 2:287, 1962.
11. Lewis, M: Blood group terminology 1990. Vox Sang 58:152, 1990.
12. Tippett, PA: A speculative model for the Rh blood groups. Ann Hum Genet 50:241, 1986.
13. Cherif-Zahar, B, Bloy, C, Le Van Kim, C, et al: Molecular cloning and protein structure of a human blood group Rh polypeptide. Proc Natl Acad Sci USA Aug;87(16):6243–6247, 1990.
14. Le van Kim, C, Mouro, I, Cherif-Zahar, B, et al: Molecular cloning and primary structure of human blood group RhD polypeptide. Proc Natl Acad Sci USA Nov 15;89(22):10925–10929,1992.
15. Arce, MA, Thompson, ES, Wagner, S, et al: Molecular cloning of RhD cDNA derived from a gene present in RhD-positive, but not RhD-negative individuals. Blood Jul 15;82(2):651–655, 1993.
16. Ridgewell, K, Spurr, NK, Laguda, B, et al: Isolation of cDNA clones for a 50 kDa glycoprotein of the human erythrocyte membrane associated with Rh (rhesus) blood group antigen expression. Biochem J 287:223–228, 1992.
17. Colin, Y, Cherif-Zahar, B, Le Van Kim, C, et al: Genetic basis of the RhD-positive and RhD-negative blood group polymorphism as determined by Southern analysis. Blood 78:2747–2752, 1991.
18. Singleton, BK, Green, CA, Avent, ND, et al: The presence of an RHD pseudogene containing a 37 base pair duplication and nonsense mutation in Africans with the RhD-negative blood group phenotype. Blood 95(1):12–18, 2000.
19. Shao, CP, Maas, JH, Su, YQ, et al: Molecular background of Rh D-positive, D-negative, D (el) and weak D phenotypes in Chinese. Vox Sang 83:156–161, 2002.
20. Blumenfeld, OO, and Patnaik, SK: Allelic genes of blood group antigens: A source of human mutations and cSNPs documented in the Blood Group Antigen Gene Mutation Database. Hum Mutat Jan;23(1):8–16, 2004.
21. Avent, ND, Butcher, SK, Liu, W et al: Localization of the C termini of the Rh (rhesus) polypeptides to the cytoplasmic face of the human erythrocyte membrane. J Biol Chem 267:15134–15139, 1992.
22. Avent, ND, Liu, W, Warner, KM, et al: Immunochemical analysis of the human erythrocyte Rh polypeptides. J Biol Chem 271:14233–14239, 1996.
23. Hughes-Jones, NC, Gardner, B, and Lincoln, PJ: Observations of the number of available c, D, and E antigen sites on red cells. Vox Sang 21:210, 1971.
24. Westhoff, CM, and Wylie, DE: Transport characteristics of mammalian Rh and Rh glycoproteins expressed in heterologous systems. Transfus Clin Biol 13:132–138, 2006.

25. Roback, JD, Combs, MR, Grossman, B, and Hillyer, C (eds): Technical Manual, 16th ed. AABB, Bethesda, MD, 2008.
26. Race, RR, Sanger, R, and Lawler, SD: The Rh antigen Du. Ann Eugen Lond 14:171, 1948.
27. Westhoff, CM: Rh complexities: Serology and DNA typing. Transfusion 47:17S–22S, 2007.
28. Beckers, EA, Faas, BH, von dem Borne, AE, et al: The R0Har RH:33 phenotype results from substitution of exon 5 of the RHCE gene by the corresponding exon of the RHD gene. Br J Haematol Mar 92(3):751–757, 1996.
29. Flegel, WA, Wagner, FF, Chen, Q, et al: The RHCE allele ceCF: The molecular basis of Crawford (RH43). Transfusion 46(8):1334–1342, 2006.
30. Ceppellini, R, Dunn, LC, and Turri, M: An interaction between alleles at the Rh locus in man which weakens the reactivity of the Rh_0 factor (D_0). Proc Natl Acad Sci 41:283, 1955.
31. Wagner, FF, Gassner, C, Muller, TH, et al: Molecular basis of weak D phenotypes. Blood 93:385–393, 1999.
32. Tippett, P, Lomas-Francis, C, and Wallace, M: The Rh antigen D: Partial D antigens and associated low incidence antigens. Vox Sang 70:123–131, 1996.
33. Shapiro, M: The ABO, MN, P and Rh blood group systems in South African Bantu: A genetic study. South Afr Med J 25:187, 1951.
34. Argall, CI, Ball, JM, and Trentelman, E: Presence of anti-D antibody in the serum of Du patient. J Clin Lab Med 41:895, 1953.
35. Wiener, AS, and Unger, LJ: Rh factors related to the Rh_0 factor as a source of clinical problems. JAMA 169:696, 1959.
36. Tippett, P, and Sanger, R: Observations on subdivisions of the Rh antigen D. Vox Sang 7:9, 1962.
37. Huang, CH, Liu, P, and Cheng, JG: Molecular biology and genetics of the Rh blood group system. Semin Hematol 37:150–165, 2000.
38. Tippett, P, Lomas-Francis, C, and Wallace, M. The Rh antigen D: Partial D antigens and associated low incidence antigens. Vox Sang 70:123–131, 1996.
39. Mollison, PL: Blood Transfusion in Clinical Medicine, 6th ed. Blackwell Scientific Publications, Oxford, 1988.
40. Diamond, LK, and Denton, RC: Rh agglutination in various media with particular reference to the value of albumin. J Clin Lab Med 30:821, 1945.
41. Romans, DG, et al: Conversion of incomplete antibodies to direct agglutinins by mild reduction. Proc Natl Acad Sci USA 74:2531, 1977.
42. Denomme, GA, Dake, LR, Vilensky, D, Ramyar, L, and Judd, WJ: Rh discrepancies caused by variable reactivity of partial and weak D types with different serologic techniques. Transfusion 48(3):473–478, 2008.
43. Queenan, JT: Modern Management of the Rh Problem, 2nd ed. Harper & Row, New York, 1977.
44. Schmidt, PJ, et al: Aberrant U blood group accompany Rh_{null}. Transfusion 7:33, 1967.
45. Schmidt, PJ, and Vos, GH: Multiple phenotypic abnormalities associated with Rh_{null} (—/—). Vox Sang 13:18, 1967.
46. Chown, B, et al: An unlinked modifier of Rh blood groups: Effects when heterozygous and when homozygous. Am J Hum Genet 24:623, 1972.
47. Daniels, G: Human Blood Groups, 2nd ed. Blackwell Scientific, Oxford, 2002.
48. Reid, MR, and Lomas-Francis, C. The Blood Group Antigen Facts Book, 2nd ed. Elsevier, San Diego, 2004.
49. Issitt, PD, and Anstee, DJ: Applied Blood Group Serology, 4th ed. Montgomery Scientific Publications, Durham, NC, 1998.
50. Callendar, ST, and Race, RR: A serological and genetic study of multiple antibodies formed in response to blood transfusion by a patient with lupus erythematosus diffuses. Ann Eugen Lond 13:102, 1946.
51. Sistonen, P, et al: MAR, a novel high-incidence Rh antigen revealing the existence of an allele sub-system including C^w (Rh8) and C^x (Rh9) with exceptional distribution in the Finnish population. Vox Sang 66:287–292, 1994.
52. Rosenfield, RE, and Haber, GV: An Rh blood factor, Rh1 (Ce) and its relationship to hr (ce). Am J Hum Genet 10:474, 1958.
53. Chen, YX, Peng, J, Novaretti, M, Reid, ME, and Huang, CH: Deletion of arginine codon 229 in the Rhce gene alters e and f but not c antigen expression. Transfusion Mar;44(3):391–398, 2004.
54. Allen, FH, and Tippett, PA: A new Rh blood type which reveals the Rh antigen G. Vox Sang 3:321, 1958.
55. Wiener, AS, and Unger, LJ: Further observations on the blood factors RhA, RhB, RhC, RhD. Transfusion 2:230, 1962.
56. Allen, FH, Jr, and Corcoran, PA: Proc 11th Ann Mtg. AABB, Cincinnati, Abstract, 1958.
57. Chown, B, et al: The Rh antigen Dw (Wiel). Transfusion 4:169, 1964.
58. Lewis, M, et al: Blood group antigen Goa and the Rh system. Transfusion 7:440, 1967.
59. Lewis, M, et al: Assignment of the red cell antigen Targett (Rh 40) to the Rh blood group systems. Am J Hum Genet 31:630, 1979.
60. Giles, CM, et al: An Rh gene complex which results in a "new" antigen detectable by a specific antibody, anti-Rh 33. Vox Sang 21:289, 1971.
61. Rosenfield, RE, et al: Problems in Rh typing as revealed by a single Negro family. Am J Hum Genet 12:147, 1960.
62. Issitt, PD: Applied Blood Group Serology, 3rd ed. Montgomery Scientific Publication, Miami, FL, 1985.
63. Vege, S, and Westhoff, CM. Molecular characterization of GYPB and RH in donors in the American Rare Donor Program. Immunohematology 22:143–147, 2006.
64. Huang, CH, Chen, Y, and Reid, M: Human D(IIIa) erythrocytes: RhD protein is associated with multiple dispersed amino acid variations. Am J Hematol. Jul;55(3):139–145, 1997.
65. DeNatale, A, et al: A "new" Rh antigen, common in Negroes, rare in white people. JAMA 159:247, 1955.
66. Sanger, R, et al: An Rh antibody specific for V and Rs. Nature (Lond) 186:171, 1960.
67. Daniels, GL, Faas, BH, Green, CA, et al: The VS and V blood group polymorphisms in Africans: A serologic and molecular analysis. Transfusion 38:951–958, 1998.
68. Contreras, M, et al: The Rh antigen Evans. Vox Sang 34:208, 1978.
69. Race, RR, and Sanger, R: Blood Groups in Man, 6th ed. Blackwell Scientific, Oxford, 1975.

Blood Group Terminology and the Other Blood Groups

Regina M. Leger, MSQA, MT(ASCP)SBB, CMQ/OE(ASQ)

OBJECTIVES

Blood Group Terminology

1. Describe how antigens, antibodies, genes, and phenotypes are correctly written.
2. List the four categories for classification of RBC surface blood group antigens used by the ISBT.
3. For each of the blood group systems described in this chapter:
   - List the major antigens and common phenotypes
   - Describe the serologic characteristics and clinical significance of the antibodies
   - Identify null phenotypes

Antigen Characteristics

4. Describe the formation of Lewis antigens and their adsorption onto RBCs.
5. Define the interaction of Lewis genes with ABO, H, and secretor genes.
6. List substances present in secretions and the Lewis phenotypes based on a given genotype.
7. Describe the reciprocal relationship of I antigen to i antigen.
8. List the antigen frequencies for the common antigens K, M, S, s, Fy^a, Fy^b, Jk^a, Jk^b, and P1.
9. Define Kp^a, Js^a, and Lu^a as low-prevalence antigens and Kp^b, Js^b, Lu^b, and I as high-prevalence antigens.
10. Define the association of M and N with glycophorin A (GPA) and S and s with glycophorin B (GPB).
11. Describe the antigen phenotypes S–s–U–, Js(a+), and Fy(a–b–) associated with blacks.
12. Define the null phenotypes M^k, p, K_o, Fy(a–b–), Jk(a–b–), and Lu(a–b–), and describe their role in problem-solving.
13. Compare dominant and recessive forms of the Lu(a–b–) and Jk(a–b–) phenotypes.
14. Explain I, P1, and Lutheran antigens as being poorly expressed on cord RBCs.
15. Describe the phenotypic relationship between LW and Rh.
16. List the Gerbich-negative phenotypes and the antibodies that can be made by each.
17. List the antigens that are denatured by routine blood bank enzymes (M, N, S, s, Fy^a, Fy^b) and antigens whose reactivity with antibody is enhanced with enzymes (I, i, P1, Jk^a, Jk^b).
18. List which antigens are destroyed by treatment with DTT (dithiothreitol).
19. Explain the prevalence of Di^a with South, Central, and North American native populations, and the consequent higher prevalence of the Di(b–) phenotype in those populations.

Antibody Characteristics

20. List the characteristics of the Lewis antibodies, including clinical significance.
21. Define antibodies to M, N, I, and P1 as being typically non-RBC-induced ("naturally occurring"), cold-reacting agglutinins that are usually clinically insignificant.
22. Describe antibodies to K, k, S, s, Fy^a, Fy^b, Jk^a, and Jk^b as usually induced by exposure to foreign RBCs ("immune"), antiglobulin-reactive antibodies that are clinically significant.
23. List the antibody specificities that commonly show dosage (anti-M, -N, -S, -s, -Fy^a, -Fy^b, -Jk^a and -Jk^b).
24. Describe the characteristic reactivity of antibodies to Ch, Rg, JMH, and Knops antigens, and their clinical significance.
25. List the antibodies in the Dombrock system that are clinically significant for transfusion (anti-Do^a and anti-Do^b).

Clinical Significance and Disease Association

26. List and correlate the common 37°C antihuman globulin–reactive antibodies K, k, S, s, Fy^a, Fy^b, Jk^a, and Jk^b with hemolytic transfusion reactions (HTR) and hemolytic disease of the fetus and newborn (HDFN).
27. Describe why the Kidd antibodies are a common cause of delayed HTR.
28. Define the relationship of autoanti-I with *Mycoplasma pneumoniae* infections and autoanti-i with infectious mononucleosis.
29. Describe the common characteristics of the McLeod syndrome, including very weak Kell antigen expression, acanthocytosis, and late onset of muscular and neurological abnormalities.
30. Describe the association of the Fy(a–b–) phenotype with *Plasmodium vivax* resistance.
31. Explain Jk(a–b–) RBCs with a resistance to lysis that normally occurs in 2M urea, a common diluting fluid used for automated platelet counters.

Introduction

The first part of this chapter covers blood group terminology and how antigens are organized into a classification scheme. Conventions for the correct use of terminology are included so that the student will be able to accurately communicate information about antigens and antibodies, **phenotypes**, and **genotypes**.

The ABO and Rh blood groups are the most significant in transfusion practice. However, there are over 300 RBC antigens that are formally recognized internationally. Blood group antigens are defined by carbohydrates (sugars) attached to glycoprotein or glycolipid structures or by amino acids on a protein. The carbohydrate blood groups Lewis, P, and I will be presented first. The antigens of these carbohydrate systems (like ABO and H) are not encoded by their genes directly. Rather, the genes encode specific **glycosyltransferases** that in turn synthesize the carbohydrate epitopes by sequential addition of sugars to a precursor.

The next blood groups discussed are MNS, Duffy, Kell, and Kidd. These are significant in routine transfusion medicine; antibodies to these antigens are more commonly encountered. The chapter then addresses the remainder of the blood groups and selected antigens. Antibodies to these latter will be rarely encountered, but it is important for clinical laboratorians to know that these other antigens and corresponding antibodies exist. While there is more information presented here than is required to work capably at the bench, students will be better prepared for those real-life situations when they encounter one of these uncommon antibodies.

Antigen and antibody characteristics are discussed for each blood group presented. Included are the effects of enzymes and chemical treatments on test RBCs. This information is a tool for antibody identification. For example, if an antibody no longer reacts with a panel of RBCs after the RBCs have been pretreated with an enzyme such as ficin or papain, then only those antibodies that don't react after enzyme treatment are considered for the specificity, and all other specificities can be excluded. These antigen and antibody characteristics are summarized on the front and back cover of the book so that students can easily access pertinent information while performing routine antibody identification.

Blood Groups and Terminology

A blood group system is one or more antigens produced by **alleles** at a single gene **locus** or at loci so closely linked that crossing over does not occur or is very rare.[1] With a few notable exceptions, most blood group genes are located on the autosomal chromosomes and demonstrate straightforward Mendelian inheritance.

Most blood group alleles are **codominant** and express a corresponding antigen. For example, a person who inherits alleles *K* and *k* expresses both K and k antigens on his or her RBCs. Some genes code for complex structures that carry more than one antigen (e.g., the glycophorin B structure, which carries S or s antigen, also carries the U antigen).

Silent, or **amorphic**, alleles exist that make no antigen, but they are rare. When paired chromosomes carry the same silent allele, a **null phenotype** results. Null phenotype RBCs can be very helpful when evaluating antibodies to unknown **high-prevalence** antigens. For example, an antibody reacting with all test cells except those with the phenotype Lu(a–b–) may be directed against an antigen in the Lutheran system or an antigen phenotypically related to the Lutheran system. In some blood group systems, the null phenotype results in RBC abnormalities.

Some blood group systems have regulator or modifying genes, which alter antigen expression. These are not necessarily located at the same locus as the blood group genes they affect and may segregate independently. For example, RBCs with the dominant type of Lu(a–b–) have suppressed expression of all the antigens in the Lutheran blood group system as well as many other antigens, including P1 and i. This modifying gene is inherited independently of the genes coding for Lutheran, P1, and i antigens.

Blood group antigens are detected by alloantibodies, which occur naturally (i.e., without a known immune stimulus) or as a response by the immune system after exposure to non-self RBC antigens introduced by blood transfusion or pregnancy. Over the last century, blood group antigens have been named using several styles of symbols: uppercase single letters, uppercase and lowercase letters to represent alleles, letters derived from the name of the system (some with superscripts to represent alleles), letter symbols followed by numbers, and finally the more recent use of all uppercase letters.

Although gene and antigen names seem confusing at first, certain conventions are followed when writing alleles, antigens, and phenotypes.[1] Some examples are given in Table 8–1. Genes are written in italics or underlined when italics are not available (e.g., when handwritten), and their allele number or letter is always superscript. Antigen names are written in regular type without italics or underlining; some antigens have numbers or superscript letters. A phenotype is a description of which antigens are present on an individual's RBCs and simply indicates the results of serologic tests on those RBCs. It is important to use subscripts, superscripts, and italics appropriately. For example, A1, A_1 and A^1 mean the antigen, the phenotype, and the allele respectively.

How the phenotype is written depends on the antigen nomenclature and whether letters or numbers are used. For letter antigens, a plus sign or minus sign written on the same line as the antigen is used to designate that the antigen is present or absent, respectively. Examples are M+ and K–. For antigens that have superscripts, the letter of the superscript is placed in parentheses on the same line as the letter defining the antigen—for example, Fy(a+) and Jk(a–). When testing for both of the antithetical antigens, both results are written within the parentheses—for instance, Fy(a–b+). For antigens that have a numerical designation, the letter(s) defining the system is followed by a colon, followed by the number representing the antigen. No plus sign is written if the antigen is present, but a minus sign is placed before the

Table 8–1 Examples of Terminology for Genes, Antigens, Antibodies, and Phenotypes

System	GENE Conventional	ISBT	ANTIGEN	ANTIBODY	PHENOTYPE Antigen Positive	Antigen Negative
Lewis	*Le* *le*	*LE*	Le^a Le^b	Anti-Le^a Anti-Le^b	Le(a+) Le(b+)	Le(a–) Le(b–)
MNS	*M* *N* *S* *s*	*MNS*1* *MNS*2* *MNS*3* *MNS*4*	M N S s	Anti-M Anti-N Anti-S Anti-s	M+ N+ S+ s+	M– N– S– s–
Kell	*K* *k*	*KEL*1* *KEL*2*	K k	Anti-K Anti-k	K+ k+	K– k–
Kidd	*Jk^a* *Jk^b*	*JK*1* *JK*2*	Jk^a Jk^b	Anti-Jk^a Anti-Jk^b	Jk(a+) Jk(b+)	Jk(a–) Jk(b–)

negative result, and multiple results are separated by a comma (e.g., Sc:–1,2). Phenotypes of more than one blood group system are separated by a semicolon—for example, S+s+; K–; Fy(a+b–).

One must remember that serologic tests determine only RBC phenotype, not genotype. A genotype is composed of the actual genes that an individual has inherited and can be determined only by family or DNA studies. Sometimes the genotype can be predicted or inferred by the phenotype. When based on results from RBC antigen typing, the genotype is a *probable interpretation* as to which genes the individual carries in order to have the observed phenotype.

Antibodies are described by their antigen notation with the prefix *anti-*, including a hyphen before the antigen symbol. Use of correct blood group terminology, especially for antibodies identified in a patient's serum, is very important so that correct information is conveyed for patient care. Some examples of correct and incorrect terminology are given in Table 8–2.

Numeric terminology was originally introduced for the Kell and Rh systems and was subsequently applied to other systems. To facilitate computer storage and retrieval of blood group information and to help standardize blood group system and antigen names, the International Society of Blood

Transfusion (ISBT) formed the Working Party on Terminology for Red Cell Surface Antigens in 1980.[2] The numeric system this group proposed was not intended to replace traditional terminology but rather to enable communication on computer systems where numbers are necessary. Each antigen is given a six-digit identification number. The first three digits represent the system, collection, or series, and the second three digits identify the antigen. The antigens within the system are numbered sequentially in order of discovery. Each system also has an alphabetical symbol. For example, using the ISBT terminology, the K antigen is 006001 with the first three numbers (006) representing the system and the second three numbers (001) representing the number assigned to K. Antigens can also be written using the system symbol followed by the antigen number; for instance, KEL1 (the redundant sinistral zeroes can be omitted). This committee's work is ongoing, and the assignment of RBC antigens to blood group systems is periodically updated. The first monograph was released in 1990, and updates are published in Vox Sanguinis[3] and on the Working Party's page of the ISBT website (www.isbtweb.org).

The ISBT assigns RBC antigens to a system, collection, or low- or high-prevalence series. This chapter uses traditional terminology, but the ISBT symbol and number are indicated for the blood group systems and collections discussed.

As defined by the ISBT, a blood group system "consists of one or more antigens controlled at a single gene locus, or by two or more very closely linked homologous genes with little or no observable recombination between them."[4] Each system is genetically distinct. To date, there are 30 blood group systems (Table 8–3).[3]

Collections are antigens that have a biochemical, serologic, or genetic relationship but do not meet the criteria for a system.[4] Antigens classified as a collection are assigned a 200 number. Some of the previously established collections have been made obsolete as criteria have been met to establish a system or incorporate antigens into an existing system. See Table 8–4 for a listing of the ISBT collections.

All remaining RBC antigens that are not associated with a system or a collection are catalogued into the 700 series of

Table 8–2 Examples of Correct and Incorrect Terminology

CORRECT	INCORRECT
Fy(a+)	Fy^a+, Fy$^{(a+)}$, Fya+, Fya(+), Duffy a-positive, Duffy^a+
Fy(a–b+)	Fy$^{a–b+}$, Fy^a(–)Fy^b(+)
Anti-Fy^a	Anti Fy^a, anti-Duffy, anti-Duffy^a
K	Kell (name of system), K1
Anti-k	Anti-Cellano, anti-K2
M+N–	M(+), MM
Ge:–2	Ge2–, Ge:2–, Ge2-negative

Table 8–3 International Society of Blood Transfusion (ISBT) Blood Group Systems

NUMBER	NAME	SYMBOL	GENE NAME ISBT (HGNC)	CHROMOSOMAL LOCATION	NO. OF AGS
001	ABO	ABO	ABO (ABO)	9q	4
002	MNS	MNS	MNS (GYPA, GYPB, GYPE)	4q	46
003	P1PK	P1PK	P1PK (A4GALT)	22q	2
004	Rh	RH	RH (RHD, RHCE)	1p	52
005	Lutheran	LU	LU (LU)	19q	20
006	Kell	KEL	KEL (KEL)	7q	32
007	Lewis	LE	LE (FUT3)	19p	6
008	Duffy	FY	FY (DARC)	1q	5
009	Kidd	JK	JK (SLC14A1)	18q	3
010	Diego	DI	DI (SLC4A1)	17q	22
011	Yt	YT	YT (ACHE)	7q	2
012	Xg	XG	XG (XG) MIC2 (CD99)	X	2
013	Scianna	SC	SC(ERMAP)	1p	7
014	Dombrock	DO	DO (ART4)	12p	7
015	Colton	CO	CO (AQP1)	7p	4
016	Landsteiner-Wiener	LW	LW (ICAM4)	19p	3
017	Chido/Rodgers	CH/RG	CH/RG (C4A, C4B)	6p	9
018	H	H	H (FUT1)	19q	1
019	Kx	XK	XK (XK)	Xp	1
020	Gerbich	GE	GE (GYPC)	2q	11
021	Cromer	CROM	CROM (CD55)	1q	16
022	Knops	KN	KN (CR1)	1q	9
023	Indian	IN	IN (CD44)	11p	4
024	Ok	OK	OK (BSG)	19p	3
025	Raph	RAPH	RAPH (CD151)	11p	1
026	John Milton Hagen	JMH	JMH (SEMA7A)	15q	6
027	I	I	IGNT (GCNT2)	6p	1
028	Globoside	GLOB	GLOB (B3GALT3)	3q	1
029	Gill	GIL	GIL (AQP3)	9p	1
030	Rh-associated glycoprotein	RHAG	RHAG (RHAG)	6p	2

HGNC = Human Gene Nomenclature Committee

Table 8–4 International Society of Blood Transfusion Blood Group Collections

COLLECTION			ANTIGEN	
Number	**Name**	**Symbol**	**Number**	**Symbol**
205	Cost	COST	205001	Cs^a
			205002	Cs^b
207	Ii	I	207002	i
208	Er	ER	208001	Er^a
			208002	Er^b
			208003	Er3
209		GLOB	209003	LKE
			209004	PX2
210			210001	Le^c
			210002	Le^d
212	Vel	VEL	212001	Vel
			212002	ABTI
213		MN CHO	213001	Hu
			213002	M$_1$
			213003	Tm
			213004	Can
			213005	Sext
			213006	Sj

Antigens in shaded boxes are discussed in text.

low-prevalence antigens or the 901 series of high-prevalence antigens. Refer to Table 8–5 for a listing of low- and high-prevalence antigens recognized by the ISBT. Antigens in these series represent those with a prevalence of less than 1% or more than 90% of most random populations, respectively. As terminology has evolved, the terms *high-* and *low-incidence*, also previously known as *high-* and *low-frequency*, are currently being replaced by the terms *high-* and *low-prevalence*, reflecting the occurrence of an inherited characteristic at the phenotypic level.[5]

The Lewis (007) System

The Lewis blood group system is unique because the Lewis antigens are not intrinsic to RBCs but are on type 1 glycosphingolipids that are passively adsorbed onto the RBC membrane from the plasma. The Lewis system was named after one of the first individuals to make the antibody, reported by Mourant in 1946.[6] This antibody, later called anti-Le^a, agglutinated RBCs from about 25% of English people.[7] In 1948, an antibody, later called anti-Le^b, was found that reacted with Le(a–) individuals. It was thought that Le^a and Le^b were antithetical antigens, but we now know this is not so because they do not result from alternative alleles of a single gene. Rather, they result from the interaction of two fucosyltransferases encoded by independent genes, *Le* and *Se*.

The Lewis blood group system has been assigned the ISBT system number 007 and the system symbol LE.

Table 8–5 International Society of Blood Transfusion Antigens of Low (700 Series) and High (901 Series) Prevalence

	NUMBER	NAME	SYMBOL	NUMBER	NAME	SYMBOL
Lows	700002	Batty	By	700039	Milne	
	700003	Christiansen	Chr^a	700040	Rasmussen	RASM
	700005	Biles	Bi	700044		JFV
	700006	Box	Bx^a	700045	Katagiri	Kg
	700017	Torkildsen	To^a	700047	Jones	JONES
	700018	Peters	Pt^a	700049		HJK
	700019	Reid	Re^a	700050		HOFM
	700021	Jensen	Je^a	700052		SARA
	700028	Livesay	Li^a	700054		REIT
Highs	901002	Langereis	Lan	901009	Anton	AnWj
	901003	August	At^a	901012	Sid	Sd^a
	901005		Jr^a	901014		PEL
	901008		Emm	901016		MAM

Antigens in shaded boxes are discussed in text.

Basic Concepts

There are several Lewis antigens, but the two of primary concern are Le^a and Le^b. The Lewis (*Le, FUT3*) gene is located on chromosome 19 (at 19p13.3), as is the **secretor** (*Se, FUT2*) gene at 19q13.3. There are two alleles at the Lewis locus, *Le* and the amorph *le*, and there are two alleles at the secretor locus, *Se* and the amorph *se*. The biochemistry and interaction of the genes at these two loci will be explained in a later section, but in short, the *Le* gene must be present for a precursor substance to be converted to Le^a, but the *Se* gene must also be present for conversion to Le^b. The four phenotypes resulting from the interaction of these two genes are shown in Table 8–6.

In 1948, it was observed that individuals with Le(a+) RBCs were mostly nonsecretors of ABH.[8] As a result, in general for adults, Le(a+b–) RBCs are from ABH nonsecretors and Le(a–b+) RBCs are from ABH secretors (refer to Chapter 6, "The ABO Blood Group System"). Individuals with the Le(a–b–) RBC phenotype are either secretors or nonsecretors.[7] The Le(a–b–) phenotype is found more frequently among Africans. The Le(a+b+) phenotype is rare among whites and Africans but is more frequent among Asians, with a prevalence of 10% to 40%.[9] The antigens of the Lewis blood group system recognized by the ISBT are listed in Table 8–7.

Lewis antigens are not expressed on cord RBCs and are often diminished on the mother's RBCs during pregnancy. Lewis antigens are found on lymphocytes and platelets and on other tissues such as the pancreas, stomach, intestine, skeletal muscle, renal cortex, and adrenal glands.[9] In addition, soluble Lewis antigens are found in saliva as glycoproteins.

Lewis antigens are resistant to treatment with the enzymes ficin and papain, dithiothreitol (DTT), and glycine-acid EDTA. Reactivity of Lewis antibodies can be greatly enhanced by testing with enzyme-treated RBCs; hemolysis of enzyme-treated RBCs may be seen if serum is tested.

Lewis Antibodies

Lewis antibodies are often naturally occurring and made by Le(a–b–) persons; that is, they occur without any known

Table 8–6   Phenotypes of the Lewis System

PHENOTYPE	ADULT PHENOTYPE PREVALENCE (%)	
	Whites	**Blacks**
Le(a+b–)	22	23
Le(a–b+)	72	55
Le(a–b–)	6	22
Le(a+b+)	Rare	Rare

Table 8–7   Antigens of the Lewis Blood Group System

ANTIGEN	ISBT NUMBER	COMMENT
Le^a	LE1	
Le^b	LE2	
Le^{ab}	LE3	Anti-Le^{ab} reacts with Le(a+b–) and Le(a–b+) RBCs from adults and with 90% cord RBCs.*
Le^{bH}	LE4	Anti-Le^{bH} reacts with group O Le(b+) and A$_2$ Le(b+) RBCs.
ALe^b	LE5	Anti-ALe^b reacts with group A$_1$ Le(b+) and A$_1$B Le(b+) RBCs.
BLe^b	LE6	Anti-BLe^b reacts with group B Le(b+) and A$_1$B Le(b+) RBCs.

*Reactive cord RBCs [serologically Le(a–b–)] are from babies with *Le* gene.

RBC stimulus. They are generally IgM and do not cross the placenta. Because of this and because the Lewis antigens are not well developed on fetal RBCs, the antibodies do not cause hemolytic disease of the fetus and newborn (HDFN). Anti-Le^a and anti-Le^b may occur together and can be neutralized by the Lewis substances present in plasma or saliva or with commercially prepared Lewis substance. Lewis antibodies occur quite frequently in the sera of pregnant women who transiently exhibit the Le(a–b–) phenotype.

Most Lewis antibodies agglutinate saline suspended RBCs, but these agglutinates are often fragile and can be easily dispersed if the cell button is not gently resuspended after centrifugation. Lewis antibodies can bind complement, and when fresh serum is tested, anti-Le^a may cause in vitro hemolysis of incompatible RBCs, though this is more often seen with enzyme-treated RBCs than with untreated RBCs.

Anti-Le^a is the most commonly encountered of the Lewis antibodies and is often detected in room temperature tests, but it sometimes reacts at 37°C and in the indirect antiglobulin test. Rare hemolytic transfusion reactions (HTR) have been reported in patients with anti-Le^a who were transfused with Le(a+) RBCs, so anti-Le^a that are reactive at 37°C, particularly those that cause in vitro hemolysis, should not be ignored.[1] It is relatively easy to find Le(a–) units since 80% of the population are secretors. Obtaining donor units that are typed Le(a–) with reagent antisera is generally not considered necessary for these patients; units that are crossmatch compatible in tests performed at 37°C are acceptable. Persons whose RBCs are Le(a–b+) do not make anti-Le^a, because small amounts of unconverted Le^a are present in their plasma and saliva.

Anti-Le^b is not as common or generally as strong as anti-Le^a. It is usually an IgM agglutinin and can bind complement. Anti-Le^b is infrequently made by Le(a+b–) individuals and can be classified into two categories: anti-Le^{bH} and anti-Le^{bL}. Anti-Le^{bH} reacts best when both the Le^b and the H antigens are present on the RBC, such as group O and A$_2$ cells. Anti-Le^{bH} represents an antibody to a compound antigen. Anti-Le[bL] recognizes any Le[b] antigen regardless of the ABO type. Anti-Le[bH] should be suspected when anti-Le[b] is identified with a panel of RBCs (group O) but most or all group A donor units are crossmatch compatible (as only about 20% of the group A RBC units will be from group A$_2$ individuals).

Lewis antigens are not intrinsic to the RBC membrane and are readily shed from transfused RBCs within a few days of transfusion. Also, Lewis blood group substance present in transfused plasma neutralizes Lewis antibodies in the recipient.[5] This is why it is exceedingly rare for anti-Le[a] or anti-Le[b] to cause hemolysis of transfused RBCs.

Genetics and Biosynthesis

Advanced Concepts

The Lewis gene (*FUT3*) is linked to *Se* (*FUT2*) and *H* (*FUT1*), all located on chromosome 19. The synthesis of Lewis antigens depends on the interaction of the **transferases** produced by the Lewis and secretor genes. The Lewis and secretor transferases preferentially fucosylate type 1 chains, whereas the *H* gene (*FUT1*) preferentially fucosylates type 2 chains. Type 1 chain refers to the beta linkage of the number 1 carbon of galactose to the number 3 carbon of *N*-acetylglucosamine (GlcNAc) residue of the precursor structure (Fig. 8–1). As shown in Figure 8–2, secretor α1,2-L-fucosyltransferase adds a terminal fucose to the type 1 chain to form type 1 H. The *Le* allele codes for α1,4-L-fucosyltransferase, which transfers L-fucose to type 1H chain on glycoprotein or glycolipid structures to form Le[b]. Small amounts of Le[a] are made before the secretor enzyme is able to add the terminal fucose. If these individuals also have *A* or *B* genes, type 1H structures will be converted to A or B structures and the *Le* fucosyltransferase will then produce ALe[b] or BLe[b] (see **Fig. 8–2**).

Individuals who are nonsecretors do not have the enzyme to convert type 1 chains in secretions to type 1H. Consequently, the type 1 precursor is available for action by the *Le* fucosyltransferase, with the result of Le[a] antigen in secretions

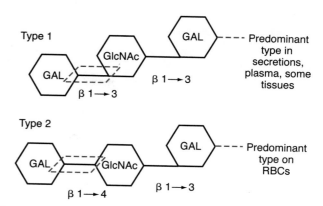

Figure 8–1.   Precursor type 1 and type 2 chains. The type 1 chain has a beta 1→3 linkage of the terminal galactose (Gal) to the *N*-acetylglucosamine (GlcNAc) of the precursor structure. The type 2 chain has a beta 1→4 linkage of the terminal galactose.

and Le(a+b−) RBCs. The Le[a] antigen cannot be converted to Le[b] because of steric hindrance from the fucose added to make Le[a]. Individuals with a weak *Se* gene, common in Asia, produce a fucosyltransferase that competes less effectively with the *Le* fucosyltransferase, resulting in RBCs with the Le(a+b+) phenotype.[7] The Le(a+b+) phenotype is rare in European populations, and it occurs in 10% to 40% of some Asian populations.[9] Mutations that result in inactivation of the fucosyltransferase, represented by the amorphic or silent *le* allele, are responsible for the Le(a−b−) phenotype.

All Le(a−b+) individuals are ABH secretors and also secrete Le[a] and Le[b]; very little Le[a] will be detected in the plasma or on the RBCs. All Le(a+b−) individuals are ABH nonsecretors, yet all secrete Le[a]. Approximately 78% to 80% of whites are secretors, and 20% are nonsecretors. In terms of Le(a−b−) individuals, 80% are ABH secretors, and 20% are ABH nonsecretors. The interaction of Lewis, secretor, and ABO genes is summarized in Table 8–8.

Lewis antigens produced in saliva and other secretions are glycoproteins, but Lewis cell-bound antigens absorbed from plasma onto the RBC membranes are glycolipids. The

Figure 8–2.   Formation of Lewis antigens. Gal = galactose; GlcNAc = *N*-acetylglucosamine; Fuc = fucose; GalNAc = *N*-acetylgalactosamine.

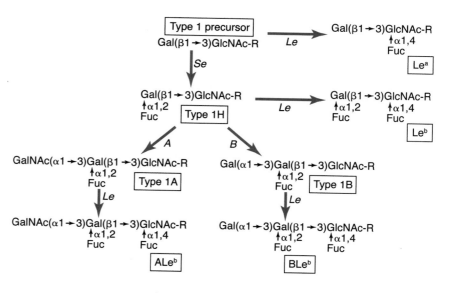

Table 8–8 Antigens and Phenotypes Resulting From Interaction of Lewis, Secretor, and ABO Genes

LEWIS, SECRETOR, AND ABO GENES

Genes	Antigens in Secretions	RBC Phenotype
Le, Se, A/B/H	Le^a, Le^b, A, B, H	A, B, H, Le(a – b+)
lele, Se, A/B/H	A, B, H	A, B, H, Le(a – b –)
Le, sese, A/B/H	Le^a	A, B, H, Le(a+b –)
lele, sese, A/B/H	None	A, B, H, Le(a – b –)
Le, sese, hh, A/B	Le^a	O$_h$, Le(a+b –)
Le, Se, hh, A/B	Le^a, Le^b, A, B, H	A*, B*, Le(a – b+)

*para-Bombay

gastrointestinal tract is thought to be the primary source of Lewis glycolipid in plasma.[5] Le(a–b–) RBCs incubated with plasma from Le(a+) or Le(b+) individuals can be converted to Le(a+b–) or Le(a–b+), respectively. With saliva as a source of Lewis substances, Le(a–b–) RBCs cannot be converted into Lewis-positive phenotypes because Lewis substances in saliva, being glycoproteins, are not adsorbed onto the RBC membranes.

Development of Lewis Antigens

Depending on the genes inherited, Le^a and Le^b glycoproteins will be present in the saliva of newborns, but Lewis glycolipids are not detectable in the plasma until about 10 days after birth. As a result, cord blood and RBCs from newborn infants phenotype as Le(a–b–). Some can be shown to be weakly Le(a+) when tested with a potent anti-Le^a or with methods more sensitive than direct agglutination. Lewis antigens will start to appear shortly after birth, with Le^a developing first when the *Le* gene is present. The Lewis fucosyltransferase is more active than the secretor fucosyltransferase in newborns, so more type 1 chains are available for conversion to Le^a. As the secretor transferase activity increases, converting type 1 to type 1H, Le^b will be detected. In children who inherit both *Le* and *Se* genes, the transformation can be followed from the Le(a–b–) phenotype at birth to Le(a+b–) after 10 days to Le(a+b+) and finally to Le(a–b+), the true Lewis phenotype, after about 6 years. In contrast, children who inherit *Le* and *sese* genes phenotype as Le(a–b–) at birth and transform to Le(a+b–) after 10 days; the Le(a+b–) phenotype persists throughout life. Individuals with *lele* genes phenotype as Le(a–b–) at birth and for the rest of their lives.

Other Lewis Antigens

Le^{ab} is present on all Le(a+b–) and Le(a–b+) RBCs and on 90% of cord RBCs. The antigen was previously known as Le^x, but in 1998 the ISBT renamed it Le^{ab}.[9] Anti-Le^{ab} is fairly

common and is frequently found with anti-Le^a or anti-Le^b. The antibody is heterogenous and occurs mainly in Le(a–b–) secretors of group A$_1$, B, or A$_1$B. The antigens now known as Le^x and Le^y are products of *FUT3* on type 2 precursor chains and are not associated with the RBC surface and are not part of the Lewis blood group.[9]

ALe^b and BLe^b result from the addition of the A or B immunodominant sugar, respectively, to type 1H chain in individuals who have at least one *Se* and one *Le* allele. *Se* converts type 1 chains to type 1H, providing a suitable acceptor for the A and B carbohydrates (see **Fig. 8–2**).

The P Blood Group: P1PK (003) and Globoside (028) Systems and Related (209) Antigens

Traditionally, the P blood group comprised the P, P1, and P^k antigens and, later, Luke (LKE). The biochemistry and molecular genetics, although not completely understood as yet, make it clear that at least two biosynthetic pathways and genes at different loci are involved in the development and expression of these antigens. Consequently, these antigens cannot be considered a single blood group system. Currently, in ISBT nomenclature, P1 and P^k are assigned to the P1PK blood group system (003, symbol P1PK), P is assigned to the Globoside blood group system (028, symbol GLOB), and LKE and PX2 are assigned to the Globoside collection (209, symbol GLOB). The reader will notice the confusing use of GLOB as the symbol for both a system and a collection. For simplicity in this chapter, these antigens will be referred to as the P blood group.

The P blood group was introduced in 1927 by Landsteiner and Levine. In their search for new antigens, they injected rabbits with human RBCs and produced an antibody, initially called *anti-P*, that divided human RBCs into two groups: P+ and P–.[7]

In 1951, Levine and colleagues[10] described anti-Tj^a (now known as anti-PP1P^k), an antibody to a high-prevalence antigen that Sanger[11] later showed was related to the P blood group. Because anti-Tj^a defined an antigen common to P+ and P– cells and was made by an apparent P null individual, the original antigen and phenotypes were renamed. Anti-P became anti-P1; the P+ phenotype became P$_1$; the P– phenotype became P$_2$; and the rare P null individual became p.

The P blood group became more complex in 1959 when Matson and coworkers[12] described a new antigen, P^k. This antigen is expressed on all RBCs except those of the very rare p phenotype, but it is not readily detected unless P is absent (i.e., in the P$_1^k$ and P$_2^k$ phenotypes).

The phenotypes, antigens, and antibodies associated with the P blood group are summarized in Table 8–9. There are two common phenotypes: P$_1$ and P$_2$, and three rare phenotypes: p, P$_1^k$, and P$_2^k$. The P$_1$ phenotype describes RBCs that react with anti-P1 and anti-P; the P$_2$ phenotype describes RBCs that do not react with anti-P1 but do react with anti-P. When RBCs are tested only with anti-P1 and not with anti-P, the phenotype should be written as P1+ (or P$_1$) or P1–. Only when P1– RBCs are tested and found to be reactive with anti-P should they be designated as phenotype P$_2$. RBCs of the p phenotype do not react with anti-P1, anti-P, or anti-P^k. RBCs of the P$_1^k$ phenotype

Table 8–9   P Blood Group: Phenotypes, Antigens, and Antibodies

PHENOTYPE	ANTIGENS PRESENT	POSSIBLE ANTIBODIES	PREVALENCE	
			Whites	Blacks
P_1	P1, P, Pk*	None	79%	94%
P_2	P, Pk*	Anti-P1	21%	6%
p	None	Anti-PP1Pk	Rare	Rare
$P_1{}^k$	P1, Pk	Anti-P	Very rare	Very rare
$P_2{}^k$	Pk	Anti-P, anti-P1	Very rare	Very rare

*Trace amounts of Pk antigen, not detectable by agglutination test

react with anti-P1 and anti-Pk but not with anti-P. RBCs of the $P_2{}^k$ phenotype react with anti-Pk but not with anti-P1 or anti-P.

Individuals with the p phenotype (P null) are very rare: 5.8 in a million. P nulls are slightly more common in Japan, North Sweden, and in an Amish group in Ohio.[1]

The antibodies generally fall into two categories: clinically insignificant or potently hemolytic.

Basic Concepts

The P blood group antigens, like the ABH antigens, are synthesized by sequential action of glycosyltransferases, which add sugars to precursor substances. The precursor of P1 can also be glycosylated to type 2H chains, which carry ABH antigens. P1, P, or Pk may be found on RBCs, lymphocytes, granulocytes, and monocytes; P can be found on platelets, epithelial cells, and fibroblasts. P and Pk have also been found in plasma as glycosphingolipids and as glycoproteins in hydatid cyst fluid.[7] The antigens have not been identified in secretions. RBCs carry approximately 14×10^6 copies of globoside, the P structure, per adult RBC and about 5×10^5 copies of P1.[9]

The P blood group antigens are resistant to treatment with ficin and papain, DTT, chloroquine, and glycine-acid EDTA. Reactivity of the antibodies can be greatly enhanced by testing with enzyme-treated RBCs.

The P1 Antigen

The P1 antigen is poorly expressed at birth and may take up to 7 years to be fully expressed.[7] Antigen strength in adults varies from one individual to another: RBCs from some P1+ individuals are P1 strong (P1+s) and others are P1 weak (P1+w). These differences may be controlled genetically or may represent homozygous versus heterozygous inheritance of the gene coding for P1. The strength of P1 can also vary with race. Blacks have a stronger expression of P1 than whites. The rare dominant gene for the In(lu) type Lu(a–b–) RBCs, discussed in the Lutheran section, inhibits the expression of P1 so that P_1 individuals who inherit this modifier gene may type serologically as P1–.

The P1 antigen deteriorates rapidly on storage. When older RBCs are typed or used as controls for typing reagents or when older RBCs are used to detect anti-P1 in serum, false-negative reactions may result.

Anti-P1

Anti-P1 is a common, naturally occurring IgM antibody in the sera of P1– individuals. Anti-P1 is typically a weak, cold-reactive saline agglutinin optimally reactive at 4°C and not seen in routine testing. Stronger examples react at room temperature, and rare examples react at 37°C and bind complement, which is detected in the antiglobulin test when polyspecific (anti-IgG plus anti-C3) reagents are used. Antibody activity can be neutralized or inhibited with soluble P1 substance. If room temperature incubation is not included, antibody activity can often be bypassed altogether. Examples of anti-P1 that react only at temperatures below 37°C can be considered clinically insignificant.

Because P1 antigen expression on RBCs varies and deteriorates during storage, antibodies may react only with RBCs that have the strongest expression and give inconclusive patterns of reactivity when antibody identification is performed. When anti-P1 is suspected, incubating tests at room temperature or lower or pretreating test cells with enzymes can enhance reactions to confirm specificity. Providing units that are crossmatch-compatible at 37°C and the antiglobulin phase, without typing for P1, is an acceptable approach to transfusion.

Rare examples of anti-P1 that react at 37°C can cause in vivo RBC destruction; both immediate and delayed HTRs have been reported.[13] Anti-P1 is usually IgM; IgG forms are rare. HDFN is not associated with anti-P1, presumably because the antibody is usually IgM and the antigen is so poorly developed on fetal RBCs.

Biochemistry

Advanced Concepts

The RBC antigens of the P blood group exist as glycosphingolipids. As with ABH, the antigens result from the sugars added sequentially to precursor structures. Biochemical analyses have shown that the precursor substance for P1 is also a precursor for type 2H chains that carry ABH antigens. However, the genes responsible for the formation of the P1 and ABH antigens are independent.

There are two distinct pathways for the synthesis of the P blood group antigens, as shown in Figure 8–3. The common precursor is lactosylceramide (or Gb2, also known as ceramide dihexose or CDH). The pathway on the figure's left results in the formation of paragloboside and P1. Paragloboside is also the type 2 precursor for ABH. The pathway shown on the figure's right side leads to the production of the globoside series: P^k, P, and Luke (LKE).

Genetics

The gene encoding the enzyme responsible for the synthesis of P^k, a 4-α-galactosyltransferase (Gb3 or P^k synthase), was cloned independently by three research groups in 2000.[14] The gene (*B3GALNT1*) encoding the 3-β-N-acetylgalactosaminyltransferase (Gb4 synthase) that is responsible for converting P^k to P was also cloned in 2000.[14] Several mutations in both genes have been identified that result in the p and P^k phenotypes. A polymorphism in the P^k synthase was recently identified that ties the P1 and P^k antigens together at the genetic level; consequently, the P system (003), to which the P1 antigen was assigned, was renamed P1PK.[3]

The *P1PK* gene (located at chromosome 22q11.2) and the *P* gene (located at chromosome 3q26.1) are inherited independently. The gene for the synthesis of LKE has not yet been cloned.

Other Sources of P1 Antigen and Antibody

The discovery of strong anti-P1 in two P1– individuals infected with *Echinococcus granulosus* tapeworms led to the identification of P1 and P^k substance in hydatid cyst fluid. This fluid was subsequently used in many of the studies that identified the biochemical structures of the P blood group. Strong antibodies to P1 have also been found in patients with fascioliasis (bovine liver fluke disease) and in bird handlers.

Soluble P1 substances have potential use in the blood bank and are commercially available. When it is necessary to confirm antibody specificity or to identify underlying antibodies, these substances can be used to neutralize anti-P1.

Anti-PP1P^k

Originally called anti-Tj^a, anti-PP1P^k was first described in the serum of Mrs. Jay, a p individual with adenocarcinoma of the stomach.[10] Her tumor cells carried P system antigens, and the antibody was credited as having cytotoxic properties that may have helped prevent metastatic growth postsurgery (the T in the Tj^a refers to *tumor*).

Anti-PP1P^k is produced by p individuals early in life without RBC sensitization and reacts with all RBCs except those of the p phenotype. Unlike antibodies made by other blood group null phenotypes, the anti-P, anti-P1, and anti-P^k components of anti-PP1P^k are separable through adsorption.[7] Components of anti-PP1P^k have been shown to be IgM and IgG.[7] They react over a wide thermal range and efficiently bind complement, which makes them potent hemolysins. Anti-PP1P^k has the potential to cause severe HTRs and HDFN.

The antibody is also associated with an increased incidence of spontaneous abortions in early pregnancy. Although the reason for this is not fully known, it has been suggested that having an IgG anti-P component is an important factor. Women with anti-P and anti-PP1P^k and a history of multiple abortions have successfully delivered infants after multiple plasmaphereses to reduce their antibody level during pregnancy.[15]

Alloanti-P

In addition to being a component of the anti-PP1P^k in p individuals (see above), anti-P is found as a naturally occurring alloantibody in the sera of P^k individuals. Its reactivity is similar to that of anti-PP1P^k in that it is usually a potent hemolysin reacting with all cells except the autocontrol and those with the p phenotype. However, it differs from anti-PP1P^k in that it does not react with cells that have the extremely rare P^k phenotype, and the individual making the antibody may type P1+. Alloanti-P is rarely seen, but because it is hemolytic with a wide thermal range of reactivity, it is very significant in transfusion. IgG class anti-P may occur and has been associated with habitual early abortion.

Autoanti-P Associated With Paroxysmal Cold Hemoglobinuria

Anti-P specificity is also associated with the cold-reactive IgG autoantibody in patients with paroxysmal cold hemoglobinuria (PCH). Historically, this rare autoimmune disorder was seen in patients with tertiary syphilis; it now more commonly presents as a transient, acute condition secondary to viral infection, especially in young children. The IgG autoantibody in PCH is described as a biphasic hemolysin: In vitro, the antibody binds to RBCs in the cold, and, via complement activation, the coated RBCs lyse as they are warmed to 37°C. The autoantibody typically does not react in routine test

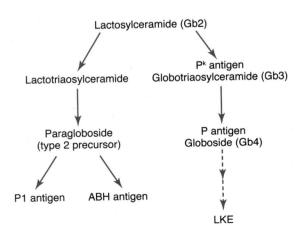

Figure 8–3.   Biosynthetic pathways of the P blood group antigens.

systems but is demonstrable only by the Donath-Landsteiner test. The etiology and diagnosis of PCH are more fully discussed in Chapter 20, "Autoimmune Hemolytic Anemias."

Antibodies to Compound Antigens

Considering the biochemical relationship of the P blood group antigens to ABH and I, it is not surprising that antibodies requiring more than one antigenic determinant have been described, including anti-IP1, -iP1, -I^{T}P1, and -IP. Most examples are cold-reactive agglutinins.

Luke (LKE) Antigen

In 1965, Tippett and colleagues[16] described an antibody in the serum of a patient with Hodgkin's lymphoma that divided the population into three phenotypes: 84% tested Luke+, 14% were weakly positive or Luke(w), and 2% were Luke–. Although this Mendelian-dominant character segregated independently of the P blood group, it was thought to be phenotypically related because the antibody reacted with all RBCs except 2% of P$_1$ and P$_2$ phenotypes and those having the rare p and P^k phenotypes. All individuals with the p and P^k phenotype are Luke–.

Disease Associations

Several pathological conditions associated with the P blood group antigens have been described: parasitic infections are associated with anti-P1, early abortions with anti-PP1P^k or anti-P, and PCH with autoanti-P. The P system antigens also serve as receptors for P-fimbriated uropathogenic E. coli—a cause of urinary tract infections. The P^k antigen is a receptor for shiga toxins, which cause shigella dysentery and E. coli–associated hemolytic uremic syndrome. In addition, P is the receptor of human parvovirus B19. Recent studies demonstrate that P^k provides some protection against HIV infection of peripheral blood mononuclear cells.[17]

The I (027) System and I Antigen

The existence of cold agglutinins in the serum of normal individuals and in patients with acquired hemolytic anemia has long been recognized. In 1956, Wiener and coworkers[2,7] gave a name to one such agglutinin, calling its antigen I for "individuality." The antibody reacted with most blood specimens tested. The few nonreactive I– specimens were thought to be from homozygotes for a rare gene producing the "i" antigen; the I– phenotype in adults is now called *adult i*. In 1960, Marsh and Jenkins[18] reported finding anti-i, and the unique relationship between I and i began to unfold.

I and i are not antithetical antigens. Rather, they are branched and linear carbohydrate structures, respectively, that are formed by the action of glycosyl transferases. The gene encoding the transferase that converts i active straight chains into I active branched chains has been cloned, and several mutations responsible for the rare adult i phenotype have been identified.[19] The synthesis of i antigen is not controlled by this same gene. Consequently, I has been raised to

blood group system status (system number 027, symbol I) and the i antigen remains in the Ii collection (collection number 207, symbol I). The reader will notice the confusing use of the same ISBT symbol, capital I, for both the I system and Ii collection; in ISBT terminology, the antigen numbers provide the distinction between the I (027001) and i (207002) antigens.

The I and i Antigens

Basic Concepts

The antigens are best introduced by classic serologic facts. Both I and i are high-prevalence antigens, but they are expressed in a reciprocal relationship that is developmentally regulated. At birth, infant RBCs are rich in i; I is almost undetectable. During the first 18 months of life, the quantity of i slowly decreases as I increases until adult proportions are reached; adult RBCs are rich in I and have only trace amounts of i antigen.

There is no true I– or i– phenotype. The strength of I and i varies from individual to individual, and the relative amount detected will depend on the example of anti-I or anti-i used. Data suggest that i reactivity on RBCs is inversely proportional to marrow transit time and RBC age in circulation.

Some people appear not to change their i status after birth. They become the rare adult i. Adult i RBCs generally express more i antigen than do cord RBCs. A spectrum of Ii phenotypes and their characteristic reactivity are shown in Table 8–10.

Treatment of RBCs with ficin and papain enhances reactivity of the I and i antigens with their respective antibodies. The I and i antigens are resistant to treatment with DTT and glycine-acid EDTA.

Anti-I

Anti-I is a common autoantibody that can be found in virtually all sera, although testing at 4°C and/or against enzyme-treated RBCs may be required to detect the reactivity.[1] Consistently strong agglutination with adult RBCs and weak or no agglutination with cord or adult i RBCs define its classic activity (see Table 8–10).

Autoanti-I, found in the serum of many normal healthy individuals, is benign—that is, not associated with in vivo

Table 8–10	I and i Antigens		
PHENOTYPE	**STRENGTH OF REACTIVITY WITH**		
	Anti-I	**Anti-i**	**Anti-I^T**
Adult I	Strong	Weak	Weak
Cord	Weak	Strong	Strong
Adult i	Weak	Strong	Weakest

RBC destruction. It is usually a weak, naturally occurring, saline-reactive IgM agglutinin with a titer less than 64 at 4°C. Stronger examples agglutinate test cells at room temperature and bind complement, which can be detected in the antiglobulin test if polyspecific reagents are used. Some examples may react only with the strongest I+ RBCs and give inconsistent reactions with panel RBCs.

Incubating tests in the cold enhances anti-I reactivity and helps confirm its identity; albumin and enzyme methods also enhance anti-I reactivity. Testing enzyme-treated RBCs with slightly acidified serum may even promote hemolysis. Occasionally, benign cold autoanti-I can cause problems in pretransfusion testing. Usually, avoiding room temperature testing and using anti-IgG instead of a polyspecific antihuman globulin help to eliminate detection of cold reactive antibodies that may bind complement at lower temperatures. Cold autoadsorption to remove the autoantibody from the serum may be necessary for stronger examples; cold autoadsorbed plasma or serum can also be used in ABO typing.

Pathogenic autoanti-I (e.g., the type associated with cold agglutinin syndrome) typically consists of strong IgM agglutinins with higher titers and a broad thermal range of activity, reacting up to 30° or 32°C. When peripheral circulation cools in response to low ambient temperatures, these antibodies attach in vivo and cause autoagglutination and peripheral vascular occlusion (acrocyanosis) or hemolytic anemia. Refer to Chapter 20 for more information.

Pathogenic anti-I typically reacts with adult and cord RBCs equally well at room temperature and at 4°C, and antibody specificity may not be apparent unless the serum is diluted or warmed to 30°C or 37°C. Potent cold autoantibodies can also mask clinically significant underlying alloantibodies and can complicate pretransfusion testing. Procedures to deal with these problems are discussed in Chapters 9 and 20.

The production of autoanti-I may be stimulated by microorganisms carrying I-like antigen on their surface. Patients with *M. pneumoniae* often develop strong cold agglutinins with I specificity and can experience a transient episode of acute abrupt hemolysis just as the infection begins to resolve. Alloanti-I exists as an IgM or IgG antibody in the serum of most individuals with the adult i phenotype. Although adult i RBCs are not totally devoid of I, the anti-I in these cases does not react with autologous RBCs. It has been traditional to transfuse compatible adult i units to these people, although such practice may be unnecessary, especially when the antibody is not reactive at 37°C.[1] Technologists must be aware that strong autoanti-I can mimic alloanti-I: if enough autoantibody and complement are bound to a patient's RBCs, blocking the antigenic sites, they may falsely type I-negative.

Anti-I is not associated with HDFN because the antibody is IgM, and the I antigen is poorly expressed on infant RBCs.

Anti-i

Alloanti-i has never been described. Autoanti-i is a fairly rare antibody that gives strong reactions with cord RBCs and adult i RBCs and weaker reactions with adult I RBCs. Most examples of autoanti-i are IgM and react best with saline-suspended cells at 4°C. Only very strong examples of autoanti-i are detected in routine testing because standard test cells (except cord RBCs) have poor i expression (see **Table 8–10**).

Unlike anti-I, autoanti-i is not seen as a common antibody in healthy individuals. Potent examples are associated with infectious mononucleosis (Epstein-Barr virus infections) and some lymphoproliferative disorders. High-titer autoantibodies with a wide thermal range may contribute to hemolysis, but because i expression is generally weak they seldom cause significant hemolysis. IgG anti-i has also been described and has been associated with HDFN.[1]

Biochemistry and Genetics

Advanced Concepts

An early association of I and i to ABH was demonstrated by complex antibodies involving both ABH and Ii specificity (see the "Antibodies to Compound Antigens" section). I and i antigens are precursors for the synthesis of ABO and Lewis antigens, and thus they are internal structures on these oligosaccharide chains.

ABH and Ii determinants on the RBC membrane are carried on type 2 chains that attach either to proteins or to lipids. See Figure 8–4 for examples of glycolipid structures for i and I antigens. The i antigen activity is defined by at least two repeating N-acetyllactosamine [Gal(β1-4)GlcNAc(β1-3)] units in linear form. I antigen activity is associated with a branched form of i antigen. The *IGnT* (also known as *GCNT2*) gene on chromosome 6p24 encodes the N-acetylglucosaminyltransferase, which adds GlcNAc to form the branches.[19,20]

In summary, fetal, cord, and adult i RBCs carry predominantly unbranched chains and have the i phenotype. Normal adult cells have more branched structures and express I antigen. The gene responsible for I antigen (*IGnT*) codes for the branching enzyme. Family studies show that the adult i phenotype is recessive. Heterozygotes (e.g., children inheriting I from one parent and i from the other parent) have intermediate I antigen expression. Several gene mutations have been identified that result in the adult i phenotype.

Antigen	Structure
(None)	Gal(β1-4)GlcNAc(β1-3)Gal(β1-4)GlcNAc(β1-3)Gal(β1-4)Glc-Cer
i	Gal(β1-4)GlcNAc(β1-3)Gal(β1-4)GlcNAc(β1-3)Gal(β1-4)Glc-Cer
I	Gal(β1-4)GlcNAc(β1-3) Gal(β1-4)GlcNAc(β1-6) ＞ Gal(β1-4)GlcNAc(β1-3)Gal(β1-4)Glc-Cer

Figure 8–4. The linear and branched structures carrying i and I activity.

Other Sources of I and i Antigen

I and i antigens are found on the membranes of leukocytes and platelets in addition to RBCs. It is quite likely that the antigens exist on other tissue cells, much like ABH, but this has not been confirmed.

I and i have also been found in the plasma and serum of adults and newborns and in saliva, human milk, amniotic fluid, urine, and ovarian cyst fluid. The antigens in secretions do not correlate with RBC expression and are thought to develop under separate genetic control. For example, the quantity of I antigen in the saliva of adult i individuals and newborns is quite high.

The I^T Antigen and Antibody

In 1965, Curtain and coworkers[21] reported a cold agglutinin in Melanesians that did not demonstrate classical I or i specificity. In 1966, Booth and colleagues[22] confirmed these observations and carefully described the agglutinin's reactivity. This agglutinin reacted strongly with cord RBCs, weakly with normal adult RBCs, and most weakly with adult i RBCs. They concluded that the agglutinin recognizes a transition state of i into I and designated the specificity I^T (T for "transition"). However, detection of I^T on fetal RBCs ranging in age from 11 to 16 weeks does not support this hypothesis.[23] This benign IgM anti-I^T was frequently found in two populations: Melanesians and the Yanomama Indians in Venezuela. Whether it is associated with an organism or parasite in these regions is unknown. Examples of IgM and IgG anti-I^T reacting preferentially at 37°C have also been found in patients with warm autoimmune hemolytic anemia, with a special association with Hodgkin's disease.[23]

Antibodies to Compound Antigens

Many other I-related antibodies have been described: anti-IA, -IB, -IAB, -IH, -iH, -IP1, -I^TP1, -IHLe^b, and -iHLe^b. Bearing in mind the close relationship of I to the biochemical structures of ABH, Lewis, and P antigens, it is not surprising to find antibodies that recognize compound antigens. These specificities are not mixtures of separable antibodies; rather, both antigens must be present on the RBCs for the antibody to react. For example, anti-IA reacts with RBCs that carry both I and A but will not react with group O, I+, or group A adult i RBCs. (Table 8–11 summarizes some common cold autoantibodies.) Anti-IH is commonly encountered in the serum of group A₁ individuals. Anti-IH reacts stronger with group O and group A₂ RBCs than with group A₁ RBCs. Anti-IH should be suspected when serum from a group A individual directly agglutinates all group O RBCs but is compatible with most group A donor units.

Disease Associations

Well-known associations between strong autoantibodies and disease or microorganisms have already been discussed: anti-I with cold agglutinin syndrome and *M. pneumoniae*, and anti-i with infectious mononucleosis.

Diseases can also alter the expression of I and i antigens on RBCs. Conditions associated with increased i antigen on RBCs include those with shortened marrow maturation time or dyserythropoiesis: acute leukemia, hypoplastic anemia, megaloblastic anemia, sideroblastic anemia, thalassemia, sickle cell disease, paroxysmal nocturnal hemoglobinuria (PNH), and chronic hemolytic anemia.[1,7] Except in some cases of leukemia, the increase in i on RBCs is not usually associated with a decrease in I antigen; the expression of I antigen can appear normal or sometimes enhanced. Chronic dyserythropoietic anemia type II or hereditary erythroblastic multinuclearity with a positive acidified serum test (HEMPAS) is associated with much greater i activity on RBCs than control cord RBCs. HEMPAS RBCs are very susceptible to lysis with both anti-i and anti-I, and lysis by anti-I appears to be the result of increased antibody uptake and increased sensitivity to complement.[1] In Asians, the adult i phenotype has been associated with congenital cataracts.[20]

The MNS (002) System

Following the discovery of the ABO blood group system, Landsteiner and Levine began immunizing rabbits with human RBCs, hoping to find new antigen specificities. Among the antibodies recovered from these rabbit sera were anti-M and anti-N, both of which were reported in 1927.[7] Data from family studies suggested that M and N were

Table 8–11 Typical Reactions of Some Cold Autoantibodies*

ANTIBODY	A₁ ADULT	A₂ ADULT	B ADULT	O ADULT	O CORD	A CORD	O_h ADULT	O i ADULT
Anti-I	++++	++++	++++	++++	0/+	0/+	++++	(0)
Anti-i	0/+	0/+	0/+	0/+	++++	++++	0/+	++++
Anti-H	0/+	++	+++	++++	+++	0/+	(0)	+++
Anti-IH	0/+	++	+++	++++	0/+	0/+	(0)	(0)
Anti-IA	++++	+++	0/+	0/+	0/+	0/+	(0)	(0)

*Reactions vary with antibody strength; very potent examples may need to be diluted before specificity can be determined.
0 = negative; + = positive

antithetical antigens. In 1947, after the implementation of the antiglobulin test, Walsh and Montgomery discovered S, a distinct antigen that appeared to be genetically linked to M and N. Its antithetical partner, s, was discovered in 1951. Family studies (and later, molecular genetics) demonstrated the close linkage between the genes controlling M, N, and S, s antigens. There is a disequilibrium in the expression of S and s with M and N. In whites, the common haplotypes were calculated to appear in the following order of relative frequency: Ns > Ms > MS > NS.[1,7] The prevalence of the common MN and Ss phenotypes are listed in Table 8–12.

In 1953, an antibody to a high-prevalence antigen, U (for almost *universal* distribution), was named by Weiner. The observation by Greenwalt and colleagues[24] that all U– RBCs were also S–s– resulted in the inclusion of U into the system.

Forty-six antigens have been included in the MNS system, making it almost equal to Rh in size and complexity (Table 8–13). Most of these antigens are of low prevalence and were discovered in cases of HDFN or incompatible crossmatch. Others are high-prevalence antigens. Antibodies to these low- and high-prevalence antigens are not commonly encountered in the blood bank. The genes encoding the MNS antigens are located on chromosome 4.

The MNS blood group system has been assigned the ISBT number 002 (symbol MNS), second after ABO.

M and N Antigens

Basic Concepts

The M and N antigens are found on a well-characterized glycoprotein called **glycophorin A** (GPA), the major RBC **sialic acid**–rich glycoprotein (sialoglycoprotein, SGP). The M and N antigens are antithetical and differ in their amino acid residues at positions 1 and 5 (Fig. 8–5). M is defined by serine at position 1 and glycine at position 5; N has leucine and glutamic acid at these positions, respectively. The antibody reactivity may also be dependent on adjacent carbohydrate chains, which are rich in sialic acid. There are about 10^6 copies of GPA per RBC.[13] The antigens are well developed at birth.

Because M and N are located at the outer end of GPA, they are easily destroyed by the routine blood bank enzymes ficin, papain, and bromelin and by the less common enzymes trypsin and pronase. The antigens are also destroyed by ZZAP, a combination of DTT and papain or ficin, but they are not affected by DTT alone, 2-aminoethylisothiouronium bromide (AET), α-chymotrypsin, chloroquine, or glycine-acid EDTA treatment. Treating RBCs with neuraminidase, which cleaves sialic acid (also known as *neuraminic acid* or *NeuNAc*), abolishes reactivity with only some examples of antibody. M and N antibodies are heterogeneous; some may recognize only specific amino acids, but others recognize both amino acids and carbohydrate chains.

Table 8–12	Prevalence of Common MN and Ss Phenotypes	
PHENOTYPE	**WHITES (%)**	**BLACKS (%)**
M+N–	28	26
M+N+	50	44
M–N+	22	30
S+s–	11	3
S+s+	44	28
S–s+	45	69
S–s–U–	0	<1

S and s Antigens

S and s antigens are located on a smaller glycoprotein called **glycophorin B** (GPB) that is very similar to GPA (see "Biochemistry" section and Fig. 8–5). S and s are differentiated by the amino acid at position 29 on GPB. Methionine defines S, whereas threonine defines s. The epitope may also include the amino acid residues at position 34 and 35 and the carbohydrate chain attached to threonine at position 25.[7] There are fewer copies of GPB (about 200,000) than GPA per RBC.[7] In addition, there are about 1.5 times more copies of GPB on S+s– RBCs than on S–s+ RBCs.[1] S and s also are well developed at birth.

S and s antigens are less easily degraded by enzymes because the antigens are located farther down the glycoprotein, and enzyme-sensitive sites are less accessible. Ficin, papain, bromelin, pronase, and chymotrypsin can destroy S and s activity, but the amount of degradation may depend on the strength of the enzyme solution, the length of treatment, and the enzyme-to-cell ratio. Trypsin does not destroy the S and s antigens, and neither does DTT, AET, chloroquine, or glycine-acid EDTA treatment.

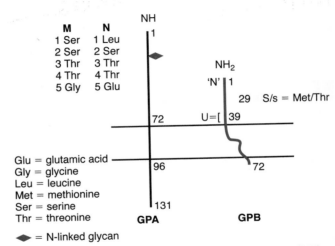

Figure 8–5.   Comparison of glycophorin A (GPA) and glycophorin B (GPB).

Table 8–13   Summary of MNS Antigens

ANTIGEN NAME	ISBT NUMBER	PREVALENCE (%)	YEAR DISCOVERED
M	MNS1	Polymorphic	1927
N	MNS2	Polymorphic	1927
S	MNS3	Polymorphic	1947
s	MNS4	Polymorphic	1951
U	MNS5	High	1953
He	MNS6	Low	1951
Mi^a	MNS7	Low	1951
M^c	MNS8	Low	1953
Vw	MNS9	Low	1954
Mur	MNS10	Low	1961
M^g	MNS11	Low	1958
Vr	MNS12	Low	1958
M^e	MNS13	Low	1961
Mt^a	MNS14	Low	1962
St^a	MNS15	Low	1962
Ri^a	MNS16	Low	1962
Cl^a	MNS17	Low	1963
Ny^a	MNS18	Low	1964
Hut	MNS19	Low	1966
Hil	MNS20	Low	1966
M^v	MNS21	Low	1966
Far	MNS22	Low	1968
s^D	MNS23	Low	1978
Mit	MNS24	Low	1980
Dantu	MNS25	Low	1982
Hop	MNS26	Low	1977
Nob	MNS27	Low	1977
En^a	MNS28	High	1969
ENKT	MNS29	High	1986
'N'	MNS30	High	1977
Or	MNS31	Low	1964
DANE	MNS32	Low	1991
TSEN	MNS33	Low	1992
MINY	MNS34	Low	1992
MUT	MNS35	Low	1992
SAT	MNS36	Low	1991

Continued

Table 8–13   Summary of MNS Antigens—cont'd

ANTIGEN NAME	ISBT NUMBER	PREVALENCE (%)	YEAR DISCOVERED
ERIK	MNS37	Low	1993
Os^a	MNS38	Low	1983
ENEP	MNS39	High	1995
ENEH	MNS40	High	1993
HAG	MNS41	Low	1995
ENAV	MNS42	High	1996
MARS	MNS43	Low	1992
ENDA	MNS44	High	2005
ENEV	MNS45	High	2006
MNTD	MNS46	Low	2006

Anti-M

Many examples of anti-M are naturally occurring saline agglutinins that react below 37°C. Although we may think of agglutinating anti-M as IgM, 50% to 80% are IgG or have an IgG component.[1] They do not bind complement, regardless of their immunoglobulin class, and they do not react with enzyme-treated RBCs. Anti-M appears to be more common in children than in adults and is particularly common in patients with bacterial infections.[7]

Because of antigen **dosage**, many examples of anti-M may react better with M+N− RBCs (genotype *MM*) than with M+N+ RBCs (genotype *MN*). Very weak anti-M may not react with M+N+ RBCs at all, making antibody identification difficult. Antibody reactivity can be enhanced by increasing the serum-to-cell ratio or incubation time, or both, by decreasing incubation temperature or by adding a potentiating medium such as albumin, low ionic strength saline solution (LISS), or polyethylene glycol (PEG).

Some examples of anti-M are pH-dependent, reacting best at pH 6.5. These antibodies may be detected in plasma (which is slightly acidic from the anticoagulant) but not in unacidified serum.[1] Other examples of anti-M react only with RBCs exposed to glucose solutions. Such antibodies react with M+ reagent RBCs or donor RBCs stored in preservative solutions containing glucose but do not react with freshly collected M+ RBCs.

As long as anti-M does not react at 37°C, it is not clinically significant for transfusion and can be ignored. When anti-M reacts at 37°C, it is sufficient to provide units that are crossmatch-compatible at 37°C and at the antiglobulin phase without typing for M antigen. Anti-M rarely causes HTRs, decreased red cell survival, or HDFN.

Anti-N

The serologic characteristics of the common anti-N (made by individuals whose RBCs type M+N− and S+ or s+) are similar to those of anti-M: a cold-reactive IgM or IgG saline agglutinin that does not bind complement or react with enzyme-treated RBCs. Anti-N can demonstrate dosage, reacting better with M−N+ (*NN*) RBCs than with M+N+ (*MN*) RBCs. Rare examples are pH- or glucose-dependent.

Also like anti-M, anti-N is not clinically significant unless it reacts at 37°C. It has been implicated only with rare cases of mild HDFN.[1] Anti-N is less common than anti-M. A potent anti-N can be made by the rare individual whose RBCs type M+N−S−s− because they lack both N and GPB that has 'N' activity (see the "Biochemistry" section).

Anti-N was also seen in renal patients, regardless of their MN type, who were dialyzed on equipment sterilized with formaldehyde. Dialysis-associated anti-N reacts with any N+ or N− RBCs treated with formaldehyde and is called anti-N^f. Formaldehyde may alter the M and N antigens so that they are recognized as foreign. The antibody titer decreases when dialysis treatment and exposure to formaldehyde stops. Because anti-N^f does not react at 37°C, it is clinically insignificant for transfusion.

Anti-S and Anti-s

Most examples of anti-S and anti-s are IgG, reactive at 37°C and the antiglobulin test. A few express optimal reactivity between 10°C and 22°C by saline indirect antiglobulin test. If anti-S or anti-s specificity is suspected but the pattern of reactivity is not clear, incubating tests at room temperature and immediately performing the antiglobulin test (without incubating at 37°C) may help in identification. Dosage effect can be exhibited by many examples of anti-S and anti-s, although it may not be as dramatic as seen with anti-M and anti-N.[1]

The antibodies may or may not react with enzyme-treated RBCs, depending on the extent of treatment and the efficiency of the enzyme. Although seen less often than anti-M, anti-S and anti-s are more likely to be clinically significant. They may bind complement, and they have been implicated in severe HTRs with hemoglobinuria. They have also caused HDFN.

Units selected for transfusion must be antigen-negative and crossmatch-compatible. Because only 11% of whites and 3% of blacks are s−, it can be difficult to provide blood for a patient with anti-s. S– units are much easier to find (45% of whites and 69% of blacks are S–). Antibodies to low-prevalence antigens are commonly found in reagent anti-S; these can cause discrepant antigen typing results.

Biochemistry

Advanced Concepts

GPA, the structure carrying the M and N antigens, is a single-pass membrane SGP that consists of 131 amino acids. The hydrophilic NH_2 terminal end, which lies outside the RBC membrane, has 72 amino acid residues, 15 O-glycosidically linked oligosaccharide chains (GalNAc-serine/threonine), and 1 N-glycosidic chain (sugar-asparagine). The portion that traverses the membrane is hydrophobic and contains 23 amino acids. The hydrophilic COOH end, which contains 36 amino acids and no carbohydrates, lies inside the membrane and interacts weakly with the membrane cytoskeleton.

GPB, the structure carrying the S, s, and U antigens, consists of 72 amino acids and 11 O-linked oligosaccharide chains and no N-glycans. It has an outer glycosylated portion of 44 amino acids, a hydrophobic portion of 20 amino acids that traverses the RBC membrane, and a short cytoplasmic "tail" of 8 amino acids.

The first 26 amino acids on GPB are identical to the first 26 amino acids on the N form of GPA (GPA^N). This N activity of GPB is denoted as 'N' (N-quotes) to distinguish it from the N activity of GPA^N. Anti-N reagents are formulated to not recognize the weak reactivity of the 'N' structure. The U antigen, expressed when normal GPB is present, is located very close to the RBC membrane (see the "U– Phenotype" section).

Most O-linked carbohydrate structures on GPA and GPB are branched tetrasaccharides containing one GalNAc, one Gal, and two NeuNAc (sialic acid). NeuNAc helps give the RBC its negative charge. About 70% of the RBC NeuNAc is carried by GPA, and about 16% is carried by GPB.

GPA associates with protein band 3, which affects the expression of the antigen Wr^b of the Diego blood group system (located on protein band 3). GPB appears to be associated with the Rh protein and Rh-associated glycoprotein complex as evidenced by the greatly reduced S and s expression on Rh_{null} RBCs.[7]

Other antigens within the MNS system have been evaluated biochemically and at the molecular level. Some are associated with altered GPA because of amino acid substitutions or changes in carbohydrate chains. Others are expressed on variants of GPA or GPB. Still others result from a genetic event that encodes a hybrid glycophorin that has parts of both GPA and GPB. The altered glycophorins are associated with changes in glycosylation, changes in molecular weight, loss of high-prevalence antigens or the appearance of novel low-prevalence antigens, or alterations in the expression of MNS antigens.[1,7,9]

RBCs that lack GPA or GPB are not associated with disease or decreased RBC survival (see the "Disease Associations" section). GPA and GPB are expressed on renal endothelium and epithelium.[9]

Genetics

The genes GYPA and GYPB, which code for GPA and GPB, respectively, are located on chromosome 4 at 4q28–q31. The known alleles for GYPA (M/N) and GYPB (S/s) are codominant. The genes are highly homologous (meaning they are very similar) and probably arose by gene duplication. GYPA is considered to be the ancestral gene.[25]

GYPA is organized into seven exons. GYPB has a size and arrangement similar to those of GYPA but has only five coding exons plus one noncoding or pseudoexon. A third highly homologous gene, GYPE, does not appear to make a glycoprotein that has been definitively recognized on the RBC surface, but it participates in gene rearrangements that result in variant alleles.

Misalignment of GYPA and GYPB during meiosis, followed by an unequal crossing over, appears to explain some of the variant glycophorins observed in the MNS system. The resulting new reciprocal GYP(A-B) and GYP(B-A) genes encode GP(A-B) and GP(B-A) hybrid glycophorins, respectively (Fig. 8–6).[7,26] The point of fusion between the GPA and GPB part in the hybrid glycophorin can give rise to novel antigens (e.g., antigen of low prevalence).

For more complex variant glycophorins, a gene conversion event probably occurs. Gene conversion involves a non-reciprocal exchange of genetic material from one gene to another homologous gene (Fig. 8–7).[7,26] As with hybrids resulting from crossing over, the new amino acid sequence at the junction of the hybrid glycophorin can give rise to novel antigens of low prevalence. Also, expected antigens may be missing if the coding exons are replaced by the inserted genetic material.

GPA- and GPB-Deficient Phenotypes

RBCs of three rare phenotypes lack GPA or GPB or both GPA and GPB; consequently, they lack all MNS antigens that are normally expressed on those structures.

U– Phenotype

The U antigen is located on GPB very close to the RBC membrane between amino acids 33 and 39 (see Fig. 8–5).

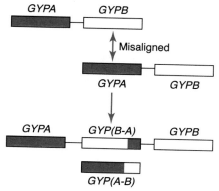

Figure 8–6. Depiction of how misalignment during meiosis can lead to a crossover and reciprocal GYP(B-A) and GYP(A–B) hybrids.

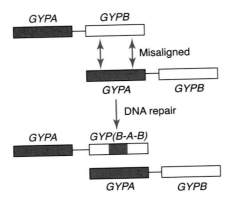

Figure 8–7. In a gene conversion event, nucleotides from one strand of DNA are transferred to the misaligned homologous gene. If this is the coding strand, a hybrid glycophorin will be formed; the partner chromosome will be repaired and carry the naïve (unaltered) *GYPA* and *GYPB* genes.

This high-prevalence antigen is found on RBCs of all individuals except about 1% of African Americans (and 1% to 35% of Africans) who lack GPB because of a partial or complete deletion of *GYPB*. The RBCs usually type S–s–U–, and these individuals can make anti-U in response to transfusion or pregnancy. Anti-U is typically IgG and has been reported to cause severe and fatal HTRs and HDFN.

The U antigen is resistant to enzyme treatment; thus, most examples of anti-U react equally well with untreated and enzyme-treated RBCs. However, there are rare examples of broadly reactive anti-U that do not react with papain-treated RBCs.[1]

Some examples of anti-U react with apparent U– RBCs, although weakly, by adsorption and elution.[7] Such RBCs are said to be U variant (U^{var}); these have an altered GPB that does not express S or s. There is a strong correlation between the low-prevalence antigen He, found in about 3% of African Americans, and U^{var} expression.[27]

Because examples of anti-U are heterogeneous, U– units selected for transfusion must be crossmatched to determine compatibility. Some patients may tolerate U^{var} units; others may not. Many examples of anti-U are actually anti-U plus anti-GPB. If the patient is U– and N–, the antibody may actually be a potent anti-N plus anti-U, making the search for compatible blood more difficult.

En(a–) Phenotype

In 1969, Darnborough and coworkers[28] and Furuhjelm and colleagues[29] described an antibody to the same high-prevalence antigen, called En^a (for *envelope*), which reacted with all RBCs except those of the propositi. In both of these cases, the En(a–) individuals appeared to be M–N– with reduced NeuNAc on their RBCs. The RBCs of the two individuals were mutually compatible.

Most En(a–) individuals produce anti-En^a, which is an umbrella term for reactivity against various portions of GPA unrelated to M or N, but not all antibodies detect the same portion. Anti-En^{a}TS recognizes a trypsin-sensitive (TS) area on GPA between amino acids 20 and 39, anti-En^{a}FS reacts with a ficin-sensitive (FS) area between amino acids 46

and 56, and anti-En^{a}FR reacts with a ficin-resistant (FR) area around amino acids 62 to 72.[1,7]

Although the gene responsible for this phenotype has been termed *En*, it is now known that the En(a–) phenotype has more than one origin. Most often, the En(a–) phenotype results from homozygosity for a rare gene deletion at the *GYPA* locus; consequently, no GPA is produced, but GPB is not affected. This type of En(a–) inheritance is called En(a–)Fin, representing the type described in the Finnish report.[29] However, the En(a–) phenotype in the English report[28] probably represents heterozygosity for a hybrid gene along with the very rare M^k gene; this type is often called En(a–)UK. Several other En(a–) phenotypes have been reported that result from homozygosity for a variant allele or inheritance of two dissimilar variant alleles.

Anti-En^a can be confused with two other specificities that react with all normal RBCs—anti-Pr and anti-Wr^b. Anti-Pr does not react with enzyme-treated RBCs and can be confused with anti-En^{a}FS; anti-Wr^b does not react with En(a–) RBCs but does react with enzyme-treated RBCs and can be confused with anti-En^{a}FR. Anti-En^a has caused severe HTRs and HDFN. It is extremely difficult and may be impossible to find units compatible for patients with anti-En^a; siblings are a potential source of compatible blood if they are also ABO and Rh compatible.

M^k Phenotype

The rare silent gene M^k was named by Metaxas and Metaxas-Buhler in 1964 when they found an allele that did not produce M or N.[7] A second family showed that M^k was also silent at the Ss locus. Several other M^k heterozygotes have been found. In 1979, two related M^kM^k blood donors were found in Japan. The RBCs of these individuals typed M–N–S–s–U–En(a–)Wr(a–b–), but they had a normal hematologic picture. More individuals have since been identified, and it is now known that the M^k gene represents a single, near-complete deletion of both *GYPA* and *GYPB*[7]; thus, M^kM^k is the null phenotype in the MNS system. The M^kM^k genotype is associated with decreased RBC sialic acid content but increased glycosylation of RBC membrane bands 3 and 4.1.

Other Antibodies in the MNS System

Antibodies to antigens other than M, N, S, and s are rarely encountered and can usually be grouped into two categories: those directed against low-prevalence antigens and those directed against high-prevalence antigens.

Antibodies to high-prevalence antigens are easily detected with antibody detection RBCs. Antibodies to low-prevalence antigens are rarely detected by the antibody detection test but are seen as an unexpected incompatible crossmatch or an unexplained case of HDFN. Few hospital blood banks have the test cells available to identify the specificity, but enzyme reactivity and MNS antigen typing may offer clues.

When antibodies to low-prevalence antigens are encountered, it is common practice to transfuse units that are crossmatch-compatible at 37°C and in the antiglobulin phase. Typing sera for MNS antigens other than M and N and S and s are not generally available, so the antigen status of compatible RBCs can seldom be confirmed. Also, when one antibody to a low-prevalence antigen is found, antibodies to other low-prevalence antigens are also frequently present in the same serum. If the antibody is directed to a high-prevalence antigen, the assistance of an immunohematology reference laboratory is generally needed to identify the antibody and obtain appropriate antigen-negative units.

Autoantibodies

Autoantibodies to M and N have been reported.[1] Not all examples of anti-M in M+ individuals or anti-N in N+ individuals are autoantibodies. Many fail to react with the patient's own RBCs. It may be that these individuals have altered GPA and that their antibody is specific for a portion of the common antigen they lack. Autoantibodies to U and En^a are more common and may be associated with warm-type autoimmune hemolytic anemia.

Disease Associations

GPA^M may serve as the receptor by which certain pyelonephritogenic strains of *E. coli* gain entry to the urinary tract. The malaria parasite *Plasmodium falciparum* appears to use alternative receptors, including GPA and GPB for cell invasion; some of these receptors also involve NeuNAc.

The Kell (006) and Kx (019) Systems

The Kell blood group system consists of 32 high-prevalence and low-prevalence antigens; it was the first blood group system discovered after the introduction of antiglobulin testing. Anti-K was identified in 1946 in the serum of Mrs. Kelleher. The antibody reacted with the RBCs of her newborn infant, her older daughter, her husband, and about 7% of the random population.[7] In 1949, anti-k, the high-prevalence antithetical partner to K, was described. Kell remained a two-antigen system until the antithetical antigens Kp^a and Kp^b were described in 1957 and 1958, respectively. Likewise, Js^a (described in 1958) and Js^b (described in 1963) were found to be antithetical and related to the Kell system. The discovery of the null phenotype in 1957, designated K$_o$, helped associate many other antigens with the Kell system. Antibodies that reacted with all RBCs except those with the K$_o$ phenotype recognized high-prevalence antigens that were phenotypically related.

The 32 antigens included in the Kell blood group system, designated by the symbol KEL or 006 by the ISBT, are listed in Table 8–14. In 1961, a numerical notation was proposed for the Kell system. As new antigens were discovered, some received only a number for the antigen name. However, the traditional notation persisted and is more useful in conveying antithetical relationships (e.g., K and Js^a). Consequently, the commonly used nomenclature for Kell antigens is a mixture of symbols using letters and numbers. The associated antigen Kx is the only antigen in the Kx system, ISBT number 019 and symbol XK.

Table 8–14 Kell System Antigens

NAME	NUMERIC TERMINOLOGY	ISBT NUMBER	PREVALENCE (%)	ANTITHETICAL ANTIGEN(S)	YEAR DISCOVERED
K	1	KEL1	9	k	1946
k	2	KEL2	99.8	K	1949
Kp^a	3	KEL3	2 (whites)	Kp^b, Kp^c	1957
Kp^b	4	KEL4	>99.9	Kp^a, Kp^c	1958
Ku	5	KEL5	>99.9		1957
Js^a	6	KEL6	<0.1 whites 20 blacks	Js^b	1958
Js^b	7	KEL7	>99.9 whites 99 blacks	Js^a	1963
Ul^a	10	KEL10	<3 Finns		1968
Côté	11	KEL11	>99.9	K17	1971
Boc	12	KEL12	>99.9		1973
SGRO	13	KEL13	>99.9		1973
San	14	KEL14	>99.9	K24	1973
k-like	16	KEL16	99.8		1976
Wk^a	17	KEL17	0.3	K11	1974
VM	18	KEL18	>99.9		1975

Continued

Table 8–14   Kell System Antigens—cont'd

NAME	NUMERIC TERMINOLOGY	ISBT NUMBER	PREVALENCE (%)	ANTITHETICAL ANTIGEN(S)	YEAR DISCOVERED
Sub	19	KEL19	>99.9		1979
Km	20	KEL20	>99.9		1979
Kp^c	21	KEL21	<0.1	Kp^a, Kp^b	1945
Ikar	22	KEl22	>99.9		1982
Centauro	23	KEL23	<0.01		1987
CL	24	KEL24	<2	K14	1985
VLAN		KEL25	<0.1		1996
TOU		KEL26	>99.9		1995
RAZ	K27	KEL27	>99.9		1994
VONG		KEL28	<0.1		2003
KALT		KEL29	>99.9		2006
KTIM		KEL30	>99.9		2006
KYO		KEL31	<0.1		2006
KUCI		KEL32	>99.9		2007
KANT		KEL33	>99.9		2007
KASH		KEL34	>99.9		2007
KELP		KEL35	>99.9		2010

Obsolete: K8, K9, K15

Basic Concepts

Kell blood group antigens are found only on RBCs. They have not been found on platelets or on lymphocytes, granulocytes, or monocytes. The associated Xk protein is found in erythroid tissues and in other tissues, such as brain, lymphoid organs, heart, and skeletal muscle.[30]

The K antigen can be detected on fetal RBCs as early as 10 weeks and is well developed at birth. The k antigen has been detected at 7 weeks. The total number of K antigen sites per RBC is quite low: only 3,500 up to 18,000 sites per RBC.[9] Despite its lower quantity, K is very immunogenic.

The antigens are not denatured by the routine blood bank enzymes ficin and papain but are destroyed by trypsin and chymotrypsin when used in combination.[7] Thiol-reducing agents, such as 100 to 200 mM DTT, 2-mercaptoethanol (2-ME), AET, and ZZAP (which contains DTT in addition to enzyme), destroy Kell antigens but not Kx. Glycine-acid EDTA (an IgG-removal agent) also destroys Kell antigens.

The prevalence of common Kell phenotypes are listed in Table 8–15. There are five sets of antithetical antigens; antithetical relationships have not been established for the other high- and low-prevalence antigens. Some of the Kell antigens (e.g., Js^b) are more prevalent in certain populations.

Table 8–15   Prevalence of Common Kell System Phenotypes

PHENOTYPE	WHITES (%)	BLACKS (%)
K–k+	91	96.5
K+k+	8.8	3.5
K+k–	0.2	<0.1
Kp(a+b–)	<0.1	0
Kp(a+b+)	2.3	Rare
Kp(a–b+)	97.7	100
Js(a+b–)	0	1
Js(a+b+)	Rare	19
Js(a–b+)	100	80

K and k Antigens

Excluding ABO, K is rated second only to D in immunogenicity. Most anti-K appear to be induced by pregnancy and transfusion.[7] Fortunately, the prevalence of K antigen is low (9% in whites), and the chance of receiving a K+ unit is small. If anti-K develops, compatible units are easy to find.

Antibodies to k antigen are seldom encountered. Only 2 in 1,000 individuals lack k and are capable of developing the antibody. The likelihood that these few individuals will receive transfusions and become immunized is even less.

Kp^a, Kp^b, and Kp^c Antigens

Alleles *Kp^a* and *Kp^c* are low-prevalence mutations of their high-prevalence partner *Kp^b*. The Kp^a antigen is found in about 2% of whites. The *Kp^a* gene is associated with suppression of other Kell antigens on the same molecule, including k and Js^b.[7] The effect appears to result from a reduced amount of the Kell glycoprotein (produced by the *Kp^a* allele) inserted in the RBC membrane. The Kp^c antigen is even more rare.

Js^a and Js^b Antigens

The Js^a antigen, antithetical to the high-prevalence antigen Js^b, is found in about 20% of blacks but in fewer than 0.1% of whites.[9] The prevalence of Js^a in blacks is almost 10 times greater than the prevalence of the K antigen in blacks. Js^a and Js^b were linked to the Kell system when it was discovered that K$_o$ RBCs were Js(a–b–).

Anti-K

Outside the ABO and Rh antibodies, anti-K is the most common antibody seen in the blood bank. Anti-K is usually IgG and reactive in the antiglobulin phase, but some examples agglutinate saline-suspended RBCs. The antibody is usually made in response to antigen exposure through pregnancy and transfusion and can persist for many years.

Naturally occurring IgM examples of anti-K are rare and have been associated with bacterial infections. Marsh and colleagues[31] studied an IgM anti-K in an untransfused 20-day-old infant with an *E. coli* O125:B15 infection whose mother did not make anti-K. The organism was shown to have a somatic K-like antigen that reacted with the infant's antibody, so the bacterial antigen was thought to have been the stimulus. The antibody disappeared after recovery.

Some examples of anti-K react poorly in methods incorporating low-ionic media, such as LISS, and in some automated systems. The most reliable method of detection is the indirect antiglobulin test. The potentiating medium, PEG, may increase reactivity.

Anti-K has been implicated in severe HTRs. Although some examples of anti-K bind complement, in vivo RBC destruction is usually extravascular via the macrophages in the spleen. Anti-K is also associated with severe HDFN. The antibody titer does not always accurately predict the severity of disease; stillbirth has been seen with anti-K titers as low as 64. Fetal anemia in anti-K HDFN is associated with suppression of erythropoiesis due to destruction of erythroid precursor cells, which can be additional to destruction of circulating antigen-positive RBCs, as seen in anti-D HDFN. Kell glycoprotein is expressed on fetal RBCs at a much earlier stage of erythropoiesis than Rh antigens.[32] When a pregnant woman is identified as making anti-K, it is prudent to type the father for the K antigen. If he's K+, the fetus should be monitored carefully for signs of HDFN.

Antibodies to Kp^a, Js^a, and Other Low-Prevalence Kell Antigens

Antibodies to the low-prevalence Kell antigens are rare because so few people are exposed to these antigens. Because routine antibody detection RBCs do not carry low-prevalence antigens, the antibodies are most often detected through unexpected incompatible crossmatches or cases of HDFN.

The serologic characteristics and clinical significance of these antibodies parallel anti-K. The original anti-Kp^a was naturally occurring, but most antibodies result from transfusion or pregnancy.

Antibodies to k, Kp^b, Js^b, and Other High-Prevalence Kell Antigens

Antibodies to high-prevalence Kell system antigens are rare because so few people lack these antigens. They also parallel anti-K in serologic characteristics and clinical significance.

The high-prevalence antibodies are easy to detect but difficult to work with, because most blood banks do not have the antigen-negative panel cells needed to exclude other alloantibodies, nor do they have typing reagents to phenotype the patient's RBCs. Testing an unidentified high-prevalence antibody against DTT- or AET-treated RBCs is a helpful technique: Reactivity that is abolished with DTT or AET treatment suggests that the antibody may be related to the Kell system and enables the technologist to exclude common alloantibodies. Caution is needed before assigning Kell system specificity until antigen-negative RBCs are tested, because DTT also denatures JMH and high-prevalence antigens in the LW, Lutheran, Dombrock, Cromer, and Knops systems. Finding compatible units for transfusion can be difficult; siblings and rare-donor inventories are the most likely sources. Patients with antibodies to high-prevalence antigens should be encouraged to donate autologous units and, if possible, to participate in a rare-donor program.

Biochemistry

Advanced Concepts

The Kell antigens are located on a glycoprotein that consists of 731 amino acids and spans the RBC membrane once. The N-terminal domain is intracellular, and the large external C-terminal domain is highly folded by disulfide linkages (Fig. 8–8). The Kell glycoprotein is covalently linked with another protein, called Xk, by a single disulfide bond. The Xk protein (440 amino acids) is predicted to span the RBC membrane ten times. Kell antigen expression is dependent upon the presence of the Xk protein.

The Kell glycoprotein is a member of the neprilysin (M13) family of zinc endopeptidases associated with the cleavage of big endothelins, but how this relates to the physiological role of the Kell glycoprotein remains unclear. The structure of the Xk protein suggests a membrane transport protein. The absence of Xk results in McLeod syndrome (see the "McLeod Phenotype and Syndrome" section below).

Genetics

The *KEL* gene, located on chromosome 7 (at 7q34), is organized into 19 exons of coding sequence. Single base mutations encoding amino acid substitutions are responsible for the different Kell antigens. Several different mutations (e.g., point, frameshift, or splice site mutations) have been found that result in the rare null phenotype K_o.[7,9]

No Kell haplotype has been shown to code for more than one low-prevalence antigen. People who test positive for two low-prevalence Kell antigens have always been found to carry the encoding alleles on opposite chromosomes. For example, someone who types Kp(a+) and Js(a+) is genetically *kKp^aJs^b* on one chromosome and *kKp^bJs^a* on the other.

The *XK* gene, which encodes the Kx antigen, is independent of *KEL* and is located on the short arm of the X chromosome at position Xp21.1.[7]

The Kx Antigen

Kx is present on all RBCs except those of the rare McLeod phenotype (see the "McLeod Phenotype and Syndrome" section below). K_o and K_{mod} phenotype RBCs have increased Kx antigen.[7] When Kell antigens are denatured with AET or DTT, the expression of Kx increases.

The K_o Phenotype and Anti-Ku(K5)

K_o RBCs lack expression of all Kell antigens. K_o RBCs have no membrane abnormality and survive normally in circulation. The phenotype is rare; data suggest a frequency of 1:25,000 in whites.[7]

Immunized individuals with the K_o phenotype typically make an antibody called anti-Ku (K5) that recognizes the "universal" Kell antigen (Ku) present on all RBCs except K_o.

Anti-Ku appears to be a single specificity and cannot be separated into components. Anti-Ku has caused both HDFN and HTRs.[7]

Because K_o RBCs are negative for k, Kp^b, Js^b, and so forth, they are very useful in investigating complex antibody problems. They can help confirm a Kell system specificity or rule out other underlying specificities. When K_o RBCs are not available, they can be made artificially by treating normal RBCs with DTT, AET, or glycine-acid EDTA.

The McLeod Phenotype and Syndrome

In 1961, Allen and coworkers[33] described a young male medical student who initially appeared to be Kell null but who demonstrated weak expression of k, Kp^b, and Js^b detectable by adsorption-elution methods. This unusual phenotype was called McLeod, after the student.

The McLeod phenotype is very rare. All who have it are male, and inheritance is X-linked through a carrier mother. McLeod phenotype RBCs lack Kx and another high-prevalence antigen, Km, and have marked depression of all other Kell antigens. The weakened expression of the Kell antigens is designated by a superscript w for "weak"—for example, K–k+^w Kp(a–b+^w). The McLeod phenotype has been associated with several mutations and deletions at the *XK* locus.

A significant proportion of the RBCs in individuals with the McLeod phenotype are acanthocytic (having irregular shapes and protrusions) with decreased deformability and reduced in vivo survival. As a result, individuals with the McLeod phenotype have a chronic but often well-compensated hemolytic anemia characterized by reticulocytosis, bilirubinemia, splenomegaly, and reduced serum haptoglobin levels.

Individuals with the McLeod phenotype have a variety of muscle and nerve disorders that, together with the serologic and hematologic picture, are collectively known as the McLeod syndrome, one of the neuroacanthocytosis syndromes. McLeod individuals develop a slow, progressive form of muscular dystrophy between ages 40 and 50 years and cardiomegaly (leading to cardiomyopathy). The associated neurological disorder presents initially as areflexia (a lack of deep tendon reflexes) and progresses to choreiform movements (well-coordinated but involuntary movements). These individuals also have elevated serum creatinine phosphokinase levels of the MM type (cardiac/skeletal muscle) and carbonic anhydrase III levels.

In 1971, Giblett and colleagues made an association between the rare Kell phenotypes, including the McLeod phenotype, and the rare X-linked chronic granulomatous disease (CGD).[34] CGD is characterized by the inability of phagocytes to make NADH oxidase, an enzyme important in generating H_2O_2, which is used to kill ingested bacteria. Afflicted children can die at an early age from overwhelming infections if not treated. Not all males with the McLeod phenotype have CGD, nor do all patients with CGD have the McLeod phenotype.

At one time it was suggested that CGD was caused by a lack of Kx on white blood cells, and several alleles at the *XK* locus were proposed to explain Kx expression on McLeod RBCs and

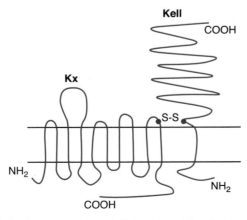

Figure 8–8.   Proposed structures for Kell and Kx proteins. The two proteins are linked through one disulfide bond. The conformation of the large external domain of the Kell glycoprotein is unknown; 15 cysteine residues suggest the presence of disulfide bonds and extensive folding.

CGD white blood cells. More recent data have shown that this theory is not valid. The *XK* gene resides on the X chromosome near deletions associated with CGD, Duchenne muscular dystrophy, and retinitis pigmentosa, in the Xp21 region.

The expression of Kx in women who are carriers of the McLeod phenotype follows the Lyon hypothesis, which states that in early embryo development, one X chromosome randomly shuts down in female cells that have two. All cells descending from the resulting cell line express only the allele on the active chromosome. Hence, McLeod carriers exhibit two RBC populations: one having Kx and normal Kell antigens, the other having the McLeod phenotype and acanthocytosis. The percentage of McLeod phenotype RBCs in carriers varies from 5% to 85%.[1]

McLeod males with CGD make anti-Kx + Km, which reacts strongly with K_o RBCs, weaker with normal Kell phenotype RBCs, and not at all with McLeod phenotype RBCs. Anti-Km is made by McLeod males without CGD. There are rare reports of a McLeod male without CGD who has made anti-Kx + Km.[35] The expression of Kell antigens on RBCs with common, McLeod, and K_o phenotypes is summarized in Table 8–16.

Altered Expressions of Kell Antigens

Weaker-than-normal Kell antigen expression is associated with the McLeod phenotype and the suppression by the Kp^a gene (cis-modified effect) on Kell antigens. Depressed Kell antigens are also seen on RBCs with the rare Gerbich-negative phenotypes Ge: –2, –3, 4 and Ge: –2, –3, –4. The phenotypic relationship between Gerbich and Kell is not understood. The umbrella term K_{mod} is used to describe other phenotypes with very weak Kell expression, often requiring adsorption-elution tests for detection. As a group, these RBCs have a reduced amount of Kell glycoprotein and enhanced Kx expression. Some K_{mod} individuals make an antibody that resembles anti-Ku but does not react with other K_{mod} RBCs (unlike anti-Ku made by K_o individuals).

Patients with autoimmune hemolytic anemia, in which the autoantibody is directed against a Kell antigen, may have depressed expression of that antigen. Antigen strength returns to normal when the anemia resolves and the DAT becomes negative. This phenomenon appears to be more common in the Kell system than in others.[1]

Finally, RBCs may appear to acquire Kell antigens. McGinnis and coworkers[36] described a K– patient who acquired a K-like antigen during a *Streptococcus faecium*

infection. Cultures containing the disrupted organism converted K– cells to K+ but bacteria-free filtrates did not.

Autoantibodies

Most Kell autoantibodies are directed against undefined high-prevalence Kell antigens, but identifiable autoantibodies to K, Kp^b, and K13 have been reported. Mimicking specificities have also been reported, such as when an apparent anti-K is eluted from DAT+ K– RBCs and the anti-K in the eluate can be adsorbed onto K– RBCs.

The Duffy (008) System

The Duffy blood group system was named for Mr. Duffy, a multiply transfused hemophiliac who in 1950 was found to have the first described example of anti-Fy^a. One year later, the antibody defining its antithetical antigen, Fy^b, was found in the serum of a woman who had had three pregnancies.

In 1955, Sanger and colleagues[37] reported that the majority of African Americans tested were Fy(a–b–). The gene responsible for this null phenotype was called *Fy*. *FyFy* appeared to be a common genotype in blacks, especially in Africa; the gene is exceedingly rare in whites.

In 1975, it was observed that Fy(a–b–) RBCs resist infection in vitro by the monkey malaria organism *Plasmodium knowlesi*. It was later shown that Fy(a–b–) RBCs also resist infection by *P. vivax* (one of the organisms causing malaria in humans).[37] This discovery provides an explanation for the predominance of the Fy(a–b–) phenotype in persons originating from West Africa.

Antibodies to other antigens in the Duffy blood group system, Fy3, Fy5, are rarely encountered. RBCs that are Fy(a–b–) are also Fy: –3, –5. Fy5 is also not present on Rh_{null} RBCs, regardless of the Fy^a or Fy^b status of those RBCs. The Duffy blood group system is designated by the symbol FY or 008 by the ISBT.

Fy^a and Fy^b Antigens

Basic Concepts

The Duffy antigens most important in routine blood bank serology are Fy^a and Fy^b. They can be identified on fetal RBCs as early as 6 weeks gestational age and are well developed at birth. There are about 13,000 to 14,000 Fy^a

PHENOTYPE	RBC ANTIGEN EXPRESSION			POSSIBLE ANTIBODY
	Kell Antigens	**Km**	**Kx**	
Common	k, Kp^b, Js^b, K11 . . .	Normal	Weak	Alloantibody
K_o	None	None	Increased	Anti-Ku
McLeod	Trace k, Kp^a, Js^b, K11 . . .	None	None	Anti-Kx + Km (CGD) Anti-Km (non-CGD)

Table 8–16 Expression of Kell Antigens on RBCs With Common, K_o, and McLeod Phenotypes

or Fy^b sites on Fy(a+b–) and Fy(a–b+) RBCs, respectively; there are half that number of Fy^a sites on Fy(a+b+) RBCs.[7] The antigens have not been found on platelets, lymphocytes, monocytes, or granulocytes, but they have been identified in other body tissues, including brain, colon, endothelium, lung, spleen, thyroid, thymus, and kidney cells.[9] The prevalence of the common phenotypes in the Duffy system are given in Table 8–17. The disparity in distribution in different races is notable.

Fy^a and Fy^b antigens are destroyed by common proteolytic enzymes, such as ficin, papain, bromelin, and chymotrypsin, and by ZZAP (which contains either papain or ficin in addition to DTT); they are not affected by DTT alone, AET, or glycine-acid EDTA treatment. Neuraminidase may reduce the molecular weight of Fy^a and Fy^b, but it does not destroy antigenic activity and neither does purified trypsin.

Anti-Fy^a and Anti-Fy^b

Anti-Fy^a is a common antibody and is found as a single specificity or in a mixture of antibodies. Anti-Fy^a occurs three times less frequently than anti-K. Anti-Fy^b is 20 times less common than anti-Fy^a and often occurs in combination with other antibodies. The antibodies are usually IgG and react best at the antiglobulin phase. Rare examples of anti-Fy^a and anti-Fy^b bind complement. A few examples are saline agglutinins. Antibody activity is enhanced in a low ionic strength medium. Because anti-Fy^a and anti-Fy^b do not react with enzyme-treated RBCs, this is a helpful technique when multiple antibodies are present.

Some examples of anti-Fy^a and anti-Fy^b show dosage, reacting more strongly with RBCs that have a double dose than RBCs from heterozygotes. It must be remembered that some reagent RBCs that appear to be from homozygotes (and have a double dose of either Fy^a or Fy^b) may actually be from heterozygotes if they are from black donors; a silent allele, *Fy*, is commonly found in blacks. For example, Fy(a+b–) RBCs will have a double dose of Fy^a if they are from a white *Fy^{a}Fy^a* donor but will have a single dose of Fy^a if they are from a black donor who is genetically *Fy^{a}Fy*. Additional phenotypic markers commonly found in black donors can give a clue to the possible presence of the silent *Fy* allele: R$_o$, S–s–, V+VS+, Js(a+), Le(a–b–).

Anti-Fy^a and anti-Fy^b have been associated with acute and delayed HTRs. Once the antibody is identified, Fy(a–) or Fy(b–) blood must be given; finding such units in a random population is not difficult. For example, one in three random units of blood is Fy(a–) and one in five random units of blood is Fy(b–). Anti-Fy^a and anti-Fy^b are associated with HDFN that ranges from mild to severe.

Rare autoantibodies with mimicking Fy^a and Fy^b specificity have been reported—for example, anti-Fy^b that can be adsorbed onto and eluted from Fy(a+b–) RBCs. Issitt and Anstee[1] suggest that these may represent alloantibodies with "sloppy" specificity made early in an immune response.

Biochemistry

Advanced Concepts

Enzymes, membrane solubilization methods, immunoblotting, radiolabeling, and amino acid sequencing have all been used to study the biochemistry of Duffy antigens.[1] Duffy antigens reside on a glycoprotein of 336 amino acids that has a relative mass of 36 kD and two *N*-glycosylation sites (Fig. 8–9).[38] The glycoprotein is predicted to traverse the cell membrane seven times and has two predicted disulfide bridges.

The amino acid at position 42 on the Duffy glycoprotein defines the Fy^a and Fy^b polymorphism: Fy^a has glycine, and Fy^b has aspartic acid. The Fy3 epitope, as defined by monoclonal antibody, is on the third extracellular loop, and Fy6 appears to involve amino acids 19 through 25.[38]

The Duffy glycoprotein is a member of the superfamily of chemokine receptors and is known as the *Duffy antigen receptor for chemokines* (DARC). Thus, in addition to being a receptor for the malaria parasite *P. vivax*, the Duffy glycoprotein binds a variety of proinflammatory cytokines.

Genetics

In 1968, the Duffy gene was linked to a visible, inherited abnormality of chromosome 1, thus becoming the first human gene to be assigned to a specific chromosome. The gene is located near the centromere on the long arm of chromosome 1 at position 1q23.2. The *Fy* locus is syntenic to the *Rh* locus, which is located near the tip of the short arm; that is, they

Table 8–17	**Prevalence of Common Duffy Phenotypes**		
PHENOTYPE	**WHITES (%)**	**AFRICAN AMERICANS (%)**	**CHINESE (%)**
Fy(a+b–)	17	9	90.8
Fy(a+b+)	49	1	8.9
Fy(a–b+)	34	22	0.3
Fy(a–b–)	Very rare	68	0

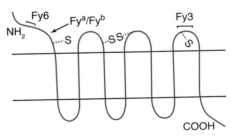

Figure 8–9. Proposed structure for the Duffy protein. Disulfide bonds probably link the NH2 terminal domain and the third loop and the first and second loop.

are on the same chromosome, but they are far enough apart that linkage cannot be demonstrated and serologically they appear to segregate independently.

There are three common alleles at the *Fy* locus: *Fy^a*, *Fy^b*, and *Fy*. *Fy^a* and *Fy^b* encode the antithetical antigens Fy^a and Fy^b, respectively, and *Fy* is a silent allele and is the major allele in blacks. The *Fy* gene in Fy(a–b–) blacks is an *Fy^b* variant with a change in the promoter region of the gene, which disrupts the binding site for mRNA transcription in the RBC.[9] Consequently, Fy(a–b–) blacks do not express Fy^b on their RBCs but express Fy^b in other tissues. The presence of Fy^b in tissues presumably precludes the recognition of Fy^b as foreign; thus, no anti-Fy^b is made by these individuals. A molecular analysis of Fy(a–b–) whites revealed different mutations. These individuals carry no Duffy protein on their RBCs or on other tissues and thus can form anti-Fy^b and anti-Fy3.

Typing for Duffy antigens has been performed on the RBCs of chimpanzees, gorillas, and old- and new-world monkeys. The results suggest that *Fy3* developed first, then *Fy^b*, and that *Fy^a* arose during human evolution.[9]

Fy^x

Fy^x was described in 1965 as a new allele at the *Fy* locus. It does not produce a distinct antigen but rather is an inherited weak form of Fy^b that reacts with some examples of anti-Fy^b. Fy^x has been described in white populations. Individuals with *Fy^x* may type Fy(b–), but their RBCs adsorb and elute anti-Fy^b. They also have depressed expression of their Fy3 and Fy5 antigens. The decreased expression of Fy^b due to *Fy^x* appears to be related to a reduced amount of Duffy glycoprotein on the surface of RBCs.[39] There is no anti-Fy^x.

Fy3 Antigen and Antibody

In 1971, anti-Fy3 was found in the serum of an Fy(a–b–) white Australian female. It reacted with all RBCs tested except those of the Fy(a–b–) phenotype. Because it was an inseparable anti-Fy^aFy^b, it was thought to react with an antigenic determinant or precursor common to both Fy^a and Fy^b and was called Fy3. Unlike Fy^a and Fy^b, the Fy3 antigen is not destroyed by enzymes.

Anti-Fy3 is a rare antibody made by Fy(a–b–) individuals who lack the Duffy glycoprotein. The Fy(a–b–) phenotype has been found in whites, Cree Indian families, and blacks.[1] Blacks with the Fy(a–b–) phenotype rarely make anti-Fy3. Some blacks who make anti-Fy3 initially make anti-Fy^a.[7]

Fy5 Antigen and Antibody

In 1973, Colledge and coworkers[40] discovered anti-Fy5 in the serum of an Fy(a–b–) black child who later died of leukemia. Initially it was thought to be a second example of anti-Fy3, because it reacted with all Fy(a+) or Fy(b+) RBCs but not with Fy(a–b–) cells. The antibody differed in that it reacted with the cells from an Fy(a–b–)Fy:–3 white female, but it did not react with Fy(a+) or Fy(b+) Rh_null RBCs and reacted only weakly with Fy(a+) or Fy(b+) D–– RBCs.

Sometimes, sera containing anti-Fy5 also contain anti-Fy^a. Several examples of anti-Fy5 have been reported in multiply transfused Fy(a–b–) sickle cell patients with a mixture of other antibodies.

The molecular structure of Fy5 is not known, but it appears to be the result of interaction between the Rh complex and the Duffy glycoprotein. People who are Fy(a–b–) or Rh_null do not make Fy5 antigen and are at risk of making the antibody, although few do. Like Fy3, Fy5 is not destroyed by enzymes.

The Kidd (009) System

The Kidd blood group is a simple and straightforward system consisting of only three antigens. In 1951, Allen and colleagues[41] reported finding an antibody in the serum of Mrs. Kidd, whose infant had HDFN. The antibody, named anti-Jk^a, reacted with 77% of Bostonians. Its antithetical partner, Jk^b, was found 2 years later. The null phenotype Jk(a–b–) was described in 1959. The propositus made an antibody to a high-prevalence antigen called Jk3, which is present on any RBC positive for Jk^a or Jk^b. No other antigens associated with the Kidd system have been described.

The Kidd system is designated by the symbol JK or 009 by the ISBT. It has special significance to routine blood banking because of its antibodies, which can be difficult to detect and are a common cause of HTRs.

Jk^a and Jk^b Antigens

Basic Concepts

Jk^a and Jk^b are antigens commonly found on RBCs of most individuals. Table 8–18 summarizes the prevalence of the four known phenotypes. There are notable differences in antigen frequency among various races: 91% of blacks and 77% of whites are Jk(a+); 57% of blacks and only 28% of whites are Jk(b–).

Jk^a and Jk^b antigens are well developed on the RBCs of neonates. Jk^a has been detected on fetal RBCs as early as 11 weeks; Jk^b has been detected at 7 weeks.[7] Although this early development of Kidd antigens contributes to the potential for HDFN, anti-Jk^a and anti-Jk^b are only rarely responsible for severe HDFN. Jk(a+b–) RBCs carry 14,000 antigen sites per cell.[7] The Kidd antigens are not very immunogenic.

Kidd antigens are not denatured by papain or ficin; treatment of RBCs with enzymes generally enhances reactivity with Kidd antibodies. Kidd antigens are also not affected by chloroquine, DTT, AET, or glycine-acid EDTA. The antigens are not found on platelets, lymphocytes, monocytes, or granulocytes.

	Table 8–18 **Prevalence of Kidd Phenotypes**		
PHENOTYPE	**WHITES (%)**	**BLACKS (%)**	**ASIANS (%)**
Jk(a+b–)	28	57	23
Jk(a+b+)	49	34	50
Jk(a–b+)	23	9	27
Jk(a–b–)	Exceedingly rare	Exceedingly rare	0.9 Polynesians

Anti-Jk[a] and Anti-Jk[b]

Kidd antibodies have a notorious reputation in the blood bank. They demonstrate dosage, are often weak, and are found in combination with other antibodies, all of which make them difficult to detect.

Anti-Jk[a] is more frequently encountered than anti-Jk[b], but neither antibody is common. The antibodies are usually IgG (antiglobulin reactive) but may also be partly IgM and are made in response to pregnancy or transfusion.

The ability of Kidd antibodies to show dosage can confound inexperienced serologists. Many anti-Jk[a] and anti-Jk[b] react more strongly with RBCs that carry a double dose of the respective antigen and may not react with Jk(a+b+) RBCs. An anti-Jk[a] that reacts only with Jk(a+b–) RBCs can give inconclusive panel results and appear compatible with Jk(a+b+) cells. Readers are urged to rule out anti-Jk[a] and anti-Jk[b] only with Jk(a+b–) and Jk(a–b+) panel cells, respectively, and to type all crossmatch-compatible units with commercial antisera. To ensure that antisera can indeed detect weak expressions of the antigen, Jk(a+b+) RBCs should be tested in parallel as the positive control.

Antibody reactivity can also be enhanced by using LISS or PEG (to promote IgG attachment), by using four drops of serum instead of two (to increase the antibody-to-antigen ratio), or by using enzymes such as ficin or papain. In vitro hemolysis can sometimes be observed with enzyme-treated RBCs if serum is tested; antigen dose may influence this hemolytic activity.[1]

Many examples of the Kidd antibodies bind complement. Rare examples are detected only by the complement they bind (i.e., they are nonreactive in antiglobulin tests using anti-IgG reagents). Testing serum (rather than plasma) and using polyspecific reagents with both anti-IgG and anti-complement can be helpful in these situations.[1]

The titer of anti-Jk[a] or anti-Jk[b] quickly declines in vivo. A strong antibody identified following a transfusion reaction may be undetectable in a few weeks or months.[1] This confirms the need to check blood bank records for previously identified antibodies before a patient is transfused. It is equally important to inform the patient that he or she has such an antibody and to provide a wallet card that notes the specificity in case the patient is transfused elsewhere.

The decline in antibody reactivity and the difficulty in detecting Kidd antibodies are reasons why they are a common cause of HTRs, especially of the delayed type. Although intravascular hemolysis has been noted in severe reactions, coated RBCs more often are removed extravascularly. The rate of clearance of incompatible RBCs can vary but is usually rapid.

Contrary to their hemolytic reputation in transfusion, most Kidd antibodies are only rarely associated with severe cases of HDFN.[42]

Biochemistry

Advanced Concepts

Heaton and McLoughlin[43] reported in 1982 that Jk(a–b–) RBCs resist lysis in 2M urea, a solution commonly used to lyse RBCs in a sample before it is used in some automated platelet-counting instruments. Urea crosses the RBC membrane, causing an osmotic imbalance and an influx of water, which rapidly lyses normal cells. With Jk(a+) or Jk(b+) RBCs, lysis in 2M urea occurs within 1 minute; with Jk(a–b–) cells, lysis is delayed by 30 minutes.[7]

The predicted Kidd glycoprotein has 389 amino acids with 10 membrane-spanning domains and two N-glycosylation sites, one of which is extracellular on the third extracellular loop (Fig. 8–10). The glycoprotein is a urea transporter.

Genetics

The *Jk* locus is on chromosome 18 at position 18q12.3. The gene *SLC14A1* (for solute carrier family 14, member 1) is a member of the urea transporter gene family. The gene is organized into 11 exons. The Jk[a]/Jk[b] polymorphism is associated with an amino acid substitution at position 280, predicted to be located on the fourth extracellular loop of the glycoprotein. Molecular studies have demonstrated the silent *Jk* allele can arise from mutations in both the *Jk[a]* and *Jk[b]* alleles. *Jk[a]* and *Jk[b]* are inherited as codominant alleles.

Jk(a–b–) Phenotype and the Recessive Allele, Jk

People with the null Jk(a–b–) phenotype lack Jk[a], Jk[b], and the common antigen Jk3. Although very rare, the Jk(a–b–) phenotype is most abundant among Polynesians, and it has also been identified in Filipinos, Indonesians, Chinese, and Japanese.[1] The null phenotype has also been reported in several European families (Finnish, French, Swiss, and English) and in the Mato Grosso Indians of Brazil. The delayed lysis

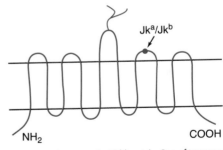

Figure 8–10.   Proposed structure for Kidd protein. One of two proposed N-glycans is extracellular and is located on the third extracellular loop; the Jk[a]/Jk[b] polymorphism is located on the fourth extracellular loop.

of Jk(a–b–) RBCs in 2M urea has proved an easy way to screen families and populations for this rare phenotype.

No clinical abnormalities have been associated with the Jk(a–b–) phenotype to date. Several unrelated Jk(a–b–) individuals had normal blood urea nitrogen, creatinine, and serum electrolytes, but studies on two individuals with this phenotype showed a marked defect in their ability to concentrate urine.

Family studies show that most Jk(a–b–) nulls are homozygous for the rare "silent" allele *Jk*. Parents of *JkJk* offspring and children of *JkJk* parents type Jk(a+b–) or Jk(a–b+) but never Jk(a+b+), because they are genetically *Jk^aJk* or *Jk^bJk*. Their RBCs also demonstrate a single dose of Jk^a or Jk^b antigen in titration studies.

Jk(a–b–) Phenotype and the Dominant In(Jk) Allele

Another genetic explanation for the Jk(a–b–) phenotype is association with a dominant gene called *In(Jk)*, for "inhibitor," that shows a dominant pattern of inheritance within a Japanese family analogous to the inhibitor gene responsible for the dominant type Lu(a–b–) phenotype in the Lutheran blood group system.[7,9] Dominant type Jk(a–b–) RBCs adsorb and elute anti-Jk3 and anti-Jk^a or anti-Jk^b (depending on which genes were inherited), indicating that the antigens are expressed but only very weakly. Individuals with the dominant type Jk(a–b–) phenotype do not make anti-Jk3. Family studies show that the *In(Jk)* gene does not reside at the *Jk* locus. The molecular basis is unknown.

Anti-Jk3

Alloanti-Jk3 is an IgG antiglobulin-reactive antibody that looks like an inseparable anti-Jk^aJk^b. Because panel cells are Jk(a+) or Jk(b+), anti-Jk3 reacts with all RBCs tested except the autocontrol. Most blood banks do not have the rare cells needed to confirm anti-Jk3; however, they can easily determine its most probable specificity by means of antigen typing. The individual making the antibody will type Jk(a–b–). Like other Kidd antibodies, anti-Jk3 reacts optimally by an antiglobulin test, and the reactivity is enhanced with enzyme pretreatment of the RBCs.

Anti-Jk3 has been associated with severe immediate and delayed HTRs and with mild HDFN. Compatible units are best found by typing siblings or searching the rare donor files.

Autoantibodies

Autoantibodies with Kidd specificity (anti-Jk^a, anti-Jk^b, and anti-Jk3) are rare, but they have been associated with autoimmune hemolytic anemia.[1] As with other blood groups, Kidd autoantibodies may have mimicking specificity or may be associated with depressed antigen expression.

The Lutheran (005) System

In 1945, anti-Lu^a was found (and described in detail a year later) in the serum of a patient with lupus erythematosus, following the transfusion of a unit of blood carrying the corresponding low-prevalence antigen.[44] (This patient also made anti-c, anti-N, the first example of anti-C^W, and anti-Levay, now known as Kp^c!) The new antibody was named Lutheran for the donor; the donor's last name was Lutteran but the donor blood sample was incorrectly labeled.[2] In 1956, Cutbush and Chanarin[45] described anti-Lu^b, which defined the antithetical partner to Lu^a.

The blood group system appeared complete until 1961, when Crawford and colleagues[46] described the first Lu(a–b–) phenotype. Unlike most null phenotypes at the time, this one demonstrated dominant inheritance. In 1963, the Lu(a–b–) phenotype inherited as a recessive silent allele was described.

Twenty antigens are part of the Lutheran system, numbered through Lu22; some antigens are also known by other common names. Two numbers (Lu10 and Lu15) are obsolete. Most of these antigens are high prevalence; four sets of antigens are antithetical. Many of the antigens were associated with the Lutheran system when their corresponding antibodies were nonreactive with the rare Lu(a–b–) RBCs. All are summarized in Table 8–19. The ISBT designation of the Lutheran blood group system is LU or 005.

Basic Concepts

Blood bankers seldom deal with the serology of the Lutheran blood group system. The antigens are either high prevalence, so only a few people lack the antigen and can make an alloantibody, or very low prevalence, so that only a few people are ever exposed. Consequently, the antibodies are seen infrequently, and there are not much data on the clinical significance of Lutheran antibodies.

Although the antigens have been detected on fetal RBCs as early as 10 to 12 weeks of gestation, they are poorly developed at birth. As a result, HDFN is rare and only mild.[9] Lutheran antigens have not been detected on platelets, lymphocytes, monocytes, or granulocytes. However, Lutheran glycoprotein is widely distributed in tissues: brain, lung, pancreas, placenta, skeletal muscle, and hepatocytes (especially fetal hepatic epithelial cells).[7] The presence of Lutheran glycoprotein on placental tissue may result in adsorption of maternal antibodies to Lutheran antigens, thus decreasing the likelihood of HDFN.[9]

Lutheran antigens are resistant to the enzymes ficin and papain and to glycine-acid EDTA treatment but are destroyed by treatment with the enzymes trypsin and α-chymotrypsin. Most Lutheran antibodies do not react with RBCs treated with the sulfhydryl reagents DTT and AET.

Lu^a and Lu^b Antigens

Lu^a and Lu^b are antigens produced by allelic codominant genes. The prevalence of common phenotypes are listed in Table 8–20. Most individuals are Lu(b+); 8% of whites and 5% of blacks are Lu(a+).[9]

Lutheran antigen expression is variable from one individual to another. The number of Lu^b sites per RBC is low, estimated to be from 1,640 to 4,070 on Lu(a–b+) RBCs and from 850 to 1,820 on Lu(a+b+) RBCs.[7]

Table 8–19   Lutheran System Antigens

CONVENTIONAL NAME	PREVALENCE (%)	YEAR DISCOVERED	COMMENTS
Lu^a	8 whites 5 blacks	1945	Antithetical to Lu^b
Lu^b	99.8	1956	Antithetical to Lu^a
Lu3	> 99.9	1963	
Lu4	> 99.9	1971	
Lu5	> 99.9	1972	
Lu6	> 99.9	1972	Antithetical to Lu9
Lu7	> 99.9	1972	
Lu8	> 99.9	1972	Antithetical to Lu14
Lu9	2	1973	Antithetical to Lu6
Lu11	> 99.9	1974	
Lu12	> 99.9	1973	
Lu13	> 99.9	1983	
Lu14	2.4	1977	Antithetical to Lu8
Lu16	> 99.9	1980	
Lu17	> 99.9	1979	
Au^a, Lu18	80 whites	1961	Antithetical to Au^b
Au^b, Lu19	50 whites	1989	Antithetical to Au^a
Lu20	> 99.9	1992	
Lu21	> 99.9	2002	
Lu22	> 99.9	2009	LURC

Table 8–20   Prevalence of Common Lutheran Phenotypes

PHENOTYPE	MOST POPULATIONS (%)
Lu (a+b–)	0.15
Lu (a+b+)	7.5
Lu (a–b+)	92.35
Lu (a–b–)	Very rare

Anti-Lu^a

Most examples of anti-Lu^a are IgM naturally occurring saline agglutinins that react better at room temperature than at 37°C. A few react at 37°C by indirect antiglobulin test. Some are capable of binding complement, but in vitro hemolysis has not been reported.

Anti-Lu^a often goes undetected in routine testing because most reagent RBCs are Lu(a–). Anti-Lu^a is more likely encountered as an incompatible crossmatch or during an antibody workup for another specificity. Experienced technologists recognize Lutheran antibodies by their characteristic loose, mixed-field reactivity in a test tube. Examples of anti-Lu^a that react only at temperatures below 37°C are clinically insignificant. There are no documented cases of immediate HTRs; there are only rare and mild delayed HTRs due to anti-Lu^a.[1]

Anti-Lu^b

Although the first example of anti-Lu^b was a room-temperature agglutinin, and IgM and IgA antibodies have been noted, most examples of anti-Lu^b are IgG and reactive at 37°C at the antiglobulin phase. The antibody is made in response to pregnancy or transfusion.

Alloanti-Lu^b reacts with all cells tested except the autocontrol, and reactions are often weaker with Lu(a+b+) RBCs and cord RBCs. Anti-Lu^b has been implicated with shortened survival of transfused cells and post-transfusion jaundice, but severe or acute hemolysis has not been reported.

Biochemistry

Advanced Concepts

The Lutheran antigens are located on a type 1 transmembrane protein. The protein exists in two forms as a result of alternative RNA splicing: the longer Lu glycoprotein and the shorter basal cell adhesion molecule (B-CAM). The longer 85-kD protein contains 597 amino acids with five extracellular domains, a hydrophobic transmembrane domain of 19 amino acids, and a cytoplasmic domain of 59 amino acids (Fig. 8–11). The smaller isoform (78 kD) is identical except for a shorter cytoplasmic domain of 59 amino acids. The external portion consists of five disulfide-bonded domains. The Lutheran glycoproteins belong to the immunoglobulin superfamily of proteins; the repeating extracellular domains are homologous to immunoglobulin variable or constant domains. The Lutheran proteins are multifunctional adhesion molecules that bind laminin, notably in sickle cell disease.[47]

The molecular basis for the four pairs of antithetical antigens and several of the high-prevalence antigens has been determined through the creation of Lutheran glycoprotein mutants and subsequent sequencing of the exons encoding the extracellular domains. For most of the antigens, expression was caused by a single nucleotide polymorphism, resulting in single amino acid changes on the protein level.[48]

Genetics

The *Lu* gene is located on chromosome 19 at position 19q13.2, along with genes that govern expression of several blood group antigens (*H, Se, Le, LW, Ok^a*) . A linkage between

Lu and the *Se* gene (*FUT2*) was the first example of autosomal linkage described in humans.

Lu(a–b–) Phenotypes

Three genetic explanations for the Lu(a–b–) phenotype have been described. These are summarized in Table 8–21.

Dominant Type Lu(a–b–)

The first Lu(a–b–) family study was reported by the propositus herself.[46] Because the phenotype was seen in successive generations in 50% of her family members and others, and because null individuals passed normal Lutheran genes to their offspring, the expression of Lutheran was thought to be suppressed by a rare dominant regulator gene later called *In(Lu)* for "inhibitor of Lutheran." Recently, mutations in the gene for Erythroid Krüppel-like Factor (EKLF), a transcription factor, were shown to be associated with the In(Lu) phenotype in 21 of 24 In(Lu) individuals studied.[49] In all cases, the mutated *EKLF* allele occurred in the presence of a normal *EKLF* allele. The authors of this study concluded that the In(Lu) phenotype is caused by inheritance of a loss-of-function mutation on one allele of *EKLF*.

Dominant-type Lu(a–b–) RBCs carry trace amounts of Lutheran antigens as shown by adsorption-elution studies. For example, the RBCs of a person with the dominant type Lu(a–b–) who inherited two normal *Lu^b* genes will type Lu(a–b–) with routine methods but will adsorb and elute anti-Lu^b. Because individuals with the dominant type Lu(a–b–) RBCs have normal Lutheran antigens, they do not make anti-Lu3.

In addition to reduced expression of Lutheran antigens, dominant type Lu(a–b–) RBCs also can have reduced expression of CD44 and a weak expression of P1, i, AnWj, MER2, and In^b blood group antigens.

Recessive Type Lu(a–b–)

In some families, the Lu(a–b–) phenotype demonstrates recessive inheritance, the result of having two rare silent alleles *LuLu* at the Lutheran locus. The parents and offspring of these nulls may type Lu(a–b–), but dosage studies and titers show them to carry a single dose of Lu^b.

Unlike the dominant type, people with recessive Lu(a–b–) RBCs truly lack all Lutheran antigens (i.e., they have the null phenotype) and can make an inseparable anti-Lu^{ab} called anti-Lu3. They also have normal antigen expression of P1, i, and the other antigens that are weakened with the dominant type. This distinction emphasizes the importance of testing an antibody against recessive Lu(a–b–) RBCs before defining the specificity phenotypically related to Lutheran.

Different inactivating mutations were recently reported for three individuals with the recessive Lu(a–b–) type.[50] In all three individuals the mutations would result in a truncated glycoprotein that would not be integrated in the RBC surface membrane.

Recessive X-Linked Inhibitor Type

An Lu(a–b–) phenotype in a large Australian family did not fit either the dominant or recessive inheritance patterns. All

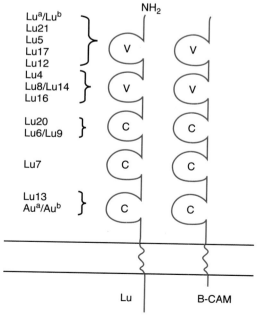

Figure 8–11. The two structures encoded by the Lu gene: the longer Lu glycoprotein and the shorter basal cell adhesion molecule (B-CAM). The five extracellular disulfide-bonded domains are homologous to immunoglobulin variable (V) or constant (C) domains.

Table 8–21   Summary of Lu(a–b–) Phenotypes

MODE OF INHERITANCE	GENE RESPONSIBLE	Lu ANTIGENS	OTHER RBC ANTIGENS AFFECTED	MAKE ANTI-Lu3?
Dominant	EKLF[49] Not at Lu locus	Extremely weak	Reduced P1, i, In[b], AnWj, MER2, CD44	No
Recessive	Lu	None	Not affected	Yes
X-linked	XS2	Extremely weak	Not affected	No

Lu(a–b–) family members were male and carried trace amounts of Lu[b] detected by adsorption-elution. The pattern of inheritance suggested an X-borne inhibitor to Lutheran. The researchers proposed calling the locus XS, XS1 being the common allele and XS2 the rare inhibitor that suppresses in a hemizygous state. There have been no other families reported with this rare X-linked Lu(a–b–) phenotype.[9]

Anti-Lu3

Anti-Lu3 is a rare antibody that reacts with all RBCs except Lu(a–b–) RBCs. The antibody looks like inseparable anti-Lu[ab] and recognizes a common antigen, Lu3, that is present whenever Lu[a] or Lu[b] is present (much like the Jk3 association with Jk[a] and Jk[b]). Anti-Lu3 is usually antiglobulin-reactive. This antibody is made only by individuals with the recessive type of Lu(a–b–).

The Diego (010) System

The Diego system is composed of 22 antigens: three sets of independent pairs of antithetical antigens—Di[a]/Di[b], Wr[a]/Wr[b], and Wu/DISK—and 17 low-prevalence antigens.[3,7] The system was named after the first antibody maker in a Venezuelan family during an investigation of HDFN. The Diego system is designated DI and number 010 by the ISBT.

The Diego antigens are carried on band 3, a major integral RBC membrane glycoprotein with about 1 million copies per RBC. Band 3 is also known as the red cell anion exchanger (AE1) or solute carrier family-4. anion exchanger, member 1 (SLC4A1). The protein crosses the membrane multiple times, and both the amino- and carboxyl-terminal domains are in the cytoplasm. A large N-glycan on the fourth external loop carries over half the RBC A, B, H, and I blood group antigens. The long amino-terminal domain of band 3 interacts with ankyrin and protein 4.2 of the membrane skeleton. The gene encoding band 3 and the Diego antigens, SLC4A1, consists of 20 exons and is located at chromosome 17q21-q22.

Reported in 1955, anti-Di[a] had caused HDFN in a Venezuelan baby. Anti-Di[b] was described 2 years later. Di[a] is rare in most populations but is polymorphic in people of Mongoloid ancestry. In South American Indians, the prevalence of Di[a] can be as high as 54%.[9] Di[a] is also present in the North and Central American native populations but is surprisingly rare in Canada and among the Alaskan Inuit.[7] The prevalence of Di[b] is generally greater than 99% but is 96% in Native Americans. The Di[a]/Di[b] polymorphism is

located on the last (seventh) extracellular loop of the protein. The Di(a–b–) phenotype has not been reported.

Wr[a], a low-prevalence antigen, and the antithetical, high-prevalence Wr[b] are associated with an amino acid substitution on the fourth external loop, close to the insertion point of the protein into the RBC membrane. However, expression of Wr[b] requires the presence of both band 3 and a normal GPA of the MNS blood group system. GPA-deficient RBCs are Wr(a–b–).[7]

Localization of Di[a] and Di[b] antigens to band 3 enabled many low-prevalence antigens to be assigned to the Diego system: Wd[a], Rb[a], WARR, ELO, Wu, Bp[a], Mo[a], Hg[a], Vg[a], Sw[a], BOW, NFLD, Jn[a], KREP, Tr[a], Fr[a], and Sw1.

Diego antigens are expressed on RBCs of newborns. The antigens are resistant to treatment with ficin and papain, DTT, and glycine-acid EDTA, with the exception of Bp[a], which is sensitive to papain.[7,9]

Diego system antibodies are sometimes IgM, but are usually IgG, reactive in the indirect antiglobulin test. Both anti-Di[a] and anti-Di[b] have caused HTRs and HDFN.[7,9] Anti-Wr[a] is a relatively common antibody in donors and patients; some are directly agglutinating, but most require the indirect antiglobulin test to be detected. Anti-Wr[a] has caused severe HTRs. Only a few examples of alloanti-Wr[b] in individuals with Wr(a–b–) RBCs have been described, so information about clinical significance is insufficient. Autoanti-Wr[b] is relatively common in the serum of patients with warm autoimmune hemolytic anemia. Little or no data are available on the clinical significance of antibodies to the low-prevalence Diego antigens, with the exception of anti-ELO, which has caused severe HDFN.[7]

The Yt (011) System

Two antigens make up the Yt system, which was named in 1956 for the first antibody maker and used the last letter "t" in the patient's last name, which was Cartwright.[51] Apparently "why T" became "Yt."[9] Yt[a] is the high-prevalence antigen in all populations; Yt[b] is the low-prevalence antigen found in about 8% of whites and 21% to 26% of Israelis, but it is not found in Japanese.[7,9] Three phenotypes are observed: the common Yt(a+b–) and Yt(a+b+) and the rare Yt(a–b+). The Yt(a–b–) phenotype has not been reported. The Yt system has the ISBT designation YT and system number 011.

The Yt antigens are antithetical and represent an amino acid substitution on the glycosylphosphatidylinositol (GPI)-linked RBC glycoprotein acetylcholinesterase (AChE). AChE is an important enzyme participating in neurotransmission, but the function of RBC-bound AChE is not known. The gene is located at chromosome 7q22.

Yt antigens are variably sensitive to ficin and papain, are sensitive to DTT, and are resistant to glycine-acid EDTA treatment. The antigens are developed at birth but are expressed more weakly on cord RBCs than on adult RBCs, and are absent from RBCs of people with paroxysmal nocturnal hemoglobinuria (PNH) III.[7]

Anti-Yt^a and anti-Yt^b are IgG and are stimulated by pregnancy or transfusion. Anti-Yt^a is not an uncommon antibody, so it appears that Yt^a is reasonably immunogenic. However, Yt^b appears to be a poor immunogen, as the antibody is rare. Yt antibodies have not caused HDFN. Some examples of anti-Yt^a have been shown to be clinically significant for transfusion while others have not.[7]

The Xg (012) System

Anti-Xg^a was discovered in 1962 in the serum of a multiply transfused man. The antibody detected an antigen with a higher prevalence in females than in males. Family studies were used to confirm the antigen Xg^a expression was controlled by an X-linked gene. The antigen was named after the X chromosome and g for "Grand Rapids," where the patient was treated.[9]

The Xg system is designated by the symbol XG and number 012. There are two antigens in the Xg system: Xg^a and CD99. CD99 is also known as 12E7 and MIC2. The gene encoding Xg^a is located on the X chromosome at Xp22.3. The gene responsible for CD99, *MIC2*, is located at Xp22.2. CD99 became part of the Xg system because the *MIC2* and *XG* genes are adjacent and homologous. Xg^a has a phenotypic relationship to CD99: all Xg(a+) individuals have a high expression of CD99 on their RBCs and all Xg(a–) females have a low expression of CD99, but 68% of Xg(a–) males have a high expression and 32% have a low expression of CD99.[7] Both Xg^a and CD99 escape X chromosome inactivation. The Xg glycoprotein crosses the RBC membrane once, with the amino terminus directed externally. There are approximately 9,000 copies of Xg^a per RBC.[9]

The prevalence of Xg^a is 66% in males and 89% in females. Because males have only one X chromosome, Xg(a+) males are hemizygotes. Females, having two X chromosomes, can be homozygotes or heterozygotes. However, homozygosity for the gene does not directly correlate to RBC antigen strength.[52] Cord RBCs express Xg^a weakly. Weak expression of Xg^a is seen on RBCs from some adult females, but weak expression on RBCs from adult males is rare.[9] The antigen is sensitive to ficin and papain but resistant to DTT treatment.

Anti-Xg^a is usually IgG; some examples are naturally occurring. Anti-Xg^a has not been implicated in HDFN or as a cause of HTRs. Two CD99– Japanese individuals have been found with alloanti-CD99.

The Scianna (013) System

The Scianna blood group system, ISBT symbol SC and number 013, currently consists of seven antigens. The system is named after the first antibody maker. In 1962, a new high-prevalence antigen was named Sm; 1 year later, a new low-prevalence antigen, Bu^a was found. After it was confirmed that these two antigens were antithetical, the Scianna blood group system was established in 1974 and the two antigens were renamed Sc1 and Sc2, respectively. The prevalence of Sc2 in Northern Europeans is 1% but is higher in the Mennonite population.

In 1980, an individual in the Marshall Islands in the South Pacific was found with the Sc:–1,–2 phenotype. He had made an antibody to an unknown high-prevalence antibody. The antibody was named anti-Sc3; separable anti-Sc1 and anti-Sc2 were not identified. The very rare Sc:–1,–2,–3 phenotype is the Scianna null type. Three examples of anti-Sc3, nonreactive with Sc:–1,–2, were found to be incompatible with the RBCs of the other anti-Sc3 makers, indicating the existence of additional high-prevalence antigens.[53]

The *SC* gene is located on chromosome 1 at 1p34. The product of the gene is a protein called erythroid membrane-associated protein (ERMAP), which is an RBC adhesion protein. Once location of Scianna to ERMAP was made, other antigens were assigned to the system. The low-prevalence antigen Rd became Sc4. Sc5 (STAR), Sc6 (SCER), and Sc7 (SCAN) are all high-prevalence antigens.[54]

The Scianna antigens are resistant to ficin and papain but are slightly weakened by DTT treatment. The antigens are expressed on cord RBCs.

Alloantibodies to Scianna antigens are rare and little is known about their clinical significance. They are usually IgG and reactive in the antiglobulin test. None have been reported to cause a severe HTR. Only mild HDFN has been reported, except for one severe case for anti-Sc4, for which the baby required exchange transfusion. Autoantibodies to Sc1 and Sc3 have been reported.

The Dombrock (014) System

The Dombrock blood group system, designated by the ISBT with the symbol DO and number 014, was named for the first antibody maker, Mrs. Dombrock, found in 1965. Anti-Do^b, which recognizes the antithetical antigen, was identified in 1973. The prevalence of the three resulting phenotypes, Do(a+b–), Do(a+b+), and Do(a–b+), varies in different populations. In whites, they are 18%, 49%, and 33%, respectively.

The high-prevalence antigens Gy^a and Hy were both described in 1967. RBCs from whites who are Gy(a–) were found to be Hy–, but Hy– RBCs from blacks were weakly Gy(a+). The high-prevalence antigen Jo^a was described in 1972, and the phenotypic relationship to Gy^a and Hy was later shown: Gy(a–) RBCs or Hy– RBCs are also Jo(a–). In 1995, it was reported that Gy(a–) RBCs were also Do(a–b–).[55] The Gy(a–) phenotype is the Dombrock null. Two additional high-prevalence antigens, DOYA and DOMR, were recently added to the system.[3] The Hy– and Jo(a–) phenotypes are not found in whites and are rare in blacks.

The Dombrock antigens are carried on a mono-ADP-ribosyltransferase 4 (ART4) attached to the RBC membrane by a GPI anchor. The gene encoding the Dombrock glycoprotein is located at chromosome 12p12.3.

The Dombrock antigens are resistant to ficin, papain, and glycine-acid EDTA, and are sensitive to 0.2 M DTT treatment. The antigens are present on cord RBCs, but are absent from PNH III RBCs. The Do[a] and Do[b] antigens are considered to be poor immunogens and the antibodies are rarely found as single specificities; Gy[a], however, is highly immunogenic.[9]

Anti-Do[a] and anti-Do[b] have caused delayed HTRs but no clinical HDFN. The Dombrock antibodies are usually IgG, reacting optimally with enzyme-treated RBCs. These antibodies are usually weakly reactive and disappear, both factors making them difficult to identify.

The Colton (015) System

The Colton blood group system, ISBT symbol CO and number 015, consists of four antigens. The system was named in 1967 for the first antibody maker; it should have been named Calton, but the handwriting on the tube was misread![9] The high- and low-prevalence antithetical antigens are Co[a] and Co[b], respectively. The Co[b] antigen is present in about 10% of most populations.[9] The third antigen, Co3, is present on all RBCs except those of the very rare Co(a–b–) phenotype. Co4, a high-prevalence antigen, has been identified on RBCs from two individuals with the Co(a–b–) phenotype.[3]

The Colton antigens are carried on an integral membrane protein, aquaporin 1 (AQP1), which accounts for 80% of water readsorption in the kidneys.[9] The glycoprotein crosses the RBC membrane multiple times. The gene (AQP1) is located at chromosome 7p14. The Colton antigens are expressed on RBCs of newborns and are resistant to treatment with ficin and papain, chloroquine, and DTT.

Antibodies are usually IgG and are enhanced with enzyme-treated RBCs. Anti-Co[a] is often seen as a single specificity and has been reported to cause HTRs and HDFN.[56] Anti-Co[b] appears more often with other specificities but has also caused HTRs and mild HDFN.[9] Anti-Co3, which reacts with all Co(a+) and Co(b+) RBCs, has been reported to cause severe HDFN.[1]

The Landsteiner-Wiener (016) System

The Landsteiner-Wiener blood group system, ISBT symbol LW and number 016, had its origins along with the discovery of the D antigen of the Rh blood group system. In 1940, Landsteiner and Wiener reported that an antibody produced in rabbits (and later, guinea pigs) after injection with RBCs of rhesus monkeys reacted with 85% of human RBCs.[57] This antibody was called anti-Rh for anti-rhesus. The reactivity of anti-Rh was similar to the human antibody reported by Levine and Stetson in 1939 in a woman who delivered a stillborn infant and had a transfusion reaction to the blood donated by her husband.[58] Both sera identified the same population of Rh+ and Rh– RBCs. The two antibodies were later shown to be different in several studies; in the 1960s, the human anti-Rh was renamed anti-D (but called anti-Rh$_o$ by some workers) and the rabbit anti-Rh was called anti-LW in honor of Landsteiner and Wiener. Examples of human anti-LW were subsequently described.

There are three LW antigens: LW[a], LW[ab], and LW[b]. The first two, LW[a] and LW[ab], are common, high-prevalence antigens, and LW[b] is of low prevalence, found in less than 1% of most Europeans but in 6% of Finns.[9] LW[ab] was originally defined by the antibody made by an individual with an inherited LW(a–b–) phenotype. Terminology for LW antigens has evolved as more information became available. The ISBT has used LW5, LW6, and LW7 as the antigen numbers for LW[a], LW[ab], and LW[b], respectively, to prevent confusion with obsolete terminology that used LW1-LW4 to designate phenotypes. The null phenotype is LW(a–b–); in one individual who made anti-LW[ab] (Mrs. Big), this phenotype resulted from a 10 base pair deletion in exon 1 of an LW[a] gene, which introduced a premature stop codon. Rh$_{null}$ RBCs also type LW(a–b–) and are considered to be the only true LW– RBCs because they fail to elicit the formation of anti-LW in animals, whereas injection of Mrs. Big's LW(a–b–) RBCs into guinea pigs caused the formation of anti-LW. The LW phenotypes are shown in Table 8–22.

As was shown by the similarity in reactivity of the original animal anti-Rh and the human anti-Rh (later called anti-D), there is a phenotypic relationship between the D antigen and anti-LW. Anti-LW usually reacts strongly with D+ RBCs, weakly (and sometimes not at all) with D– RBCs from adults, and not at all with Rh$_{null}$ RBCs. A weak anti-LW may react only with D+ RBCs and may appear to be anti-D unless enhancement techniques are used. This is because there are more LW antigen sites on D+ RBCs from adults than on D– RBCs.[9] However, anti-LW reacts equally well with cord RBCs regardless of their D type. Distinguishing anti-LW

Table 8–22	**LW Phenotypes**				
PHENOTYPE	**REACTIVITY WITH**			**PREVALENCE**	
	Anti-LW[a]	**Anti-LW[b]**	**Anti-LW[ab]**	**Most Europeans**	**Finns**
LW(a+b–)	+	–	+	97%	93.9%
LW(a+b+)	+	+	+	3%	6%
LW(a–b+)	–	+	+	Rare	0.1%
LW(a–b–) Big	–	–	–		
LW(a–b–) Rh$_{null}$	–	–	–		

from anti-D is most easily accomplished by testing DTT-treated D+ RBCs: the D antigen is not denatured by DTT, so anti-D would still be detected; however, LW antigen is destroyed by DTT, so anti-LW would no longer react. LW antigens are resistant to treatment of RBCs with enzymes and glycine-acid EDTA.

The structure that carries the LW antigens is a glycoprotein known as intracellular adhesion molecule 4 (ICAM-4), a member of the immunoglobulin superfamily. The LW glycoprotein is part of the band 3/Rh macrocomplex[59]; Rh_{null} RBCs lack the LW glycoprotein. The *LW* gene is located on chromosome 19 at 19p13.3.

LW antigens may be depressed during pregnancy and in some diseases, such as lymphoma and leukemia.[9] Autoanti-LW made by these patients can appear to be an alloantibody; as the antigen strength returns the antibody diminishes. Autoanti-LW is also common in serum from patients with warm autoimmune hemolytic anemia. No anti-LW has been shown to cause serious HDFN or transfusion reactions. Many patients with anti-LW have successfully been transfused with D– RBCs. Only two examples of alloanti-LW[ab] have been described, the antibodies of the only two known propositi with an inherited LW(a–b–) phenotype.[7]

The Chido/Rodgers (017) System

The Chido/Rodgers blood group system, designated by the ISBT with symbol CH/RG and number 017, was named after the first two antibody producers, Ch for Chido and Rg for Rodgers. These two antibodies were described in 1967 and 1976, respectively. Serologically, they were both characterized as nebulous because antigen strength on different samples of RBCs was variable.[1] It was also appreciated that both anti-Ch and anti-Rg could be neutralized by plasma.

Ch and Rg antigens are not intrinsic to the RBC membrane. Rather, they are on the fourth component of complement (C4), and are adsorbed onto RBCs from plasma.[1] The C4 glycoprotein has two isoforms: C4B carries the Ch antigens and C4A expresses Rg antigens. Genes at two closely linked loci located at chromosome 6p21.3 encode these isoforms. The Chido/Rodgers system consists of nine antigens: Ch1 to Ch6, Rg1, and Rg2 are all high prevalence; WH has a prevalence of about 15%.[9] Differentiation of the determinants is not made for routine serology.

Ch is present in 96% to 98% of most populations.[1,9] Rg is present in 97% to 98% of most populations.[1,9] The antigens are destroyed by ficin and papain but are resistant to treatment with DTT and glycine-acid EDTA.[9]

Anti-Ch and anti-Rg are usually IgG and react weakly, often to moderate or high titration endpoints. Neutralization of anti-Ch and anti-Rg with pooled plasma is often used as part of the identification of these antibodies in a patient's serum. Anti-Ch and anti-Rg are clinically insignificant for transfusion.[1]

The Gerbich (020) System

The Gerbich blood group system was named in 1960 after Mrs. Gerbich, the first antibody producer. Gerbich became a system in 1990, designated by the ISBT as GE and number 020. There are currently six high-prevalence Gerbich antigens (Ge2, Ge3, Ge4, GEPL, GEAT, and GETI) and five low-prevalence antigens (Wb, Ls[a], An[a], Dh[a], and GEIS). The antigens are carried on sialoglycoprotein structures GPC and GPD. The glycoproteins help to maintain the RBC membrane integrity through interaction with protein band 4.1, and because they are rich in sialic acid, they contribute to the net negative charge of the RBC membrane (as do GPA and GPB of the MNS system). There are about 135,000 copies of GPC and 50,000 copies of GPD per RBC.[9] GPC and GPD are both encoded by the *GYPC* gene, located on chromosome 2 at 2q14.3.

There are three Gerbich-negative phenotypes in which the RBCs lack one or more of the high-prevalence antigens: Ge:–2,3,4 (Yus type), Ge:–2,–3,4 (Gerbich type), and Ge:–2,–3,–4 (Leach type). The Leach type is the Gerbich null phenotype. These are summarized in Table 8–23. Outside of Papua, New Guinea, the Gerbich-negative phenotypes are very rare, but they have been found in diverse populations. The Yus phenotype has been found in Mexicans, Israelis, and others but has not been found in Papua, New Guinea and other Melanesians.[9] The Gerbich phenotype is polymorphic in certain areas of Papua, New Guinea and has also been found among Europeans, Africans, Native Americans, Japanese, and Polynesians.[9]

Gerbich antigens are expressed at birth. RBCs of the Gerbich or Leach phenotypes have weak expression of Kell blood group antigens, and some anti-Vel fail to react with Ge:–2,–3,4 RBCs.[9] Gerbich antigens are resistant to treatment with DTT and glycine-acid EDTA; Ge2 and Ge4 are ficin and papain sensitive, but Ge3 is ficin resistant.

Some Gerbich antibodies may be IgM, but most are IgG. Gerbich antibodies are sometimes clinically significant for transfusion and sometimes not. Gerbich antibodies can be eluted from DAT+ cord bloods, but only three cases of serious HDFN due to anti-Ge3 have been reported, and two were children of the same mother.[60,61] In these cases, the severe anemia was late onset, after birth, associated with inhibition of erythroid cell growth; in one case there was also early onset of hemolysis.

Anti-Ge2 is the most common of the Gerbich antibodies.[7] It is the antibody made by the Ge:–2,3,4 phenotype individuals, but it is also the more common antibody made by the Ge:–2,–3,4 phenotype and Ge:–2,–3,–4 phenotype individuals. Anti-Ge3 is less frequently made by the Ge:–2,–3,4 and Ge:–2,–3,–4 phenotype individuals. Anti-Ge4 is a very rare antibody.

Table 8–23	Gerbich-Negative Phenotypes	
PHENOTYPE	**TYPE**	**ANTIBODY**
Ge: –2, 3, 4	Yus	Anti-Ge2
Ge: –2, –3, 4	Gerbich	Anti-Ge2 or anti-Ge3
Ge: –2, –3, –4	Leach type	Anti-Ge2 or anti-Ge3

The Cromer (021) System

In 1965, an antibody was found in a black prenatal patient, Mrs. Cromer, that reacted with all RBCs except her own and two siblings. It was originally thought her antibody recognized an antigen antithetical to Go[a] of the Rh blood group system. The antibody was named anti-Cr[a] in 1975.[7,9]

The antigens of the Cromer system are carried on decay accelerating factor (DAF, CD55), a complement regulatory protein. The *CD55* gene is located at chromosome 1q32. The glycoprotein encoded by the gene is attached to the RBC membrane through a GPI linkage. PNH III RBCs are deficient in DAF so they also lack Cromer antigens.

The Cromer system has 16 antigens: 13 high-prevalence antigens and 3 low-prevalence antigens.[62,63] All these antigens are absent from Inab phenotype RBCs, the Cromer null phenotype, which is very rare. The Cr(a−) phenotype is typically found in blacks and is not found in whites. Three Cromer antigens, Tc[a], Tc[b], and Tc[c], are antithetical; Tc[a] is the high-prevalence antigen and the other two are low prevalence. The Dr[a] antigen is of high prevalence; Dr(a−) RBCs have weakened expression of all other high-prevalence Cromer antigens due to a markedly reduced copy number of DAF.

Cromer system antigens are resistant to treatment with ficin and papain but are destroyed by α-chymotrypsin, which is used to distinguish specificities in this system from other blood group antibodies. Cromer antigens are weakened with DTT treatment and are resistant to glycine-acid EDTA.

Antibodies in the Cromer system are usually IgG, but do not cause HDFN. DAF is strongly expressed on placental tissue and will adsorb Cromer antibodies.[9,63] Anti-Cr[a] and anti-Tc[a] have been implicated in HTRs, but other examples of these specificities have not caused clinical reactions after transfusion of incompatible units.[62] Anti-IFC is the antibody made by individuals with the Cromer null Inab phenotype.

The Knops (022) System

There are nine antigens in the Knops blood group system, designated by the ISBT as KN and number 022. The system was established when the antigens were shown to be located on complement receptor 1 (CR1) and was named after Mrs. Knops, the first antibody maker. The gene is located at chromosome 1q32.

With the exception of the low-prevalence antigens Kn[b] and McC[b], the Knops antigens have a prevalence of more than 90% in most populations; however, ethnic differences exist. Sl[a] is present on RBCs of only about 60% of African Americans. Among West Africans, Sl[a] has a prevalence of 30% to 38%, and KCAM has a prevalence of only 20%.[64] The antithetical pairs of antigens are Kn[a] and Kn[b], McC[a] and McC[b], and Sl[a] and Vil. Knops antigens are weakly expressed on cord RBCs and weaken upon storage of adult RBCs (e.g., older units of blood). The antigens are weakened by treatment with ficin and papain and are destroyed by DTT; the antigens are resistant to glycine-acid EDTA.[9]

Serologically, these antigens have been grouped together because their corresponding antibodies demonstrate variable reactions, are not neutralized by pooled normal serum (unlike anti-Ch and anti-Rg), and are difficult to adsorb and elute.[64] Antibody reactivity is enhanced with longer incubation (e.g., 1 hour, at 37°C). Weak and variable reactivity is due to variable expression of CR1 on different samples of RBCs. The "Helgeson phenotype" represents the serologic null phenotype for the Knops blood group; these RBCs type Kn(a−b−), McC(a−), Sl(a−), and Yk(a−) because of the low copy number of CR1, but they are not truly devoid of Knops antigens.[9,64]

The antibodies are usually IgG, reactive in the antiglobulin test, but are clinically insignificant for both transfusion and HDFN. Of the Knops antibodies, anti-Kn[a] is frequently found in multiply transfused individuals and multispecific sera; anti-Sl[a] is more frequently found in blacks.

CR1 binds the complement component fragments C3b and C4b and processes immune complexes for transportation to the liver and spleen and subsequent clearance from the circulation.[7,64] CR1 has also been identified as a receptor for several pathogenic organisms.

The Indian (023) System

The Indian blood group system was named because the first In(a+) individuals were from India. There are now four antigens in the system, designated IN and number 023 by the ISBT. The antigen In[a] was reported in 1973 and is present on RBCs of 4% of Indians, 11% of Iranians, and 12% of Arabs.[9] In[b] is the antithetical high-prevalence antigen. These and two other high-prevalence antigens are located on CD44, an adhesion molecule. The gene encoding CD44 is located at chromosome 11p13. The extremely rare In(a−b−) phenotype has been found in only one individual who presented with congenital dyserythropoietic anemia and whose RBCs also typed Co(a−b−).[65]

CD44 is reduced on RBCs of dominant type Lu(a−b−) individuals. In[a] and In[b] are weakly expressed on cord RBCs and are sensitive to treatment with ficin, papain, and DTT but are resistant to glycine-acid EDTA.[9]

Antibodies are usually IgG and reactive in the antiglobulin test and they do not bind complement. Positive DATs but no clinical HDFN have been reported for anti-In[a] and anti-In[b]; decreased cell survival with anti-In[a] and an immediate HTR due to anti-In[b] have been reported.[9]

The Ok (024) System

Currently, there are three high-prevalence antigens in the Ok system, designated by the ISBT symbol OK and number 024. Anti-Ok[a] was identified in 1979 and was named after the antibody maker, Mrs. Kobutso. Because *Ko* was already in use, the first two letters were switched to *Ok*.[2] Her parents were cousins from a small Japanese island. Two of three siblings of the proposita were also Ok(a−).[7] RBCs from 400 individuals from the same island were all Ok(a+).[1] Two additional antigens, OKGV and OKVM, were recently added to the system.

The OK antigens are carried on CD147, a member of the immunoglobulin superfamily that mainly functions as receptors and adhesion molecules. The gene locus is at chromosome 19p13.3.

Ok^a is well developed on RBCs from newborns and is resistant to treatment with ficin and papain, DTT, and glycine-acid EDTA.[9]

The original anti-Ok^a was IgG, reactive in the antiglobulin test. At least one other example of the antibody has been found. The antibody caused reduced survival of ^{51}Cr-labeled Ok(a+) RBCs injected into the original antibody maker.[1] Anti-Ok^a has not been reported to cause HDFN.

The Raph (025) System

The only antigen in the Raph system is MER2, which was originally defined by two monoclonal antibodies; it has since been recognized by human polyclonal antibodies. The antigen name is derived from *monoclonal*, and *Eleanor Roosevelt*, the laboratory where the antibody was produced. When MER2 was raised to system status, the system was named Raph for the first patient to make the alloanti-MER2. MER2 is encoded by a gene located at chromosome 11p15.

Three examples of alloanti-MER2 were found in Jews originating from India and living in Israel; two were related. All three had end-stage renal disease. A fourth example of anti-MER2 was found in a healthy Turkish blood donor. Blood samples from these four individuals were studied. It was shown that MER2 is located on CD151, a tetraspanin, which appears to be essential for the assembly of basement membranes in the kidney and skin.[66]

The polymorphism identified by the monoclonal antibodies indicated that 8% of the English blood donor population is MER2–. Subsequent studies suggest the antigen-negative status represents the low end of antigen expression on RBCs.[66] MER2 is abundant on platelets and is expressed on erythroid precursors of individuals with either MER2+ or MER2– RBCs. MER2 expression decreases over time with increasing maturation of erythroid cells.[66] It has been suggested that most people whose RBCs type MER2– have MER2 expressed on other cells and tissues and will not make anti-MER2, and those individuals who have made alloanti-MER2 are true MER2–. Those individuals who have made anti-MER2 showed mutations in *CD151*. In the patients with renal disease, a truncated CD151 protein would be predicted, but in patients without renal disease, mutations would result in an altered CD151 that appears to be present and functional at the cell surface.[66,67]

The antigen is resistant to treatment with ficin and papain but is sensitive to treatment with trypsin, α-chymotrypsin, pronase, and AET.

Little is known about the clinical significance of anti-MER2, but one patient with the antibody showed signs of a transfusion reaction after transfusion with 3 units. As 8% of the population is expected to be MER2–, it would be prudent to transfuse with crossmatch compatible units.[67]

The John Milton Hagen (026) System

JMH is a high-prevalence antigen. Numerous examples of anti-JMH have been seen, especially in patients 50 years and older. In 1978, a large number of samples with this antibody were characterized and the antibody was named anti-JMH

for the first antibody maker, John Milton Hagen. The system (ISBT symbol JMH and number 026) was established after it was shown that the JMH protein is the GPI-linked glycoprotein CD108 and the gene *SEMA7A* was cloned. The gene is located at chromosome 15q24.1.

Five other antigens were recently added to the system, JMH2 through JMH6; these are JMH variants associated with amino acid substitutions in the protein.[68] JMH1 represents the antigen recognized by antibodies made by individuals lacking the JMH protein.

Most examples of anti-JMH are not found in patients who lack the JMH protein or who have one of the variant JMH phenotypes. Rather, the patient's JMH– status is acquired and can be transient.[1] It is widely accepted that JMH levels decline during the later years of life, sometimes to the point of not being detected serologically.[1] Once JMH expression is reduced, anti-JMH can be made. In some cases with anti-JMH, the DAT is positive and some JMH is detected on the patient's RBCs. This autoanti-JMH with a positive DAT has never been associated with autoimmune RBC destruction.[1]

JMH is weakly expressed on cord RBCs and is destroyed by treating RBCs with ficin and papain, and DTT; the antigen is resistant to treatment with glycine-acid EDTA.[9]

Anti-JMH is usually IgG (predominantly IgG4 in acquired JMH-negative people).[9] The antibodies are often high titer but weakly reactive, even when tested without dilution, and they are not neutralized with pooled plasma. JMH antibodies are generally considered clinically insignificant. Rare examples of alloanti-JMH in individuals whose RBCs express variant forms of CD108 may be clinically significant.[1]

The Gill (029) System

Anti-GIL was first identified in 1980, but the antigen was not raised to system status until 2002 when it was shown that GIL is genetically discrete from all other blood group systems. The ISBT Gill system symbol is GIL and number 029. There is only one antigen, GIL.

This antigen is found on the glycerol transporter aquaporin 3 (AQP3), a member of the major intrinsic protein family of water channels. *AQP3* is located at chromosome 9p13. The GIL$_{null}$ phenotype results from a frameshift and a premature stop codon.

Reactivity with anti-GIL is enhanced with ficin and papain treatment of RBCs; the antigen is resistant to DTT and glycine-acid EDTA treatment.

RBCs of two babies born to mothers with anti-GIL have had a positive DAT but no clinical HDFN.[7] One example of anti-GIL was found following a hemolytic transfusion reaction.

The RH-Associated Glycoprotein (030) System

Rh-associated glycoprotein is the newest blood group system (IBST symbol RHAG and number 030).[3] The Rh-associated glycoprotein (RhAG) does not have Rh blood group antigens; however, its presence in a complex with the Rh proteins is essential for Rh antigen expression. Absence of RhAG due to inactivating mutations in *RHAG* results in the Rh$_{null}$ phenotype; some missense mutations in RHAG result in the Rh$_{mod}$ phenotype.[69] Unlike the RhD and RhCcEe proteins, RhAG is glycosylated on the first extracellular loop. RhAG is encoded by *RHAG*, located at chromosome 6p11-21.

Two antigens have been definitively assigned to the RHAG system: Duclos (RHAG1), previously 901013 in the high-prevalence series, and Ol^a (RHAG2), previously 700043 in the low-prevalence series. Two antigens, DSLK (for Duclos-like) and RHAG4, have been provisionally assigned to the system.

Miscellaneous Antigens

Vel

Vel, a high-prevalence antigen, is in the Vel collection, along with another high-prevalence antigen ABTI. Anti-Vel was first described in 1952 and was named after the first antibody maker. Anti-Vel is characterized by its ability to activate complement and cause in vitro and in vivo hemolysis. The antibody is most often IgG but can be IgM, and it has caused severe, immediate HTRs.[1,7] Anti-Vel has also caused one case of severe HDFN in which the mother had previously been transfused.[9]

Vel antigen expression is weak on cord RBCs and can be variable on RBCs of different adult individuals. RBCs with weak expression of Vel can be mistyped as Vel–. This is one of the reasons why anti-Vel can be a difficult antibody to work with and identify. Reactivity with anti-Vel can be enhanced with enzyme-treated RBCs. The antigen is also resistant to glycine-acid EDTA and DTT treatment, though some examples of anti-Vel do not react with DTT-treated RBCs.[70]

At^a

Anti-At^a was first described in 1967 in the serum of a black woman named Mrs. Augustine.[1] At^a is a high-prevalence antigen, and all At(a–) individuals have been black. The antigen is fully developed at birth and is resistant to treatment with ficin and papain, DTT, and glycine-acid EDTA. The antibody is usually IgG, reactive in the antiglobulin test. Anti-At^a has caused severe HTRs and one reported mild case of HDFN.[7,9]

Jr^a

Jr^a is a high-prevalence antigen in most populations; the Jr(a–) phenotype is found more commonly in Japanese. The first anti-Jr^a was described in 1970; several examples have since been found. The antigen is fully developed at birth and is resistant to treatment with ficin and papain, DTT, and glycine-acid EDTA.

Anti-Jr^a is usually IgG. Clinical significance of anti-Jr^a is not well established since it is a rare antibody. One fatal case of HDFN was recently reported; in this case, the mother had previously been massively transfused, whereas in previous cases of no to mild HDFN, the mothers had not been transfused.[71] Some patients with anti-Jr^a have received Jr(a+) incompatible units for transfusion and have had no ill effect, but in other cases, incompatible transfusions have resulted in HTRs.[72]

Sd^a

The Sd^a antigen is a high-prevalence antigen named for Sid, who was the head of the maintenance department at the Lister Institute in London. His RBCs had been used for many years as a panel donor, and they reacted strongly with examples of a new antibody. The soluble form of Sd^a is Tamm-Horsfall glycoprotein found in urine. The antigen is not expressed on RBCs of newborns but is in their saliva, urine, and meconium. The strength of Sd^a on adult RBCs varies and is markedly reduced in pregnancy. The antigen is found on 91% of RBC samples, and Sd^a substance is found in 96% of urine samples. Only 4% of people are Sd(a–).[9] Strong examples of Sd^a are noted as Sd(a++).

Anti-Sd^a can naturally occur (i.e., without known stimulation by transfusion or pregnancy) in the sera of individuals who are Sd(a–). Anti-Sd^a is usually an IgM agglutinin that is reactive at room temperature, but it can be detected in the indirect antiglobulin test and does not react with cord RBCs. Reactivity is described as small, refractile (shiny) agglutinates in a sea of free RBCs. Because the soluble antigen is present in urine of Sd(a+) individuals, neutralization of the refractile agglutinates by urine is a technique used to identify anti-Sd^a. The Sd^a antigen is resistant to treatment with ficin, papain, DTT, and glycine-acid EDTA. Reactivity of the antibody is enhanced with enzyme-treated RBCs. Anti-Sd^a is generally considered clinically insignificant for transfusion, though there are two reports of transfusion reactions associated with the transfusion of Sd(a++) RBCs.

Applications to Routine Blood Banking

The major blood group systems outside of ABO and Rh become important only after patients develop unexpected antibodies. Then a fundamental knowledge of antibody characteristics, clinical significance, and antigen frequency is needed to help confirm antibody specificity and to select appropriate units for transfusion.

Only a few antibody specificities are commonly seen: M, P1, and I antibodies react at room temperature and are considered clinically insignificant; K, S, s, Fy^a, Fy^b, Jk^a, and Jk^b antibodies react in the antiglobulin phase and are clinically significant. These and selected others are summarized in Table 8–24.

Not all antibody problems are easily solved; panel reactions are sometimes inconclusive. As described in this chapter, the existence of silent, regulator, and inhibitor genes can affect antigen expression. Hopefully the reader will find that the information in this chapter provides a starting point for serologic problem-solving. For further detailed information about the RBC antigens and antibodies described here, see Issitt and Anstee[1] and Daniels.[7] Resolution of antibody problems involving the unusual specificities described here may require the assistance of an immunohematology reference laboratory.

Table 8–24   Summary of Antibody Characteristics

ANTIBODY	REACTIVITY			ENZYMES	BIND COMPLEMENT	IN VITRO HEMOLYSIS	HTR	HDFN	COMPATIBLE IN U.S. POPULATION (%)
	≤RT	37	AHG						
M*	Most	Few	Few	Destroy	No	No	Few	Mild–severe	22
N*	Most	Few	Few	Destroy	No	No	Rare	Moderate	2B
S	Some	Some	Most	Variable effect	Some	No	Yes	Mild	45 W
									69 B
s	Few	Few	Most	Variable effect	Rare	No	Yes	Mild–severe	11 W
									3 B
U	Rare	Some	Most	No change	No	No	Yes	Mild–severe	< 1 B
P1*	Most	Some	Rare	Enhance	Rare	Rare	Rare	No	21
PP1Pk†	Most	Some	Some	Enhance	Most	Most	Yes	Mild	< 0.1
P‡	Most	Some	Some	Enhance	Most	Some	Yes	Mild–severe	< 0.1
I*	Most	Few	Few	Enhance	Most	Few	Rare	No	See text
i*	Most	Few	Few	Enhance	Most	Few	No	Mild	See text
K	Some	Some	Most	No change	Rare	No	Yes	Mild–severe	91
k	Few	Few	Most	No change	No	No	Yes	Mild	0.2
Kpa	Some	Some	Most	No change	No	No	Yes	Mild	99.7
Kpb	Few	Few	Most	No change	No	No	Yes	Mild	< 0.1
Jsa	Few	Few	Most	No change	No	No	Yes	Moderate	100 W
									80 B
Jsb	No	No	Most	No change	No	No	Yes	Mild–moderate	1 B
Fya	Rare	Rare	Most	Destroy	Rare	No	Yes	Mild–severe	34 W
Fyb	Rare	Rare	Most	Destroy	Rare	No	Yes	Mild	17 W
									77 B
Jka‡	Few	Few	Most	Enhance	Yes§	Some	Yes	Mild	23
Jkb‡	Few	Few	Most	Enhance	Yes§	Some	Yes	Mild	28 W
									57 B
Lua	Most	Few	Few	Variable effect	Some	No	No	Mild	92
Lub	Few	Few	Most	Variable effect	Some	No	Yes	Mild	0.15

B = blacks; HDFN = hemolytic disease of the newborn; HTR = hemolytic transfusion reactions; ≤ RT = room temperature or colder; W = whites.
*Usually clinically insignificant
†Potent hemolysins may be associated with early abortions
‡Associated with severe delayed HTR
§Provided IgM is present

SUMMARY CHART

Blood Group Terminology

✓ The ISBT terminology for RBC surface antigens provides a standardized numeric system for naming authenticated antigens that is suitable for electronic data processing equipment. This terminology was not intended to replace conventional terminology.

✓ In the ISBT classification, RBC antigens are assigned a six-digit identification number: The first three digits represent the system, collection, or series, and the second three digits identify the antigen. All antigens are catalogued into one of the following four groups:

- A blood group system if controlled by a single gene locus, or by two or more closely linked genes
- A collection if shown to share a biochemical, serologic, or genetic relationship
- The high-prevalence series (901) if found in more than 90% of most populations
- The low-prevalence series (700) if found in less than 1% of most populations

Lewis Blood Group

✓ Lewis blood group antigens are not synthesized by the RBCs. These antigens are adsorbed from plasma onto the RBC membrane.

✓ The *Le* gene codes for L-fucosyltransferase, which adds L-fucose to type 1 chains.

✓ The *Le* gene is needed for the expression of Le^a substance, and *Le* and *Se* genes are needed to form Le^b substance.

✓ The *lele* genotype is more common among blacks than among whites and results in the Le(a–b–) phenotype.

✓ Lewis antigens are poorly expressed at birth.

✓ Lewis antibodies are generally IgM (naturally occurring) made by Le(a–b–) individuals.

✓ Lewis antibodies are frequently encountered in pregnant women.

✓ Lewis antibodies are not considered significant for transfusion medicine.

The P Blood Group

✓ The P blood group consists of the biochemically related antigens P, P1, P^k and LKE.

✓ P1 antigen expression is variable; P1 antigen is poorly developed at birth.

✓ Anti-P1 is a common naturally occurring IgM antibody in the sera of P1– individuals; it is usually a weak, cold-reactive saline agglutinin and can be neutralized with soluble P1 substance found in hydatid cyst fluid.

✓ Anti-PP1P^k is produced by the rare p individuals early in life without RBC sensitization and reacts with all RBCs except those of other p individuals. Antibodies may be a mixture of IgM and IgG, efficiently bind complement, may demonstrate in vitro hemolysis, and can cause severe HTRs. Anti-PP1P^k is associated with spontaneous abortions.

✓ Alloanti-P is found as a naturally occurring alloantibody in the sera of P^k individuals and is clinically significant.

✓ Autoanti-P is most often the specificity associated with the cold-reactive IgG autoantibody in patients with paroxysmal cold hemoglobinuria (PCH).

✓ The autoanti-P of PCH usually does not react by routine tests but is demonstrable as a biphasic hemolysin only in the Donath-Landsteiner test.

The I and i Antigens

✓ I and i antigens are not antithetical; they have a reciprocal relationship.

✓ Most adult RBCs are rich in I and have only trace amounts of i antigen.

✓ At birth, infant RBCs are rich in i; I is almost undetectable; over the next 18 months of development, the infant's RBCs will convert from i to I antigen.

✓ Anti-I is typically a benign, weak, naturally occurring, saline-reactive IgM autoagglutinin, usually detectable only at 4°C.

✓ Pathogenic anti-I is typically a strong cold autoagglutinin that demonstrates high-titer reactivity at 4°C and reacts over a wide thermal range (up to 30°–32°C).

✓ Patients with *M. pneumoniae* infections may develop strong cold agglutinins with autoanti-I specificity.

✓ Anti-i is a rare IgM agglutinin that reacts optimally at 4°C; potent examples may be associated with infectious mononucleosis.

The MNS Blood Group System

✓ Anti-M and anti-N are cold-reactive saline agglutinins that do not bind complement or react with enzyme-treated cells; both anti-M and anti-N may demonstrate dosage.

✓ Anti-S and anti-s are IgG antibodies, reactive at 37°C and the antiglobulin phase. They may bind complement and have been associated with HDFN and HTRs.

✓ The S–s–U– phenotype is found in blacks.

✓ Anti-U is usually an IgG antibody and has been associated with HTRs and HDFN.

The Kell Blood Group System

✓ The Kell blood group antigens are well developed at birth and are not destroyed by enzymes.

✓ The Kell blood group antigens are destroyed by DTT, ZZAP, and glycine-acid EDTA.

✓ Excluding ABO, the K antigen is rated second only to D antigen in immunogenicity.

SUMMARY CHART—cont'd

- ✔ The k antigen is high prevalence.
- ✔ Anti-K is usually an IgG antibody reactive in the antiglobulin phase and is made in response to pregnancy or transfusion of RBCs; it has been implicated in severe HTRs and HDFN.
- ✔ The McLeod phenotype, affecting only males, is described as a rare phenotype with decreased Kell system antigen expression. The McLeod syndrome includes the clinical manifestations of abnormal RBC morphology, compensated hemolytic anemia, and neurological and muscular abnormalities. Some males with the McLeod phenotype also have the X-linked chronic granulomatous disease.

The Duffy Blood Group System

- ✔ Fy^a and Fy^b antigens are destroyed by enzymes and ZZAP; they are well developed at birth. The Fy(a–b–) phenotype is prevalent in blacks but virtually nonexistent in whites.
- ✔ Fy(a–b–) RBCs resist infection by the malaria organism *P. vivax*.
- ✔ Anti-Fy^a and anti-Fy^b are usually IgG antibodies and react optimally at the antiglobulin phase of testing; both antibodies have been implicated in delayed HTRs and HDFN.

The Kidd Blood Group System

- ✔ Anti-Jk^a and anti-Jk^b may demonstrate dosage, are often weak, and found in combination with other antibodies; both are typically IgG and reactive in the antiglobulin test.
- ✔ Kidd system antibodies may bind complement and are made in response to foreign RBC exposure during pregnancy or transfusion.
- ✔ Kidd system antibodies are a common cause of delayed HTRs.
- ✔ Kidd system antibody reactivity is enhanced with enzymes, LISS, and PEG.

The Lutheran Blood Group System

- ✔ Lu^a and Lu^b are antigens produced by codominant alleles; they are poorly developed at birth.
- ✔ Anti-Lu^a may be a naturally occurring saline agglutinin that reacts optimally at room temperature.
- ✔ Anti-Lu^b is usually an IgG antibody reactive at the antiglobulin phase; it is usually produced in response to foreign RBC exposure during pregnancy or transfusion.
- ✔ The Lu(a–b–) phenotype is rare and may result from three different genetic backgrounds; only individuals with the recessive type Lu(a–b–) can make anti-Lu3.

Other Blood Groups and Antigens

- ✔ The Diego system antigens are located on a major RBC protein, band 3, also known as the RBC anion exchanger (AE1).
- ✔ Anti-Di^a, anti-Di^b, and anti-Wr^a are generally considered to be clinically significant; all have caused severe HTRs and HDFN. Anti-Wr^a is a relatively common antibody.
- ✔ Wr^b expression requires the presence of a normal GPA (MNS system); alloanti-Wr^b is extremely rare.
- ✔ Anti-Yt^a is a fairly common antibody to a high-prevalence antigen that is sometimes clinically significant and sometimes insignificant.
- ✔ The Xg^a antigen is found on the short arm of the X chromosome and is of higher prevalence in females (89%) than in males (66%). Although it is usually IgG, anti-Xg^a has not been implicated in HDFN or as a cause of HTRs.
- ✔ Antibodies to Scianna system antigens are rare and little is known about their clinical significance. The rare null phenotype, Sc:–1,–2,–3, has been observed in the Marshall Islands and New Guinea.
- ✔ In addition to the Do^a and Do^b antigens, the Gy^a, Hy, Jo^a antigens are assigned to the Dombrock system. Anti-Do^a and anti-Do^b have caused HTRs but no clinical HDFN; these antibodies are usually weak and difficult to identify.
- ✔ The Colton system is composed of the antithetical Co^a and Co^b antigens as well as the high-prevalence Co3 antigen; the antigens are carried on aquaporin 1, a red cell water channel. The Colton antibodies have caused HTRs and HDFN.
- ✔ LW has a phenotypic relationship with the D antigen; Rh_{null} RBCs type LW(a–b–).
- ✔ Anti-LW reacts strongly with D+ RBCs and can look like anti-D. DTT treatment of test RBCs will distinguish between these two antibodies because the LW antigen is denatured by DTT, but the D antigen is not. In other words, anti-LW does not react with DTT-treated D+ RBCs but anti-D does.
- ✔ The antigens in the Chido/Rodgers system are located on the complement fragments C4B and C4A, respectively, that are adsorbed onto RBCs from plasma.
- ✔ The clinically insignificant anti-Ch and anti-Rg react weakly, often to moderate or high-titer endpoints in the antiglobulin test and may be tentatively identified by plasma inhibition methods.
- ✔ Gerbich-negative phenotypes are very rare outside of Papua, New Guinea.

Continued

SUMMARY CHART—cont'd

✔ Gerbich antibodies are sometimes clinically significant for transfusion and sometimes insignificant. Only three cases of serious HDFN due to anti-Ge3 have been reported.

✔ The Cromer antigens are carried on the decay accelerating factor and are distributed in body fluids and on RBCs, WBCs, platelets, and placental tissue.

✔ The rare anti-Cr^a and anti-Tc^a have been found only in black individuals; some examples have caused HTRs.

✔ The Knops antigens are located on complement receptor 1 (CR1). Knops antibodies are clinically insignificant and have weak and "nebulous" reactivity at the antiglobulin phase; they are not inhibited by plasma.

✔ The In^a antigen is more prevalent in Arab and Iranian populations, with In^a and In^b antigen expression being depressed on the dominant type Lu(a–b–) RBCs.

✔ JMH antibodies most often occur in individuals with acquired JMH– status. Anti-JMH in these individuals is not clinically significant.

✔ Anti-Vel is most often IgG but can be IgM, and has caused severe immediate HTRs and HDFN. When serum is tested, anti-Vel characteristically causes in vitro hemolysis.

✔ Anti-At^a has been found only in blacks; the antibody is usually IgG and has caused severe HTRs.

✔ Anti-Jr^a is found more commonly in Japanese, but clinical significance is not well established, since it is a rare antibody; it has caused HTRs and a fatal case of HDFN.

✔ Anti-Sd^a has characteristic shiny and refractile agglutinates under the microscope and is inhibited with urine from Sd(a+) individuals.

Review Questions

1. The following phenotypes are written incorrectly except for:
   a. Jk^a+
   b. Jka+
   c. Jk^a(+)
   d. Jk(a+)

2. Which of the following characteristics best describes Lewis antibodies?
   a. IgM, naturally occurring, cause HDFN
   b. IgM, naturally occurring, do not cause HDFN
   c. IgG, in vitro hemolysis, cause hemolytic transfusion reactions
   d. IgG, in vitro hemolysis, do not cause hemolytic transfusion reactions

3. The *Le* gene codes for a specific glycosyltransferase that transfers a fucose to the N-acetylglucosamine on:
   a. Type 1 precursor chain.
   b. Type 2 precursor chain.
   c. Types 1 and 2 precursor chain.
   d. Either type 1 or type 2 in any one individual but not both.

4. What substances would be found in the saliva of a group B secretor who also has *Lele* genes?
   a. H, Le^a
   b. H, B, Le^a
   c. H, B, Le^a, Le^b
   d. H, B, Le^b

5. Transformation to Le^b phenotype after birth may be as follows:
   a. Le(a–b–) to Le(a+b–) to Le(a+b+) to Le(a–b+)
   b. Le(a+b–) to Le(a–b–) to Le(a–b+) to Le(a+b+)
   c. Le(a–b+) to Le(a+b–) to Le(a+b+) to Le(a–b–)
   d. Le(a+b+) to Le(a+b–) to Le(a–b–) to Le(a–b+)

6. In what way do the Lewis antigens change during pregnancy?
   a. Le^a antigen increases only
   b. Le^b antigen increases only
   c. Le^a and Le^b both increase
   d. Le^a and Le^b both decrease

7. A type 1 chain has:
   a. The terminal galactose in a 1-3 linkage to subterminal N-acetylglucosamine.
   b. The terminal galactose in a 1-4 linkage to subterminal N-acetylglucosamine.
   c. The terminal galactose in a 1-3 linkage to subterminal N-acetylgalactosamine.
   d. The terminal galactose in a 1-4 linkage to subterminal N-acetylgalactosamine.

8. Which of the following best describes Lewis antigens?
   a. The antigens are integral membrane glycolipids
   b. Le^a and Le^b are antithetical antigens
   c. The Le(a+b–) phenotype is found in secretors
   d. None of the above

9. Which of the following genotypes would explain RBCs typed as group A Le(a+b–)?
   a. *A/O Lele HH Sese*
   b. *A/A Lele HH sese*
   c. *A/O LeLe hh SeSe*
   d. *A/A LeLe hh sese*

10. Anti-Le^{bH} will not react or will react more weakly with which of the following RBCs?
    a. Group O Le(b+)
    b. Group A$_2$ Le(b+)
    c. Group A$_1$ Le(b+)
    d. None of the above

11. Which of the following best describes MN antigens and antibodies?
    a. Well developed at birth, susceptible to enzymes, generally saline reactive
    b. Not well developed at birth, susceptible to enzymes, generally saline reactive
    c. Well developed at birth, not susceptible to enzymes, generally saline reactive
    d. Well developed at birth, susceptible to enzymes, generally antiglobulin reactive

12. Which autoantibody specificity is found in patients with paroxysmal cold hemoglobinuria?
    a. Anti-I
    b. Anti-i
    c. Anti-P
    d. Anti-P1

13. Which of the following is the most common antibody seen in the blood bank after ABO and Rh antibodies?
    a. Anti-Fy^a
    b. Anti-k
    c. Anti-Js^a
    d. Anti-K

14. Which blood group system is associated with resistance to *P. vivax* malaria?
    a. P
    b. Kell
    c. Duffy
    d. Kidd

15. The null K$_o$ RBC can be artificially prepared by which of the following treatments?
    a. Ficin and DTT
    b. Ficin and glycine-acid EDTA
    c. DTT and glycine-acid EDTA
    d. Glycine-acid EDTA and sialidase

16. Which antibody does *not* fit with the others with respect to optimum phase of reactivity?
    a. Anti-S
    b. Anti-P1
    c. Anti-Fy^a
    d. Anti-Jk^b

17. Which of the following Duffy phenotypes is prevalent in blacks but virtually nonexistent in whites?
    a. Fy(a+b+)
    b. Fy(a–b+)
    c. Fy(a–b–)
    d. Fy(a+b–)

18. Antibody detection cells will *not* routinely detect which antibody specificity?
    a. Anti-M
    b. Anti-Kp^a
    c. Anti-Fy^a
    d. Anti-Lu^b

19. Antibodies to antigens in which of the following blood groups are known for showing dosage?
    a. I
    b. P
    c. Kidd
    d. Lutheran

20. Which antibody is most commonly associated with delayed hemolytic transfusion reactions?
    a. Anti-s
    b. Anti-k
    c. Anti-Lu^a
    d. Anti-Jk^a

21. Anti-U will not react with which of the following RBCs?
    a. M+N+S+s–
    b. M+N–S–s–
    c. M–N+S–s+
    d. M+N–S+s+

22. A patient with an *M. pneumoniae* infection will most likely develop a cold autoantibody with specificity to which antigen?
    a. I
    b. i
    c. P
    d. P1

23. Which antigen is destroyed by enzymes?
    a. P1
    b. Js^a
    c. Fy^a
    d. Jk^a

24. The antibody to this high-prevalence antigen demonstrates mixed-field agglutination that appears shiny and refractile under the microscope:
    a. Vel
    b. JMH
    c. Jr^a
    d. Sd^a

25. Which of the following has been associated with causing severe immediate HTRs?

    a. Anti-JMH

    b. Anti-Lu[b]

    c. Anti-Vel

    d. Anti-Sd[a]

26. Which of the following antibodies would more likely be found in a black patient?

    a. Anti-Cr[a]

    b. Anti-At[a]

    c. Anti-Hy

    d. All of the above

27. Which of the following antigens is not in a blood group system?

    a. Do[a]

    b. Vel

    c. JMH

    d. Kx

28. A weakly reactive antibody with a titer of 128 is neutralized by plasma. Which of the following could be the specificity?

    a. Anti-JMH

    b. Anti-Ch

    c. Anti-Kn[a]

    d. Anti-Kp[a]

29. An antibody reacted with untreated RBCs and DTT-treated RBCs but not with ficin-treated RBCs. Which of the following antibodies could explain this pattern of reactivity?

    a. Anti-JMH

    b. Anti-Yt[a]

    c. Anti-Kp[b]

    d. Anti-Ch

30. The following antibodies are generally considered clinically insignificant because they have not been associated with causing increased destruction of RBCs, HDFN, or HTRs.

    a. Anti-Do[a] and anti-Co[a]

    b. Anti-Ge3 and anti-Wr[a]

    c. Anti-Ch and anti-Kn[a]

    d. Anti-Di[b] and anti-Yt

References

1. Issitt, PD, and Anstee, DJ: Applied Blood Group Serology, 4th ed. Montgomery Scientific, Durham, NC, 1998.
2. Garratty, G, Dzik, W, Issit, PD, et al: Terminology for blood group antigens and genes—historical origins and guidelines in the new millennium. Transfusion 40:477–489, 2000.
3. Storry, JR, Castilho, L, Daniels, G, et al: International Society of Blood Transfusion Working Party on red cell immunogenetics and blood group terminology: Berlin report. Vox Sang 101: 77–82, 2011.
4. Daniels, GL, Fletcher, A, Garratty, G, et al: Blood group terminology 2004: From the International Society of Blood Transfusion committee on terminology for red cell surface antigens. Vox Sang 87:304–316, 2004.
5. Roback, JD, Combs, MR, Grossman, BJ, and Hillyer, CD (eds): Technical Manual, 16th ed. Bethesda, MD: AABB, 2008.
6. Mourant, AE. A "new" human blood group antigen of frequent occurrence. Nature 158:237–238,1946.
7. Daniels, G: The Human Blood Groups, 2nd ed. Blackwell Science, Oxford, 2002.
8. Grubb R. Correlation between Lewis blood group and secretor character in man. Nature 162:933,1948.
9. Reid, ME, and Lomas-Francis, C: The Blood Group Antigen Facts Book, 2nd ed. Academic Press, San Diego, CA, 2003.
10. Levine, P, Bobbitt, OB, Waller, RK, et al: Isoimmunization by a new blood factor in tumor cells. Proc Soc Exp Biol Med 77:403–405, 1951.
11. Sanger, R: An association between the P and Jay systems of blood groups. Nature 176:1163–1164, 1955.
12. Matson, GA, Swanson J, Noades, J, et al: A "new" antigen and antibody belonging to the P blood group system. Am J Hum Genet 11:26–34, 1959.
13. Arndt, PA, Garratty, G, Marfoe, RA, et al: An acute hemolytic transfusion reaction caused by an anti-P$_1$ that reacted at 37°C. Transfusion 38:373–377, 1998.
14. Hellberg, A, Poole, J, and Olsson, ML: Molecular basis of the globoside-deficient P[k] blood group phenotype. J Biol Chem 277:29455–29459, 2002.
15. Yoshida, H, Ito, K, Kusakari, T, et al: Removal of maternal antibodies from a woman with repeated fetal loss due to P blood group incompatibility. Transfusion 34:702–705,1994.
16. Tippett, P, Sanger, R, Race, RR, et al: An agglutinin associated with the P and the ABO blood group systems. Vox Sang 10:269–280, 1965.
17. Lund, N, Olsson, ML, Ramkumar, S, et al: The human P[k] histo-blood group antigen provides protection against HIV-1 infection. Blood 113:4980–4991, 2009.
18. Marsh, WL, and Jenkins, WJ: Anti-i: A new cold antibody. Nature 188:753, 1960.
19. Yu, L, Twu, Y, Chang, C, et al: Molecular basis of the adult i phenotype and the gene responsible for the expression of the human blood group I antigen. Blood 98:3840–3845, 2001.
20. Yu, L, Twu, Y, Chou, M, et al: The molecular genetics of the human I locus and molecular background explain the partial association of the adult i phenotype with congenital cataracts. Blood 101:2081–2088, 2003.
21. Curtain, CC, Baumgarten, A, Gorman, J, et al: Cold haemagglutinins: Unusual incidence in Melanesian populations. Br J Haematol 11:471–479, 1965.
22. Booth, PB, Jenkins, WL, and Marsh, WL: Anti-I[T]: A new antibody of the I blood group system occurring in certain Melanesian sera. Br J Haematol 12:341–344, 1966.
23. Garratty, G, Petz, LD, Walerstein, RO, et al: Autoimmune hemolytic anemia in Hodgkin's disease associated with anti-I[T]. Transfusion 14:226–231, 1974.
24. Greenwalt, TJ, Sasaki, T, Sanger, R, et al: An allele of the S(s) blood group genes. Proc Natl Acad Sci 40:1126–1129, 1954.
25. Fukuda, M: Molecular genetics of the glycophorin A gene cluster. Semin Hematol 30:138–151, 1993.
26. Palacajornsuk, P: Review: Molecular basis of MNS blood group variants. Immunohematology 22:171–182, 2006.
27. Reid, ME, Storry, JR, Ralph, H, et al: Expression and quantitative variation of the low-incidence blood group antigen He on some S–s– red cells. Transfusion 36:719–724, 1996.
28. Darnborough, J, Dunsford, I, and Wallace, JA: The En[a] antigen and antibody: A genetical modification of human red cells affecting their blood grouping reactions. Vox Sang 17:241–255, 1969.
29. Furuhjelm, U, Myllylä, G, Nevanlinna, HR, et al: The red cell phenotype En(a-) and anti-En[a]: Serological and physiochemical aspects. Vox Sang 17:256–278, 1969.
30. Jung, HH, Danek, A, and Frey, BM: McLeod syndrome: A neurohaematological disorder. Vox Sang 93:112–121, 2007.

31. Marsh, WL, Nichols, ME, Øyen R, et al: Naturally occurring anti-Kell stimulated by *E. coli* enterocolitis in a 20-day-old child. Transfusion 18:149–154, 1978.

32. Daniels, G, Hadley, A, and Green, CA: Causes of fetal anemia in hemolytic disease due to anti-K [letter]. Transfusion 43: 115–116, 2003.

33. Allen, FH, Krabbe, SMR, and Corcoran, PA: A new phenotype (McLeod) in the Kell blood group system. Vox Sang 6: 555–560, 1961.

34. Giblett, ER, Klebanoff, SJ, Pincus, SH, et al: Kell phenotypes in chronic granulomatous disease: A potential transfusion hazard [letter]. Lancet 1:1235–1236, 1971.

35. Bansal, I, Jeon, H, Hui, SR, et al: Transfusion support for a patient with McLeod phenotype without chronic granulomatous disease and with antibodies to Kx and Km. Vox Sang 94:216–220, 2008.

36. McGinnis, MH, MacLowry, JD, and Holland, PV: Acquisition of K:1-like antigen during terminal sepsis. Transfusion 24: 28–30, 1984.

37. Sanger, R, Race, RR, and Jack, J: The Duffy blood groups of New York Negroes: The phenotype Fy(a–b–). Br J Haematol 1:370–374, 1955.

38. Pogo, AO, and Chaudhuri, A: The Duffy protein: A malarial and chemokine receptor. Semin Hematol 37:122–129, 2000.

39. Yazdanbakhsh, K, Rios, M, Storry, JR, et al: Molecular mechanisms that lead to reduced expression of Duffy antigens. Transfusion 40:310–320, 2000.

40. Colledge, KI, Pezzulich, M, and Marsh, WL: Anti-Fy5, an antibody disclosing a probable association between the Rhesus and Duffy blood group genes. Vox Sang 24:193–199, 1973.

41. Allen, FH, Diamond, LK, and Niedziela, B: A new blood group antigen. Nature 167:482, 1951.

42. Fernando, M, Martinez-Cañabate, S, Luna, I, et al: Severe hemolytic disease of the fetus due to anti-Jk^b [letter]. Transfusion 48:402–403, 2008.

43. Heaton, DC, and McLoughlin, K: Jk(a–b–) red blood cells resist urea lysis. Transfusion 22:70–71, 1982.

44. Callender, STE, and Race, RR: A serological and genetical study of multiple antibodies formed in response to blood transfusion by a patient with lupus erythematosus diffusus. Ann Eugen 13:102, 1946.

45. Cutbush, M, and Chanarin, I: The expected blood-group antibody, anti-Lu^b. Nature 178:855–856, 1956.

46. Crawford, MN, Greenwalt, TJ, Sasaki, T, et al: The phenotype Lu(a–b–) together with unconventional Kidd groups in one family. Transfusion 1:228–232, 1961.

47. Eyler, CE, and Telen, MJ: The Lutheran glycoprotein: A multifunctional adhesion receptor. Transfusion 46:668–677, 2006.

48. Karamatic Crew, V, Green, C, and Daniels, G: Molecular bases of the antigens of the Lutheran blood group system. Transfusion 43:1729–1737, 2003.

49. Singleton, BK, Burton, NM, Green, C, et al: Mutations in *EKLF/KLF1* form the molecular basis of the rare blood group In(Lu) phenotype. Blood 112:2081–2088, 2008.

50. Karamatic Crew, V, Mallinson, G, Green, C, et al: Different inactivating mutations in the *LU* genes of three individuals with the Lutheran-null phenotype. Transfusion 47:492–498, 2007.

51. Eaton, BR, Morton, JA, Pickles, MM, et al: A new antibody, anti-Yt^a, characterizing a blood-group antigen of high incidence. Br J Haematol 2:333–341, 1956.

52. Byrne, KM, and Byrne, PC: Review: Other blood group systems—Diego, Yt, Xg, Scianna, Dombrock, Colton, Landsteiner-Wiener, and Indian. Immunohematology 20:50–58,2004.

53. Devine, P, Dawson, FE, Motschman, TL, et al: Serologic evidence that Scianna null (Sc:–1,–2) red cells lack multiple high-frequency antigens. Transfusion 28:346–349, 1988.

54. Flegel, WA, Chen, Q, Reid, ME, et al: SCER and SCAN: Two novel high-prevalence antigens in the Scianna blood group system. Transfusion 45:1940–1944, 2005.

55. Banks, JA, Hemming, N, and Poole, J: Evidence that the Gy^a, Hy and Jo^a antigens belong to the Dombrock blood group system. Vox Sang 68:177–182, 1995.

56. Michalewska, B, Wielgos, M, Zupanska, B, et al: Anti-Co^a implicated in severe haemolytic disease of the foetus and newborn. Transfus Med 18:71–73, 2008.

57. Landsteiner, K, and Wiener, AS: An agglutinable factor in human blood recognized by immune sera for rhesus blood. Proc Soc Exp Biol NY 43:223, 1940.

58. Levine, P, and Stetson, RE: An unusual case of intragroup agglutination. J Am Med Ass 113:126–127, 1939.

59. Bruce, LJ: Hereditary stomatocytosis and cation leaky red cells—recent developments. Blood Cells Mol Dis 42:216–222, 2009.

60. Arndt, PA, Garratty, G, Daniels, G, et al: Late onset neonatal anaemia due to maternal anti-Ge: Possible association with destruction of erythroid progenitors. Transfus Med 15: 125–132, 2005.

61. Blackall, DP, Pesek, GD, Montgomery, MM, et al: Hemolytic disease of the fetus and newborn due to anti-Ge3: Combined antibody-dependent hemolysis and erythroid precursor cell growth inhibition. Am J Perinatol 25:541–545, 2008.

62. Storry, JR, and Reid, ME: The Cromer blood group system: A review. Immunohematology 18:95–103, 2002.

63. Hue-Roye, K, Lomas-Francis, C, Belaygorod, L, et al: Three new high-prevalence antigens in the Cromer blood group system. Transfusion 47:1621–1629, 2007.

64. Moulds, JM: The Knops blood group system: A review. Immunohematology 26:2–7, 2010.

65. Parsons, SF, Jones, J, Anstee, DJ, et al: A novel form of congenital dyserythropoietic anemia associated with deficiency of erythroid CD44 and a unique blood group phenotype [In(a–b–), Co(a–b–)]. Blood 83:860–868, 1994.

66. Karamatic Crew, V, Burton, N, Kagan, A, et al: CD151, the first member of the tetraspanin (TM4) superfamily detected on erythrocytes, is essential for the correct assembly of human basement membranes in kidney and skin. Blood 104: 2217–2223, 2004.

67. Karamatic Crew, V, Poole, J, Long, S, et al: Two MER2-negative individuals with the same novel *CD151* mutation and evidence for clinical significance of anti-MER2. Transfusion 48: 1912–1916, 2008.

68. Seltsam, A, Strigens, S, Levene, C, et al: The molecular diversity of Sema7A, the semaphorin that carries the JHM blood group antigens. Transfusion 47:133–146, 2007.

69. Tilley, L, Green, C, Poole, J, et al: A new blood group system, RHAG: Three antigens resulting from amino acid substitutions in the Rh-associated glycoprotein. Vox Sang 98:151–159, 2010.

70. Rainer, T, Israel, B, Caglioti, S, et al: The effects of dithiothreitol-treated red blood cells with anti-Vel [abstract]. Transfusion 44:122A, 2004.

71. Peyrard, T, Pham, B, Arnaud, L, et al: Fatal hemolytic disease of the fetus and newborn associated with anti-Jr^a. Transfusion 48:1906–1911, 2008.

72. Kwon, MY, Su, L, Arndt, PA, et al: Clinical significance of anti-Jr^a: Report of two cases and review of the literature. Transfusion 44:197–201, 2004.

Chapter 9

Detection and Identification of Antibodies

Kathleen S. Trudell, MLS (ASCP)[CM], SBB[CM]

OBJECTIVES

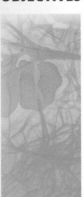

1. Differentiate between the following antibodies: expected and unexpected, immune, naturally occurring, passive, autoantibody and alloantibody, warm and cold.
2. Explain what factors make an antibody clinically significant.
3. Describe which patient populations require an antibody screen.
4. Select appropriate cells to include in a screen cell set.
5. Describe the impact of various enhancement media on antibody detection.
6. Compare and contrast antibody detection methods.
7. Interpret the result of an antibody screen.
8. List the limitations of the antibody screen.
9. Interpret the results of an antibody identification panel.
10. Summarize the exclusion and inclusion methods.
11. Correlate knowledge of the serologic characteristics of commonly encountered antibodies with antibody identification panel findings.
12. Identify the situations in which additional panel cells should be tested and select appropriate cells.
13. Describe antigen-typing techniques.
14. Calculate the number of red blood cell (RBC) units that must be antigen-tested to fulfill a physician's request for crossmatch.
15. Explain the principles behind enzyme and neutralization techniques.
16. Given a patient's history and initial results, choose the correct method for performing an adsorption.
17. Describe elution methods and give an example of when each would be used.
18. List three chemicals used in performing a partial elution and the advantages of use.

OBJECTIVES—cont'd

19. Outline the procedure for determining the antibody titer level, including reporting of results.
20. Given a patient scenario, identify additional steps that could be employed to resolve a complex antibody identification problem, including investigating a warm autoantibody.

Introduction

The detection of antibodies directed against red blood cell antigens is critical in pretransfusion compatibility testing. It is one of the principle tools for investigating potential hemolytic transfusion reactions and immune hemolytic anemias. In addition, it aids in detecting and monitoring patients who are at risk of delivering infants with hemolytic disease of the fetus and newborn (HDFN).

The focus of antibody detection methods is on "irregular" or "unexpected" antibodies, as opposed to the "expected" antibodies of the ABO system. The **unexpected antibodies** of primary importance are the **immune alloantibodies**, which are produced in response to red blood cell (RBC) stimulation through transfusion, transplantation, or pregnancy. Other unexpected antibodies may be "naturally occurring" (i.e., produced without RBC stimulation). **Naturally occurring antibodies** may form as a result of exposure to environmental sources, such as pollen, fungus, and bacteria, which have structures similar to some RBC antigens. Antibodies produced in one individual and then transmitted to another via plasma-containing blood components or derivatives such as intravenous immunoglobulin (IVIG) are known as **passively acquired antibodies**, a third category of unexpected antibody. The presence of naturally occurring and passive antibodies may complicate the detection and identification of immune, clinically significant antibodies.

Clinically significant antibodies are those that cause decreased survival of RBCs possessing the target antigen. These antibodies are typically IgG antibodies that react at 37°C or that react in the antihuman globulin (AHG) phase of the indirect antiglobulin test. **Autoantibodies** may also complicate the detection of clinically significant antibodies. Autoantibodies are directed against antigens expressed on one's own RBCs. Because they react with all RBCs tested, autoantibodies may mask the presence of clinically significant alloantibodies.

After detection, an antibody identification panel is performed to determine the specificity of the antibody (or antibodies) present. Once identified, the antibody's clinical significance can be ascertained and the appropriate transfusion considerations put into place. This chapter describes antibody detection and identification methods and the resolution of complex antibody cases.

Antibody Screen

Only a small percentage of the population (between 0.2% and 2%) has detectable RBC antibodies.[1,2] However, certain populations require careful screening. The AABB's *Standards*

for Blood Banks and Transfusion Services requires the use of an antibody screen to detect clinically significant antibodies in both the blood donor and the intended recipient as part of pretransfusion compatibility testing.[3] The donors may be used as a source of antigen-typing sera and antigen-negative RBC units. An antibody screen may be included when evaluating the compatibility of hematopoietic progenitor cell (HPC) and bone marrow donors with the intended transplant recipient.[4] Antibodies detected in these donors may indicate that additional processing steps are required to reduce the plasma in the product. An antibody screen is included in standard prenatal testing for obstetric patients to evaluate the risk of HDFN in the fetus and to assess the mother's candidacy for Rh-immune globulin (RHIG) prophylaxis.[5]

Tube Method

The traditional method for detecting antibodies is an **indirect antiglobulin test** performed in a test tube. RBC reagents, enhancement reagents, and AHG reagents are used to sensitize the reagent RBCs with the patient's antibodies, followed by formation of visible RBC agglutinates.

Method Overview

In the test tube method, the patient's serum or plasma is mixed with RBCs that have known antigen content (Fig. 9–1). The test may include an immediate spin phase to detect antibodies reacting at room temperature. This phase is not required and may lead to the detection of clinically insignificant cold antibodies.

The test must include a 37°C incubation phase during which IgG molecules sensitize any RBCs that possess the target antigen, coating those RBCs with antibody. Enhancement media may be added to increase the degree of sensitization. Depending on the enhancement added, the tubes may be centrifuged and observed for **hemolysis** and **agglutination** following incubation. To observe for hemolysis, the tube is carefully removed from the centrifuge so as not to dislodge the RBC button. The supernatant is observed for pink or red discoloration. To observe for agglutination, the tube is gently tilted or rolled to dislodge the cell button. The degree of reactivity is graded as 0 (no agglutination present) to w+ (agglutination barely visible to the naked eye) to 4+ (one solid agglutinate). See **Color Plate 1**.

The degree of agglutination should be judged only after all of the RBCs have been dislodged from the bottom of the test tube. The tubes are then washed with 0.9% saline a minimum of three times to remove all antibodies that remain unbound. AHG reagent, also known as Coombs' serum, is added to each tube. The tubes are centrifuged and examined for hemolysis and agglutination. In this phase, hemolysis

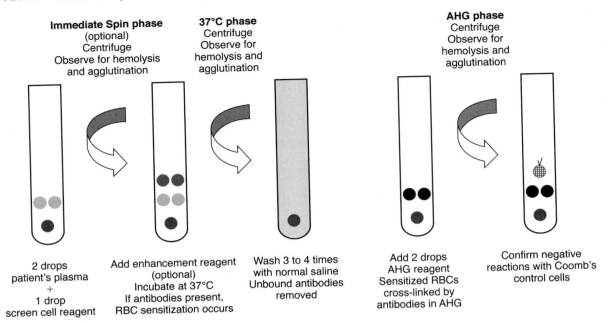

Figure 9–1. Steps for performing the tube antibody screen test.

may appear as a loss of cell button mass. If the RBCs are coated with IgG antibodies, the anti-IgG antibody in the AHG reagent will create a bridge between sensitized RBCs, resulting in observable agglutination. If there are no antibodies directed against any of the antigens present on the screen cell RBCs, the RBCs will not be sensitized, and there will be no agglutination. Again, depending on the enhancement media used, the agglutination reactions may be observed macroscopically only or may include a microscopic examination. All negative tests will have Coombs' control cells (also known as *check cells*) added to confirm the negative result.

RBC Reagents

The RBC reagents used in the antibody screen come from group O individuals who have been typed for the most common, and the most significant, RBC antigens. Group O cells are used so that anti-A and anti-B will not interfere in the detection of antibodies to other blood group systems. The RBCs are suspended at a concentration between 2% and 5% in a preservative diluent, which maintains the integrity of the antigens and prevents hemolysis. The **screen cells** are packaged in sets of two or three cell suspensions, each having a unique combination of antigens. Within the set, there

should be one cell that is positive for each of the following antigens: D, C, c, E, e, K, k, Fy^a, Fy^b, Jk^a, Jk^b, Le^a, Le^b, P_1, M, N, S, and s. Other antigens will be expressed as well. Each set of screen cells will be accompanied by an antigen profile sheet, detailing which antigens are present in each vial of cells. These profiles are lot-specific and should not be interchanged. Figure 9–2 shows an example of a three-cell profile.

Ideally, there will be **homozygous** expression of many of the antigens within the screen cell set, allowing for detection of antibodies that show dosage. A cell with homozygous antigen expression is from an individual who inherited only one allele at a given genetic locus. Therefore, the cell surface has a "double dose" of that antigen. A cell with **heterozygous** antigen expression is from a person who inherited two different alleles at a locus. The alleles "share" the available antigen sites on the cell surface. In Figure 9–3, the pair of chromosomes on the left both possess the same allele, giving rise to the "homozygous" RBC. The pair of chromosomes on the right each possess a different allele, resulting in the "heterozygous" cell.

Certain antibodies, such as those of the Kidd system, may be detected only when tested against RBCs expressing one allele (homozygous). Antibodies that react more strongly with cells having homozygous antigen expression are said to show **dosage**. Box 9–1 lists the antibodies that

CELL	Rh								MNS				Lutheran		P	Lewis		Kell		Duffy		Kidd				
	D	C	E	c	e	f	V	C^w	M	N	S	s	Lu^a	Lu^b	P_1	Le^a	Le^b	K	k	Fy^a	Fy^b	Jk^a	Jk^b			
R1R1-29	+	+	0	0	+	0	0	0	+	0	+	0	0	+	+	+	0	0	+	+	0	+	0			
R2R2-45	+	0	+	+	0	0	0	0	+	+	0	+	0	+	+	0	+	+	+	+	0	0	+			
rr-86	0	0	0	+	+	+	0	0	0	+	0	+	0	+	+	+	0	0	+	0	+	+	+			

Figure 9–2. Antigen profile of three-cell screen set.

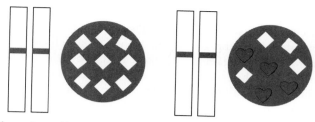

Figure 9–3. Homozygous inheritance versus heterozygous inheritance.

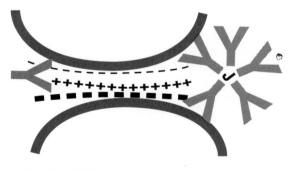

Table 9–1	Examples of RBC Phenotypes From Homozygous and Heterozygous Individuals	
PHENO-TYPE	**ANTIGENS PRESENT**	**HOMOZYGOUS VS HETEROZYGOUS**
Jk(a–b+)	Jk^b only	Homozygous
Jk(a+b+)	Both Jk^a and Jk^b	Heterozygous
Fy(a+b–)	Fy^a only	Homozygous
Fy(a+b+)	Both Fy^a and Fy^b	Heterozygous
M+ N-	M only	Homozygous
M+N+	Both M and N	Heterozygous

may show dosage, and Table 9–1 gives an example of RBC phenotypes, comparing homozygous and heterozygous antigen expression.

When testing blood donors, it is acceptable to use a pooled screening reagent that contains RBCs from at least two different individuals. These reactions should be carefully observed for mixed-field agglutination, as the target antigen may be expressed on only one cell in the pool.

Using commercially prepared screen cells to detect antibodies is superior to relying on the crossmatch alone to ensure compatibility with a donor RBC unit. The screen cell sets will test for most clinically significant antigens, whereas the crossmatched unit of blood will possess only some of those antigens. The screen cell sets will have cells with homozygous expression of many antigens, making it more reliable in detecting weakly reacting antibodies. Donor units may or may not have homozygous antigen expression, so it is possible that weak antibodies may not be detected by crossmatch alone. As RBCs age, antigen expression begins to weaken. Commercially prepared screen cell sets are diluted in a preservative to maintain antigen integrity, whereas donor RBCs may have reduced antigen expression.

Enhancement Reagents

Various **enhancement reagents**, or **potentiators**, may be added to the cell/serum mixture before the 37°C incubation phase to increase the sensitivity of the test system. These reagents may also allow for a shortened incubation time.

22% Albumin. In an electrolyte solution, negatively charged RBCs are surrounded by cations, which in turn are surrounded by anions. The effect is to produce an ionic cloud around each RBC, forcing the cells apart. The difference in electrical potential between the surface of the RBC and the outer layer of the ionic cloud is called the **zeta potential**. Albumin works by reducing the zeta potential and dispersing the charges, thus

allowing the RBCs to approach each other and increasing the chances of agglutination. The top section of Figure 9–4 demonstrates the repulsion of RBCs due to the surrounding electrical charges. The bottom of the figure illustrates that once those charges are dispersed by an enhancement reagent, the RBCs may approach each other more closely.

Low Ionic Strength Solution. Low Ionic Strength Solution (LISS) contains glycine in an albumin solution. In addition to lowering the zeta potential, LISS increases the uptake of antibody onto the RBC during the sensitization phase. This increases the possibility of agglutination.

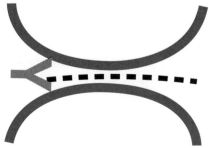

Electrical charges surrounding RBCs in a saline test system repel neighboring RBCs. IgM antibodies are able to span the distance between RBCs causing agglutination. IgG antibodies are too small to crosslink RBCs.

With the addition of an enhancement reagent, charges surrounding the RBCs are reduced, allowing the RBCs to approach each other. IgG antibodies may now be able to crosslink neighboring RBCs.

Figure 9–4. Use of enhancement reagents can lower the zeta potential, allowing for better interaction between RBCs and increasing the possibility of agglutination.

BOX 9–1

Common Blood Group Systems With Antibodies That Exhibit Dosage

- Rh (except D)
- Kidd
- Duffy
- MNSs
- Lutheran

Polyethylene Glycol. Polyethylene glycol (PEG) in a LISS solution removes water from the test system, thereby concentrating any antibodies present. This increases the degree of RBC sensitization. PEG can cause nonspecific aggregation of cells, so centrifugation after the 37°C incubation is not performed. Generally, PEG test systems are more sensitive than LISS, albumin, or saline systems. However, in patients with elevated levels of plasma protein, such as in multiple myeloma, PEG is not appropriate for use due to increased precipitation of proteins.[6]

AHG Reagents

Adding AHG reagent allows for the agglutination of incomplete antibodies. Polyspecific AHG reagent (also called *polyvalent* or *broad spectrum* **Coombs' serum**) contains antibodies to both IgG and complement components, either C3 and C4 or C3b and C3d (refer to Chapter 5, "The Antiglobulin Test"). It has been suggested that antibodies to the C3 components, especially C3d, are more desirable in the reagent, as these are more abundant on the RBC surface during complement activation and lead to fewer false-positive reactions.[7] The presence of anticomplement in the AHG reagent may lead to the detection of clinically insignificant antibodies. Relatively few examples of clinically significant antibodies, most notably Jk[a], react with complement alone.[8] As AABB's *Standards* requires only the detection of clinically significant antibodies when performing donor antibody screening and pretransfusion testing in the recipient,[9] many technologists use monospecific AHG reagent containing anti-IgG only. This also avoids time-consuming investigations of insignificant antibodies.

Any test that is negative after adding the AHG reagent should be controlled by adding Coombs' control cells. These are Rh-positive RBCs that have been coated with anti-D. In a negative antiglobulin test, these antibody-coated cells will react with the anti-IgG in the AHG reagent that remains free, resulting in visible agglutination. The addition of the Coombs' control cells proves that adequate washing was performed to remove unbound antibodies before the AHG reagent was added, that the AHG reagent was added to the test tube, and that the AHG reagent was working properly. If the Coombs' control cells fail to agglutinate, the antibody screen must be repeated from the beginning.

Use of the tube test remains popular, due to the flexibility of the test system, use of commonly available laboratory equipment, and relative low cost. The disadvantages include the instability of the reactions and subjective nature of grading by the technologist, the amount of hands-on time for the technologist, and problems related to the failure of the washing phase to remove all unbound antibody.

Gel Method

The antibody screen may also be performed using a microtubule filled with a dextran acrylamide gel (refer to Chapter 12, "Other Technologies and Automation"). The screen cells used for this technique meet the same criteria as for the tube test but are suspended in LISS to a concentration of 0.8%. With this technique, the patient's serum or plasma specimen and screen cells are added to a reaction chamber that sits above the gel. There are up to six chamber/gel microtubules contained in a plastic card, about the size of a credit card. The card is incubated at 37°C for 15 minutes to 1 hour,[10] thus allowing sensitization to occur. The card is then centrifuged for 10 minutes. During this time, the RBCs are forced out of the reaction chamber down into the gel. The gel contains anti-IgG. If sensitization occurred, the anti-IgG will react with the antibody-coated RBCs, resulting in agglutination. The agglutinated cells will be trapped within the gel because of the action of the anti-IgG and because the agglutinates are too large to pass through the spaces between gel particles. If no agglutination occurred, the RBCs will form a pellet at the bottom of the microtubule (Fig. 9–5).

There are numerous advantages to the gel technique. It is reported to be as sensitive as the PEG tube test method.[11,12] The omission of the washing and Coombs' control steps results in fewer hands-on steps for the technologist to perform. Reactions are stable for up to 24 hours and may be captured electronically, leading to standardized grading of reactions and facilitating review by a supervisor. Mixed-field reactions may be more apparent in gel. One of the greatest advantages is the ability to automate many of the pipetting and reading steps, thereby allowing increased productivity. Disadvantages include the need for incubators and centrifuges that can accommodate the gel cards.

Solid Phase Adherence Method

A third method that is commonly used to perform the antibody screen is solid phase adherence (refer to Chapter 12). One example of this method is Immucor's Capture-R. With Capture-R, RBC antigens coat microtiter wells rather than being present on intact RBCs (Fig. 9–6A). The patient's serum or plasma is added to each well in the screen cell set along with LISS. Incubation at 37°C allows any antibodies present to react with the antigens (Fig. 9–6B). The wells are then washed to remove unbound antibodies. Rather than traditional AHG reagent, indicator red blood cells that have

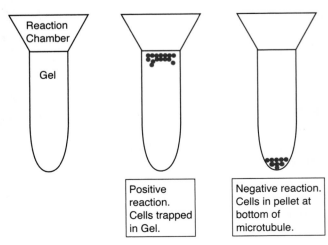

Reaction Chamber		
Gel		
	Positive reaction. Cells trapped in Gel.	Negative reaction. Cells in pellet at bottom of microtubule.

Figure 9–5.   The gel test system.

been coated with anti-IgG are added. The wells are then centrifuged for several minutes. If sensitization occurred, the indicator cells react with the antibodies bound to the antigens coating the microtiter well, forming a diffuse pattern in the well (Fig. 9–6C). If no sensitization occurred (a negative reaction), the indicator cells form a pellet in the bottom of the well (Fig. 9–6D).

The solid phase adherence test has been successfully automated. Such instruments may perform pipetting steps and determine the degree of reactivity by taking multiple readings of light transmission through each well. Other advantages include a smaller sample size (when compared with the tube test), making it ideal in a pediatric setting, and a LISS reagent that changes color when added to serum or plasma. This ensures that an adequate sample is present in the test system. Among the disadvantages is the need for careful pipetting when performing the test manually, due to the small sample and reagent volume. An inadequate volume of indicator cells may result in a pattern similar to that of a weak positive reaction. Interpretations made by automated instruments should be carefully evaluated when the specimen is hemolyzed, icteric, or lipemic, as this may interfere with the light measurement used to determine reactivity. Staff should be carefully trained to visually interpret results if automation is not used. Those who have primarily used the tube test may interpret the diffuse positive pattern as a negative reaction and the dense pellet of the negative reaction as a positive (4+) reaction. Incubators, washers, and centrifuges that can hold the microtiter wells are among the special equipment needed for this method.

A method currently being investigated is erythrocyte-magnetized technology (EMT). In this method, microtiter wells are coated with anti-IgG. Paramagnetic polymer beads have been adsorbed onto the screen cells by the manufacturer. These screen cells are incubated in the microtiter wells along with the patient's plasma at 37°C for 20 minutes.[13] A high-density liquid separates the screen cell/plasma mixture from the anti-IgG until the microtiter plate is placed on a magnetized shaker. At that point, the magnet "pulls" the screen cells through the high-density liquid. Screen cells that have been sensitized with antibody will react with the anti-IgG coating the well, yielding a diffuse pattern throughout the well. Screen cells that have not been coated with antibody will form a pellet at the bottom of the well. Unbound antibodies will remain in a layer above the high-density liquid, eliminating the wash step that is necessary in solid phase adherence.

Interpretation

Agglutination or hemolysis at any stage of testing is a positive test result, indicating the need for antibody identification studies. However, evaluation of the antibody screen results (and autologous control, if tested at this time) can provide clues and give direction for the identification and resolution of the antibody or antibodies. The investigator should consider the following questions:

1. **In what phase(s) did the reaction(s) occur?**
   Antibodies of the IgM class react best at room temperature or lower and are capable of causing agglutination

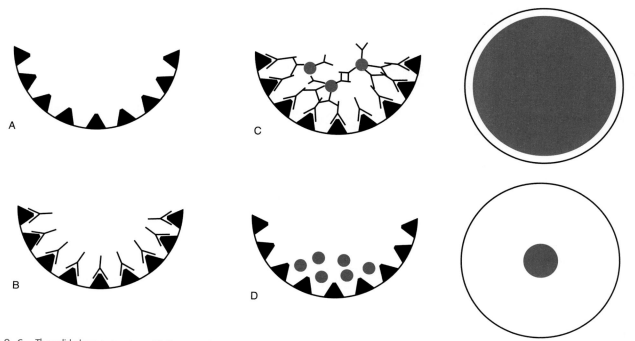

Figure 9–6. The solid phase test system. (A) illustrates the microtiter well coated with RBC antigens. (B) The patient's antibody has attached to the RBC antigens in the microtiter well. (C and D) The figure on the left is a detailed side view of what is taking place in the well, on a cellular level, and the figure on the right is the view looking down into the well, as the technologist would view it for grading purposes. C illustrates the reaction between the patient's antibodies and the indicator cells. In D, when no patient antibody is present, the indicator cells form a pellet at the bottom of the well.

of saline-suspended RBCs (immediate spin reaction). Antibodies of the IgG class react best at the AHG phase. Of the commonly encountered antibodies, anti-N, anti-I, and anti-P_1 are frequently IgM, whereas those directed against Rh, Kell, Kidd, Duffy, and Ss antigens are usually IgG. Lewis and M antibodies may be IgG, IgM, or a mixture of both.

2. **Is the autologous control negative or positive?**
The **autologous control** is the patient's RBCs tested against the patient's serum or plasma in the same manner as the antibody screen. A positive antibody screen and a negative autologous control indicate that an alloantibody has been detected. A positive autologous control may indicate the presence of autoantibodies or antibodies to medications. If the patient has been recently transfused (i.e., in the previous 3 months), the positive autologous control may be caused by alloantibody coating circulating donor RBCs. Evaluation of samples with positive autologous control or **direct antiglobulin test** (DAT) results is often complex and may require a great deal of time and experience on the part of the investigator. Some technologists choose to omit the autologous control when performing the antibody screen and include it only when performing antibody identification studies.

3. **Did more than one screen cell sample react? If so, did they react at the same strength and phase?**
More than one screen cell sample may be positive when the patient has multiple antibodies, when a single antibody's target antigen is found on more than one screen cell, or when the patient's serum contains an autoantibody. A single antibody specificity should be suspected when all screen cells yielding a positive reaction react at the same phase and strength. Multiple antibodies are most likely when screen cells react at different phases or strengths, and autoantibodies should be suspected when the autologous control is positive. Figure 9–7 provides several examples of antibody screen results with possible causes.

4. **Is hemolysis or mixed-field agglutination present?**
Certain antibodies, such as anti-Le^a, anti-Le^b, anti-PP1P^k, and anti-Vel, are known to cause in vitro hemolysis. Mixed-field agglutination is associated with anti-Sd^a and Lutheran antibodies.

5. **Are the cells truly agglutinated, or is rouleaux present?**
Serum from patients with altered albumin-to-globulin ratios (e.g., patients with multiple myeloma) or from those who have received high-molecular-weight plasma expanders (e.g., dextran) may cause nonspecific aggregation of RBCs, known as **rouleaux**. Rouleaux is not a significant finding in antibody screening tests but is easily confused with antibody-mediated agglutination. Knowing the following characteristics of rouleaux helps in differentiating between rouleaux and agglutination:
   - Cells have a "stacked coin" appearance when viewed microscopically (see **Color Plate 2**).
   - Rouleaux is observed in all tests containing the patient's serum, including the autologous control and the reverse ABO grouping.

   - Rouleaux does not interfere with the AHG phase of testing because the patient's serum is washed away prior to the addition of the AHG reagent.
   - Unlike agglutination, rouleaux is dispersed by adding one to three drops of saline to the test tube.

Limitations

Screening reagents and methods are designed to detect as many clinically significant antibodies as possible and to avoid detecting those antibodies that are insignificant. When using a three-cell screen set, a negative result with all three cells gives the technologist 95% confidence that there are no clinically significant antibodies are present.

Despite this, there are limitations to the antibody screen. The screen will not detect antibodies when the antibody titer has dropped below the level of sensitivity for the screening method employed. One study, which reviewed antibodies detected over a 20-year period, showed that 26% of antibodies became undetectable over time, with a median time of 7 months.[14] Another study of antibodies formed in response to transfusion found that two-thirds of antibodies were no longer detectable 5 years after formation.[15] The screen also cannot detect antibodies directed against low-prevalence antigens that are not present on any of the RBCs in the screen cell set. Antibodies showing dosage may not be detected if none of the screen cells have homozygous expression of the target antigen.

Several factors may influence the sensitivity of the antibody screen. These include cell-to-serum ratio, temperature and phase of reactivity, length of incubation, and pH.

Cell-to-Serum Ratio

When antibody is present in the test system in excess (when compared to antigen concentration), false-negative reactions occur as a result of prozone. When the antigen is in excess, false-negative reactions occur due to postzone. A ratio of two drops of serum to one drop of the RBC suspension typically gives the proper balance between antigen and antibody to allow sensitization and agglutination to occur. (This ratio may be altered, depending on the test method employed.) Occasionally, when an antibody is weak, the amount of serum in the test system may be increased to four to ten drops, providing more antibodies to react with the available antigens. This should be done only when potentiators have not been included in the test system.

Temperature and Phase of Reactivity

The optimal temperature at which an antibody reacts can provide useful clues to antibody identity. When performing pretransfusion compatibility testing, the focus is on clinically significant antibodies, which generally react at 37°C or with the anti-IgG in the AHG reagent. Technologists may omit the immediate spin and room temperature phases to limit the detection of insignificant cold antibodies. Should it be necessary to identify an antibody reacting at room

			Results	**Possible Interpretation**
cell	IS	37°	AGT (poly)	1. Single alloantibody
SC I	neg	neg	neg	2. Two alloantibodies, antigens only present on cell II
SC II	neg	neg	2+	
auto	neg	neg	neg	3. Probably IgG antibody

cell	IS	37°	AGT	1. Multiple antibodies
SC I	neg	1+	3+	2. Single antibody (dosage)
SC II	neg	neg	1+	3. Probable IgG
auto	neg	neg	neg	

cell	IS	37°	AGT	1. Single or multiple antibodies
SC I	1+	neg	neg	2. Probably IgM antibodies
SC II	2+	neg	neg	
auto	neg	neg	neg	

cell	IS	37°	AGT	1. Multiple antibodies, warm and cold
SC I	2+	neg	1+	
SC II	3+	1+	2+	2. Potent cold antibody binding complement in AGT
auto	neg	neg	neg	

cell	IS	37°	AGT	1. Single warm antibody, antigen present on both cells
SC I	neg	neg	1+	
SC II	neg	neg	1+	2. Antibody to high-prevalence antigen
auto	neg	neg	neg	3. Complement binding by a cold antibody not detected at IS

cell	IS	37°	AGT	1. Warm antibodies
SC I	neg	neg	3+	2. Transfusion reaction
SC II	neg	neg	3+	3. Probable IgG antibody
auto	neg	neg	3+	4. Warm autoantibody

Figure 9–7. Examples of reactions that may be obtained in antibody screening tests.

temperature, it may be useful to incubate the screen at 18°C or 4°C to enhance reactivity. In such cases, an autocontrol should be included to aid in the detection of common cold autoantibodies, such as anti-I or anti-IH. Table 9–2 summarizes the optimal phase of reactivity for some of the most common antibodies.

Length of Incubation

Antigen-antibody reactions are in dynamic equilibrium. If too little contact time is allowed, too few RBCs will be sensitized to be detected by routine methods. If the incubation time is allowed to continue for too long, bound antibody may begin to dissociate from the RBCs. Incubation time is dependent on the medium in which the reaction takes place. A saline environment may require an incubation time of 30 minutes to 1 hour, whereas potentiators may shorten the incubation time to as little as 10 minutes.

pH

Most antibodies react best at a neutral pH between 6.8 and 7.2;[16] however, some examples of anti-M demonstrate enhanced reactivity at a pH of 6.5.[17] Acidifying the test system may aid in distinguishing anti-M from other antibodies.

Antibody Identification

Once an antibody has been detected, additional testing is necessary to identify the antibody and determine its clinical

| Table 9–2 | **Optimal Phase of Reactivity for Some Common Antibodies** | | |

PHASE	IMMEDIATE SPIN (ROOM TEMPERATURE)	37°C INCUBATION	ANTIGLOBULIN PHASE
Antibodies	Cold autoantibodies (I, H, IH)	Potent cold (IgM) antibodies (especially those causing hemolysis)	Rh antibodies
	Le^a, Le^b	Some warm antibodies, if high in titer (e.g., D, E, and K)	Kell
	M, N		Duffy
	P$_1$		Kidd
	Lu^a		S,s
			Lu^b
			Xg^a
Immunoglobulin Class	IgM	Usually IgG IgM that activate complement	IgG
Clinically Significant	No	Yes	Yes

significance. The patient's serum or plasma is tested against additional RBCs possessing known antigens. The test method used should be as sensitive as that used for detection.

Patient History

Information concerning the patient's age, sex, race, diagnosis, transfusion and pregnancy history, medications, and intravenous solutions may provide valuable clues in antibody identification studies, particularly in complex cases. Knowing the patient's race may be valuable, as some antibodies are associated with a particular race. For example, anti-U is more frequently associated with persons of African descent because most U-negative individuals are found in this population.

Transfusion and pregnancy history are also helpful, as patients who have been exposed to "non-self" RBCs via transfusion or pregnancy are more likely to have produced immune antibodies. Naturally occurring antibodies (e.g., anti-M, anti-Le^b) should be suspected in patients with no transfusion or pregnancy history. Medications such as IVIG, RhIG, and antilymphocyte globulin may passively transfer antibodies such as anti-A or anti-B, anti-D, and antispecies antibodies, respectively. This will result in the presence of an unexpected serum antibody that is likely to confound the interpretation of antibody identification.

The patient's history is especially important when the autologous control or DAT is positive. Certain infectious and autoimmune disorders are associated with production of RBC autoantibodies, and some medications are known to cause positive DATs. Furthermore, in a patient transfused within the past 3 months, a positive DAT result may indicate a delayed hemolytic transfusion reaction.

Information regarding recent transfusions is also important when antigen-typing the patient's RBCs. Antigen-typing

results must be interpreted carefully when the patient has recently received a transfusion, because positive reactions may be caused by the presence of donor RBCs remaining in the patient's circulation. Positive reactions caused by donor RBCs usually show mixed-field agglutination, but this depends on how recently the transfusion was given and how much blood was transfused.

Reagents

An **antibody identification panel** is a collection of 11 to 20 group O RBCs with various antigen expression. The pattern of antigen expression should be diverse so that it will be possible to distinguish one antibody from another and should include cells with homozygous expression of Rh, Duffy, Kidd, and MNSs antigens. A profile sheet specifying the antigens on each cell and providing a place to record reactions accompanies each panel (Fig. 9–8). As with the screen cells, the profile sheet is lot-specific and should not be interchanged with that of another panel. The profile sheet will often indicate the presence of rare cells, which are positive for low-prevalence antigens or negative for high-prevalence antigens.

Exclusion

When interpreting panel results, the first step is to exclude antibodies that could not be responsible for the reactivity seen. To perform exclusions or "rule-outs," the RBCs that gave a negative reaction in all phases of testing are examined. The antigens on these negatively reacting cells probably will not be the antibody's target. Generally, it is advisable to perform this rule-out technique only if there is homozygous expression of the antigen on the cell. This avoids excluding a weak antibody that is showing dosage. Exceptions are

Donor	Cell number	D	C	c	E	e	Cw	K	k	Kpa	Kpb	Jsa	Jsb	Fya	Fyb	Jka	Jkb	Lea	Leb	P1	M	N	S	s	Lua	Lub	Xga
R1R1	1	+	+	0	0	+	0	0	+	0	+	0	+	+	+	+	+	0	0	+	+	+	+	+	0	+	+
R1r	2	+	+	+	0	+	+	+	+	0	+	0	+	+	0	+	+	0	+	0	+	0	+	+	0	+	+
R1R1	3	+	+	0	0	+	0	0	+	0	+	0	+	0	+	+	+	0	+	+	0	+	0	+	0	+	+
R2R2	4	+	0	+	+	0	0	0	+	0	+	0	+	+	0	+	+	0	+	+	+	0	0	0	0	+	+
r'r	5	0	+	+	0	+	0	0	+	0	+	0	+	0	0	0	+	+	0	+	+	0	+	0	0	+	+
r"r"	6	0	0	0	+	+	0	0	+	0	+	0	+	+	0	+	0	0	+	0	+	0	+	0	0	+	0
rr K	7	0	0	+	0	+	0	+	+	0	+	0	+	+	0	0	+	0	+	+	0	+	0	+	0	+	+
rr	8	0	0	+	0	+	0	0	+	0	+	0	+	0	+	0	0	0	+	0	+	0	+	0	0	+	+
rr	9	0	0	+	0	+	0	0	+	0	+	0	+	+	0	+	0	0	0	+	+	+	+	0	0	+	+
R1r	10	+	+	+	0	+	0	0	+	0	+	0	+	+	0	+	+	0	+	+	+	0	0	0	0	+	+
R0	11	+	0	+	0	+	0	0	+	0	+	0	+	+	+	0	+	0	+	+	+	0	0	+	0	+	+
	Patient Cells																										

Figure 9–8.   Antibody identification profile sheet: + indicates the antigen is present on the cell; 0 indicates the antigen is not present.

made for low-prevalence antigens that are rarely expressed homozygously, such as K, Kpa, Jsa, and Lua. In the sample panel shown in Figure 9–9, cell numbers 1, 3, 4, 6, 7, 10, and 11 reacted positively and cannot be used for exclusions. Cell number 2 reacted negatively and can be used to exclude D, C, e, Cw, K, Kpb, Jsb, Fyb, Jka, P1, M, S, Lub, and Xga. Cell number 5 can be used to exclude k, Jkb, and Leb. Cell number 8 is used to rule out c, Lea, and Lua, and cell number 9 eliminates N and s. This leaves anti-E, anti-Kpa, anti-Jsa, and anti-Fya as possible antibodies present.

Evaluation of Panel Results

After each negatively reacting cell has been evaluated, the remaining antigens should be examined to see if the pattern of reactivity matches a pattern of antigen-positive cells (inclusion technique). Evaluation of panel results should be carried out in a logical step-by-step method to ensure proper identification and to avoid missing antibody specificities that may be masked by other antibodies. A logical approach to antibody identification is outlined below, using a series of questions and the example illustrated in Figure 9–9.

1. **In what phase(s) and at what strength(s) did the positive reactions occur?** Do all of the positive cells react to the same degree? Carefully grading the observed reactions may aid in antibody identification. The strength of the reaction does not indicate the significance of the antibody, only the amount of antibody available to participate in the reaction. A stronger reaction may be due

Donor	Cell number	D	C	c	E	e	Cw	K	k	Kpa	Kpb	Jsa	Jsb	Fya	Fyb	Jka	Jkb	Lea	Leb	P1	M	N	S	s	Lua	Lub	Xga	IS	37	AHG	CC
R1r	1	+	+	+	0	+	0	0	+	0	+	0	+	+	+	+	+	0	+	+	+	+	+	+	0	+	+	0	0	2+	
R1R1	2	+	+	0	0	+	+	+	+	0	+	0	+	0	+	+	0	0	0	+	+	0	+	0	0	+	+	0	0	0	3+
R2R2	3	+	0	+	+	0	0	0	+	0	+	0	+	+	0	0	+	0	+	+	0	+	0	+	0	+	+	0	0	3+	
R0r	4	+	0	+	0	+	0	0	+	0	+	0	+	+	0	+	+	+	0	0	+	0	+	+	0	+	0	0	0	3+	
r'r	5	0	+	+	0	+	0	0	+	0	+	0	+	0	0	0	+	0	+	+	+	0	+	0	0	+	0	0	0	0	3+
r"r	6	0	0	+	+	+	0	0	+	0	+	0	+	+	+	+	0	+	0	+	+	0	+	0	+	0	+	0	0	3+	
rr K	7	0	0	+	0	+	0	+	+	0	+	0	+	+	+	+	+	0	+	0	+	0	+	0	+	+	+	0	0	2+	
rr	8	0	0	+	0	+	0	0	+	0	+	0	+	0	+	0	+	0	+	+	0	+	0	+	0	+	+	0	0	0	3+
r'r"	9	0	+	+	+	+	0	0	+	0	+	0	+	0	+	+	0	0	+	+	0	+	0	+	0	+	0	0	0	0	3+
rr	10	0	0	+	0	+	0	0	+	0	+	0	+	+	0	+	+	0	+	+	0	+	0	0	0	+	+	0	0	3+	
R1r	11	+	+	+	0	+	0	0	+	0	+	0	+	+	+	+	+	0	+	+	+	+	+	+	0	+	+	0	0	2+	
	Patient Cells																											0	0	0	3+

Figure 9–9.   Sample panel demonstrating anti-Fya.

to dosage (cells with homozygous antigen expression reacting more strongly than cells with heterozygous antigen expression). Different reaction strengths could also indicate the presence of more than one antibody. A cell that possesses more than one of the target antigens may react more strongly than a cell possessing only one of the target antigens. A third possibility is an antigen with variable expression. I, P_1, Le^a, Le^b, Vel, Ch/Rg, and Sd^a antigens are expressed more strongly on some RBCs than on others; antibodies to these antigens may react more strongly with one panel cell than another.

2. **Do all of the positive cells react at the same phase, or do any react at different or multiple phases?** Reactions of certain cells at one phase and different cells at another phase may indicate the presence of multiple antibodies. Cells that react at multiple phases may also be a sign of an antibody showing dosage, with the cells having homozygous antigen expression reacting at an earlier phase than those with heterozygous antigen expression.

   Phase of reactivity may be helpful in establishing the clinical significance of an antibody. IgM antibodies, which are usually not significant, most often react at the immediate spin phase, room temperature or colder. Clinically significant IgG antibodies are most often detected during the AHG phase. Some potent IgG antibodies, such as D, E, and K, may become evident following the 37°C incubation phase. In the case presented in **Figure 9–9**, all reactions occurred in the AHG phase with strengths of both 2+ and 3+. Multiple antibodies or a single antibody showing dosage should be considered.

3. **Does the serum reactivity match any of the remaining specificities?** When a single alloantibody is present, the pattern of reactivity usually matches a pattern of antigen expression exactly. In our example, the serum reactivity matches the Fy^a pattern exactly. The serum gave uniform positive results with all Fy^a-positive cells (1, 3, 4, 6, 7, 10, and 11) and negative results with all of the Fy^a-negative cells (2, 5, 8, and 9). The reason for the variation in strength in the AHG phase is due to dosage; all cells yielding 2+ reactions were heterozygous for Fy^a, and all cells yielding 3+ reactions were homozygous for Fy^a.

4. **Are all commonly encountered RBC antibodies excluded?** As previously mentioned, in this case anti-E, anti-Kp^a, and anti-Js^a were not ruled out. None of the RBCs on this panel were positive for Kp^a or Js^a, so they cannot be the cause of the observed reactions. These two antigens are characterized as low prevalence, occurring in less than 5% of the population. Antibodies to low-prevalence antigens are uncommon because the chance of being exposed to the antigen is low; therefore, it may not be necessary to pursue additional testing to exclude these specificities. In contrast, if a commonly encountered antibody is not ruled out, it is important to test selected cells that will rule out the presence of the antibody. In this example, additional testing should be performed to exclude anti-E. A negative result when testing an E+ e– Fy^a- RBC sample would exclude anti-E (see the "Selected Cell Panels" section).

5. **Is the autologous control (last row in panel antigen profile) positive or negative?** In the example shown, the autocontrol is negative, indicating that the positive reactions are caused by alloantibody, not by autoantibody. The presence of autoantibodies may mask the presence of alloantibodies, and complicates the process of antibody identification. Resolution of autoantibody problems is discussed briefly in the case studies at the end of this chapter.

6. **Is there sufficient evidence to prove the suspected antibody?** Conclusive antibody identification requires testing the patient's serum with enough antigen-positive and antigen-negative RBC samples to ensure that the pattern of reactivity is not the result of chance alone. Testing the patient's serum with at least three antigen-positive and three antigen-negative cells (also known as the *3 and 3 rule*) will result in a probability (*P*) value of 0.05.[18] A *P* value is a statistical measure of the probability that a certain set of events will happen by random chance. A *P* value of 0.05 or less is required for identification results to be considered valid, and it means that there is a 5% (1 in 20) chance that the observed pattern occurred for reasons other than a specific antibody reacting with its corresponding antigen. Stated another way, it means that the interpretation of the data will be correct 95% of the time. When multiple antibodies are present, the 3 and 3 rule must be applied to each specificity separately. For example, if anti-K and anti-E are both suspected, the 3 and 3 rule would be fulfilled if three K–E– cells reacted negatively, three K+E– cells reacted positively, and three K–E+ cells reacted positively. Other researchers have derived formulas where *P* 0.05 is fulfilled with two positive cells and three negative cells[19] or two positive cells and two negative cells.[20]

   Testing of RBCs selected from other panels is necessary when inadequate numbers of antigen-positive or antigen-negative cells have been tested initially. In our example, the patient's serum reacted with seven Fy^a-positive cells (1, 3, 4, 6, 7, 10, and 11) but did not react with four Fy^a-negative cells (2, 5, 8, and 9). As a result, additional cells need not be tested to increase the confidence level to 95%, and the identification of anti-Fy^a is conclusive.

7. **Does the patient lack the antigen corresponding to the antibody?** Individuals cannot make alloantibodies to antigens that they possess on their own RBCs; therefore, the last step in identification studies is to test the patient's RBCs for the corresponding antigen. A negative result is expected, providing additional evidence that identification results are correct. If the patient's RBCs are positive for the corresponding antigen, misidentification of the antibody or a false-positive typing are the most likely explanations. Antigen typing can also help resolve complex cases, as it may eliminate possible specificities. For example, an R_1R_1, K-negative, Fy(a–b+), Jk(a+b+), M+N+S+s+ patient could form only anti-c, anti-E, anti-K, or anti-Fy^a. It is not practical to do extended typing on all patients with antibodies; however, judicious use of this procedure can be useful, especially in patients who chronically receive transfusions and are at risk for alloimmunization, such as patients with sickle cell disease or thalassemia.

Phenotyping may be complicated when a patient has a positive DAT or has been transfused in the last 3 months. When the DAT is positive due to IgG coating the RBCs, typing reagents employing the indirect antiglobulin test (IAT) may give invalid results. The coating antibody blocks the antigen sites, preventing the typing serum from reacting. The AHG reagent will react with the coating antibody, yielding false-positive results. Removal of the antibody coating (elution) will be necessary to get an accurate phenotype. Two reagents useful in stripping antibody from the RBC surface, while leaving the membrane intact to allow phenotyping, are chloroquine diphosphate and acid glycine/EDTA.[21] In the chloroquine diphosphate method, washed RBCs are incubated with the reagent at room temperature for 30 minutes to 2 hours. The cells are washed to remove the chloroquine diphosphate. When the treated cells yield a negative DAT, they may then be phenotyped. Rh antigens may show diminished reactivity with this method. Acid glycine/EDTA (EGA) is a rapid method for removing antibody. Kell antigens are denatured when using this method, so patient cells cannot be reliably typed for these antigens.

In cases where the coating antibody resists elution, an absorption method has been described.[22] RBCs to be phenotyped are incubated with diluted antiserum. Following incubation, the cell/antiserum mixture is centrifuged. The supernatant is harvested and tested against a cell with heterozygous antigen expression. If the patient's RBCs are positive for the target antigen, the antibody will have been absorbed from the diluted antiserum, and the supernatant will react negatively. If the patient's RBCs are negative for the target antigen, the antibody will remain in the antiserum, and the supernatant will be positive when tested against the heterozygous cell.

Recently transfused patients present a different challenge. Mixed-field reactions are common when phenotyping these patients; the donor cells that stimulated antibody formation react with the typing serum, whereas the patient's autologous cells do not react. To get an accurate phenotype of the patient's autologous cells, reticulocyte typing can be performed. For this technique, the patient's RBCs are drawn into microhematocrit tubes and centrifuged. Because reticulocytes are less dense than mature RBCs, the patient's reticulocytes should be at the top of the RBC layer. These cells can be harvested and used for antigen typing.[23]

Positive and negative control cells should be tested with each antisera used for antigen typing, on the day of use. The positive control cell should have heterozygous antigen expression to ensure that the antiserum has the sensitivity to detect small quantities of the antigen. The negative control cell should lack the target antigen to confirm reactivity with only the target antigen.

Antigen typing is routinely performed using the tube, solid phase adherence,[24] or gel methods.[25] Flow cytometry has been used to detect minute quantities of antigens. Various molecular methods based on polymerase chain reaction (PCR) are being used to examine DNA for the single-nucleotide polymorphisms (SNPs) that give rise to various red blood cell antigens.[26–29] Advantages of molecular testing include the ability to screen for multiple antigens at one time and to screen large numbers of donors in a relatively short time. There is no interference from a recent transfusion or positive DAT on the RBCs. In addition, there are no limitations due to the lack of rare antisera or the expense in purchasing these reagents. Several of these methods have been automated to reduce the amount of hands-on time required of the technologist.

Additional Techniques for Resolving Antibody Identification

There may be times when the initial antibody identification panel does not reveal a clear-cut specificity. When multiple specificities remain following the exclusion and inclusion process, additional testing is necessary.

Selected Cell Panels

Perhaps the simplest step to take is to test additional cells from a different panel. The cells selected for testing should have minimal overlap in the antigens they possess. Figure 9–10 shows the results of an initial panel in which anti-E, anti-Kp^a, anti-Js^a, anti-Fy^a, and anti-Jk^b are not excluded. The lower section of the figure shows a selected cell panel that could be used to differentiate between those antibodies. Anti-Jk^b appears to be present in the sample. Anti-Fy^a is eliminated by selected cell number 1, and anti-E is eliminated by selected cell number 3. Finding cells that are positive for low-prevalence antigens such as C^w, Kp^a, Js^a, and Lu^a may not be possible in many cases.

Selected cell panels are also useful when a patient has a known antibody and the technologist is attempting to determine if additional antibodies are present. Figure 9–11 is an example of a selected cell panel for a patient with a history of anti-Fy^a. As it is not necessary to demonstrate the presence of anti-Fy^a, the panel cells selected are each negative for Fy^a but possess examples of other common, significant antigens. In this case, the remaining major clinically significant antibody specificities have been excluded.

Enzymes

When it appears that multiple antibodies may be present in a sample, treating the panel cells with enzymes may help separate the specificities and allow for identification. Ficin is commonly used to treat RBCs; however, papain, bromelin, or trypsin may also be used. Enzymes modify the RBC surface by removing sialic acid residues and by denaturing or removing glycoproteins. The effect is to destroy certain antigens and enhance expression of others. Table 9–3 reviews how enzymes affect some common antigens.

Enzymes may be utilized in place of enhancement media, such as LISS or PEG, in a one-step enzyme test method. A second, more sensitive method uses enzymes to treat the panel RBCs first, and then the antibody identification panel is performed using the treated cells. Because enzymes

Donor	Cell number	D	C	c	E	e	Cw	K	k	Kpa	Kpb	Jsa	Jsb	Fya	Fyb	Jka	Jkb	Lea	Leb	P1	M	N	S	s	Lua	Lub	Xga	IS	37	AHG	CC
R1r	1	+	+	+	0	+	0	0	+	+	0	+	0	+	+	+	+	0	+	+	+	+	+	+	0	+	+	0	0	1+	
R1R1	2	+	+	0	0	+	+	+	+	0	+	0	+	0	+	+	0	0	0	+	+	0	+	0	0	+	+	0	0	0	3+
R2R2	3	+	0	+	+	0	0	0	+	0	+	0	+	+	0	+	+	0	+	+	0	+	0	+	0	+	+	0	0	1+	
R0r	4	+	0	+	0	+	0	0	+	0	+	0	+	+	0	+	+	+	0	0	+	0	+	+	0	+	0	0	0	1+	
r'r	5	0	+	+	0	+	0	0	+	0	+	0	+	0	0	+	0	0	+	+	+	+	0	+	0	+	0	0	0	0	3+
r"r	6	0	0	+	+	+	0	0	+	0	+	0	+	+	+	0	+	0	+	+	0	+	0	+	0	+	+	0	0	2+	
rr K	7	0	0	+	0	+	0	+	+	0	+	0	+	+	+	+	+	0	+	0	+	0	+	0	+	0	+	+	0	0	1+	
rr	8	0	0	+	0	+	0	0	+	0	+	0	+	0	+	+	0	+	0	+	+	+	0	+	+	0	+	0	0	0	3+
r'r"	9	0	+	+	+	0	0	0	+	0	+	0	+	0	+	+	0	0	+	+	0	+	0	+	0	+	+	0	0	0	3+
rr	10	0	0	+	0	+	0	0	+	0	+	0	+	+	0	+	+	0	+	+	0	+	+	0	+	0	+	+	0	0	1+	
R1r	11	+	+	+	0	+	0	0	+	0	+	0	+	+	+	0	+	0	+	+	+	+	+	+	0	+	+	0	0	2+	
	Patient Cells																											0	0	0	3+

Selected Cell Panel

Donor	Cell number	D	C	c	E	e	Cw	K	k	Kpa	Kpb	Jsa	Jsb	Fya	Fyb	Jka	Jkb	Lea	Leb	P1	M	N	S	s	Lua	Lub	Xga	IS	37	AHG	CC
R1R1	SS1	+	+	0	0	+	0	+	+	0	+	0	+	+	0	+	0	0	+	+	0	+	+	+	0	+	0	0	0	0	3+
rr	SS2	0	0	+	0	+	0	0	+	0	+	0	+	+	+	0	+	0	+	0	+	+	0	0	+	+	0	0	0	3+	
R2R2	SS3	+	0	+	+	0	0	0	+	0	+	0	+	+	+	0	0	+	0	+	0	+	0	+	0	+	0	0	0	0	3+

Figure 9–10.   Selected cell panel.

Donor	Cell number	D	C	c	E	e	Cw	K	k	Kpa	Kpb	Jsa	Jsb	Fya	Fyb	Jka	Jkb	Lea	Leb	P1	M	N	S	s	Lua	Lub	Xga	Peg/ IgG	CC		
	1	+	+	0	0	+	0	0	+	0	+	0	+	0	+	+	0	0	+	+	+	+	+	0	0	+	+	0	2+		
	2	+	+	0	0	+	+	0	+	+	+	0	+	0	+	+	+	0	+	+	+	0	+	0	0	+	0	0	2+		
	3	+	0	+	+	0	0	+	+	0	+	0	+	0	+	0	+	0	0	0	0	+	0	+	0	+	+	0	2+		
	4	0	+	+	0	+	0	0	+	0	+	0	+	0	0	+	+	+	0	+	+	0	+	+	0	+	+	0	2+		
	Patient Cells																											0	2+		

Figure 9–11.   Selected cell panel for a patient with known antibody.

Table 9–3	The Effect of Proteolytic Enzymes on Select Antigen-Antibody Reactions
ENHANCED	**INACTIVATED**
Rh	Duffy
Kidd	MNS
Lewis	Xga
P1	
I	
ABO	

destroy some antigens, not all specificities can be excluded using the enzyme panel alone. When possible, the reactivity of cells on the enzyme treated panel should be compared to the reactivity of the same cells before enzyme treatment. Observing which cells reacted positively in the untreated panel but did not react (or gave weaker reactions) with the treated panel will aid the technologist in identification. Similarly, observation of cells that reacted more strongly or at an earlier phase in the enzyme panel than in the untreated panel may lead to identification.

Neutralization

Other substances in the body and in nature have antigenic structures similar to RBC antigens. These substances can be used to neutralize antibodies in serum, allowing for separation of antibodies or confirmation that a particular antibody is present. The patient's serum is first incubated with the neutralizing substance, allowing the soluble antigens in that substance to bind with the antibody. An antibody identification panel is performed using the treated serum. The neutralizing substance inhibits reactions between the antibody and panel RBCs. Use of a control (saline and serum) is necessary to prove that the loss of reactivity is due to **neutralization** and not to dilution of antibody strength by the added substance. In Figure 9–12, positive reactions are seen in cells 1 through 4, 7, and 8. When the serum is incubated with Lewis' substance, positive reactions are seen in only cells 3, 4, and 7, which matches the pattern of anti-Kell. Anti-Le^b activity has been inhibited by Lewis' substance. This technique is helpful when multiple antibodies are suspected. Table 9–4 lists some of the antibodies that can be neutralized and the source of corresponding neutralizing substance. Lewis and P$_1$ substances are available commercially.

Adsorption

Antibodies may be removed from serum by adding the target antigen and allowing the antibody to bind to the antigen, in a manner similar to the neutralization technique. In the **adsorption** method, the antigen-antibody complex is composed of solid precipitates and is removed from the test system

Table 9–4	Sources of Substances for Neutralization of Certain Antibodies
ANTIBODY	**SOURCE OF NEUTRALIZING SUBSTANCE**
Anti-P$_1$	Hydatid cyst fluid, pigeon droppings, turtledoves' egg whites
Anti-Lewis	Plasma or serum, saliva
Anti-Chido, anti-Rodgers	Serum (contains complement)
Anti-Sd^a	Urine
Anti-I	Human breast milk

by centrifugation. The absorbed serum is tested against an RBC panel for the presence of unabsorbed alloantibodies. The adsorbent is typically composed of RBCs but may be another antigen-bearing substance.

Commercial Reagents for Adsorption

Human platelet concentrate is used to adsorb Bg-like antibodies from serum. The HLA antigens present on platelets bind the HLA-related Bg antibodies,[30] leaving other specificities in the serum. Antibody identification can be performed on the adsorbed serum.

CELL	D	C	E	c	e	f	V	Cw	M	N	S	s	Lua	Lub	P1	Lea	Leb	K	k	Fya	Fyb	Jka	Jkb	Albumin 37 C	Albumin AHG	Control: Serum + Saline AHG	Serum + Lewis Substance AHG
1. r'r-2	0	+	0	+	+	+	0	0	+	+	0	+	0	+	0	0	+	0	+	+	0	+	+	0	2+	2+	0
2. R1wR1-1	+	+	0	0	+	0	0	+	+	+	+	0	+	+	+	0	+	0	+	0	+	+	0	0	2+	2+	0
3. R1R1-6	+	+	0	0	+	0	0	0	0	+	0	+	0	+	+	+	0	+	0	0	+	+	0	0	2+	2+	2+
4. R2R2-8	+	0	+	+	0	0	0	0	+	+	+	+	0	+	+	0	+	+	0	0	+	0	+	0	2+	2+	2+
5. r"r-3	0	0	+	+	+	+	0	0	+	+	+	0	0	+	+	+	0	0	+	0	+	+	0	0	0	0	0
6. rr-32	0	0	0	+	+	+	0	0	+	0	+	0	0	+	+	+	0	0	+	+	+	+	0	0	0	0	0
7. rr-10	0	0	0	+	+	+	0	0	+	+	+	+	0	+	0	0	+	+	+	+	+	+	0	0	2+	2+	2+
8. rr-12	0	0	0	+	+	+	0	0	0	+	0	+	0	+	+	0	+	0	+	+	0	0	+	0	2+	2+	2+
9. Ro-4	+	0	0	+	+	+	0	0	+	0	0	+	0	+	0	0	0	0	+	0	0	0	+	0	0	0	0
Cord cell	/	/	/	/	/	/	/	/	/	/	/	/	/	/	/	0	0	/	/	/	/	/	/	0	0	0	0
Patient																								0	0	0	0

DIRECT ANTIHUMAN GLOBULIN TEST

Poly	negative
IgG	
C3	

Figure 9–12. Neutralization using Lewis' substance in a serum containing anti-Le^b and anti-Kell.

Rabbit erythrocyte stroma (RESt) performs a similar function with some cold-reacting autoantibodies. RESt possesses I, H, and IH-like structures. Incubating the patient's serum at 4°C with RESt will remove these insignificant antibodies, which may interfere with the detection of clinically significant warm-reacting antibodies. Most other antibody specificities remain unaffected by RESt adsorption.[31] However, RESt also possesses structures similar to B and P_1 antigens. Because RESt may absorb anti-B, reverse grouping and crossmatching with RESt-adsorbed serum is not recommended.

Autoadsorption

Autoantibodies are commonly removed through adsorption techniques. Perhaps the simplest method is adsorption using the patient's own RBCs. The autologous cells are first washed thoroughly to remove unbound antibody. They may then be treated to remove any autoantibody coating the RBCs. Next, the cells are incubated with the patient's serum for up to 1 hour. Temperature of incubation depends on the thermal range of the autoantibody being removed, generally 4°C for cold-reacting autoantibodies and 37°C for warm-reacting autoantibodies. The sample is inspected for signs of agglutination throughout the incubation period. If agglutination appears, all the RBC binding sites are saturated with autoantibody. The serum is harvested and incubated with a new aliquot of autologous RBCs. When no agglutination is apparent during incubation, the harvested serum is tested against the patient's RBCs. If no reactivity is observed, the absorption is complete. However, if a reaction is observed, autoantibody remains in the serum, and further absorption is necessary. It is not unusual for three to six aliquots of RBCs to be used for autoadsorption. With some powerful warm autoantibodies, the technologist may be unable to remove the autoantibody completely and must settle for diminished reactivity.

Figure 9–13 illustrates the steps in performing an autoadsorption. In the first set of figures, the patient's RBC is coated with autoantibody. Autoantibody can be seen free in the serum, along with an alloantibody. The cells are washed and then treated to remove the autoantibody. They are incubated with the patient's serum (middle figure). The autoantibody

begins to adsorb onto the patient's RBC and is removed from the serum. In the last set of figures, the autoantibody has once again coated the patient's RBC, leaving only the alloantibody in the serum. The serum is separated from the autologous RBCs, and an antibody identification panel is performed to reveal any alloantibodies that had previously been masked by the autoantibody. Figure 9–14 shows an example of an antibody identification panel before and after warm autoadsorption. Anti-K is apparent in the postadsorption panel.

Homologous Adsorption

When a patient is so anemic that there are not enough autologous RBCs available to perform an adequate number of adsorptions or when a patient has been recently transfused (donor RBCs in the specimen may adsorb alloantibodies), homologous or differential adsorptions may be employed in place of autoadsorption. For homologous adsorption, the patient is phenotyped, and then phenotypically matched RBCs are used for the adsorption in place of autologous cells. If an exact match cannot be made, the focus is on finding cells that lack the antigens to which the patient may form antibodies. For example, if the patient types as R_1R_1, K–, Fy^a+, Fy^b+, Jk^a–, Jk^b+, S+, s–, then he or she may form anti-E, anti-c, anti-K, anti-Jk^a, and anti-s. The homologous donor cells used for adsorption must be negative for E, c, K, Jk^a, and s antigens in order for those antibodies to remain in the adsorbed serum.

Differential Adsorption

When phenotyping the patient is difficult because of a positive DAT or recent transfusion, differential absorption may be performed. For this method, the patient's serum sample is divided into a minimum of three aliquots. Each aliquot is adsorbed using a different cell. One cell is usually R_1R_1, one is usually R_2R_2, and the third is usually rr. Among the three, one must be negative for K, another negative for Jk^a, and the third negative for Jk^b. The cells are treated with an enzyme to render them negative for antigens of the Duffy and MNSs systems. Following adsorption, antibody identification panels are performed separately on each aliquot, and the reactivities are compared to reveal underlying alloantibodies.

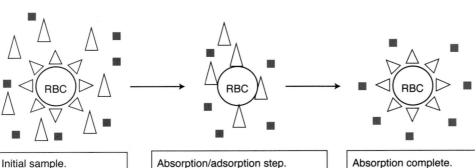

Figure 9–13. Steps for performing an autoadsorption.

Initial sample. Autoantibody (triangle) is coating patient's cells, and is free in patient's serum. Alloantibody (square) is also present in serum.

Absorption/adsorption step. Patient's cells have been treated to remove autoantibody. Treated cells are incubated with patient's serum. Autoantibody from serum begins to adsorb onto patient's cells. Alloantibody remains in serum.

Absorption complete. Autoantibody has been removed from the serum. The absorbed serum may be harvested and tested to identify the remaining alloantibody.

Donor	Cell number	D	C	c	E	e	Cw	K	k	Kpa	Kpb	Jsa	Jsb	Fya	Fyb	Jka	Jkb	Lea	Leb	P1	M	N	S	s	Lua	Lub	Xga	Peg/ IgG	CC	Absorbed serum	CC
R1R1	1	+	+	0	0	+	0	0	+	0	+	0	+	+	0	+	+	+	0	+	+	+	+	0	+	+	+	2+		0	3+
R1R1	2	+	+	0	0	+	+	+	+	+	0	+	0	+	+	+	0	+	0	+	+	+	+	0	+	+	+	2+		0	3+
R2R2	3	+	0	+	+	0	0	0	+	0	+	0	+	0	+	0	+	0	+	+	+	+	+	0	0	+	+	3+		2+	
R0r	4	+	0	+	0	+	0	0	+	0	+	0	+	0	+	0	0	+	+	0	+	+	+	0	+	+	0	2+		0	3+
r'r	5	0	+	+	0	+	0	0	+	0	+	0	+	0	+	+	0	0	0	0	0	+	0	+	0	+	0	2+		0	3+
r"r	6	0	0	+	+	+	0	+	+	0	+	0	+	0	+	+	+	+	0	+	+	+	+	+	0	+	+	3+		2+	
rr	7	0	0	+	0	+	0	0	+	0	+	0	+	+	+	+	+	+	0	0	+	0	+	0	+	+	+	2+		0	3+
rr	8	0	0	+	0	+	0	0	+	0	+	0	+	0	+	0	+	0	+	+	+	0	0	+	0	+	+	2+		0	3+
rr	9	0	0	+	0	+	0	0	+	0	+	0	+	0	+	0	0	+	0	+	+	+	+	0	+	0	+	2+		0	3+
rr	10	0	0	+	0	+	0	+	0	+	0	+	0	+	0	+	+	+	0	+	+	0	+	0	+	0	+	3+		2+	
R0r	11	+	0	+	0	+	0	0	+	0	+	0	+	+	0	+	0	+	0	+	+	0	+	0	+	+	+	2+		0	3+
	Patient Cells																											2+		0	3+

Figure 9–14.   Panel using warm autoadsorption technique.

See Chapter 20, "Autoimmune Hemolytic Anemias" for a more complete discussion.

Adsorption may also be performed when multiple alloantibodies are present in order to separate the specificities. The adsorbing cell must be antigen-positive for one suspected specificity but negative for others. Following adsorption, the serum is tested to see which, if any, additional alloantibodies have been unmasked.

Direct Antiglobulin Test and Elution Techniques

Detection of antibodies coating RBCs is valuable when investigating suspected hemolytic transfusion reactions, HDFN, and autoimmune and drug-induced hemolytic anemias. The direct antiglobulin test (DAT) is used to detect in vivo sensitization of RBCs. In the tube method, the patient's RBCs are washed thoroughly to remove any unbound antibody, and then AHG reagent is added. If IgG antibodies or complement are coating the RBCs, agglutination will be observed. If neither is present, no agglutination will be observed. Coombs' control cells are added to validate the negative test. The DAT may also be performed using solid phase adherence and gel methods.

When IgG antibodies are detected, the next step is to dissociate the antibodies from the RBC surface to allow for identification. **Elution** techniques are used to release, concentrate, and purify antibodies. The methods used to remove the antibody change the thermodynamics of the environment, change the attractive forces between antigen and antibody, or change the structure of the RBC surface. The antibody is then freed into a solution known as an **eluate**. The eluate may be tested against an RBC panel to identify the antibody. A total elution, in which antibody is released and the RBC antigens are destroyed, is usually necessary when performing antibody identification. Partial elution, in which antibody is removed but RBC antigens remain intact, is useful to prepare RBCs for phenotyping and to use in autoadsorption procedures. Chloroquine diphosphate, EGA, and ZZAP are examples of chemicals used for these purposes.

Temperature-Dependent Methods

The simplest elution methods involve changing the temperature of the antigen-antibody environment. Heat may be used to remove antibody. After washing with saline, coated RBCs are suspended in an equal volume of saline or albumin. The gentle heat method, performed at 45°C, allows for antibody removal while leaving the RBC intact.[32] Elution performed at 56°C is a total elution method, allowing for antibody identification.[33] The Lui freeze method[34] also performs a total elution. With this method, washed, coated RBCs suspended in saline or albumin are frozen at –18°C or colder until solid. The mixture is then thawed rapidly, causing the RBCs to burst, freeing the bound antibody. Temperature-dependent elutions are best at detecting IgG antibodies directed against antigens of the ABO system.

pH

A common and relatively quick and easy method for total elution in order to detect non-ABO antibodies is acid elution.[35,36] In this method, the washed antibody-coated cells are mixed with a glycine acid solution at a pH of 3. The antigen-antibody bond is disrupted, and the antibody is released into the acidic supernatant. The supernatant is harvested, and the pH is neutralized so that antibody identification testing can take place. Citric acid and digitonin acid are also used in similar methods.

Organic Solvents

Several organic solvents have been used in total elution methods, including dichloromethane, xylene, and ether.

These solvents act on the lipids in the RBC membrane to reduce surface tension and lead to the reversal of the van der Waals forces that hold antigens and antibodies together.[37,38] Organic eluates are very potent as compared with the temperature-dependent eluates and are best for detecting non-ABO antibodies. However, these procedures are time-consuming, and the chemicals pose several health and safety hazards, as they may be carcinogenic or flammable. Organic solvents are rarely used in the clinical laboratory.

The most critical step in preparing any eluate is the original washing, which is used to remove unbound immunoglobulins. If allowed to remain in the test system, these antibodies will contaminate the final eluate and yield false-positive results. As a control, the last wash supernatant should be tested in parallel with the eluate to detect the presence of unbound antibody. The last wash should be nonreactive, or the eluate results will be invalid.

Antibody Titration

Once an antibody is identified, it is sometimes useful to quantify the amount that is present. While techniques employing flow cytometry, radioimmunoassay, or enzyme-linked immunoassay may give more precise results, these methods are not readily available in every laboratory. Performing an antibody titration can help determine antibody concentration levels. Twofold serial dilutions of serum containing an antibody are prepared and tested against a suspension of RBCs that possesses the target antigen. The **titer** level is the reciprocal of the greatest dilution in which agglutination of 1+ or greater is observed. A score may also be assigned, based on the strength of reactivity. Each reaction is given a value, and the score is determined by adding up the individual values.

After determining the initial titer, the specimen should be frozen. When new specimens are submitted for titer determinations, the initial titer specimen should be tested in parallel to control variability among technologists' technique (e.g., pipetting, grading reactions) and the relative strength of the target antigen on the cells used in testing. A comparison of the current specimen's results and the initial specimen's current results should be made. A fourfold or greater increase in titer (reactivity in two or more additional tubes) or an increase in score of 10 or more is considered to be significant. Table 9–5 shows an example of titer-level results that indicate a significant increase in antibody levels.

When performing the antibody titer, careful preparation of dilutions is necessary. Contamination from a tube with a higher antibody concentration can lead to falsely elevated titer-level results. Changing pipette tips between each tube when preparing the dilutions and working or reading from the most diluted tube to the least diluted can help avoid this problem.

The phenotype of the RBCs selected for use in testing should be consistent throughout the series of titer-level studies. If a cell with homozygous antigen expression was used for the initial titer, then all subsequent titer specimens should be tested against a homozygous cell. The method used must also be consistent. It has been reported that titers using the gel method are more sensitive than those using the tube method and therefore result in a higher titer level.[39] The technologist must make the test systems as identical as possible in order to make valid comparisons between samples.

Titer-level studies are useful in monitoring the obstetric patient who has an IgG antibody that may cause HDFN. An increase in antibody titer level during pregnancy suggests that the fetus is antigen-positive and therefore at risk of developing HDFN. An increasing titer level may indicate the need for intrauterine exchange transfusion. An antibody titer may also be used to help differentiate immune anti-D from passively acquired anti-D due to RhIG administration. The titer level in RhIG is rarely above 4.[40]

Performing a titer is one way to confirm the presence of antibodies that have previously been known as HTLA (high titer, low avidity). These antibodies, directed against high-prevalence antigens, are observed at the AHG phase of testing with weakly positive reactions. The weak reactions persist through extensive dilutions (as high as 2048).[41] Examples of these antibodies include anti-Ch, anti-Rg, anti-Cs^a, anti-Yk^a, anti-Kn^a, anti-McC^a, and anti-JMH. These antibodies usually are not clinically significant but may mask significant antibodies.

Providing Compatible Blood Products

The relative difficulty in providing compatible blood products is determined by the frequency of the antigen in the population and by the clinical significance of the antibody. If the antibody does not cause decreased survival of antigen-positive RBCs, then use of random blood products that are crossmatch-compatible is acceptable. Examples of such antibodies include anti-M, anti-N, anti-P$_1$, anti-Le^a, and anti-Le^b.[42]

Table 9–5 **Titer and Score of Anti-D***								
DILUTION	**1:2**	**1:4**	**1:8**	**1:16**	**1:32**	**1:64**	**1:128**	**TITER AND SCORE**
Previous sample	2+	2+	1+	0	0	0	0	Titer 8
Score	8	8	5	0	0	0	0	Score 21
Current sample	3+	3+	2+	2+	1+	0	0	Titer 32
Score	10	10	8	8	5	0	0	Score 41

*Score values: 4+ = 12, 3+ = 10, 2+ = 8, 1+ = 5

When the patient sample contains clinically significant antibodies or the patient has a history of clinically significant antibodies, units for transfusion must be antigen-negative. The crossmatch technique must demonstrate compatibility at the AHG phase.[43] If the patient sample is plentiful, the technologist may choose to crossmatch units, then antigen-type those that are crossmatch-compatible. If sample quantity is limited or if the antibody is no longer detectable in the serum, units should be antigen-typed first, then crossmatched.

Knowing the frequency of the antigen in the population is helpful when determining the number of units that must be antigen-typed to find a sufficient number to fill the crossmatch request. The number of units requested is divided by the frequency of antigen-negative individuals. For example, if a crossmatch for two units of RBCs is ordered on a patient whose serum contains anti-E, the calculation would be 2 (units requested)/0.70 (the frequency of E-negative individuals). The result is 2.8, meaning that three units would need to be typed for E antigen in order to find two E-negative units. When multiple specificities are present, the frequencies of antigen negative are multiplied together. If E-negative, c-negative units were required in the above example, the calculation would be 2/(0.70 × 0.20) = 14.3. Fourteen or 15 units would have to be antigen-typed for E and c in order to find two units that are negative for both antigens.

In certain cases, knowing the donor's race is helpful when selecting units for antigen testing because the frequency of some antigens varies between races. For example, when searching for units that are Fy^a-negative, it may be prudent to screen black donors, as 90% will be negative for Fy^a compared with only 34% of whites.

Some transfusion medicine experts have proposed that certain populations, particularly sickle cell and beta-thalassemia patients, receive units that are phenotypically matched.[44,45] These patients, who are transfused repeatedly, seem more likely to make alloantibodies than the general population; if they are immunized, it may be difficult to find compatible blood. When the number of antigens that must be negative makes it difficult to find suitable units, rare-donor registries may be consulted. These registries maintain lists of donors and may provide frozen units of rare phenotypes. Another approach is to transfuse units that are phenotypically matched for Rh antigens and K, as these antigens are the most immunogenic.[46]

CASE STUDIES

Case 9-1

Multiple Antibodies

Suspect multiple antibodies when all or most of the screen and panel cells are positive but reactions are at different strengths or in different phases and the autocontrol is negative. When using inclusion techniques, it may appear that no single antibody accounts for all of the positive reactions observed.

Resolution may include performing a selected cell panel to exclude certain specificities. Several sets of cells may need to be tested to narrow the list of possible antibodies (see **Fig. 9–10**). Alternatively, the use of enzyme enhancement may allow for separation of antibodies if one antigen is destroyed by enzymes and another has enhanced expression or is unaffected by enzyme treatment. In other cases, neutralization or absorption techniques may prove useful in separating multiple antibodies. Refer to Figure 9–15.

1. Looking at the original testing (PEG/IgG column), is there reactivity that suggests that this specimen may contain more than one antibody?
2. Of the specificities not excluded in the original testing, which antigens are destroyed by enzymes and which are enhanced?

Donor	Cell number	D	C	c	E	e	C^w	K	k	Kp^a	Kp^b	Js^a	Js^b	Fy^a	Fy^b	Jk^a	Jk^b	Le^a	Le^b	P$_1$	M	N	S	s	Lu^a	Lu^b	Xg^a	Peg/ IgG	CC	Ficin/ IgG	CC
R$_1$r	1	+	+	+	0	+	0	0	+	0	+	0	+	+	+	+	+	0	+	+	+	+	+	+	0	+	+	1+		0	3+
R$_1$R$_1$	2	+	+	0	0	+	+	+	+	0	+	0	+	0	+	+	0	0	0	+	+	0	+	0	0	+	+	3+		2+	
R$_2$R$_2$	3	+	0	+	+	0	0	0	+	0	+	0	+	+	0	0	0	+	0	+	0	+	0	+	0	+	+	0	3+	0	3+
R$_0$r	4	+	0	+	0	+	0	0	+	0	+	0	+	+	0	+	+	+	0	0	+	0	+	+	0	+	0	0	3+	0	3+
r'r	5	0	+	+	0	+	0	0	+	0	+	0	+	0	0	0	+	0	+	+	+	0	+	+	0	+	0	0	3+	0	3+
r"r	6	0	0	+	+	+	0	0	+	0	+	0	+	+	+	0	+	0	+	+	0	+	0	+	0	+	+	1+		0	3+
rr K	7	0	0	+	0	+	0	+	+	0	+	0	+	+	+	+	+	0	+	0	+	+	0	+	0	+	+	2+		2+	
rr	8	0	0	+	0	+	0	0	+	0	+	0	+	0	+	0	+	0	+	0	+	+	+	0	+	+	0	2+		0	3+
r'r"	9	0	+	+	+	+	0	0	+	0	+	0	+	0	+	0	+	0	+	0	+	0	+	0	+	0	+	2+		0	3+
rr	10	0	0	+	0	+	0	0	+	0	+	0	+	+	0	+	+	0	+	+	+	0	+	0	0	+	+	0	3+	0	3+
R$_1$r	11	+	+	+	0	+	0	0	+	0	+	0	+	+	+	+	+	0	+	+	+	+	+	+	+	0	+	1+		0	3+
	Patient Cells																											0	3+	0	3+

Figure 9–15. Enzyme panel.

3. Comparing the original reactions to those of the enzyme panel, which antibodies appear to be present in this specimen?
4. What additional testing could be performed to eliminate anti-C?

Case 9-2

Antibody to a High-Prevalence Antigen

High-prevalence antigens are those that are present in almost all individuals (98% or more). Suspect an antibody to a high-prevalence antigen when all or most screen and panel cells are positive, with reactions in the same phase and at the same strength, along with a negative autocontrol (Fig. 9–16). Panel cells that are negative for these high-prevalence antigens are usually indicated on the antigen profile sheet or may be indicated on the manufacturer's extended typing list, which usually accompanies the panel set.

Among the antibodies included in this category are the so-called HTLA. Although these antibodies are usually not clinically significant themselves, up to 25% of patients with an HTLA antibody also make clinically significant antibodies.[47] It is not necessary to determine the specificity of the HTLA antibody, but removing these antibodies is usually necessary to identify any underlying alloantibodies. Some HTLA antibodies, notably anti-Ch and anti-Rg, may be neutralized by normal serum, which contains complement. Routine blood bank enzymes will destroy anti-Ch, anti-Rg, and anti-JMH, whereas anti-Kn^a and anti-McC^a are destroyed by dithiothreitol (DTT).

Finding compatible blood for patients with an antibody to a high-prevalence antigen may be a challenge.

Autologous donations should be encouraged. Other sources of antigen-negative blood may include family members and the rare donor registry. Fortunately, because these antigens do occur so frequently, it is rare to find a patient with an antibody to one of them. Refer to **Figure 9–16.**

1. What antibody appears to be present in this specimen?
2. What additional testing needs to be performed to confirm this identification?
3. What additional patient information would be useful when resolving a case such as this?

Case 9-3

Antibody to a Low-Prevalence Antigen

Low-prevalence antigens are present in less than 10% of the population. Antibodies to these antigens are uncommon because exposure to the antigen is rare. The antibody screen will most likely be negative; therefore, no panel will have been performed. Antibodies to these antigens should be suspected when an antiglobulin crossmatch is incompatible and other reasons for reactivity, such as ABO incompatibility or positive donor DAT, have been eliminated. These antibodies may also be suspected when an infant has a positive DAT and there is no known blood group discrepancy between mother and infant. Because these antigens are infrequent, finding antigen-negative units for crossmatch is usually not difficult. Refer to Figure 9–17.

1. What low-prevalence antigen is found on cell 4?
2. What additional testing should be performed to confirm the identity of the antibody?

Donor	Cell number	D	C	c	E	e	Cw	K	k	Kpa	Kpb	Jsa	Jsb	Fya	Fyb	Jka	Jkb	Lea	Leb	P1	M	N	S	s	Lua	Lub	Xga	Peg/IgG	CC
R1R1	1	+	+	0	0	+	0	0	+	0	+	0	+	+	0	+	+	+	0	+	+	+	+	+	0	+	+	2+	
R1R1	2	+	+	0	0	+	+	+	+	0	+	0	+	+	+	0	+	0	+	+	+	0	+	+	0	+	+	2+	
R2R2	3	+	0	+	+	0	0	0	+	0	+	0	+	0	+	0	+	0	+	+	+	+	+	0	0	+	+	2+	
R$_0$r	4	+	0	+	0	+	0	0	+	0	+	0	+	0	0	+	+	0	+	+	+	0	+	0	0	+	0	2+	
r'r	5	0	+	+	0	+	0	0	+	0	+	0	+	+	0	+	0	0	0	0	0	+	0	+	0	+	0	2+	
r"r	6	0	0	+	+	+	0	+	+	0	+	0	+	+	+	+	+	0	+	+	+	+	+	0	+	+	2+	
rr Co^b +	7	0	0	+	0	+	0	0	+	0	+	+	+	+	+	+	+	0	0	+	+	0	+	0	+	+	2+	
rr	8	0	0	+	0	+	0	0	+	0	+	0	+	0	+	0	+	0	+	+	+	0	0	+	0	+	+	2+	
rr	9	0	0	+	0	+	0	0	+	0	+	0	+	0	+	+	0	0	+	0	+	+	+	+	0	+	0	2+	
rr Yt(a)−	10	0	0	+	0	+	0	+	+	0	+	0	+	0	+	+	+	0	+	+	0	+	0	+	0	+	+	0	3+
R$_0$r	11	+	0	+	0	+	0	0	+	0	+	0	+	+	+	0	+	0	+	+	0	+	0	+	0	+	+	2+	
	Patient Cells																												0	3+

Figure 9–16.   Panel performed on a patient with an antibody to a high-prevalence antigen.

Donor	Rh-Hr					Kell				Duffy		Kidd		Lewis		P	MNS				Lutheran		Reactions			
	D	C	c	E	e	K	k	Jsa	Jsb	Fya	Fyb	Jka	Jkb	Lea	Leb	P1	M	N	S	s	Lua	Lub	IS	37	IgG	CC
1	+	+	+	0	+	0	+	0	+	0	+	0	+	+	0	+	+	+	0	+	0	+	0	0	0	3+
2	+	+	0	0	+	0	+	0	+	0	+	0	+	+	0	+	+	+	+	+	0	+	0	0	0	3+
3	+	0	0	+	+	0	+	0	+	+	+	0	+	+	+	0	+	+	+	+	0	+	0	0	0	3+
4	+	+	+	0	+	0	+	+	+	+	+	+	+	+	+	0	+	+	+	0	0	+	0	1+	2+	NT
5	+	+	+	0	+	0	+	0	+	+	0	+	+	0	0	+	0	+	0	+	0	+	0	0	0	3+
6	0	0	+	0	+	0	+	0	+	+	0	+	0	+	+	+	+	0	+	+	0	+	0	0	0	3+
7	0	0	+	0	+	+	+	0	+	+	0	+	0	+	+	+	+	0	+	+	0	+	0	0	0	3+
8	0	0	+	+	0	0	+	0	+	+	0	0	+	0	+	+	0	+	0	0	0	+	0	0	0	3+
9	0	0	+	0	+	0	+	0	+	0	0	0	+	0	+	+	+	+	0	0	0	+	0	0	0	3+
10	+	0	+	0	+	0	+	0	+	0	+	+	+	0	+	+	+	0	+	0	+	0	+	0	0	0	3+
11	+	+	0	+	0	0	+	0	+	0	+	+	0	+	0	+	+	0	+	+	0	+	0	0	0	3+
12	+	+	0	0	+	0	+	0	+	+	+	+	0	+	+	+	+	0	0	+	0	+	0	0	0	3+
PC																							0	0	0	3+

Figure 9–17. Panel performed on a patient with an antibody to a low-prevalence antigen.

Case 9-4

Cold-Reacting Autoantibodies

Most adult sera contain low titers of cold-reacting autoantibodies, most notably autoanti-I, autoanti-H, and autoanti-IH. These antibodies are usually IgM and of no clinical significance. They are troublesome in that they may interfere with the detection of significant antibodies, resulting in prolonged workups and delayed transfusions.

Cold-reacting autoantibodies may be suspected when the screen cells, panel cells, and the autocontrol are all positive at the immediate spin phase and reactivity gets weaker or disappears with incubation at 37°C (Fig. 9–18).

Certain cold autoantibodies activate complement and may be detected at the AHG phase when using complement-containing AHG reagent. These autoantibodies may be mistaken for weakly reacting IgG antibodies.

Although it is not usually necessary to determine the specificity of the cold autoantibody, testing against additional cells may confirm its presence. Cord blood cells that lack the I antigen are of particular value for this

Donor	Cell number	D	C	c	E	e	Cw	K	k	Kpa	Kpb	Jsa	Jsb	Fya	Fyb	Jka	Jkb	Lea	Leb	P1	M	N	S	s	Lua	Lub	Xga	IS	37	AHG	CC
R1R1	1	+	+	0	0	+	0	0	+	0	+	0	+	+	0	+	+	+	0	+	+	+	+	+	0	+	+	2+	W+	0	3+
R1R1	2	+	+	0	0	+	+	+	+	0	+	0	+	+	0	+	+	0	+	0	+	+	+	0	+	0	+	2+	W+	0	3+
R2R2	3	+	0	+	+	0	0	0	+	0	+	0	+	0	+	0	+	0	+	+	+	+	+	0	0	+	+	2+	W+	0	3+
R0r	4	+	0	+	0	+	0	0	+	0	+	0	+	0	0	+	+	0	+	+	+	+	0	0	0	+	0	2+	W+	0	3+
r'r	5	0	+	+	0	+	0	0	+	0	+	0	+	+	0	+	0	0	0	0	0	+	0	+	0	+	0	2+	W+	0	3+
r"r	6	0	0	+	+	+	0	+	+	0	+	0	+	+	+	+	0	+	+	+	+	+	0	+	0	+	+	2+	W+	0	3+
rr	7	0	0	+	0	+	0	0	+	0	+	0	+	+	+	+	+	0	0	+	0	+	0	+	0	+	0	2+	W+	0	3+
rr	8	0	0	+	0	+	0	0	+	0	+	0	+	0	+	0	+	0	+	+	+	+	0	0	+	0	+	2+	W+	0	3+
rr	9	0	0	+	0	+	0	0	+	0	+	0	+	+	0	+	0	0	+	0	+	+	+	+	0	+	0	2+	1+	0	3+
rr	10	0	0	+	0	+	0	+	+	0	+	0	+	0	+	0	+	0	+	+	0	+	0	+	0	+	+	2+	1+	0	3+
R0r	11	+	0	+	0	+	0	0	+	0	+	0	+	+	0	+	0	+	+	0	+	0	+	0	+	0	+	2+	1+	0	3
I neg	Cord Cell																											0	0	0	3+
	Patient Cells																											2+	1+	0	3+

Figure 9–18. Panel performed on a patient with a cold autoantibody.

CELL	IS	RT	18°C	4°C
A₁	0	0	1+	2+
A₂	1+	2+	4+	4+
B	0	0	2+	3+
O adult	2+	3+	4+	4+
O cord	0	0	1+	2+
Auto	0	0	1+	2+

Figure 9–19. Cold antibody screen performed on an AB patient with autoanti-IH.

purpose. A cold panel consisting of group O adult cells (H and I antigens), group O cord cells (H and i antigens), group A₁ adult cells (I antigen), and an autocontrol may be tested at 4°C to determine the specificity of the cold autoantibody (see Figs. **9–18** and **9–19**).

1. Why is a cold autoantibody suspected in this case?
2. Why may a technologist test cord blood cells in a case such as this?
3. How might a technologist avoid interference from cold autoantibodies?

Case 9-5

Warm-Reacting Autoantibodies

Warm-reacting autoantibodies are some of the most challenging to work up. Warm autoantibodies are uncommon, but they may occur secondary to chronic lymphocytic leukemia, lymphoma, systemic lupus erythematosus, and other autoimmune diseases or as a result of drug therapy. Suspect a warm autoantibody when all cells, including the autocontrol, are reactive at the AHG phase and at the same strength. If an underlying alloantibody is present, cells that possess that antigen may react stronger than those that are antigen-negative. It is of

primary importance to remove the warm autoantibody to detect the alloantibody. It is not necessary to determine the specificity of the autoantibody, although many seem to be directed against Rh antigens.

Warm autoantibodies are IgG antibodies that are found coating the patient's RBCs and that are free in the patient's serum. Adsorption techniques are used to remove the antibody from the serum.

Finding RBC units that are compatible with a patient who has a warm autoantibody may be difficult. If after the absorption no clinically significant antibodies are detected, an immediate spin crossmatch to detect ABO incompatibility is all that is necessary. If clinically significant antibodies are present, then antigen-negative units should be crossmatched using an antiglobulin technique. The warm autoantibody frequently interferes with this testing, making interpretation of results difficult.

Some transfusion medicine experts believe that repeating the full warm autoantibody workup is unnecessary if the patient's serologic picture has remained unchanged when compared with previous results.[48,49] They advocate transfusing the patient with units that are phenotypically matched for Rh and K antigens in order to minimize the risk of alloimmunization. Refer to **Figure 9–14**.

This panel was performed on a male lymphoma patient who was last transfused 2 years ago. He has not received any transplants and is not currently on any medications.

1. What does the pattern of reactivity in the original panel (PEG/IgG column) suggest?
2. How can you differentiate this pattern from that of an antibody to a high-prevalence antigen?
3. What type of adsorption procedure is recommended in this case?
4. Are any alloantibodies present in this specimen?
5. How would you prepare red blood cell products for this patient?

SUMMARY CHART

✔ The purpose of the antibody screen is to detect *unexpected* antibodies, which may be found in approximately 0.2% to 2% of the general population. The antibodies may be classified as immune (the result of RBC stimulation in the patient), passive (transferred to the patient through blood products or derivatives), or naturally occurring (the result of environmental factors). Antibodies may also be classified as alloantibodies, directed at foreign antigens, or autoantibodies, directed at one's own antigens.

✔ A clinically significant antibody is one that results in the shortened survival of RBCs possessing the target antigen. Clinically significant antibodies are IgG antibodies that react best at 37°C or in the AHG phase of testing. They are known to cause hemolytic transfusion reactions and HDFN.

✔ Screen cells are commercially prepared group O red blood cell suspensions obtained from individual donors who are phenotyped for the most commonly encountered and clinically important RBC antigens.

✔ RBCs from a homozygous individual have a double dose of a single antigen, which results from the inheritance of two genes that code for the same antigen, whereas heterozygous individuals carry only a single dose each of two different antigens. (Each gene codes for a different antigen.)

✔ Antibodies in the Kidd, Duffy, Lutheran, Rh, and MNSs blood group systems show *dosage* and yield stronger reactions against RBCs with homozygous expression of their corresponding antigen.

SUMMARY CHART—cont'd

✔ Enhancement reagents, such as LISS and PEG, are solutions added to serum and cell mixtures in the IAT to promote antigen-antibody binding or agglutination.

✔ Coombs' control cells are RBCs coated with human IgG antibody, which are added to all AHG-negative tube tests to ensure that there was an adequate washing step performed and that the AHG reagent is present and functional in the test system.

✔ Gel and solid phase adherence methods are alternatives to tube testing. These methods may be automated to increase efficiency.

✔ The antibody exclusion method rules out possible antibodies based on antigens that are present on negatively reacting cells.

✔ Conclusive antibody identification is achieved when the serum containing the antibody is reactive with at least three antigen-positive cells (i.e., reagent cells that express the corresponding antigen), negative with at least three antigen-negative cells (i.e., reagent cells that do not express the corresponding antigen), and the patient's RBCs phenotype negative for the corresponding antigen.

✔ The DAT detects RBCs that were sensitized with antibody in vivo. Elution methods are used to free antibody from the cell surface to allow for identification.

✔ The calculation used to determine the number of random donor units that should be antigen typed in order to provide the requested number of antigen-negative RBC units for patients with an antibody involves dividing the number of antigen-negative units requested by the frequency of antigen-negative individuals in the donor population.

✔ The relative quantity of an RBC antibody can be determined by testing serial twofold dilutions of serum against antigen-positive RBCs; the reciprocal of the highest serum dilution showing agglutination is the antibody titer.

Review Questions

1. Based on the following phenotypes, which pair of cells would make the best screening cells?
   a. Cell 1: Group A, D+C+c–E–e+, K+, Fy(a+b–), Jk(a+b–), M+N–S+s–
      Cell 2: Group O, D+C–c+E+e–, K–, Fy(a–b+), Jk(a–b+), M–N+S–s+
   b. Cell 1: Group O, D–C–c+E–e+, K–, Fy(a–b+), Jk(a+b+), M+N–S+s+
      Cell 2: Group O, D+C+c–E–e+, K–, Fy(a+b–), Jk(a+b–), M–N+S–s+
   c. Cell 1: Group O, D+C+c+E+e+, K+, Fy(a+b+), Jk(a+b+), M+N–S–s+
      Cell 2: Group O, D–C–c+E–e+, K–, Fy(a+b–), Jk(a+b+), M+N+S–s+
   d. Cell 1: Group O, D+C+c–E–e+, K+, Fy(a–b+), Jk(a–b+), M–N–S+s+
      Cell 2: Group O, D– C–c+E+e–, K–, Fy(a+b–), Jk(a+b–), M+N–S+s–

2. Antibodies are excluded using RBCs that are homozygous for the corresponding antigen because:
   a. Antibodies may show dosage
   b. Multiple antibodies may be present
   c. It results in a P value of .05 for proper identification of the antibody
   d. All of the above

3. A request for 8 units of packed RBCs was received for patient LF. The patient has a negative antibody screen, but one of the 8 units was 3+ incompatible at the AHG phase. Which of the following antibodies may be the cause?
   a. Anti-K
   b. Anti-Le^a
   c. Anti-Kp^a
   d. Anti-Fy^b

4. The physician has requested 2 units of RBCs for patient DB, who has two antibodies, anti-L and anti-Q. The frequency of antigen L is 45%, and the frequency of antigen Q is 70% in the donor population. Approximately how many units will need to be antigen-typed for L and Q to fill the request?
   a. 8
   b. 12
   c. 2
   d. 7

5. Anti-Sd^a has been identified in patient ALF. What substance would neutralize this antibody and allow detection of other alloantibodies?
   a. Saliva
   b. Hydatid cyst fluid
   c. Urine
   d. Human breast milk

6. Patient JM appears to have a warm autoantibody. She was transfused 2 weeks ago. What would be the next step performed to identify any alloantibodies that might be in her serum?
   a. Acid elution
   b. Warm autoadsorption using autologous cells
   c. Warm differential adsorption
   d. RESt™ adsorption

7. What is the titer and score for this prenatal anti-D titer? (Refer to Figure 9–20.)
   a. Titer = 64; score = 52
   b. Titer = 1:32; score = 15
   c. Titer = 64; score = 21
   d. Titer = 32; score = 52

For Questions 8 through 10, refer to Figure 9–21.

8. Select the antibody(ies) most likely responsible for the reactions observed:
   a. Anti-E and anti-K
   b. Anti-Fy^a
   c. Anti-e
   d. Anti-Jk^b

9. What additional cells need to be tested to be 95% confident that the identification is correct?
   a. Three e-negative cells that react negatively and one additional e-positive cell that reacts positively
   b. One additional E-positive cell to react positively and one additional K-positive cell to react positively
   c. Two Jk^b homozygous positive cells to react positively and one Jk^b heterozygous positive cell to react negatively
   d. No additional cells are needed

10. Using the panel in **Figure 9–21**, select cells that would make appropriate controls when typing for the C antigen.
    a. Cell number 1 for the positive control and cell number 2 for the negative control
    b. Cell number 1 for the positive control and cell number 6 for the negative control
    c. Cell number 2 for the positive control and cell number 4 for the negative control
    d. Cell number 4 for the positive control and cell number 5 for the negative control

Dilution	1:1	1:2	1:4	1:8	1:16	1:32	1:64	1:128	1:256	1:512	1:1024	Saline control
Results	4+	4+	3+	2+	1+	1+	0	0	0	0	0	0

Figure 9–20. Anti-D titer results for Question 7.

Donor	Cell number	D	C	c	E	e	C^w	K	k	Kp^a	Kp^b	Js^a	Js^b	Fy^a	Fy^b	Jk^a	Jk^b	Le^a	Le^b	P$_1$	M	N	S	s	Lu^a	Lu^b	Xg^a	IS	37	AHG	CC
R$_1$R$_1$	1	+	+	0	0	+	0	0	+	0	+	0	+	+	+	+	+	0	0	+	+	+	+	+	0	+	+	0	0	0	3+
R$_1$r	2	+	+	+	0	+	+	+	+	0	+	0	+	+	0	0	+	0	+	0	+	0	+	+	0	+	+	0	0	3+	
R$_1$R$_1$	3	+	+	0	0	+	0	0	+	0	+	0	+	0	+	+	+	0	+	+	0	+	0	+	0	+	+	0	0	0	3+
R$_2$R$_2$	4	+	0	+	+	0	0	0	+	0	+	0	+	+	0	+	+	0	+	+	+	0	+	0	0	+	+	0	2+	3+	
r'r	5	0	+	+	0	+	0	0	+	0	+	0	+	0	0	0	+	+	0	+	+	0	+	+	0	+	0	0	0	0	3+
r"r"	6	0	0	+	+	0	0	0	+	0	+	0	+	+	0	0	+	0	0	+	0	+	0	+	0	+	+	0	2+	3+	
rr K	7	0	0	+	0	+	0	+	+	0	+	0	+	+	0	0	0	+	0	+	0	+	0	+	0	+	+	0	0	3+	
rr	8	0	0	+	0	+	0	0	+	0	+	0	+	0	+	+	0	0	+	0	+	0	+	0	0	+	+	0	0	0	3+
rr	9	0	0	+	0	+	0	0	+	0	+	0	+	+	+	0	+	0	0	+	+	+	+	0	+	+	0	0	0	0	3+
R$_1$r	10	+	+	+	0	+	0	0	+	0	+	0	+	+	0	+	+	0	+	+	+	0	0	+	0	+	+	0	0	0	3+
R$_0$	11	+	0	+	0	+	0	0	+	0	+	0	+	+	+	0	+	0	+	+	+	0	0	+	0	+	+	0	0	0	3+
	Patient Cells																											0	0	0	3+

Figure 9–21. Panel study for Questions 8–10.

11. Which of the following methods may be employed to remove IgG antibodies that are coating a patient's red blood cells?
    a. Adsorption
    b. Elution
    c. Neutralization
    d. Titration

12. A technologist has decided to test an enzyme-treated panel of RBCs against a patient's serum. Which of the following antibody pairs could be separated using this technique?
    a. Anti-Jk^a and anti-Jk^b
    b. Anti-S and anti-Fy^a
    c. Anti-D and anti-C
    d. Anti-Jk^a and anti-Fy^a

13. An antibody demonstrates weak reactivity at the AHG phase when using a tube method with no enhancement reagent and monospecific anti-IgG AHG reagent. When repeating the test, which of the following actions may increase the strength of the positive reactions?
    a. Adding an enhancement reagent, such as LISS or PEG
    b. Decreasing the incubation time from 30 minutes to 10 minutes
    c. Employing the prewarm technique
    d. Decreasing the incubation temperature to 18°C

References

1. Giblett, ER: Blood group alloantibodies: An assessment of some laboratory practices. Transfusion 17:299, 1977.
2. Boral, L, and Henry, IB: The type and screen: A safe alternative and supplement in selected surgical procedures. Transfusion 17:163, 1977.
3. Standards for Blood Banks and Transfusion Services, 26th ed. American Association of Blood Banks, Bethesda, MD, 2009.
4. International Standards for Cellular Therapy Product Collection, Processing, and Administration Accreditation Manual, 4th ed. Foundation for the Accreditation of Cellular Therapy/Joint Accreditation Committee—ISCT and EBMT, Omaha, NE, and Barcellona, Spain, 2008, p 183.
5. Judd, WJ, Luban, NLC, Ness, PM, et al: Prenatal and perinatal immunohematology: Recommendations for serologic management of the fetus, newborn infant, and obstetric patient. Transfusion 30:175, 1990.
6. Issitt, PD, and Anstee, DJ: Applied Blood Group Serology, 4th ed. Montgomery Scientific Publications, Durham, NC, 1998, p 47.
7. Klein, HG, and Anstee, DJ: Mollison's Blood Transfusion in Clinical Medicine, 11th ed. Blackwell Scientific Publications, Oxford, England, 2005, p 312.
8. Issitt, PD, and Anstee, DJ: Applied Blood Group Serology, 4th ed. Montgomery Scientific Publications, Durham, NC, 1998, p 132.
9. Standards for Blood Banks and Transfusion Services, 26th ed. American Association of Blood Banks, Bethesda, MD, 2009.
10. Kosanke, J, Dickstein, B, and Davis, K: Evaluation of incubation times using the ID-Micro Typing system (abstract). Transfusion 42:108S, 2000.
11. Ciavarella, D, Pate, L, and Sorenson, E: Serologic comparisons of antibody detection and titration methods: LISS, PeG, gel (abstract). Transfusion 42:108S, 2002.
12. Yamada, C, Serrano-Rahman, L, Vasovic, LV, Mohandas, K, and Uehlinger, J: Antibody identification using both automated solid-phase red cell adherence assay and a tube polyethylene glycol antiglobulin method. Transfusion 48:1693, 2008.
13. Bouix, O, Ferrera, V, Delamaire, M, Redersdorff, JC, and Roubinet, F: Erythrocyte-magnetized technology: An original and innovative method for blood group serology. Transfusion 48:1878, 2008.
14. Schonewille, H, Haack, HL, and van Zijl, AM: RBC antibody persistence. Transfusion 40:1127, 2000.
15. Tormey, CA, and Stack, G: The persistence and evanescence of blood group alloantibodies in men. Transfusion 49:505, 2009.
16. South, SF: Use of the direct antiglobulin test in routine testing. In Wallace, ME, and Levitt, JS (eds): Current Application and Interpretation of the Direct Antiglobulin Test. American Association of Blood Banks, Arlington, VA, 1988, p 25.
17. Issitt, PD, and Anstee, DJ: Applied Blood Group Serology, 4th ed. Montgomery Scientific Publications, Durham, NC, 1998, p 470.
18. Fisher, RA: Statistical methods and scientific inference, 2nd ed. Oliver and Boyd, Edinburgh, Scotland, 1959.
19. Harris, RE, and Hochman, HG: Revised p values in testing blood group antibodies. Transfusion 26:494, 1986.
20. Kanter, MH, Poole, G, and Garretty, G: Misinterpretation and misapplication of p values in antibody identification: The lack of value of a p value. Transfusion 37:816, 1997.
21. Roback, J (ed): Technical Manual, 16th ed. American Association of Blood Banks, Bethesda, MD, 2008, p 894.
22. Kosanke, J, and Arrighi, S: Antigen typing red cells that are resistant to IgG reduction (abstract). Transfusion 40:119S, 2000.
23. Roback, J (ed): Technical Manual, 16th ed. American Association of Blood Banks, Bethesda, MD, 2008, p 896.
24. Morelati, F, Revelli, N, Musella, A, et al: Automated red cell phenotyping (abstract). Transfusion 41:110S, 2001.
25. Lowe, L: Use of MTS IgG gel cards for red blood cell antigen typing (abstract). Transfusion 42:109S, 2002.
26. Bennett, PR, Le Van Kim, C, Dolon, Y, et al: Prenatal determination of fetal RhD type by DNA amplification. N Engl J Med 329:607–610, 1993.
27. Palacajornsuk, P, Halter, C, Isakova, V, et al: Detection of blood group genes using multiplex SNaPshot method. Transfusion 49:740, 2009.
28. Wagner, FF, Bittner, R, Petershofen, EK, Doescher, A, and Müller, TH: Cost-efficient sequence-specific priming–polymerase chain reaction screening for blood donors with rare phenotypes. Transfusion 48:1169, 2008.
29. Karpasitou, K, Drago, F, Crespiatico, L, et al: Blood group genotyping for Jk^a/Jk^b, Fy^a/Fy^b, S/s, K/k, Kp^a/Kp^b, Js^a/Js^b, Co^a/Co^b, and Lu^a/Lu^b with microarray beads. Transfusion 48:505, 2008.
30. Aster, RH, Miskovich, BH, and Rodey, GE: Histocompatibility antigens of human plasma; localization to HLD-3 lipoprotein fraction. Transplantation 16:205, 1973.
31. Yuan S: Immunoglobulin M red blood cell alloantibodies are frequently adsorbed by rabbit erythrocyte stroma. Transfusion 50(5):1139–1143, 2010.
32. Roback, J (ed): Technical Manual, 16th ed. American Association of Blood Banks, Bethesda, MD, 2008, p 893.
33. Landsteiner, K, and Miller, CP: Serologic studies on the blood of primates: II. The blood group of anthropoid apes. J Exp Med 42:853, 1925.

34. Feng, CS, Kirkley, KC, Eicher, CA, et al: The Lui elution technique: A simple and efficient method for eluting ABO antibodies. Transfusion 25:433, 1985.

35. Rekkvig, OP, and Hannestad, K: Acid elution of blood group antibodies from intact erythrocytes. Vox Sang 33:280, 1977.

36. Judd, WJ, Johnson, ST, and Storry, J: Judd's methods in immunohematology, 3rd ed. AABB Press, Bethesda, MD, 2008.

37. van Oss, CJ, Absolom, DR, and Neumann, AW: The "hydrophobic effect": Essentially a van der Waals interaction. Colloid Polymer Sci 1:424, 1980.

38. van Oss, CJ, Absolom, DR, and Neumann, AW: Applications of net repulsive van der Waals forces between different particles, macromolecules, or biological cells in liquids. Colloid Polymer Sci 1:45, 1980.

39. Ciavarella, D, Pate, L, and Sorenson, E: Serologic comparisons of antibody detection and titration methods: LISS, PeG, gel (abstract) Transfusion 42:108S, 2002.

40. Roback, J (ed): Technical Manual, 16th ed. American Association of Blood Banks, Bethesda, MD, 2008, p 633.

41. Schulman, IA, and Petz, LD: Red cell compatibility testing: Clinical significance and laboratory methods. In Petz, LD, Swisher, SN, and Kleinman, S (eds): Clinical Practice of Transfusion Medicine, 3rd ed. Churchill Livingstone, New York, 1996, p 199.

42. Roback, J (ed): Technical Manual, 16th ed. American Association of Blood Banks, Bethesda, MD, 2008, p 454.

43. Standards for Blood Banks and Transfusion Services, 26th ed. American Association of Blood Banks, Bethesda, MD, 2009.

44. Tahhan, HR, Holbrook, CT, Braddy, LR, et al: Antigen-matched donor blood in the transfusion management of patients with sickle cell disease. Transfusion 34:562, 1994.

45. Matteocci, A, Palange, M, Dionisi, M, et al. Retrospective study on the red cell alloimmunization after multiple blood transfusions (abstract). Transfusion 41:112S, 2001.

46. Vichinsky, EP, Luban, NLC, Wright, E, et al: Prospective RBC phenotype matching in a stroke-prevention trial in sickle cell anemia: A multicenter transfusion trial. Transfusion 41:1086, 2001.

47. Moulds, MK: Special serologic techniques useful in resolving high-titer, low-avidity antibodies. In Recognition and Resolution of High-Titer, Low-Avidity Antibodies: A Technical Workshop. American Association of Blood Banks, Washington, DC, 1979.

48. Sanguin, J, Angus, N, and Sutton, DM: Repeated serological testing of patients with warm autoimmune hemolytic anemia may not be necessary (abstract). Transfusion 41:106S, 2001.

49. Judd, WJ: Investigation and management of immune hemolysis: Autoantibodies and drugs. In Wallace, ME, and Levitt, JS (eds): Current Applications and Interpretations of the Direct Antiglobulin Test. American Association of Blood Banks, Arlington, VA, 1988, p 47.

50. Cheng, CK, Wong, ML, and Lee, AW: PEG adsorption of autoantibodies and detection of alloantibodies in warm autoimmune hemolytic anemia. Transfusion 41:13, 2001.

51. Leger, RM, and Garratty, G: Evaluation of methods for detecting alloantibodies underlying warm autoantibodies. Transfusion 39:11, 1999.

Chapter 10

Pretransfusion Testing

William B. Zundel, MS, MLS^{CM}, SBB

OBJECTIVES

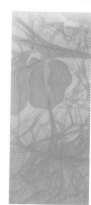

1. Describe appropriate methods for proper patient identification in sample collection.
2. Outline the procedure for testing donor and patient specimens.
3. Select appropriate donor units based on availability, presence, or absence of unexpected alloantibody in the patient.
4. Compare and contrast crossmatch procedures.
5. Resolve incompatibilities in the crossmatch.
6. Explain compatibility testing procedures and protocols in special circumstances.
7. State the limitations of compatibility testing procedures.
8. Describe a scheme for effective blood utilization.
9. List the steps necessary to reidentify the patient before transfusion.
10. Discuss future issues of compatibility testing.

Introduction

Under the umbrella of pretransfusion testing is a series of serologic and nonserologic protocols and testing procedures with the ultimate objective of preventing an immune mediated hemolytic transfusion reaction. Much of this textbook thus far has described how to perform serologic testing procedures (e.g., ABO, Rh, and antibody detection) and has explained processes of pretransfusion testing. This chapter is a comprehensive examination of how testing procedures enhance the safety of blood transfusion.

Testing Standards

Transfused red blood cells (RBCs) should have an acceptable survival rate, and there should not be significant destruction of the recipient's own RBCs. Table 10–1 outlines the steps in pretransfusion testing and associated AABB standards from the AABB's *Technical Manual*, 16th edition.[1] Strict adherence to and application of each parameter of pretransfusion testing is imperative in managing safe blood transfusion therapy. Each parameter must also be considered in any comprehensive review of the process used to select blood for a recipient.

Pretransfusion testing cannot guarantee normal survival of transfused RBCs in the recipient's circulation. The potential benefits of RBC transfusion should always be weighed against the potential risks any time this form of therapy is considered. Although adverse responses to transfusion cannot always be avoided, results are much more likely to be favorable if pretransfusion testing is carefully performed and if results of laboratory testing show no incompatibility between donor and recipient.

The Clinical Laboratory Improvement Amendments of 1988 (CLIA '88) gives the United States federal government authority to regulate pretransfusion testing. Testing regulated via CLIA '88 includes ABO group, Rh type, antibody detection and identification, and crossmatch testing.

Identification, Collection, and Preparation of Samples

Pretransfusion testing begins and ends with the proper identification and collection of the patient sample. Those responsible for identifying the patient and collecting recipient blood must adhere to the strict standards set forth to ensure recipient safety and acceptable survival rates.

Positive Recipient Identification

A major cause of transfusion-associated fatalities is clerical error resulting in incorrect ABO groupings and transfusion of ABO incompatible blood. In a study of transfusion errors in New York State over a 10-year period, 47% of errors involved misidentification of the patient or the blood at bedside.[2] Clerical error is the greatest threat to safe transfusion therapy. The most common cause of error is misidentification of the recipient. Examples include misidentification of the recipient when the blood sample is drawn, mix-up of samples during handling in the laboratory, and misidentification of the recipient when the transfusion is given. Exact procedures for proper identification of the recipient, recipient sample, and donor unit must be established and utilized by all staff responsible for each aspect of transfusion therapy.

To prevent collecting samples from the wrong patient, a facility-generated recipient ID wristband must always be compared with the blood requisition form (blood request form). The blood request form must state the recipient's full name and unique hospital identification number.[3] Other information such as age, date of birth, address, sex, and name of requesting physician can be used to further

---

Table 10–1 Steps in Pretransfusion Testing and AABB Standards

STEPS IN PRETRANSFUSION TESTING	RELEVANT AABB STANDARD(S)
Request for transfusion	5.11.1 and 5.11.1.1
Identification of transfusion recipient and blood specimen collected	5.11, 5.11.1, 5.11.2, 5.11.2.1, 5.11.2.2, 6.2.3.1, and 8.2
Testing of transfusion recipient's blood specimen: • Blood specimen acceptability • ABO group and Rh type • Antibody detection testing • Antibody identification • Comparison of current and previous test results	5.11.2.3 and 5.11.3 5.13, 5.13.1, and 5.13.2 5.13.3, 5.13.3.1, 5.13.3.2, 5.13.3.3, and 5.13.3.4 5.13.3, 5.13.3.1, 5.13.3.2, 5.13.3.3, and 5.13.3.4 5.13.5, 5.13.5.1, and 5.13.5.2
Donor RBC unit testing: • ABO group confirmation and Rh type confirmation for Rh-negative RBC units	5.12 and 5.12.1
Donor red cell unit selection: • Selection of components of ABO group and Rh type that are compatible with the transfusion recipient and with any unexpected allogeneic antibodies	5.14, 5.14.1, 5.14.2, 5.14.2.1, 5.14.3, 5.14.4, and 5.14.5
Compatibility testing (crossmatch): • Serologic • Computer or electronic	5.15, 5.15.1, and 5.15.1.1 5.15.2, 5.15.2.1, 5.15.2.2, 5.15.2.3, 5.15.2.4, and 5.15.2.5
Labeling of blood or blood components with the recipient's identifying information and issue	5.1.6, 5.10, 5.18, 5.18.1, 5.18.2, 5.18.2.1, and 5.18.3

Reprinted with permission bfrom Roback, J (ed): Technical Manual, 16th ed. American Association of Blood Banks, Bethesda, MD, 2008.

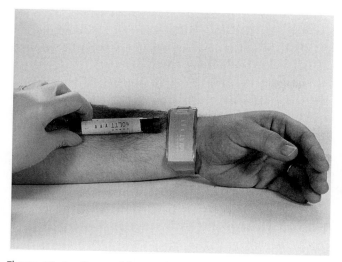

Figure 10–1.   Commercially manufactured identification systems. Compare preprinted label with the patient armband.

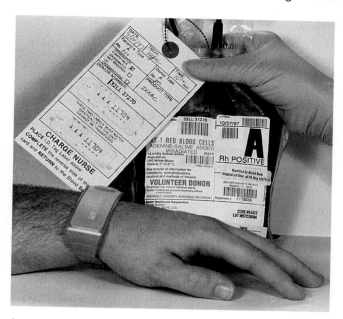

Figure 10–3.   Commercially manufactured identification systems. Pretransfusion comparison of recipient armband and donor unit bag.

verify patient identity but is not required on the form. Printing must be legible, and indelible nameplate impressions or computer printouts are preferable to handwritten forms. Any discrepancies must be completely resolved before the sample is taken. Nameplates on the wall or bed labels must never be used to verify identity, as the patient specified may no longer occupy that bed. If the patient does not have a wristband or if the patient's identity is unknown, some form of positive identification must be attached to the patient before collecting the samples. This may be a temporary tie tag or a wristband or ankle band; it should not be removed until proper identification has been attached to the patient and the person collecting the recipient sample verifies identity.

In some transfusion facilities, if the patient does not have a wristband and is coherent, it is permissible to ask the patient to state his or her full name and to spell it out. If the date of birth or home address is printed on the requisition form, the patient might be asked to state this information. Occasional errors can result from two patients with the same name being mistaken for each other. The phlebotomist should never offer a name and ask the patient to confirm that it is correct (e.g., "Are you Mr. Jones?"). Some disoriented patients may answer yes to any question. If the patient is very young or is incoherent, some other reliable professional individual who knows the patient must confirm the identity and document this on the requisition form.

Commercially manufactured identification systems using preprinted tags and numbers (Figs. 10–1, 10–2, and 10–3) are useful in verifying patients and donors. Emerging systems include bar-code readers and radio frequency identification (RFID). Whatever procedure is adopted, it must be an integral part of the blood bank's standard operating procedure (SOP) manual, thus resulting in the requirement that all blood bank personnel demonstrate competency in the process.[4]

Collection of Patient Samples

After positive identification has been made, blood samples should be drawn, carefully using a technique that avoids hemolyzing the sample. In vitro hemolysis of recipient samples for pretransfusion testing cannot be used because it can mask hemolysis caused by antigen–antibody complexes that activate complement to completion. There are patients experiencing in vivo hemolytic processes (such as hemolytic anemia) who will do so no matter how well the collection procedure is performed. The hemolysis occurs in the patient

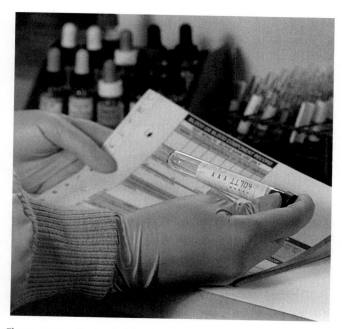

Figure 10–2.   Confirm that sample and requisition form agree.

prior to collection and cannot be avoided. In these circumstances, care must be taken to note the extent of hemolysis present in the patient serum or plasma and observe for any increases during each stage of testing.

Serum or plasma may be used for pretransfusion testing. Disadvantages to using plasma include the possible formation of small fibrin clots, which may be difficult to distinguish from true agglutination. Also, plasma anticoagulants may inactivate complement so that some antibodies may not be detected. Having said this, more transfusion services are using plasma today than ever before due to the ease of handling. About 10 mL of blood is usually sufficient for all testing procedures if there are no known serologic problems.

Tubes must be labeled before they leave the recipient's bedside. If imprinted labels are used, they must be compared with the recipient's wristband and requisition form before the tubes are used. Labels must be attached to the tubes at the bedside in a tamper-proof manner that will make removal and reattachment impossible. All writing must be legible and indelible, and each tube must be labeled with the patient's full name, unique identification number, and date of sample collection.[5] The phlebotomist must initial or sign the label and add additional pertinent information as required by the facility's SOP.

To avoid contamination with materials that may cause confusing serologic results, blood samples should not be taken from intravenous (IV) tubing lines. Venous samples are to be drawn only from below the infusion site, not above it. For example, if a patient has an IV line in the antecubital area of the arm, any vein below the angle of the arm to the hand can be used. If a sample must be taken from an IV line, the line should be disconnected for 5 to 10 minutes, the first 10 mL of blood drawn should be discarded, and then the sample should be obtained.

When a specimen is received in the laboratory, blood bank personnel must confirm that the information on the sample and requisition form agree. All discrepancies must be resolved before the sample is accepted, and if any doubt exists, a new sample must be drawn. Receipt of an unlabeled specimen requires that a new sample be obtained.[6]

Recipient samples should be tested as soon as possible after collection. If using a serum sample, the recipient serum should be separated from the RBCs as soon as possible after the sample has clotted. If testing cannot be performed immediately, samples should be kept at 1°C to 6°C.

As noted in Chapter 3, "Fundamentals of Immunology," recent pregnancy or transfusion indicates an opportunity for a humoral immune response. Antibody production occurs over a predictable range of time, which varies from patient to patient. Specimens used in pretransfusion testing should ideally be collected during the critical phases of the immune response. In an attempt to capture this important time for each patient, serum obtained from samples fewer than 72 hours after collection must be used for antibody screening and crossmatch testing if the patient was pregnant or received RBC products by transfusion within the last 3 months, or if these histories are unknown.[7]

Patient RBCs can be obtained from either clotted or anticoagulated samples. They can be washed with physiological saline before use to remove plasma or serum, which may interfere with some testing procedures. A 2% to 5% saline suspension of RBCs is used for most serologic testing procedures; however, the manufacturer's directions should be consulted for the proper cell concentration to use for typing tests performed with licensed reagents.

 A method for preparing a button of washed RBCs suitable for performing one test is outlined in Procedure 10-1 on the textbook's companion website.

Collection of Donor Samples

Samples for donor testing must be collected at the same time as the full donor unit. Depending on the method used for testing, clotted or anticoagulated pilot samples are obtained. The donor information and medical history card, the pilot samples for processing, and the collection bag must be labeled with the same unique number before starting the phlebotomy, and the numbers must be verified again immediately after collection.[8] The donor unit identification number is used to identify all records of testing and eventual disposition of all component parts of the unit of blood. More detailed information on donor samples can be found in Chapter 13, "Donor Screening and Component Preparation."

RBCs for donor pretransfusion testing can be prepared from the segmented tubing through which the donor blood was collected. The tubing or segment is attached to the collection bag, and each segment is imprinted with the same number. These numbers are different from the donor unit identification number but nonetheless are a positive means of sampling a given unit of blood.

Donor RBCs can be obtained from the segments in many ways that permit several procedures to be performed from the same segment. One technique that works well for sampling is using a lancet to make a tiny hole in the segment through which a single drop of blood can be expressed and then disposing the lancet in a biohazard sharps container. The hole is essentially self-sealing, so the rest of the blood in the segment remains uncontaminated. Another technique is to cut the RBC end of the segment tubing with scissors and use an applicator stick to remove cells or squeeze the tubing to express a drop.

Commercially manufactured segment puncture devices eliminate the need for scissors and lancets, thus enabling the dispensing of the RBCs into a test tube in one motion. The segment may be stored with the cut end down in a properly labeled test tube and covered or stoppered to minimize contamination and maintain RBC integrity. The contents of the segment should not be emptied into a test tube for storage because of the increased risk of contamination. Regardless of the method used to harvest cells from a segment, it is important that engineering or work practice controls be used to eliminate or minimize aerosol production when the segment is cut or opened.

Refer to Chapter 25, "Transfusion Safety and Federal Regulatory Requirements" for additional information on safety procedures.

Both donor and recipient samples must be stored for a minimum of 7 days following transfusion.[9] The samples should be stoppered, carefully labeled, and refrigerated at 1°C to 6°C. They should be adequate in volume so they can be reevaluated if the patient experiences any adverse reaction to the transfusion.

Compatibility Testing Protocols

Compatibility testing refers to the serologic aspect of pretransfusion testing. It includes every serologic facet, beginning with donor blood and ending with the recipient blood sample.

Testing the Donor Sample

According to the *Code of Federal Regulations*[10] and the AABB *Standards for Blood Banks and Transfusion Services*,[11] ABO grouping and Rh typing (including a test for weak D) and tests intended to prevent disease transmission must be performed on a sample of donor blood taken at the time of collection. AABB *Standards* requires a screening test for unexpected antibodies to RBC antigens on samples from donors who have a history of transfusion or pregnancy.[12] Testing is performed by the facility collecting the donor unit, and results must be clearly indicated on all product labels appearing on the unit.

AABB *Standards*[13] also requires that the transfusing facility confirm the ABO cell grouping on all units and Rh typing on units labeled Rh-negative. Repeat weak-D testing is not required. The transfusing facility is not required to repeat any other testing procedure on donor blood. The sample used for this testing must be obtained from an attached segment on the donor unit.

All testing must be performed using in-date licensed reagents according to manufacturers' directions and protocol established in the facility's written SOP. A detailed explanation of the processing of donor blood can be found in Chapter 13.

Testing the Patient Sample

A record must be maintained of all results obtained in testing patient samples. Some large transfusion services keep this information on a computerized retrieval system for ready access. However, when computer records are not available, these transfusion services must have another system that permits retrieval of patient testing results.[14]

Ideally, the same unique identification number should be assigned each time a patient is admitted to a health-care facility for treatment. The number can then be used as a method for positive identification by comparing results of previous and current testing. Verification of previous results helps establish that the current samples were collected from the correct individual. Any discrepancies between previous and current results must be resolved before transfusion is initiated. A new sample should be collected from the patient, if necessary, to resolve the problem.

ABO, Rh, and unexpected antibody screening test results should be included in the record. Notations concerning unusual serologic reactions and the identity of unexpected antibodies in the patient's serum should also be included in the record. This may be the most important information. Sometimes an unexpected antibody can drop below detectable levels in a patient's serum, and previous records are the only source of information regarding its presence, identity, and clinical significance.

ABO, Rh grouping, and antibody screening of the patient's serum can be performed in advance of or at the same time as the crossmatch. If the patient has had a transfusion or has been pregnant within the last 3 months or if the history is unavailable or uncertain, the sample must be obtained from the patient within 3 days of the scheduled transfusion.[15] An accurate medical history, including information on medications, recent blood transfusions, and previous pregnancies, may help to explain unusual results.

ABO Grouping

Determining the patient's correct ABO group is the most critical pretransfusion serologic test. ABO grouping can be performed on slides or in tubes, using solid-phase RBC adherence or column gel technology. Testing is performed in a manner similar to that described in Chapter 6, "The ABO Blood Group System," using potent licensed reagents according to the manufacturer's directions. If the ABO forward and reverse grouping results do not agree, additional testing must be conducted to resolve the discrepancy. Useful information on resolving ABO grouping discrepancies has also been presented in Chapter 6. If the patient's ABO group cannot be satisfactorily determined and immediate transfusion is required, group O–packed RBCs should be used.

Rh Typing

Rh typing is performed using anti-D blood typing reagents. Tube or slide tests should be performed according to the manufacturer's directions for the reagent, which may include the use of a suitable diluent control. When indicated, these controls must be run in parallel when Rh typing tests are performed on patient samples to avoid incorrectly designating Rh-negative patients as Rh-positive. If the diluent control is positive, the result of the Rh typing test is invalid. In such a case, a direct antiglobulin test (DAT) should be performed on the patient's RBCs to determine whether uptake of autoantibodies or alloantibodies (if the recipient has been recently transfused) is responsible for the positive control. If the DAT is positive, accurate Rh typing can sometimes be performed using saline-active or chemically modified Rh blood typing serum with an appropriate diluent or 8% albumin control. If the Rh type of the recipient cannot be determined and transfusion is essential, Rh-negative blood should be given. Currently, most monoclonal or monoclonal blend anti-D reagents are room temperature–reactive and do not require the use of a control. See Chapter 7, "The Rh Blood Group System," for more in-depth discussion.

The test for weak D is unnecessary when testing transfusion recipients.[16] Individuals typing as Rh-negative in direct testing should receive Rh-negative blood, and those typing as Rh-positive in direct testing should receive Rh-positive blood. There are those in the blood bank community who prefer complete Rh typing of all recipients to conserve Rh-negative blood for Rh-negative patients. Female patients whose RBCs type as weak D are considered Rh-positive and may receive Rh-positive blood during transfusion.

Some patients who type as Rh-positive, whether by direct or indirect testing, may produce anti-D following transfusion of Rh-positive RBC components. This occurs rarely and does not justify the routine transfusion of Rh-negative blood to these Rh-positive patients until the antibody is detected.

Antibody Screening

The recipient's serum or plasma must be tested for clinically significant unexpected antibodies. The object of the antibody screening test is to detect as many clinically significant unexpected antibodies as possible. In general, "clinically significant unexpected antibody" refers to antibodies that are reactive at 37°C or in the antihuman globulin test and are known to have caused a transfusion reaction or unacceptably short survival of transfused RBCs. Table 10–2 outlines these antibodies and their clinical significance as "usually," "rarely," or "sometimes" causing obvious clinical symptoms.[17]

The incidence of unexpected alloantibodies depends on the fact that antibody formation is the result of exposure to a foreign RBC antigen and the patient's ability to respond to that exposure. This occurs by allogeneic transfusion of RBCs, pregnancy, or transplantation. Therefore, the incidence of unexpected antibodies in the general patient population is low: 1.64% in one large study[18] and 0.78% in another.[19] It follows, then, that the more frequently a patient is exposed to foreign RBC antigens, the more likely that patient will produce unexpected alloantibodies. This is evidenced by a study of multiply transfused sickle cell patients in which 29% of pediatric and 47% of adult patients developed clinically significant alloantibodies.[20]

Detection of unexpected antibodies is important for the selection of donor RBCs that will have the best survival rate in the patient's circulation and reduce the risk of hemolytic transfusion reaction. Refer to Chapter 9, "Detection and Identification of Antibodies," for a complete discussion of the detection and identification of unexpected clinically significant alloantibodies.

Antibody screening tests should demonstrate the presence of all potentially clinically significant alloantibodies in the recipient's serum or plasma and indicate the need for further studies. All antibodies encountered in the screening test must be identified to determine potential clinical significance and to decide whether there is a need to select antigen-negative units for transfusion.

Table 10–2   Clinical Significance of 37°C-Reactive Antibodies

USUALLY*	VERY UNUSUAL (IF EVER)†	SOMETIMES
ABO	Bg (HLA)	Cartwright (e.g., Yt^a)‡
Rh	Ch/Rg (complement C4)	Lutheran (e.g., Lu^b+)‡
Kidd	Le^b	Gerbich‡
Duffy	JMH	Dombrock‡
S, s, U	Xg^a	M, N‡
P		Le^a
		Vel
		LW
		Ii
		H
		At^a
		In^b
		Mi^a
		Cs^a

* These antibodies usually cause obvious clinical symptoms and decreased RBC survival. Sometimes no obvious clinical symptoms occur.
† These antibodies rarely (if ever) cause clinically obvious symptoms, but there are some data to suggest that some unusual examples of Bg,[36,39–41] anti-Kn/Mc/Yk,[36,42] and JMH[36,43] cause shortened RBC survival.
‡ These antibodies rarely cause acute severe HTR, but when they are "clinically significant," they may cause obvious clinical symptoms (e.g., jaundice); they more often cause only shortened RBC survival.
Reprinted with permission from Garratty, G: Evaluating the clinical significance of blood group alloantibodies that are causing problems in pretransfusion testing. Vox Sanguinis 74: 285–290, 1998. Table 1, p 289.

Selection of Appropriate Donor Units

In almost all cases, the first choice for transfusion is blood and blood components of the patient's own ABO and Rh group. This is defined as ABO group–specific. When blood and blood components of the patient's ABO blood group are not available or some other reason precludes their use, units selected must lack any antigen against which the recipient has a clinically significant antibody. However, it is completely acceptable to use blood and blood components that do not contain all of the antigens carried on the patient's own RBCs (e.g., group A– or B–packed RBCs can be safely given to a group AB recipient).

When a recipient must be given blood of a different ABO group, only packed RBCs can be given. Whole blood cannot be administered in these situations because incompatible, preformed ABO antibodies are present in the whole-blood plasma. For example, group A whole blood cannot be transfused into a group AB recipient, because the plasma of the group A whole blood has anti-B antibodies present. Group O packed RBCs can be safely used for all patients; however, conservation of a limited supply of group O blood should dictate its use for recipients of other ABO types only in special circumstances. If ABO group–specific blood is not available or is in low supply, alternative blood groups are chosen, as summarized in Table 10–3.

Rh-negative blood can be given to Rh-positive patients; however, good inventory management should conserve this limited resource for use in Rh-negative recipients. But if the Rh-negative unit is near expiration, the unit should be given rather than wasted. Rh-positive blood should not be given to Rh-negative female patients of childbearing age. Transfusion of Rh-negative male patients and female patients beyond menopause with Rh-positive blood is acceptable as long as no preformed anti-D is demonstrable in their sera. About 80% of Rh-negative patients who receive 200 mL or more of Rh-positive blood respond to such a transfusion by producing anti-D.[21] However, this outcome must sometimes be weighed against the alternatives of not transfusing at all if the supply of Rh-negative blood has been exhausted. If the formation of anti-D is unlikely to be of great significance (e.g., in an Rh-negative elderly surgical patient), many technologists feel the use of Rh-positive blood is judicious. In these situations, approval by or notification of the blood bank's medical director is necessary, according to the laboratory's SOP.

When an unexpected antibody is found in the patient's serum during an antibody screening test, donor units selected at random are crossmatched with the patient's serum and shall include incubation at 37°C and the AHG test.[22] This should not be assumed to be the standard, although this may help identify the unexpected antibody. If a clinically significant antibody is identified, the serologically compatible units are then phenotyped with commercial antiserum to verify that they are antigen-negative for the corresponding antibody. For example, if a recipient has an anti-K1 antibody, the crossmatch-compatible donor RBC unit is tested with commercial anti-K1 antisera for the presence of the K1 antigen.

There is no need to provide antigen-negative RBCs for patients whose sera contain antibodies that are reactive only below 37°C, because these antibodies are incapable of causing significant RBC destruction in vivo.

Potent examples of IgG, warm reactive antibodies in patients' serum can also be used to select suitable donor units by direct crossmatch testing. Commercially prepared typing reagents must be used to select blood for patients whose serum contains weak examples of antibodies active at 37°C or whose antibodies react well only with panel cells carrying homozygous expression of the corresponding antigens. It must also be used for patients whose serum no longer exhibits demonstrable in vitro reactivity, but that previously was known to contain clinically significant IgG antibodies such as anti-Jk[a], anti-K1, or anti-E.

Donor units should be selected so that the RBCs are of appropriate age for the patient's needs and will not expire before use. For efficient inventory management, units that will definitely be transfused should be selected from units close to their expiration date based on the needs of the recipient.

Before compatibility testing, donor units should be examined visually for unusual appearance, correct labeling, and hermetic seal integrity. Donor units showing abnormal color, turbidity, clots, incomplete or improper labeling information, or leakage of any sort should be returned to the collecting facility.

Crossmatch Testing

The crossmatch test has traditionally meant the testing of the patient's serum with the donor RBCs, including an antiglobulin phase or simply an immediate spin phase to confirm ABO compatibility. The terms *compatibility test* and *crossmatch* are sometimes used interchangeably, but they should be clearly differentiated. A crossmatch is only one part of pretransfusion testing (see Table 10–1).

Originally the serologic crossmatch preceded antibody screening as part of pretransfusion compatibility testing to check for unexpected alloantibodies. Considering that over 99% of clinically significant unexpected antibodies in patients' sera can be detected by adequate antibody screening procedures, many blood banks abbreviate or even eliminate the serologic crossmatch. What, then, is the value of performing serologic crossmatching between patient and donor samples? Two main functions of the serologic crossmatch test can be cited:

1. It is a final check of ABO compatibility between donor and patient.
2. It may detect the presence of an antibody in the patient's serum that will react with antigens on the donor RBCs but that was not detected in antibody screening because the corresponding antigen was lacking from the screening cells.

The current AABB *Standards*[23] state that tests to detect ABO incompatibility are sufficient if no clinically significant

RECIPIENT ABO GROUP	1st CHOICE	2nd CHOICE	3rd CHOICE	4th CHOICE
AB	AB	A	B	O
A	A	O		
B	B	O		
O	O			

Table 10–3   **Suggested ABO Group Selection Order for Transfusion of RBCs**

Reprinted with permission from AABB Technical Manual, 14th ed, p 454, Table 21.1 Suggested ABO Group Selection Order for Transfusion of RBCs.

antibodies were detected in the antibody screening process and if no historical record exists of clinically significant unexpected antibodies being detected.

Elimination of advanced crossmatch testing—for patients undergoing surgical procedures, in which blood is unlikely to be used—has been implemented successfully in many facilities. This is accomplished by using the "type and screen" in conjunction with the maximum surgical blood order schedule (MSBOS) approach or the abbreviated crossmatch. This leads to the next generation of crossmatch decisions: the computer crossmatch.

Serologic Crossmatch Tests

The serologic crossmatch test consists of mixing the recipient's serum with donor RBCs. Several procedures can be used for serologic crossmatch testing, including the immediate spin and antiglobulin crossmatch. The objective of testing is to select donor units that can provide maximal benefit to the patient, which should be kept in mind when developing the test protocol. Crossmatch methods can generally be categorized by the test phase in which the procedure ends.

 A sample procedure for a one-tube crossmatch test is given in Procedure 10-2 on the textbook's companion website.

Immediate Spin Crossmatch

When no clinically significant unexpected antibodies are detected and there are no previous records of such antibodies, a serologic test to detect ABO incompatibility is sufficient.[24] This is accomplished by mixing the recipient's serum with donor RBCs and centrifuging immediately(i.e., immediate spin). Absence of hemolysis or agglutination indicates ABO compatibility.

The type-and-screen procedure involves testing the patient's blood sample for ABO, Rh, and clinically significant unexpected antibodies. The patient sample is then stored in the blood bank refrigerator for future crossmatch if blood is needed for transfusion. The type-and-screen procedure has application for patients undergoing many elective procedures who may need blood; because the process may not always require transfusion, the crossmatch is not performed until necessary. The type and screen, coupled with an immediate spin crossmatch, is referred to as an *abbreviated crossmatch*. Studies of abbreviated crossmatch use show that it is a safe and effective method of pretransfusion testing. It has been calculated to be 99.9% effective in preventing occurrence of an incompatible transfusion.[25] Walker[26] showed that the frequency with which an incompatible antiglobulin crossmatch follows a negative screen is very low: 0.06%. Other studies confirm its safety with similar statistics.[27–30]

However, the immediate spin does not detect all ABO incompatibilities.[31] False reactions may be seen in the presence of other immediate spin-reactive antibodies (e.g., autoanti-I) or in patients with hyperimmune ABO antibodies, or may be seen when the procedure is not performed correctly (e.g., delay in centrifugation or reading), when rouleaux is observed, or when infants' specimens are tested. Adding ethylenediaminetetraacetic to the test system reportedly eliminates some of the false-positive reactions, thus improving the sensitivity of the immediate spin crossmatch.[32]

Antiglobulin Crossmatch

The antiglobulin crossmatch procedure begins in the same manner as the immediate spin crossmatch, continues to a 37°C incubation, and finishes with an antiglobulin test. Several enhancement media may be applied to boost antigen-antibody reactions. These may include albumin, low ionic strength solution (LISS), polyethylene glycol, and polybrene (as discussed in Chapter 5, "The Antiglobulin Test"). For greatest sensitivity, an antihuman globulin (AHG) reagent containing both anti-IgG and anticomplement may be selected for the final phase of this crossmatch method. However, many laboratories routinely use monospecific anti-IgG AHG reagents.

An autocontrol, consisting of the patient's own cells and serum, may be tested in parallel with the crossmatch test. Although current AABB *Standards* no longer requires an autocontrol, some technologists still find it useful. Perkins[33] calculated the predictive value of a positive autocontrol (3.6%) when the antibody screen was negative and decided to continue using the autocontrol in pretransfusion testing. Results of the autocontrol help clarify possible explanations for positive results in the crossmatches and are discussed later in this chapter.

Interpretation of Results

Tubes (gel cards, etc.) should be carefully labeled so that the contents can be identified at any stage of the procedure. After centrifugation of tubes, the supernatant should be examined for hemolysis, which, if present, must be interpreted as a positive result. Results should be read against a white or lighted background, and a magnifying mirror or hand lens can be used to facilitate reading. The button of RBCs should be gently resuspended. A "tilt and wiggle" method of resuspension is ideal. The initial tilt, when the clear supernatant sweeps over the button of RBCs, immediately indicates a positive or negative reaction. A jagged or firm button edge is indicative of a positive agglutination reaction, whereas a smooth swirling of free cells off the RBC button indicates a negative reaction.

Violent or excessive shaking or tapping of the tubes may yield false-negative results, because weak reactions or fragile agglutinates may be shaken loose and misread as negative. After the button has been completely resuspended, the contents of the tube should be interpreted and positive results graded according to a scale used by all technologists in the facility according to the SOP. Uniform grading of reactions allows retrospective analysis of results by supervisory staff as well as comparison of serial results obtained on samples collected from the same patient. Results can be examined microscopically for verification, if desired. Review the **Color Plate** on red cell antigen-antibody reactions in the front of the book for typical grading of agglutination reactions.

According to the *Code of Federal Regulations*,[34] all results must be recorded immediately in a permanent ledger by means of a logical system that allows them to be easily recalled; actual observations and interpretations must be recorded. All work should be signed or initialed by the technologist performing the test. If an incompatibility is found, the record should clearly show the location of results of the follow-up studies, and additional testing should be performed.

Resolution of Incompatibilities in the Serologic Crossmatch

The primary objective of the crossmatch test is to detect the presence of antibodies in the recipient's serum, including anti-A and anti-B, that could destroy transfused RBCs. A positive result in the crossmatch test requires explanation, and the recipient should not receive a transfusion until the cause of the incompatibility has been determined. When the crossmatch test result is positive, the results of the autocontrol and antibody screening test should be reviewed to identify patterns that may help determine the cause of the problem.

Causes of Positive Results in the Serologic Crossmatch

A positive result in the serologic crossmatch test may be caused by any of the following:

1. **Incorrect ABO grouping of the patient or donor.** ABO grouping should be immediately repeated, especially if strong incompatibility is observed in a reading taken after immediate spin. Samples that bear undisputable identity with the original patient sample and the donor bag should be used for retesting.
2. **An alloantibody in the patient's serum reacting with the corresponding antigen on donor RBCs.** The autocontrol tube will be negative unless the patient has been recently transfused with incompatible RBCs. If the antibody screening test is positive, antibody identification panel studies should allow identification of antibody specificity, which then permits selection of units lacking the antigens for compatibility testing. Chapter 9 provides further discussion of antibody detection and identification and has examples for study.
   - If RBCs of all donors tested are incompatible with the patient's serum and the antibody screening test is positive, suspect either an antibody directed against an antigen of high incidence or multiple antibodies in the patient's serum. Consult a reference laboratory if you are unable to identify the specificity. *Note:* If the patient has ABO-compatible siblings, the siblings may lack the antigen(s) to which the patient has been sensitized and may be excellent potential donors in an emergency.
   - If the antibody screening test is negative and only one donor unit is incompatible, an antibody in the patient's serum may be directed against an antigen of relatively low incidence that is present on that donor's RBCs.
   - If the antibody screening test is negative, the patient's serum may contain either naturally occurring (e.g., anti-A1) or passively acquired ABO agglutinins. Passive acquisition of anti-A, anti-B, or anti-A,B may occur after transfusion of non-ABO-specific blood products (e.g., platelets) or after organ (e.g., liver) or bone marrow transplantation. Checking the serum grouping result to confirm the presence of an unexpected reaction with A1 cells or checking the patient's transfusion and transplant histories is helpful when investigating these cases.

3. **An autoantibody in the patient's serum reacting with the corresponding antigen on donor RBCs.** The autocontrol tube will be positive. The antibody screening test and tests of the patient's serum with donor cells will show positive results. Most autoantibodies have specificity for antigens of relatively high incidence. Panel adsorption and elution studies are important to assess whether underlying alloantibodies are also present. Techniques for management of patients with autoantibodies include, among other tests, autoadsorption of the patient's serum to remove autoantibody activity. Compatibility testing could then be performed using the autoabsorbed serum. Chapter 20, "Autoimmune Hemolytic Anemias" provides further discussion of autoantibodies and their serologic activity.
4. **Prior coating of the donor RBCs with protein, resulting in a positive antihuman globulin test.** If one isolated positive result is obtained, a DAT should be performed on the donor's RBCs. Donor cells that demonstrate a positive DAT will be incompatible with all recipients tested in the AHG phase, because the cells are already coated with immunoglobulin or complement.
5. **Abnormalities in the patient's serum.**
   - Imbalance of the normal ratio of albumin and gamma globulin (A/G ratio), as in diseases such as multiple myeloma and macroglobulinemia, may cause RBCs to stick together on their flat sides, giving the appearance of stacks of coins when viewed microscopically. This is called rouleaux formation (see **Color Plate 2**). This property of the serum will affect all tests, including the autocontrol. Strong rouleaux may mimic true agglutination. Rouleaux are usually strongest after 37°C incubation but do not persist through washing before the AHG test.

    Problems with rouleaux can often be resolved using the saline replacement technique (see Procedure 10-3 on the textbook's companion website).[35]

   - The presence of high-molecular-weight dextrans or other plasma expanders may cause false-positive results in pretransfusion testing. However, Bartholomew[36] raised doubt that the use of dextran interferes with pretransfusion testing. In scenarios in which plasma expanders interfere, all tests, including the autocontrol, are generally affected equally. Saline replacement may be useful to resolve the problem.
   - An antibody against additives in the albumin reagents may cause false-positive results in compatibility tests. Rarely, a patient's serum reacts against the albumin in testing reagents. This occurs when the patient has antibodies to the stabilizing substances, such as caprylate, added to the albumin reagents.[37] Thus, caprylate-free albumin solutions should be used in testing.

6. **Contaminants in the test system.** Dirty glassware, bacterial contamination of samples, chemical or other contaminants in saline, and fibrin clots may produce false-positive compatibility test results. Refer to Table 10–4 for suggestions on investigating causes of pretransfusion tests.

Computer Crossmatch

A report by Judd[38] indicated that an electronic (computer) crossmatch to detect ABO incompatibilities was as safe as the serologic immediate spin test. Many believe that the computer crossmatch is safer than the immediate spin because of the integrity of the computer software to detect ABO incompatibility between the sample submitted for pretransfusion testing and the donor unit.[39] The computer crossmatch compares recent ABO serologic results and interpretations on file for both the donor and the recipient being matched and determines compatibility based on this comparison. Butch and colleagues[40] provide an excellent model of the computer crossmatch SOP. Also helpful is the "Computer Crossmatch" (Electronic Based

Table 10–4   Causes of Positive Pretransfusion Tests*

Negative Antibody Screen, Incompatible Immediate-Spin Crossmatch

- Donor red cells are ABO incompatible.
- Donor red cells are polyagglutinable.
- Anti-A1 is the serum of an A$_2$ or A$_2$B individual.
- Other alloantibodies reactive at room temperature (e.g., anti-M).
- Rouleaux formation.
- Cold autoantibodies (e.g., anti-I).
- Passively acquired anti-A or anti-B.

Negative Antibody Screen, Incompatible Antiglobulin Crossmatch

- Donor red cells have a positive direct antiglobulin test.
- Antibody reacts only with red cells having strong expression of a particular antigen (e.g., dosage) or variation in antigen strength (e.g., P1).
- Antibody to a low-incidence antigen on the donor red cells.
- Passively acquired anti-A or anti-B.

Positive Antibody Screen, Compatible Crossmatches

- Autoanti-IH (autoanti-H) or anti-Le^{bH} and nongroup O units are selected.
- Antibodies dependent on reagent red cell diluent.
- Antibodies demonstrating dosage and donor red cells are from heterozygotes (i.e., expressing a single dose of antigen).
- Donor unit is lacking corresponding antigen.

Positive Antibody Screen, Incompatible Crossmatches, Negative Autocontrol

- Alloantibody(ies)

Positive Antibody Screen, Incompatible Crossmatches, Positive Autocontrol, Negative Direct Antiglobulin Test

- Antibody to ingredient in enhancement media or enhancement dependent autoantibody.
- Rouleaux formation.

Positive Antibody Screen, Incompatible Crossmatches, Positive Autocontrol, Positive DAT

- Alloantibody causing either a delayed serologic or hemolytic transfusion reaction.
- Passively acquired autoantibody (e.g., intravenous immune globulin).
- Cold- or warm-reactive autoantibody.
- Rouleaux formation.

*Causes depend on serologic methods used.
Reprinted with permission from Roback, J (ed): Technical Manual, 16th ed. American Association of Blood Banks, Bethesda, MD, 2008.

Testing for the Compatibility between the Donor's Cell Type and the Recipient's Serum or Plasma Type) Draft Guidance, CBER June 2007. Additional benefits of using the computer crossmatch include annual savings, reduced sample requirements, reduced handling of biological materials, and elimination of false reactions associated with the immediate spin crossmatch. Although the advantages outweigh the disadvantages, a compilation of the College of American Pathologists' interlaboratory comparison program survey data[41] indicates that as of 2004, only 2.1% of labs participating in the CAP survey use a computer crossmatch.

Figure 10–4 is a flowchart that illustrates the necessary steps for a computer crossmatch to meet the AABB *Standards*.[42] The AABB *Standards* specifies that the computer crossmatch can be used only for the purpose of detecting an ABO incompatibility between the donor unit and the recipient sample that was submitted for pretransfusion testing. Current testing for unexpected antibodies must be nonreactive, and there must not be any history of such antibodies. Also, at least

two concordant patient ABO/Rh types must be on file or the computer crossmatch is not permissible.[43]

One of the ABO determinations must be done on the current sample. Having a previous ABO result on file may serve as the second occasion. When there are no results on file, testing of the same sample by a second technologist, if possible, or testing of a second current sample is indicated. The computer system must have logic to notify the user of the following: discrepancies between the donor ABO group and Rh type on the unit label, and those determined by blood group confirmatory tests, and ABO incompatibility between the recipient and the donor unit. Additionally, the computer system must be validated to show that it can detect data entry discrepancies and ABO incompatibilities between patient and donor.[44]

Pretransfusion Testing in Special Circumstances

As with all things, there are special circumstances that just don't fit into the rigid regulatory world of pretransfusion testing. There are circumstances associated with emergency transfusion needs that take precedence over standard protocols such as waiving pretransfusion testing in trauma situations. This is just one of the following special circumstances discussed.

Emergencies

Blood component needs sometimes exceed pretransfusion testing requirements. In other words, the recipient may require the transfusion of RBC components prior to the completion of pretransfusion testing. Several approaches can be utilized in these circumstances. Some laboratories use an "emergency" pretransfusion testing procedure that employs a shortened incubation time, often with addition of LISS, to accelerate antigen–antibody reactions. Others maintain that regular procedures should be used in all circumstances and that blood should be issued before completing the standard pretransfusion testing procedure, if necessary. They believe that there is greater danger in using an unfamiliar procedure under pressure than in releasing blood without completed testing. Although both lines of reasoning have merit, the ideal compromise may be to develop regular testing procedures that are most efficient so that they can be used in emergency and routine situations alike. Whatever the approach, the protocol for handling emergencies must be decided in advance of the situation and be familiar to all staff in the transfusion service. Adequate pretransfusion samples should be collected before transfusion of any donor blood, if possible, so that pretransfusion testing, if necessary, can subsequently be performed.

If blood must be issued in an emergency, the patient's ABO and Rh group should be determined so that ABO group–specific blood can be given. In extreme emergencies, when there is no time to obtain and test a pretransfusion sample, group O Rh-negative packed cells can be used. If the patient is Rh-negative and large amounts of blood are likely to be needed, a decision should be made rapidly whether inventory allows and the situation demands transfusion of Rh-negative blood. Conversion to Rh-positive is best made immediately if

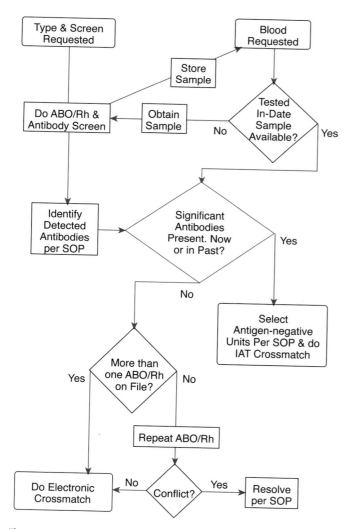

Figure 10–4. Flowchart for the electronic crossmatch that meets the requirements set forth by the AABB. *(Reprinted with permission from Judd, JW: Requirements for the electronic crossmatch. Vox Sanguinis 74:409–417, 1998, Figure 1, p 410.)*

the patient is a man or is a woman beyond childbearing age. Injections of Rh immunoglobulin to prevent formation of anti-D may sometimes be appropriate after the crisis has been resolved. This product is discussed in detail in Chapter 19, "Hemolytic Disease of the Fetus and Newborn."

Accurate records of all units issued in the emergency must be maintained. A conspicuous tie tag or label must be placed on each unit that indicates compatibility testing was not completed before release of the unit, and the physician must sign a waiver authorizing and accepting responsibility for using blood products prior to completion of pretransfusion testing, according to the *Code of Federal Regulations*.[45] Subsequent pretransfusion testing should be completed according to the chosen protocol, and any incompatible result should be reported immediately to the recipient's physician and the blood bank medical director.

Transfusion of Non-Group-Specific Blood

When donor units of an ABO group other than the recipient's own type have been transfused, such as giving a group A recipient large volumes of group O RBCs, testing the recipient's serum in a freshly drawn sample for the presence of unexpected anti-A or anti-B must be performed prior to giving any additional RBC transfusions. When serum from the freshly drawn sample is compatible with donor RBCs of the recipient's own ABO group, ABO group–specific blood may be given for the transfusion. If the serologic crossmatch reveals incompatibility, additional transfusions should be of the alternative blood group.

For example, if a group B patient has been given a large number of units of group O packed cells, anti-B may be present in adequate amounts to result in a positive reaction in an immediate spin crossmatch. Group O units should therefore be used for any additional transfusions.

Compatibility Testing for Transfusion of Plasma Products

Compatibility testing procedures are not required for transfusion of plasma products. However, for transfusion of large volumes of plasma and plasma products, a crossmatch test between the donor plasma and patient RBCs may be performed, although current *Standards* does not require a crossmatch test. The primary purpose for testing is to detect ABO incompatibility between donor and patient; therefore, an immediate spin crossmatch is sufficient.

Intrauterine Transfusions

Blood for intrauterine transfusion must be compatible with maternal antibodies capable of crossing the placenta. If the ABO and Rh groups of the fetus have been determined, group-specific blood could be given provided that there is no fetomaternal ABO or Rh incompatibility. If the ABO and Rh groups of the fetus are not known, then group O Rh-negative RBCs should be selected for the intrauterine transfusion. The group O Rh-negative cells must lack any antigens against which the mother's serum contains unexpected antibodies (e.g., anti-K1, anti-Jk^a). Crossmatch testing is performed using the mother's serum sample.

Neonatal Transfusions

Blood for an exchange or regular transfusion of a neonate (younger than 4 months of age) should be compatible with any maternal antibodies that have entered the infant's circulation and are reactive at 37°C or AHG. Blood of the infant's ABO and Rh group can be used, as long as the ABO and Rh groups are not involved in the fetomaternal incompatibility. An initial pretransfusion specimen from the infant must be typed for ABO and Rh groups (only anti-A and anti-B reagents are required for ABO grouping, omitting the testing of the infant's serum with reagent RBCs).[46] Antibody detection testing can be performed using the maternal serum, the infant's serum (e.g., cord serum), or an eluate prepared from the infant's RBCs. In addition, when cells selected for transfusion are not group O, the infant's serum or plasma must be tested to demonstrate the absence of anti-A (using A1 cells) and anti-B. This testing must include an antiglobulin phase.[47]

It is unnecessary to repeat these pretransfusion tests during any one hospital admission, provided that the infant received only ABO-compatible and Rh-compatible transfusions and had no unexpected antibodies in the serum or plasma.[48] The presence of clinically significant antibodies, including anti-A and anti-B, indicates that cells lacking the corresponding antigen must be selected for transfusion until the antibody is no longer demonstrable in the infant's serum.[49] A crossmatch does not have to be performed in these situations. Box 10–1 summarizes

---

BOX 10–1

Compatibility Tests for Infants Once per Admission

Routine

ABO
Rh
Antibody screen
- Using maternal serum *or*
- Using infant's serum, especially when:
  - No maternal specimen is available
  - Mother has clinically insignificant antibodies *or*
- Using infant's eluate

Additional

IAT using infant serum and A$_1$ *or* B cells
- Cells can be reagent or donor (i.e., major crossmatch)
- Must be done if non-group O cells will be transfused
- Antigen typing donor unit
- While infant antibody screen is positive
- Donor units must lack antigen corresponding to antibody

Every 3 Days

Same tests as above when:
- ABO- or Rh-incompatible units are transfused *or*
- Unexpected antibodies are demonstrating via antibody screen

the compatibility tests for infants (younger than 4 months old) and how frequently they must be performed.

For both intrauterine and infant (younger than 4 months) transfusions, blood should be as fresh as possible and no older than 7 days. Refer to Chapters 15 and 19 for additional information on neonatal transfusion.

Massive Transfusions

When the amount of whole blood or packed cell components infused within 24 hours approaches or exceeds the patient's total blood volume, the compatibility testing procedure may be shortened or eliminated at the discretion of the transfusion service physician following written policy guidelines.[50] The current technical manual uses the following guideline: "Massive transfusion is arbitrarily defined either as the administration of 8 to 10 RBC units to an adult patient in less than 24 hours, or as the acute administration of 4 to 5 RBC units in 1 hour." If the patient is known to have a clinically significant unexpected antibody, all infused units should be tested for and lack the corresponding antigen, if time permits. The antibody in the patient's serum may not be demonstrable because of dilution with large volumes of plasma and other fluids. However, a rapid rise in antibody titer level and subsequent destruction of donor RBCs may occur if antigen-positive units are infused. The transfusion service physician may decide that it is better to give antigen-untested units than to hold up transfusion by waiting for the test results. The rationale is that it is important to give the patient a chance to survive and then to treat the immune-mediated anemia induced by massive transfusion of antigen-untested units. Again, the physician must sign a waiver of testing or a release form for all untested units for transfusion.

Specimens with Prolonged Clotting Time

Testing difficulties may be observed in blood samples from patients who have prolonged clotting times caused by coagulation abnormalities associated with disease or medications (such as heparin). A fibrin clot may form spontaneously when partially clotted serum is added to saline-suspended screening or donor RBCs. Complete coagulation of these samples can often be accelerated by adding thrombin. One drop of thrombin, 50 U/mL, to 1 mL of plasma (or the amount of dry thrombin that will adhere to the end of an applicator stick) is usually sufficient to induce clotting.[51] A small amount of protamine sulfate can be added to counteract the effects of heparin in samples of blood collected from patients on this anticoagulant.[52]

Preoperative Autologous Blood

Autologous transfusion refers to the removal and storage of blood or components from a donor for the donor's possible use at a later time, usually during or after an elective surgical procedure. The ABO and Rh groups of the units must be determined by the facility collecting the blood. Tests for unexpected antibodies and tests designed to prevent disease transmission are not required when the blood will be used within the collecting facility.[53] These units must be labeled "For autologous use only."[54] According to AABB *Standards*, the pretransfusion testing and identification of the recipient and the blood sample are required and must conform to the protocols mentioned earlier in this chapter. However, tests for unexpected antibodies in the recipient's serum or plasma and a crossmatch test are optional.[55]

Limitations of Compatibility Testing Procedures

As mentioned in the introduction to this chapter, no current testing procedure can guarantee the fate of a unit of blood that is to be transfused. Even a compatible crossmatch cannot guarantee that the transfused RBCs will survive normally in the recipient. Despite careful and meticulous in vitro testing, some compatible units will be hemolyzed in the patient. In some cases, even limited survival of donor cells may help to maintain a patient until the patient can begin to produce his or her own cells. Certainly no patient should be denied a transfusion if he or she needs one to survive, and donor cells that appear incompatible by in vitro testing procedures may, in fact, survive quite well in vivo. Refer to Table 10–5 for suggestions on streamlining pretransfusion testing processes.

In vivo compatibility can be determined using donor RBCs labeled with radioactive chromium (^{51}Cr) or technetium (^{99m}Tc) to measure the likelihood of successful transfusion when standard in vitro testing procedures are inconclusive.[56,57] If a transfusion is needed to save a patient's life and all units are incompatible and if the ^{51}Cr studies indicate adequate survival of donor RBCs, then transfusion of an in vitro incompatible unit may need to be considered. This decision should be made in consultation with the blood bank medical director and the patient's physician. The blood should be transfused slowly, and the patient should be monitored carefully.[58]

Blood Inventory Management

Many blood bankers are acutely aware of the need to use blood efficiently due to limited blood supplies and increasing demands for blood. Technologists have observed that there have been many surgical procedures, such as dilatation and curettage and cholecystectomy, for which blood was routinely ordered but rarely used. Blood bankers also pointed out that for many other surgical procedures, more units were being ordered than were used.

The Maximum Surgical Blood Order Schedule (MSBOS) was developed to promote more efficient utilization of blood. The goal of the MSBOS is to establish realistic blood ordering levels for certain procedures. Because variation exists in the surgical requirements of institutions, the standard blood orders should be based on the transfusion pattern of each institution and should be agreed upon by the staff surgeons, anesthesiologists, and the blood bank medical director. (See Chapter 24, "Utilization Management.")

Table 10–5 Pretransfusion Testing Schemes

TEST SCHEME	TESTS PERFORMED	ADVANTAGES	LIMITATIONS
No order	None		No specimen has been collected. ABO, Rh, and antibody detection testing are *not* performed.
Hold clot	None	A specimen has been collected.	ABO, Rh, and antibody detection testing are *not* performed.
Type Type and hold	ABO, Rh	A specimen has been collected; patient's ABO/Rh are known.	Antibody detection testing is *not* performed.
Type and screen	ABO, Rh, antibody detection test/identification	Most of the pretransfusion testing has been performed; compatible blood can be provided in most situations.	Does not include crossmatch.
Type and crossmatch	ABO, Rh, antibody detection test/identification, RBC unit selection or phenotyping, crossmatch	Routine pretransfusion testing has been performed; compatible blood can be provided in most situations.	Units are removed from inventory and may not be available for use by other patients in a timely manner.

Reprinted with permission from Roback, J (ed): Technical Manual, 16th ed. American Association of Blood Banks, Bethesda, MD, 2008.

Utilization of a type and screen policy is another method to manage blood inventory levels efficiently and to reduce blood banking operating costs.[59–61] The type and screen method involves testing the recipient's blood sample for ABO, Rh, and unexpected antibodies. The specimen is refrigerated and kept available for immediate crossmatching if the need arises. If transfusion becomes necessary, then an immediate spin or computer crossmatch may be performed. The blood bank must ensure that the appropriate donor blood is available in case it is needed. The type and screen policy does not apply to patients with existing clinically significant unexpected alloantibodies, because donor blood lacking the corresponding antigens must be available and should be fully crossmatched prior to surgery or transfusion.

A type and screen policy applies to a recipient who does not have any clinically significant unexpected alloantibodies present or any abnormal serologic results in the ABO or Rh testing. If blood is needed quickly, the blood bank is then prepared to perform the immediate spin (or computer) crossmatch and release blood of the same ABO and Rh group as that of the recipient before releasing the unit to the hospital floor. Once the blood is issued, both a 37°C incubation and AHG crossmatch can be performed using the same tube employed for the immediate spin crossmatch, if the antiglobulin crossmatch is the standard protocol used by the laboratory. If either the 37°C incubation or AHG phase of testing is positive, the patient's physician is notified immediately, and the transfusion of the unit of blood is stopped.

The application of the type and screen in combination with the MSBOS can greatly enhance the effectiveness of the blood inventory management program in a health-care facility by minimizing the crossmatch-to-transfusion ratio, reducing blood bank personnel workload, and using the blood inventory efficiently.

Reidentification of the Patient Before Transfusion

Reestablishing the intended recipient's identity and the selected donor product is the final step in the transfusion process. The same careful approach used to properly identify the patient before sample collection must now be applied to verify that the recipient is indeed the same person who provided the initial blood sample for testing. In addition, the actual product and accompanying record of testing must be verified as relating to the same donor unit number. The bedside check just prior to blood administration is the most critical step for preventing mistransfusion.[62] Mistransfusion, in which the wrong blood is transfused to the recipient, is the single most frequent error resulting in ABO-incompatible transfusions and is one of the leading causes of morbidity and death resulting from blood transfusion.[63]

After pretransfusion testing is completed, two records must be prepared. A statement of compatibility must be retained as part of the patient's permanent medical record if the blood is transfused, and a label or tie tag must be attached to the unit stating the intended recipient's identity, the results of pretransfusion testing, and the donor unit number.[64] This identification must remain on the donor unit throughout the transfusion.

The original blood transfusion request form can be used conveniently to accomplish one or both of these record-keeping requirements. Some facilities use a multipart form to record the history of pretransfusion testing and transfusion of the unit. Useful information might include the initials or signature of the phlebotomist taking the sample, donor numbers, results of pretransfusion testing, initials or signature of the technologist performing the testing, and signatures of the persons who verify the recipient's identity before transfusion and those (two) who start the transfusion. One copy of the form can be placed on the recipient's chart after the transfusion is completed, and the other is returned to the blood bank, if desired, for filing. The last copy of the form might be printed on card stock and perforated so that it can be easily removed and attached to the donor unit in the laboratory. The most important feature of this system is that the patient's nameplate impression rather than a handwritten transcription indicates all forms used to identify the patient-donor combination. Most facilities now use computer-generated labels to attach to each form.

Recognizing the complexity of the process, other useful systems are emerging throughout the transfusion center and throughout health care as a whole, including for administering patient medications. Machine-readable, bar-code patient–blood unit identification is ideally suited to bedside check requirements and has been recently reported to significantly improve transfusion practice.[65] In addition to bar codes on patient identification wristbands, radio frequency identification devices (RFID) are being integrated. RFID consists of at least two parts: an integrated circuit for storing, processing, and sending information (i.e., patient number, ABO group, Rh type, etc.) and an antenna or receiver to collect or transmit the information. For example, on the patient wristband is the RFID or bar code that can now be used for identification purposes at every stage of pretransfusion testing.

Whatever system is used, the information should be verified at least twice before the blood product is transfused. A copy of the original blood requisition form, placed on the recipient's chart after samples are collected, can be used as the request for release of the units from the blood bank. This allows another check of the nameplate impressions on all forms. Before blood is taken from the blood bank to the patient treatment area, the following records must be checked: ABO and Rh results, clinically significant unexpected antibodies, and adverse reactions to transfusion.[66] In addition, the person releasing and the person accepting the units should verify agreement between the donor numbers and ABO and Rh groups on the compatibility form and on the products themselves. The unit should also be inspected visually for any abnormalities in appearance, indicating contamination. If any abnormality is seen, the unit should not be issued unless specifically authorized by the medical director.[67]

Before transfusion is initiated, a reliable professional (preferably two) must once again verify identity of the patient and donor products. A system of positive patient identification by comparison of wristband identification and compatibility forms must be followed strictly. This is the most critical check and yet the most fallible, because the transfusion may take place in the operating suite or emergency room where the person responsible for identification may be involved with many other duties as well.

If a unit is returned to the blood bank for any reason within the specified time for that laboratory, it should not be reissued if the container closure was opened or if the unit was allowed to warm above 10°C or to cool below 1°C.[68]

The Future of Pretransfusion Testing

Automation with pretransfusion testing instruments, such as continuous-flow and batch analyzers, has streamlined compatibility testing, especially in large blood centers. Two of the most successful approaches have used microplates to perform either liquid agglutination tests or solid-phase RBC adherence tests. In addition to microplates is the column agglutination technology, whether using gel or glass beads in the column to capture agglutinates.[69,70] These methods provide efficient and economic compatibility tests for processing large numbers of donor specimens. Similar innovations are emerging to streamline blood banking testing in hospital transfusion services.

The use of column gel technology is on the rise in hospital and transfusion services. Utilization of the column gel method for antibody detection has risen dramatically from 26.1% in 2001 to 42% in 2004.[71] The gel test is sensitive for both antigen testing and antibody detection and identification and ABO and Rh typing.[72,73] Advantages of the gel system include standardizing pipetting of reagents and specimens, reading of agglutination reactions, reviewing stable reaction endpoints up to 24 hours, and significantly reducing specimen volume. Disadvantages include longer turnaround time for ABO determinations and less sensitive detection of ABO antibodies in patient serum or plasma when compared with the tube method.[74]

The emergence of molecular biology techniques in blood bank testing is just now beginning. Nucleic acid amplification techniques, often based on polymerase chain reaction, have demonstrated application in blood typing[75] and in screening blood for hepatitis C. This testing process goes beyond detecting antigenic determinants on the RBC membrane and goes directly into the genetic foundation of those antigens. Molecular testing is currently one of the hottest topics in pretransfusion testing.[76–78]

As a result of the French requirement to perform a final check of the ABO compatibility of the recipient and donor, several methods are available, including:

- A card with four columns containing reagent anti-A and anti-B (two for recipient and two for donor)
- A card with six wells, two for recipient and donor samples, and four with dried anti-A and anti-B for testing of the recipient and donor.[79]

Preparing for clinical care in space, National Aeronautics and Space Administration (NASA) scientists showed that ABO and Coombs-sensitized standard blood grouping tests can be performed under microgravity. This was done using a closed self-operating system that automatically performed the tests and fixed the results onto filter paper for analysis on Earth. Agglutinates were smaller than usual; however, reaction endpoints were clear.[80] Although these researchers noted that additional experiments in space were needed to confirm and quantify their results, these preliminary findings indicate yet another method for performing compatibility testing.

Finally, an automated flow cytometry system is currently being developed and investigated for pretransfusion compatibility testing. A study comparing flow cytometry with column agglutination and standard tube testing for ABO, Rh typing, and antibody detection revealed a system equivalent for each methodology. It is also quite comparable in many aspects, including sensitivity, accuracy, and specimen turnaround time.[81,82]

As information technology continues to grow, all aspects of patient care, including compatibility testing, may be computerized. In addition to performing an electronic crossmatch, computer systems now include electronic identification of the patient, automated testing, and electronic transfer of data. The success of these systems depends on interfacing automated testing instruments with bar-code readers and a laboratory computer.[83]

Our knowledge of compatibility testing is in a dynamic state, and we look forward to continuing developments in technical procedures to streamline and safeguard transfusion practice. The challenge of modern blood banking will be to merge new technology with the assurance of beneficial results and positive outcomes for the patient.

CASE STUDIES

Case 10-1

Labor and delivery orders 4 units of packed red blood cells stat on a 32-year-old white female with the following results: ABO/Rh—A-positive; antibody screen—no unexpected antibodies detected; history—no unexpected antibodies in two previous deliveries at this facility, and no previous red cell transfusions recorded.

1. What crossmatch options do you have?
2. Which do you choose and why?

Case 10-2

Pretransfusion testing results on a presurgical patient with a 3-unit crossmatch order are as follows: ABO/Rh—B-positive; unexpected antibody screen—no unexpected antibodies detected; 3 RBC units crossmatched—unit 1, compatible at AHG; unit 2, compatible at AHG; and unit 3, incompatible at AHG using gel column methodology.

1. What can account for the incompatible unit? Explain?
2. How would you resolve this situation?

SUMMARY CHART

- ✔ Most fatal transfusion reactions are caused by clerical errors.
- ✔ Samples and forms must contain patient's full name and unique identity number.
- ✔ Writing must be legible and indelible.
- ✔ Date of collection must be written on sample.
- ✔ Sample must be collected within 3 days of scheduled transfusion.
- ✔ A blood bank specimen must have two unique patient identifiers—the date of collection and initials or signature of the person who collected the sample.
- ✔ Confirm blood type of donor.
- ✔ Check patient records (history) for results of previous tests. Perform ABO grouping, Rh typing, and antibody screening on patient.
- ✔ Select donor unit based on ABO group and Rh type of patient; further consider presence of antibodies in patient by antigen-typing donor unit for the corresponding antigen.
- ✔ Perform immediate spin or antiglobulin crossmatch based on current or historical serologic results.
- ✔ Electronic crossmatch can replace immediate spin crossmatch when two blood types are on file for the patient and antibody screen is negative.
- ✔ Positive results in the crossmatch may be caused by incorrect ABO grouping of patient or donor, alloantibody or autoantibody in patient reacting with the corresponding antigen on the donor RBCs, donor having a positive DAT, abnormalities in patient serum such as increased protein concentration (rouleaux) or contaminants in test system.
- ✔ Emergencies:
  - May have to select uncrossmatched, group O, Rh-negative packed RBCs.
  - May want to give uncrossmatched, group O, Rh-positive packed RBCs if male patient or female patient is beyond childbearing years.
  - May be able to provide type-specific, uncrossmatched RBCs.
- ✔ Plasma products units:
  - No compatibility testing required.
- ✔ Transfusion to fetus:
  - Compatibility testing performed using mother's sample.
  - Donor unit must lack antigen against maternal antibody.
  - Group O Rh-negative donor selected when fetal type is unknown or when type is known but is not compatible with mother's type.
- ✔ Transfusion to infant:
  - Maternal sample can be used for compatibility testing.
  - Initial sample from infant typed for ABO (front type) and Rh.
  - Donor unit selected should be compatible with both mother and baby.

Review Questions

1. Pretransfusion testing:
   a. Proves that the donor's plasma is free of all irregular antibodies
   b. Detects most irregular antibodies on the donor's RBCs that are reactive with patient's serum
   c. Detects most errors in the ABO groupings
   d. Ensures complete safety of the transfusion

2. Which is not true of rouleaux formation?
   a. It is a stacking of RBCs to form aggregates.
   b. It can usually be dispersed by adding saline.
   c. It can appear as an ABO incompatibility.
   d. It cannot cause a false-positive immediate spin crossmatch.

3. What type of blood should be given in an emergency transfusion when there is no time to type the recipient's sample?
   a. O Rh_0 (D)-negative, whole blood
   b. O Rh_0 (D)-positive, whole blood
   c. O Rh_0 (D)-positive, packed cells
   d. O Rh_0 (D)-negative, packed cells

4. A patient developed an anti-Jk^a antibody 5 years ago. The antibody screen is currently negative. To obtain suitable blood for transfusion, which procedures apply?
   a. Type the patient for the Jk^b antigen as an added part to the crossmatch procedure.
   b. Crossmatch random donors with the patient's serum, and release the compatible units for transfusion to the patient.
   c. Type the patient and donor units for the Jk^a antigen, and then crossmatch the Jk^a negative units with the patient serum.
   d. Computer-crossmatch Jk^a negative donor units.

5. A 26-year-old B Rh_0 (D)-negative female patient requires a transfusion. No B Rh_0 (D)-negative donor units are available. Which should be chosen for transfusion?
   a. B Rh_0 (D)-positive RBCs
   b. O Rh_0 (D)-negative RBCs
   c. AB Rh_0 (D)-negative RBCs
   d. A Rh_0 (D)-negative RBCs

6. Having checked the patient's prior history after having received the specimen and request, you:
   a. Do not have to repeat the ABO and Rh if the name and hospital number agree
   b. Do not have to repeat the indirect antiglobulin test (IAT) if the previous IAT was negative
   c. Have to perform a crossmatch only if one has not been done within the last 2 weeks
   d. Have to compare the results of your ABO, Rh, and IAT with the previous results

7. The purpose of the immediate spin crossmatch is to:
   a. Ensure survival of transfused RBCs
   b. Determine ABO compatibility between donor and recipient
   c. Detect cold-reacting unexpected antibodies
   d. Meet computer crossmatch requirements

8. Which does not represent requirements set forth by the AABB for the performance of a computer crossmatch?
   a. Computer system must be validated on-site.
   b. Recipient antibody screen must be positive.
   c. Two determinations of the recipient ABO and Rh must be performed.
   d. Computer system must have logic.

9. You have just received a request and sample for pretransfusion testing. Which is the *most* appropriate to do *first*?
   a. Perform the ABO grouping and Rh typing
   b. Complete the crossmatch
   c. Perform the IAT to see if the patient is going to be a problem
   d. Check the records for prior type and screen results on the patient

10. Blood donor and recipient samples used in crossmatching must be stored for a minimum of how many days following transfusion?
    a. 2
    b. 5
    c. 7
    d. 10

11. Which is true regarding compatibility testing for the infant younger than 4 months old?
    a. A DAT is required.
    b. A crossmatch is not needed with the infant's blood when unexpected antibodies are present.
    c. Maternal serum cannot be used for antibody detection.
    d. To determine the infant's ABO group, RBCs must be tested with reagent anti-A, anti-B, and anti-A,B.

12. A nurse just called to request additional RBC units for a patient for whom you performed compatibility testing 4 days ago. She would like you to use the original specimen, as you keep it for 7 days anyway. Your *most* appropriate course of action would be to:
    a. Check to see if there is enough of the original specimen
    b. Perform the compatibility testing on the original specimen
    c. Request more information in case the patient has developed a clinically significant unexpected antibody
    d. Indicate that a new specimen is necessary because the patient has been recently transfused

13. A crossmatch is positive at AHG phase with polyspecific AHG reagent but is negative with monospecific anti-IgG AHG reagent. This may indicate the antibody:

a. Is a weak anti-D

b. Is a clinically insignificant Lewis antibody

c. Can cause decreased survival of transfused RBCs

d. Is a Duffy antibody

14. The emergency room requests 6 units of packed RBCs for a trauma patient prior to collection of the patient's specimen. The *most* appropriate course of action is to:

a. Release group O RBCs to ER with trauma patient identification on each unit sent

b. Refuse to release units until you get a patient sample

c. Indicate necessity for signed patient waiver for incomplete pretransfusion testing

d. Explain need of patient's ABO group prior to issuing blood

15. Which is not an example of the most common form of error associated with fatal transfusion reactions?

a. Phlebotomist labels patient A tubes with patient B information

b. Technologist enters results of patient A testing into patient B field

c. Wrong RBC unit is tagged for transfusion

d. Antibody below detectable levels during pretransfusion testing

References

1. Roback, J (ed): Technical Manual, 16th ed, American Association of Blood Banks, Bethesda, MD, 2008.

2. Linden, JV, et al: Transfusion error in New York State: An analysis of 10 years experience. Transfusion 40:1207, 2000.

3. Carson, TH: Standards for Blood Banks and Transfusion Services, 26th ed. American Association of Blood Banks, Bethesda, MD, 2009, p 32, 5.11.2.

4. Ibid, p 3, 2.1.2

5. Ibid, pp 32, 33, 5.11.2–4.

6. Ibid, p 33, 5.11.2.3, 5.11.3.

7. Ibid, p 34, 5.13.3.2.

8. Ibid, p 21, 5.6.3.

9. Ibid, p 33, 5.11.4.

10. Code of Federal Regulations (CFR), Title 21, Food and Drugs. Office of the Federal Register, National Archives and Records Service, General Services Administration, Part 610, section 40, revised June 11, 2001, and Part 640, section 5 revised August 6, 2001.

11. Standards, op cit, pp 29–31, 5.8, and pp 33, 34, 5.13.

12. Ibid, p 29, 5.8.3.1.

13. Ibid, p 33, 5.12.

14. Ibid, p 63, 6.2.5.

15. Ibid, p 34, 5.13.3.2

16. Ibid, p 33, 5.13.2.

17. Garratty, G: Evaluating the clinical significance of blood group alloantibodies that are causing problems in pretransfusion testing. Vox Sang 74:285, 1998.

18. Giblett, ER: Blood group alloantibodies: An assessment to some laboratory practices. Transfusion 17:299, 1977.

19. Spielmann, W, and Seidl, S: Prevalence of irregular red cell antibodies and their significance in blood transfusion and antenatal care. Vox Sang 26:551, 1974.

20. Aygun B, et al: Clinical significance of RBC alloantibodies and autoantibodies in sickle cell patients who received transfusion. Transfusion 42:37, 2002.

21. Mollison, PL: Blood Transfusion in Clinical Medicine, 9th ed. Blackwell Scientific, Oxford, England, 1993, p 225.

22. Roback, J (ed): Technical Manual, 16th ed. American Association of Blood Banks, Bethesda, MD, 2008, p 453.

23. Standards, op cit, p 35, 5.15.1.1.

24. Roback, J. (ed): Technical Manual, 16th ed. American Association of Blood Banks, Bethesda, MD, 2008, p 453

25. Alexander, D, and Henry, JB: Immediate spin crossmatch in routine use: A growing trend in compatibility testing for red cell transfusion therapy. Vox Sang 70:48, 1996.

26. Walker, RH: On the safety of the abbreviated crossmatch. In Polesky, HF, and Walker, RH (eds): Safety in Transfusion Practices; CAP Conference, Aspen, 1980. College of American Pathologists, Skokie, IL, 1982, p 75.

27. Shulman, IA, et al: Experience with the routine use of an abbreviated crossmatch. Am J Clin Pathol 82:178, 1984.

28. Dodsworth, H, and Dudley, HAF: Increased efficiency of transfusion practice in routine surgery using pre-operative antibody screening and selective ordering with an abbreviated crossmatch. Br J Surg 72:102, 1985.

29. Garratty, G: Abbreviated pretransfusion testing. Transfusion 26:217, 1986.

30. Freidberg, RC, et al: Type and screen completion for scheduled surgical procedures. Arch Pathol Lab Med 127, 2003.

31. Judd, WJ: Are there better ways than the crossmatch to demonstrate ABO incompatibility? Transfusion 31:192, 1991.

32. Shulman, IA, and Calderon, C: Effect of delayed centrifugation or reading on the detection of ABO incompatibility by the immediate-spin crossmatch. Transfusion 31:197, 1991.

33. Perkins, JT, et al: The relative utility of the autologous control and the antiglobulin test phase of the crossmatch. Transfusion 30:503, 1990.

34. CFR, op cit, part 606, section 160.

35. Green, TS: Rouleaux and autoantibodies (or things that go bump in the night). In Treacy, M (ed): Pre-Transfusion Testing for the 80s. American Association of Blood Banks, Washington, DC, 1980, p 93.

36. Bartholomew, JR, et al: A prospective study of the effects of dextran administration on compatibility testing. Transfusion 26:431, 1986.

37. Golde, DW, et al: Serum agglutinins to commercially prepared albumin. In Weisz-Carrington, P: Principles of Clinical Immunohematology. Year Book Medical, Chicago, 1986, p 214.

38. Judd, JW: Requirements for the electronic crossmatch. Vox Sang 74:409, 1998.

39. Ibid.

40. Butch, SH, et al: Electronic verification of donor-recipient compatibility: The computer crossmatch. Transfusion 34:105, 1994.

41. Shulrman, IA, et al: North American Pretransfusion Testing Practices, 2001–2004. Results from the College of American Pathologists Interlaboratory Comparison Program Survey Data, 2001–2004, p 986.

42. Judd, JW: Requirements for the electronic crossmatch. Vox Sang 74:409, 1998.

43. Ibid p 36, 5.15.2.

44. Standards, op cit p 36, 5.15.2.1–5.

45. CFR, op cit, part 606, section 160.

46. Standards, op cit, p 37, 5.16.

47. Ibid.

48. Ibid.

49. Ibid.

50. Ibid, p 38, 5.17.5.

51. Roback, J (ed): Technical Manual, 16th ed. American Association of Blood Banks, Bethesda, MD, 2008, p 441.

52. Ibid.

53. Standards, op cit, pp 30, 31, 5.8.5.

54. Ibid, p 45, 5.1.6A.

55. Ibid, p 29, 5.8

56. Garratty, G: Evaluating the clinical significance of blood group alloantibodies that are causing problems in pretransfusion testing. Vox Sang 74:285, 1998.

57. Marcus CS, et al: Radiolabeled red cell viability II. ^{99m}Tc and ^{111}In for measuring the viability of heterologous red cells in vivo. Transfusion 7:420, 1986.

58. Garratty, G: Evaluating the clinical significance of blood group alloantibodies that are causing problems in pretransfusion testing. Vox Sang 74:285, 1998.

59. Shulman, IA, et al: Experience with a cost-effective crossmatch protocol. JAMA 254:93, 1985.

60. Davis, SP, et al: Maximizing the benefits of type and screen by continued surveillance of transfusion practice. Am J Med Technol 49:579, 1983.

61. Issitt, PD: Applied Blood Group Serology, 4th ed. Montgomery Scientific, Durham, NC, 1998, pp 892, 893.

62. Dzik, WH: Emily Cooley lecture 2002: Transfusion safety in the hospital. Transfusion, 43:181–190, 2003.

63. Dzik, WH: New technology for transfusion safety. Br J Haematol, 136:181–190, 2006.

64. Standards, op cit, pp 11, 12, 5.1.6.3.

65. Ohsaka, A, et al: Causes of failure of a barcode-based pretransfusion check at the bedside: Experience in a university hospital. Transfusion Medicine, 18:216–222, 2008.

66. Ibid, pp 39, 40, 5.18.

67. Ibid.

68. Ibid.

69. Sandler, SG: A fully automated blood typing system for hospital transfusion services. ABS2000 Study Group. Transfusion 40:201, 2000.

70. Morelati, R, et al: Evaluation of a new automated instrument for pretransfusion testing. Transfusion 38:959, 1998.

71. Shulrman, IA, et al: North American Pretransfusion Testing Practices, 2001–2004. Results from the College of American Pathologists Interlaboratory Comparison Program Survey Data, 2001–2004, p 986.

72. Weisbach, V, et al: Comparison of the performance of four microtube column agglutination systems in the detection of red cell alloantibodies. Transfusion 39:1045, 1999.

73. Dittmar, K, et al: Comparison of DATs using traditional tube agglutination to gel column and affinity column procedures. Transfusion 41:1258, 2001.

74. Langston, JL, et al: Evaluation of the gel system for ABO grouping and D typing. Transfusion 39:300, 1999.

75. Anstee, DJ: Red cell genotyping and the future of pretransfusion testing. Blood 114(2): 2009.

76. Reid, ME: Overview of molecular methods in immunohematology. Transfusion 47(suppl): 2007.

77. Klapper, E, et al: Toward extended phenotype matching: A new operational paradigm for the transfusion service. Transfusion 50: 2010.

78. Hillyer, D, et al: Integrating molecular technologies for the red blood cell typing and compatibility testing into blood centers and transfusion services. Transfus Med Rev 22(2): 2008, pp 117–132.

79. Migeot, V, et al: Reliability of bedside ABO testing before transfusion. Transfusion 42:1348, 2002.

80. Morehead, RT, et al: Erythrocyte agglutination in microgravity. Aviat Space Environ Med 60:235, 1989.

81. Stussi, G, et al: Isotype-specific detection of ABO blood group antibodies using a novel flow cytometric method. Br J Haematol, 130:954–963, 2005.

82. Roback, JD, et al: An automatable format for accurate immunohematology testing by flow cytometry. Transfusion 43:918, 2003.

83. Dzik, WH: New technology for transfusion safety. Br J Haematol, 136:181–190, 2006.

Chapter 11

Overview of the Routine Blood Bank Laboratory

Darlene M. Homkes, MT(ASCP); Cara L. Calvo, MS, MT(ASCP)SH, CLS(NCA); and Burlin Sherrick, MT(ASCP)SBB

OBJECTIVES

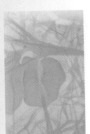

1. Describe a modern blood bank laboratory in terms of its operations, personnel, facilities, and equipment.
2. Explain the purpose of the following equipment used in a blood bank laboratory: apheresis machine, flatbed agitator, sterile docking device, and leukoreduction filter.
3. Summarize blood bank laboratory services in terms of policies, procedures, and tests performed.
4. Compare and contrast testing performed on donor units and recipient blood samples.
5. Apply knowledge of immunohematology theory and skills developed in classroom practice to actual work situations in a blood bank laboratory.

Introduction

The American Association of Blood Banks (AABB) estimates that 9.5 million volunteers donate blood each year.[1] About 17 million units of whole blood in the United States were donated in 2008. In addition, in the United States, approximately 24 million blood products were transfused in 2008.[2] The blood bank laboratory is one of the most specialized and challenging workplaces in the field of laboratory medicine and is the most highly regulated. Scientific discovery, technological innovation, advances in medical informatics, and changing regulations are played out on a daily basis against a backdrop of work routines unfamiliar to the newcomer. Underlying theories and principles of antigen–antibody reactions and their effects on blood are translated into clinical practice. The blood bank laboratory is a place of business where donated blood and blood products undergo extensive testing, and every task associated with the work performed is scrutinized to ensure the quality and safety of both the services and the products provided. The regulating agency is the Food and Drug Administration (FDA), and the accrediting organization is usually the American Association of Blood Banks (AABB).

This chapter will serve as a tour through the typical blood bank and will describe the various sections within the department and the procedures that are performed. Although every blood bank may not contain all of the sections described in this chapter, it is important for the reader to understand and appreciate the complete scope of transfusion medicine.

Organization

For this discussion, a **blood bank laboratory** is defined as a facility involved in the collection, storage, processing, and distribution of human blood and blood products for transfusion. Typically, it functions as a unit of a larger organization, such as a hospital department or community blood center, and follows the general operational guidelines of that organization. The larger organization stipulates the conditions under which the blood bank conducts business, such as hours of operations, and provides necessary facilities, equipment, and personnel. However, the blood bank laboratory also functions as a component of the heavily regulated health-care industry. This means that the blood bank laboratory also operates under constraint of laws administered by various governmental agencies and in accordance with standards established by nonregulatory accrediting organizations such as the AABB.[3,4] (Refer to Chapter 25, "Transfusion Safety and Federal Regulatory Requirements" for additional information.)

Blood bank laboratories are located in a variety of settings, and the extent of services that a blood bank offers varies accordingly. For example, hospital blood banks may choose to collect and process blood components for their own use, or they may choose to contract to receive blood products from a blood center. For ease of discussion, it is assumed that the blood bank is divided into distinct areas, each with its own purpose and function: component preparation and storage, donor processing, product labeling, main laboratory, and reference laboratory areas (Table 11–1). With the exception of very large transfusion services, these areas are not physically separated but overlap within the overall structure of the blood bank laboratory.

Component Preparation and Storage

Depending on the needs of a hospital, blood components may be acquired from external sources such as the American Red Cross or other regional blood centers, or components may be processed in-house.

Blood Banks With Collection Facilities

Blood banks that collect their own units of whole blood can use their blood resources more efficiently by separating them into a variety of components, including packed red blood cells (RBCs), platelets, fresh frozen plasma (FFP), frozen plasma prepared within 24 hours of collection (FP24), and cryoprecipitate (Table 11–2; see also see Chapter 13, "Donor Screening and Component Preparation").

After collection, whole blood is allowed to cool to room temperature (20°C to 24°C) if platelets are to be prepared from the unit, or cooled to 1°C to 10°C if the unit is to be processed for frozen plasma. FFP must be prepared within 8 hours of collection of the whole blood unit, whereas FP24 may be prepared up to 24 hours following collection of the whole blood unit. Platelets may be prepared from whole blood stored at room temperature for up to 24 hours after the whole blood unit is collected.[4]

The blood is centrifuged to pack the red cells using large, floor-model temperature-controlled centrifuges, and the components (packed cells, plasma, platelets) are separated (Fig. 11–1). Additionally, through a controlled thawing process, the frozen plasma can be further manipulated to yield cryoprecipitate.

Some blood components may also be prepared through a procedure known as **apheresis**. A donor's blood is removed, anticoagulated, and transported directly to an apheresis machine. The blood is separated into specific components (platelets, plasma, granulocytes, red blood cells) by centrifugation within the machine, and the desired component(s) is removed. The remaining portion of the blood is returned to the donor. (Apheresis is described in detail in Chapter 14, "Apheresis.")

Table 11–1	**Blood Bank Areas and Functions**	
AREA	**FUNCTIONS**
Component preparation and storage	• Separation of whole blood into packed RBCs, plasma, platelets, and cryoprecipitate
	• Storage of blood products at appropriate temperatures
	• Apheresis procedures
Donor processing	• Donor units tested for:
	– ABO and Rh
	– Antibody screen
	– Serologic test for syphilis
	– Transfusion-transmitted viruses
Product labeling	• RBCs and any other components are labeled
	• Products are stored at their proper temperatures
Main laboratory	• Patient samples tested for:
	– ABO and Rh
	– Antibody screen
	– Crossmatch
	– DAT
	– Prenatal evaluation
	– Postpartum evaluation
	– Cord blood studies
	• Issue blood products
Reference laboratory	• Resolution of:
	– ABO and Rh discrepancies
	– Antibody identification
	– Positive DAT
	– Warm autoantibodies
	– Cold autoantibodies
	– Transfusion reactions

Blood Banks Without Collection Facilities

Blood banks that depend on an outside source for their blood supplies usually receive their products in component form. However, situations do arise in which products must be modified (Fig. 11–2). For example, a patient who is deficient in IgA may require washed RBCs. **Automated cell washers** are used to prepare this product. A unit of blood is introduced into a sterile disposable bowl that has tubing connected to a normal saline solution. A portion of this saline is added

Table 11–2	Components Made from Whole Blood and Processes of Component Preparation
COMPONENT	**PROCESSES OF PREPARATION**
Granulocytes	Apheresis
RBCs	Leukoreduction filtration, centrifugation, apheresis
Platelets	In-line filtration, centrifugation, apheresis
Cryoprecipitated	Frozen plasma cryoprecipitation antihemophilic factor (slow thaw)
Fresh frozen plasma FP24	Heavy spin centrifugation followed by freezing (−18°C) or colder

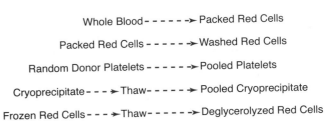

Whole Blood - - - - - ➤ Packed Red Cells

Packed Red Cells - - - - - ➤ Washed Red Cells

Random Donor Platelets - - - - - ➤ Pooled Platelets

Cryoprecipitate - - - ➤ Thaw - - - - - ➤ Pooled Cryoprecipitate

Frozen Red Cells - - - ➤ Thaw - - - - - ➤ Deglycerolyzed Red Cells

Figure 11–2. Additional modifications that blood banks without collection facilities can make to various blood components.

to the bowl, the cells and saline are mixed, the mixture is centrifuged, and the supernatant is removed through waste tubing. Multiple washes can be performed in this manner, using a machine like the one shown in Figure 11–3.

Blood components such as platelet concentrates and cryoprecipitate may be received as individual units but are more easily administered if pooled before infusion. Such product manipulation is common in most blood banks.

Sterile connecting devices (STCDs) have also become commonplace in some blood banks (Fig. 11–4). These devices produce sterile welds between two pieces of compatible tubing.

This procedure permits sterile connection of a variety of containers and tube diameters. Sterile connecting devices can be used in many settings; for example, transplant patients often require a specific type of RBCs and a specific type of plasma, depending on the ABO type of the donor and the recipient. If apheresis platelets are ordered for a transplant patient and the plasma contained in this product is incompatible, an STCD can be used to replace the incompatible plasma with sterile saline in the apheresis unit. Other applications of STCDs are listed in Box 11–1.

If freezers capable of maintaining temperatures at or below −65°C are available, blood banks may freeze rare or autologous units in 40% glycerol for long-term storage. The same automated cell washers used for patients deficient in IgA can be used to remove the glycerol from these units before transfusion by adding increasingly diluted concentrations of saline to thawed cells.

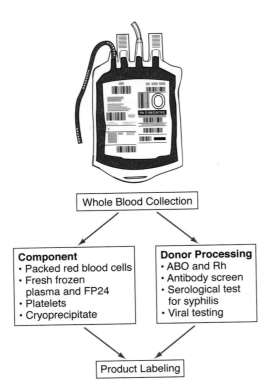

Figure 11–1. Processing of whole blood units from collection to labeling. Note that component preparation and donor processing may occur concurrently. FP24 = frozen plasma prepared within 24 hours of collection.

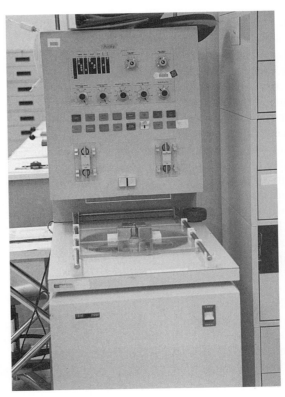

Figure 11–3. Automated cell washers such as this may be used to prepare washed RBCs or to deglycerolize frozen RBCs. *(Courtesy National Institutes of Health, Bethesda, MD.)*

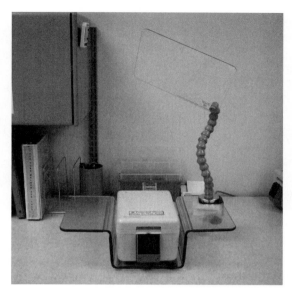

Figure 11–4. This sterile docking device allows for entry into donor units without affecting the expiration date of the product.

A patient who is immunosuppressed (e.g., bone marrow transplant recipient) may have a restriction in the record to **irradiate** all cellular products prior to transfusion. Irradiation renders donor lymphocytes nonfunctional and protects against **graft-versus-host disease**. Usually, irradiators are housed only in large transfusion services so that if such a product is required in a small hospital, an external resource is used. An irradiated product is usually labeled with an irradiation sticker showing the date and time of irradiation. The expiration date of the unit may change depending on the product irradiated (see Chapter 13).

Regardless of the method used to obtain blood and blood components, all blood banks must follow certain requirements for storing blood products.[3–5] Therefore, the following equipment is common to most blood banks:

- Refrigerators maintained at 1°C to 6°C for the storage of packed RBCs and whole blood
- Freezers maintained at –18°C or lower for the storage of FFP and cryoprecipitate

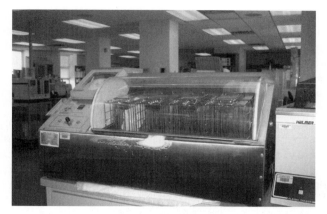

Figure 11–5. Platelet rotators prevent the formation of platelet aggregates and optimize the exchange of gases required for platelet survival.

- Freezers maintained at –65°C or lower for the storage of RBCs frozen in 40% glycerol
- Platelet rotators (Fig. 11–5) or flatbed agitators (Fig. 11–6) that provide constant gentle agitation at room temperature for the storage of apheresis and random donor platelets

Many blood banks also serve as **tissue banks** (see Chapter 28, "Tissue Banking: A New Role for the Transfusion Service") and have temperature-monitored storage areas for tissues and blood. Tissue storage areas include room temperature, refrigerator, and freezer with temperature ranges and required monitoring devices much the same as for blood. Some tissues require storage in an ultralow freezer at –80°C or below.

Donor Processing

Before a unit of blood can be placed into the general inventory (rendering it available to be used for crossmatching purposes), testing must be performed to determine its suitability for transfusion. This is the responsibility of the donor processing area. These tests must be performed at each donation regardless of the number of times a donor has previously donated. Separate tubes of blood are collected from the donor at the time of donation for this

---

Applications of Sterile Connecting Devices

- Adding a fourth bag to a whole blood collection triple pack for the production of cryoprecipitated antihemophilic factor AHF from fresh frozen plasma
- Connecting an additive solution to an RBC unit
- Adding an in-line filter for leukocyte reduction
- Adding a third storage container to a plateletpheresis harness
- Pooling of blood components
- Preparing aliquots for pediatric transfusion
- Attaching processing solutions such as: additive solutions for RBCs, glycerol for frozen RBCs, and normal saline to replace incompatible plasma

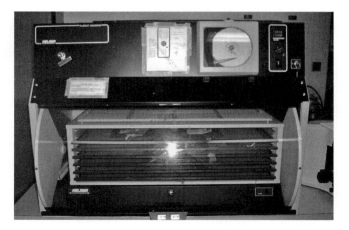

Figure 11–6. Flatbed agitators like this one provide optimal environmental conditions for platelet viability during storage.

purpose. Box 11–2 lists the required tests that are performed on blood after donation. Blood processing centers utilize the testing methods that will provide the safest blood product for patients. For instance, **nucleic acid amplification testing** (NAT) is being used to detect HIV-1 and HCV, and this technology is under investigation for detecting other infectious disease agents.[1]

Automation has greatly increased the efficiency and productivity of this section of the blood bank. Description of these tests and of the automation is provided in Chapter 13.

Product Labeling

Labeling of blood products may occur only after a careful review of all test results shows the unit to be suitable for transfusion. Suitability requirements include:

- No discrepancies in the ABO and Rh testing
- Absence of detectable antibodies in plasma-containing components
- Nonreactive viral marker tests
- Nonreactive syphilis test

When the established criteria are met, the RBCs and any other components are labeled with the appropriate ABO, Rh, and expiration date, and the products are stored at their proper temperatures (Fig. 11–7).

Units received from outside sources would have undergone the required testing and been deemed suitable for transfusion by the shipping facility. However, according to AABB *Standards*, the blood bank to which this blood is shipped is required to reconfirm the labeled ABO of each RBC-containing product received.[3] As a cost-containment measure, many blood banks confirm group O units using a commercially available mixture of monoclonal anti-A and anti-B in a single reagent (anti-A,B) and confirm other blood groups using separate anti-A and anti-B reagents (Table 11–3). Because of the potential sensitization that may occur if Rh-positive blood is transfused to an Rh-negative patient, the Rh type of all Rh-negative units must be reconfirmed.

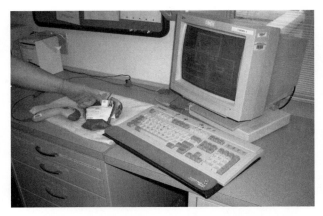

Figure 11–7.   When all testing requirements are complete and discrepancies are resolved, a packed RBC unit is labeled prior to storage.

Main Laboratory

Patient care is the primary mission of the main laboratory. Here the testing is performed that determines the **compatibility** between a patient requiring transfusion and the unit of blood to be transfused. Severe adverse reactions are possible if the wrong unit of blood is transfused; thus, strict adherence to all policies involving sample collection, testing, and identification of patient sample and donor unit, and all steps in the actual transfusion process are essential. Common approaches are evident in the pretransfusion testing protocols that are established by different blood banks to ensure the orderly, timely, and accurate processing of patient samples (Fig. 11–8).

Sample Collection and Acceptance

Proper patient identification is crucial for any specimen used in blood bank testing. A minimum of two identifiers is required for patient samples used for blood bank testing. The patient's full name is required, as is date of birth or medical record number. The patient's location or room number may not be used as an identifier. Many hospitals utilize a separate blood bank patient identification bracelet in addition to the

---

BOX 11–2

Required Tests for Donor Blood

- ABO and Rh
- Antibody screen
- Serologic test for syphilis
- Hepatitis B surface antigen (HBsAg)
- Antibodies to HIV (anti-HIV-1/2)
- Antibodies to human T-cell lymphotropic virus (anti-HTLV-I/II)
- Antibodies to hepatitis C virus (anti-HCV)
- Antibodies to hepatitis B core antigen (anti-HBc)
- Hepatitis C virus (HCV RNA)
- Human immunodeficiency virus (HIV-1 RNA)
- West Nile virus (WNV) RNA

Table 11–3	Abbreviated ABO and Rh Retype Protocol
BLOOD TYPE	**TEST PERFORMED**
A-positive	Anti-A, anti-B
B-positive	Anti-A, anti-B
AB-positive	Anti-A, anti-B
O-positive	Anti-A,B
A-negative	Anti-A, anti-B, anti-D
B-negative	Anti-A, anti-B, anti-D
AB-negative	Anti-A, anti-B, anti-D
O-negative	Anti-A,B, anti-D

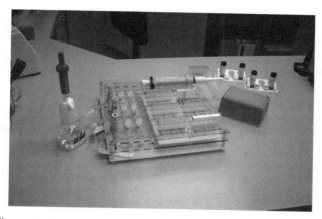

Figure 11–8. Patient samples received by the blood bank laboratory are identified, and a sample tube is carefully organized prior to testing.

hospital identification bracelet. This blood bank bracelet is applied at the time the sample for potential compatibility testing is collected. The blood bank bracelet includes the patient identification and a separate blood bank number that is unique to that blood sample collection. The blood bank number will also be applied to the blood sample and will be included in the record of any compatibility testing performed on that sample and on any donor units transfused based on results from that sample.

Consequences may be fatal if a blood specimen is labeled with the wrong patient's name or other identification. Thus, each specimen and request form the blood bank receives is carefully examined for proper spelling of the patient's name, correct identification number(s), correct date of collection, and identity of the phlebotomist. All of the identifying information on the request must be identical to that on the sample label. If there is any discrepancy, another sample must be obtained.[3]

Routine Testing

Once a patient sample has been judged acceptable, the testing requested by the patient's physician can be performed. Tests are usually requested as a group, and for ease in ordering, a "shorthand notation" designates a group. These may include:

- Type and screen
- Type and crossmatch
- Prenatal evaluation
- Postpartum evaluation
- Cord blood studies

Some hospitals may have an additional "test" available for use when it is not certain if any actual blood bank testing is needed, but it is desired that a sample is collected using any required blood bank labeling and patient banding protocol. This "test" may be called a "blood bank hold" (BB HOLD) and can be quickly converted to a "type and screen" or a "type and crossmatch" if the need arises. No testing will be performed on this sample unless the blood bank is notified. This "test" is commonly utilized by the obstetrical department or by the emergency department when the patient's possible need for transfusion is not initially known.

Type and Screen. Many surgical procedures have a very low probability of requiring blood transfusion. To better utilize their blood supplies, blood bankers may choose not to cross-match units of blood for these procedures but may instead use a type-and-screen protocol. ABO and Rh testing and antibody screening are performed using a current patient specimen. The patient's historical record is also checked for past history of atypical antibodies and for sample identification verification by comparing current blood type with prior records.

To increase the sensitivity of the antibody screen, some blood banks use a three-cell antibody screening set that provides homozygous antigen expression in all major blood group systems. In the absence of a positive antibody screen, if blood is needed on an emergency basis during surgery, it can be released using an abbreviated crossmatch if the patient has no history of significant antibodies. If an antibody is detected, identification of that antibody is performed, and compatible units are reserved for the patient. Compatible units are also reserved for the patient if there is previous history of significant antibodies, even though these antibodies may not be detectable in the current sample. Refer to Chapter 10, "Pretransfusion Testing."

Type and Crossmatch. When a physician orders units to be crossmatched for a patient, more testing is necessary than the order itself implies. ABO and Rh testing and antibody screening must be performed on a current patient specimen. The same specimen is also used to crossmatch with a segment of the unit intended for transfusion. In the absence of extreme emergency, the unit of blood can be issued for transfusion only if all testing discrepancies are resolved and the crossmatch is compatible. If the result of the antibody screen is positive, the antibody must be identified. If the antibody is clinically significant, antigen-negative units must be chosen for transfusion. Antigen-negative units must also be chosen if there is previous history of a significant antibody, even though the antibody may not be detected in the current sample.

Abbreviated crossmatch protocols have been adopted by some blood banks for routine crossmatching and by others for emergency situations only. In these protocols, ABO and Rh testing and antibody screening are performed. In the absence of clinically significant antibodies, blood is issued after an immediate spin crossmatch that serves as a confirmation of ABO compatibility.

An **electronic** or **computer crossmatch** is another method of crossmatching donor and patient that is intended to replace serologic compatibility testing. Two separate ABO and Rh tests are performed on a patient's RBCs and entered into a validated computer system; the ABO confirmatory test on a unit of blood is also entered. At the time when the blood is to be issued to the patient for transfusion, the computer verifies the ABO compatibility between the donor unit and the patient and allows the release of the blood. If ABO incompatibilities between the recipient and the donor unit are discovered, the computer alerts the user to the discrepancy so that the blood will not be released.

Prenatal Evaluation. Accurate serologic testing of obstetric patients is an essential component in the prevention and treatment of hemolytic disease of the fetus and newborn (HDFN). Maternal blood samples are evaluated during pregnancy to determine the ABO group and Rh type of the mother and the presence of serum antibodies that can potentially cause HDFN. If the woman is classified as Rh-D negative, she may be a candidate for antenatal Rh-immune globulin unless her serum contains actively acquired anti-D. **Weak D** testing is not required as part of a prenatal evaluation. It is not possible to differentiate weak D from **partial D** serologically. Since patients who are partial-D positive may still develop anti-D, many hospital blood banks consider all prenatal patients who test D-negative initially as "negative" without further testing. (See Chapter 7, "The Rh Blood Group System.")

If the result of the antibody screen is positive, the antibody must be identified. **Serial titrations** may be performed during the course of the pregnancy if the antibody is considered potentially harmful to the fetus. The obstetrician uses these laboratory results together with other methods for evaluating the fetal condition and the need for clinical intervention (see Chapter 19, "Hemolytic Disease of the Fetus and Newborn").

Postpartum Evaluation. All women admitted for delivery are required to be tested to determine their Rh status. Weak-D testing is not required. If the mother is Rh-negative and her baby is Rh-positive, the maternal sample is further evaluated to detect a **feto-maternal hemorrhage** (FMH) in excess of 30 mL of whole blood. (One 300-µg dose of RhIg prevents maternal Rh immunization from exposure of up to 30 mL of fetal whole blood.[4]) Commercial kits utilizing rosetting techniques are commonly used for this purpose. Once an FMH in excess of 30 mL of whole blood has been detected, quantification is performed using a **Kleihauer-Betke** test, **flow cytometry**, or **enzyme-linked antiglobulin** test. This may be performed in the blood bank or in a separate laboratory. If HDFN is suspected, an antibody screen is performed on the mother's serum, and if the result is positive, attempts are made to identify the antibody.

Cord Blood Studies. Protocols to evaluate cord blood specimens can vary widely from blood bank to blood bank. Cord blood from infants born to Rh-negative mothers is tested for D and for weak D to determine the mother's candidacy for RhIg prophylaxis. ABO and Rh typing and **direct antiglobulin testing** (DAT) are performed on cord samples from infants born to women with clinically significant antibodies. Additional testing may also be performed. Many blood banks follow published guidelines stating that beyond these circumstances, routine testing of cord blood is not necessary unless the clinical situation warrants it. If an infant develops symptoms that suggest HDFN, a full cord blood study is performed that may include ABO and Rh typing (including a test for weak D) and DAT. If the DAT result is positive, an eluate and subsequent antibody identification are performed. Note that only forward testing is performed in the ABO test.

Requests for Other Blood Components

When components containing large amounts of RBCs (e.g., granulocyte concentrates) are requested, pretransfusion testing is identical to that performed for RBC requests. There are no such requirements for platelets or FFP.

Issue of Blood Products

After all pretransfusion testing has been completed, blood components may be released for transfusion to the designated recipient. It is essential that all serologic discrepancies be resolved before issuing blood products, except in extreme emergency. The individual who obtains the blood product from the blood bank for delivery to the nursing unit is usually required to present a written request for the blood product containing a minimum of two patient identifiers. The individual in the blood bank who will issue the blood product inspects the unit for any abnormal appearance (Box 11–3) and verifies that all required transfusion forms and labels are complete and that they adequately identify the transfusion recipient. If another individual is responsible for delivering the blood product to the appropriate location, he or she may also verify that all information is complete. A computer crossmatch may also be performed at this time, and if there are no discrepancies, the component can be released for transfusion. Some form of documentation is used to record the transaction.

Some component preparation or modification may be necessary before the issue of blood products. FFP may be thawed in a constant-temperature (30°C to 37°C) water bath, individual platelet concentrates may be pooled into a single bag for ease of transfusion, and a packed RBC may need to be irradiated (Fig. 11–9). These modifications may shorten the expiration date of the products and must be reflected on the unit itself and in the computer system.

Reference Laboratory

Whether it is an entity separate from the main laboratory or, as in most cases, an integrated part, the reference laboratory is the problem-solving section of the transfusion service. The reference laboratory's goal is to ensure that any discrepancies detected in routine testing are resolved in an accurate and time-efficient manner. Other chapters in this book discuss in depth the various problems encountered in serologic testing and the strategies for resolving them. Here is a brief summary

---

BOX 11–3

Reasons to Quarantine Blood Components Before Shipment or Transfusion

- Plasma of RBC unit is brown, red, murky, or purple
- Zone of hemolysis is above RBC mass
- Inadequate sealing of RBC segments in tubing
- Hemolysis of RBCs
- Grossly lipemic units
- Unusual cloudy or turbid appearance of platelet unit

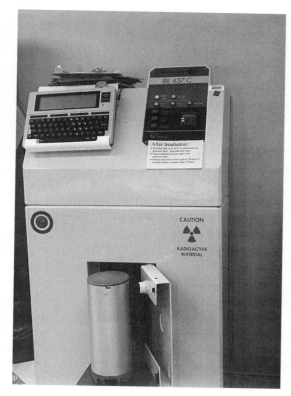

Figure 11–9. Irradiators are used to prevent lymphocytes in RBC products from causing graft-versus-host disease in susceptible patient populations. *(Courtesy National Institutes of Health, Bethesda, MD.)*

of some situations and common methods used in their investigation. It should be noted that before any serologic testing is performed, special testing should always include an investigation of patient's diagnosis, age, pregnancy, drug, and transfusion history.

ABO Discrepancies

All inconsistencies between forward and reverse grouping must be resolved before an ABO interpretation can be made (see Chapter 6, "The ABO Blood Group System"). ABO investigations may include:

- Variations in incubation times and temperatures
- Testing with A_2 cells or **anti-A_1 lectin**
- Room temperature antibody identification
- **Adsorption and elution** using human sources of anti-A or anti-B
- **Autoadsorption**
- Removal of RBC-bound cold autoantibodies
- **Secretor studies**

Rh Discrepancies

Problems in Rh typing may occur because of certain clinical conditions or inherited characteristics (see Chapter 7). Rh investigations may include:

- Rh phenotyping
- Adsorption and elution using Rh antisera
- Isolation of cell populations
- Use of rare antisera and RBCs

Antibody Identification

A positive antibody screen in the absence of a positive auto-control or DAT result indicates possible **alloantibody immunization** by means of blood transfusion or pregnancy (see Chapter 9, "Detection and Identification of Antibodies"). To establish the identity and clinical significance of an antibody and to provide appropriate blood for transfusion, antibody investigation may include:

- Antibody identification panels using various **enhancement media** (albumin, low ionic strength solution, polyethylene glycol) and test systems (such as tubes, gel, or solid phase technologies)
- Antibody identification panels pretreated with reagents such as enzymes, dithiothreitol (DTT), or 2-aminoethylisothiouronium bromide
- **Neutralization** using such substances as plasma, saliva, urine, or human milk
- Antigen typing
- Titration
- Adsorption and elution studies
- Treatment of serum with DTT or 2-mercaptoethanol
- IgG subclassing
- Monocyte monolayer assay
- Use of rare sera and cells

Positive DAT

A positive DAT may be the result of an immune reaction to a drug, a disease state, or a **delayed hemolytic transfusion reaction** (see Chapter 16, "Adverse Effects of Blood Transfusion"). The investigation of a positive DAT may include:

- Use of monospecific reagents (anti-IgG, anti-C3)
- Elution techniques
- Antibody identification
- Removal of cell-bound antibody using chloroquine diphosphate
- RBC phenotyping
- Drug studies
- Cell separation techniques

Warm Autoantibodies

In addition to causing a positive DAT, the presence of a **warm autoantibody** in a patient's serum may mask the presence of clinically significant alloantibodies (see Chapter 20, "Autoimmune Hemolytic Anemias"). Tests performed in the investigation of warm autoantibodies may include:

- Removal of RBC-bound autoantibody followed by serum **autoadsorption**
- Heterologous or differential serum adsorptions
- Elution techniques
- Autoantibody identification
- Reticulocyte enrichment or other cell separation techniques

Cold Autoantibodies

Potent cold autoantibodies may cause discrepancies in ABO testing and a positive DAT result and may mask the presence of clinically significant alloantibodies (see Chapter 20). The management of cold autoantibodies may include:

- Removal of RBC-bound autoantibody using 37°C saline
- Prewarmed technique
- Antibody identification
- Autoadsorption
- Adsorption using rabbit erythrocyte stroma
- Treatment of serum or cells with DTT or 2-ME

Transfusion Reactions

Any adverse reactions to transfusion must be investigated to determine if the reaction is antibody-mediated (see Chapter 16). The extent of transfusion reaction investigations varies widely, depending on the policies established by a particular blood bank and the result of initial testing. At a minimum, an investigation of a suspected hemolytic reaction to transfusion should include an ABO, Rh, DAT, and visual checkfor hemolysis using a post-transfusion sample.[3] If there is strong evidence of an antibody-mediated transfusion reaction, further investigation may include:

- Elution followed by antibody identification
- Use of more sensitive techniques for antibody detection in serum and eluates, including enzymes, polybrene, polyethylene glycol, or enzyme-linked antiglobulin test
- Cell separation techniques

Personnel Requirements

The pursuit of quality begins with people. This is no less true for the blood bank laboratory, where the essence of service is all about quality: providing blood and blood products that are safe for transfusion. Like all complex organizations, the blood bank laboratory is staffed by a variety of individuals with various credentials and qualifications. Blood bank laboratory work centers on labor-intensive tasks and sophisticated analyses often performed under stressful conditions complicated by emergency requests for blood. Work demands like these can only be met by an educated, well-trained, and highly skilled labor force.

In recognition that quality laboratory testing is in part a function of the people performing the analyses, the U.S. government included personnel requirements in the **Clinical Laboratory Improvement Amendments of 1988 (CLIA '88)**. Subpart M of these regulations establishes personnel qualifications for laboratories performing certain types of testing. Blood bank laboratories are engaged in both moderately and highly complex testing. Manual tube testing has long been the standard method for the testing done in the blood bank laboratory. More recently, however, less labor-intensive methods have been employed. These include manual or automated gel technologies (Fig. 11–10) and solid phase RBC adherence (see Chapter 12, "Other Technologies and Automation"). These methods allow for workload consolidation and facilitate ease of cross-training testing personnel.

Under CLIA, blood bank laboratories must employ personnel who are qualified by education, training, or experience.[3] In addition, most blood banks will have specific written

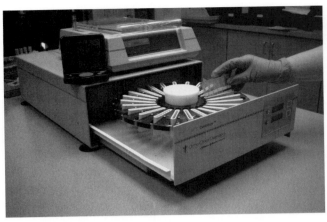

Figure 11–10.   A gel card is loaded into a centrifuge. The gel test employs the principle of controlled centrifugation of RBCs through a dextran-acrylamide gel/reagent matrix contained in a specially designed microtube.

procedures outlining the training program for new hires in their institution. In all cases, the blood bank laboratory must have a qualified director to manage the personnel and the operations. However, the director may delegate to a qualified supervisor the day-to-day work-related activities that include managing personnel and reporting test results.

Standard Operating Procedures

Orientation to a blood bank laboratory begins with reading the **standard operating procedure** (SOP) manuals. These manuals, usually located at the workbench and accessible to all personnel, contain information outlining the operations of the laboratory; details on how, when, and why particular activities are done; and procedures for all tests performed. SOP manuals are integral components of any blood bank laboratory's quality-assurance program (see Chapter 23, "Quality Management"). They are reviewed at least annually and updated on a regular basis to reflect changes in operations and implementation of new regulations.

Transfusion Process Oversight

The blood bank staff is familiar with regulations involving the transfusion process, from sample collection to blood administration and observation of the patient following transfusion; thus, the blood bank often is involved in providing the required training for staff who administer and monitor blood and blood component transfusions. Training may be done in a variety of ways such as Web-based training, seminars, or lectures that include questions to assess the staff members' comprehension. This training and verification of competency must be documented.[6]

In addition, an audit system should be in place in which a blood bank technologist (or other assigned patient safety staff member) observes a predetermined number of transfusions to verify that proper procedure is being followed. It is important to perform audits in all nursing units where transfusions are performed. A "check-off" form, such as that shown in Figure 11–11, should be utilized to verify such

BLOOD ADMINISTRATION OBSERVATION

Process Control

Assessor's Survey (Data Collection)

Associate's Name: _____

Date Assessed: _____

Floor: _____

Unit Number: _____

PRETRANSFUSION	YES	NO	N/A
1. Was there a written order for transfusion on the chart?			
2. Was the transfusion initiated within the institution's defined time limit?			
3. Was the blood component placed or found in an unmonitored ward or refrigerator?			
4. Is the transfusionist aware of the location of the current blood administration SOP online?			
5. Was the signed blood consent form on the patient's chart?			

PATIENT AND COMPONENT IDENTIFICATION	YES	NO	N/A
1. Was the patient wearing the correct identification band at the start of and during the transfusion?			
2. Was the nursing verification performed at bedside?			
3. At the bedside, was institutional policy followed for:			
a. Checking the ID band of the patient with the patient ID on the unit tag?			
b. Did both the transfusionist and witness check the patient's blood bank and hospital ID band?			
c. Comparing the unit number and blood type of the blood component with that shown on the unit tag?			
4. Did the information on the patient ID band, blood component, and unit tag agree?			
5. Were any discrepancies reported to the transfusion service?			

ADMINISTRATION TECHNIQUES AND MONITORING	YES	NO	N/A
1. Were pretransfusion vital signs obtained and recorded?			
2. Did the transfusionist document the transfusion start time on the transfusion record?			
3. Was the initial start time documented as the time when blood reached the patient's skin/vein?			
4. Were any medications or IV solutions other than normal saline (0.9N) being infused through the filter tubing while the transfusion was taking place? If yes, what was given? _____			
5. Were vital signs obtained per institutional policy and recorded?			
6. Did the unit tag remain attached to the unit during transfusion?			
7. Was the transfusion completed within the time appropriate for the blood component being administered?			
8. Did the transfusionist record the transfusion stop time on the transfusion record?			
9. Did the transfusionist document any adverse effects, if applicable?			
10. If an adverse effect was observed:			
a. Did transfusionist (or designee) notify physician?			
b. Did transfusionist (or designee) notify transfusion service?			
c. Was an investigation of the suspected transfusion effect initiated?			
d. Was a current copy of nursing procedure for adverse reaction investigations available?			
11. Was blood warmer (Hot Lines) used in accordance with manufacturer's instructions and institutional policy?			
12. If outpatient, were written instructions for possible adverse effects provided?			

DISPOSITION	YES	NO	N/A
1. Was the requisition completed according to institutional policy?			
2. Was the medical record copy of the requisition charted?			
3. Was a copy of the requisition returned to the transfusion service in a biohazard bag along with the empty blood bag?			

GENERAL COMMENTS ON ASSESSMENT: _____

_____

_____

_____

_____

Figure 11–11.   Sample Blood Administration Observation Form. This form is used to document direct observations of transfusions. Audits such as this are performed to verify compliance with transfusion process regulations and policies.

things as presence of a signed patient consent form, a properly documented order to transfuse, proper patient identification, a correct patient and unit verification process was followed, and other process items as determined by hospital policy. A report should be prepared from this audit data, usually quarterly, and this report should be presented to the blood bank medical director and the hospital patient safety or risk management team for evaluation (Fig. 11–12). See Chapter 23 for more information.

The blood bank supervisor will usually prepare a monthly or quarterly blood bank report listing such things as the number of physicians whose crossmatch versus transfusion (C:T) ratio exceeds the hospital's target, the number of transfusion reaction investigations, patients transfused who may not meet hospital transfusion triggers, or any other parameter the blood bank medical director deems necessary to monitor (Fig. 11–13). This report is given to the blood bank medical director and often a medical review committee for evaluation.

BLOOD AUDIT SUMMARY

			YEAR	
Quarter	**# Audits**	**# Failures**	**Failure description**	**# Transfusions**
1				
2				
3				
4				
Total for year			**Total % failures =** **Patient safety failures* =**	

			YEAR	
Quarter	**# Audits**	**# Failures**	**Failure description**	**# Transfusions**
Total for year			**Total % failures =** **Patient safety failures* =**	
Note: Patient safety failures indicated with *				

Figure 11–12. Sample Blood Audit Summary Form. This form is used to summarize the data collected from transfusion process observations over a period of time, most often quarterly. This form is then presented for review by the medical director or transfusion oversight committee.

BLOOD UTILIZATION REVIEW REPORT
PERIOD:

Parameter	Result	Goal	Comment
Statistics			
C:T Ratio		1.5	Concern at ≥ 2.0
# Physicians C:T ≥ 1.5		0	See attached for physician names
Patients transfused		NA	
Patients receiving > 1 component		NA	
Massive transfusions		NA	
Breakdown of units given:	RBC –	NA	
	PLT -		
	FFP –		
	CRYO -		
Tissue products implanted		NA	
T&S converted for surgery		< 5% of TYSC	
Wasted units		0	
ABO and/or RH type change	(POS units to NEG patients)	< 5%	
	(NEG units to POS patients)	NA	
	ABO change	NA	
Lookback investigations	1	NA	
Reactions			
Transfusion reaction workups		3% total transfusions	
Inventory control			
Units received/units transfused		< 2	
Returned to supplier		NA	
Expired units		0	
Component usage			
__ patients receiving red cells were reviewed.	Did not meet screening criteria of HGB ≤ 8.0	NA	Chart reviews being performed by medical director
All patients receiving components were reviewed	Did not meet screening criteria of PT ≥ 13; PTT ≥ 30; PLT ≤ 20	NA	Chart reviews being performed by medical director

Figure 11–13.   Sample Blood Utilization Report. This report helps the blood bank monitor effective use of blood products, including the number of physicians whose C:T ratio exceeds the hospital standard, and possible inappropriate transfusions. This report is typically reviewed by the blood bank medical director and a medical peer review committee.

SUMMARY CHART

✔ The goal of every blood bank laboratory is to provide quality service and safe blood products.

✔ All blood bank laboratory operations are regulated by law.

✔ Personnel employed by blood bank laboratories must be qualified by education, training, or experience.

✔ A primary source of operational information is the SOP manual.

✔ Hemapheresis is a process that uses an apheresis machine to selectively remove components from donor blood.

✔ Blood and blood components must be stored and shipped under conditions that ensure their viability.

✔ Every donor unit is tested to determine ABO group and Rh type, including weak D when indicated. Units are also tested for selected viral markers.

✔ The type of Rh-negative units must be confirmed because of potential sensitization that may occur if Rh-positive blood is transfused to an Rh-negative recipient.

✔ Manual tube procedures are being replaced by emerging technologies, including gel-based methods and automation.

Review Questions

1. What is the shipping temperature requirement for plasma?
   a. 1°F to 6°F or higher
   b. 1°C to 6°C or lower
   c. −18°F or higher
   d. −18°C or lower

2. Antibody serial titration studies are most often associated with which of the following blood bank test groupings?
   a. Prenatal evaluation
   b. Type and screen
   c. Type and crossmatch
   d. Blood unit processing

3. The prewarm technique is most useful in investigating which types of blood bank problems?
   a. ABO discrepancies
   b. Rh discrepancies
   c. Warm antibodies
   d. Cold antibodies

4. It is most important to perform weak-D testing in which of the following blood bank test groupings?
   a. Type and screen
   b. Type and crossmatch
   c. Cord blood evaluation
   d. Prenatal evaluation

5. Which of the following is a method for determining approximate volume of fetal-maternal bleed?
   a. Kleihauer-Betke test
   b. Eluate testing
   c. Nucleic acid amplification testing
   d. Antibody screening

6. Which of the following may not be used as a patient identifier?
   a. Patient's full name
   b. Patient's date of birth
   c. Patient's medical record number
   d. Patient's room number

7. Which of the following is not an enhancement media that may be used in antibody screening and identification?
   a. Albumin
   b. Low ionic strength solution (LISS)
   c. Normal saline
   d. Polyethylene glycol

8. Which of the following methods may be useful in investigating a positive DAT?
   a. Elution techniques
   b. Removal of cell-bound antibody using chloroquine diphosphate
   c. Drug studies
   d. All of the above

References

1. American Association of Blood Banks: "About Blood and Cellular Therapies." Available at www.aabb.org.
2. United States Department of Health and Human Services: 2009 National Blood Collection and Utilization Survey Report, 2011. Available at www.hhs.gov/bloodsafety.
3. Standards for Blood Banks and Transfusion Services, 27th ed. American Association of Blood Banks, Bethesda, MD, 2011.
4. Roback, John D, et al: Technical Manual, 16th ed. American Association of Blood Banks, Bethesda, MD, 2008.
5. Code of Federal Regulations, Title 21 CFR Parts 640. Washington, DC: US Government Printing Office, 2009 (revised annually).
6. The Joint Commission Edition, Quality System Assessment for Nonwaived Testing, January 2010.

Chapter 12

Other Technologies and Automation

Phyllis S. Walker, MS, MT(ASCP)SBB and Denise M. Harmening, PhD, MT(ASCP)

OBJECTIVES

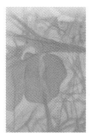

1. Explain the principles of gel, solid-phase red cell adherence (SPRCA), protein A, and enzyme-linked immunosorbent assay (ELISA) technology.
2. Describe the test reactions and how the results are interpreted for each technology.
3. List the advantages and disadvantages of each technology.
4. Describe the automated equipment that is available for each technology.
5. Compare the gel and SPRCA technologies in terms of equipment, test reactions, procedures, sensitivity and specificity, and quality control.

Introduction

Previous chapters have discussed ABO and Rh typing, direct **antiglobulin** testing (DAT), and antibody detection and identification procedures based on routine test tube testing techniques. In response to the pressures of current good manufacturing practices, two other technologies, the **gel test** and **solid-phase** assays, have emerged to provide accurate, reproducible blood bank testing. These technologies provide the increased safety offered by plasticware and reduce biohazardous waste. In addition, these technologies have been automated, decreasing the opportunities for human error and freeing laboratory personnel to perform other tasks. Surveys indicate that there is an ongoing trend toward adopting these other technologies in clinical laboratories.[1,2] This chapter presents the history, applications, basic principles, and advantages and disadvantages of each technology, and describes currently available automated equipment.

Blood banks and transfusion services are the last areas of the clinical laboratory to move to **automation**. Chemistry, hematology, and immunology have been using automation for many years, but blood services have been hampered by the complexity of the testing and the subjectivity of the test interpretation. In recent years, new pressure has been applied to this area of the laboratory. Personnel shortages, turnaround time requirements, and the need for cost containment because of increased managed care and greater regulatory demands have provided the incentive for blood services to seek automation. By using walk-away automation, laboratory personnel are able to perform multiple tasks simultaneously. Automated equipment provides the level of quality assurance required by current regulatory standards. Bar-coding reduces identification errors by providing accurate patient and reagent identification, and standardized techniques reduce testing errors.

Automation in blood centers was first applied to infectious disease testing. Assays for infectious disease are easier to automate because they are less subjective than serologic tests. Although automated viral marker testing is performed in all blood centers, this chapter focuses on equipment that automates serologic testing in blood centers and transfusion services.

Gel Technology

In 1985, Dr. Yves Lapierre of Lyon, France, developed the gel test.[3] Using various media, including gelatin, acrylamide gel, and glass beads, Dr. Lapierre investigated ways to trap red blood cell (RBC) agglutinates during standardized sedimentation or centrifugation. Gel particles were found to be the ideal material for trapping the agglutinates, and this discovery led to a patented process for separating agglutinated red blood cells. In addition, it was discovered that antiglobulin testing could be performed without multiple saline washes to remove unbound immunoglobulin and that antiglobulin control cells were not needed to confirm the presence of antiglobulin reagent in negative tests. Compared with traditional tube technology, the gel test provides a more stable endpoint and more reproducible results. This improvement reduces the variability associated with the physical resuspension of RBC buttons after centrifugation and the subsequent interpretation of **hemagglutination** reactions.

History

In 1988, Dr. Lapierre worked with DiaMed A.G. to develop and produce the gel test in Europe. In September 1994, the FDA granted Micro Typing Systems (MTS) a license to manufacture and distribute an antiglobulin **anti-IgG gel card** and a buffered gel card in the United States. In January 1995, Ortho Diagnostic Systems Inc. (ODSI) and MTS signed an agreement giving ODSI exclusive rights to distribute the gel test in North America. In March 2002, Ortho Clinical Diagnostics fully acquired MTS and became known as Micro Typing Systems. This gel-based test is named the ID-Micro Typing System.[4]

Applications

In the United States, the FDA has approved gel technology for ABO forward and reverse grouping, Rh typing, direct antiglobulin testing, antibody screening, identifying antibodies, and compatibility testing. The ABO blood grouping card has gels that contain anti-A, anti-B, and anti-A,B for forward grouping. **Microtubes** with buffered gel are used for ABO reverse grouping.[5] The Rh typing card uses microtubes filled with gel containing anti-D.[6] The Rh phenotype card has gels that contain anti-D, anti-C, anti-E, anti-c, anti-e, and a control.[7] Microtubes filled with gel containing anti-IgG are used for compatibility testing, antibody detection, and identification.[8]

Principle

The gel test, which is performed in a specially designed microtube, is based on the controlled centrifugation of RBCs

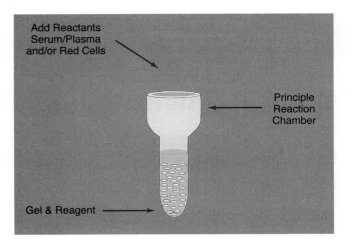

Figure 12–1.   Gel microtube. Microtubes filled with gel containing anti-IgG are used for compatibility testing, antibody detection, and identification.

through a dextran-acrylamide gel that contains predispensed reagents. Each microtube is composed of an upper reaction chamber that is wider than the tube itself and a long, narrow portion referred to as the *column* (Fig. 12–1). In the gel test, a plastic card with microtubes is used instead of test tubes (Fig. 12–2). A gel card measures approximately 5 × 7 centimeters and consists of six microtubes. Each microtube contains predispensed gel, diluent, and reagents, if applicable. Measured volumes of serum or plasma or RBCs are dispensed into the microtube's reaction chamber (Fig. 12–3). If appropriate, the card is incubated (Fig. 12–4) and then centrifuged (Fig. 12–5).

The reaction chamber is where RBCs may be **sensitized** (antigen-antibody binding) during incubation. The column of each microtube contains dextran-acrylamide gel particles suspended in a diluent with reagents added, if applicable. The shape and length of the column provides a large surface area for prolonged contact of the RBCs with the gel particles during centrifugation.

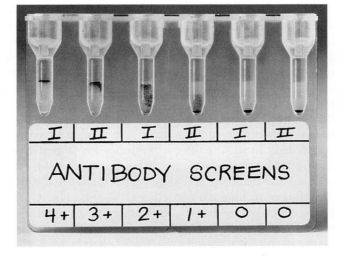

Figure 12–2.   The gel card. Each measures approximately 5 x 7 centimeters and consists of six microtubes (instead of test tubes).

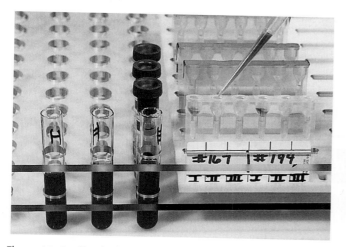

Figure 12–3. Pipetting into gel card microtubes. Measured volumes of serum or plasma or RBCs are dispensed into the reaction chamber of the microtube.

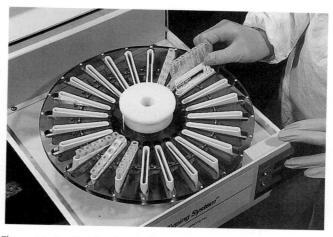

Figure 12–5. Centrifugation of gel cards.

The gel particles, composed of beads of dextran-acrylamide, make up 75% of the gel-liquid mixture that is preloaded by the manufacturer into each microtube.[4] The gel particles are porous, and they serve as a reaction medium and filter, sieving the RBC agglutinates according to size during centrifugation. Large agglutinates are trapped at the top of the gel and are not allowed to travel through the gel during the centrifugation of the card (Fig. 12–6). Agglutinated RBCs remain trapped in the gel, whereas unagglutinated RBCs travel unimpeded through the length of the microtube, forming a pellet at the bottom after centrifugation.

Agglutination reactions in the gel test are graded from 1+ to 4+ (including **mixed-field**), just like the reactions in the test tube hemagglutination technique[4] (Fig. 12–7). In the gel test, a 4+ reaction is characterized by a solid band of agglutinated RBCs at the top of the gel column. Usually, no RBCs are visible at the bottom of the microtube. In a 3+ reaction, most of the agglutinated RBCs remain near the top of the gel column, with a few agglutinates staggered below the thicker band. The majority of agglutinates are observed in the top half of the gel column. In a 2+ reaction, RBC agglutinates are distributed throughout the upper and lower halves of the gel column, with a few agglutinates at the bottom of the microtube. In a 1+ reaction, RBC agglutinates are predominantly seen in the lower half of the gel column, with some RBCs at the bottom of the microtube. These reactions may be weak, with only a few agglutinates remaining in the gel area just above the RBC pellet at the bottom of the microtube. In a negative reaction, the RBCs form a well-delineated pellet at the bottom of the microtube. The gel above the RBC pellet is clear and free of agglutinates. In a mixed-field (mf) reaction, the layer of agglutinated RBCs is at the top of the gel and a pellet of unagglutinated cells is at the bottom of the microtube.

False-positive mixed-field reactions can occur when incompletely clotted serum is used in the gel test. Fibrin strands in such serum may trap unagglutinated RBCs, forming a thin line at the top of the gel. Other unagglutinated cells pass through the gel during centrifugation and travel to the bottom of the microtube. Before interpreting a reaction as mixed-field, the patient's clinical history should be considered. For example, recently transfused patients or bone marrow transplant recipients are expected to have mixed populations of RBCs, and their RBCs commonly produce mixed-field reactions.

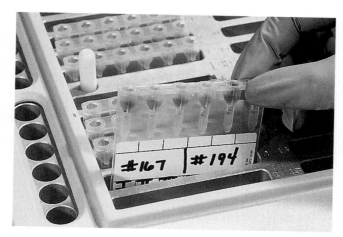

Figure 12–4. Incubation of gel cards.

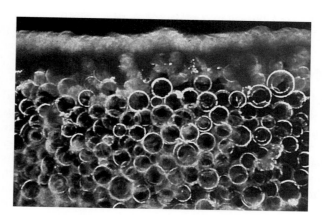

Figure 12–6. Magnified photograph of agglutinated RBCs trapped above the gel matrix.

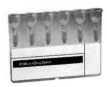

ID-Micro Typing System™

Gel Technology Reaction Grading Chart

Agglutinated cells form a cell layer at the top of the gel media.

4+

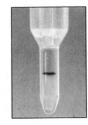

Agglutinated cells disperse throughout the gel media and may concentrate toward the bottom of the microtube.

1+

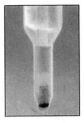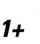

Agglutinated cells begin to disperse into gel media and are concentrated near the top of the microtube.

3+

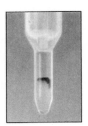

All cells pass through the gel media and form a cell button at the bottom of the microtube.

Negative

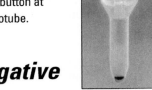

Agglutinated cells disperse into the gel media and are observed throughout the length of the microtube.

2+

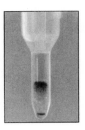

Agglutinated cells form a layer at the top of the gel media. Unagglutinated cells pass to the bottom of the microtube.

Mixed-Field

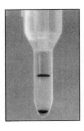

Figure 12–7. Gel technology reaction grading chart. *(Courtesy of Ortho Clinical Diagnostics, Raritan, New Jersey.)*

Advantages and Disadvantages

Gel technology, which is applicable to a broad range of blood bank tests, offers several advantages over routine tube testing.[9] **Standardization** is one of the major advantages, since there is no tube shaking to resuspend the RBC button. Tube-shaking technique varies among technologists, which results in variations in reading, grading, and interpreting the test. The gel technique provides stable, well-defined endpoints of the agglutination reaction that can be observed or reviewed for up to 3 days. It includes simple standardized procedures, no wash step, and no need for antiglobulin control cells.

These factors combine to produce more objective, consistent, and reproducible interpretation of the test results.

Because the gel technology offers objective, consistent results, it is ideally suited to individuals who have been cross-trained to work in the blood bank. Other advantages include the decreased sample volume needed for testing and the enhanced **sensitivity** and **specificity** of the results. Finally, gel technology offers improved productivity when compared with traditional tube testing.[10]

The major disadvantages of the gel technology are the sample restrictions and the need for special equipment. **Hemolyzed** or grossly **icteric** blood samples should not be used, because the results may be difficult to interpret visually in the ID Micro Typing System.[5] Grossly **lipemic** samples containing particulates that clog the gel, as indicated by diffuse blotches of RBCs, must be clarified by centrifugation or filtration and retested. **Rouleaux** caused by serum or plasma with abnormally high concentrations of protein (such as in patients with multiple myeloma or Waldenström's macroglobulinemia or from patients who have received plasma expanders of high molecular weight) may produce hazy reactions or false-positive results.[5] Special incubators and centrifuges are needed to accommodate the microtube cards, and a specific pipette must be used to measure and dispense the 25 µL of plasma or serum and the 50 µL of 0.8% RBCs into the reaction chambers of the microtubes. Finally, the **calibration** on the special pipette must be checked on a regular schedule.[11,12]

Automation

Automated equipment for serologic testing using the gel test is being performed successfully for ABO and Rh testing, antibody screening, compatibility testing, and antibody identification in both the United States and Europe. The ORTHO ProVue™ Analyzer (Fig. 12–8) is a walk-away instrument with a capacity for testing 48 samples and 16 reagents. Instrument safety features include a bar-code tracking system and three cameras that record sample, reagent, and card identification. A camera in the instrument performs image analysis and uses a mathematical algorithm to interpret the results.

Solid-Phase Technology

Solid-phase immunoassays have been used for many years in immunology and chemistry laboratories. In these test systems (immunoassays), one of the test reactants (either antigen or antibody) is bound to a solid support (usually a microtiter well) before the test is started. The ability of plastics, such as polystyrene, to absorb proteins from solution and to bind them irreversibly makes plastic **microplate** wells ideal for

solid-phase serologic assays. In 1978, Rosenfield and coworkers[13] were the first to apply the principle of solid-phase immunoassay to RBC typing and antibody screening tests.

Solid-phase technology relevant to serologic testing in blood centers and transfusion services include **solid-phase red cell adherence** (SPRCA), solid-phase **protein A**, and solid-phase enzyme-linked immunosorbent assay (**ELISA**).

Solid-Phase Red Cell Adherence

History

In 1984, Plapp and coworkers reported using solid-phase red cell adherence (SPRCA) for detecting RBC antigens and antibodies.[14,15] The first SPRCA assays to be developed commercially were manufactured by Immucor under the trade name of Capture for the detection of RBC and platelet antibodies. Currently, Capture immunoassays are available to detect antibodies to RBCs, platelets, and cytomegalovirus.[16]

Applications

SPRCA assays are either first- or second-generation tests. In first-generation tests, the user adds the target antigen (RBCs, platelets, or platelet proteins, etc.) to the microplate wells before starting the test. In second-generation tests, the manufacturer binds the target antigen (RBC, platelet glycoproteins, or CMV) to the microplate test wells during the manufacturing process.

First- and second-generation SPRCA assays are currently approved by the FDA for antibody screening, antibody identification, weak-D testing, IgG **autologous** control, and compatibility testing. Second-generation assays use **microwells** that are preloaded with antibody screening cells, in either a set of two-cells (I and II), a set of three cells, a set of four cells, or a pool of two cells. The two- and four-cell sets are recommended for antibody detection in transfusion recipients. Pooled cells are used for donor antibody detection when increased sensitivity is undesirable. Reagent panels of preloaded cells are also available for RBC antibody identification. When it is desirable to test selected cells, intact reagent RBCs are added by the user to chemically modified microwells (i.e., a first-generation test).

Principle

SPRCA assays may be performed with either plasma or serum, but plasma is preferable. If a clotted sample is incompletely clotted, the serum is difficult to remove during the wash cycle, which allows residual unbound serum to clot and make the endpoint of the test unreadable. For best results, the manufacturer recommends adding a pH-stabilizing buffer to the isotonic saline that is used to wash the microplates. A suitable buffer is available from the manufacturer.[17]

Capture technology offers both first- and second-generation SPRCA tests, which are performed in microplate wells—in either full 96-well U-bottomed plates or in 1 × 8 or 2 × 8 U-bottomed strips.[18] To perform second-generation tests, patient serum or plasma and low ionic strength saline (**LISS**) are added to microwells that are coated with the target antigen, and the

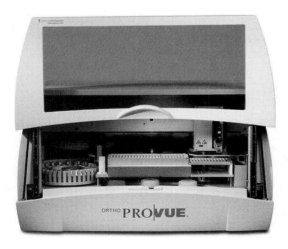

Figure 12–8.   ORTHO ProVue™ Analyzer. *(Courtesy of Ortho Clinical Diagnostics, Raritan, New Jersey.)*

wells are incubated at 37°C, to allow time for possible antibodies to attach to the antigens in the well. After incubation, the wells are washed with pH-buffered isotonic saline to remove unbound serum proteins. Next, anti-IgG-coated indicator RBCs are added, and the microwells are centrifuged. Centrifugation forces the indicator RBCs into close contact with **IgG** antibodies from the test serum or plasma that are bound to the immobilized target antigen (i.e., the sandwich technique). If antibody is attached to the antigen during the incubation phase, the indicator cells form a **monolayer** of RBCs. If no antibody is present, nothing is attached to the antigen, and the indicator cells form a clearly delineated button at the center of the microplate well during centrifugation (Fig. 12–9).

Figure 12–10 compares test results from solid-phase technology with traditional tube testing reactions. Positive tests show adherence of indicator RBCs to part or all of the well bottom, depending on the reaction's strength. Capture-R

Select, which identifies RBC antibodies, and Capture-P, which detects platelet antibodies, are examples of first-generation solid-phase tests, whereas Capture-R Ready-Screen, Capture-R Ready-ID, and Capture-P Ready Screen are second-generation tests.[18]

The laboratory equipment that is needed to perform SPRCA testing includes a microplate centrifuge capable of holding 96-well microplates or strip wells, a microplate incubator, and a microplate washer. Also, an illuminated surface for reading manual microplates is very desirable. (Fig. 12–11).

Advantages and Disadvantages

Standardization is the major advantage of SPRCA technology. SPRCA provides stable, well-defined endpoints of the reaction. Objective, consistent, reproducible test results facilitate technologist training or cross-training. SPRCA is convenient

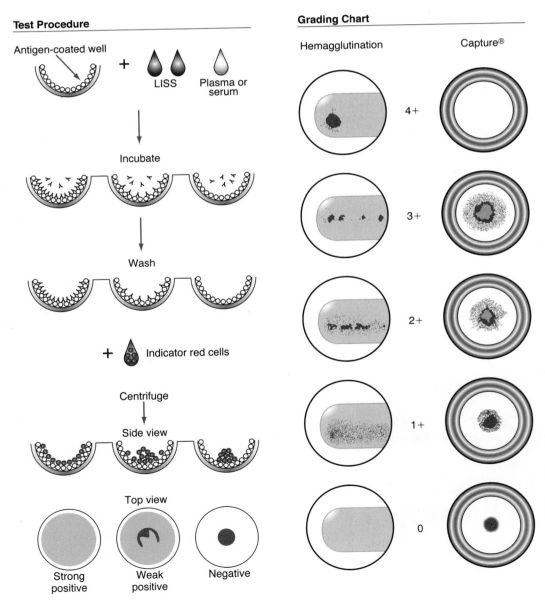

Figure 12–9. Solid-phase test procedure. (*Courtesy of Immucor, Norcross, Georgia.*)

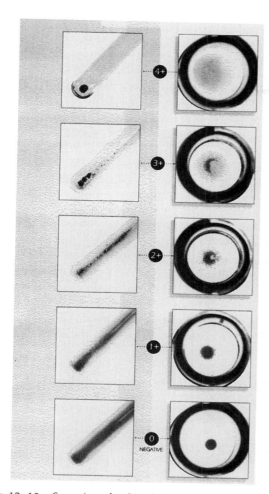

Figure 12–10. Comparison of traditional tube test reactions with solid-phase reactions.

because no predilution of reagents is required. It is possible to test hemolyzed, lipemic, or icteric samples, and the enhanced sensitivity makes detecting weak alloantibodies easier. Also, the Immucor Capture technology includes a LISS reagent that changes color when serum or plasma is added; this safety feature ensures that the patient sample is added to the test system when manual testing is performed.

The major disadvantage of SPRCA is the need for specialized equipment—a microplate centrifuge, a 37°C incubator for microplates, and a light source for reading the final results. In addition, the increased sensitivity may also be a disadvantage since SPRCA may detect weak autoantibodies that other systems miss.

Automation

Full automation of the solid-phase technology is available from Immucor using an FDA-cleared, walk-away instrument called Galileo Echo™[19] (Fig. 12–12). Echo™ is the third-generation instrument for automating the Capture solid-phase technology. Echo™ can be continuously loaded and unloaded and can hold 20 samples, 16 reagents, and 32 microstrips. The tests that are available on Echo™ include ABO/Rh type, donor confirmation–ABO retype, weak D, RBC phenotype, antibody screen (three-cell), antibody identification (three panels), DAT (IgG only), and an IgG crossmatch. Echo™ provides multiple quality control features, including bar-code readers to ensure proper identification of samples and reagents, liquid level sensors, clot detectors, controlled temperature settings, and incubation timers. A fourth-generation instrument called Galileo Neo is currently awaiting FDA clearance.[20] This instrument will allow 224 samples to be loaded at once.

Solid-Phase Protein A Technology

History

In 1992, Biotest AG developed a test in Europe for detecting IgG antibodies, using microplate wells that are coated with protein A. Protein A is a component of the cell wall of *Staphylococcus aureus* that has a very high affinity for the Fc portion of most immunoglobulin classes.[21] In 2005, the FDA approved the distribution of the Solidscreen II assay in the United States, and in 2010, Bio-Rad Laboratories acquired this test from Biotest AG. Solidscreen II and the automated equipment for performing the assay, TANGO™ optimo, are currently available from Bio-Rad Laboratories.

Applications

Solidscreen II is an assay that uses traditional antiglobulin technique to detect and identify red cell antibodies, perform compatibility tests, detect IgG on patients' red blood cells, and type red cells for weak D and partial D antigens (DVI and DVII).[22]

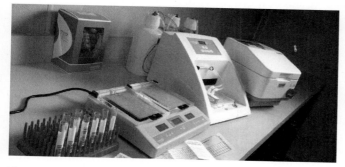

Figure 12–11. Equipment for manual SPRCA technology. *(Courtesy of Immucor, Norcross, Georgia.)*

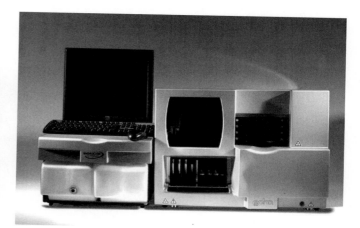

Figure 12–12. Galileo Echo™ instrument. *(Courtesy of Immucor, Norcross, Georgia.)*

Principle

The Solidscreen II assay is performed in the automated TANGO™ optimo[23] (Fig. 12–13). To perform the indirect test, 50 μL of patient serum or plasma, typing serum, or control reagents is combined in a microwell with a 1% suspension of reagent red blood cells (antibody screen and identification), patient or donor cells (antigen typing), or donor red cells (crossmatch), depending on which test is being performed. A low ionic strength solution (MLB 2) is added to the microwells. The contents of the microwell are mixed and allowed to incubate at 37°C.

For the direct test, a 1% suspension of the unknown red blood cells is prepared, but no incubation is required. For both direct and indirect tests, the mixture is then centrifuged, the supernatant is aspirated, and the microwell is washed with phosphate buffered saline (PBS). Next, 100 μL of anti-IgG anti-human globulin (AHG) is added. The microwell is remixed and centrifuged. Any antibodies attached to the red blood cells are captured by protein A on the microwell's surface and form a **homogeneous** layer on the bottom of the microwell (positive reaction). If no antibodies are attached to the RBCs, a compact red blood cell button is formed in the center of the well (negative reaction). The reaction patterns are recorded as a digital image and interpreted by the TANGO™ optimo, using decision logic programmed into the instrument. Positive and negative controls are performed each day before testing, whenever reagents are changed, or after service or repair of the TANGO™ optimo. Figure 12–14 illustrates the Solidscreen II test principle.

Advantages and Disadvantages

The Solidscreen II assay provides a standardized method for performing antiglobulin testing using a unique solid-phase capture method. A study by Heintz and colleagues showed that the detection of **clinically significant** antibodies by TANGO™ optimo was similar to Capture-R Ready-Screen.[24] Because the assay uses microwells that are coated with protein A, the microplates have a long product and onboard shelf-life. The assay uses intact red cells as opposed to red cell fragments that are used in other solid-phase methods. Also, the TANGO™ optimo captures a high-resolution digital image of the endpoint that the user can review and store. The TANGO™ optimo interprets all results as positive or negative and grades the reaction strength on a scale of 0 to 4+. This is an advantage in antibody identification where the strength of a reaction may offer clues to dosage or an antibody mixture.

In the United States, the TANGO™ optimo is not cleared by the FDA to test enzyme-treated or frozen or deglycerolized cells, although such cells can be used outside the United States. Finally, the Solidscreen II assay is FDA licensed only for use with anti-IgG reagent, and it does not detect complement-coated cells as a positive result. Outside the United States, both polyspecific AHG and anti-IgG are available for use on the TANGO™ optimo.

Automation

Solid-phase protein A testing is available only in the United States as an automated technology on the TANGO™ optimo instrument. Although many of the TANGO™ reagents used for antibody detection and identification can be used off-line in traditional tube tests, there is no manual Solidscreen II method to use as a backup in the United States. Outside the United States, a manual workstation is available for use with the Solidscreen II method.

Solid-Phase Enzyme-Linked Immunosorbent Assay (ELISA)

History

In 1994, GTi Diagnostics (acquired by Gen-Probe in 2011 and now known as Gen-Probe GTi Diagnostics) developed an ELISA assay to test for antibodies to platelet glycoproteins. By using separate microwells for each glycoprotein, it was possible to identify antibodies to specific platelet glycoproteins. The first assay to be developed, PAK1, detects antibodies such as anti-HPA-1a that react with platelet antigens that occur on glycoprotein IIb/IIIa. This assay was followed by PAK2 that detects antibodies to antigens on platelet glycoproteins IIb/IIIa, Ia/IIa, Ib/IX, IV, and class I HLA. Also, PAK1 and PAK2 have been combined into a single assay called PAKPLUS®. Other variations of the original two ELISA-based assays followed, including PAK12 and PAK2-LE.

In addition, Gen-Probe GTi Diagnostics has developed ELISA assays to detect and identify HLA (human leukocyte antigen) antibodies (both class I and class II). They have also developed a new Luminex-based assay for platelet and HLA antibodies. Luminex is a bead-based assay that uses fluorescence and flow cytometry to achieve a high level of sensitivity. The Luminex assay uses a mixture of up to 100 different colored beads; each bead is coated with a different protein. The flow cytometer distinguishes between each of the 100 beads by the amount and color of the internal dyes. This simple assay will make it possible for high-complexity laboratories to identify multiple antibodies with a single assay.

Applications

The solid-phase ELISA assay is used by Gen-Probe GTi Diagnostics in two product lines, MACE® (MACE1 and MACE2) and PAK® (PAK1, PAK2-LE, PAK12, PAK12G, and PAKPLUS®), to screen and identify platelet antibodies.[25]

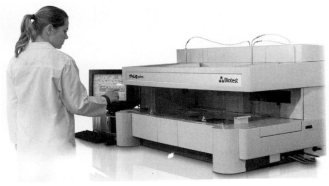

Figure 12–13. TANGO™ optimo instrument. *(Courtesy of Bio-Rad Laboratories, Hercules, California.)*

Solidscreen II test principle

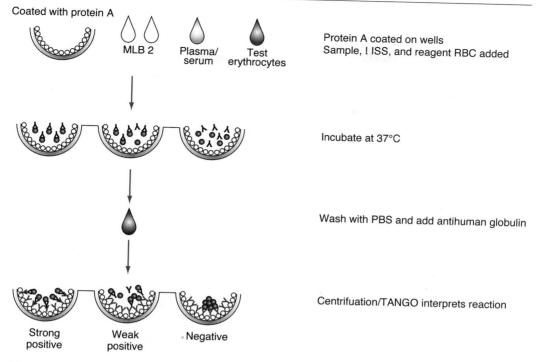

Coated with protein A

MLB 2
Plasma/serum
Test erythrocytes

Protein A coated on wells
Sample, LISS, and reagent RBC added

Incubate at 37°C

Wash with PBS and add antihuman globulin

Centrifuation/TANGO interprets reaction

Strong positive   Weak positive   Negative

Figure 12–14.   Solidscreen II test procedure. *(Courtesy of Bio-Rad Laboratories, Hercules, California.)*

The MACE® products provide well-characterized **monoclonal** antibodies immobilized in microwells that are used to capture glycoproteins from platelets supplied by the user.[26] The MACE® products allow a user to detect and differentiate between antibodies that bind to platelet-specific glycoproteins (IIb/IIIa, Ib/IX, Ia/IIa, and IV) and class I HLA. The MACE® kits provide a test that can be used for either antibody identification, if previously typed platelets are used, or a platelet crossmatch, if potential donor platelets are used.

The PAK® products provide well-characterized platelet glycoproteins that are either immobilized directly or captured by monoclonal antibodies to wells of a microwell plate.[27] The available formats allow a user to detect and differentiate between antibodies that bind to platelet-specific glycoproteins (IIb/IIIa, Ib/IX, Ia/IIa, and IV) and class I HLA.

PAKAUTO® is designed to detect platelet autoantibodies eluted from a patient's platelets using **elution** methods already well established in the blood bank. An elution is first performed on washed patient platelets. The **eluate** and a serum sample are tested side by side against the platelet glycoproteins Ib/IX, Ia/IIa, and IIb/IIIa, which are individually presented in different wells of the ELISA assay. Unlike the PAIgG assay (flow assay using intact platelets), which detects all antibodies bound to a platelet's surface, PAKAUTO® detects only platelet-specific autoantibodies. This is useful in the diagnosis of autoimmune thrombocytopenic purpura (AITP).

Principle

The solid-phase ELISA test (MACE®) is used primarily for compatibility testing.[26] To perform MACE® tests, patient serum or plasma is incubated with intact platelets to allow antibody, if present, to bind to the platelet glycoproteins. Unbound antibodies are washed from the platelets, and the antibody-sensitized platelets are solubilized by the addition of a lysis buffer that contains a nonionic detergent. Next, the platelet **lysate** containing soluble glycoproteins is transferred to the microwells. This allows the platelet glycoproteins (sensitized or unsensitized with patient antibody) to be captured by immobilized monoclonal antibodies. Control samples are handled similarly. After a brief incubation, unbound glycoproteins are washed away. An alkaline phosphatase labeled AHG reagent (anti-IgG) is added to the wells and incubated. The unbound anti-IgG is washed away, and the substrate PNPP (p-nitrophenyl phosphate) is added.

Next, a 30-minute incubation period allows the conjugated anti-IgG to produce a color change in the substrate. After the incubation period, the reaction is stopped by a sodium hydroxide solution. The optical density of the color that develops is measured in a spectrophotometer at 405 or 410 nm using a reference filter of 490 nm. A positive result indicates the presence of glycoprotein-specific antibody in the patient's plasma. The amount of color change (strength of the reaction) depends on the amount of conjugated anti-IgG that was bound to the platelets, which depends on the amount of antibody in the patient's serum.

The solid-phase ELISA test (PAK®) is used to detect and differentiate between antibodies that bind to platelet-specific glycoproteins (IIb/IIIa, Ib/IX, Ia/IIa, and IV) and class I HLA.[27] (PAK® tests may be used to test for alloantibody in patient's serum or autoantibody on patent's autologous platelets.) To perform PAK® tests, patient serum or plasma is added to microwells that are coated with platelet glycoproteins, allowing antibody, if present, to bind. Unbound antibodies are then washed away. Then, similar to the procedure described above, an alkaline phosphatase labeled AHG reagent (anti-IgG/A/M) is added to the wells and incubated. The unbound AHG reagent is washed away and the substrate PNPP (p-nitrophenyl phosphate) is added. After a 30-minute incubation period, the reaction is stopped by a sodium hydroxide solution. Finally, the optical density of the color that develops is measured in a spectrophotometer. Figure 12–15 illustrates the results of an antibody test on two samples, as well as a positive and negative control. Sample 1 reacts with platelet alloantigen HPA-5b/5b, suggesting the sample contains antibody to HPA-5b antigens. Sample 2 reacts with HLA class I antigens.

Advantages and Disadvantages

The solid-phase ELISA (MACE® and PAK®) technology is more complex than some assays performed in the blood bank. An assay takes approximately 2 hours to perform; however, ELISA is a well-established mainstay in the immunology laboratory that provides increased sensitivity and specificity. These commercially available assays make it possible to characterize and quantify platelet antibodies.

Specialized laboratory equipment that is needed to perform ELISA solid-phase testing includes adjustable micropipettes to deliver 10 to 100 μL and 100 to 1,000 μL and disposable tips, a microplate reader capable of measuring optical density (OD) at 405 or 410 and 490 nm, a microplate washer, a 37°C waterbath or incubator and a microcentrifuge for centrifuging patient samples.

Automation

Currently, no dedicated automation is available for the Gen-Probe GTi solid-phase ELISA assays, although some

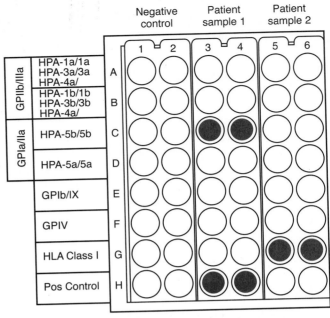

Figure 12–15.   Illustration of PAKPLUS® assay showing patient sample 1 with anti-HPA-5b pattern and patient sample 2 with anti-HLA class I pattern. *(Courtesy of GTi Diagnostics, Waukesha, Wisconsin.)*

laboratories have incorporated automation for portions of the assay, such as sample handling and plate washing.

Comparison of Gel and SPRCA Technologies

This section compares the gel and SPRCA technologies in terms of equipment, procedures, test reactions, sensitivity, specificity, quality control, and automation. Table 12–1 compares the procedural steps of the two technologies, and Table 12–2 compares the features of the two technologies for routine blood bank testing.

Table 12–1	**Procedural Steps of Gel and Solid-Phase Red Cell Adherence Technologies**		
PROCEDURAL STEPS	**GEL TEST**	**SOLID-PHASE RED CELL ADHERENCE TEST**	
	ID-MTS	**Capture-R Select**	**Capture-R Ready Screen, Capture-R Ready-ID**
1. Add RBCs to wells or tubes	Yes	Yes	N/A
2. Centrifuge plate to form monolayer	N/A	Yes	N/A
3. Wash away unbound RBCs	N/A	Yes	N/A
4. Add test serum or plasma	Yes	Yes	Yes
5. Incubation	15 min	15 min	15 min
6. Wash cycle	N/A	Yes	Yes
7. Add indicator cells	N/A	Yes	Yes
8. Centrifuge	10 min	2 min	2 min

Capture solid-phase; ID-MTS gel test; RBC = red blood cells; N/A = not applicable.

Table 12–2   Comparison of Features of the Gel and SPRCA Techniques

TESTS AND FEATURES	ID-MTS	CAPTURE
ABO forward	Yes	Yes
ABO reverse	Yes	Yes
Rh	Yes	Yes
Antibody screen	Yes	Yes
Antibody identification	Yes	Yes
Crossmatch	Yes	Yes
Direct antiglobulin test	No C3d detection	No C3d detection
Autocontrol (IgG)	Yes	Yes
Washing required	No	Yes
pH of wash critical	N/A	Yes
Centrifugation critical	Yes	Yes
Detects:	IgG and IgM	IgG
Media	LISS	LISS Enzyme DTT
Incubation time	15 min	15 min
Minimum tests	6	8
Sensitivity (antibodies detected)	↑ LISS (tube) Gel ↓ SPRCA	↑ LISS (tube) SPRCA ↑ gel
Specificity		
Clinically significant antibodies Insignificant/nonspecific antibodies	Similar to SPRCA Gel ↓ SPRCA	Similar to gel SPRCA ↑ gel
Stability	Yes (2 to 3 days)	Yes (2 days)
Standardized reproducible results	Yes	Yes
Quantitation of reactions	Neg, 1+ to 4+ Mixed-field	Neg, 1+ to 4+ No mixed-field
Quality control	Daily QC	LISS color change +s, +w & neg controls
Safety increased over tubes?	Yes	Yes
Hazardous waste decreased?	Yes	Yes
Special equipment needed?	Yes	Yes
Automation (FDA approved)	Yes ORTHO ProVue	Yes Galileo Echo

DTT = dithiothreitol; IgG = immunoglobulin G; IgM = immunoglobulin M; N/A = not applicable; ↑ = increased; ↓ = decreased; LISS = low ionic strength saline; neg = negative control; SPRCA = solid-phase red cell adherence; +s = strong positive control; +w = weak positive control.

Equipment

The gel technology requires a special incubator and a centrifuge that accommodates the cards. The solid-phase technology requires a centrifuge that can spin microplates, a 37°C incubator for microplates, and a light source for reading the final results. Automated and semiautomated equipment, approved by the FDA, is currently available for both the gel and solid-phase technologies.

Both technologies improve safety and decrease hazardous waste, because using plastic eliminates the danger associated with broken glass, and miniaturized reaction chambers reduce the quantity of hazardous waste.

Test Reactions and Procedures

Both technologies provide stable, reproducible endpoints. The gel test uses a special pipette to precisely measure the quantity of test cells and sera, whereas the solid-phase technology uses conventional drops of cells and sera. By standardizing the reactants in the assay and eliminating variation in the tube-shaking technique, both technologies eliminate the subjectivity associated with interpreting the endpoint of test tube agglutination tests.

The gel test is read as 4+, 3+, 2+, 1+, mixed-field (mf), or negative, and it is based on agglutination reactions. The ease of quantitating reactions with the gel test is an advantage when evaluating an antibody identification for multiple antibodies or dosage effects, whereas the solid-phase assays are read as weak positive, positive, or negative.

Mixed-field agglutination produces a characteristic pattern in the gel technology. In this technology, the agglutinated population of RBCs is trapped in the gel, and the unagglutinated population is pelleted at the bottom of the microtube following centrifugation. The ability to recognize mixed-field reactions is particularly valuable in evaluating a possible transfusion reaction or evaluating the survival of a minor population of transfused cells.

The endpoints of both technologies are stable, and they can be read 2 to 3 days after the test is performed. Such stability is a distinct advantage when less experienced technologists are cross-trained to work in the transfusion service. Whenever the interpretation of an assay is uncertain, the test results can be retained until a supervisor can review them.

The procedures for both technologies parallel steps performed in routine blood bank tube testing, including pipetting, incubating, spinning, and reading. The washing cycle step has been eliminated with the gel technology. The endpoint of both assays detects IgG, and it is possible to perform an **autocontrol** to detect IgG-coated cells; however, an autocontrol cannot be substituted for a DAT because neither of the technologies detects C3d complement–coated cells.

Sensitivity and Specificity

Before gel and SPRCA were licensed by the FDA for use in the United States, studies were performed to show that the new technologies were as effective in detecting antibodies as traditional test tube methods.

Ideally, a technique should detect antibodies that are considered clinically significant and should avoid detecting antibodies that are considered clinically insignificant, such as benign autoantibodies and cold agglutinins. Studies have shown that although these technologies are both LISS-based, they are both more sensitive than LISS test tube technique.[28] Also, differences in sensitivity have been reported when gel is compared with SPRCA. Ramsey and colleagues reported that SPRCA was more sensitive than gel for detecting RBC alloantibodies, particularly for detecting antenatal RhIg in Rh-negative mothers. However, he also reported that SPRCA had a higher rate of nonspecific reactions.[29] These conclusions were confirmed by Garozzo and coworkers[30] and Yamada and others.[31]

Because these assays are designed to detect IgG, they avoid detecting clinically insignificant **IgM** antibodies such as cold agglutinins. However, they may fail to detect clinically significant IgM antibodies that are forming during a primary immune response. The gel technique detects IgM antibodies when incompatible cells form a lattice in the reaction chamber and are trapped at the top of the gel during centrifugation. Increased sensitivity is an advantage when a weak, clinically significant antibody is present, but it is a disadvantage when weak autoantibodies are present.

Finally, the question of specificity is complex. Both of the technologies demonstrated the ability to detect the majority of clinically significant antibodies before they were licensed by the FDA; however, there are many isolated reports of method-dependent antibodies that are only demonstrable by one technique. Combs and coworkers reported missing eleven antibodies in nine patients (three anti-K, two anti-c, two anti-E, two anti-Fy^a, one anti-D, and one anti-Jk^a) using the gel technique.[32] Callahan and colleagues reported a severe transfusion reaction caused by anti-Jk^b that was only demonstrable by SPRCA.[33] Barker and coworkers reported a delayed transfusion reaction caused by anti-Fy^a that was not detected in the pretransfusion sample by LISS, **PEG**, or gel tests.[34] The post-transfusion sample demonstrated anti-Fy^a using only PEG-AHG technique; LISS-AHG and gel were negative. In a review article by Casina that compared antibody screening methods, he concluded that there is no one method that will detect all clinically important antibodies.[35]

Quality Control

In addition to routine quality control (QC) for the 37°C incubator, centrifuge, pipette tips, and pipette dispenser used in testing, the new technologies have other QC features. The gel test uses special dispensers to prepare the RBC suspensions and special pipettes to add a measured volume of plasma or serum and RBCs. Each lot number of cards and diluent should be tested on the day of use to confirm that the test cards and the diluted reagent RBCs are reacting as expected. The manufacturer of the solid-phase technology recommends including a positive and a negative control with each batch of tests. In addition, the LISS used in the solid-phase system is formulated to detect the addition of serum or plasma by a color change from purple to blue when plasma is added. This feature protects the user from failing to add plasma to a well during manual testing.

SUMMARY CHART

- ✔ Advantages of gel and solid-phase technologies over routine tube testing are:
  - Standardization: There is no tube shaking or resuspension of an RBC button to cause subjectivity in the interpretation of the test.
  - Stability: There are well-defined endpoints of the reaction.
  - Decreased sample volume needed for testing
  - Enhanced sensitivity and specificity
- ✔ Gel test points to remember:
  - The principle of the gel test is hemagglutination.
  - In the gel test, RBCs and serum or plasma are allowed to incubate together in a reaction chamber.
  - Following incubation, controlled centrifugation drives the RBCs through a specially designed microtube filled with beads of dextran-acrylamide gel.
  - Agglutinated cells remain at the top of the tube or are trapped in the gel, depending on the size of the agglutinates.
  - Unagglutinated cells move through the gel to the bottom of the tube.
  - The gel test reactions are stable for observation or review for 2 to 3 days.
  - Gel technology is currently approved for ABO forward and reverse grouping, Rh typing, DAT, antibody screening, antibody identification, and compatibility testing.
  - The major disadvantage of the gel technology is the need to purchase special equipment: a centrifuge to accommodate the microtube cards used for testing and a pipette for dispensing plasma or serum and RBC suspensions into the reaction chambers of the microtubes.
- ✔ SPRCA assay points to remember:
  - The principle of SPRCA is based on solid-phase technology.
  - In SPRCA tests, the target antigen is affixed to the bottom of the microplate wells.
  - If the test plasma contains antibodies to the antigen, they attach to the fixed antigen, and indicator cells detect the attached antibodies by forming a monolayer of RBCs.
  - If the test plasma contains no antibodies to the antigen, there is no attachment to the fixed antigen, and the indicator cells form a clearly delineated button at the center of the microplate well.
  - Solid-phase reactions are stable for observation or review for 2 days.

- Solid-phase technology is currently approved for antibody screening, antibody identification, and compatibility testing.
- Advantages of solid-phase technology include the ease of use, because no predilution of reagents is required, and the ability to test hemolyzed, lipemic, or icteric samples. Enhanced sensitivity increases the detection of weak alloantibodies.
- The major disadvantage of solid-phase technology is the need to purchase special equipment: a centrifuge that can spin microplates, a 37°C incubator for microplates, and a light source for reading the final results.
- ✔ Solid-phase protein A technology points to remember:
  - IgG antibodies are captured in microwells that are coated with protein A.
  - Solidscreen II, which uses solid-phase protein A technology, is an assay that uses traditional antiglobulin technique.
  - Solid-phase protein A testing is available only in the United States as an automated technology on the TANGO optimo instrument.
- ✔ Solid-phase immunosorbent assay (ELISA) points to remember:
  - The MACE products provide well-characterized monoclonal antibodies immobilized in microwells that are used to capture glycoproteins from platelets supplied by the user.
  - MACE is used primarily for compatibility testing.
  - The PAK products provide well-characterized platelet glycoproteins that are either immobilized directly or captured by monoclonal antibodies to wells of a microwell plate.
  - PAK is used to detect and differentiate between antibodies that bind to platelet-specific glycoproteins (IIb/IIIa, Ib/IX, Ia/IIa, and IV) and class I HLA, primarily for compatibility testing.
- ✔ Luminex-based assay points to remember:
  - Luminex-based assay is a bead-based assay that uses florescence and flow cytometry to test for platelet/HLA antibodies.
  - Luminex assay uses a mixture of 100 different colored beads, each bead coated with a different protein.
  - The flow cytometer distinguishes between each of the 100 beads by the amount and color of the internal dyes.

Review Questions

1. The endpoint of the gel test is detected by:

a. Agglutination
b. Hemolysis
c. Precipitation
d. Attachment of indicator cells

2. The endpoint of the SPRCA test is detected by:

a. Agglutination
b. Hemolysis
c. Precipitation
d. Attachment of indicator cells

3. The endpoint of the solid-phase protein A assay is:

a. Agglutination
b. Hemolysis
c. Precipitation
d. Attachment of cells to microwell

4. Protein A captures antibodies by binding to:

a. Fab portion of immunoglobulin
b. Fc portion of immunoglobulin
c. Surface of test cells
d. Surface of indicator cells

5. The endpoint of the solid-phase immunosorbent assay (ELISA) is:

a. Agglutination
b. Hemolysis
c. Color change in the substrate
d. Attachment of indicator cells

6. Mixed-field reactions can be observed in:

a. Gel
b. SPRCA
c. Protein A technology
d. Luminex

7. The endpoint of the luminex assay is change of:

a. Electrical charge on the RBCs
b. Color of the liquid substrate
c. Color of indicator on beads
d. Density of the indicator substrate

8. An advantage for both gel and solid-phase technology is:

a. No cell washing steps
b. Standardization
c. Use of IgG-coated control cells
d. Specialized equipment

9. A disadvantage for both gel and solid-phase technology is:

a. Decreased sensitivity
b. Inability to test hemolyzed, lipemic, or icteric samples
c. Inability to detect C3d complement–coated cells
d. Large sample requirement

10. A safety feature in the SPRCA test is:

a. Air bubble barrier
b. Viscous barrier
c. Color change of the LISS
d. Use of IgG-coated control cells

References

1. Shulman, IA, Maffei, LM, and Downes, KA: North American pretransfusion testing practices, 2001–2004: Results from the College of American Pathologists Interlaboratory Comparison Program survey data, 2001–2004. Arch Path Lab Med 129:984–989, 2005.
2. College of American Pathologists. CAP survey final critique J-B, 2005.
3. Lapierre, Y, Rigal, D, Adams, J, et al: The gel test: A new way to detect red cell antigen-antibody reactions. Transfusion 30:109–113, 1990.
4. ID-Micro Typing System. Question and answer guide. Ortho Diagnostic Systems, Raritan, NJ, 1996.
5. Package insert for MTS buffered gel card. Pompano Beach, FL. Micro Typing Systems, 2008.
6. Package insert for MTS Anti-D (Monoclonal)(IgM) card. Pompano Beach, FL. Micro Typing Systems, 2008.
7. Package insert for MTS Monoclonal Rh phenotype card. Pompano Beach, FL. Micro Typing Systems, 2009.
8. Package insert for MTS Anti-IgG card, Pompano Beach, FL. Micro Typing Systems, 2008.
9. Chan, A, Wong, HF, Chiu, CH, et al: The impact of a gel system on routine work in a general hospital blood bank. Immunohematology 12:30–32, 1996.
10. A new era begins: Introducing ID-MTS, ID-Micro Typing System (product brochure). Ortho Diagnostics Systems, Raritan, NJ, November 1995.
11. Package insert for ID-Tipmaster Repetitive Dispense Pipetor, Pompano Beach, FL. Micro Typing Systems, 2011.
12. Package insert for Biohit/MTS Electronic Pipettor. Biohit, Neptune, NJ. Ortho-Clinical Diagnostics, 2011.
13. Rosenfield, RE, Kochwa, SE, and Kaczera, Z: Solid phase serology for the study of human erythrocyte antigen-antibody reactions. Proceedings, Plenary Session, 25th Congress, International Society Blood Transfusion, Paris, 1978.
14. Plapp, FV, et al: Blood antigens and antibodies: Solid phase adherence assays. Lab Manage 22:39, 1984.
15. Moore, HH: Automated reading of red cell antibody identification tests by a solid phase antiglobulin technique. Transfusion 24:218–221, 1985.
16. Capture (solid phase technology). Product brochure, Immucor, Norcross, GA, 2009.
17. Capture (solid phase technology). Package insert for Capture-R Ready-ID Extend I & II. Immucor, Norcross, GA, 2008.
18. Rolih, S, et al: Solid phase red cell adherence assays. La Transfusione del Sangue 36:4, 1991.
19. Galileo Echo instrument (solid phase automation). Product brochure, Immucor, Norcross, GA, 2007.
20. Galileo Neo instrument (solid phase automation). Product brochure, Immucor, Norcross, GA, 2010.
21. King, BF, and Wilkinson, BJ: Binding of human immunoglobulin G to protein A in encapsulated Staphylococcus aureus. Infect Immun 33:666–672, 1981.
22. Solidscreen II (solid phase protein A technology), package insert, Biotest AG, 2008.

23. TANGO optimo instrument (solid phase protein A automation), product brochure, Biotest AG, 2009.
24. Heintz, M, Bahl, M, Mann, J, Yohannes, M, and Levitt, J: Evaluation of blood group antisera and antibody screening with the TANGO™ automated blood bank analyzer. Transfusion 44:125A, 2004.
25. ELISA products designed to detect antibodies reactive with platelet glycoproteins. Product brochure, GTI Diagnostics, Waukesha, WI, 2006.
26. MACE1. Package insert, GTI Diagnostics, Waukesha, WI, 2008.
27. PAK1. Package insert, GTI Diagnostics, Waukesha, WI, 2007.
28. Weisbach, V, Kohnhäuser, T, Zimmermann, R, et al: Comparison of the performance of microtube column systems and solid-phase systems and the tube low-ionic-strength solution additive indirect antiglobulin test in the detection of red cell alloantibodies. Trans Med 16:276–284, 2006.
29. Ramsey, G, Sumugod, RD, Garland, FD, et al: Automated solid-phase RBC antibody screening in a transfusion service. Transfusion 45:123A, 2005.
30. Garozzo, G, Licitra, V, Criscione, R, et al: A comparison of two automated methods for the detection and identification of red blood cell alloantibodies. Blood Transfus 5:33–40, 2007.
31. Yamada, C, Serrano-Rahman, L, Vasovic, LV, et al: Antibody identification using both automated solid-phase red cell adherence assay and a tube polyethylene glycol antiglobulin method. Transfusion 48:1693–1698, 2008.
32. Combs, MR, and Bredehoeft, SJ: Selecting an acceptable and safe antibody detection test can present a dilemma. Immunohematol 17:86–89, 2001.
33. Callahan, DL, Kennedy, MS, Ranalli, MA, et al: Delayed hemolytic transfusion reaction caused by Jk^b antibody detected by only solid phase technique. Transfusion 40:113S, 2000.
34. Barker, JM, Scillian, J, Spindler, BJ, and Cruz, MC: A delayed transfusion reaction due to anti-Fy^a not detected by LISS-tube or gel techniques. Transfusion 44:119A, 2004.
35. Casina, TS: In search of the holy grail: Comparison of antibody screening methods. Immunohematol 22:196–202, 2006.

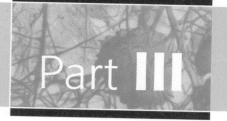

Donor Screening and Component Preparation

Patricia A. Wright, BA, MT(ASCP)SBB, and Virginia C. Hughes, PhD(ABD), MT(ASCP)SBB, CLS(NCA)I

OBJECTIVES

1. Identify the organizations that regulate or accredit the immunohematology laboratory.
2. State the minimum acceptable levels for the following tests in allogeneic and autologous donation:
   - Weight
   - Temperature
   - Pulse

Continued

OBJECTIVES—cont'd

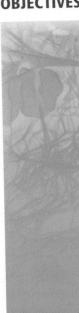

- Blood pressure
- Hemoglobin
- Hematocrit

3. Differentiate between acceptable donation and permanent deferral given various medical conditions.
4. Differentiate among the four different types of autologous donations.
5. Describe the procedure for a whole blood donation, including arm preparation, blood collection, and postphlebotomy care instructions for the donor.
6. Differentiate among mild, moderate, and severe donor reactions and list recommended treatments for each.
7. List the tests required for allogeneic, autologous, and apheresis donation.
8. State the acceptable interval of donation for allogeneic donors.
9. State the acceptable interval of donation for apheresis donors.
10. List the labeling criteria for a unit of allogeneic and autologous blood.
11. Identify the storage conditions, shelf life, quality-control requirements, and indications for use for the following:
    - Whole blood
    - Red blood cells, including irradiated, leukoreduced, and saline washed
    - Random and apheresis platelets, including irradiated, leukoreduced, and washed
    - Pooled random platelets
    - Frozen, deglycerolized RBCs
    - Fresh frozen plasma and plasma frozen within 24 hours
    - Liquid plasma
    - Cryoprecipitate and pre-pooled cryoprecipitate
    - Granulocyte concentrates
    - Factor concentrates, including activated factor VII, VIII, IX, and XIII concentrates
    - $Rh_o(D)$ immunoglobulin
    - Normal serum albumin
    - Immune serum globulin
    - Plasma protein fraction
    - Antithrombin III concentrates

Introduction

The selection of potential blood donors and the subsequent collection and processing of those donor units are the first stages of the blood banking process that eventually lead to the transfusion of lifesaving blood products to a patient.

Governing Agencies

Guidelines and regulations for these initial processes have long been established by several organizations or agencies.

U.S. Food and Drug Administration

The U.S. Food and Drug Administration (FDA) is a regulating agency. Its regulations for donor screening are outlined in the *Code of Federal Regulations (CFR)*, parts 211, 600–799. Under the auspices of the FDA, blood is regarded both as a biologic and a drug. In 1988, the Center for Biologics Evaluation and Research (CBER) was formed. CBER is responsible for regulating the collection of blood and blood components used for transfusion and for the manufacture of pharmaceuticals derived from blood and blood components. CBER develops and enforces quality standards; inspects blood establishments; and monitors reports of errors, accidents, and adverse clinical events. In the early 1990s, the FDA began to treat blood establishments the same as any drug manufacturer, requiring strict compliance toward all aspects of transfusion medicine, including donor selection and screening. In addition, they establish and maintain the regulations and inspect blood-collection and processing centers. The FDA is also responsible for licensing the collection and processing facilities, the blood products and derivatives, and the reagents used in the processing and testing of those products. (See Chapter 25, "Transfusion Safety and Federal Regulatory Requirements.")

AABB

The AABB, formerly known as the American Association of Blood Banks, was established in 1947. It is an international association of blood centers, transfusion and transplantation services, and individuals involved in transfusion medicine. It provides a voluntary inspection and accreditation program for its member institutions that meets the requirements of CMS (Centers for Medicare and Medicaid Services) and the CLIA '88 (Clinical Laboratory Improvement Amendments of 1988). The mission of the AABB is to establish and provide the highest standard of care for patients and donors in all aspects of transfusion medicine. The AABB has published books on transfusion medicine throughout its existence; two resources that are vital to donor screening procedures are *AABB Standards for Blood Banks and Transfusion Services* and *AABB Technical Manual*. The specific guidelines for donor screening and component preparation are discussed in these publications and will be referred to throughout this chapter.

College of American Pathologists

The College of American Pathologists (CAP) also provides a voluntary inspection and accreditation program for its member institutions. Since most transfusion services are part of the clinical laboratory departments in a hospital, they are included in a CAP inspection. As with the AABB inspections, CAP inspections are approved by CMS and meet the CLIA requirements.

Donor Screening

Donor screening encompasses the medical history requirements for the donor, the (mini) physical examination, and serologic testing of the donor blood. Any one of these areas may preclude a potential donor from the donation process. The medical history information and physical examination are designed to answer two questions: (1) Will a donation of approximately 450 mL of whole blood at this time be harmful to the donor? (2) Could blood drawn from this donor at this time potentially transmit a disease to the recipient?

Registration

As outlined in *AABB Standards*, blood collection facilities must confirm donor identity and link the donor to existing donor records.[1] Most facilities require a photographic identification such as a driver's license, passport, or school identification card. In addition, to prevent an ineligible donor from donating again, every donor must be checked against a permanent record of previously deferred donors.[2] The following is a list of information used by the collection facility in the registration process and is kept on record as a single donation record form (Fig. 13–1) or electronically:

- **Name (first, last, MI)**
- **Date and time of donation**
- **Address**
- **Telephone**
- **Gender**
- **Age or date of birth:** The minimum age for an allogeneic donation is between 16 and 17 years, depending on individual state requirements (see applicable state laws). There is no upper age limit. For **autologous** donation (donating blood to be used for oneself), there is no age

restriction; however, each donor-patient must be evaluated by the blood bank medical director.
- **Consent to donate:** Donors should be informed of the procedure for donating blood and its potential risks. They must also be given educational materials informing them of the signs and symptoms associated with HIV (human immunodeficiency virus) infection and AIDS (acquired immune deficiency syndrome), behaviors that put them at high risk of infection, and a caution not to donate blood as a means of getting an HIV test. At some point in the interview process, donors must sign a statement documenting that they have given consent to the donation. This is typically done at the end of the donor history questionnaire. (Blood donor education materials are shown in Fig. 13–2.)
- **Additional information:** The following additional information may be helpful in some cases:
  - The name of the patient for whom the blood is intended (directed donation)
  - Race of the donor for unique phenotypes
  - Cytomegalovirus (CMV) status (some patient groups, such as neonates, require CMV-negative blood in certain circumstances)

Medical History Questionnaire

Obtaining an accurate medical history of the donor is essential to ensure protection of the donor and benefit to the recipient. A standardized medical history questionnaire was developed by a task force that included representatives from the AABB, the FDA, and the blood and plasma industry (Fig. 13–3). The questionnaire was designed to be self-administered by the donor but if preferred may be administered by a trained donor historian.[3] Self-administered questionnaires must be reviewed by trained personnel before completing the screening process and prior to collecting blood. The interviewer should be familiar with the questions, and the interview should be conducted in a secluded area of the blood center or donor site. The questions are designed so that a simple "yes" or "no" can be answered but elaborated if indicated. The medical history is conducted on the same day as the donation. The currently approved version of the Donor History Questionnaire (DHQ) can be downloaded from the FDA website.

Medical History Questions

The following is a summary of the DHQ questions with elaboration and explanation. For more in-depth information on the questionnaire and interpretations of the questions, please refer to the AABB *Technical Manual* and the FDA website.

- **Are you feeling healthy and well today?** Donors should appear to be in good health without obvious signs or symptoms of colds, flu, or other illness.
- **Are you currently taking an antibiotic or taking any other medication for an infection?** Donors currently taking antibiotics for an infection or for **prophylaxis** after

Text continued on page 296

JAN 2003

SINGLE DONATION RECORD

Community Blood Centers

Location:

4039 West Newberry Road · Gainesville, Florida 32607 · (352) 334-1000

SEX:	ETHNIC:	STUDENT:	NEW CARD:	DATE DRAWN:

CALL OK?	BIRTH DATE:	# PREV. DONATIONS:	PREVIOUS REACTION:

CALL STATUS:	HLA TYPING:

CALL OK?	HLA TYPING DATE:	LAST DONATION DATE:

CREDIT FOR:

COMMENTS:

REMARKS:

DEFERRAL INFO:	NUMBER	NEXT DONATION DATE:	INITIALS:
DEFERRAL ◯ PD ◯			

LAB ONLY

POSITIVE ANTIBODIES:

POSITIVE ANTIGENS:

NEGATIVE ANTIGENS:

ABO Prescreening (First Time Donor)

ABO SLIDE TYPE:	PER DONOR TYPE:	INITIALS:
◯ 0 ◯ 1	◯ A ◯ B	
◯ 2 ◯ 1,2	◯ O ◯ AB	

Collection Information

Donor Reaction: ◯ Type 1   ◯ Type 2   ◯ Type 3

◯ Apheresis RBC Loss (if > 50ml):   mL

◯ Enter/Remove Donor Comment:

DRAWN UNIT INFORMATION

◯ QNS <= 50 mL   ◯ QNS > 50 mL   ◯ Long Draw Discard

◯ Low Volume   ◯ Overdraw   ◯ Air Contaminated

First Stick Information

BAG INFO: ◯ ASA	BAG LOT NUMBER:	BAG EXPIRATION:

BAG TYPE:		SCALE NUMBER:
CPDA-1: ◯	1 ◯	
Additive: ◯	2 ◯	◯ Fenwal ◯ Donormatic
ACD-A: ◯	3 ◯	VENIPUNCTURE: START TIME:
_____ ◯	4 ◯	
	5 ◯	DISCONNECT: END TIME:

FRONT DESK	COMMENTS:	AMOUNT DRAWN:
		mL

CRBCIS Lab Information

CMV:	CMV DATE:	BLOOD TYPE:	FIRST UNIT NUMBER

LAB CMV:	INITIALS	LAB TYPE	INITIALS

Second Stick Information

BAG INFO: ◯ ASA	BAG LOT NUMBER:	BAG EXPIRATION:

BAG TYPE:		SCALE NUMBER:
CPDA-1: ◯	1 ◯	
Additive: ◯	2 ◯	◯ Fenwal ◯ Donormatic
ACD-A: ◯	3 ◯	VENIPUNCTURE: START TIME:
_____ ◯	4 ◯	
	5 ◯	DISCONNECT: END TIME:

COMMENTS:	AMOUNT DRAWN:
	mL

SECOND UNIT NUMBER

Figure 13–1.   Single donation record form. *(LifeSouth Blood Center, Montgomery, AL, with permission.)*

Blood Donor Educational Materials:
MAKING YOUR BLOOD DONATION SAFE

Thank you for coming in today! This information sheet explains how **YOU** can help us make the donation process safe for yourself and patients who might receive your blood. **PLEASE READ THIS INFORMATION BEFORE YOU DONATE! If you have any questions now or anytime during the screening process, please ask blood center staff.**

ACCURACY AND HONESTY ARE ESSENTIAL!
Your **complete honesty** in answering all questions is very important for the safety of patients who receive your blood. **All information you provide is confidential.**

DONATION PROCESS:
To determine if you are eligible to donate we will:
- Ask questions about health, travel, and medicines
- Ask questions to see if you might be at risk for hepatitis, HIV, or AIDs
- Take your blood pressure, temperature and pulse
- Take a small blood sample to make sure you are not anemic

If you are able to donate we will:
- Cleanse your arm with an antiseptic. **(If you are allergic to Iodine, please tell us!)**
- Use a new, sterile, disposable needle to collect your blood

DONOR ELIGIBILITY – SPECIFIC INFORMATION
Why we ask questions about sexual contact:
Sexual contact may cause contagious diseases like HIV to get into the bloodstream and be spread through transfusions to someone else.

Definition of "sexual contact":
The words "have sexual contact with" and "sex" are used in some of the questions we will ask you, and apply to <u>any</u> of the activities below, whether or not a condom or other protection was used:
1. Vaginal sex (contact between penis and vagina)
2. Oral sex (mouth or tongue on someone's vagina, penis, or anus)
3. Anal sex (contact between penis and anus)

HIV/AIDS RISK BEHAVIORS AND SYMPTOMS
AIDS is caused by HIV. HIV is spread mainly through sexual contact with an infected person OR by sharing needles or syringes used for injecting drugs.

DO NOT DONATE IF YOU:
- **Have AIDS or have ever had a positive HIV test**
- Have ever used needles to take drugs, steroids, or anything not prescribed by your doctor
- Are a male who has had sexual contact with another male, even once, since 1977
- Have ever taken money, drugs or other payment for sex since 1977
- Have had sexual contact in the past 12 months with anyone described above
- Have had syphilis or gonorrhea in the past 12 months
- In the last 12 months have been in juvenile detention, lockup, jail or prison for more than 72 hours
- Have any of the following conditions that can be signs or symptoms of HIV/AIDS:
  - Unexplained weight loss or night sweats
  - Blue or purple spots in your mouth or skin
  - Swollen lymph nodes for more than one month
  - White spots or unusual sores in your mouth
  - Cough that won't go away or shortness of breath
  - Diarrhea that won't go away
  - Fever of more than 100.5°F for more than 10 days

Remember that you <u>CAN</u> give HIV to someone else through blood transfusions even if you feel well and have a negative HIV test. This is because tests cannot detect infections for a period of time after a person is exposed to HIV. **If you think you may be at risk for HIV/AIDS or want an HIV/AIDS test, please ask for information about other testing facilities.** *PLEASE DO NOT DONATE TO GET AN HIV TEST!*

Travel to or birth in other countries
Blood donor tests may not be available for some contagious diseases that are found only in certain countries. If you were born in, have lived in, or visited certain countries, you may not be eligible to donate.

What happens after your donation:
To protect patients, your blood is tested for hepatitis B and C, HIV, certain other infectious diseases, and syphilis. If your blood tests positive it will not be given to a patient. You will be notified about test results that may disqualify you from donating in the future. **Please do not donate to get tested for HIV, hepatitis, or any other infections!**

Thank you for donating blood today!
(Donor Center Name)
(Telephone Number)

DHQ v. 1.3

eff. May 2008

Figure 13–2. Blood Donor Educational Materials. *(U.S. Food and Drug Administration, "Guidance for industry: Implementation of acceptable full-length Donor History Questionnaire and accompanying materials for use in screening donors of blood and blood components," October 2006.)*

Full-Length Donor History Questionnaire

	YES	NO
Are you		
1. Feeling healthy and well today?		
2. Currently taking an antibiotic?		
3. Currently taking any other medication for an infection?		
Please read the Medication Deferral List.		
4. Are you now taking or have you ever taken any medications on the Medication Deferral List?		
5. Have you read the educational materials?		
In the past 48 hours		
6. Have you taken aspirin or anything that has aspirin in it?		
In the past 6 weeks		
7. Female donors: Have you been pregnant or are you pregnant now? (Males: check "I am male.") I am male ☐		
In the past 8 weeks have you		
8. Donated blood, platelets, or plasma?		
9. Had any vaccinations or other shots?		
10. Had contact with someone who had a smallpox vaccination?		
In the past 16 weeks		
11. Have you donated a double unit of red cells using an apheresis machine?		
In the past 12 months have you		
12. Had a blood transfusion?		
13. Had a transplant such as organ, tissue, or bone marrow?		
14. Had a graft such as bone or skin?		
15. Come into contact with someone else's blood?		
16. Had an accidental needle-stick?		
17. Had sexual contact with anyone who has HIV/AIDS or has had a positive test for the HIV/AIDS virus?		
18. Had sexual contact with a prostitute or anyone else who takes money or drugs or other payment for sex?		
19. Had sexual contact with anyone who has ever used needles to take drugs or steroids, or anything not prescribed by their doctor?		
20. Had sexual contact with anyone who has hemophilia or has used clotting factor concentrates?		
21. Female donors: Had sexual contact with a male who has ever had sexual contact with another male? (Males: check "I am male.") I am male ☐		
22. Had sexual contact with a person who has hepatitis?		
23. Lived with a person who has hepatitis?		
24. Had a tattoo?		
25. Had ear or body piercing?		
26. Had or been treated for syphilis or gonorrhea?		
27. Been in juvenile detention, lockup, jail, or prison for more than 72 hours?		
In the past three years have you		
28. Been outside the United States or Canada?		
From 1980 through 1996,		
29. Did you spend time that adds up to three (3) months or more in the United Kingdom? (Review list of countries in the UK)		
30. Were you a member of the U.S. military, a civilian military employee, or a dependent of a member of the U.S. military?		

Continued

Figure 13–3. Donor History Questionnaire. (*U.S. Food and Drug Administration, "Guidance for industry: Implementation of acceptable full-length Donor History Questionnaire and accompanying materials for use in screening donors of blood and blood components," October 2006.*)

Full-Length Donor History Questionnaire — Continued

	YES	NO
From **1980 to the present,** did you		
31. Spend time that adds up to five (5) years or more in Europe? (Review list of countries in Europe.)		
32. Receive a blood transfusion in the United Kingdom or France? (Review list of countries in the UK.)		
From **1977 to the present,** have you		
33. Received money, drugs, or other payment for sex?		
34. Male donors: had sexual contact with another male, even once?		
(Females: check "I am female.") I am female ☐		
Have you **EVER**		
35. Had a positive test for the HIV/AIDS virus?		
36. Used needles to take drugs, steroids, or anything <u>not</u> prescribed by your doctor?		
37. Used clotting factor concentrates?		
38. Had hepatitis?		
39. Had malaria?		
40. Had Chagas' disease?		
41. Had babesiosis?		
42. Received a dura mater (or brain covering) graft?		
43. Had any type of cancer, including leukemia?		
44. Had any problems with your heart or lungs?		
45. Had a bleeding condition or a blood disease?		
46. Had sexual contact with anyone who was born in or lived in Africa?		
47. Been in Africa?		
48. Have any of your relatives had Creutzfeldt-Jakob disease?		
Use this area for additional questions		

Figure 13–3.   cont'd

dental surgery may be deferred temporarily until the donor has completed the prescribed antibiotic regimen and the infection has cleared up. Donors who have taken tetracyclines or other antibiotics used to treat acne are acceptable for donation. All drugs and medications must be cleared by the blood collection facility or blood bank medical director. If the donor's response is a "yes" the interviewer must investigate further. Types and descriptions of deferrals are listed in Box 13–1.

- **Are you now taking or have you ever taken any medications on the Medication Deferral List** (Fig. 13–4)? The Medication Deferral List was developed along with the DHQ and is recommended to be used in conjunction with the DHQ. It can be found on the FDA website along with other donor history documents. Each facility's medical director is responsible for determining if any other medications require a deferral. Most centers have a predetermined list of medications and their deferral requirements.

- **Have you read the educational materials (see Fig. 13–2)?** Prior to beginning the Donor History Questionnaire, prospective donors must be provided information about the collection procedure and any risks involved. They must also be informed (in a language they can understand) about high-risk behavior related to the AIDS virus and must be given the opportunity to ask questions regarding any aspect of the collection procedure. The donor needs to acknowledge that they have read and understand all of the material. This is generally done by having the donor sign a statement indicating they have read and understand the materials, they have answered the health history questions honestly, and they have been informed of the risks of donation and give their consent to the donation. This meets the requirements for documentation of informed consent.

BOX 13–1

Types of Deferral

Temporary Deferral: Prospective donor is unable to donate blood for a limited period of time.

   EXAMPLE: Donor has received a blood transfusion; defer for 12 months from date of transfusion. Donor received vaccination for yellow fever; defer for 2 weeks from date of vaccination.

Indefinite Deferral: Prospective donor is unable to donate blood for someone else for an unspecified period of time due to current regulatory requirements. This donor would not be able to donate blood until the current requirement changes. These donors may be eligible to donate autologous blood.

   EXAMPLE: Donor states they have lived in England for 1 year in 1989; defer indefinitely.

Permanent Deferral: Prospective donor will never be eligible to donate blood for someone else. These donors may be eligible to donate autologous blood. Some permanent deferrals may result from the testing performed on a previous donation.

   EXAMPLE: Donor states that he or she has hepatitis C; defer permanently.

   From: Donor History Questionnaire user brochure, FDA May 2008. Available at www.fda.gov.

- **In the past 48 hours, have you taken aspirin or anything with aspirin in it?** Donors who have taken piroxicam, aspirin, or anything with aspirin in it within 3 days of donation may not be a suitable donor for platelet pheresis; these medications inhibit platelet function. There is no restriction for whole blood donation.

- **In the past 6 weeks, have you been pregnant or are you pregnant now?** Female donors should be temporarily deferred for 6 weeks following termination of pregnancy. Exceptions can be made by the blood bank medical director for an autologous donation if complications are anticipated at delivery. A first-trimester or second-trimester abortion or miscarriage is not cause for deferral. A 12-month deferral would apply if the woman received a transfusion during her pregnancy.

- **In the past 8 weeks, have you donated blood, platelets, or plasma? In the past 16 weeks, have you donated a double unit of red cells using an apheresis machine?** The time interval between allogeneic whole blood donations is 8 weeks or 56 days. If the prospective donor has participated in an apheresis donation (platelets, leukocytes, granulocytes), at least 48 hours must pass before donating whole blood.[1] (FDA limits plateletpheresis procedures to no more than 24 in a calendar year.) Infrequent plasma apheresis requires a 4-week deferral. The deferral time for a double red cell unit apheresis is 16 weeks due to the additional volume of red cells that are donated.

- **In the past 8 weeks, have you had any vaccinations or other shots? Have you had contact with someone who had a smallpox vaccination?** If a potential donor has received a live attenuated or bacterial vaccine such as measles (rubeola), mumps, oral polio, typhoid, or yellow fever, there is a 2-week deferral; if the donor has received a live attenuated vaccine for German measles (rubella) or chickenpox, there is a 4-week deferral.[1] However, there is no deferral for toxoids or killed or synthetic viral, bacterial, or rickettsial vaccines such as diphtheria, hepatitis A, hepatitis B, influenza, Lyme disease, pneumococcal polysaccharide, polio injection (Salk), anthrax, cholera, pertussis, plague, paratyphoid, rabies, Rocky Mountain spotted fever, tetanus, or typhoid injection, if the donor is symptom-free and afebrile.[2] Deferral for smallpox vaccination is 14 to 21 days or until the scab has fallen off. In addition, donors who have been in close contact with someone who was recently vaccinated are at risk of possible infection as well.[4] The FDA defines *close contact* as exposure to the vaccination site or bandages, clothing, towels, or bedding that have been in contact with the vaccination site. Determine if the donor developed any active *Vaccinia virus* infection symptoms (new rash or skin sores since the time of contact[7]) from the vaccine.

- **In the past 12 months, have you had a blood transfusion; a transplant such as organ, tissue, or bone marrow; or a graft such as bone or skin?** Donors who during the preceding 12 months have received a transfusion of blood or its components or other human tissues (organ, tissue, bone marrow transplant, or bone or skin graft) known to be possible sources of blood-borne pathogens should be

---

MEDICATION DEFERRAL LIST

Please tell us if you are now taking or if you have EVER taken any of these medications:

☐ **Proscar© (finasteride)** – usually given for prostate gland enlargement

☐ **Avodart© (dutasteride)** – usually given for prostate enlargement

☐ **Propecia© (finasteride)** – usually given for baldness

☐ **Accutane© (Amnesteem, Claravis, Sotret, isotretinoin)** – usually given for severe acne

☐ **Soriatane© (acitretin)** – usually given for severe psoriasis

☐ **Tegison© (etretinate)** – usually given for severe psoriasis

☐ **Growth Hormone from Human Pituitary Glands** – used usually for children with delayed or impaired growth

☐ **Insulin from Cows (Bovine, or Beef, Insulin)** – used to treat diabetes

☐ **Hepatitis B Immune Globulin** – given following an exposure to hepatitis B.
   NOTE: This is different from the hepatitis B vaccine which is a series of 3 injections given over a 6 month period to prevent future infection from exposures to hepatitis B.

☐ **Plavix (clopidogrel) and Ticlid (ticlopidine)** – inhibits platelet function; used to reduce the chance for heart attack and stroke.

☐ **Feldene** – given for mild to moderate arthritis pain

☐ **Experimental Medication or Unlicensed (Experimental) Vaccine** – usually associated with a research protocol

---

IF YOU WOULD LIKE TO KNOW WHY THESE MEDICINES AFFECT YOU AS A BLOOD DONOR, PLEASE KEEP READING:

• If you have taken or are taking **Proscar, Avodart, Propecia, Accutane, Soriatane, or Tegison**, these medications can cause birth defects. Your donated blood could contain high enough levels to damage the unborn baby if transfused to a pregnant woman. Once the medication has been cleared from your blood, you may donate again. Following the last dose, the deferral period is one month Proscar, Propecia and Accutane, six months for Avodart and three years for Soriatane. Tegison is a permanent deferral.

• **Growth hormone from human pituitary glands** was prescribed for children with delayed or impaired growth. The hormone was obtained from human pituitary glands, which are found in the brain. Some people who took this hormone developed a rare nervous system condition called Creutzfeldt-Jakob Disease (CJD, for short). The deferral is permanent.

• **Insulin from cows (bovine, or beef, insulin)** is an injected material used to treat diabetes. If this insulin was imported into the US from countries in which "Mad Cow Disease" has been found, it could contain material from infected cattle. There is concern that "Mad Cow Disease" is transmitted by transfusion. The deferral is indefinite.

• **Hepatitis B Immune Globulin (HBIG)** is an injected material used to prevent infection following an exposure to hepatitis B. HBIG does not prevent hepatitis B infection in every case, therefore persons who have received HBIG must wait 12 months to donate blood to be sure they were not infected since hepatitis B can be transmitted through transfusion to a patient.

• **Feldene** is a non-steroidal anti-inflammatory drug that can affect platelet function. A donor taking Feldene will not be able to donate platelets for 2 days; however, its use will not affect whole blood donations.

• **Plavix and Ticlid** are medications that can decrease the chance of a heart attack or stroke in individuals at risk for these conditions. Since these medications can affect platelets, anyone taking Plavix or Ticlid will not be able to donate platelets for 14 days after the last dose. Use of either medication will not prohibit whole blood donations.

• **Experimental Medication or Unlicensed (Experimental) Vaccine** is usually associated with a research protocol and the effect on blood donation is unknown. Deferral is one year unless otherwise indicated by Medical Director.

Figure 13–4. Medication Deferral List. *(U.S. Food and Drug Administration, "Guidance for industry: Implementation of acceptable full-length Donor History Questionnaire and accompanying materials for use in screening donors of blood and blood components," October 2006.)*

---

deferred for 12 months from the time of receiving the blood product or graft.

• **In the past 12 months, have you come in contact with someone else's blood or had an accidental needle-stick injury? Had a tattoo? Had ear or body piercing?** Deferral is 12 months due to exposure to substances known to be sources of blood-borne pathogens. Exposure is assumed if the blood came in contact with an open wound, any broken skin, or mucous membranes (nose, mouth, eyes, etc.).

Skin-penetrating injuries from instruments, equipment, needles, and so on, that are nonsterile and contaminated with blood or body fluids other than the donor's own are also cause for deferral. This includes tattoos, permanent makeup, and ear and body piercings unless applied by a state-regulated organization where sterile needles and ink are not reused.[2]

• **In the past 12 months, have you had sexual contact with anyone who has HIV/AIDS or has had a positive** test for HIV/AIDS? Deferral is for 12 months from the time of sexual contact with a person with clinical or laboratory evidence of HIV infection or who is at high risk for infection.

- **In the past 12 months, have you had sexual contact with a prostitute or anyone else who takes money or drugs or other payment for sex?** Persons who have engaged in sex with such people are deferred from donating blood or its components for 12 months from the time of sexual contact.
- **In the past 12 months, have you had sex with anyone who has ever used a needle to take drugs or steroids or anything not prescribed by their doctor? In the past 12 months, have you ever had sex with anyone who has hemophilia or has used clotting factor concentrates?** The FDA mandates persons who have had sex with any person who is a past or present IV drug user should be deferred for 12 months; additionally, persons who have had sex with any person with hemophilia or related blood disorder who has received factor concentrates should be deferred for 12 months.
- *Female donors:* **Have you had sexual contact with a male who has ever had sexual contact with another male?** Women who have had sex with men who have had sex with another man, even once since 1977, should be deferred for 12 months.[5] There is no tangible evidence of HIV being transmitted by close contact (living in the same house, working with, shaking hands, kissing, etc.); therefore, potential donors who meet the definition of being in close contact with someone with AIDS or an HIV-positive individual need not be deferred.[6]
- **In the past 12 months, have you had sexual contact with a person who has hepatitis? Have you lived with a person who has hepatitis?** Sexual contact or living with a person ("close contact") who has acute or chronic hepatitis B (test positive for HBsAg or HBV) or who has symptomatic hepatitis C or other hepatitis virus requires a 12-month deferral following discontinuation of the "close contact." FDA defines "living with" as residing in the same dwelling (house, apartment, or dormitory).[3]
- **In the past 12 months, have you been treated for syphilis or gonorrhea?** Prospective donors with a history of syphilis or gonorrhea, of treatment for either, or of a reactive screening test for syphilis, or where no confirmatory test was performed, should be deferred for 12 months after completion of therapy. The agent that causes syphilis, *Treponema pallidum*, may live for 1 to 5 days in cold storage so that only a fresh unit of RBCs may transmit infection. At room temperature, however, this agent thrives very well, placing platelet concentrates above RBCs as potentially supporting transfusion-transmitted syphilis. To date, though, only three cases of transfusion-transmitted syphilis have been documented.[7-10]
- **Have you been in juvenile detention, lockup, or prison for more than 72 hours?** Deferral is 12 months from the last date of the incarceration.[11]
- **In the past 3 years, have you been outside of the United States or Canada?** This question is general and is used to detect a donor who may have an increased risk of exposure to malaria, Creutzfeldt-Jakob disease (CJD or vCJD), and more recently leishmaniasis.

- **Malaria:** Travelers to areas the CDC (Centers for Disease Control and Prevention) considers to be endemic for malaria should be deferred for 1 year following departure from the endemic area, provided the donor has showed no signs or symptoms of malaria infection, with or without antimalarial prophylactic drug therapy. Immigrants, refugees, citizens, or persons who have resided in the endemic area for at least 5 consecutive years should be deferred for 3 years from the time of departure from the area provided they have remained symptom free.
- **CJD and vCJD:** Creutzfeldt-Jakob disease and variant Creutzfeldt-Jakob disease are members of a group of neurological disorders known as the *transmissible spongiform encephalopathies* or *prion diseases*, which affect sheep, cows, and humans. CJD results in progressive dementia and spongiform alterations in the brain and is rapidly fatal. CJD may be transmitted by corneal transplants, human dura mater grafts, pituitary-derived human growth hormone, and neurosurgical instruments.[12] Donors who are at higher risk for CJD or vCJD should be indefinitely deferred.
- **Leishmaniasis:** *Leishmania spp.* are intracellular protozoan parasites that cause leishmaniasis. They are endemic tropical and subtropical areas in the Middle East, Mediterranean coast, Africa, Central and South America, and Asia. In 2003, with the deployment of military and National Guard troops in Iraq, a 12-month deferral from the date of departure from the area was instituted for any military personnel stationed in Iraq and any civilian and contract personnel who have visited the country. This same deferral was in place between 1990 and 1993 as a result of Operation Desert Storm.
- **From 1980 through 1996:**
  - **Did you spend time that adds up to 3 months or more in the United Kingdom? (Review list of countries in the UK.)** FDA recommendations state that potential donors who have spent 3 or more months, cumulatively, in the UK from 1980 and 1996 are to be deferred indefinitely (Box 13–2).
  - **Were you a member of the U.S. military, a civilian military employee, or a dependent of a member of the U.S. military?** U.S. military personnel and their dependents and civilian military employees who spent a total of 6 months or more at a U.S. military base in Europe (United Kingdom, Belgium, Netherlands, Germany) from 1980 through 1990 or who were at a base in Spain, Portugal, Turkey, Italy, or Greece from 1980 through 1996 are deferred indefinitely.
- **From 1980 to the present, did you:**
  - **Spend time that adds up to 5 years or more in Europe? (Review the list of countries in Europe; see Box 13–2.)** Individuals who have spent at least 5 years, cumulatively, in Europe between 1980 and the present should be indefinitely deferred as donors of whole blood, blood components, or source leukocytes intended for

BOX 13–2

European Countries with BSE or Increased Risk of BSE (CJD and vCJD; used for deferral of donors based on geographic risk of BSE)

Albania	United Kingdom
Greece	Denmark
Romania	Netherlands
Austria	Federal Republic of Yugoslavia
Hungary	Finland
Slovak Republic	Norway
Belgium	France
Republic of Ireland	Poland
Slovenia	Germany
Bosnia-Herzegovina	Portugal
Italy	**Countries Included in the United Kingdom**
Spain	England
Bulgaria	Northern Ireland
Liechtenstein	Scotland
Sweden	Wales
Croatia	the Isle of Man
Luxembourg	the Channel Islands
Switzerland	Gibraltar
Czech Republic	Falkland Islands
Macedonia	

Data from Guidance for industry revised preventive measures to reduce the possible risk of transmission of Creutzfeldt-Jakob disease (CJD) and variant Creutzfeldt-Jakob disease (vCJD) by blood and blood products. FDA, Rockville, MD, May 2010.

transfusion. However, they may donate source plasma if not otherwise deferred.[12]

- **Receive a blood transfusion in the United Kingdom or France? (Review the list of countries in the UK; see Box 13–2.)** Those who have received a transfusion of blood, platelets, plasma, cryoprecipitate, or granulocytes in the UK or France since 1980 should be indefinitely deferred as a blood donor.
- From 1977 to the present, have you:
  - **Received money, drugs, or other payment for sex?** Men or women who engage in sex for money or drugs since 1977 are permanently deferred.
  - **Male Donors: Have you had sexual contact with another male, even once?** Male-to-male sexual contact, even once, since 1977 is cause for permanent deferral.
- Have you ever:
  - **Had a positive test for HIV/AIDS virus?** Indefinite deferral for any person with clinical or laboratory diagnosis of HIV infection.
  - **Used needles to take drugs, steroids, or anything not prescribed by your doctor?** Donors' arms should be checked for evidence of scars or punctures indicating addiction to self-injected drugs or for presence of any skin lesions in the venipuncture site. Donors with evidence of past or present nonprescription drug use should be indefinitely deferred.
  - **Used clotting factor concentrates?** Prospective donors with hemophilia or other bleeding disorders and who

receive clotting factor concentrates should be deferred from donating blood or components unless otherwise approved by the medical director, because there is a high risk of bleeding following venipuncture. Receipt of clotting factor concentrates, like receipt of blood transfusions, requires a 12-month deferral.

- **Had hepatitis?** Donors with a history of hepatitis after their 11th birthday or a confirmed positive test for hepatitis B surface antigen (HBsAg) or a repeatedly reactive test for anti-HBc should be indefinitely deferred. Donor suitability with regard to the age restriction for hepatitis can be assessed by the medical director; recollections of symptoms, diagnoses, and laboratory data can be helpful in deciding if the donor is suitable for whole blood donation. The FDA stipulates that a history of an elevated alanine aminotransferase or a reactive test for antibodies to hepatitis A virus or to hepatitis B surface antigen should not exclude a potential donor without additional clinical evidence of viral hepatitis. If viral hepatitis before the age of 11 years is suspected, the donor should be deferred temporarily until the circumstances are investigated and medical opinion concludes there is no history or diagnosis of viral hepatitis after age 11.
- **Had malaria?** Prospective donors with a history of malaria are deferred for 3 years following treatment and being asymptomatic.
- **Had Chagas' disease? Had babesiosis?** A history of Chagas' disease or babesiosis is cause for indefinite

deferral. Chagas' disease, also known as *American trypanosomiasis*, is caused by the protozoan parasite *Trypanosoma cruzi*. The vector responsible for transmitting the parasite is the hematophagous bug belonging to the family *Reduviidae*. Transmission occurs when mucous membranes or breaks in the skin are contaminated with the feces of infected hematophagous bugs.[19] Chagas' disease is endemic in parts of Central and South America and Mexico, where an estimated 16 to 18 million persons are infected with *T. cruzi*. Approximately 25,000 to 100,000 Latin American immigrants living in the United States are infected with *T. cruzi*. Chagas' disease may be transmitted congenitally by breastfeeding, organ transplants, or blood transfusion.[13]

In the United States and Canada, there have been seven documented cases of transfusion-associated transmission of Chagas' disease in the past 20 years, all occurring in immunosuppressed recipients.[14] There are 70 known species of *Babesiai*, and at least 5 are identified as infecting humans. *Babesia microti* utilizes the vector *Ixodes scapularis* to infect the human and transmit the parasite. The *Babesia* organism penetrates the erythrocyte where the trophozoite multiplies; upon lysis of the RBC, merozoites are released into the blood where they are free to infect other RBCs. Transfusion-associated infection with *Babesia* carries an incubation period of 2 to 8 weeks; symptoms may include **malaise**, fatigue, **anorexia**, **arthralgias**, nausea, vomiting, abdominal pain, and fever reaching temperatures of 40°C.

- **Received a dura mater (or brain covering) graft?** Due to an increased risk of exposure to CJD or vCJD, prospective donors with history of a dura mater graft require an indefinite deferral.
- **Had any type of cancer, including leukemia?** A history of cancer, leukemia, or lymphoma is generally a cause for indefinite deferral. Any donor presenting with a history of cancer should be reviewed by the blood bank medical director. The exceptions include basal or squamous cell cancer, carcinoma in situ of the cervix, and papillary thyroid carcinoma that has been surgically removed.
- **Had any problems with your heart or lungs?** A history of cardiovascular, coronary, or rheumatic heart disease is usually a cause for deferral; however, in the absence of disability or restrictions by the patient's physician, the donor may be accepted on a case-by-case basis by the blood bank director. Active pulmonary tuberculosis or other active pulmonary disease is cause for deferral.
- **Had a bleeding condition or a blood disease?** Donors indicating a history of a bleeding problem following surgery, invasive dental procedures, cuts, or abrasions must be further evaluated by the blood bank director. Diseases of the blood such as hemophilia, von Willebrand disease, sickle cell anemia, thalassemia, Kaposi's sarcoma, or polycythemia, or a history of receiving clotting factor concentrates are causes for indefinite deferral.

- **Been in Africa?** HIV-1 group O virus is endemic to the central and west regions of Africa. Anyone who was born or lived in any of the African countries on the FDA list of countries with HIV-1 group O risk (Box 13–3) since 1977 should be deferred indefinitely. In addition, if the prospective donor has traveled to any of the countries on the list since 1977 and received a blood transfusion or other medical treatment with a blood product, they should be deferred indefinitely.[15]
- **Had sexual contact with anyone who was born in or lived in Africa?** The FDA recommends indefinite deferral for any prospective donor who indicates having had sex with a person who was born in any of the African countries on the list of those with increased risk of HIV-1 group O infection (see **Box 13–3**).
  - If the collecting facility has implemented testing for HIV-1/2 that has been licensed for use in detecting antibodies to HIV-1 group O, the questions concerning residence in or travel to specific African countries or sexual contact with persons from those countries may be omitted. In addition, donors who were previously deferred prior to the availability of the HIV-1 group O testing may be reentered provided it has been at least 1 year since the last potential exposure to HIV-1 group O and the screening test results are non-reactive.[15]
- **Have any of your relatives had Creutzfeldt-Jakob disease?** The FDA recommends prospective donors with a family history of CJD be permanently deferred unless the diagnosis of CJD was confidently excluded.

The Physical Examination

The donor center representative evaluates the prospective donor with regard to general appearance, weight, temperature, pulse, blood pressure, hemoglobin, and presence of

---

BOX 13–3

African Countries at Increased Risk of HIV-1 Group O Infection

Cameroon
Benin
Central African Republic
Chad
Congo
Equatorial Guinea
Kenya
Gabon
Niger
Nigeria
Senegal
Togo
Zambia

Data from Guidance for industry recommendations for management of donors at increased risk for human immunodeficiency virus type 1 (HIV-1) group O infection. FDA, Rockville, MD, August 2009.

skin lesions. A blood bank physician should be available to evaluate any special considerations.

- **General appearance**: The donor center representative should observe the prospective donor for presence of excessive anxiety, drug or alcohol influence, or nervousness. If possible, this should be done in a gentle manner so as to not deter the donor from donations in the future.
- **Weight**: *Standards* mandates a maximum of 10.5 mL of blood/kg of donor weight for whole blood collection inclusive of pilot tubes for testing. If the donor weighs less than 100 pounds, the amount of blood collected must be proportionately reduced as well as that of the anticoagulant. The following formulas can be used to calculate the adjusted volume of blood to be collected and anticoagulant to be used.

  Volume to collect = (donor's weight in kg/50) × 450 mL

  Volume to collect/450 × 63 mL = reduced volume of anticoagulant

  63 mL − above calculated volume = amount of solution to be removed
- **Temperature**: *Standards* mandates the donor temperature must be less than or equal to 37.5°C or 99.5°F.[28] Donors are asked not to drink coffee or hot beverages while waiting to donate, as this may sometimes affect their temperature. Oral temperatures that are lower than normal are not cause for deferral.
- **Pulse**: The donor's pulse should be between 50 and 100 bpm. Often, a donor who is athletic will have a pulse less than 50 bpm, which is not cause for deferral. The pulse should be counted for at least 15 seconds; any irregularities should be evaluated by a blood bank physician.
- **Blood pressure**: A potential donor's systolic blood pressure should be less than or equal to 180 mm Hg and the diastolic less than or equal to 100 mm Hg. Blood pressure readings above these levels should be evaluated by a blood bank physician.
- **Hemoglobin**: The donor's hemoglobin level should be greater than or equal to 12.5 g/dL and the hematocrit level greater than or equal to 38% for allogeneic donation. For autologous donation, the hemoglobin and hematocrit level should be greater than or equal to 11 g/dL and 33%, respectively.[1] The methods used for measuring hemoglobin include copper sulfate or point-of-care instruments using spectrophotometric methodology. A hematocrit or packed cell volume can be determined manually by centrifugation. The blood is usually acquired via a finger stick.
- **Skin lesions**: Prior to donation, the donor's arms should be inspected for skin lesions. Evidence of skin lesions (e.g., multiple puncture marks) is cause for indefinite deferral. Skin disorders that are not cause for deferral include poison ivy and other rashes; these, however, should not be present in the area of the venipuncture site and may need to be evaluated by a blood bank physician.

Informed Consent

AABB Standards mandates that informed consent of allogeneic, autologous, and apheresis donors be obtained before donation. The donor must be informed of the risks of the procedure and of the tests that are performed to reduce the risk of infectious disease transmission to the recipient. The donor must be able to ask questions concerning any element of the collection or testing process. If the donor is a minor or is unable to comprehend the informed consent protocol, applicable state law provisions will intercede. An example of an informed consent is shown in Figure 13–5.

Autologous Donors

An autologous donor is one who donates blood for his or her own use; thus, such a donor is referred to as the donor-patient. Most autologous blood is used to treat surgical blood loss in very specific situations where there is a reasonable opportunity to avoid homologous transfusions or when compatible allogeneic blood is not available. The potential advantage of using autologous blood over allogeneic blood includes a decreased risk of disease transmission, transfusion reactions, and alloimmunization. However, there is still a risk of bacterial contamination, circulatory overload, cytokine-mediated reactions, and misidentification of the product or patient.[16] The patients for whom autologous donation or

Donor Release:

I have read and I understand the information contained in the *Responsibilities of a Blood Donor and Important Information About Donating Blood* Information sheet. I understand that if my behavior or physical condition puts me at risk to transmit AIDS or any other disease, I should not donate blood. The medical history I have given is truthful and accurate to the best of my knowledge. I have not participated in activities considered high risk for acquiring and transmitting AIDS.

I give my permission for all laboratory testing necessary to provide safe blood to the recipient including tests to detect exposure to hepatitis, AIDS, and other transfusion-transmitted diseases. Some of these tests may be unlicensed and for research only. Some positive test results are routinely reported to the State Health Department as required by law for notification of sexual partners. I realize that LifeSouth is not a testing center and that by giving blood I am not guaranteed that disease testing will be performed.

Although donating blood is normally a pleasant experience, I realize that short-term side effects can occur, such as bruising, dizziness, or fainting, and that, in rare cases, a donor may experience infection or nerve damage.

I voluntarily donate my blood to the LifeSouth Community Blood Centers to be used as the blood center deems advisable.

Donor: _____   Date: _____

Figure 13–5. Sample informed consent. (*LifeSouth Blood Center, Montgomery, AL, with permission.*)

transfusion holds the greatest advantage are those with very rare blood types and those with multiple antibodies where compatible units in the general blood supply may be difficult or impossible to find.

The disadvantages of autologous donation or transfusion include a higher cost due to added administrative processes and special labeling requirements to ensure that units get transfused to the proper patient. It should be noted that there is a high percentage of wasted units (30% to 50%), because patients end up not requiring any or all of the units donated.[16] In addition, the *AABB Standards* do not permit "crossing over" of unused autologous units into the general inventory, except in exceptional circumstances. The decision must be approved by the medical director on a case-by-case basis.[17]

Although the use of autologous blood has decreased in the past several years, it is still a viable and common alternative therapy for select patients. There are various methods and techniques for obtaining autologous blood, including:

- Preoperative collection
- Acute normovolemic hemodilution
- Intraoperative collection
- Postoperative collection

Preoperative Collection

Preoperative collection occurs during the 5 to 6 weeks immediately preceding a scheduled, elective surgical procedure unless the red blood cells and plasma are scheduled to be frozen. Procedures that typically might use preoperative autologous blood include orthopedic procedures, vascular surgery, cardiac or thoracic surgery, and radical prostatectomy. Although some women do participate in an autologous collection program during pregnancy for unforeseen complications, blood is seldom needed except in cases in which the mother has multiple antibodies to high-frequency antigens or risk for placenta previa or intrapartum hemorrhage.[2]

The decision to use preoperative autologous blood requires both an order from the patient's physician (Fig. 13–6) and an approval from the blood bank medical director. The maximal surgical blood order schedule (MSBOS) can provide guidance for surgical procedures to estimate the number of units needed for transfusion. The last blood collection should occur no later than 72 hours (3 days) before the scheduled surgery to allow for volume replacement.

Medical history and physical exam requirements for autologous donation are less stringent than those for allogeneic donations. There is no minimum or maximum age requirement; however, the donor must be able to tolerate the donation, and for younger donors, most centers limit the age to children whose veins can accommodate the phlebotomy needle and who can understand the procedure. The minimum hemoglobin/hematocrit level is 11 g/dL and 33%, respectively. Blood pressure and pulse are the same as with allogeneic donors unless otherwise defined by the blood bank medical director, and the donor's temperature should not be elevated or indicate any sign of possible infection. Medical history questions can

be limited to those needed to ensure the safety of the donor, including cardiac history, bleeding disorders, major illness, previous donor reactions, fainting problems, and so on. In addition, there should be questions to rule out the possibility of bacteremia in the donor or patient. This would include information on current medications, antibiotics, recent infections, fever, recent minor procedures such as dental procedures, gastrointestinal problems, or diarrhea.

Most autologous donor units are a standard 450 or 500 mL ± 10%; however, if the donor weighs less than 50 kg (110 lb), the total amount of blood collected must be reduced proportionately. If the amount of blood to be collected is determined to be 300 to 405 mL, the unit must be labeled as low volume. There is no requirement to reduce the volume of anticoagulant-preservative solution; however, the plasma is not suitable for transfusion. If the unit must be less than 300 mL, the anticoagulant-preservative solution must be adjusted, and approval by the blood bank medical director is required. See the earlier section "The Physical Examination" for formulas to calculate the volume and anticoagulant adjustments.

Testing requirements for autologous donor units are somewhat less stringent than with allogeneic units. The collecting facility must determine the ABO and Rh of the blood, but antibody screening is optional. If the collection facility and the transfusion facility are the same, then viral marker testing is not required; however, if they are different, the collecting facility must test for HBsAg, anti-HBc, anti-HCV, HCV RNA, anti-HIV-1/2, HIV-1 RNA, anti-HTLV-I/II, WNV RNA, and STS on at least the first unit collected from the donor in every 30-day period. If any of the markers yield a positive or reactive result, the patient's physician and transfusing facility must be notified of the result.[1]

The transfusing facility must reconfirm the ABO and Rh of the unit, but a crossmatch is optional; however, an immediate spin crossmatch would be a good safety check that the selected unit is identified properly.

Units collected for autologous use must be labeled appropriately. The label should include the patient's full name, medical record number or ID number, expiration date of the unit, and the name of the facility where the donor-patient will be transfused. The label must also clearly state "For Autologous Use Only" (Fig. 13–7). Autologous units also generally have a distinct green label and tag (Fig. 13–8). This is done both to ensure the unit is linked correctly with the donor-patient and to make the blood bank technologists aware that certain patients have autologous units on the shelf that must be transfused before allogeneic units; more specifically, the oldest units should be transfused first. Blood banks should have a system in place to ensure autologous units are selected first.

Acute Normovolemic Hemodilution

Acute normovolemic hemodilution (ANH) results in the collection of whole blood with the concurrent infusion of crystalloid or colloid solutions, thus maintaining a normal blood

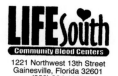

Branch Location:

*An appointment is recommended for this service. Please contact your local blood bank for information.

[Reset Form]

1221 Northwest 13th Street
Gainesville, Florida 32601
(352) 334-1000

Request For Autologous Collections

Patient's Name _____ SS# _____ Birth Date _____

Patient's Phone Number _____ Patient's Address _____

Date of Surgery/Transfusion _____ Diagnosis _____ Hospital _____

If patient is also under treatment for, or has any, preexisting medical condition(s), please indicate below.

_____, MD   Condition _____

_____, MD   Condition _____

_____, MD   Condition _____

Please list all medications prescribed for this patient: _____

_____

LifeSouth Community Blood Centers will process and store this blood for subsequent replacement transfusion. The number of units drawn and the interval between donations will be determined by the patient's hemoglobin and anticipated blood requirements, and will be at the discretion of the blood center's Medical Director. Units will be held only until outdate (42 days from the date drawn) unless specific arrangements are made with the blood center prior to that date. Blood should not be drawn from the donor-patient within 72 hours of the time of anticipated surgery or transfusion. A cardiac release is required for all patients with a history of cardiac problems; units will not be collected until the blood center has received written release from the patient's cardiologist.

Physicians will be notified in writing of abnormal test results as soon as possible. It is the responsibility of the ordering physician to notify the patient.

Physicians, please complete:
I have explained the reasons for and risks involved in autologous collection to this patient and have considered the need for iron supplementation:

#Units _____

- Packed Cells   Signature, MD _____ Date _____
- Whole Blood   Physician (printed name) _____
- Fresh Frozen Plasma   Phone _____
- Cryoprecipitated AHF

················ **Blood Center Use Only** ················

Verbal Order _____ Taken by _____ Date _____

Donation Date _____ Unit Number _____ Donation Date _____ Unit Number _____

Donation Date _____ Unit Number _____ Donation Date _____ Unit Number _____

Apr 99   ver 1.0

Figure 13–6.   Autologous donation permission form. *(LifeSouth Blood Center, Montgomery, AL, with permission.)*

volume but decreasing the patient's hematocrit. The ratio of replacement is 3:1 for crystalloids and 1:1 for colloids.[15] The number of units collected depends of the patient's ability to tolerate the decrease in hemoglobin/hematocrit. A limited hemodilution will reduce the hematocrit to 28%; severe dilution will reach 21% or less. It is recommended that the patient start with a hemoglobin of at least 12 g/dL. The procedure is performed in surgery immediately prior to beginning the surgical procedure and is managed by anesthesiology. The blood is collected in standard blood bags

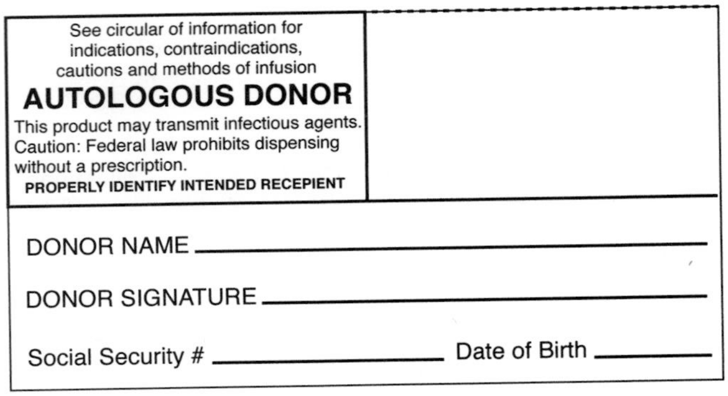

See circular of information for
indications, contraindications,
cautions and methods of infusion

AUTOLOGOUS DONOR

This product may transmit infectious agents.
Caution: Federal law prohibits dispensing
without a prescription.
PROPERLY IDENTIFY INTENDED RECEPIENT

DONOR NAME _____

DONOR SIGNATURE _____

Social Security # _____ Date of Birth _____

Figure 13–7. Autologous donation label. *(LifeSouth Blood Center, Montgomery, AL, with permission.)*

containing anticoagulant or preservative and is stored in the room at room temperature. The blood is normally reinfused to the patient during or immediately following the surgery, but within 8 hours of collection, thus maintaining the viability of both platelets and coagulation factors.

Blood units are reinfused in the reverse order of collection so that the last unit reinfused carries the highest hematocrit level. Because the blood generally does not leave the operating room (OR), the units generally are not tested, labeled, or tracked, and the blood bank is generally not involved. However, if the blood is not transfused during surgery, it can be stored for up to 24 hours in a monitored blood bank refrigerator if refrigerated within the first 8 hours. If the units leave the OR and are stored, they must be appropriately tested and labeled as with predeposit autologous units.

Intraoperative Collection

Intraoperative autologous collection involves collecting shed blood from the surgical site; processing the blood through an instrument that washes it with saline to remove tissue debris, free hemoglobin, and plasma that may contain activated coagulation factors; concentrating the residual red cells (to a hematocrit of 50% to 60%); and then reinfusing those cells immediately. This process is repeated continually during the surgical procedure. This type of collection has been used in cardiothoracic, major orthopedic, and cardiac surgeries, in addition to vascular surgeries, such as liver transplantation. The advantage of using intraoperative autologous blood collection is that it may be used in cases where preoperative donation is not possible due to the

urgency of the surgery or the patient cannot be scheduled for multiple preoperative donations. In addition, the risk of misidentifying the patient and blood product is minimized, and there are no labeling, testing, and storing costs.

The disadvantages include the high cost of the instrumentation involved and training of the personnel to run the instrument. In addition, frequently the amount of blood that is collected is not sufficient for the patient's total needs, and allogeneic blood may still need to be given. The procedure is counterindicated if there is potential for contamination of the surgical site by bowel contents, amniotic fluid, urine, clotting agents, and so on, or where there is a risk of bacterial contamination or activation of coagulation factors.

As with ANH, the blood generally does not leave the OR; however, if some of the blood is to be stored postoperatively, it must be labeled with the patient's full name, medical record number, date and time of collection, and with "For Autologous Use Only." The blood may be stored at room temperature for up to 6 hours or at 1°C to 6°C for up to 24 hours, as long as the latter temperature has begun within 4 hours from the end of collection. Hospitals should establish their own policies and procedures for this type of collection.

Postoperative Blood Salvage

Postoperative blood salvage is collected from a drainage tube placed at the surgical site. It is reinfused, with or without processing, via a microaggregate filter to screen out any debris. This blood is characterized as being dilute, partially hemolyzed, and defibrinated. It is recommended that no more than 1,400 mL be reinfused.[2] Procedures that have used postoperative blood collection include orthopedic (e.g., arthroplasty) and cardiac surgeries. Blood must be reinfused within 6 hours of collection or it is to be discarded. Hospitals should establish their own policies and procedures for this type of collection.

The advantage of this procedure is that it has a very low cost, and it can be used in conjunction with other autologous blood collection procedures to avoid the need for allogeneic blood transfusions. Because the blood does not leave the patient's bedside, there is no risk of the blood being transfused to the wrong person. The disadvantage of post-op salvage is that generally it does not yield a large volume of blood and by itself would not generally produce enough blood for the patient's needs. In addition, it carries a significant risk of producing transfusion reactions due to the presence of activated coagulation factors, fibrin degradation products, and cytokines.

Although the blood bank is frequently not responsible for managing ANH intraoperative recovery and post-op salvage collection procedures, both the AABB and the College of American Pathologists (CAP) have recommendations and guidelines that require the blood bank medical director or supervisor to assist in the development and implementation of the programs. This includes assisting with the development of procedures, maintaining the equipment, monitoring quality control, and training personnel and assessing competency.

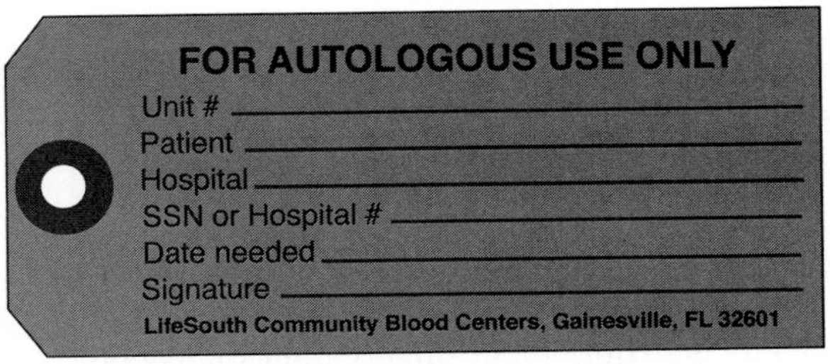

FOR AUTOLOGOUS USE ONLY

Unit # _____
Patient _____
Hospital _____
SSN or Hospital # _____
Date needed _____
Signature _____
LifeSouth Community Blood Centers, Gainesville, FL 32601

Figure 13–8. Autologous donation tag. *(LifeSouth Blood Center, Montgomery, AL, with permission.)*

Directed Donation

A directed donation is a unit collected under the same requirements as those for allogeneic donors, except that the unit collected is *directed* toward a specific patient. Often, when a friend or family member needs blood, the donor center will accommodate these directed donations so that the required testing may be done as soon as possible; if the blood is compatible, it can be used by the patient. The tag for the directed unit is a distinct color (e.g., yellow, salmon) to differentiate it from autologous tags (Fig. 13–9). If the donor is a blood relative, the unit must be irradiated to prevent graft versus host disease so that viable T cells from the donor that enter the patient's circulation do not mount an attack against patient's cells and tissue.[18] A system should be in place to ensure directed units from blood relatives are irradiated.

Apheresis Donation

Apheresis collection is an effective mechanism for collecting a specific blood component while returning the remaining whole blood components back to the patient. Most apheresis instrumentation use an automated cell separator device whose centrifugal force separates blood into components based on differences in density. (Refer to Chapter 14, "Apheresis.")

Apheresis can be used to collect platelets, plasma, white cells (leukocytes), red cells, and stem cells. It is designed to collect large volumes of the intended component and is the only effective method for collecting leukocytes and stem cells. The donor requirements for apheresis donation are generally the same as for whole blood donation; however, there are some differences, depending on the component that is to be collected. As with whole blood donation, the process is regulated by the FDA, and both the AABB and the American Society for Apheresis (ASFA) provide comprehensive guidelines and standards.

Plateletpheresis

Today the majority (more than 75%) of platelet transfusions are pheresis-derived platelets.[2] A pheresis platelet unit is equivalent to six to eight random donor platelets, so a single product is a typical therapeutic dose for most adult patients. This significantly reduces the recipient's donor exposure, makes routine leukoreduction of the product practical, and allows compatibility matching of

the donor and patient possible in cases where the patient has become alloimmunized and refractory to random donor platelets. Plateletpheresis donors may donate more often. The interval between donations is at least 2 days, not to exceed more than twice a week or more than 24 times a year.[1]

Donors who have ingested aspirin, Feldene, or aspirin-containing medications should be deferred for 48 hours, because these medications interfere with platelet adhesion, and all of the platelets in a given therapeutic dose would be affected. In addition, donors on Plavix (clopidogrel) or Ticlid (ticlopidine) should be deferred for 14 days, which is the time required for the medication to clear the system and the platelet function to return to normal. If the donor has donated whole blood, or if 100 mL or more of red cells were not able to be returned to the donor on the previous pheresis procedure, the donor must be deferred for 8 weeks to allow time for the donor to replenish the lost red cell mass. Certain exceptions can be made for compelling medical reasons, provided a physician certifies that the donor will not be harmed and the blood bank medical director agrees.

Although a platelet count is not required on the first donation, it is required if the interval between donations is less than 4 weeks; in that case, the platelet count must be above 150,000/μL. The total amount of plasma that can be removed along with the platelets is limited to 500 mL (600 mL for donors weighing more than 175 lb) or the amount of plasma stated in the directions circular for the automated instrument being used for the collection. Each pheresis platelet unit is required to contain at least 3×10^{11} platelets. The automated instruments used today are very efficient, and a single donor collection frequently yields a high enough platelet count to allow the collection to be split into two or three individual products. (Refer to Chapter 14.) Donor reactions to platelet pheresis collections are most commonly a reaction to the citrate or anticoagulant used in the procedure. Vasovagal and hypovolemic reactions are very rare but have been reported.[2]

Testing requirements are the same as for other allogeneic blood products, ABO group/Rh type, antibody screen, and infectious disease markers. If the donor is donating repeatedly for a specific patient, repeat testing need only be done every 30 days. In addition, the platelet count on each product is determined and recorded but does not have to be recorded on the product label. If there are visible red cells in the finished product, the amount of red cells must be determined. If the product contains more than 2 mL of red cells, a pilot sample must be attached to the product and used by the transfusing facility to crossmatch the product with the intended recipient. FDA guidelines require that the donation records of regular platelet pheresis donors be reviewed by a physician at least every 4 months.[19]

Plasmapheresis

Plasma was the first product to be collected by apheresis methods and was primarily used as a method for collecting "source plasma," which is further manufactured into plasma

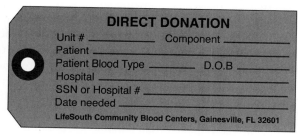

Figure 13–9. Directed donation tag. *(LifeSouth Blood Center, Montgomery, AL, with permission.)*

derivatives. Today plasma apheresis is also used to collect transfusable fresh frozen plasma. Plasmapheresis donors are classified as either "infrequent/occasional" or "serial," depending on the frequency of donations. An infrequent donor undergoes no more than one procedure in a 4-week period. Serial donors may donate more frequently than 4 weeks but no more than every 48 hours and no more than two donations in a 7-day period.

The donor requirements for both infrequent and serial donors are the same as for allogeneic whole blood donors, although serial donors have some additional requirements to protect the donor from excessive red cell and plasma protein loss. The red cell loss must not exceed 25 mL/week or 200 mL in an 8-week period. As with any pheresis procedure, if the donor's red cells cannot be returned, the donor must be deferred for 8 weeks before returning to a plasma pheresis program. At the start of a serial pheresis program and at 4-month intervals, the donor must be tested for total serum/plasma protein levels and quantitative immunoglobulin levels, and protein electrophoresis must be performed. The levels must remain in the normal range, or the donor must be removed from the program until the levels return to normal.

If the plasmapheresis procedure is being performed manually, there must be a mechanism in place to ensure positive donor and product identification, as well as safe return of the donor's cells. There should be two separate forms of identification so that both the donor and the phlebotomist can verify the ID. Full names, signatures, unique numbers, or pictures may all be used.

Leukapheresis

Apheresis is the only effective method for collecting leukocytes or, more specifically, granulocytes. The therapeutic effectiveness of granulocyte transfusions is still somewhat controversial, but they have been shown to be effective in specific cases. A typical therapeutic dose is at least 1×10^{11} granulocytes each day for 5 consecutive days.

In order to collect a large enough volume of leukocytes (more than 1×10^{11} granulocytes), the donor must be given certain drugs or sedimenting agents, and specific informed consent must be obtained from the donor prior to administering these drugs. AABB *Standards* states that any of these drugs or agents used to facilitate leukapheresis will not be used on donors whose medical history suggests that such a drug will exacerbate previous disease.[1]

One of the drugs typically given is hydroxyethyl starch (HES), which is a common sedimenting agent. It enhances the separation of the white cells from the red cells during centrifugation, which increases the amount of leukocytes collected and decreases the amount of red cell contamination in the final product. The disadvantage is that HES is a colloid; it expands the donor's blood volume and remains in the circulation for extended periods of time. As a result, caution must be taken to control the amount of HES given to a donor and its accumulation in the donor's circulation.

Corticosteroids such as prednisone or dexamethasone can also be used. These drugs are given to the donor prior to the collection procedure. They work by pulling the granulocytes from the marginal pool into the general circulation, thus increasing the supply of cells available for collection. Careful scrutiny must be used to obtain an accurate health history on the donor to identify any medical condition that could be exaggerated by the presence of corticosteroids.

Finally, the newest agents are growth factors. Now that recombinant hematopoietic growth factors are available, they are being used in leukapheresis procedures. The advantages of these growth factors is that they can produce four to eight times the volumes of cells in each collection compared with other agents. In addition, these growth factors appear to be quite well tolerated by the donor. Each collection facility should develop policies outlining maximal doses of stimulating agents used in leukapheresis with appropriate contraindications for donors.

Each leukapheresis product must be tested for ABO group and Rh type as well as the HLA type of the leukocytes. Most leukocyte concentrates are contaminated with some red cells. As stated for platelet concentrates, if the amount of contaminating red cells exceeds 2 mL, the product should be crossmatched with the recipient, and a pilot tube sample must accompany the product.

Double RBC Pheresis

In the 1990s, double units of red cells were collected using the apheresis equipment. The FDA finalized the guidance recommendations for this procedure in 2001. Double red cell pheresis can be used to collect either allogeneic or autologous units. The donor must meet the requirements for whole blood donation and the recommendations established by the equipment manufacturer. The hemoglobin level must be determined by a quantitative method; copper sulfate method is not acceptable. If the donor's weight or hemoglobin level are at the minimum level, it is recommended that the donor be further evaluated by the blood bank physician to ensure the procedure is safe for the donor. If the procedure method used calls for saline infusion to minimize volume depletion, then male donors must weigh at least 130 pounds and be at least 5'1" tall. Female donors must weigh at least 150 pounds and be at least 5'5" tall. The hematocrit level for both sexes must be a minimum of 40%.[2]

Donors participating in double red cell pheresis programs are deferred for 16 weeks following successful completion of the donation procedures. They should not participate in platelet or plasma pheresis during that period. If the procedure is discontinued prior to completion and the total red cell loss is less than 200 mL, the donor can donate again within 8 weeks provided all other donation criteria are met. If the red cell loss is greater than 200 mL but less than 300 mL, the donor should be deferred for 8 weeks. If the total red cells lost is greater than 300 mL, the donor must be deferred for the full 16 weeks.

Whole Blood Collection

Once the donor has satisfied requirements of the screening process and has been registered, whole blood collection can proceed. This procedure must be performed only by trained personnel working under the direction of a qualified licensed physician. This section describes donor identification, aseptic technique, venipuncture, collection of pilot tubes and whole blood unit, postdonation instructions, and adverse donor reactions.

Donor Identification

A numeric or alpha numeric system is used to link the donor to the donor record, pilot tubes, blood container, and all components made from the original collection. Care must be taken to avoid duplicate numbers, voided numbers, or other mistakes in the labeling system. These issues must be investigated and kept on record.

AABB *Standards* require that the trained phlebotomist must identify the donor record and ensure that the donor name and identification numbers match. The phlebotomist should ask the donor to state or spell his or her name. At this time, the phlebotomist can attach all labels to blood bags, donor record, and pilot tubes.

Aseptic Technique

For blood collection, most blood centers use an iodine compound such as PVP-iodine or polymer iodine complex. Using a tourniquet or blood pressure cuff, the venipuncture site is identified, and the area is scrubbed at least 4 cm in all directions from the site for a minimum of 30 seconds. The area is then covered with a dry sterile gauze pad until the venipuncture is performed. Donors who are allergic or sensitive to iodine compounds may use chlorhexidine gluconate and isopropyl alcohol. All methods must be approved by the FDA (Box 13–4).

Collection Procedure

The collection procedure for whole blood is outlined in Box 13–5.

Postdonation Instructions

Most donor reactions will occur during or shortly after the donation. It is recommended that donors remain in an area where they can be observed by the donation center staff and be given instructions to follow for the next 24 hours. Most blood centers have a designated postdonation area where donors can sit and replenish their fluids. An example of postdonation instructions is shown in Figure 13–10.

Donor Reactions

Most donors tolerate the withdrawal of a unit of blood without incident; however, in the event an adverse reaction does occur, the donor room staff must be well trained and able to react immediately to the donor's needs. Donor reactions cover a wide spectrum, from nervousness and hematomas at the phlebotomy site to convulsions and loss of consciousness. The donor staff should be trained in CPR. Reactions can generally be divided into three categories: mild, moderate, and severe.

Mild Reactions

Reactions in this category encompass one or more of the following: syncope or fainting, nausea or vomiting, hyperventilation, twitching, and muscle spasm. Syncope may be idiopathic or may be brought about by the sight of blood. The donor may show signs of sweating, dizziness, pallor, or convulsions. The following instructions apply for a donor who has fainted:

1. Remove the tourniquet and withdraw needle
2. Place cold compresses on the donor's forehead

BOX 13–4

Arm Preparation Methods

Method I

1. Scrub the site (2 × 2 inches) for 30 seconds using an aqueous iodophor scrub solution (0.7%). Iodophor is a polyvinyl pyrrolidone-iodine or poloxamer iodine complex.
2. Apply iodophor complex and let stand for 30 seconds. Use a concentric spiral motion, starting in the center and moving outward. Do not go back to the center. Removal of the iodophor solution is not necessary.
3. Site is now ready for venipuncture. Cover with sterile gauze until ready for needle insertion.
4. If the donor bends the arm, or the prepared site is touched with the fingers or other nonsterile object, the arm preparation must be repeated.

Method II

1. Apply a minimum of 1 mL of One Step Gel directly to the venipuncture site by squeezing the gel bottle directly over the intended area.

2. Using a sterile applicator and while holding it at an approximate 30° angle, begin scrubbing in a circular motion in about a 1-inch area directly over the venipuncture site. Continue this for a minimum of 30 seconds.
3. After scrubbing for 30 seconds, use the same applicator to begin at intended site of venipuncture, and move gradually outward in concentric circles to form a total prepared area measuring at least 3 inches in diameter.
4. Using a second sterile applicator and starting from the center of the 3-inch prepared area, remove excess gel by moving gradually outward in concentric circles.
5. Allow site to air-dry according to manufacturer's instructions.
6. If the donor bends the arm or the prepared site is touched with the fingers or with any other nonsterile object, the arm preparation must be repeated.

BOX 13–5

Whole Blood Collection Procedure

1. Confirm donor identity, and make the donor as comfortable as possible.
2. Using a tourniquet or blood pressure cuff, select a large, firm vein in the antecubital space that is free of any skin lesions or scarring. Inspect both arms.
3. Prepare the site using an FDA-approved cleansing method. When finished, cover site with sterile gauze.
4. Inspect the blood bags for any defects or discoloration.
5. Ensure the balance system is adjusted to the volume being drawn; ensure counterbalance is level. Place hemostats on the tubing to prevent air from entering the line.
6. Reapply tourniquet or blood pressure cuff (40 to 60 mm Hg) to increase distention of the vein.
7. Uncover the sterile gauze, and perform the venipuncture immediately. Check the position of the needle, and tape the tubing to the donor's arm to hold the needle in place. Cover with a sterile gauze.
8. Release the hemostat, and ask the donor to open and close the hand every 10 to 12 seconds during collection procedure.
9. Reduce the pressure on the cuff to approximately 40 mm Hg.
10. Continue to monitor the patient throughout the entire collection process. The donor should never be left unattended. Mix blood and anticoagulant periodically during the procedure (e.g., every 45 seconds).
11. When the primary bag has tripped the scale, the donor can stop squeezing and tubing can be clamped. A unit containing a volume of 405 to 550 mL should weigh between 429 to 583 g, plus the weight of the container and anticoagulant. The conversion 1.06 g/mL is used to convert grams to milliliters. If the volume collected is in the low volume range (300 to 404 mL in a 450-mL collection or 333 to 449 mL in a 500-mL collection), the unit must be labeled as a "low volume unit," and fresh frozen

plasma (FFP) cannot be made from this unit, as it would not contain adequate levels of coagulation factors.

12. Before the needle is removed from the donor's arm, pilot tubes are filled. The pressure is reduced to 20 mm Hg or less and, depending on the tubing of the bag, the tubes are filled:
    - *In-line needle.* A hemostat or metal clip is used to seal tubing distal to the needle. The connector is opened, the needle is inserted into the pilot tube, the hemostat is removed, and tubes are filled. The donor needle can now be removed.
    - *Straight-tubing assembly.* Place hemostats approximately four segments from the needle. Tighten the loose knot made previously in the tubing; release the hemostats, and strip a segment of tubing between knot and needle. Secure hemostat and cut tubing in stripped area of segment. Fill required tubes by releasing hemostats. This is an open system, and appropriate biohazard precautions should be followed. Reapply hemostats and remove needle from donor's arm.
13. Once the needle has been removed from the donor's arm, apply pressure over gauze, and ask the donor to raise his or her arm, continuing to exert pressure over the site. When the bleeding has stopped, the donor can lower his or her arm, and an appropriate bandage can be applied.
14. The needle assembly should be discarded into an appropriate biohazard receptacle. The tubing should be stripped to allow proper mixing of anticoagulant/preservative with blood.
15. Heat seal the filled tubing into segments, and apply an appropriate identification label to one segment and detach from the blood bag for storage. Place blood at the appropriate temperature. Units in which platelets will be made must be maintained at room temperature (20°C to 24°C) until the platelet concentrate has been prepared; all others can be stored at 1°C to 6°C.

---

3. Raise the donor's legs above the level of the head
4. Loosen tight clothing and secure airway
5. Monitor vital signs

Donors who are extremely nervous may exhibit sudden twitching or muscle spasms. If this happens, try to disengage the hyperventilation sequence by conversing with the donor and having the donor breathe into a paper bag, if necessary. It is not advised to give oxygen to these donors.

If the donor starts to feel nauseated or vomits, the following instructions apply:

1. Instruct the donor to breathe slowly
2. Apply cold compresses to the forehead
3. Turn the donor's head to one side and provide an appropriate receptacle
4. The donor may be given water after vomiting has ceased

Moderate Reactions

A moderate reaction can include any of the reactions listed above in addition to loss of consciousness. The donor may have a decreased pulse rate, may hyperventilate, and may

exhibit a fall in systolic pressure to 60 mm Hg. The following instructions apply:

1. Check vital signs frequently
2. Administer 95% oxygen and 5% carbon dioxide

Severe Reactions

A donor experiencing convulsions defines a severe reaction. Convulsions can be caused by cerebral ischemia, marked hyperventilation, or epilepsy. The former is associated with vasovagal syncope or reduced blood flow to the brain owing to the shock symptoms, and hyperventilation is caused by marked depletion of carbon dioxide. The following should be followed by the donor room personnel:

1. Call for help immediately; notify blood bank physician
2. Try and restrain the donor to prevent injury to self or others
3. Ensure an adequate airway

In the event of cardiac or respiratory difficulties, the donor room staff should perform CPR until medical help arrives.

LifeSouth Community Blood Centers
1221 NW 13th Street
Gainesville, FL 32601

Post Donation Recommendations

Date:	Location:	Branch:

Donor Recommendations

Please read the following instructions and sign at the bottom.

1. Contact the blood center:

   - If any illness arises after your donation.

   - If you develop a headache and fever of 101°F or higher within 14 days following your donation or if you become diagnosed with West Nile Virus infection.

   - If you have any questions about your donation or if you remember something about your medical or personal history that may affect your blood donation.

2. Do not smoke for one-half hour.

3. Eat and drink something before leaving.

4. Do not leave until released by the donor technician.

5. Drink more fluids (nonalcoholic) than usual in the next four hours, especially fruit juices.

6. Leave the bandage on for a few hours, and then you may remove it. If there is any bleeding from the puncture site, raise arm, and apply direct pressure.

7. If you feel faint or dizzy, either lie down or sit down with head between the knees.

8. Do not perform strenuous activities or engage in critical work where safety requires your maximum abilities.

9. If any symptoms persist, either return to blood center or see your doctor.

Signatures

Thank you for your blood donation.

Figure 13–10.   Sample postdonation instructions. *(LifeSouth Blood Center, Montgomery, AL, with permission.)*

Hematomas

A hematoma is a localized collection of blood under the skin, resulting in a bluish discoloration. It is caused by the needle going through the vein, with subsequent leakage of blood into the tissue. If a hematoma develops, the following instructions apply:

1. Remove the tourniquet and needle from donor's arm
2. Apply pressure with sterile gauze pads for 7 to 10 minutes, with the donor raising his or her arm above the heart
3. Apply ice to the area for 5 minutes

Donor Records

Donor records must be retained by the blood collection facility as mandated by the FDA and AABB. There must be a system to ensure that the donor's confidentiality is not compromised and that donor records are not altered. There must be policies on record-keeping and storage, and the blood bank staff should be well trained on these policies and procedures.

The minimum retention time for donor records varies from 5 to 10 years to indefinitely. Table 13–1 lists minimum retention times for various donor records.

Donor Processing

The donor unit collected must be tested and processed by blood bank technologists before it can be made available for

Table 13–1   Retention of Donor Records

DONOR RECORD	RETENTION TIME (YEARS)
Donor ABO/Rh	10
Donor antibody screen	10
Informed consent for donation	10
Medical director approval for donation interval	5
Physical examination	10
Medical history information	10
Identification number of donor unit	10
Viral marker testing results	10
Quarantine of donor unit	10
Repeat testing of donor blood	10
ID of donor processing tech	10
Plt count for frequent platelet pheresis	10
Sedimenting agent of leukapheresis	10
Notification of abnormal results	10/indefinite

Modified from AABB *Standards*, American Association of Blood Banks, Bethesda, MD 2009, p. 74.

transfusion. The tests performed on donor blood include those detailed in the following sections.

ABO/Rh

Testing for the donor's ABO group must include both forward and reverse grouping. The ABO group must be determined by testing the donor RBCs with anti-A and anti-B reagents and by testing the donor serum or plasma with reagent A_1 cells and B cells. (Refer to Chapter 6, "The ABO Blood Group System.")

The donor's Rh type should be determined by testing with anti-D reagent at the immediate spin phase. In the event the initial testing is negative, a test for weak D should be performed. This involves a 37°C incubation and an antihuman globulin (AHG) phase. If both the immediate spin and weak-D test results are negative, label the donor as Rh-negative; however, if any part of the testing yields a positive test for D, the donor unit should be labeled as Rh-positive. (Refer to Chapter 7, "The Rh Blood Group System.") Some automated testing systems do not require an antiglobulin test phase for the detection of the weak-D variants.

Antibody Screen

AABB *Standards* requires that donors with a history of pregnancy or transfusion be tested for unexpected antibodies to RBC antigens. Most blood centers choose to perform the antibody screen test on all donors, not just those with a history of pregnancy or transfusion. Unlike the antibody screen performed on a recipient prior to transfusion, which uses two or three individual reagent cells, the testing of donor units generally uses a pooled cell reagent. This reagent contains two or three individual cells pooled into a single reagent. The pooled screening cell reagent contains all of the required antigens and is capable of detecting the presence of the clinically significant alloantibodies. (Refer to Chapter 9, "Detection and Identification of Antibodies.") A control system must be in place for the method used. For example, in the tube system, cells sensitized with IgG are added to all negative tubes after the AHG phase. If the gel system or an automated instrument is used, the manufacturer's guidelines must be followed (see Chapter 12, "Other Technologies and Automation").

HBsAg

Screening for hepatitis B surface antigen (HBsAg) began in 1972. The methods currently available include enzyme immunoassay (EIA), chemiluminescence (ChLIA), and nucleic acid amplification (NAT). If the EIA or ChLIA tests are initially positive, they must be repeated in duplicate and a confirmatory (neutralization) test must be performed. If the confirmatory test is positive, the donor is considered to be infected (acute or chronic) with the hepatitis B virus (HBV) and must be permanently deferred. NAT testing for HBV, although available and approved by the FDA, is not mandated for donor screening and has not been widely implemented in the United States at this time. If the initial HBsAg testing is reactive but the confirmatory testing is not (unconfirmed positive), all the current products are discarded but the donor need not be permanently deferred, provided the antibody to hepatitis B core (anti-HBc) testing is also nonreactive. The donor is deferred for 8 weeks and may be reinstated if the next HBsAg testing is nonreactive.

If the donor unit is needed in an emergency that precludes completion of viral marker testing, a notation indicating testing is not yet completed must be conspicuously attached to the unit. If tests are subsequently found to be reactive or positive, the transfusion service must be notified as soon as possible.

Anti-HBc

Antibody to the core or interior protein on the hepatitis B virus has been implicated in hepatitis C disease. This test was once part of surrogate testing, along with its counterpart alanine transferase (ALT). In 1995, a National Institutes of Health consensus panel voted to discontinue the ALT test for blood donors because of the increased sophistication and sensitivity for anti-HCV testing;[22] however, testing for anti-HBc has remained a requirement of blood donors in the prevention of post-transfusion hepatitis B. The methods employed are similar to those for HBsAg. Presence of HBc antibody in the donor serum suggests the possibility of HBV infection, either acute or chronic. A positive result for anti-HBc along with a positive HBsAg would place the donor in a permanently deferred category. A positive test for anti-HBc without an accompanying positive test for HBsAg or HBC is not cause for donor deferral unless it occurs on more than one occasion or on two consecutive tests. The products will not be used for transfusion even if the donor is not deferred for a positive result.

Anti-HCV and NAT

The hepatitis C virus (HCV) was identified in 1988[21] and was initially referred to as non-A, non-B hepatitis. Screening tests for anti-HCV involve EIA and ChLIA methods. In 1999, NAT for HCV RNA was introduced and in 2002 the tests were licensed by FDA and mandated for routine donor screening in addition to the EIA or ChLIA methods. NAT is able to detect small amounts of viral nucleic acid in blood before antibodies or viral proteins such as HCV core antigen are detectable by current methods. Implementation of HCV NAT testing effectively reduced the window period for detection of HCV by approximately 70%, from a mean of 82 days to 25 days.

Confirmatory methods include the RIBA (recombinant immunoblot assay) and HCV RNA. The test is reported as positive, negative, or indeterminate. An individual who is positive by RIBA is considered to have the HCV antibody and would be indefinitely deferred as a blood donor. Donors who test repeat reactive for HCV screening tests must be deferred, and the components or products prepared are discarded. If the confirmatory RIBA or NAT testing are nonreactive, the donor may be considered for reentry.

Anti-HIV-1/2 and NAT

All donor units must be screened for the presence of the human immunodeficiency virus (HIV-1/2) antibody using an FDA-approved method. If the initial screening test is negative, the unit is suitable for transfusion; if it is positive, the test must be repeated in duplicate. If any one of the duplicate tests is reactive, the unit must be discarded as well as any in-date components from prior donations. Screening tests include EIA, ChLIA, and NAT. NAT testing is run using 16 to 24 donation samples per pool. Confirmation tests for HIV include the Western blot (Wb) and the immunofluorescence assay (IFA). Results are expressed as positive, negative, or indeterminate.

Anti-HTLV-I/II

The HTLV-I virus or human T-cell lymphotrophic virus type I is the causative agent of adult T-cell leukemia and has been associated with a neurological disorder called HTLV-associated myelopathy. HTLV-II has been shown to have about 60% homology with type I and is prevalent among intravenous drug users in the United States.[22] Persons can contract both viruses from transfusion via infected lymphocytes. Screening for HTLV-I began in 1988; a combined HTLV-I/II was approved 10 years later in 1998. Screening test methodologies include both EIA and ChLIA. In recipients of blood infected by HTLV-I and II, 20% to 60% will develop infection. Myelopathy can occur in a person infected with these viruses as a result of blood transfusion.[23]

As with the other viral markers, a donation that is repeatedly reactive may not be used for transfusion. It is recommended that if another kit is used by another manufacturer and that test is also positive, the donor should be indefinitely deferred. Confirmatory tests include Western blot, RIPA, and NAT testing.

WNV RNA

Testing for West Nile virus (WNV) began in 2003, and in 2009 the FDA published their final guidelines for testing whole blood and component donor samples. It is recommended that units be tested year-round using either a mini-pool (MP-NAT) or individual donor (ID-NAT) method.[41] MP-NAT uses pools of 6 to 16 donor samples and is routinely used when risk of WNV infection in the geographical area is low. A switch to the ID-NAT format is recommended when the risk is high. This generally coincides with mosquito season during the summer months. Each blood collection facility must define the trigger point and have established procedures to switch from MP-NAT to ID-NAT testing and when to switch back again. If a mini-pool is reactive, each sample in the pool should be retested individually. Those that remain nonreactive may be released for transfusion. Any individual units that test reactive should be discarded, and the donor should be deferred from further donations for 120 days. In addition, any currently in-date products from the same donor during the previous 120 days should be retrieved and quarantined. The donor should be notified and counseled. Repeat testing with the same or another individual NAT test and a test for WNV antibodies is recommended.

Syphilis

A serologic test for syphilis is required by both the AABB and the FDA. Screening tests include the rapid plasma regain (RPR) and the Venereal Disease Research Laboratory (VDRL). Both tests are based on reagin, or antibody directed toward cardiolipin particles. Cardiolipin-like antibodies have been documented in persons with untreated syphilis infections. Antibody will agglutinate cardiolipin carbon particles in the form of visible flocculation.

The confirmatory test for syphilis is the FTA-ABS or fluorescent treponemal antibody absorption test. In this test, indirect immunofluorescence is used to detect antibodies to the spirochete *T. pallidum*, the agent that causes syphilis. If the STS or VDRL screening test is reactive or indeterminate, the components from that donation must be discarded and the donor deferred unless a confirmatory FTA-ABS test is nonreactive. If the FTA-ABS test is nonreactive, the donor may be reentered and the components labeled as reactive with the screening test. The donor of a confirmed reactive test may be reentered into the donor pool after 12 months and documentation of completion of treatment.

There have only been three documented cases of transfusion-transmitted syphilis. The spirochete that causes syphilis, *T. pallidum*, cannot survive more than 72 hours in citrated blood stored at 1°C to 6°C, which would make platelets the only component capable of transmitting infection. A serologic test for syphilis is also done because the disease is characterized as being sexually transmitted and places the donor at higher risk for possible exposure to hepatitis and HIV.

T. Cruzi (Chagas' Disease)

Chagas' disease is a parasitic infection that is endemic to Mexico and Central and South America. The infection is generally mild but persists, without symptoms, throughout the infected individual's life and can be transmitted through blood transfusions. The FDA first recommended testing donors for antibodies to *T. Cruzi* in 1989, but it wasn't until December of 2007 that an EIA test was licensed. In 2007, some donor centers began testing, and in 2010 the FDA released their final recommendations for donor screening.

All donors (allogeneic and autologous) are to be tested once. If the results are nonreactive, the donor need not be retested with each donation. This was reasoned because most donors who are infected in the United States have a chronic infection that was acquired when residing in a country where the disease is endemic. Repeat reactive donors must be deferred indefinitely and the products quarantined and destroyed. No approved confirmatory tests are available, so there are no mechanisms for reentry for deferred donors. The donor should be notified and counseled, and a "look-back" procedure should be performed, looking back to all donations from that donor for the prior 10 years. If the donor had been previously tested with a licensed test, "look back" 12 months from the last nonreactive test.

Platelet Bacterial Detection

Bacterial contamination of platelet concentrates whether pheresis or whole blood derived has been an issue for many years. Platelet components are particularly at risk because they are stored at room temperature. In 2011, AABB, in a revised interim standard, outlined the acceptable methods that could be used by donor centers or transfusion services to detect possible bacterial contamination in both leukocyte reduced or non-leukocyte-reduced platelets.

For apheresis-derived platelets, it is recommended that a culture method be used that would usually be performed by the collecting facility. For whole blood–derived platelets, there are two choices. For platelets that are pooled within 4 hours of transfusion, a new PGD test (Verax) can be used. It is a relatively easy test to perform, requires about 45 minutes, and can be done by a transfusion service at the time of issue. For platelets that are pooled and stored as a pre-pooled product, a culture-based test is recommended. This would typically be performed by the collection facility. If a facility wishes to use a method that has not been approved by the FDA, documentation of validation must be available and it must demonstrate that the procedure performs equal to or greater than a method already approved by the FDA. Any product that is found to be initially positive must be quarantined and destroyed. Any products that have already been issued should be recalled and the transfusion service or recipient's physician notified.

Component Preparation

A single blood donation can provide transfusion therapy to multiple patients in the form of RBCs, platelets, fresh frozen plasma, and cryoprecipitate. Other products such as derivatives of plasma (e.g., immune serum globulin) also benefit patients in various diseases or conditions. This section describes the manufacturing process of all components used in transfusion therapy.

Whole Blood

Whole blood contains RBCs and plasma, with a hematocrit level of approximately 38%. Whole blood transfusions provide both oxygen-carrying capacity and volume expansion. However, this same benefit can be obtained with concentrated red blood cells and either a manufactured volume expander such as saline or albumin or frozen plasma that would contain viable clotting factors. The platelets, white cells, and labile clotting factors do not survive in stored whole blood, so whole blood is rarely used for transfusion today with the exception of autologous units in some transfusion facilities.[24] Most whole blood donations are made into components, red cells, platelets, plasma, cryoprecipitate or some combination of these components. If the donation remains as whole blood, it must be stored at 1°C to 6°C, and the shelf-life is dependent on the preservative used. If collected in ACD or CPD, shelf-life is 21 days and CPDA-1 is 35 days.

Whole blood units can be irradiated to inhibit T-cell proliferation in the recipient. Irradiation will decrease the shelf-life to 28 days from the date of irradiation or the original outdate of the unit, whichever is sooner. The dose of radiation is a minimum of 25 Gy, delivered to the center of the container, and 15 Gy at any other point of the container. Cesium-137 or cobalt-60 may be used. Irradiated whole blood is also stored at 1°C to 6°C.

Red Blood Cells

RBCs are prepared from whole blood by centrifugation or sedimentation. In addition, they may be obtained directly by apheresis. Although RBCs may be prepared at any time during the normal storage time, they are typically prepared shortly after donation to allow the manufacture of platelet concentrates, frozen plasma, or cryoprecipitate, which must be prepared within 8 hours of collection. The amount of plasma removed from the whole blood unit will vary depending on the anticoagulant-preservative solution used. If CPDA-1 is used, 200 to 250 mL of plasma can be removed, leaving the RBC product with a hematocrit of 65% to 80%. If additive solutions (AS) are employed, an additional 50 mL of plasma can be removed, because 150 mL of adenine-saline is added back to the cells, achieving the desired hematocrit level of less than 80%. Typically, RBCs with AS added will have a hematocrit of 55% to 65%. RBCs typically have a final red cell volume of 160 to 275 mL or 50 to 80 g of hemoglobin suspended in the residual plasma or additive solution.[24] RBC transfusions are indicted in patients who require an increase in RBC mass and oxygen-carrying capacity. They are particularly useful when the patient is also at risk of circulatory overload; for example, patients with anemia in addition to cardiac failure. Box 13–6 outlines a general procedure for RBC production using centrifugation.

RBC Aliquots

Aliquotted red cells is the product most often transfused during the neonatal period or in infants younger than 4 months of age. Indications for transfusion include anemia caused by spontaneous fetomaternal or fetoplacental hemorrhage, twin-twin transfusion, obstetric accidents, and internal hemorrhage. Blood drawn from infants for laboratory testing (iatrogenic anemia) also may warrant a neonatal transfusion if more than 10% of the blood volume has been removed. Transfusions for neonates require only small

BOX 13–6

Procedure for RBC Production Using Centrifugation

1. Weigh and balance each unit.
2. Load units into a swinging bucket apparatus, making sure each unit is balanced. An assortment of rubber weights is generally used.
3. Centrifuge whole blood using a heavy spin (5,000 × g for 5 minutes in a refrigerated centrifuge). Temperature setting should be 4°C. If also preparing platelet concentrates, the initial spin will be light (2 to 3 minute at 3,200 rpm).
4. When the centrifuge has stopped completely, place the unit carefully onto an expressor and release the spring.
5. Express the plasma into the attached satellite bag. If more than one satellite bag is attached, apply hemostats to one of the bags so that the plasma will flow into only one bag. Remove the appropriate amount of plasma by using a scale. Approximately 230 to 256 g of plasma will yield a hematocrit level between 70% and 80%.[4] If additive solutions are to be added to the red cell product, virtually all of the plasma may be removed (90% to 95% hematocrit).
6. When the appropriate amount of plasma has been removed, hemostats can again be applied to the satellite bag until such time as a dielectric heat sealer can separate the tubing. Always ensure the satellite bags have the same donor number as the primary bag. Follow the manufacturer's instructions for adding the attached additive solution if applicable.
7. Store the RBCs at 4°C. The plasma is stored depending on the product desired (FFP, liquid plasma, etc.).
8. Quality control on the hematocrit level of the RBCs is performed monthly; 75% of samples tested must yield a hematocrit level of 80% or less.

volumes of RBCs (10 to 25 mL); several aliquots may be prepared from a single-donor unit.

A multiple-pack system or a quad pack is available for use when a single unit of whole blood is collected in a bag with four integrally attached containers; such a system can increase the number of transfusions an infant can receive from one donor. Each pack retains the original outdate of the primary bag within a closed system. Sterile connecting devices can be used to maintain a closed system in attaching Pedi-Paks to a unit of RBCs. The precise volume of blood desired can be aspirated into a syringe through a large-bore needle inserted through an injection site coupler. The filled syringe should be closed securely with a sterile cap and labeled with expiration date, patient identification, volume transfused, preservative, and ABO type. The aliquotted blood has an expiration time of 24 hours and should be stored at 1°C to 6°C until issued. In some institutions, the blood bank will issue the Pedi-Pak to the neonatal ICU or floor rather than preparing a syringe. The syringe, if used, will be filled by the patient care staff.

Initial testing for neonates includes ABO, Rh, and antibody screen for unexpected antibodies, which can be performed on serum or plasma from the infant or mother. AABB *Standards*[1] states that repeat ABO and Rh typing may be omitted for the remainder of the neonate's hospital admission; in the event the initial screen for RBC antibodies is negative, it is not necessary to crossmatch donor RBCs for the initial or subsequent transfusions. If the antibody screen is positive for clinically significant RBC antibodies, the neonate must receive blood that does not contain the corresponding antigen or is compatible by the antiglobulin crossmatch.

The anticoagulant most often used for neonate transfusions is CPDA-1. A transfusion of 10 mL/kg in a unit with a hematocrit level of 80% should raise the hemoglobin by 3 g/dL.[25] Some institutions, however, have begun using additive solutions for neonatal transfusions when the volume transfused is minimal. Concerns with additive solutions involve the constituents adenine and mannitol and their toxic effects on the renal system. Most physicians advocating the use of additive solutions do so in the limited setting of small-volume transfusions. Blood units with additive solutions are contraindicated for use in exchange transfusions.

RBCs Irradiated

Patients who are immunocompromised or who are receiving a bone marrow or stem cell transplant, fetuses undergoing an intrauterine transfusion, and recipients of blood from relatives must receive irradiated blood. Irradiation inhibits the proliferation of T cells and subsequent transfusion-associated graft-versus-host disease. RBCs, platelets, and granulocyte concentrates contain viable T lymphocytes that can become engrafted when transfused if the host's immune system is not capable of identifying or defending against the foreign cells.

Both the FDA and AABB recommend a minimum dose of gamma irradiation of 25 Gy to the central portion of the blood unit, with no less than 15 Gy delivered to any part of the blood unit.[2] Irradiation is generally performed using cesium-137 or cobalt-60. To confirm a product was irradiated, a radiochromic film label is affixed to the component before it is placed into the metal canister of the irradiator. Darkening of the film confirms irradiation requirements. Each facility should have a protocol and procedure for irradiating blood components, training of personnel using the irradiator, and issuing of irradiated components. The expiration date of irradiated RBCs is 28 days from the time of irradiation or the original outdate, whichever is sooner.

RBCs Leukoreduced

According to AABB *Standards*, leukoreduced red cells is a product in which the absolute WBC count in the unit is reduced to less than 5×10^6 and contains at least 85% of the original RBC mass.[1] There are two major categories of leukoreduced RBCs: prestorage and poststorage.

In prestorage leukoreduction, special filters procure at least a 99.9% (a 2- to 4-log) removal of leukocytes by employing multiple layers of polyester or cellulose acetate nonwoven fibers that trap leukocytes and platelets but that allow RBCs to flow through. These filters provide a leukocyte-reduced product with normal shelf-life and meet the requirement for 85% retention of original RBCs. The impetus for prestorage leukoreduction involved biological response modifiers (BRMs) released from leukocytes during storage of the component that were found to promote febrile transfusion reactions. Examples of BRMs include proinflammatory cytokines (interleukin-1, interleukin-6, and tumor necrosis factor) and complement fragments (C5a and C3a).[26]

There are three methods available in prestorage leukoreduction. In the first method, an in-line filter can be attached to the whole blood unit and filtered via gravity; RBCs and plasma can then be prepared. In the second method, plasma is initially removed from the whole blood unit, and then the packed cells are passed through an in-line reduction filter. In both these methods, random-donor platelets cannot be prepared, as they would have been trapped in the filter. In the third method, a sterile docking device can be used to attach a leukocyte reduction filter to a unit of RBCs, which is allowed to flow via gravity. Today, many institutions maintain 100% of their red cell inventory as prestored leukoreduced products.

In poststorage leukoreduction, leukocytes are removed in the blood bank prior to issuing blood or at the bedside before transfusion. Whereas centrifugation can procure counts less than 5×10^8, which can prevent most febrile hemolytic reactions to RBC concentrates, third-generation filters reduce leukocytes to levels of 5×10^6 or lower. Removing leukocytes by centrifugation or filtration just before transfusion of blood should prevent reactions that are caused by leukocyte antibodies in patient's plasma and leukocytes present in the transfused blood; however, it won't prevent reactions caused by BRMs that originate from the leukocytes present in the component during storage. Studies suggest that the age of the RBC unit is a predictor of a febrile reaction and that the cytokine involvement may be cumulative.[27]

RBCs that have been frozen, thawed, deglycerolized, and washed also produce a leukoreduced product. Arnaud and Meryman[28] recently discovered that removing the buffy coat at the time of collection lowered the level of leukocytes to acceptable limits (1.9×10^6) after freezing and deglycerolization and could provide a possible economic alternative to leukocyte filtration after freezing. This product has a shelf-life of 24 hours, because it is an open system and requires special equipment to carry out the procedure. Leukoreduced RBCs have been useful in trying to avoid the following reactions associated with products containing leukocytes: febrile nonhemolytic transfusion reactions; transfusion-related acute lung injury; and transmission of Epstein-Barr virus, CMV, and human T-cell lymphotrophic virus.

Frozen, Deglycerolized RBCs

Freezing RBCs with glycerol dates back to the 1950s.[29] Frozen RBCs can be stored for up to 10 years for those patients with rare phenotypes, for autologous use, and for the military to maintain blood inventories around the world for U.S. military use. The resulting deglycerolized product is free of leukocytes, platelets, and plasma due to the washing process. Since all donor plasma is deglycerolized when removed, washed red cells can be used for patients with paroxysmal nocturnal hemoglobinuria and IgA deficiency with circulating anti-IgA.

Cryoprotective agents can be categorized as penetrating and nonpenetrating. A penetrating agent involves small molecules that cross the cell membrane into the cytoplasm. The osmotic force of the agent prevents water from migrating outward as extracellular ice is formed, preventing intracellular dehydration. An example of a penetrating agent is glycerol. An example of a nonpenetrating agent is hydroxyethyl starch (HES). This comprises large molecules that do not enter the cell but instead form a shell around it, preventing loss of water and subsequent dehydration. HES, as well as dimethylsulfoxide, is used to freeze hematopoietic progenitor cells. Two procedures used for freezing and deglycerolizing RBCs are the high-glycerol and low-glycerol methods. The methods differ in the equipment used, the temperature of storage, and the rate of freezing. Most blood centers practice the high-glycerol method, which is outlined in Table 13–2.

High Glycerol (40% Weight per Volume)

This method increases the cryoprotective power of the glycerol, thus allowing a slow, uncontrolled freezing process. The freezer is generally a mechanical freezer that provides storage at –80°C. This particular procedure is probably the one most widely used, because the equipment is fairly simple and the products require less delicate handling. It does, however, require a larger volume of wash solution for deglycerolization. RBCs are frozen within 6 days of collection when the preservative is CPD or CPDA-1 and up to 42 days when preserved in AS-1, AS-3, and AS-5. AABB *Standards*[1] states that RBCs must be placed in the freezer within 4 hours of opening the system. It is advisable to freeze a sample of donor serum in the event additional testing is required for donor screening.

The thawing process takes approximately 30 minutes and involves immersing units into a 37°C waterbath and washing the RBCs with solutions of decreasing osmolarity (e.g., 12% NaCl, 1.6% NaCl, 0.9% NaCl, + 0.2% dextrose). An exception to this rule is a donor with sickle trait in which RBCs would hemolyze upon suspension in hypertonic solutions; in this case, the cells would be washed in 12% NaCl and then 0.9% NaCl with 0.2% dextrose, omitting the 1.6% solution. Automated continuous-flow instruments can be utilized for washing. Once the RBCs have been deglycerolized, the unit is considered an open system with an expiration date of 24 hours and is stored at 1°C to 6°C.

Low Glycerol (20% Weight per Volume)

In this method, the cryoprotection of the glycerol is minimal, and a very rapid, more controlled freezing procedure is required. Liquid nitrogen (N_2) is routinely used for this method. The frozen units must be stored at about –120°C, which is the temperature of liquid N_2 vapor. Because of the minimal amount of protection by the glycerol, temperature fluctuations during storage can cause RBC destruction.

The quality-control procedures necessary for RBC freezing include all of the standard procedures for monitoring refrigerators, freezers, water baths, dry thaw baths, and centrifuges. They also include procedures to ensure good RBC recovery (80%), good viability (70% survival at 24 hours post-transfusion), and adequate glycerol removal (less than 1% residual intracellular glycerol; Box 13–7). Valeri and colleagues[30] froze RBCs for up to 37 years by using the high-glycerol method (40 w/v) and yielded an average RBC recovery of 75%, with 1% hemolysis. Although researchers are attempting to freeze cells for more than 10 years, the FDA has not yet been swayed to change the maximum storage time. Studies have also shown that irradiated (25 Gy) red cells that are subsequently frozen and deglycerolized yield similar results in RBC recovery, post-transfusion survival, and residual hemoglobin as nonirradiated units.[31] Cells should be frozen within 6 hours of collection unless they have been rejuvenated. Rejuvenation serves to increase the levels of 2,3-DPG and ATP in RBCs stored in citrate/phosphate/dextrose (CPD) or CPDA-1 using an FDA-approved solution. RBCs can be rejuvenated up to 3 days after expiration and then glycerolized and frozen.

Table 13–2 Key Steps in Freezing Red Cells Using High-Glycerol Concentration

PREPARATION	GLYCEROLIZATION	DEGLYCEROLIZATION
Weigh RBCs	Place cells on a shaker and add 100 mL glycerol	Thaw frozen cells at 37°C in water bath
Adjust to 260–400 g 0.9% NaCl	Stop agitation and allow cells to equilibrate 5–30 min	Deglycerolize cells using a continuous flow washer
Prewarm RBCs and glycerol to 25°C		
Set glycerol bottles in a water bath for 15 min at 25–37°C	Let partially glycerolized cells flow into freezing bag; slowly add glycerol	Apply a deglycerolize label to transfer pack; ABO, Rh, WB unit #s and expiration date
Label the freezing bag with name of facility, whole blood unit #s, ABO, Rh, date collected, date frozen, cryoprotective agent, expiration, and "red blood cells frozen"	Maintain glycerolized cells at 24–32°C until ready to freeze (not to exceed 4 hours)	Dilute unit with hypertonic 12% NaCl and let equilibrate for 5 min
	Freeze at ≤ 65°C	Wash with 1.6% NaCl until residual glycerol is less than 1%; wash with 0.9% NaCl plus 0.2% dextrose; store at 1–6°C

Quality Control Procedures for Deglycerolization

1. RBC recovery can be determined by estimating the recovered RBC mass:

$$\% \text{ Recovery} = \frac{\text{wt. of DRBC (g)} \times \text{Hct of DRBC} \times 100}{\text{wt. of liquid RBC (g)} \times \text{Hct of liquid RBC}}$$

DRBC = deglycerolized RBCs

2. A post-transfusion survival study should be done when the program is first being set up to ensure the proper use of the equipment and procedure. If the procedure being used is standard, with data already published in the literature, these survival studies are not required.

3. Glycerol must be removed to a level of less than 1% residual. The published procedures should accomplish this. However, it is important to perform this check on each unit before releasing it for transfusion.
   - Measure the osmolarity of the unit using an osmometer. The osmolarity should be about 420 mOsm (maximum 500 mOsm).
   - Perform a simulated transfusion. Place one segment (approximately 3 inches) of deglycerolized cells into 7 mL of 0.7% NaCl. Mix, centrifuge, and check for hemolysis.
   - Compare with a standard hemoglobin color comparator. If the hue exceeds the 500 mOsm level, hemolysis is too great, and the unit is not suitable for transfusion.

4. Postdeglycerolized tests include confirmation of ABO, Rh, and a direct antiglobulin test.

Platelet Concentrates

Platelet concentrates can be produced during the routine conversion of whole blood into concentrated RBCs or by apheresis; more and more blood centers are producing apheresis platelets because of the high yield and minimal RBC contamination. Platelets have widespread use for a variety of patients: actively bleeding patients who are thrombocytopenic (less than 50,000/µL) due to decreased production or decreased function, cancer patients during radiation and chemotherapy because of induced thrombocytopenia (less than 20,000/µL), and thrombocytopenic preoperative patients (less than 50,000/µL). Prophylactic platelet transfusion is not usually indicated or recommended in disseminated intravascular coagulation (DIC) or idiopathic thrombocytopenic purpura (ITP). In both cases, there is an induced thrombocytopenia owing to increased destruction in ITP and consumption in DIC.

Platelet concentrates prepared from whole blood are generally referred to as random-donor platelets to distinguish them from single-donor platelets produced by apheresis. Random-donor platelet concentrates should contain at least 5.5×10^{10} platelets, are stored at 20°C to 24°C with continuous agitation, contain sufficient plasma (typically 40 to 70 mL) to yield a pH of greater than or equal to 6.2, and have a shelf-life of 5 days.[1] Apheresis or single-donor platelets contain at least 3×10^{11} platelets (therapeutic equivalent of four to six random donor platelets), are stored at 22°C to 24°C with continuous agitation, contain approximately 300 mL of plasma, and have a shelf-life of 5 days.

Single-donor platelets are generally indicated for patients who are unresponsive to random platelets due to HLA alloimmunization or to limit the platelet exposure from multiple donors. In 2005, the FDA approved the PASSPORT (Post Approval Surveillance Study of Platelet Outcomes, Release Tested) study of leukoreduced apheresis platelets stored for 7 days rather than the currently approved 5-day storage. The study required that all platelet units in the study be tested for bacterial contamination prior to testing. A total of 388,903 apheresis platelets were accrued during the study period (September 2005 to January 2008). The testing revealed an unacceptably high risk of bacterial contamination in the units, and the study and the use of 7-day stored apheresis platelets was stopped based upon the results.[32]

Whole blood used to prepare platelet concentrates must be drawn by a single nontraumatic venipuncture, and the concentrate must be prepared within 4 hours of collection. Whole blood–derived platelet concentrates are generally prepared as part of the production of red blood cells and frozen plasma (Box 13–8).

The quality-control procedures must include a platelet count (5.5×10^{10} for random donor, 3×10^{11} for single donor), pH (6.2 or greater), and volume (must be sufficient to maintain an acceptable pH until the end of the dating period). A new standard, included in the 26th edition of *Standards*, requires transfusion services to have methods in place to limit and detect or inactivate bacterial contamination in all platelet components. The interim standard for bacterial detection, 5.1.5.1.1, states that detection methods shall either be approved by the FDA or validated to provide sensitivity equivalent to FDA-approved methods. To satisfy quality-control requirements, one to four units are tested per month. Ninety percent of all units tested must meet or exceed the minimum standards. Temperature monitoring must be performed during each major stage of production, and records must be maintained of all procedures performed.

Platelets, either random donor or single donor, can be irradiated if the patient's diagnosis indicates that it is appropriate or the platelets have been HLA matched. The irradiation requirements are the same as for RBCs and do not affect the shelf-life of the platelet product. Some institutions have implemented programs to irradiate all platelet inventories.

Platelet Aliquots

As with RBCs, platelet transfusions for neonates require only small volumes, and several aliquots may be prepared from a single unit with the use of a sterile docked/connected quad bag (Pedi-Pak). This system can increase the number of transfusions an infant can receive from one donor, limiting the number of donor exposures, or it can be used to supply transfusions to several neonates or infants, providing better utilization of the product during the short dating period. Each pack retains the original outdate of the primary bag, because the sterile docking processes are considered a closed system. Transfusion of platelet concentrates is indicated

Procedure for Preparing Random-Donor Platelets and Plasma from Whole Blood

1. Maintain the whole blood at 20°C to 24°C before and during platelet preparation.

2. Set the centrifuge temperature at 22°C. The rpm and time must be specifically calculated for each centrifuge. It will generally be a short (2 to 3 minute), light (3,200 rpm) spin. This spin should separate most of the RBCs but leave most of the platelets suspended in the plasma.

3. Platelet preparation should be done in a closed, multibag system.

4. Express off the platelet-rich plasma into one of the satellite bags. Enough plasma must remain on the RBCs to maintain a 70% to 80% hematocrit level.

5. Seal the tubing between the RBC and the plasma. Disconnect the RBC and store it at 4°C.

6. Recentrifuge the platelet-rich plasma at 22°C using a heavy spin (approximately 3,600 rpm for 5 minutes). This will separate the platelets from the plasma.

7. Express the majority of the plasma into the second satellite bag, leaving approximately 50 to 70 mL on the platelets. The volume is important to maintain the pH above 6.2 during storage.

8. Seal the tubing between the bags and separate. Make segments for both the platelets and the plasma for testing purposes.

9. Allow the platelets to rest undisturbed for 1 to 2 hours at 20°C to 24°C or until all platelet clumps have been resuspended in the residual plasma. Be sure the platelet button is covered with the plasma. Gentle manipulation can be used if needed.

10. Weigh the plasma bag and determine the volume. Record the volume on the bag.

11. Place the plasma in a protective container and freeze. The plasma must be frozen in such a way that evidence of thawing can be determined. Freezing some sort of indentation into the bag, which is visible as long as the plasma remains frozen, is an easy way to accomplish this. The freezing container is important because the plastic bag becomes quite brittle when frozen at low temperatures and can be cracked or broken easily.

12. The plasma must be frozen solid within 8 hours or 24 hours, depending on which frozen plasma product is to be made. The rate of freezing for the plasma will depend on the temperature of the freezer and the amount of air circulation around the plasma.

13. Before freezing, be sure that any tubing segments and the transfusion ports (ears) of the bag are tucked in or placed in such a manner as to prevent or minimize possible breakage.

14. The label on the frozen plasma must include all of the standard information. (See the following section on labeling).

15. The plasma can be stored as FFP, single-donor plasma frozen within 24 hours (PF24), or liquid recovered plasma. Be sure to record the plasma volume on the bag. Shelf-life is 12 months when stored at −18°C or colder.

16. Once the platelet concentrate has rested, the unit should be placed on an agitator to maintain gentle agitation during storage.

17. Platelet concentrate shelf-life is 5 days from the date of collection. If the system is opened, transfusion must occur within 6 hours. The volume, expiration date, and time (if indicated) must be on the label.

18. All of the units for a single platelet dose (typically 6 to 8 units for an adult) can be pooled into a single bag before transfusion. Once pooled, the product must be transfused within 4 hours of pooling. The pooled unit must be given a unique pool number, which must be placed on the label.

for neonates whose counts fall below 50,000/μL and who are experiencing bleeding. Factors that may be associated with thrombocytopenia include immaturity of the coagulation system, platelet dysfunction, increased platelet destruction, dilution effect secondary to massive transfusion, or exchange transfusion and intraventricular hemorrhage. Either random or apheresis platelets may be transfused and should increase the platelet count by 50,000 to 100,000, given a dose of 5 to 10 mL/kg.[2]

A procedure for the preparation of platelet aliquots for neonates is outlined in Box 13–9.

Platelets Leukoreduced

Platelets can be leukoreduced to help prevent febrile non-hemolytic reactions. Random-donor platelets can be leukoreduced by using a leukoreduction filter designed for platelets. Some apheresis equipment is designed to produce a leukoreduced product with or without an integrated filter. Random donor platelets must contain less than 8.3×10^5 leukocytes, and at least 95% of units sampled should meet this criterion.[1] If random donor platelets have been pooled, a method must be used that results in a leukocyte count of less than 5×10^6 in the final pooled product. Single-donor or apheresis platelets that have been leukoreduced must contain less than 5×10^6 leukocytes in at least 95% of units tested.

Single-Donor Plasma

Frozen plasma from single donors may be made into fresh frozen plasma (FFP), plasma frozen within 24 hours (PF24), or plasma cryoprecipitate-reduced. Frozen plasma may be

Preparation of Platelet Aliquots for Neonates

1. Select a unit to be aliquotted. Either AB or group-specific units should be selected. CMV-negative or volume-reduced platelets may be requested by the physician. For volume-reduced platelets, when infants cannot tolerate large intravenous infusions of plasma, stored platelets are centrifuged and the plasma is removed. The platelets remain undisturbed at room temperature for 20 to 60 minutes before being resuspended in residual plasma.

2. If platelets are shipped from another facility, they should rotate for at least 30 minutes at room temperature following volume reduction.

3. Remove cap from stopcock apparatus and attach to end of blood set. Use a filter 170 to 260 μm.

4. Remove second cap from stopcock and cap from syringe to be filled and place them on a piece of sterile gauze. Attach syringe to stopcock.

5. Close the roller clamps at the spike end of the blood set above the filter, and spike the platelet unit.

6. Open the roller clamp on the spike, and draw the platelets through the filter and into the syringe. Remove the syringe from the filter set, and force the excess air back out of the syringe.

7. Label the syringe properly. Indicate volume of aliquot on platelet product label.

8. The expiration is 4 hours from the time the unit was spiked.

produced from whole blood or apheresis collections. FFP must be frozen within 8 hours of collection if the anticoagulant used was CPD, CD2D, or CPDA-1 and within 6 hours if the preservative was ACD. FFP is stored at –18°C or colder for 1 year or at –65°C for 7 years, with FDA approval. FFP will contain the maximum levels of both stable and labile clotting factors, about 1 international unit (IU) per mL. PF24 is frozen within 8 to 24 hours of collection and is stored at –18°C or colder. It contains all stable proteins found in FFP, has normal levels of factor V, and has only slightly reduced levels of factor VIII.

Both PF24 and FFP are thawed at temperatures between 30°C and 37°C or in an FDA-approved microwave device. If a waterbath is used, the product must be placed in a protective lining or overwrap so that the ports of the unit are not contaminated by contact with the water. Once thawing is complete, the product may be stored at 1°C to 6°C for 24 hours. If not transfused within the initial 24-hour period, the thawed plasma may be stored for up to 5 days, but the product label must be changed to "thawed plasma." A single unit of FFP or PF24, from whole blood collection, should contain 150 to 250 mL of plasma, approximately 400 mg of fibrinogen, and 1 unit of activity per mL of each of the stable clotting factors. FFP also contains the same level (1 unit/mL) of factors V and VIII. FFP or PF24 prepared from apheresis collections may contain from 400 to 600 mL.

The use of FFP or PF24 is indicated in patients who are actively bleeding and have multiple clotting factor deficiencies. Examples may include massive trauma, routine surgical bleeding, liver disease, DIC, and when a specific disorder cannot be or has not yet been identified. They may also be used when a patient on warfarin must undergo surgery and there is not sufficient time for vitamin K to reverse the effect. Either product may also be used for transfusion or therapeutic plasma exchange in patients with thrombotic thrombocytopenic purpura (TTP). FFP or PF24 are contraindicated in patients with specific, known coagulation disorders that can be better treated with specific factor concentrates or vitamin K and should not be used as a volume expander when other, safer products are adequate and available.

Cryoprecipitate-reduced plasma is prepared from FFP after thawing and centrifugation to prepare cryoprecipitate. In addition to removing factor VIII, the process also removes fibrinogen, factor XIII, von Willebrand factor (vWF), cryoglobulin, and fibronectin.[24] The resulting cryo-poor plasma must be refrozen within 24 hours and stored at –18°C or colder for 1 year from the time of collection. This product still contains albumin; factors II, V, VII, IX, X, XI; and ADAMTS13. This product is most often used for transfusion or plasma exchange in patients with TTP but could also be used as a source of those factors that remain. This product cannot be used as a substitute for FFP, PF24, or thawed plasma.[24]

Thawed Plasma and Liquid Plasma

Thawed plasma contains stable coagulation factors such as fibrinogen and prothrombin but reduced amounts of factor V, VII, VIII, and X.[24] Thawed plasma is prepared from FFP and PF24 thawed at 30°C to 37°C and maintained at 1°C to 6°C for up to 4 days after the initial 24-hour post-thaw period has elapsed. Thawed plasma may be indicated in all of the same situations as FFP or PF24, and like FFP and PF24, it should not be used to treat specific factor deficiencies where other products with higher factor levels are available, and it should not be used purely as a volume expander. Many institutions now have programs to routinely maintain a thawed plasma inventory to facilitate emergency and trauma situations and to convert all nontransfused FFP or PF24 into thawed plasma to prevent outdate.

Liquid plasma is separated no later than 5 days after the expiration date of whole blood, is stored at 1°C to 6°C, and can be transfused for up to 5 days after the whole blood's expiration date. Levels of coagulation factors are poorly characterized and depend upon storage conditions and cellular interactions over time. Indications include patients undergoing massive transfusion with concurrent coagulation deficiencies. Because very little blood is stored as whole blood, this product is not often produced or available.

Cryoprecipitated Antihemophilic Factor

Cryoprecipitate is the cold-precipitated concentration of factor VIII, the antihemophilic factor (AHF). It is prepared from FFP thawed slowly between 1°C and 6°C. The product is prepared from a single whole blood unit collected into CPDA-1 or CPD and suspended in approximately 15 mL of plasma. The product contains most of the factor VIII and part of the fibrinogen from the original plasma. It contains at least 80 units of AHF activity and at least 150 mg of fibrinogen.[25] Other significant factors found in cryoprecipitate are factor XIII, von Willebrand factor, and fibronectin. Cryoprecipitate has a shelf-life of 12 months in the frozen state and must be transfused within 6 hours of thawing or within 4 hours of pooling. Like FFP and PF24, cryoprecipitate should be thawed quickly at 37°C. Once cryoprecipitate is thawed, the FDA recommends storing at room temperature (22°C to 24°C) until transfused. Cryoprecipitate is indicated in the treatment of factor XIII deficiency, as a source of fibrinogen for hypofibrinogenemia, and as a secondary line of treatment for classic hemophilia (hemophilia A) and von Willebrand disease. Cryoprecipitate should not be used to treat hemophilia A or von Willebrand disease if virus-inactivated or recombinant factor preparations are available.[24]

In recent years, cryoprecipitate has also been used to make fibrin glue, a substance composed of cryoprecipitate (fibrinogen) and topical thrombin. Generally, 1 to 2 units of cryoprecipitate are thawed and drawn into a syringe. Topical thrombin with or without calcium is drawn into a second syringe. The contents of the two syringes are simultaneously applied to the bleeding surface, where fibrinogen is converted to fibrin.[2] Fibrin glue is also available as commercially prepared products that are viral-inactivated and licensed to control bleeding in cardiovascular surgeries.

The whole blood donor requirements and preparation requirements for cryoprecipitate are the same as those for platelets and FFP. The quality-control requirements mandate that the volume and AHF activity of the final product must be tested on at least 4 units monthly. The volume should not exceed 25 mL, and 75% of all units tested must show a minimum of 80 IU of AHF activity. Records must be maintained of all quality-assurance testing performed.

A procedure for producing cryoprecipitate is outlined in Box 13–10.

Granulocyte Concentrates

See information on leukapheresis in Chapter 14.

Plasma Derivatives

The following products are different from blood components because they are prepared by further manufacture of pooled, human source, and recovered plasma; **recombinant**

DNA technology; or monoclonal antibody purification. Source plasma is defined as plasma collected by plasmapheresis and intended for further manufacture into plasma derivatives. Recovered plasma is plasma recovered from whole blood donations. The plasma is frozen when sent to the manufacturer. The manufacturing process usually begins with a separation of the cryoprecipitate from the plasma. The cryoprecipitate is then used to produce factor VIII concentrate. The residual plasma is separated into various proteins by manipulating the pH, alcohol content, and temperature and then is viral inactivated by any of several methods, including heat, solvent-detergent treatment, and nanofiltration.[2] Most derivative plasma is also further tested for hepatitis A and parvovirus.

Activated Factor VII (Factor VIIa)

Activated factor VII (rFVIIa) is produced by recombinant DNA technology and has been approved for use in patients with hemophilia A who have circulating antibodies or inhibitors to factor VIII and in patients with congenital factor VII deficiency. It has also been used in other situations such as trauma, massive transfusion, and liver transplantation, where bleeding has proved difficult to control and the patient's life is threatened. In these other situations, it has been most successful in controlling intracranial bleeding in patients with major head trauma and cerebral hematomas.[2] In addition, the administration of rFVIIa has seen promising results in uncontrolled nonsurgical hemorrhages after implanting VADs (ventricular assist devices) to treat end-stage cardiac failure.[33] VADs are frequently used in cardiac surgery procedures if weaning from cardiopulmonary bypass is refractory due to poor cardiac performance. The disadvantage to using rFVIIa is that it has been associated with an increased risk of spontaneous thrombosis and thromboemboli. In addition, the product is very expensive and should used with caution and restraint.

One theory for the mechanism of factor VIIa is that rFVIIa binds to tissue factor that is released from injured tissue and then activates factor IX and X. Factor X's presence on the surface of platelets leads to the generation of thrombin. Studies have shown that full thrombin generation occurred after the addition of up to 150 nm of recombinant FVIIa.[34]

Factor VIII Concentrates (FVIII)

Factor VIII concentrates are used to treat patients with hemophilia A or classical hemophilia and have almost completely replaced cryoprecipitate as the product of choice. Factor VIII concentrates may be prepared from large volumes of pooled plasma, but more commonly they are prepared by recombinant DNA technology. If prepared from pooled plasma, the plasma must be treated by pasteurization, solvent/detergent treatment, or monoclonal purification to inactivate or eliminate viral contamination. In pasteurization, stabilizers such as albumin, sucrose, or

---

glycine are added to the factor VIII concentrate to prevent denaturation of the product. The product is heated to 60°C for 10 hours. The stabilizers are removed, and the product is lyophilized. This product is safe from HIV-1 and hepatitis transmission.

In solvent/detergent treatment, ethyl ether and tri(*n*-butyl) phosphate and the detergent sodium cholate and Tween 80 are effective in disrupting the viral coat membrane, preventing the transmission of lipid-envelope viruses like HIV and hepatitis B. The solvent and detergent are removed, and the final product is lyophilized. Combinations of TnBP (tri-n-butyl phosphate) and polysorbate 20 during the manufacture of FVIII/vWF concentrate Optivate® resulted in inactivation of most enveloped viruses over a wide range of conditions, including solvent/detergent concentration, protein concentration, and temperature.

For monoclonal purification, immunoaffinity chromatography is used to positively select out the vWF:FVIII complex from the plasma pool. Briefly, a murine monoclonal antibody directed at the vWF:FVIII complex is bound to a solid-phase matrix. On addition of pooled plasma, the complex will attach to the monoclonal antibody. The product is in lyophilized form and is safe from viral transmission.[36]

Porcine Factor VIII

This xenographic form of factor VIII is made from porcine plasma and is beneficial for patients with hemophilia A who have developed inhibitors or antibodies to human factor VIII. Porcine factor VIII has been shown to provide effective hemostatic control for patients with intermediate FVIII inhibitor levels. Other studies have shown that residual porcine vWF in the preparation of the product induces platelet activation, thus providing a mechanism for enhancing hemostasis apart from the action of circulating FVIII.[35]

Recombinant Factor VIII

The gene for FVIII was sequenced nearly 16 years ago and led to the production of recombinant human FVIII (rFVIII). The first generation rFVIII products are synthesized by introducing human FVIII gene into BHK (baby hamster kidney) cells. The rFVIII is released into culture medium and harvested, isolated, and purified using a combination of ion-exchange chromatography, gel filtration, and immunoaffinity chromatography. The purification and final formulation of rFVIII (BHK) uses human albumin as a stabilizer. The next-generation product is referred to as rFVIII:FS; it is formulated using sucrose as a final stabilizer instead of albumin and is available in three doses (250, 500, and 1,000 IU).

When compared with the first-generation rFVIII, rFVIII-FS demonstrated a predictable clinical hemostatic response with an efficacy among previously treated patients and previously untreated patients with hemophilia A. In one study with previously untreated patients, inhibitors to rFVIII-FS were present in 15% of patients, which was lower than the

percentage of the first-generation product (20%).[37] To date, no transmission of hepatitis or HIV has been reported in association with this product. The next-generation native recombinant FVIII has included a solvent/detergent step as well as a purification step to help ensure a safe and effective product.

Factor IX Concentrates

Factor IX concentrates are available in three forms: prothrombin complex concentrates, factor IX concentrates, and recombinant FIX. The first contains significant levels of vitamin K–dependent factors: II, VII, IX, and X. The complex concentrate is prepared from large volumes of pooled plasma by absorbing the factors out using barium sulfate or aluminum hydroxide. The concentrate is then lyophilized and virally inactivated by methods previously described (e.g., solvent/detergent). The prothrombin complex concentrates may contain activated vitamin K–dependent factors.

Factor IX concentrate is developed by monoclonal antibody purification and is less thrombogenic than prothrombin complex concentrates. This product contains approximately 20% to 30% of FIX and is stored in the refrigerator in lyophilized form. Prothrombin complex concentrates should be used with caution in patients with liver disease due to reports of DIC and thrombosis.[25] This is most likely due to failure of the liver to produce adequate amounts of antithrombin III and a decreased hepatic clearance of activated factors.

Recombinant factor IX (rFIX) has been commercially available in Europe and in the United States since 1997. It is produced in a Chinese hamster ovary cell line and not thought to transmit human infectious disease. In 2001, Roth and colleagues[38] published a study evaluating this product in the treatment of patients with hemophilia B. Based on this study and other data accumulated by physicians using rFIX for hemophilia B patients, the Committee for Proprietary Medicinal Products (CPMP) considered the benefit–risk balance for rFIX for the treatment and prophylaxis of bleeding in previously treated patients with hemophilia B to be favorable. However, there were concerns regarding some aspects of the study, as there was the possibility of inhibitors to rFIX and allergic reactions to this product. As a result, a new clinical trial will be conducted.

Factor XIII Concentrates

Factor XIII deficiency is a severe autosomal-recessive bleeding disorder associated with a characteristic pattern of neonatal hemorrhage and a lifelong bleeding diathesis. There are currently two plasma-derived virus-inactivated factor XIII concentrates. One is available in Europe, South America, South Africa, Japan, and the United States as an investigational new drug under the FDA. The second is available only on a "named patient" basis in the UK.

Immune Serum Globulin

Immune serum globulin is a concentrate of plasma gamma globulins in an aqueous solution. It is prepared from pooled plasma by cold ethanol fractionation. Preparations are in the form of intravenous (IV) or intramuscular (IM) solutions. The IV preparation generally contains more IgG protein than the IM preparation, with a half-life of 18 to 32 days.

Immune globulin preparations are indicated for patients with immunodeficiency diseases (i.e., severe combined immunodeficiency and Wiskott-Aldrich syndrome) and for providing passive antibody prophylaxis against hepatitis and herpes. IVIg is also used in patients with idiopathic thrombocytopenic purpura, post-transfusion purpura, HIV-related thrombocytopenia, and neonatal alloimmune thrombocytopenia. Individuals with a history of IgA deficiency or anaphylactic reactions should not receive immune globulin because of the presence of trace amounts of IgA.

Whereas there are no documented cases of HIV or hepatitis B transmission, transmission of hepatitis C has been reported with IVIg preparations. This has led to preparations of immune globulin treated with solvent/detergent for viral inactivation.

Normal Serum Albumin (NSA)

NSA is prepared from salvaged plasma, pooled and fractionated by a cold alcohol process, then treated with heat inactivation (60°C for 10 hours), which removes the risk of hepatitis or HIV infection. It is composed of 96% albumin and 4% globulin. It is available in 25% or 5% solutions. NSA is indicated in patients who are hypovolemic and hypoproteinemic and in clinical settings for shock and burn patients. The 25% preparation is contraindicated in patients who are dehydrated, unless it is followed with crystalloid infusions (e.g., normal saline) for volume expansion.

Plasma Protein Fraction

The preparation of plasma protein fraction (PPF) is similar to that of NSA, with fewer purification steps. PPF contains 83% albumin and 17% globulins. PPF is available in a 5% preparation; its uses parallel that of NSA. PPF, however, is contraindicated for infusion during cardiopulmonary bypass procedures. Both PPF and NSA can be stored for 5 years at 2°C to 10°C and have not been reported to transmit HIV or hepatitis.

Rh₀(D) Immune Globulin

Rh immune globulin (RhIg) is a solution of concentrated anti-Rh₀(D). It is prepared from pooled human plasma of patients who have been hyperimmunized and contains predominantly IgG anti-D. RhIg has two primary uses: treatment of ITP and prevention of Rh HDN.

The FDA has approved two doses for treatment of ITP and immunization against the D antigen: a 120-μg dose and a 300-μg dose.[25,39] These are IV preparations that have been heat-treated. An IM preparation is available as a 50-μg dose and a 300-μg dose. The latter is considered a full dose protective against 15 mL of D-positive RBCs.

In preventing immunization to the D antigen during gestation, a number of scenarios with varying dosages apply. During the first 12 weeks of pregnancy, a 50-μg dose of RhIg is indicated for D-negative females for abortion or miscarriage. After 12 weeks' gestation, a full dose (300 μg) is indicated for abortion or miscarriage in D-negative women. The 120-μg dose is advised after 34 weeks' gestation when amniocentesis is performed or in the event of obstetric complication or following termination of pregnancy.

An antepartum dose (300 μg IM or IV) should be given to nonimmunized D-negative females at 28 weeks' gestation. Following delivery, a postpartum blood sample is drawn from the mother. The sample undergoes a screening test for fetomaternal hemorrhage (FMH) in which D-positive RBCs from the newborn are detected. Additionally, the newborn's Rh status is determined. If the newborn is D-positive or if the Rh type cannot be determined on the newborn (i.e., positive DAT), the mother should receive a full dose of RhIg unless she has demonstrated previous active immunization to the D antigen. If the screening test is negative for the presence of D-positive RBCs of fetal origin, the mother should receive a full dose of RhIg within 72 hours of delivery. If the screening test is positive, the FMH must be quantified using the Kleihauer-Betke test.

RhIg is also used in the event Rh-positive platelet concentrates are transfused to an Rh-negative patient. A 300-μg dose IM (120-μg dose IV) is sufficient to protect against D-positive RBCs contained in up to 10 units of random platelets or 1 pheresis product.

Synthetic Volume Expanders

There are two categories of the synthetic volume expanders: crystalloids and colloids. Ringer's lactate and normal isotonic saline comprise the crystalloids; dextran and HES make up the colloid solutions. Normal saline consists only of sodium and chloride ions; Ringer's lactate consists of sodium, chloride, potassium, calcium, and lactate ions. These solutions are useful in burn patients because of their ability to rapidly cross the capillary membrane and increase the plasma volume. Colloids are used as volume expanders in hemorrhagic shock and burn patients. Dextran is prepared in a 6% and 10% solution with a half-life of 6 hours. HES is available in a 6% solution with an IV half-life of more than 24 hours. Both colloids and crystalloids are free from viral transmission. Table 13–3 provides a comparison of crystalloids and colloids.

Antithrombin III Concentrates

Antithrombin III (AT-III) concentrates, or antithrombin (AT) as it is now called, is prepared from pooled human

Table 13–3 Comparison of Crystalloid and Colloid Solutions

CHARACTERISTIC	CRYSTALLOID	COLLOID
Intravascular retention	Poor	Good
Peripheral edema	Common	Possible
Pulmonary edema	Possible	Possible
Easily excreted	Yes	No
Allergic reactions	Absent	Rare
Cost	Inexpensive	Expensive
Examples	Ringer's lactate solution	Albumin
	7.5% normal saline	Dextran
		Hydroxyethyl starch

plasma and heat-treated to prevent viral transmission. This product, pdAT, has been approved in the United States for treating patients with hereditary AT deficiency in connection with surgical or obstetrical procedures or for those suffering from thromboembolism.[40] AT-III is an inhibitor of clotting factors IX, X, XI, XII, and thrombin. Patients with plasma levels of AT-III less than 50% of normal are at risk of thrombosis.

A new recombinant AT (rhAT) concentrate produced using transgenic technology has been developed on a compassionate-use basis. It is produced by transgenic goats expressing recombinant human AT in their milk, under the control of the beta-casein promoter. It is purified from the milk and concentrated. Initial studies using rhAT have indicated effective support for AT-deficient patients who undergo surgery and that it is a suitable alternative to pdAT. No antibodies have been produced against rhAT in studies to date, and adverse events, which are minimal, include spontaneously resolving skin hyperpigmentation at the site of drug infusion. Table 13–4 provides a comprehensive list of blood component characteristics.

Labeling of Components

Once the component has been made, it must be labeled in accordance with AABB *Standards*, FDA regulations, and ISBT (International Society of Blood Transfusion) Code 128. The latter system is an adaptation of the conventional coding system known as Code 128. This code has been adapted for use in blood transfusion services throughout the world by the ISBT—hence ISBT 128. The precursor to ISBT 128 was Codabar. In the 1970s, the Committee for Commonality in Blood Banking Automation appointed by the American Blood Commission (ABC) published a seven-volume report for labeling recommendations leading to adoption of ABC Codabar to improve and simplify the labeling of blood and its components. In 1985, the FDA published the Guideline for the Uniform Labeling

of Blood and Blood Components supporting Codabar in the United States.

As time progressed and complexities of the transfusion medicine industry heightened, the ISBT working group designed a totally new system based upon the bar code symbology known as Code 128. This allowed for multidimensional bar codes and nonrepetitiveness of the DIN (donor identification number) in not less than 100 years. ISBT 128 is managed by ICCBBA (International Council for Commonality in Blood Banking Automation). ICCBBA was established in 1994 and is a not-for-profit organization whose mission is to support ISBT 128 and assist in its implementation from blood establishments. Each blood center or transfusion service must register with ICCBBA when using ISBT 128 coding labels.

The donor identification number (DIN) is comprised of 14 characters that contain information relating to the country, the center of origin, the year of collection, a sequential number, and a check character. Each ISBT 128 donation number is unique on a worldwide basis. Each blood bank or transfusion service should have its own protocol for labeling components. The original unit, its components, or any modifications thereof must be identified; serologic results of the unit must be reviewed and the appropriate labels attached in such a way that is clear and readable to the naked eye. If a change must be made to the unit, such as a modification of the expiration date, the handwritten change must be legible.

The unique identifier of the unit, the ABO and Rh type, expiration date, and component labels must be checked with a second person. There must be a method in place linking the respective donor to the unit. The donor must be classified as autologous (Fig. 13–11) or volunteer (Fig. 13–12). The maximum number of unique identifiers that may be affixed to the unit is two; this may be in numeric or alphanumeric form. If the unit is shipped to a transfusion facility that applies its own unique identifier for the unit, the original identifier of the collecting facility must not be removed. There must be a method in place for tracing the unit from its origin to its final disposition.

Table 13–4 Blood Component Characteristics

COMPONENT	SHELF-LIFE	STORAGE TEMPERATURE	QUALITY CONTROL	VOLUME	INDICATIONS FOR USE	CONTENT	DOSAGE	TRANSFUSION CRITERIA
Whole blood	CPD-21 d CPDA-1 35 d CP2D-21 d ACD-21 d	1–6°C	Hct approx. 40%	450–500 mL	Volume expansion, ↑O$_2$	RBC Plasma Platelets WBCs	↑ hgb 1g/dL ↑ hct 3%	ABO, Rh
Whole blood irradiated	Original expiration or 28 days from irradiation	1–6°C	25 Gy to center of canister	450–500 mL	Prevent GVHD volume expansion ↑O$_2$	RBC Plasma Platelets	↑ hgb 1 g/dL ↑ hct 3%	ABO, Rh
RBCs	CPD-21 d CPDA-1 35 d CP2D-21 d ACD-21 d AS-42 d	1–6°C	Hct ≤ 80%	250–300 mL	↑O$_2$	RBC	↑ hgb 1 g/dL ↑ hct 3%	ABO, Rh
RBC aliquots	CPDA-1 35 d (closed system)	1–6°C	Hct ≤ 80%	varies	↑O$_2$	RBC	10 mL/kg ↑ hgb 2 g/dL	ABO, Rh
RBC irradiated	Original outdate or 28 days from irradiation	1–6°C	25 Gy to center of canister	250–300 mL	Prevent GVHD ↑O$_2$	RBC	↑ hgb 1 g/dL ↑ hct 3%	ABO, Rh
RBC leukoreduced	Closed system: same Open system: 24 hours	1–6°C	< 5 × 10^6 WBCs ≥ 85% RBC recovery	250–300 mL	Febrile rxn, ↑O$_2$	RBC Few platelets; residual plasma	↑ hgb 1 g/dL ↑ hct 3%	ABO, Rh
Washed RBCs	24 hours	1–6°C	Hct 70–80%	180 mL	IgA-negative persons PNH	RBC WBC < 5 × 10^8	↑ hgb 1 g/dL ↑ 3%	ABO, Rh
Frozen RBCs	10 years	≤ –65°C			Rare phenotypes	RBC Glycerol		
RBC deglycerolized	24 hr	1–6°C	80% RBC recovery < 1% glycerol < 300 mg hgb	180 mL	Rare phenotypes ↑O$_2$	RBC Saline Dextrose < 1% WBC, platelets	↑ hgb 1 g/dL ↑ hct 3%	ABO, Rh
Platelets, RD	5 d	20–24°C	≥ 5.5 × 10^{10} plts pH ≥ 6.2	50–70 mL	Thrombocytopenia DIC, bleeding	Platelets	↑5k–10k/µL	

Continued

Table 13–4 Blood Component Characteristics—cont'd

COMPONENT	SHELF-LIFE	STORAGE TEMPERATURE	QUALITY CONTROL	VOLUME	INDICATIONS FOR USE	CONTENT	DOSAGE	TRANSFUSION CRITERIA
Platelets, SD	5 d	20–24°C	$\geq 3 \times 10^{11}$ pH ≥ 6.2	200–400 mL	Platelet refractoriness	Platelets	↑30k–60k/µL	HLA compatible
Platelets, irradiated	5 d	20–24°C	25 Gy to center of canister	Same	Prevent GVHD	Platelets	Same	Same
Platelets, pooled	4 hr	20–24°C	pH ≥ 6.2	Varies	Thrombocytopenia DIC, bleeding	Platelets	Varies	
Platelets, leukoreduced	5 d	20–24°C	$<5 \times 10^{6}$ SD $<8.3 \times 10^{5}$ RD	pH ≥ 6.2	Febrile rxns	Platelets	RD: ↑ 5–10k SD: ↑ 30–60k	SD: HLA
FFP	1 yr 7 yr	–18°C –65°C	8 hr CPD, CPDA-1, CP2D 6 hr ACD	200–250 mL	Coagulation deficiency Liver disease DIC Massive trx	1 U/mL clotting factors	↑Factor 20–30% 10–20 mL/kg	ABO
PF24	1 yr 7 yr	–18°C –65°C	24 hr WB	150–250 mL	Same	↓Labile factors	Same	Same
SDP	1–6°C liquid	5 days after WB expiration Frozen: 5 yr	Frozen 6 hr	150–250 mL		Stabile clotting factors	Same	Same
Cryoprecipitate	Frozen: 1 yr Thawed: 6 hr Pooled: 4 hr	–18°C 20–24°C	FVIII:C 80 IU	10–25 mL	Hemophilia A VWD FXIII deficiency Fibrin sealant Hypofibrinogene-mia	FVIII:C (80–120U) VWF (40–70%) FXIII (20–30%) Fibrinogen (150 mg/dL)	↑Fibrinogen 5–10 mg/dL	ABO
FVIII concentrates	Check vial	1–6°C		10–30 mL	Hemophilia A	FVIII Trace other clotting factors	1U FVIII/kg body wt ↑ 2%	Reconstitute before infusion
FIX concentrates	Check vial	1–6°C		20–30 mL	Hemophilia B	FIX Trace other clotting factors	1U FIX/kg body wt ↑ 1.5%	Reconstitute before infusion

	Shelf life	Temperature	Count	Volume	Indication	Contents	Dose	Compatibility
Granulocytes	24 hr	20–24°C	$\geq 1.0 \times 10^{10}$	200–600 mL	Neutropenia <500 PMN/uL	WBC RBC Plts plasma	$1\text{–}2 \times 10^{10}$/infusion four daily doses	ABO, Rh, HLA
Granulocytes, irradiated	24 hr	20–24°C	$\geq 1.0 \times 10^{10}$	200–600 mL	Prevent GVHD neutropenia	Same	Same	Same
ISG	3 yr IM / 1 yr IV			Varies	Prophylaxis Immunodeficiency Hypogammaglobulinemia	Gamma globulins IgG, IgM, IgA		IM or IV
NSA	5 yr, 25%	2–10°C		50 mL / 250 mL	Plasma volume expansion	96% albumin 4% globulin		
PPF, 5%	5 yr	2–10°C		250 mL	Plasma volume expansion	Albumin 80–85% Globulin 15–20%		
Dextran	6% (dex 40) / 10% (dex 70)				Volume expansion burns			
HES	6%				Volume expansion burns			
Rhlg	2 yr	1–6°C		1 mL	Rh HDN	Anti-D IgG	300 µg / 120 µg / 50 µg	Mother Rh-negative; baby Rh-positive, Rh-unknown

Figure 13–11.   Autologous labeled RBCs. *(LifeSouth Blood Center, Montgomery, AL, with permission.)*

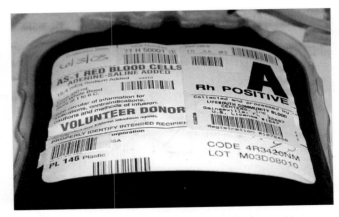

Figure 13–12.   Volunteer labeled RBCs. *(LifeSouth Blood Center, Montgomery, AL, with permission.)*

CASE STUDIES

Case 13-1

A 79-year-old woman was admitted to a community hospital for sepsis/anemia in January 2010. Transfusion history included 2 units of leukocyte reduced red blood cells (LR RBC) on December 2, 2009; 2 units of LR RBCs on December 5, 2009; and 2 units of LR RBCs on December 17, 2009. Parasitemia was observed on her peripheral blood smear on January 3, 2010. Serology confirmed the parasitemia was due to *Babesia* with a titer greater than 1,024. The woman resided in the northeast region of the United States.

1. Is the transfusion history consistent with the incubation period for *Babesia microti*?
2. What symptoms are associated with *Babesia* infection?

The blood supplier conducted a look-back study to identify if any of the donors had risk factors associated with *Babesia* or had serologic or symptomatic evidence of infection. It was determined that one donor had an IgG titer with *Babesia* specificity of greater than 1,024 (transfused on December 5, 2009) and one donor was not tested (transfused on December 17, 2009).

3. Should the donor with the high titer be permanently deferred?
4. Should the donor who was not tested be permanently deferred?

Case 13-2

An 89-year-old white male with a history of cholecystectomy and aortic valve replacement was admitted to the community hospital complaining of right upper quadrant abdominal pain. His lab work demonstrates hyperbilirubinemia, decreased platelets, elevated PT and INR, and increased white blood cell count. His ABO/Rh type is O positive with no recent history of transfusion. Current medications include prednisone and warfarin. The attending physician withheld further doses of warfarin to stabilize coagulopathy. Radiographic studies suggest an increased bile duct and bile duct stone.

Lab Results: Current Admission

Test	5-21-10	5-22-10	5-23-10	5-24-10	5-25-10
WBC (x10⁹/L)	25.8	23.1	20.4	25.8	23.1
Hgb (g/dL)	14	15.4	14	13.5	10.6
Hct (%)	42.4	47	43.6	42.5	32.3
Platelets (x10⁹/L)	106	90	72	103	88
PT (sec)	25.6	31.7	22.7	18	37.2
INR	2.7	3.3	2.3	1.8	3.8
Total Bili (mg/dL)	8.9	10.1	9.2	8.4	8.1

Transfused Products

5-21-2010: 8 units of FFP, 1 unit of PF24
5-22-2010: 3 units of PF24, 1 unit of FFP
5-23-2010: 1 unit of FFP, 1 unit of single donor platelets
5-25-2010: 1 unit of leukoreduced RBCs

1. What would you expect the patient's hemoglobin and hematocrit to be after receiving the leukoreduced RBCs?
2. Was the increase in platelet count from May 23 to May 24 consistent with general guidelines for apheresis platelets?
3. What is the difference in the preparation of FFP and PF24, and should only one type of plasma have been transfused to this patient?

SUMMARY CHART

- An allogeneic blood donor should weigh at least 110 lb (50 kg).
- The pulse rate of a potential blood donor should be between 50 and 100 beats per minute.
- The hemoglobin/hematocrit level of an allogeneic blood donor should be at least 12.5/38%.
- A donor must be permanently deferred if he or she has had a confirmed positive test for HBsAg after the 11th birthday.
- The deferral period for persons who have been treated for malaria is 3 years following therapy.
- Persons who have had a blood transfusion are deferred for 12 months owing to risk of exposure to hepatitis, HIV, or other viral diseases.
- A platelet pheresis donor should not have taken aspirin for 3 days before donation because it decreases platelet function.
- The interval between whole blood donations is 8 weeks or 56 days.
- A person with a history of hemophilia A or B, von Willebrand disease, or severe thrombocytopenia must be permanently deferred from donating blood.
- Attenuated live viral vaccines such as smallpox, measles, mumps, yellow fever, and influenza (live virus) carry a 2-week deferral.
- Attenuated live viral vaccines such as German measles (rubella) and chickenpox (varicella zoster) carry a 4-week deferral.
- A blood donor who has a positive serologic test for syphilis must be deferred for 12 months.
- Donors who have tested positive for the HIV antibody must be indefinitely deferred.
- *Predeposit autologous donation* refers to blood for the donor-patient that is drawn before an anticipated transfusion (e.g., surgery) and stored until use.
- An autologous donor must have a hemoglobin of at least 11 g/dL and a hematocrit level of at least 33%.
- Intraoperative autologous transfusion occurs when blood is collected during a surgical procedure and is usually reinfused immediately.
- Acute normovolemic hemodilution takes place in the operating room when 1 to 3 units of whole blood are collected and the patient's volume is replaced with colloid or crystalloid. The blood is reinfused during the surgical procedure.
- Postoperative salvage is an autologous donation in which a drainage tube is placed in the surgical site and postoperative bleeding is salvaged, cleaned, and reinfused.
- All whole blood units should be stored at 1°C to 6°C; those units destined for platelet production should be stored at 20°C to 24°C until platelets have been removed.
- Donor units must be tested for the following viral markers: STS, anti-HIV-1/2, HIV-antigen, anti-HTLV I/II, HBsAg, anti-HBc, and anti-HCV.
- RBCs must be prepared by a method that separates the RBCs from the plasma and results in a hematocrit level of less than or equal to 80%.
- Irradiated RBCs must be given a radiation dose of at least 25 Gy to the midplane of the canister, after which the expiration date of the product changes to 28 days from the time of irradiation or maintains the original outdate, whichever comes first.
- Leukocyte-reduced RBCs are products in which the absolute leukocyte count is less than 5×10^6.
- Random-donor platelets must contain at least 5.5×10^{10} platelets; single-donor platelets must contain at least 3×10^{11} platelets; each carries a shelf-life of 5 days.
- FFP must be prepared within 8 hours of collection for CPD, CPDA-1, and CP2D; it is stored at −18°C for 12 months.
- Cryoprecipitate is prepared from FFP and contains at least 80 units of antihemophilic factor and 150 to 250 mg of fibrinogen; this product is indicated for hemophilia A, factor XIII deficiency, and hypofibrinogenemia.
- RhIg is a solution of concentrated anti-$Rh_o(D)$, which is manufactured from pooled hyperimmunized donor plasma. It is used to prevent $Rh_o(D)$ immunization of an unsensitized Rh-negative mother after an abortion, miscarriage, amniocentesis, or delivery of an Rh-positive or Rh-unknown infant.
- One unit of random-donor platelets typically increases the platelet count in a 70-kg adult by 5,000 to 10,000/µL; 1 unit of apheresis platelets should increase the platelet count in a 70-kg adult by 30,000 to 60,000/µL.

Review Questions

1. Which of the following information is not required for whole blood donors?
   a. Name
   b. Address
   c. Occupation
   d. Sex
   e. Date of birth

2. Which of the following would be cause for deferral?
   a. Temperature of 99.2°F
   b. Pulse of 90 beats per minute
   c. Blood pressure of 110/70 mm Hg
   d. Hematocrit level of 37%
   e. None of the above

3. Which of the following would be cause for permanent deferral?
   a. History of hepatitis after 11th birthday
   b. Positive hepatitis C test result
   c. Positive HTLV-I antibody
   d. Positive anti-HBc test result
   e. All of the above

4. Immunization for rubella would result in a temporary deferral for:
   a. 4 weeks
   b. 8 weeks
   c. 6 months
   d. 1 year
   e. no deferral required

5. Which of the following donors is acceptable?
   a. Donor who had a first-trimester therapeutic abortion 4 weeks ago
   b. Donor whose husband is a hemophiliac who regularly received cryoprecipitate before 1989
   c. Donor who was treated for gonorrhea 6 months ago
   d. Donor who had a needlestick injury 10 months ago

6. Which of the following tests is not required as part of the donor processing procedure for allogeneic donation?
   a. ABO
   b. Rh
   c. STS
   d. Anti-HTLV I
   e. Anti-CMV

7. Which of the following lists the correct shelf-life for the component?
   a. Deglycerolized RBCs—24 hours
   b. RBCs (CPD)—35 days
   c. Platelet concentrate—7 days
   d. FFP—5 years
   e. RBCs (CPDA-1)—21 days

8. Each unit of cryoprecipitate prepared from whole blood should contain approximately how many units of AHF activity?
   a. 40 IU
   b. 80 IU
   c. 120 IU
   d. 160 IU
   e. 180 IU

9. Platelet concentrates prepared by apheresis should contain how many platelets?
   a. 5.5×10^{10}
   b. 6×10^{10}
   c. 3×10^{11}
   d. 5.5×10^{11}
   e. 6×10^{11}

10. The required storage temperature for frozen RBCs using the high-glycerol method is:
    a. 4°C
    b. −20°C
    c. −18°C
    d. −120°C
    e. −65°C

11. How does irradiation affect the shelf-life of red blood cells?
    a. Irradiation has no effect on the shelf-life.
    b. The expiration date is 28 days from the date of irradiation or the original outdate, whichever is later.
    c. The expiration date is 28 days from the date of irradiation or the original outdate, whichever is sooner.
    d. The expiration date is 25 days from the date of irradiation or the original outdate, whichever is later.
    e. The expiration date is 25 days from the date of irradiation or the original outdate, whichever is sooner.

12. Once thawed, FFP must be transfused within:
    a. 4 hours
    b. 6 hours
    c. 8 hours
    d. 12 hours
    e. 24 hours

13. Quality control for RBCs requires a maximum hematocrit level of:
    a. 75%
    b. 80%
    c. 85%
    d. 90%
    e. 95%

14. AHF concentrates are used to treat:
    a. Thrombocytopenia
    b. Hemophilia A
    c. Hemophilia B
    d. von Willebrand disease
    e. Factor XIII deficiency

15. Prothrombin complex concentrates are used to treat which of the following?

a. Factor IX deficiency
b. Factor VIII deficiency
c. Factor XII deficiency
d. Factor XIII deficiency
e. Factor V deficiency

16. How is the antibody screen test different for donors than for patients?

a. In donors, a 2-cell screen is used.
b. In donors, a 3-cell screen is used.
c. In donors, a pooled cell is used.
d. There is no difference in testing.

17. RBCs that have been leukoreduced must contain less than _____ and retain at least _____ of original RBCs.

a. 8×10^6/85%
b. 8×10^6/90%
c. 5×10^6/85%
d. 5×10^6/80%

18. Random-donor platelets that have been leukoreduced must contain less than _____ leukocytes.

a. 8.3×10^5
b. 8×10^6
c. 5×10^6
d. 3×10^{11}

19. A single unit of FFP or PF24 should contain _____ mL of plasma.

a. 100–150
b. 200–400
c. 150–250
d. 50–150

20. Cryoprecipitate that has been pooled must be transfused within _____ hours.

a. 24
b. 6
c. 4
d. 8

References

1. Price, TH (ed): Standards for Blood Banks and Transfusion Services, 26th ed. AABB, Bethesda, MD, 2009.
2. Roback, JD (ed): Technical Manual, 16th ed. AABB, Bethesda, MD, 2008.
3. Food and Drug Administration. Donor History Questionnaire user brochure. DHQ v1.3 May 2008. Available at www.fda.gov/BiologicsBloodVaccines/BloodBloodProducts/Questions.
4. Food and Drug Administration. Guidance for Industry. Recommendations for deferral of donors and quarantine and retrieval of blood and blood products in recent recipients of smallpox vaccine (Vaccinia virus) and certain contacts of smallpox vaccine recipients. December 2002. Available at www.fda.gov/cber/guidelines.htm.
5. Kleinman, S: Blood donor screening and transfusion safety. In Linden, JV, and Bianco, C (eds): Blood Safety and Surveillance. Marcel Dekker, New York, 2001.
6. Friedland, GH, et al: Lack of transmission of HTLV-III/LAV infection to household contacts of patients with AIDS or AIDS related complex with oral candidiasis. N Engl J Med 314:344, 1986.
7. Kaur, P, and Basu, S: Transfusion-transmitted infections: Existing and emerging pathogens. J Post Grad Med 51:146, 2005.
8. Soendjojo, A, et al: Syphilis d'emblee due to a blood transfusion. Br J Veneral Dis 58:149, 1982.
9. Risseeuw-Appel, IM, and Kothe, FC: Transfusion syphilis: A case report. Sex Transm Dis 10:200, 1983.
10. Chambers, RW, et al: Transfusion of syphilis by fresh blood components. Transfusion 9:32, 1969.
11. Director, Center for Biologics Evaluation and Research, Food and Drug Administration: Recommendations for the deferral of current and recent inmates of correctional institutions as donors of whole blood, blood components, source leukocytes, and source plasma. Memorandum to all registered blood and plasma establishments, June 8, 1995.
12. Food and Drug Administration. Guidance for Industry. Revised preventive measures to reduce the possible risk of transmission of Creutzfeldt-Jakob disease (CJD) and variant Creutzfeldt-Jakob disease (vCJD) by blood and blood products. May 2010. Available at www.fda.gov/cber/guidelines.htm.
13. Zayas, CF, et al: Chagas disease after organ transplantation—United States, 2001. MMWR Weekly 51:210, 2002.
14. Stramer, SL, et al: Blood donor screening for Chagas disease—United States, 2006–2007. MMWR 56: 141, 2007.
15. Food and Drug Administration. Guidance for Industry. Recommendations for management of donors at increased risk for human immunodeficiency virus type 1 (HIV-1) group O infection. August 2009. Available at www.fda.gov/cber/guidelines.htm.
16. Petrides, M, Stack, G, Cooling, L, and Maes, LY: Practical Guide to Transfusion Medicine, 2nd ed. Bethesda, MD, 2007.
17. Walther, WG: Incidence of bacterial transmission and transfusion reactions by blood components. Clin Chem Lab Med 46:919, 2008.
18. Thaler, M, et al: The role of blood from HLA-homozygous donors in fatal transfusion-associated graft vs. host disease. N Engl J Med 321:25, 1989.
19. Food and Drug Administration. Guidance for Industry and FDA review staff: Collection of platelets by automated methods. December 2007. Available at www.fda.gov/cber/guidelines.htm.
20. Allain, JP, et al: Transfusion-transmitted infectious diseases. Biologicals 37:71, 2009.
21. Alter, HJ: Detection of antibody to hepatitis C virus in prospectively followed transfusion recipients with acute and chronic non-A, non-B hepatitis. N Eng J Med 321:1494, 1989.
22. Hjelle, B: Transfusion-transmitted HTLV-I and HTLV-II. In Rossi, EC, et al: Principles of Transfusion Medicine, 2nd ed. Williams & Wilkins, Baltimore, MD, 1995.
23. Centers for Disease Control and Prevention. Detection of West Nile Virus in blood donations—United States, 2003. MMWR 52:769, 2003.
24. Food and Drug Administration Guidelines for Industry: An Approved Circular of Information for the use of human blood and blood components, 2009. (available at www.fda.gov/cber/guidelines.htm)
25. King, KE (ed): Blood Transfusion Therapy: A Physician's Handbook, 9th ed. American Association of Blood Banks, Bethesda, MD, 2008.
26. Heddle, NM, and Kelton, JG: Febrile nonhemolytic transfusion reactions. In Popovsky, MA: Transfusion Reactions. American Association of Blood Banks, Bethesda, MD, 1996.
27. Heddle, NM, et al: A prospective study to identify the risk factors associated with acute reactions to platelet and red cell transfusions. Transfusion 33:794, 1993.

28. Arnaud, FG, and Meryman, HT: WBC reduction in cryopreserved RBC units. Transfusion 43:517, 2003.

29. Smith, AU: Prevention of haemolysis during freezing and thawing of red blood cells. Lancet 2:910, 1950.

30. Valeri, CR, et al: An experiment with glycerol-frozen red blood cells stored at −80 degrees C for up to 37 years. Vox Sang 79:168, 2000.

31. Suda, BA, et al: Characteristics of red cells irradiated and subsequently frozen for long-term storage. Transfusion 33:389, 1993.

32. Dumont, LJ, et al: Screening of single-donor apheresis platelets for bacterial contamination: The PASSPORT study results. Transfusion 50:589, 2010.

33. Heise, D, Brauer, A, and Quintel, M: Recombinant activated factor VII (Novo7®) in patients with ventricular assist devices: Case report and review of current literature. J Cardiothor Surg 2:47, 2007.

34. Hoffman, M, and Monroe, DM: The action of high-dose factor VIIa in a cell-based model of hemostasis. Dis Mon 49:14, 2003.

35. Freedman, J, et al: Platelet activation and hypercoagulability following treatment with porcine factor VIII (HYATE:C). Am J Hematol 69:192, 2002.

36. Roberts, PL, Lloyd, D, and Marshall, PJ: Virus inactivation in a factor VII/vWF concentrate treated using a solvent/detergent procedure based on polysorbate 20. J Biologicals 37(1): 26, 2009.

37. Suiter, TM: First and next generation native rFVIII in the treatment of hemophilia A. What has been achieved? Can patients be switched safely? Semin Thromb Hemost 28:277, 2002.

38. Roth, DA, et al: Human recombinant factor IX: Safety and efficacy studies in hemophilia B patients previously treated with plasma-derived factor IX concentrates. Blood 98:3600, 2002.

39. George, JN: Initial management of adults with idiopathic (immune) thrombocytopenic purpura. Blood Rev 16:37, 2002.

40. Konkle, BA, et al: Use of recombinant human antithrombin in patients with congenital antithrombin deficiency undergoing surgical procedures. Transfusion 43:390, 2003.

41. Food and Drug Administration (CBER). Guidance for industry. Recommendations for the assessment of donor suitability and blood and blood product safety in cases of known or suspected West Nile Virus infection. June 2005.

Chapter 14

Apheresis

Beth A. Hartwell, MD, MT(ASCP), SBB and Paul J. Eastvold, MD, MT(ASCP)

OBJECTIVES

1. Define *apheresis* and describe the physiology of the process.
2. Define leukapheresis, plateletpheresis, plasmapheresis, and erythrocytapheresis.
3. Compare and contrast the procedures of continuous flow centrifugation and intermittent flow centrifugation.
4. Describe the use of membrane technology for the collection of plasma.
5. List the components that can be collected using apheresis technology.
6. State the regulatory requirements for apheresis donations, including the frequency of donation.
7. Explain the rationale for the basic types of therapeutic apheresis.
8. List the indications for therapeutic apheresis, differentiating between conditions requiring plasma exchange and those requiring cytapheresis.
9. List the different types of adsorbents and their clinical application.
10. Identify the factors that can be removed by plasmapheresis.
11. Describe the use of cytapheresis to collect hematopoietic progenitor (stem) cells.
12. Identify the possible adverse effects of apheresis.

Introduction

Apheresis (plural *aphereses*; from the ancient Greek *aphairesis*, "a taking away") is a procedure in which whole blood is removed from the body and passed through an apparatus that separates out one (or more) particular blood constituent. It then returns the remainder of the constituents to the individual's circulation. Through the use of sophisticated automation, an apheresis procedure can be performed on either a blood donor or a patient. It represents a significant advance in blood component collection and the treatment of specific disease states. Rather than collecting only a single unit of whole blood from a donor, apheresis allows a larger volume of specific components to be collected, such as platelets or red blood cells. This increases the ability to produce the optimal components for patients and prevents wastage.

The use of apheresis on a therapeutic basis permits the removal of disease-causing or unwanted cellular or plasma constituents from a patient. Importantly, apheresis is also used to harvest stem cells from the peripheral blood of donors and patients, avoiding the need for extraction from the bone marrow. Apheresis technology continues to evolve, and the procedure is now commonplace in blood donor centers and many hospitals and acute care settings.[1]

History and Development

Early developments in apheresis began some 60 years ago when Harvard biochemist Dr. Edwin J. Cohn devised a large-scale method, based on a simple dairy centrifuge (the "Cohn centrifuge"), for purifying albumin from pooled human plasma. This procedure, along with pasteurization, provided a safer therapeutic agent for resuscitating wounded soldiers than using lyophilized pooled plasma, which had an alarming risk of hepatitis transmission.

The device Dr. Cohn invented was ultimately not practical for its intended purpose; however, later modifications led to its use in deglycerolizing frozen red blood cells. In the 1960s, A. Solomon and J. L. Fahey used centrifugation technology to separate whole blood into plasma and red blood cells to perform the first reported therapeutic plasmapheresis procedure. In 1965, collaboration between Emil J. Freireich, a physician with the National Cancer Institute, and George Judson, a research engineer with the IBM Corporation, led to the development of the first continuous flow apheresis machine. Later on in the same decade, plasmapheresis was introduced as a means of collecting plasma for fractionation. As we entered the 1970s, apheresis was used to extract one cellular component and return the remainder of the blood to the donor. In 1978, the primary membrane plasma separator was introduced as a method for performing therapeutic plasma exchange. Since these early pioneering processes were developed, many different companies have developed apheresis technology based on the same principles.[2]

Although the technology is much more advanced than in the early years of development, an apheresis procedure performed today still consists of withdrawing a small volume of whole blood from a donor or patient and separating into its components. One (or more) of the components is collected and retained, and the remaining components are recombined and returned to the individual. Apheresis can be performed on a donor to collect a specific blood component (**donor apheresis**), or it can be performed on a patient to remove a particular blood component for therapeutic purposes (**therapeutic apheresis**).[3] The process of removing plasma is termed **plasmapheresis**. In a similar manner, platelets (**plateletpheresis**), red blood cells (**erythrocytapheresis**), or leukocytes (**leukapheresis**) can be removed (or collected) using apheresis technology. Table 14–1 outlines the types of apheresis procedures and their applications.

PROCEDURE	COMPONENT REMOVED	APPLICATION	
		Donor	**Patient**
Plasmapheresis	Plasma	√	√
Plateletpheresis	Platelets	√	√
Leukapheresis	White blood cells (WBC)	√*	√**
Erythrocytapheresis	Red blood cells (RBC)	√	√
HPC apheresis	Hematopoietic progenitor cells (HPC)***	√	√

Table 14–1 **Types of Apheresis Procedures and Their Application**

* Typically granulocytes are the primary component collected
** Removal of granulocytes and/or lymphocytes
*** Also called peripheral blood stem cells (PBSC)

The separation of blood components is based on the specific gravity or weight of each individual blood constituent (Fig. 14–1). If a tube of anticoagulated blood is centrifuged, distinct layers develop with the heavier red blood cells (RBCs) at the bottom and the lighter plasma portion at the top. Between these two prominent layers is a smaller layer composed of white blood cells (WBCs) and platelets (the buffy coat/layer). If a pipette is placed at the appropriate level in the test tube, any of these components can be removed.

Apheresis technology utilizes this same principle for separating blood components. Blood is removed from an individual (usually with a large-bore needle), mixed with an anticoagulant, and transported directly to the separation device (typically a machine with a centrifuge bowl or belt). There it is separated into specific components. Once the components have been separated, any component can be withdrawn. The remaining portions of the blood are then mixed and returned to the donor or patient (Fig. 14–2).

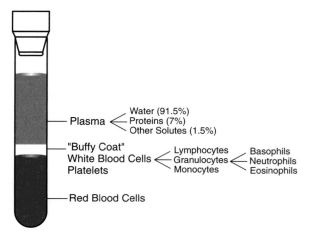

Figure 14–1. Sedimented blood sample.

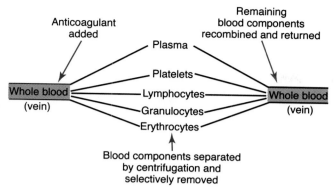

Anticoagulant
added

Remaining
blood components
recombined and returned

Plasma

Platelets

Whole blood — Lymphocytes — Whole blood
(vein)   Granulocytes   (vein)

Erythrocytes

Blood components separated
by centrifugation and
selectively removed

Figure 14–2.   Principles of apheresis.

Physiology of Apheresis

Apheresis collection of a blood component, whether for therapeutic or nontherapeutic purposes, is obviously different than the routine collection of a unit of whole blood. Since apheresis involves removing whole blood from an individual, manipulating the removed blood, and subsequently reinfusing portions of the blood, it is not surprising that the human body can be impacted in varying ways.

Anticoagulation

Citrate is used as the primary anticoagulant in apheresis procedures. The binding of calcium ions by citrate inhibits the calcium-dependent coagulation cascade; if calcium ions are not available, coagulation cannot proceed to its normal endpoint. Citrate is mixed with the blood immediately as it is removed from the donor's (or patient's) vein, and effectively anticoagulates the blood before it enters the apheresis machine. In normal situations, the infused citrate is not only actively metabolized by the liver, kidneys, and muscles, but is also diluted throughout the intra- and extracellular fluids of the body. As the citrate-calcium complex is metabolized, the previously bound calcium ions are released back into the bloodstream. In addition, parathyroid hormone (PTH) is released in response to the decreased ionized calcium levels. This results in mobilization of calcium from bone,[4] increased intestinal absorption of calcium, and increased reabsorption of calcium by the kidneys, thereby helping to maintain adequate circulating calcium levels. Despite these compensatory mechanisms, in some individuals the decrease in ionized calcium levels can result in symptomatic transient hypocalcemia.[5] This is described in more detail in the "Adverse Effects" section at the end of this chapter.

Fluid Shifts

During an apheresis procedure, changes in intravascular volume occur secondary to removal of blood into the extracorporeal circuit. During donor apheresis procedures, the total volume of components collected may be more than the simple whole blood donation. If additional fluid is not infused during the apheresis procedure, the donor may experience hypotension due to the depletion of intravascular volume. The sympathetic nervous system attempts to compensate for the hypovolemia by increasing cardiac output; this results in an increase in heart rate. Hypovolemic reactions are not common among apheresis donors, as regulatory restrictions limit the extracorporeal volume to 10.5 mL/kg. Most modern instruments have an extracorporeal volume well below this, except in the smallest of donors.

Hypotension may also occur during an apheresis procedure due to a vasovagal reaction.[6] During a vasovagal reaction, the parasympathetic nervous system overrides the output of the sympathetic nervous system, resulting in hypotension and a slowing of the heart rate. Factors that have been associated with vasovagal reactions in apheresis donors include younger age and the sex of the donor. Teenaged donors have higher vasovagal reaction rates compared with adults, and female donors have a higher incidence of these reactions than male apheresis donors.[7] However, vasovagal reaction rates are significantly lower in apheresis donors when compared with whole blood donors.

Cellular Loss

For both donor and patient apheresis procedures, the goal is to intentionally remove a specific cellular component. This would be expected to decrease circulating levels of the specific cells; however, other cellular components may be affected as well. Accordingly, the FDA and the AABB have requirements regulating how much time must elapse between donor apheresis procedures, depending on the particular blood component being collected.

A platelet donor typically experiences an acute fall in platelet count of 20% to 29% following apheresis donation. Among females, this decrease tends to be greater. Interestingly, the fall in platelet count does not correlate with the yield of the plateletpheresis procedure, as more platelets are collected than anticipated due to the mobilization of platelets from the spleen during apheresis collection. No adverse effects of the transient decrease in platelet counts have been demonstrated, and platelet counts normalize within a few days of donation.

In granulocyte collections, in addition to WBCs, platelets and significant numbers of RBCs are present in the leukapheresis product. Typically, a drop in hematocrit of 7% and a fall in platelet count of 22% occurs after each granulocyte donation. This fall is due to the loss of these cells in the product and the dilutional effects of volume expansion caused by the sedimenting agent, hydroxyethyl starch (HES), used during the procedure.

Varying numbers of RBCs are lost during each donor apheresis procedure, depending on the equipment used for collection and the specific component being collected. Each collection facility must have procedures in place to ensure that the cumulative annual red cell loss for apheresis donors is not exceeded. This must take into account all red cell losses, including those associated with the actual donation of whole blood, RBCs, and other apheresis components, as well as losses due to sample collection.

Methodology

Apheresis is performed using automated technology, and separation is typically performed by centrifugation. Apheresis instruments in use today have a computerized control panel, allowing the operator to select the desired component to be collected or removed. On-board optical sensors detect specific plasma-cell or cell-cell interfaces and divert the specific component to a collection bag. Currently available machines use disposable equipment, which includes sterile single-use tubing sets, bags, and collection chambers unique to the machine. The donor or patient remains attached to the apheresis instrument for the duration of the procedure; the amount of time for a particular procedure can range from 45 to 120 minutes. Collection of hematopoietic progenitor cells takes considerably longer.

Depending on the goal of the individual apheresis procedure (e.g., collecting platelets or removing plasma or RBCs), the appropriate apheresis instrument must be selected.[8] Each commercially available instrument has specific performance characteristics. Some instruments are suitable only for donor apheresis; others can be used for donor or therapeutic apheresis. By manipulating certain variables on an apheresis instrument, the operator can harvest plasma, platelets, WBCs, or RBCs for commercial or therapeutic purposes. The variables that are considered during an apheresis procedure include:

- Centrifuge speed and diameter
- Duration of dwell time of the blood in the centrifuge
- Type of solutions added, such as anticoagulants or sedimenting agents
- Cellular content or plasma volume of the patient or donor

Methods of Centrifugation

The most commonly used instruments employ one of two methods of centrifugation: intermittent flow centrifugation (IFC) and continuous flow centrifugation (CFC).

Intermittent Flow Centrifugation

In an intermittent flow centrifugation (IFC) procedure, blood is processed in batches or cycles, hence the term *intermittent*. Whole blood is drawn from an individual with the assistance of a pump. To keep the blood from clotting, an anticoagulant is mixed with the blood as it is pumped into a centrifuge bowl through the inlet port. The bowl rotates at a fixed speed, separating the components according to their specific gravities. A rotary seal is used, resulting in a closed system. The RBCs, which have greater mass, are packed against the outer rim of the bowl, followed by the WBCs, platelets, and plasma. Once separated, the pump is reversed and the desired component(s) are pumped through the outlet port into a collection bag (Fig. 14–3). The undesired components are pumped into a reinfusion bag and returned to the individual, constituting one cycle (or pass). The cycles are repeated until the desired quantity of product is obtained (e.g., a plateletpheresis procedure usually takes six to eight cycles to collect a therapeutic dose).

The IFC procedure can be performed as a single-needle procedure with only one venipuncture (blood is drawn and

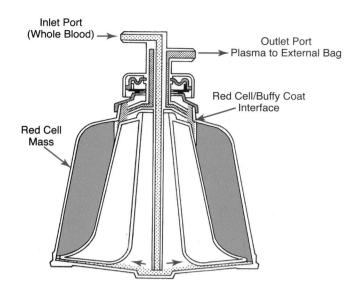

Figure 14–3. Cross-section of Haemonetics centrifuge bowl (IFC procedure). (*Courtesy Haemonetics Corporation, Braintree, MA.*)

reinfused through the same needle). This is advantageous when collecting apheresis products from blood donors. If both arms are used (double-needle procedure: one for phlebotomy and one for reinfusion), the amount of time for the apheresis can be reduced. The currently available systems are versatile, portable, fully automated, and capable of efficient component collections (Fig. 14–4).

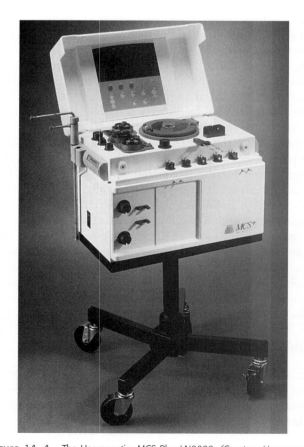

Figure 14–4. The Haemonetics MCS Plus LN9000. (*Courtesy Haemonetics Corporation, Braintree, MA.*)

Continuous Flow Centrifugation

In a continuous flow centrifugation (CFC) procedure, the processes of blood withdrawal, processing, and reinfusion are performed simultaneously in a ongoing manner. This is in contrast to IFC procedures, which complete a cycle before beginning the next one. Because blood is drawn and returned continuously during a procedure, two venipuncture sites are necessary. Alternatively, especially with therapeutic procedures, a dual-lumen central venous catheter can be used. Blood is drawn from the phlebotomy site with the assistance of a pump, mixed with anticoagulant, and collected in a specially designed chamber or belt, depending on the instrument. Separation of the components is performed by centrifugation, and the specific component is diverted and retained in a collection bag. The remainder of the blood is reinfused to the individual via the second venipuncture site.

Examples of machines employing this concept are the Baxter/Fenwal CS-3000 Plus and the Amicus (Fig. 14–5), the CaridianBCT COBE® Spectra (Fig. 14–6) and Spectra Optia® (Fig. 14–7), and the Fresenius AS-104 (Fig. 14–8).

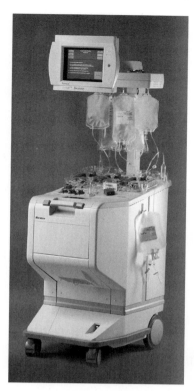

Figure 14–5. Baxter/Fenwal Amicus. *(Courtesy Baxter Healthcare Corporation, Deerfield, IL.)*

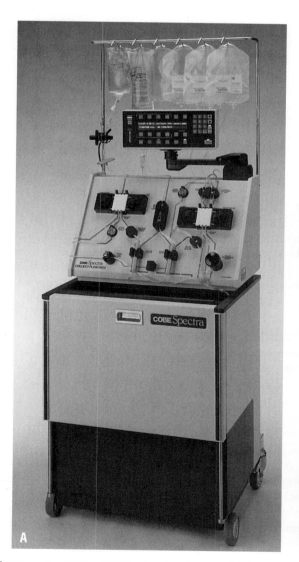

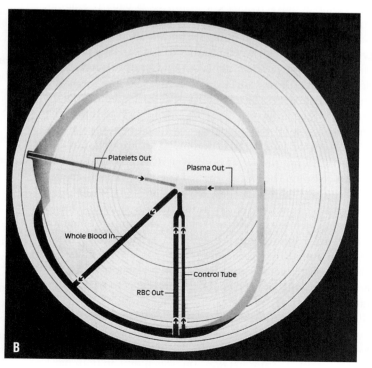

Figure 14–6. (A) The COBE Spectra apheresis system. (B) The separation chamber uses a unique asymmetric design to minimize contamination from RBCs and WBCs. *(Courtesy CaridianBCT, Lakewood, CO.)*

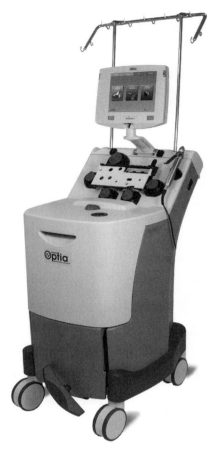

Figure 14–7. The Spectra Optia. *(Courtesy CaridianBCT, Lakewood, CO.)*

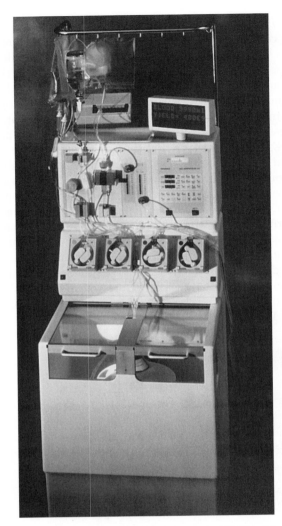

Figure 14–8. The Fresenius AS-104. *(Courtesy Fresenius USA, Walnut Creek, CA.)*

The IFC and CFC machines have individual advantages and disadvantages. The IFC equipment is usually smaller and more mobile, lending itself for use on mobile donor collections. A single venipuncture may be used with the IFC procedures, whereas two venipunctures are usually required with the CFC procedures. However, new protocols have been developed to allow some CFC machines to operate using single-needle access (e.g., the Amicus and Spectra). Based on AABB *Standards*, the extracorporeal blood volume (the amount of blood out of the individual in the centrifuge bowl/chamber and tubing) for blood donors should not exceed 10.5 mL per kg of body weight at any time during the procedure.[9] The extracorporeal volume is usually greater with the IFC than with the CFC machines. This can be an important consideration in individuals with small blood volumes, such as children and elderly individuals, since the additional volume removed may leave the patient hypovolemic during the procedure.

In the last several years, improvements in apheresis technology have allowed IFC and CFC processes to be incorporated into a single platform. Examples of this platform are the Trima from CaridianBCT (Fig. 14–9) and the Baxter/Fenwal Alyx. The Trima uses intermittent flow technology to draw and reinfuse blood to the donor, while the centrifuge operates with continuous flow. Improvements in both hardware and software allow the collection of concurrent components (e.g., each of these apheresis machines can collect two units of RBCs; the Trima can also collect several different combinations of RBCs, plasma, or platelets during a single apheresis procedure). Another important improvement allows the cellular products to be leukoreduced at the time of collection.

Membrane Filtration

Advanced Concepts

Membrane filtration technology can also be used to separate blood components.[10] Membrane separators are typically composed of bundles of hollow fibers or flat plate membranes with specific pore sizes. As whole blood flows over the fibers or membrane, plasma passes through the pores and is collected, while the remainder of the cellular components is returned to the donor. This technology lends itself well to the collection of plasma, since pores can be sized to prevent the passage of even small cellular elements. Filtration has several advantages over centrifugation, including the collection of a cell-free product and the ability to selectively remove specific plasma proteins by varying the pore size. The Fenwal Autopheresis-C

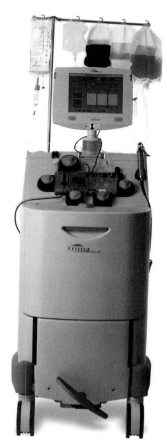

Figure 14–9. The Trima Accel automated collection system. *(Courtesy CaridianBCT, Lakewood, CO.)*

instrument combines centrifugation and membrane filtration technology through the use of a small rotating cylindrical filter. Like other filtration technology, it is used only for plasma collection.

Component Collection

In component collection by apheresis, a healthy donor undergoes an automated procedure to obtain a specific blood component that will be transfused to a patient.[11] In general, most of the requirements for whole blood donation must be met; however, apheresis donors must meet additional requirements established by the AABB *Standards for Blood Banks and Transfusion Services*[9] and the FDA *Code of Federal Regulations*.[12] Exceptions to the apheresis donation criteria and donation frequency may be approved by the facility medical director.

Collection of each apheresis blood component carries with it a different deferral period; a brief synopsis is provided in Table 14–2. For example, if RBCs are not one of the components collected, apheresis collections can be done more often than would be possible for whole blood donation. However, the red cell loss for each apheresis procedure must be closely monitored and tracked to ensure that a donor's cumulative annual red cell loss does not exceed the maximum permitted by regulations.

Table 14–2	**Donation Frequency**
APHERESIS COMPONENT COLLECTED	**FREQUENCY OF DONATION***
2RBC	16 weeks
Plasma (frequent)	Every 2 days (no more than two times in 7 days)
Plasma (infrequent)	Every 4 weeks (no more than 13 times/year)
Platelets, single apheresis unit	Every 2 days (no more than 2 times in 7 days; no more than 24 times in 12 months)
Platelets, double or triple apheresis unit	Every 7 days
Granulocytes	Every 2 days

2RBC = double unit of red blood cells.
* Donation frequency will vary, based on red cell loss and if more than one type of component is collected concurrently. Donation frequency may be often if for a specific medical reason and is approved by the blood bank medical director.

A qualified, licensed physician must be responsible for all aspects of the apheresis program. Good equipment and a well-trained, motivated staff are essential. Operators of apheresis instruments may be medical technologists (clinical laboratory scientists), nurses, or technicians trained on the job and should be friendly and outgoing. Because the apheresis procedure is more lengthy than whole blood donation, complications may be avoided by the operator's ability to relieve the first-time donor's boredom and anxiety. Although serious complications are unusual, it is essential to have another qualified individual immediately available to assist in case of emergencies.[13]

Written, informed consent must be obtained from the donor. The apheresis procedure, the testing to be performed, and the possible risks and benefits must be explained in understandable language.[14] Collection of an apheresis blood component does not provide specific medical benefit to the donor; however, there may be a psychological benefit, particularly if the donor is of a rare type or is donating for a particular patient need. The apheresis procedure itself may be more comfortable for the donor since the needle used for venous access is typically of a larger gauge (i.e., smaller size) than for whole blood collection. In addition, the infusion of saline during the procedure helps reduce donor reactions due to hypovolemia. There are special risks associated with apheresis donation, including side effects of the anticoagulant, hypovolemia, and fainting. The FDA has provided guidance on statements of risk that must be provided to donors of platelets, plasma, and red cells.[15] The donor must be given the opportunity to accept or reject the apheresis procedure.

There are a variety of apheresis instruments on the market that can be used for component collection. Examples of instruments used for donor apheresis, along with the specific blood components that can be collected with each, are listed in Table 14–3. Several of these instruments provide integral leukocyte reduction filters for RBC components.

Table 14–3	Examples of Instruments Used for Donor Apheresis and Component(s) Collected				
INSTRUMENT	**2RBC**	**PLASMA**	**PLATELETS**	**WBC**	**COMBINATION**
Haemonetics					
• MCS+ LN8150	√				RBC/P
• MCS+ LN9000			√		PLT/P
• PCS-2		√			
• Cymbal	√				
CaridianBCT					
• COBE Spectra			√	√	PLT/P
• Trima Accel	√	√	√		RBC/PLT/P
Fenwal					
• ALYX	√				RBC/P
• Amicus			√		RBC/PLT/P
• Autopheresis C		√			
Fresenius AS104		√	√	√	

RBC = red blood cells; WBC = white blood cells (granulocytes); PLT = platelets; P = plasma

Red Blood Cells

RBCs collected by apheresis are typically collected as a double unit (termed a 2RBC or double RBC procedure). Depending on the instrument used, the plasma and platelets are returned to the donor, or one or both of these components may be collected as a concurrent apheresis product. A clinical advantage to the collection of apheresis RBCs is reduced donor exposure for the recipient since the patient can potentially receive two units from the same individual.

An FDA guidance issued in 2001 requires the collection facility to follow specific donor selection criteria outlined in each apheresis instrument manufacturer's operator's manual.[16] Donors must meet the appropriate collection criteria for a whole blood donation; however, many instruments have minimum gender-specific height and weight standards as well. Since the volume of RBCs being collected during a 2RBC procedure is greater than it would be for a whole blood donation, the requirements for donor hematocrit are more stringent. The hematocrit must be at least 40% regardless of gender, and the level (hemoglobin or hematocrit) must be determined by a quantitative method; the use of copper sulfate is not acceptable.[9,16]

If two units of RBCs are collected by apheresis, the donor must wait 16 weeks before providing another donation that includes RBCs. If one RBC and one plasma and/or platelet unit are collected, the donor must wait 56 days before donating another red cell product. These procedures may be performed on both allogeneic and autologous donors. The RBC apheresis procedure is well tolerated by donors, and several collection facilities have noted a decreased incidence of donor reactions compared with collection of whole blood.[9] Some of this may be attributed to the infusion of saline during the procedure to replace lost volume.

Plasma

Collection of plasma by apheresis is termed *plasmapheresis*. In a plasmapheresis procedure, whole blood from the donor is centrifuged, the plasma is diverted into a collection bag, and the cellular components (RBCs, platelets, WBCs) are returned to the donor. This allows a larger volume of plasma to be collected from a donor, such that each apheresis unit ("jumbo" plasma) is the volume equivalent of at least two whole-blood-derived plasma units. In addition to direct patient use, collection of apheresis plasma can serve a variety of purposes. It can be used to augment the inventory of fresh frozen plasma (FFP) of a particular ABO group, especially group AB. Plasma can be collected from donors with high titers of antibodies directed against specific infectious agents (hepatitis B, cytomegalovirus, varicella zoster) to prepare immune globulin. These preparations are used to provide prophylaxis against infectious organisms in exposed individuals. Finally, apheresis is used commercially to collect plasma for further manufacturing into such products as intravenous immune globulin (IVIG), hepatitis immune globulin, and Rh-immune globulin.

For donor purposes, collection is divided into frequent and infrequent plasmapheresis. With infrequent plasmapheresis, donation occurs no more than once every 4 weeks, and the donor requirements are the same as for whole blood.[17] With frequent, or serial, plasmapheresis, donation occurs more frequently than once every 4 weeks. There must be at least 2 days between procedures and no more than two procedures in a 7-day period. In addition, these donors must be evaluated periodically by a physician and must undergo specific laboratory testing (total protein and serum protein electrophoresis or measurement of immunoglobulin levels).[9] RBC loss must not be greater than 25 mL per week. FDA guidelines recommend 12 L (14.4 L for donors weighing more than 175 pounds) as the maximum allowable plasma volume donated per year.[17]

Platelets

Platelets obtained by an apheresis procedure provide the equivalent of six to eight whole-blood-derived platelets (random-donor platelets). This significantly decreases the donor exposure for a patient. In a plateletpheresis procedure, platelets along with a portion of plasma are removed, and the remaining RBCs, WBCs, and majority of the plasma are returned to the donor. The platelets are suspended in donor plasma in a collection bag specifically designed for platelet storage. A routine plateletpheresis procedure typically takes 45 to 90 minutes. Like other donor apheresis procedures, additional blood components may be collected concurrently, including a single RBC and/or plasma product. Furthermore, depending on the donor's platelet count and the apheresis instrument used, a high-yield product can be obtained that is subsequently divided into two or three platelet products, each containing an acceptable number of platelets.[18,19]

Donor selection criteria for the plateletpheresis donor are the same as for whole blood donation, with two additional requirements.[20] Prior to each plateletpheresis procedure, a sample must be collected to determine the donor's platelet count. The regulations concerning donor qualification can be somewhat confusing. The platelet count must be at least 150,000/μL in order to provide an adequate platelet collection and for the donor to safely undergo the collection procedure. If the donor's platelet count is less than 150,000/μL, he or she is deferred from platelet donation until a subsequent count is at least 150,000/μL. In some collection centers, the platelet count can be measured immediately and used to qualify the donor. However, if the platelet count is not immediately available, then the most recent platelet count can be used for qualification.[21] If it is the initial plateletpheresis collection for the donor, or if 4 weeks have elapsed since the prior platelet donation, it is not necessary that the platelet count be determined prior to beginning the procedure as long as it is evaluated after the platelet collection.

Plateletpheresis collections should not be performed on potential donors taking medications that interfere with platelet function, as this would result in production of a suboptimal and therapeutically ineffective patient product. Antiplatelet medications have differing deferral time periods: 48 hours for aspirin, aspirin-containing medications, and the anti-inflammatory drug Feldene, and 14 days for clopidogrel (Plavix), ticlopidine (Ticlid), ticagrelor (Brilinta), and prasugrel (Effient).[9]

The interval between plateletpheresis procedures must be at least 2 days with no more than two procedures in a 7-day period. However, to protect the donor, if a double or triple apheresis platelet is collected, 7 (rather than 2) days must elapse before the donor is again eligible to provide apheresis platelets. A donor may undergo no more than 24 plateletpheresis procedures in a rolling 12-month period. Exceptions to any of these time periods can be made in unusual circumstances (HLA-matched platelets for a specific patient) but must be approved by the blood bank medical director. Finally, the total volume of plasma collected during any one procedure cannot exceed 500 mL (or 600 mL if the donor weighs 175 lb or more) or the volume of plasma cleared by the FDA for the instrument.[9,20]

Apheresis platelets produced on newer instruments are typically leukocyte-reduced and contain less than 5×10^6 WBCs per unit, which meets the regulatory guidelines established by the FDA and the AABB.[9,20]

Granulocytes

The patient population that can benefit from granulocyte transfusions is very limited.[22,23] Patients who undergo aggressive chemotherapy may develop profound neutropenia during the course of their treatment. The decrease in neutrophils places these patients at risk for acquiring bacterial and fungal infections, which may become life-threatening. Granulocyte transfusions have been shown to be beneficial in some severely neutropenic patients (neutrophil count less than 500/μL) who meet the following criteria: documented (clinically or by culture) infection for 24 to 48 hours that is unresponsive to standard antibiotic or antifungal therapy, bone marrow demonstrates myeloid hypoplasia, and there is a reasonable chance of bone marrow recovery (i.e., the neutropenia is reversible).[24,25] Granulocyte transfusions have also shown favorable results in the treatment of neutropenic neonates with sepsis.[26,27]

Although granulocytes can be prepared from a whole blood donation,[28] the yield is insufficient for treating a pediatric or adult patient. Collection of granulocytes by apheresis provides a higher yield product.[29] Apheresis collection requires close communication between the blood center or apheresis center, the blood bank physician, and the patient's physician. Since granulocytes must be transfused as soon as possible after collection for optimal therapeutic effectiveness, typically there is insufficient time to perform all infectious disease testing on the donor. Therefore, advance planning can allow one or more donors to be prescreened prior to the actual collection procedure.

A minimum therapeutic dose is 1×10^{10} granulocytes per day.[24,25] The granulocyte yield is influenced by the donor's neutrophil count and the collection process. In general, most collection facilities stimulate the donor with corticosteroids or a colony stimulating factor prior to the procedure and utilize a red cell sedimenting agent during the collection process.[30]

During centrifugation of whole blood, granulocytes are found in the buffy coat between the RBC and plasma layers (see **Fig. 14–2**). Adding the red cell sedimenting agent, hydroxyethyl starch (HES), allows better separation of layers, resulting in an improved yield with reduced RBC contamination.[31,32] Since HES is added directly to the apheresis circuit, some amount will enter the donor's circulation during the collection procedure and ultimately be removed by the reticuloendothelial system. Immediate side effects of HES are due to its colloid properties, including circulatory volume expansion, with headaches and peripheral edema. Residual

HES has been reported in donors up to 1 year after granulocyte apheresis; therefore, collection facilities are required to control the maximum cumulative dose of HES (or any other sedimenting agent) given to a donor during a specified time interval.[9]

A number of granulocytes are normally present in the marginal, or noncirculating, pool. The administration of oral corticosteroids, such as prednisone or dexamethasone, can mobilize these granulocytes and significantly increase the number of circulating granulocytes. The use of steroids in donors prior to granulocyte collection may exacerbate certain medical conditions, such as diabetes, peptic ulcer, or hypertension, and should be used under the guidance of the blood bank physician.[26]

The administration of granulocyte colony-stimulating factor (GCSF), a recombinant hematopoietic growth factor, to granulocyte donors has resulted in marked increases in granulocyte yield. Although mild side effects, such as muscle and skeletal pain, have been reported with the use of these growth factors, they are usually well tolerated by donors.[30]

Advanced Concepts

Apheresis granulocytes contain a large number of viable lymphocytes. If transfused to a severely immunocompromised patient, there is a significant risk for graft-versus-host disease (GVHD). Therefore, the product should be irradiated prior to administration. Granulocyte function will not be affected. Even with the use of sedimenting agents, granulocyte preparations contain a significant number of RBCs (the component resembles a diluted RBC rather than a platelet concentrate). Compatibility testing is typically performed, since the apheresis granulocyte product contains greater than 2 mL of RBCs.[9] Leukocyte depletion filters must not be used; a standard blood administration filter is sufficient.

Therapeutic Procedures

The rationale of therapeutic apheresis (TA) is based on the following:

- A pathogenic substance exists in the blood that contributes to a disease process or its symptoms.
- The substance can be more effectively removed by apheresis than by the body's own homeostatic mechanisms.

Therefore, therapeutic apheresis, like donor apheresis, involves the removal of a specific blood component, with return of the remaining blood constituents to the patient. However, with TA, since the component being removed is considered pathological (or contributing to the patient's underlying disease state), significantly larger volumes of blood must be processed in order to remove as much of the offending agent as possible. The TA procedure is classified according to the blood component removed: a cytapheresis procedure may be used to selectively remove RBCs, WBCs, or platelets; a plasmapheresis procedure is used to remove plasma when the pathological substance is found in the circulation. Therapeutic apheresis has become an accepted and standard therapy for many hematologic, neurological, renal, metabolic, autoimmune, and rheumatic diseases, among others.[33,34]

General Considerations

Therapeutic apheresis has placed blood banks and transfusion services in the position of providing direct medical care for a patient. This situation has necessitated a change in the perspective of the medical director and the technical staff. Clearly defined policies must delineate the responsibility of the blood bank and attending physicians; typically the blood bank physician provides TA as a consultative service. It is imperative that the blood bank medical director be closely involved with the attending physician in deciding whether there are clinical indications for the TA procedure requested. Issues such as who makes the decision about vascular access, who orders laboratory tests to evaluate and monitor the patient, and who chooses replacement fluids must be clearly defined. The technical staff must be properly trained in the care of very ill patients and be able to handle emergency situations. As with donor apheresis, written informed consent must be properly obtained from the patient, outlining risks and benefits. Obviously, the number and type of risks will vary depending on the type of TA procedure being performed and the anticipated duration of treatment. Proper documentation of all facets of the procedure is required.[35]

Numerous studies performed during the last decade, many of them randomized, controlled clinical trials, have provided clinicians with sufficient data to more realistically evaluate apheresis as a form of therapy and to define its role in the treatment of numerous disorders. The American Society for Apheresis (ASFA) has developed guidelines for therapeutic apheresis based on a systematic review of information from clinical trials, case studies, and anecdotal reports and has designed a series of categories denoting the likely effectiveness of apheresis in the treatment of various clinical disorders.

The indication categories for therapeutic apheresis are as follows:

- **Category I.** Apheresis is standard and acceptable, either as primary therapy or as a first-line adjunct to other initial therapies. Efficacy is based on well-designed randomized controlled clinical trials or a broad base of published experience.
- **Category II.** Apheresis is generally accepted in a supportive role or as second-line therapy, rather than first-line therapy.
- **Category III.** Apheresis is not clearly indicated based on insufficient evidence, conflicting results, or inability to document a favorable risk-to-benefit ratio. Decision-making should be individualized.
- **Category IV.** Apheresis has been demonstrated to lack efficacy or be harmful, and should be discouraged in these disorders. Clinical applications should be undertaken only under an approved research protocol.

These guidelines are published and periodically updated (Table 14–4).[34,36] It should be noted that this text is not intended to provide detailed information on using TA to manage specific diseases. If needed, more thorough reviews should be consulted.[30,34,35]

Vascular Access

Adequate vascular access is mandatory during TA, as larger volumes of blood are processed and the duration of the procedure is longer than for donor apheresis. Vascular access can be obtained via peripheral veins, central veins, or a combination of both. If only one to two TA procedures are to be performed, peripheral access can be used. In such instances, two venous sites are necessary—one for removal and one for return. Therefore, the patient must have adequate veins at two sites capable of accommodating a 16- to 18-gauge needle. If several or frequent TA procedures are required, central venous access with a double-lumen catheter is desirable.

Table 14–4   Indication Categories for Therapeutic Apheresis

DISEASE	PROCEDURE	INDICATION CATEGORY
Renal and Metabolic Diseases		
Antiglomerular basement membrane disease	Plasma exchange	I
Rapidly progressive glomerulonephritis	Plasma exchange	III
Hemolytic uremic syndrome (atypical)	Plasma exchange	I, II
Renal transplantation	Plasma exchange	
Antibody-mediated rejection	Plasma exchange	I
HLA desensitization	Plasma exchange	II
Recurrent focal glomerulosclerosis	Plasma exchange	I
Heart transplant rejection	Plasma exchange	III
	Photopheresis	II
Acute liver failure	Plasma exchange	III
Familial hypercholesterolemia	Selective adsorption	I
	Plasma exchange	II
Overdose or poisoning	Plasma exchange	II-III
Phytanic acid storage disease	Plasma exchange	II
Sepsis, with multiorgan failure	Plasma exchange	III
Thyrotoxicosis	Plasma exchange	III
Autoimmune and Rheumatic Diseases		
Cryoglobulinemia	Plasma exchange	I
Autoimmune hemolytic anemia (warm)	Plasma exchange	III
Rheumatoid arthritis, refractory	Immunoadsorption	II
Scleroderma (progressive systemic sclerosis)	Plasma exchange	III
	Photopheresis	IV
Systemic lupus erythematosus, severe	Plasma exchange	II
Hematologic Diseases		
ABO-incompatible hematopoietic stem cell transplant	Plasma exchange	II
ABO-incompatible solid organ transplant		
Kidney	Plasma exchange	II
Heart (infants)	Plasma exchange	II

Continued

Table 14–4   Indication Categories for Therapeutic Apheresis—cont'd

DISEASE	PROCEDURE	INDICATION CATEGORY
Hematologic Diseases		
Liver	Plasma exchange	III
Erythrocytosis/polycythemia vera	Erythrocytapheresis	III
Leukocytosis and thrombocytosis, symptomatic	Cytapheresis	I, II
Thrombotic thrombocytopenia purpura	Plasma exchange	I
Post-transfusion purpura	Plasma exchange	III
Sickle cell disease	RBC exchange	I-II
Hyperviscosity associated with monoclonal gammopathy	Plasma exchange	I
Coagulation factor inhibitors	Plasma exchange	IV
	Immunoadsorption	III
Aplastic anemia	Plasma exchange	III
Cutaneous T-cell lymphoma	Photopheresis	I
Red cell alloimmunization in pregnancy (if intrauterine transfusion not available)	Plasma exchange	II
Malaria or babesiosis	RBC exchange	I, II
Neurological Disorders		
Acute inflammatory demyelinating polyneuropathy (Guillain-Barré syndrome)	Plasma exchange	I
Chronic inflammatory demyelinating polyradiculoneuropathy (CIDP)	Plasma exchange	I
Lambert-Eaton myasthenic syndrome	Plasma exchange	II
Multiple sclerosis		
Acute CNS inflammatory disease	Plasma exchange	II
Chronic progressive	Plasma exchange	III
Myasthenia gravis	Plasma exchange	I
Paraneoplastic neurological syndromes	Plasma exchange	III
	Immunoadsorption	III
Paraproteinemic polyneuropathy		
Due to IgG, IgA, or IgM	Plasma exchange	I
Due to multiple myeloma	Plasma exchange	III
Rasmussen's encephalitis	Plasma exchange	II
PANDAS*	Plasma exchange	I

- **Category I.** Apheresis is standard and acceptable, either as primary therapy or as a first-line adjunct to other initial therapies. Efficacy is based on well-designed randomized controlled clinical trials or a broad base of published experience.

- **Category II.** Apheresis is generally accepted in a supportive role or as a second-line therapy, rather than first-line therapy.

- **Category III.** Apheresis is not clearly indicated based on insufficient evidence, conflicting results, or inability to document a favorable risk-to-benefit ratio. Decision-making should be individualized.

- **Category IV.** Apheresis has been demonstrated to lack efficacy or be harmful, and should be discouraged in these disorders. Clinical applications should be undertaken only under an approved research protocol.

*PANDAS = pediatric autoimmune neuropsychiatric disorders associated with streptococcus
Source: Szczepiorkowski, Z (ed): Clinical applications of therapeutic apheresis: An evidence based approach, 5th ed. J Clin Apheresis 25:81, 2010.

Catheters designed for hemodialysis are preferable; standard intravenous lines or central catheters are not designed to provide the flow rates required with apheresis.

Physiological Considerations

The patient's extracorporeal blood volume (ECV) should be less than 15% of the total blood volume (TBV) in order to minimize the risk of hypovolemia. Current instruments used for TA typically calculate the patient's TBV based on height and weight. Calculating the patient's plasma volume (PV) is often necessary when performing a plasma exchange in order to appropriately remove sufficient amounts of plasma during the TA procedure. This is easily calculated from the patient's TBV and hematocrit. The lower the patient's hematocrit, the higher the PV.

Attention must be given to the patient's medication schedule. Plasmapheresis in particular may dangerously lower plasma levels of medications as the drug is removed during the procedure. Removal of a drug is based on its vascular distribution (drugs that are present primarily in the intravascular space are most vulnerable), its half-life in the circulation, the timing of the drug's administration, the amount of plasma removed, and the duration of the procedure. A few studies have evaluated the removal of specific medications,[37] and a clinical pharmacist can often offer additional information on the possible extracorporeal removal of various drugs.

The number of TA procedures performed varies with the disease or disorder being treated and the individual patient. For plateletpheresis and leukapheresis, one to two TA procedures may be sufficient. For erythrocytapheresis (RBC exchange), only one TA procedure may be needed; however, some patients benefit from an RBC exchange on a more frequent basis. Almost all diseases treated by plasmapheresis require several TA procedures in order to remove sufficient amounts of the pathological substance.

A blood warmer is often used as part of the apheresis circuit to avoid hypothermia due to the rapid infusion of room temperature fluids.

Plasmapheresis (Plasma Exchange)

Therapeutic plasma exchange (TPE) is the removal and retention of the plasma, with return of all cellular components to the patient. This is the most common TA procedure performed. The purpose is to remove the agent in the plasma, such as an antibody, toxin, or abnormal protein, that is causing the clinical symptoms.[38–43] TPE is also used to replace a normal factor or substance that may be missing or deficient in the patient's plasma.[44–47] Regardless of the purpose, a large volume of plasma must be removed during TPE and replaced with sufficient physiological fluid to maintain the intravascular compartment. It has been postulated that beneficial effects of the procedure, particularly in diseases that involve malfunction of the immune system, may be attributed to the removal of factors listed in Box 14–1.[48]

The effectiveness of TPE is related to the volume of plasma removed and the concentration of the pathological substance in the blood. Apheresis is most efficient at removing the substance at the beginning of the procedure and least

> **BOX 14–1**
>
> ### Factors Removed by Therapeutic Plasmapheresis
>
> - Immune complexes (e.g., systemic lupus erythematosus)
> - Alloantibodies (e.g., antibody-mediated transplant rejection)
> - Autoantibodies (e.g., Guillain-Barré syndrome, Goodpasture's syndrome)
> - Immunoglobulins causing hyperviscosity (e.g., Waldenström's macroglobulinemia)
> - Protein-bound toxins or drugs (e.g., Amanita mushroom poisoning, barbiturate poisoning)
> - Lipoproteins (e.g., familial hypercholesterolemia, hypertriglyceridemia)
> - Phytanic acid (e.g., Refsum's disease)

efficient at the end. A one-volume exchange removes an amount of plasma equal to the patient's plasma volume, approximately 3 liters for the average-size adult patient. However, a one-volume exchange does not reduce the unwanted plasma component to 0% as might be expected. There are several reasons this occurs. Physiologically, there is varying transfer of plasma proteins between the intravascular and extravascular spaces; some plasma proteins are primarily partitioned in the extravascular compartment; and synthesis or catabolism of the protein may occur.

In addition, during the TPE procedure, replacement fluids are being administered to maintain the patient's intravascular volume, resulting in dilution of plasma proteins. Mathematical models depicting the theoretical removal of substances from plasma by TPE show that a one-volume exchange should reduce the unwanted plasma component to approximately 30% of its initial value. If a two-volume exchange is performed, the procedure becomes less efficient, reducing the unwanted component from 30% to only 10%.[30,49] Because of the diminishing effect of increased plasma removal, it is recommended that approximately 1 to 1.5 plasma volumes be exchanged per procedure.[30,35]

As mentioned, synthesis and catabolism of the pathological protein and its distribution between the extravascular and intravascular space are factors affecting the efficiency of TPE. Disorders characterized by overproduction of a specific monoclonal or polyclonal antibody (e.g., Waldenström's macroglobulinemia, cryoglobulinemia) can result in hyperviscosity syndromes. If the antibody is IgM, TPE can be an effective therapeutic tool, since IgM antibodies tend to be located primarily in the intravascular space. However, IgG antibodies are often distributed equally in the intravascular and extravascular spaces, requiring a series of TPE procedures as the intravascular and extravascular pools equilibrate. Because of these characteristics, TPE performed to remove IgG antibodies is most effective when combined with immunosuppressive drugs.

Plateletpheresis

Therapeutic plateletpheresis can be used to treat patients who have abnormally elevated platelet counts with related symptoms.[30] Thrombocytosis (at least 500,000/μL) can occur in myeloproliferative disorders (essential thrombocythemia, polycythemia vera, chronic myelogenous leukemia) or as a reactive process in response to splenectomy, infection, chronic inflammation, or malignancy. Should the platelet count reach levels above 1,000,000/μL, the patient is at risk for developing thrombotic or hemorrhagic complications. The preferred method for lowering the platelet count is medication;[50] however, therapeutic apheresis may be indicated during an acute event to rapidly reduce the platelet count until pharmacological therapy takes effect. During a plateletpheresis procedure, the platelet count will be decreased by 30% to 60%. More than one procedure may be required until the platelet count normalizes to desired levels (usually less than 600,000/μL).[34] There are no specific guidelines as to the level the platelet count must be reduced to or a standardized procedure to reach a particular target platelet count.

Leukapheresis

Therapeutic leukapheresis has been used to treat patients with hyperleukocytosis, defined as a WBC or circulating blast count of over 100,000/μL.[34] These elevated levels place the patient at risk for complications associated with leukostasis, including organ dysfunction due to the formation of microthrombi in the pulmonary and cerebral microvasculature.[51] Leukostasis is more common in patients with acute myelogenous leukemia (AML) than with acute lymphocytic leukemia (ALL).[30] It is difficult to predict how much blood volume should be processed to permit a sufficient reduction in WBCs or blast cells to prevent leukostasis, and WBC counts should be monitored during the procedure. A single procedure should reduce the WBC count by 30% to 60%; however, more than one procedure may be necessary due to rapid mobilization of cells from the extravascular compartment. To achieve an adequate reduction in the WBC count, up to 1 liter of fluid may be removed, necessitating the use of a replacement fluid. Use of a red cell sedimenting agent, such as HES, may be of benefit during a leukapheresis procedure.[30,52]

Erythrocytapheresis (Red Cell Exchange)

Erythrocytapheresis, or red cell exchange, removes a large number of RBCs from the patient and returns the patient's plasma and platelets along with compatible allogeneic donor RBCs. The procedure is most commonly performed in patients with sickle cell disease in order to decrease the number of hemoglobin S–containing RBCs, thereby treating or preventing the complications (acute chest syndrome, impending stroke, unrelenting painful crisis) associated with the disease.[30,34,53]

The therapeutic goal is to decrease the level of hemoglobin S to less than 30%. This is usually accomplished with a single red cell exchange procedure, requiring from six to ten RBC units, depending on the patient's age and red cell volume. The donor RBCs selected for transfusion should be ABO- and Rh-compatible, relatively fresh (less than 10 days is preferable to allow maximum in vivo survival), leukocyte-reduced, negative for hemoglobin S (donor does not have sickle cell trait), and partially phenotype-matched for the Rh (C, c, E, e) and K1 antigens to avoid future alloimmunization.[26,35] Some patients may be placed on a long-term program of prophylactic red cell exchange to decrease the risk of complications associated with the disease.

Other indications for red cell exchange are much less common. The procedure can be considered for treatment of overwhelming malaria or *Babesia* infections.[54–56] Both of these protozoa infect red blood cells, and a pronounced parasitemia can occur. Red cell exchange has been shown to be beneficial for treating these patients when the parasite load is greater than 10%. A 1.5- to 2-volume red cell exchange should significantly decrease the parasite load.[30,34] It is important to note that these patients are often extremely ill and must be closely monitored during the procedure.

Finally, red cell exchange can be used to remove incompatible RBCs from a patient's circulation; for example, the emergent transfusion of Rh-positive RBCs to an Rh-negative female of child-bearing potential or an ABO-mismatched transfusion.[35]

Fluid Replacement

In TA procedures, the extracorporeal circuit (tubing, collection chamber, blood warmer) is primed with normal saline, providing the patient with an initial bolus of crystalloid. During therapeutic cytapheresis procedures, additional fluid replacement is often not necessary, since the majority of the patient's plasma is being returned. Should hypovolemia become a concern, normal saline can be infused during the procedure.

In therapeutic plasmapheresis procedures, however, large volumes of the patient's plasma are retained. This fluid must be replaced to maintain appropriate intravascular volume and oncotic pressure. Several options are available, and the choice is determined by the disease being treated, the condition of the patient, and the preference of the institution. The most common replacement fluid for TPE is human serum albumin (HSA) as a 5% solution.[34,57] Although 5% HSA can be used to replace the entire volume removed, a crystalloid such as normal saline may be used for up to one-third of the replacement volume. The availability of sufficient HSA has been challenging in recent years, leading to the use of pentastarch as a portion of the replacement solution in addition to HSA.[58,59]

Fresh frozen plasma (FFP) contains all the constituents of the removed plasma and thus would appear to be the optimal replacement fluid for TPE procedures. However, the use of FFP is not without risk, including transmission of infectious disease, additive effect contributing to citrate toxicity, and sensitization to plasma proteins. Therefore, the use of FFP is usually reserved for treatment of thrombotic thrombocytopenic purpura (TTP) and related disorders. For patients with TTP who do not respond in a timely manner to replacement with FFP, cryoprecipitate-reduced plasma is an alternative.[35] FFP may also be used as replacement during TPE on patients with a preexisting coagulopathy (severe liver disease) or on those who are scheduled to undergo an invasive procedure (such as a pretransplant antibody reduction).

Special Procedures

Expanding on the basic principles of separation employed by apheresis, new technology has allowed the collection of very specialized components, as well as the removal of specific plasma constituents.

Hematopoietic Progenitor Cells

Hematopoietic progenitor cells (HPCs), also referred to as *peripheral blood stem cells* (PBSCs), can be collected by apheresis from an autologous or allogeneic donor.[30] The procedure is much like donor leukapheresis, with the selective collection of mononuclear cells, since HPCs are found in the upper portion of the buffy coat during centrifugation. At least one, and sometimes two to three, apheresis collections are usually needed to produce an acceptable "dose." Each collection procedure lasts 4 to 6 hours, since very large blood volumes are processed in order to obtain the required yield. The number and frequency of procedures are determined by the yield of HPCs and the patient's condition.

Hematopoietic growth factors, in particular GCSF, are commonly used prior to the collection procedure to increase the number of circulating stem cells in the peripheral circulation. HPCs express the cell surface glycoprotein CD34, and measurement of CD34+ cells in the peripheral blood prior to collection is typically performed to ensure adequate mobilization has occurred.[30,60,61] In contrast to use in the routine granulocyte donor, four to five daily injections of GCSF are typically required to mobilize sufficient HPCs for collection. Therefore, it is not uncommon for individuals to experience headache and musculoskeletal pain.

There are several advantages to using HPCs collected by apheresis over traditional bone marrow collection. Anesthesia is avoided, and the procedures can be performed safely in the outpatient setting. For the autologous HPC donor, other advantages include a shorter period of cytopenia, decreased transfusion requirements, fewer infectious complications, and decreased length of hospitalization.[35] Although peripheral venous access is preferred (two venous sites are required), a small number of allogeneic donors will require central venous line placement for adequate access and return. Autologous HPC donors often have an existing central venous line.

There have been remarkable advances in the field of HPC collection and transplantation over the last several years. Donor or patient selection and care; laboratory testing; and the collection, storage, and infusion of HPCs are regulated by the FDA,[62] the AABB,[63] and the Foundation for the Accreditation of Cellular Therapy (FACT).[64] The enormous complexity of this practice is beyond the scope of this chapter; the regulations and standards as well as other relevant literature should be consulted.[30,35]

Advanced Concepts
Immunoadsorption/Selective Absorption

Therapeutic plasma exchange is used to treat a variety of immunological disorders. In the TPE procedure, 5% HSA is typically used as replacement fluid. Although HSA is a relatively safe fluid, there are disadvantages to its long-term use on a daily or slightly less frequent basis. Most significant are the depletion of coagulation factors (e.g., fibrinogen) and reduction in immunoglobulin levels.[30] This led to the development of methods to selectively remove pathological substances, in particular antibodies.

Immunoadsorption refers to a method in which a specific ligand is bound to an insoluble matrix in a column or filter. Plasma is separated from anticoagulated whole blood by means of centrifugation or filtration, using a routine plasmapheresis procedure. The sequestered plasma is then perfused through the column or filter, with selective removal of the pathogenic substance and subsequent reinfusion of the patient's own plasma and cellular components. The removal is usually mediated by an antigen–antibody or chemical reaction. This abrogates the need for a volume-replacement fluid such as 5% HSA. Figure 14–10 is a diagrammatic representation of this process.

Staphylococcal protein A is a cell wall component of *Staphylococcus aureus*. It has an affinity for IgG classes 1, 2, and 4 and for IgG immune complexes. When plasma is passed through a small column containing staphylococcal protein A, a significant amount of IgG is removed, as well as lesser amounts of IgM and IgA. The mechanism of action of these columns is not well established, and the removal of IgG and immune complexes alone cannot explain the treatment's clinical benefit. There appears to be a significant immunomodulatory effect of this treatment, with enhanced anti-idiotypic antibody regulation and activated cellular immune function.[30,65]

Initially licensed to treat patients with either refractory idiopathic thrombocytopenic purpura (ITP)[34] or rheumatoid arthritis,[66] it was also used off-label to treat a variety of other disease processes.[67–69] Several adverse reactions, including fever, chills, hypo- and hypertension, and allergic reactions were reported, including death.[70] In 2006, manufacturing of the columns ceased in the United States, and they are no longer available for use.

Familial hypercholesterolemia is an autosomal-dominant disorder associated with abnormal clearance of low-density lipoproteins (LDL), resulting in markedly elevated cholesterol levels. Both homozygotes and heterozygotes experience significant morbidity and mortality from premature atherosclerotic cardiovascular disease. TPE is only partially effective in this disorder. Several selective removal systems have been developed; the Kaneka Liposorber and Braun Plasmat Secura systems have both been approved for use in the United States.[34] LDL-apheresis selectively removes LDL and has been associated with regression of cardiovascular disease.[70] Since the underlying disorder cannot be

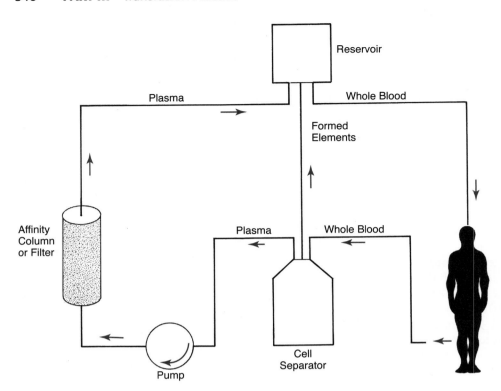

Figure 14–10. Perfusion of plasma over columns or filters. *(From Berkman, EM, and Umlas, J [eds]: Therapeutic Hemapheresis: A Technical Workshop. American Association of Blood Banks, Washington, DC, 1980, p 142, with permission.)*

treated, LDL-apheresis must be performed indefinitely, typically at 2- to 3-week intervals.[26]

Numerous adsorptive matrices have been developed with varying clinical usefulness. These include charcoal for removal of bile acids, polymyxin B for removal of endotoxin, and cellulose acetate for removal of granulocytes or monocytes, to mention a few. The majority of the adsorbent systems are not available or in clinical use in the United States.[30]

Photopheresis

Photopheresis utilizes leukapheresis to collect the buffy coat layer from whole blood. These cells are treated with 8-methoxypsoralen (8-MOP), exposed to ultraviolet A (UVA) light, and then reinfused into the patient. The combination of 8-MOP and UVA irradiation results in crosslinking of leukocyte DNA, ultimately leading to apoptosis (cell death).[30] Photopheresis has been shown to be efficacious and has been approved by the FDA for the treatment of cutaneous T-cell lymphoma.[71] It has subsequently been used successfully to treat acute and chronic graft-versus-host disease,[72] solid organ transplant rejection,[73] and selected immunologically mediated diseases.[30,74,75]

Adverse Effects

Apheresis is accepted as a relatively safe procedure, but complications do occur, especially for donors at higher risks for presyncopal or syncopal reactions associated with component collections due to donor factors such as younger age, female sex, and small total blood volume.[6,7,76] Adverse effects may be observed in therapeutic procedures as well.[77] In this case, it is

sometimes difficult to evaluate whether the deleterious effects were caused by the procedure or by the underlying disease. Some of the problems encountered are listed in Box 14–2. Some of the more common reactions and complications of donor and therapeutic apheresis are discussed here.[76–79]

Citrate Toxicity

Citrate toxicity is usually observed during cytapheresis component collections when anticoagulated plasma is returned at a rapid rate. It is also relatively common during therapeutic apheresis procedures. Citrate is the anticoagulant used in apheresis and is normally metabolized quickly in the liver. If the amount of citrate infused exceeds the

BOX 14–2

Adverse Effects of Apheresis

- Citrate toxicity
- Vascular access complications (hematoma, sepsis, phlebitis, neuropathy)
- Vasovagal reactions
- Hypovolemia
- Allergic reactions
- Hemolysis
- Air embolus
- Depletion of clotting factors
- Circulatory and respiratory distress
- Transfusion-transmitted diseases
- Lymphocyte loss
- Depletion of proteins and immunoglobulins

body's ability to metabolize it, the level of ionized calcium will decrease, and the donor may feel numbness or tingling around the mouth (paresthesias).[35] This can be clinically detected using the Chvostek's sign or Trousseau's sign. To prevent this complication, calcium is infused intravenously while the patient is undergoing the therapeutic plasmapheresis. Intravenous calcium is not recommended on a routine basis. If unattended, the symptoms can lead to tetany and cardiac arrhythmia. Calcium supplementation by mouth may also be given. If FFP is used as replacement fluid during a therapeutic plasma exchange, this phenomenon is more likely to occur because of the combined effects of the anticoagulant in the FFP and the citrate used in the apheresis procedure itself.

Vascular Access

Though plasmapheresis is helpful in certain medical conditions, like any other therapy, there are potential risks and complications that should be discussed with the patient before the procedure. Insertion of a rather large intravenous catheter can lead to bleeding, lung puncture (depending on the site of catheter insertion), and, if the catheter is left in too long, infection.

Vasovagal Reactions

A vasovagal episode (also called a vasovagal response, vasovagal attack, and neurocardiogenic syncope) is a malaise mediated by the vagus nerve. When it leads to syncope or "fainting," it is called *vasovagal syncope*, which is the most common type of fainting. Another mechanism causing hypotension during apheresis procedures is the vasovagal reaction.[76,78] In this reaction, hypovolemia results in a decrease in blood pressure. The compensatory response for this volume depletion is to increase sympathetic nervous system output with physiological compensation as previously described. During a vasovagal reaction, however, parasympathetic output that normally counteracts sympathetic output increases, resulting in a slowing of heart rate and decreased vascular tone. This results in hypotension. Factors that have been associated with vasovagal reactions in whole blood donors include younger age, low weight, first-time donation, and inattentive collection staff.[6,7]

Miscellaneous Reactions

Hypovolemia is observed more frequently with IFC instruments. Careful monitoring of the volume in and out is necessary to prevent hypovolemia and hypervolemia. **Allergic reactions** are related to the replacement fluids. This type of reaction is generally observed in patients in whom FFP is being administered (such as during a TPE procedure for TTP), but it has also been reported during infusion of albumin. **Hemolysis** is usually caused by a mechanical problem with the equipment, such as a kink in the plastic tubing. Observing the return line is critical in avoiding this problem. **Air embolism** and clotting factor deficiencies are not commonly observed.

Plasma Protein Interactions

The concentration of most plasma substances is reduced by 50% to 60% after one standard plasmapheresis treatment, with the rate of return to steady state concentrations varying among analytes. Plasma lipids, total protein, immunoglobulins, and transferrin recover to steady state concentrations by 8 days postplasmapheresis, whereas ceruloplasmin concentrations take longer to reach prepheresis levels.

Fatalities

Rare fatalities occurring during therapeutic apheresis procedures have been reported. The majority of these have been caused by circulatory (cardiac arrest or arrhythmia) or respiratory complications (acute pulmonary edema or adult respiratory distress syndrome). Of the cases reported, about half had received plasma as part or all of the replacement fluid. Because plasma has been associated with fatalities, its use is recommended only in cases of TTP or hemolytic uremic syndrome (HUS) in which there is a specific indication for its use. Plasma is also capable of transmitting diseases such as hepatitis and the human immunodeficiency viruses.

CASE STUDY

Case 14–1

A 72-year-old man presented to the emergency department at approximately 10:00 a.m. after waking during the night with confusion and expressive dysphasia. These symptoms initially appeared to improve and then progressively worsened. Apart from a recent 3-week history of left shoulder pain on abduction, his previous medical history was significant for excision of melanoma in situ and multiple basal cell carcinomas, mild gastroesophageal reflux, and an appendectomy 52 years earlier. He was a nonsmoker, did not drink alcohol, used no regular medications, and had no known drug allergies.

Physical examination findings:

- Expressive dysphasia
- Cranial nerves intact
- Vital signs: BP 150/90 mm Hg, heart rate (HR) 82 bpm, respiratory rate (RR) 12, temperature 101.4°F.
- All extremities moved equally, with normal strength.
- Multiple petechiae over both lower extremities and abdomen.
- Computerized tomography (CT) of the brain showed no abnormalities.
- Carotid duplex ultrasound revealed no significant carotid or vertebral artery disease.
- Twelve-lead electrocardiograph (ECG) was normal.
- Chest x-ray showed normal heart size and no abnormalities.

Laboratory findings during the first 48 hours:

- Anemia
- Thrombocytopenia
- Normal prothrombin time (PT) and partial thromboplastin time (PTT)
- Normal D-dimer and fibrinogen
- Elevated LDH
- Decreased haptoglobin

Hospital Course

Overnight, the patient became increasingly agitated, refused oral intake, and pulled out his intravenous catheter. His urine output decreased significantly and he became anuric. He was then transferred to the intensive care unit (ICU).

Negative direct antiglobulin test (DAT)

Peripheral smear: decreased platelets, rare nucleated RBC, 2+ schistocytes.
    Decreased ADAMTS 13

1. What are the top five possible diagnoses for this case?
2. What is the most likely diagnosis for this patient and why?
3. What are the main symptoms in cases of this type?
4. What is the main treatment for this disease?

SUMMARY CHART

- ✔ In an apheresis procedure, blood is withdrawn from a donor or patient and separated into its components. One or more of the components is retained, and the remaining constituents are recombined and returned to the individual.

- ✔ The process of removing plasma from the blood is termed *plasmapheresis*; removing platelets is termed *plateletpheresis* or *thrombocytopheresis*; removing RBCs is termed *erythrocytapheresis*; removing leukocytes is known as *leukapheresis*.

- ✔ Apheresis equipment that uses intermittent flow centrifugation (IFC) requires only one venipuncture, in which the blood is drawn and reinfused through the same needle. Once the desired component is separated, the remaining components are reinfused to the donor, and one cycle is complete. Apheresis procedures performed on patients usually require many cycles to reach an acceptable therapeutic endpoint.

- ✔ Continuous flow centrifugation (CFC) procedures withdraw, process, and return the blood to the individual simultaneously. Two venipuncture sites are necessary. The process of phlebotomy, separation, and reinfusion is uninterrupted.

- ✔ Membrane filtration technology uses membranes with specific pore sizes, allowing plasma to pass through the membrane while the cellular portion passes over it.

- ✔ The most common anticoagulant used in apheresis is acid citrate dextrose.

- ✔ Therapeutic apheresis is used to remove a pathological substance, to supply an essential or missing substance to alter the antigen–antibody ratio, or to remove immune complexes.

- ✔ The American Society for Apheresis (ASFA) has developed categories to define the effectiveness of therapeutic apheresis in treating a particular condition or disease. Therapeutic apheresis is most appropriate for treating category I or II disorders.

- ✔ In therapeutic plasmapheresis procedures, the replacement fluids used to maintain appropriate intravascular volume and oncotic pressure include normal saline, FFP, cryo-reduced plasma, and 5% human serum albumin.

- ✔ Complications of apheresis include vascular access issues, alteration of pharmacodynamics of medications, citrate toxicity, fluid imbalance, allergic reactions, equipment malfunction (hemolysis), and infection. Fatalities have occurred (primarily patient rather than donor).

Review Questions

1. The most common anticoagulant used for apheresis procedures is:
   a. Heparin.
   b. Sodium fluoride.
   c. Warfarin.
   d. Citrate.

2. Therapeutic cytapheresis has a primary role in treatment of patients with:
   a. Sickle cell disease and acute chest syndrome.
   b. Systemic lupus erythematosus to remove immune complexes.
   c. Leukemia to help increase granulocyte production.
   d. Myasthenia gravis to increase antibody production.

3. The minimum interval allowed between plateletpheresis component collection procedures is:

   a. 1 day.
   b. 2 days.
   c. 7 days.
   d. 8 weeks.

4. In plasma exchange, the therapeutic effectiveness is:

   a. Greatest with the first plasma volume removed
   b. Affected by the type of replacement fluid used
   c. Enhanced if the unwanted antibody is IgG rather than IgM
   d. Independent of the use of concomitant immunosuppressive therapy

5. The replacement fluid indicated during plasma exchange for TTP is:

   a. Normal (0.9%) saline.
   b. Hydroxyethyl starch (HES).
   c. FFP.
   d. Albumin (human) 5%.

6. The most common adverse effect of plateletpheresis collection is:

   a. Allergic reaction.
   b. Hepatitis.
   c. Hemolysis.
   d. Citrate effect.

7. Apheresis technology can be used to collect each of the following components except:

   a. Leukocytes.
   b. Macrophages.
   c. Hematopoietic progenitor cells.
   d. Platelets.

8. The anticoagulant added to blood as it is removed from a donor or patient during an apheresis procedure acts by:

   a. Binding calcium ions.
   b. Increasing intracellular potassium.
   c. Binding to antithrombin III.
   d. Inactivating factor V.

9. Peripheral blood stem cells are:

   a. Responsible for phagocytosis of bacteria.
   b. Removed during erythrocytapheresis.
   c. Pluripotential hematopoietic precursors that circulate in the peripheral blood.
   d. Lymphocytes involved with the immune response.

10. Which of the following can be given to an apheresis donor to increase the number of circulating granulocytes?

    a. DDAVP
    b. Hydroxyethyl starch (HES)
    c. Immune globulin
    d. G-CSF

References

1. McLeod, B: Therapeutic apheresis: History, clinical application, and lingering uncertainties. Transfusion (in press), 2009.
2. Hester, J: Apheresis: The first 30 years. Transfus Apher Sci 24:155, 2001.
3. Malchesky, PS, et al: Apheresis technologies and clinical applications: The 2007 international apheresis registry. Ther Apher Dial 14(1):52, 2009.
4. Chen, Y, et al: Effect of acute citrate load on markers of bone metabolism in healthy volunteers. Vox Sang 97:324, 2009.
5. Bell, AM, et al: Severe citrate toxicity complicating volunteer apheresis platelet donation. J Clin Apheresis 22:15, 2007.
6. Tomita, T, et al: Vasovagal reactions in apheresis donors. Transfusion 42(12):1561–1566, 2002.
7. Reiss, RF, Harkin, R, Lessig, M, et al: Rates of vaso-vagal reactions among first time teenaged whole blood, double red cell, and platelet pheresis donors. Ann Clin Lab Sci 39(2):138–143, 2009.
8. Price, TH: Centrifugal equipment for the performance of therapeutic hemapheresis procedures. In MacPherson, JL, and Kaspirisin, DO (eds): Therapeutic Hemapheresis, vol 1. CRC Press, Boca Raton, FL, 1985: 123.
9. Price, TH (ed): Standards for Blood Banks and Transfusion Services, 26th ed. American Association of Blood Banks, Bethesda, MD, 2009.
10. Rock, G, Tittley, P, and McCombie, N: Plasma collection using an automated membrane device. Transfusion 26:269, 1986.
11. Burgstaler, EA: Blood component collection by apheresis. J Clin Apheresis 21:142, 2006.
12. Code of federal regulations. Title 21 Parts CFE 606, 610. Washington, DC: US Government Printing Office, 2006 (revised annually).
13. Balint, B, et al: Apheresis in donor and therapeutic settings: Recruitments vs. possibilities—a multicenter study. Transfus Apher Sci 33:181, 2005.
14. Eder, AF, and Benjamin, RF: Safety and risks of automated collection of blood components. In Eder, AF, and Goldman, M (eds): Blood Donor Health and Safety. AABB Press, Bethesda, MD, 2009, pp 103–121.
15. Rossmann, SN: Talking with the donor: Information, consent, and counseling. In Eder, AF, and Goldman, M (eds): Blood Donor Health and Safety. AABB Press, Bethesda, MD, 2009, pp 1–20.
16. FDA Guidance for Industry and FDA Review Staff, February 13, 2001, Technical correction: Recommendations for collecting red blood cells by automated apheresis methods.
17. FDA Memorandum, March 10, 1995, Revision of FDA memorandum of August 27, 1982: Requirements for infrequent plasmapheresis donors.
18. Moog, R: Feasibility and safety of triple dose platelet collection by apheresis. J Clin Apheresis 24:238, 2009.
19. Picker, SM, et al: Prospective comparison of high-dose plateletpheresis with the latest apheresis systems on the same donors. Transfusion 46:1601–1608, 2006.
20. FDA Guidance for Industry and FDA Review Staff, December 17, 2007, Collection of platelets by automated methods.
21. Alex, J, Roberts, B, and Raife, T: Postdonation platelet counts are safe when collecting platelets with the Trima Accel using a postdonation platelet count target of ≥50,000 platelets/μL. J Clin Apheresis 24:215, 2009.
22. Atallah, E, and Schiffer, CA: Granulocyte transfusion. Curr Opin Hematol 13:45-49, 2006.
23. Price, TH: Granulocyte transfusion therapy. J Clin Apheresis 21:65–71, 2006.
24. King, KE (ed): Blood Transfusion Therapy: A Physician's Handbook, 9th ed. AABB, Bethesda, MD, 2008.

25. Vamvkas, EC, and Pineda, AA: Determinants of the efficacy of prophylactic granulocyte transfusions: A meta-analysis. J Clin Apheresis 12:74, 1997.

26. Roback, JD (ed): Technical Manual, 16th ed. American Association of Blood Banks, Bethesda, MD, 2008.

27. Sachs, UJ, et al: Safety and efficacy of therapeutic early onset granulocyte transfusions in pediatric patients with neutropenia and severe infections. Transfusion 46(11):1909–1914, 2006.

28. Kikuta, et al: Therapeutic transfusions of granulocytes collected by simple bag method for children with cancer and neutropenic infections: Results of a single-centre pilot study. Vox Sang 91:70, 2006.

29. Leitner, G, et al: Preparation of granulocyte concentrates by apheresis. Vox Sanguinis 98:567–575, 2010.

30. McLeod, BC (ed): Apheresis: Principles and Practice, 2nd ed. AABB Press, Bethesda, MD, 2003.

31. Bryant, BJ, et al: Gravity sedimentation of granulocytapheresis concentrates with hydroxyethyl starch efficiently removes red blood cells and retains neutrophils. Transfusion 50:1203, 2009.

32. Lee, JH, et al: A controlled study of the efficacy of hetastarch and pentastarch in granulocyte collections by centrifugal leukapheresis. Blood 86:4662, 1995.

33. McLeod, BC (ed): Clinical application of therapeutic hemapheresis. J Clin Apheresis 14(4): 1999.

34. Szczepiorkowski, Z (ed): Clinical applications of therapeutic apheresis: An evidence based approach, 5th ed. J Clin Apheresis 25:81, 2010.

35. Winters, JL (ed): Therapeutic Apheresis: A Physician's Handbook, 2nd ed. AABB, Bethesda, MD, 2008.

36. Smith, JW, Weinstein, R, and Hillyer, KL: Therapeutic apheresis: A summary of current indication categories endorsed by the AABB and the American Society for Apheresis. Transfusion 43:820, 2003.

37. Kintzel, PE, Eastlund, T, and Calis, KA. Extracorporeal removal of antimicrobials during plasmapheresis. J Clin Apheresis 18:67–70, 2003.

38. Boga, C, et al: Plasma exchange in critically ill patients with sickle cell disease. Transfus Apher Sci 37:17, 2007.

39. Hastings, D, et al: Plasmapheresis therapy for rare but potentially fatal reaction to rituximab. J Clin Apheresis 24:28, 2009.

40. Gore, EM, Jones, BS, and Marques, MB: Is therapeutic plasma exchange indicated for patients with gemcitabine-induced hemolytic uremic syndrome? J Clin Apheresis 24:209, 2009.

41. Sivakumaran, P, et al: Therapeutic plasma exchange for desensitization prior to transplantation in ABO-incompatible renal allografts. J Clin Apheresis 24:155, 2009.

42. Wu, SG, Kuo, PH, and Yang, PC: Successful weaning after plasma exchange for polyneuropathy related to POEMS syndrome. J Clin Apheresis 24:170, 2009.

43. Ezer, A, et al: Preoperative therapeutic plasma exchange in patients with thyrotoxicosis. J Clin Apheresis 24:111, 2009.

44. George, JN, et al: Lessons learned from the Oklahoma thrombotic thrombocytopenic purpura-hemolytic uremic syndrome registry. J Clin Apheresis 23:129, 2008.

45. Scully, M: Thrombotic thrombocytopenic purpura and pregnancy. ISBT Sci Series 2:226, 2007.

46. Lalmuanpuii, J, et al: Hypersensitivity to plasma exchange in a patient with thrombotic thrombocytopenic purpura. J Clin Apheresis 24:18, 2009.

47. Park, YA, et al: Is it quinine TTP/HUS or quinine TMA? ADAMTS 13 levels and implications for therapy. J Clin Apheresis 24:115, 2009.

48. Patten, E: Pathophysiology of the immune system. In Kilins, J, and Jones, JM (eds): Therapeutic Apheresis. American Association of Blood Banks, Arlington, VA, 1983.

49. Klein, HG: Effect of plasma exchange on plasma constituents: Choice of replacement solutions and kinetics of exchange. In MacPherson, JL, and Kaspirisin, DO (eds): Therapeutic Hemapheresis, vol 2. CRC Press, Boca Raton, FL, 1985.

50. Cortelazzo, S, et al. Hydroxyurea for patients with essential thrombocythemia and a high risk of thrombosis. N Engl J Med, 332:1132–1136, 1995.

51. Procu, P, et al: Hyperleukocytic leukemias and leukostasis: A review of pathophysiology, clinical presentation and management. Leuk Lymphoma 39:1–18, 2000.

52. Fenger-Eriksen, C, et al: Mechanisms of hydroxyethyl starch-induced dilutional coagulopathy. J Thrombosis Hemostases 7:1099–1105, 2009.

53. National Heart, Lung, and Blood Institute. The management of sickle cell disease, 4th ed. NIH Publication No. 02-2117. Bethesda, MD: National Institutes of Health, 2002.

54. Spaete, J, et al: Red cell exchange transfusion for babesiosis in Rhode Island. J Clin Apheresis 24:97, 2009.

55. Yarrish, RL, et al: Transfusion malaria: Treatment with exchange transfusion after delayed diagnosis. Arch Intern Med 142:187, 1982.

56. Cahill, KM, et al: Red cell exchange: Treatment of babesiosis in a splenectomized patient. Transfusion 21:193, 1981.

57. Pusey, C, et al: Experience of using human albumin solution 4.5% in 1195 therapeutic plasma exchange procedures. Transfusion Med 20(4):244–299, 2010.

58. Goss, GA, and Weinstein, R: Pentastarch as partial replacement fluid for therapeutic plasma exchange: Effect on plasma proteins, adverse events during treatment, and serum ionized calcium. J Clin Apheresis, 14:114–121, 1999.

59. Agreda-Vásquez, GP, et al: Starch and albumin mixture as replacement fluid in therapeutic plasma exchange is safe and effective. J Clin Apheresis 23:163, 2008.

60. Itoh, T, et al: Predictive value of the original content of CD34+ cells for enrichment of hematopoietic progenitor cells from bone marrow harvests by the apheresis procedure. J Clin Apheresis 21:176, 2006.

61. Bishop, MR, et al: High-dose therapy and peripheral blood progenitor cell transplantation: Effects of recombinant human granulocyte-macrophage colony-stimulating factor on the autograft. Blood 83:610, 1994.

62. Food and Drug Administration: Current good tissue practice for manufacturers of human cellular and tissue-based products: Inspection and enforcement; proposed rule. 21 CFR 1271. Federal Register 66:1507, 2001.

63. Padley, D (ed): Standards for Cellular Therapy Product Services, 4th ed. AABB, Bethesda, MD, 2010.

64. FACT-JACIE: International Standards for Cellular Therapy Product Collection, Processing, and Administration, 4th ed. Online (factwebsite.org), 2008.

65. Pineda, AA: Immunoaffinity apheresis columns: Clinical applications and therapeutic mechanisms of action. In Sacher, RA, et al: Cellular and Humoral Immunotherapy and Apheresis. American Association of Blood Banks, Arlington, VA, 1991.

66. Felson, DT, et al: The Prosorba column for treatment of refractory rheumatoid arthritis: A randomized, double-blind, sham-controlled trial. Arthritis Rheum 42:2153, 1999.

67. Mittelman, A, et al: Treatment of patients with HIV thrombocytopenia and hemolytic uremic syndrome with protein A (Prosorba® Column) immunoadsorption. Semin Hematol 26 (Suppl 1):15, 1989.

68. Snyder, HW, Jr, et al: Successful treatment of cancer-chemotherapy–associated thrombotic thrombocytopenic purpura/hemolytic uremic syndrome (TTP/HUS) with protein A immunoadsorption. Blood 76(Suppl 1):4679, 1990.

69. Doesch, AO, et al: Effects of protein A immunoadsorption in patients with advanced chronic dilated cardiomyopathy. J Clin Apheresis 24:141, 2009.

70. Heustis, DW, and Morrison, FS: Adverse effects of immune adsorption with staphylococcal protein A columns. Transfus Med Rev 10:62, 1996.

71. Edelson, R, et al: Treatment of cutaneous T-cell lymphoma by extracorporeal photochemotherapy—preliminary results. N Engl J Med 316:297, 1987.

72. Rossetti F, et al: Extracorporeal photochemotherapy for the treatment of graft-vs-host disease. Bone Marrow Transplant 18(Suppl 2):175, 1996.

73. Constanza-Nordin, MR, et al: Successful treatment of heart transplant rejection with photopheresis. Transplantation 53:808, 1992.

74. Malawista, SE, Trock, DH, and Edelson, RL: Treatment of rheumatoid arthritis by extracorporeal photochemotherapy: A pilot study. Arthritis Rheum 34:646, 1991.

75. Rook, AH, et al: Treatment of systemic sclerosis with extracorporeal photochemotherapy. Arch Dermatol 128:337, 1992.

76. Winters, J: Complications of donor apheresis. J Clin Apheresis 21:132, 2006.

77. Bramlage, CP, et al: Predictors of complications in therapeutic plasma exchange. J Clin Apheresis 24:225, 2009.

78. Yuan, S, et al: Moderate and severe adverse events associated with apheresis donations: incidences and risk factors. Transfusion 50(2):478, 2010.

79. Shemin, D, Briggs, D, and Greenan, M: Complications of TPE. J Clin Apheresis 22: 270, 2007.

Transfusion Therapy

Melanie S. Kennedy, MD

OBJECTIVES

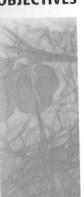

1. Describe the blood products that are currently available for therapeutic use.

2. List the indications for each blood product, including the approximate volume of each product.

3. Select the appropriate blood product for patients with specific disorders.

4. State the expected incremental increase of a patient's hematocrit level following transfusion of each unit of red blood cells (RBCs) and platelet count following transfusion of each unit of platelets.

5. List the required procedures for preparing each blood component for transfusion.

6. Identify the groups of recipients who are at highest risk of infection from transfusion of cytomegalovirus-positive RBCs or platelets.

7. Explain the role of irradiation in the prevention of transfusion-associated graft-versus-host disease (GVHD).

8. State the purpose of the surgical blood order schedule.

9. List the main advantages and disadvantages of autologous transfusion.

10. Identify the most important factors to consider when emergency transfusion is indicated.

11. Define *massive transfusion*.

12. Describe the various transfusion requirements of oncology patients.

13. Compare and contrast hemophilia A and von Willebrand's disease.

14. State the respective blood products of choice for treating von Willebrand's disease and hemophilia B.

15. Specify the steps involved in the proper administration of blood.

Introduction

Transfusion therapy is a broad term that encompasses all aspects of the transfusion of patients. Each blood component has specific indications for use, expected outcomes, and other considerations. In addition, patients with special conditions require strategies and decisions to optimize therapy. This chapter describes the selection and use of blood components and the strategies for transfusion in special conditions.

Blood Products

Blood and blood products are considered drugs because of their use in treating diseases. As with drugs, adverse effects may occur, necessitating careful consideration of therapy. The transfusion of blood cells is also transplantation, in that the cells must survive and function after transfusion to have a therapeutic effect. The transfusion of red blood cells (RBCs), the best tolerated form of transplantation, can cause rejection, as in a hemolytic transfusion reaction. The rejection of platelets, as shown by refractoriness to platelet transfusion, is relatively common in multiply transfused patients.

Transfusion therapy is used primarily to treat two conditions: inadequate oxygen-carrying capacity because of anemia or blood loss and insufficient coagulation proteins or platelets to provide adequate hemostasis. Each patient requires an individualized plan that reflects his or her changing clinical condition, anticipated blood loss, capacity for compensatory mechanisms, and laboratory results. Some patients do not require transfusion, even in anemia or thrombocytopenia, because their clinical conditions are stable and they have little or no risk of adverse outcomes. An example is a patient with iron-deficiency anemia with minor symptoms.

Appropriate blood therapy is the transfusion of the specific blood product needed by the patient. By selecting blood products, several patients can be treated with the blood from one donor, giving optimal use of every blood donation. Table 15–1 provides a summary of the blood products discussed in this chapter.[1,2]

Whole Blood

When compared with the circulating blood in the donor's blood vessels, the product of whole blood is diluted in the proportion of eight parts circulating blood to one part anticoagulant. The citrate in the anticoagulant chelates ionized calcium, preventing activation of the coagulation system. The glucose, adenine, and phosphate (if present) serve as substrates for RBC metabolism during storage (see Chapter 1, "Red Blood Cell and Platelet Preservation: Historical Perspectives and Current Trends").

Table 15–1   Blood Components and Plasma Derivatives

CATEGORY	MAJOR INDICATIONS	COMPOSITION	VOLUME
Whole blood	Symptomatic anemia with large-volume deficit	Approx. Hct 40%	570 mL
Red blood cells: RBCs (adenine-saline added), RBC pheresis	Symptomatic anemia	Approx. Hct 55%	330 mL
Red blood cells: deglycerolized, washed	Severe allergic reactions Rare donors	Approx. Hct 75%	180 mL
Red blood cells: leukocyte-reduced	Symptomatic anemia Febrile reactions due to leukocyte antibodies Reduce CMV transmission Reduce HLA alloimmunization	$< 5 \times 10^6$ WBC	330 mL
Platelets: platelets pooled	Bleeding due to thrombocytopenia or platelet function abnormality Prevention of bleeding from marrow hypoplasia	$\geq 3 \times 10^{11}$ platelets/unit	300 mL
Platelets pheresis	see Platelets; platelets pooled (above) Crossmatched or HLA-matched	see Platelets	300 mL
Platelets or platelets pheresis, leukocyte-reduced	see Platelets Prevention of febrile reactions and HLA-alloimmunization	see Platelets	300 mL
Granulocytes pheresis	Neutropenia with infection unresponsive to appropriate antibiotics	$\geq 1 \times 10^{10}$ PMN/unit	220 mL
Plasma	Deficiency of labile and stable plasma coagulation factors; TTP	All coagulation factors ADAMTS 13	250 mL
Cryoprecipitate pooled	Hypofibrinogenemia Factor XIII deficiency	Fibrinogen, vWF, factors VIII and XIII	300 mL

Source: Circular of information for the use of human blood and blood components, American Association of Blood Banks, America's Blood Centers, American Red Cross, Washington, DC, 2010.

The transfusion of whole blood is limited to a few clinical conditions. Whole blood should be used to replace the loss of both RBC mass and plasma volume.[1,2] Thus, rapidly bleeding patients can receive whole blood, although RBCs and plasma are more commonly used and are equally effective clinically.

A definite contraindication to the use of whole blood is severe chronic anemia. Patients with chronic anemia have a reduced amount of RBCs but have compensated by increasing their plasma volume to restore their total blood volume. Thus, these patients do not need the plasma in the whole blood and, in fact, may adversely respond by developing pulmonary edema and heart failure because of volume overload. This is more likely to occur in patients with kidney failure or preexisting heart failure.

For a 70-kg (155-lb) adult, each unit of whole blood should increase the hematocrit level 3% or hemoglobin 1 g/dL. After transfusion, the increase may not be apparent until 48 to 72 hours when the patient's blood volume adjusts to normal. For example, a patient with a 5,000-mL blood volume and 20% hematocrit level has 1,000-mL RBCs. With transfusion of 500-mL whole blood containing 200-mL RBCs, the blood volume will be 5,500 mL and will result in 21.8% hematocrit. When the patient's blood volume readjusts to 5,000 mL, the hematocrit level will be 24% (1,200 mL divided by 5,000 mL). The increase is greater in a smaller person and less in a larger one.

Red Blood Cells

RBCs are indicated for increasing the RBC mass in patients who require increased oxygen-carrying capacity.[1,2] These patients typically have pulse rates greater than 100 beats per minute; have respiration rates greater than 30 breaths per minute; and may experience dizziness, weakness, angina (chest pain), and difficulty thinking. The decreased RBC mass may be caused by decreased bone marrow production (leukemia or aplastic anemia), decreased RBC survival (hemolytic anemia), or surgical or traumatic bleeding.

The human body compensates for anemia by increasing plasma volume, heart rate, respiratory rate, and oxygen extraction from the RBCs. Normally, only about 25% of the oxygen is extracted, but with increased demand at the organ and tissue level, up to 50% of the oxygen can be extracted. When the demand exceeds 50% of the oxygen content, the compensatory mechanisms fail, and the patient requires transfusion.

No set hemoglobin levels indicate a need for transfusion. The critical level is 6 g/dL or less. Consensus committees suggest trigger values of hemoglobin of less than 7 g/dL for most patients and less than or equal to 8 g/dL for certain patients with heart disease.[3] Most patients can tolerate 7 g/dL, especially if on bed rest or at decreased levels of activity and given supplemental oxygen.[4] In fact, healthy individuals can tolerate hemoglobin levels as low as 5 g/dL with minimal effects.

Transfusion of RBCs is contraindicated in patients who are well compensated for the anemia. RBCs should not be used to treat nutritional anemia, such as iron deficiency or pernicious anemia, unless the patient shows signs of decompensation (need for increased oxygen-carrying capacity). RBC transfusion is not to be used to enhance general well-being, promote wound healing, prevent infection, expand blood volume when oxygen-carrying capacity is adequate, or prevent future anemia.

Each unit of transfused RBCs is expected to increase the hemoglobin level 1 g/dL and the hematocrit level 3% in the typical 70-kg (154-lb) human, the same as whole blood. In pediatric patients, a dose of 10 to 15 mL/kg will increase the hemoglobin about 2 to 3 g/dL or the hematocrit 6% to 9%.

The increase in hemoglobin and hematocrit is evident more quickly than with 1 unit of whole blood, because the adjustment in blood volume is less. As in the example for whole blood, the RBC volume is increased to the same amount, 1,200 mL, but the blood volume is increased only 330 mL to 5,330 mL. The hematocrit level is increased immediately to 22.5%.

RBCs prepared with additive solutions such as AS-1 or AS-3 have greater volume than with citrate phosphate dextrose (CPD) or citrate phosphate dextrose adenine (CPDA-1), 330 mL versus 250 to 275 mL (see Chapter 1), but the additive solution units have less plasma. The RBC mass is the same. Therefore, the hematocrit differs from 65% to 80% for CPDA-1 RBCs to 55% to 65% for additive solution RBCs (see **Table 15–1**).

Leukocyte-Reduced RBCs

The average unit of RBCs contains approximately 2×10^9 leukocytes. Donor leukocytes may cause febrile nonhemolytic transfusion reactions, transfusion-associated graft-versus-host disease (TA-GVHD), and transfusion-related immune suppression. In addition, human leukocyte antigens (HLA) are responsible for HLA alloimmunization. Leukocytes may harbor cytomegalovirus (CMV).

To reduce HLA alloimmunization and CMV transmission, the leukocyte content must be reduced to less than 5×10^6, which can be achieved by using one of several leukocyte reduction filters.[5] With these filters, most RBC units are less than 1×10^6; some are 1×10^4 leukocytes. In the United States, the standard leukocyte content is less than 5×10^6; in Europe, the standard is less than 1×10^6. Controversial is the effect of leukocyte-reduced blood on length of hospital stay and postsurgical wound infection. However, febrile nonhemolytic transfusion reactions, CMV transmission, and HLA alloimmunization are decreased by the use of leukocyte-reduced RBCs and platelets.[6] The indications for transfusion of leukocyte-reduced RBCs and platelets are outlined in Table 15–2.

Washed RBCs and Frozen/Deglycerolized RBCs

Patients who have severe allergic (anaphylactic) transfusion reactions to ordinary units of RBCs may benefit from receiving washed RBCs.[1] The washing process removes plasma proteins, the cause of most allergic reactions. Washed RBCs are used for the rare patient who has had moderate to severe allergic transfusion reactions and has anti-IgA antibodies because of IgA deficiency.

Table 15–2 Indications for Leukocyte-Reduced RBCs and Platelets

ACCEPTED	CONTROVERSIAL
Decrease febrile nonhemolytic transfusion reactions	Decrease hospital length of stay
Decrease alloimmunization to white blood cell antigens	Decrease incidence of wound infections postsurgery
Decrease transmission of cytomegalovirus (CMV)	Decrease incidence of cancer recurrence postsurgery

Freezing RBCs allows the long-term storage of rare blood donor units, autologous units, and units for special purposes, such as intrauterine transfusion. Because the process needed to deglycerolize the RBCs removes nearly all the plasma, these units, although more expensive, can be used interchangeably with washed RBCs. However, the 24-hour outdate of washed or deglycerolized RBCs severely limits the use of these components. The expected hematocrit increase for washed or deglycerolized RBCs is the same as that for regular RBC units.

Platelets and Plateletpheresis

Platelets are essential for the formation of the primary hemostatic plug and maintenance of normal hemostasis. Patients with severe thrombocytopenia (low platelet count) or abnormal platelet function may have petechiae, ecchymoses, and mucosal or spontaneous hemorrhage. The thrombocytopenia may be caused by decreased platelet production (e.g., after chemotherapy for malignancy) or increased destruction (e.g., disseminated intravascular coagulation [DIC]). Massive transfusion, which is discussed later in this chapter, may also cause thrombocytopenia because of the rapid consumption of platelets for hemostasis and the dilution of the platelets by resuscitation fluids and RBC transfusion.

Platelet transfusions are indicated for patients who are bleeding because of thrombocytopenia or abnormally functioning platelets (Box 15–1). In addition, platelets are indicated as prophylaxis for patients who have platelet counts under 5,000 to 10,000/μL.[7]

BOX 15–1

Indications for Platelet Transfusion

- Thrombocytopenia with bleeding or invasive procedure
- Chemotherapy for malignancy (decreased production, less than 5,000 to 10,000/μL)
- Disseminated intravascular coagulation (increased destruction, less than 50,000/μL)
- Massive transfusion (platelet dilution, less than 50,000 to 100,000/μL)

Bacterial testing is required for each platelet product. Plateletpheresis products and pooled platelets (from whole blood) are cultured by the blood center. However, individual platelet products from whole blood are difficult to culture because of their small volume and thus are less commonly used for transfusion.

A plateletpheresis component is prepared from one donor and must contain a minimum of 3×10^{11} platelets.[5] One plateletpheresis should increase the adult patient's platelet count to 20,000 to 60,000/μL. Each unit of platelets from whole blood must contain at least 5.5×10^{10} platelets[5] and should increase the platelet count by 5,000 to 10,000/μL in a 70-kg human. A pool of 5 units, then, will contain roughly 3×10^{11} platelets and should give a platelet count increase similar to plateletpheresis.

Refractory Patients

Advanced Concepts

Massive splenomegaly, high fever, sepsis, disseminated intravascular coagulation (DIC), and platelet or HLA antibodies can cause less-than-expected platelet count increment and survival. The 10-minute to 1-hour post-transfusion platelet count increment is less affected by splenomegaly, high fever, and DIC than by the presence of platelet or HLA antibodies.[1] If the 10-minute increment is less than 50% of that expected on two occasions, the patient is considered refractory. Positive platelet crossmatch or positive HLA antibody screen is considered evidence of alloimmunization. Platelet crossmatching with available inventory can speed the provision of platelets for transfusion, as HLA-typing the patient and recruiting HLA-compatible platelet donors can be time-consuming. HLA-matched platelets should be irradiated.

A corrected count increment using a 10-minute to 1-hour post-transfusion platelet count can provide valuable information about patient response to a platelet component.[1] The platelet count increment is corrected for differences in body size so that more reliable estimates of expected platelet increment can be determined. The expected corrected platelet increment is greater than 10,000/μL per m². One formula for corrected count increment is:

$$\frac{\text{Absolute platelet increment/}\mu\text{L} \times \text{body surface area (m}^2)}{\text{Number of platelets transfused (}10^{11})}$$

in which the absolute platelet increment is the post-transfusion platelet count minus the pretransfusion platelet count, the body surface area is expressed as square meters, and the number of platelets transfused is 3 for plateletpheresis or pooled platelets (the number of platelets in each unit expressed in 10^{11}).

For example, a patient with a 10,000/μL platelet count has a body surface area of 1.3 m². One unit of plateletpheresis is given. The 1-hour post-transfusion platelet count is 50,000/μL. Put these into the formula:

$$\frac{(50,000/\mu\text{L} - 10,000/\mu\text{L}) \times 1.3}{}$$

The answer, 17,333, shows that the patient has a good increment (greater than 10,000/μL) and is not refractory to platelets. An answer less than 5,000/μL indicates refractoriness.

In addition to HLA- and platelet-specific antigens, ABO antigens are also expressed on the platelet membrane. Sometimes platelets are selected for transfusion without regard to ABO; however, group O recipients may have a lower increment when given group A platelets than when group-identical platelets are selected.[7] Group A, B, and AB patients may also develop a positive direct antiglobulin test owing to passive transfer of anti-A, anti-B, or anti-A,B when several ABO-incompatible platelet transfusions are given.

Although platelet membranes do not express Rh antigens, platelet products contain small amounts of RBCs and thus can immunize patients to Rh antigens. Rh-immune globulin can be given to girls and women of childbearing potential to prevent Rh sensitization. Each 300-μg vial of Rh immune globulin is adequate for about 30 platelet-phereses or 4 platelet pools of 5.

For the same reasons as RBCs, platelet components may also be leukocyte-reduced or washed. Washing platelet components removes some platelets and plasma proteins and, if using an open method, requires a 4-hour expiration time. Therefore, platelet components should be washed only to prevent severe allergic reactions or to remove alloantibodies in cases of neonatal alloimmune thrombocytopenia.

Granulocyte Pheresis

Patients who have received intensive chemotherapy for leukemia or bone marrow transplant or both may develop severe neutropenia and serious bacterial or fungal infection. Without neutrophils (granulocytes), the patient may have difficulty controlling an infection, even with appropriate antibiotic treatment. Criteria have been developed to identify patients who are most likely to benefit from granulocyte transfusions: those with fever, neutrophil counts less than 500/μL, septicemia or bacterial infection unresponsive to antibiotics, reversible bone marrow hypoplasia, and a reasonable chance for survival.[1] Prophylactic use of granulocyte transfusions is of doubtful value for those patients who have neutropenia but no demonstrable infection.

Newborn infants may develop overwhelming infection with neutropenia because of their limited bone marrow reserve for neutrophil production. In addition, neonatal neutrophils have impaired function. Studies show granulocyte transfusions to be beneficial for these patients. For an adult or a child, the usual dose is one granulocyte pheresis product daily for 4 or more days. For neonates, a portion of a granulocyte pheresis unit is usually given once or twice.

Granulocyte components should be administered as soon as possible and within 24 hours of collection.[5] The granulocyte pheresis needs to be crossmatched because of the significant content of RBCs. The patient must be monitored for resolution of symptoms and clinical evidence of efficacy.

The neutrophil count will increase to 1,000/μL or more in response to infusion of granulocyte colony-stimulating factor (GCSF)–mobilized granulocyte pheresis.

Plasma

Plasma includes fresh frozen plasma, plasma 24 (frozen within 24 hours), and thawed plasma. Plasma and plasma 24 contain all coagulation factors. After fresh frozen plasma and plasma 24 are thawed, they can become thawed plasma and stored for 5 days at 4°C. The 5-day storage reduces outdating and allows rapid response to urgent orders for bleeding patients. Thawed plasma after 5-day storage has less factor V and VIII but is still therapeutic.

Plasma can be used to treat multiple coagulation deficiencies occurring in patients with liver failure, DIC, vitamin K deficiency, warfarin overdose, or massive transfusion.[8] Sometimes, plasma is used to treat patients with single factor deficiencies, such as factor XI deficiency.

Vitamin K deficiency or warfarin overdose should be treated with vitamin K orally, intravenously, or intramuscularly if liver function is adequate and with an adequate interval (4 to 24 hours) before a major or minor hemostatic challenge such as surgery. Plasma is given if the patient is actively bleeding or if time is not available for warfarin reversal before surgery.

Patients with liver disease or liver failure frequently develop clinical coagulopathy due to impaired hepatic synthesis of all coagulation factors and antithrombotic factors. Plasma is the product of choice for patients with multiple-factor deficiencies and hemorrhage or impending surgery. Usually 4 to 6 units of plasma will effectively control hemostasis. Even so, plasma may not correct coagulation tests to normal range because of dysfibrinogenemia. Mild hemostatic abnormalities do not predict bleeding, so correction is not indicated for minor procedures, such as liver biopsy.[9] In addition, plasma is not a concentrate so that volume overload may be a serious complication of transfusion.

Congenital coagulation factor deficiencies are rarely treated with plasma, because the dose requirement for surgical procedures and serious bleeding is so great as to cause pulmonary edema as a result of volume overload, even in a young individual with a healthy cardiovascular system. Factor concentrates (see the "Factor VIII" and "Factor IX" sections below) offer more effective modes of therapy. Factor XI deficiency, however, is still treated by plasma infusion, requiring 20% to 30% factor XI levels for adequate hemostasis. This disease is milder than hemophilia A (factor VIII deficiency) or hemophilia B (factor IX deficiency). Factor XI also has a long half-life, so treatment is not needed on a daily basis.

A coagulation factor unit is defined as the activity in 1 mL of pooled normal plasma, so 100% activity is 1 unit/mL or 100 units/dL. About 30% activity of each of the coagulation factors is required for adequate hemostasis. Thus, less than half of the plasma volume, or about 4 to 6 plasma units, is required to correct a coagulopathy such as in liver disease or DIC. With continued hemorrhage, additional doses are usually needed if the prothrombin time is more than 1.5 times normal or if the international normalized ratio is greater than 1.5. Because several key clotting factors, such as factor VII, VIII, or IX, have half-lives less than 24 hours, repeated transfusions are required to control post-operative bleeding or to maintain hemostasis. For example, factor IX has a half-life of 18 to 24 hours, requiring daily transfusions.

Plasma is sometimes used as a replacement fluid during plasma exchange (therapeutic plasmapheresis; see Chapter 14, "Apheresis"). In cases of thrombotic thrombocytopenic purpura, plasma provides a metalloprotease (ADAMTS13) and removes inhibitors, thus reversing the symptoms. Plasma should not be used for blood volume expansion or protein replacement because safer products are available for these purposes—serum albumin, synthetic colloids, and balanced salt solutions—none of which transmit disease or cause severe allergic reactions or transfusion-associated acute lung injury.

Plasma should be ABO-compatible with the recipient's RBCs, but the Rh type can be disregarded.

Cryoprecipitate

Cryoprecipitate is used primarily for fibrinogen replacement. The AABB requires that at least 150 mg of fibrinogen be in each unit of cryoprecipitate,[5] although quality control levels are often over 250 mg. Generally, 5 cryoprecipitate units are pooled, rinsing each bag with saline, at the blood center. These pools are frozen and shipped to transfusion services where the pools can be thawed and issued. Each pool contains 750 to 1,250 mg of fibrinogen.

Fibrinogen replacement may be required in patients with liver failure, DIC, or massive transfusion and in rare patients with congenital fibrinogen deficiency. A fibrinogen plasma level of about 100 mg/dL is recommended for adequate hemostasis with surgery or trauma. For example, a patient's fibrinogen must be increased from 30 mg/dL to 100 mg/dL, or an increment of 70 mg/dL (100 − 30 mg/dL):

- To calculate the amount to be infused, first convert milligrams per deciliter to milligrams per milliliter by dividing by 100 (100 mL/dL).
- Multiplying the answer 0.7 mg/mL by the plasma volume, 3,000 mL, we thus require 2,100 mg (0.7 mg/mL × 3,000 mL).
- To calculate the number of pools needed, divide 2,100 mg by 750 mg/pool, which equals 2.8 or almost 3 pools.
- Instead, plasma volume can be converted to deciliters by dividing by 100 mL/dL or 70 mg/dL × 30 dL.

Cryoprecipitate was used as a source for fibrin sealant, which uses cryoprecipitate as the source of fibrinogen. FDA-approved fibrin sealants, which have been treated to reduce viral transmission, are preferred.

Cryoprecipitate was originally prepared as a source of factor VIII. Each unit of cryoprecipitate must contain at least 80 units of factor VIII. However, mild or moderate factor VIII deficiency (hemophilia A) is now treated with desmopressin acetate (1-deamino-[8-D-arginine]-vasopressin [DDAVP]) or factor VIII, or both, whereas severe factor VIII deficiency is treated only with factor VIII.

Cryoprecipitate was used to treat patients with von Willebrand's disease, a deficiency of vWF. Cryoprecipitate is no longer considered the product of choice for factor VIII deficiency or von Willebrand's disease. Virus-safe factor VIII with assayed amounts of factor VIII and vWF is available.

Factor VIII

Patients with hemophilia A or factor VIII deficiency have spontaneous hemorrhages that are treated with recombinant or human plasma–derived factor VIII replacement.[10] Plasma derived factor VIII is prepared from plasma obtained from paid donors by plasmapheresis or from volunteer whole blood donors. Factor VIII is treated by different methods, such as pasteurization, nanofiltration, and solvent detergent, to ensure sterility for HIV, hepatitis B virus, and hepatitis C virus (HCV).[11] The recombinant human product is virus-safe. Recombinant human products and their indications are listed in Table 15–3.

Both the plasma derived and recombinant factor VIII are stored at refrigerator temperatures and are reconstituted with saline at the time of infusion. This ease of handling allows self-therapy for individuals with hemophilia.

The following example illustrates the calculation of a factor VIII dose:

A 70-kg hemophiliac patient with a hematocrit level of 30% has an initial factor VIII level of 4% (4 units/dL, 0.04 units/mL). How many units of factor VIII concentrate should be given to raise his factor VIII level to 50%?

$$\{\text{desired factor VIII (units/mL)} - \text{initial factor VIII (units/mL)}\} \times \text{plasma volume (mL)} = \text{units of factor VIII required.}$$

- Blood volume = weight (kg) × 70 mL/kg
- 70 kg × 70 mL/kg = 4,900 mL
- Plasma volume = blood volume (mL) × (1.0 − Hct)
- 4,900 mL × (1.0 − 0.30) = 3,430 mL
- Solution: 3,430 mL × (0.50 − 0.04) = 1,578 units
- The assayed value on the label can be divided into the number of units required to obtain the number of vials to be infused.

Table 15–3	Recombinant Human Products
PRODUCT	**INDICATIONS**
Factor VIII	Hemophilia A, von Willebrand's disease
Factor IX	Hemophilia B
Factor VIIa	Inhibitors in hemophilia A or B Factor VII deficiency Acquired factor VII deficiency* • Liver disease • Warfarin overdose Massive hemorrhage*

*Randomized controlled trials needed

Only factor VIII products labeled as containing vWF should be used for patients with von Willebrand's disease.

Factor IX

Factor IX complex (prothrombin complex) is prepared from pooled plasma using various methods of separation and viral inactivation. The prothrombin complex contains factors II, VII, IX, and X; however, the product is recommended for factor IX–deficient patients (hemophilia B), patients with factor VII or X deficiency (rare), and selected patients with factor VIII inhibitors or reversal of warfarin overdose.[10] Activated coagulation factors present in prothrombin complex may cause thrombosis, especially in patients with liver disease. Recombinant human factor IX (see **Table 15–3**) is effective only in the management of factor IX deficiency.

The dose is calculated in the same manner as that for factor VIII concentrate, using the assayed value of factor IX on the label, with the caveat that half the dose of factor IX rapidly diffuses into tissues, and half remains within the intravascular space, so the initial dose must be doubled.

Antithrombin and Other Concentrates

Antithrombin is a protease inhibitor with activity toward thrombin. Heparin accelerates the binding and inactivation of thrombin by antithrombin. The hereditary deficiency of antithrombin is associated with venous thromboses, whereas the acquired deficiency is seen most frequently with DIC. **Antithrombin concentrates** are licensed for use in the United States for patients with hereditary deficiency of antithrombin. The product is pasteurized to eliminate the risk of HIV or HCV infections. Antithrombin has been shown to provide no significant clinical benefit in acquired deficiency. Thawed plasma is an alternative source of antithrombin.

Protein C and protein S are vitamin K–dependent proteins synthesized in the liver. **Protein S** functions as a cofactor for activated **protein C**, which, in turn, inactivates factors V and VIII, thus preventing thrombus formation. Deficiency (hereditary or acquired) leads to a hypercoagulable state (i.e., the tendency for thrombosis). Human plasma–derived protein C concentrates are approved for use in hereditary deficiency states. Recombinant-human activated protein C has been used for DIC and sepsis.

Recombinant human activated factor VII (rFVIIa; see Table 15–3) has been used to control bleeding episodes in hemophilia A and B patients with inhibitors.[10,12] rFVIIa has been used in patients with a wide variety of bleeding disorders. However, large randomized controlled trials are needed to define dose, indications, and adverse effects. Reports of use for liver disease, massive transfusion, and other bleeding disorders have been promising.[13]

Albumin

Albumin is prepared by chemical and physical fractionation of pooled plasma. Albumin is available as a 5% or a 25% solution, of which 96% of the protein content is albumin. The product is heat-treated and has proved to be virus-safe over many years of use.

Albumin may be used to treat patients requiring volume replacement. Whether albumin or colloids other than crystalloid (i.e., saline or electrolyte) solutions are better for treating hypovolemia with shock is controversial. In many plasmapheresis procedures, albumin is used routinely as the replacement fluid for the colloid that is removed during the procedures. Albumin can also be used in the treatment of burn patients to replace colloid pressure.

Albumin, with diuretics, can induce diuresis in patients who have low total protein because of severe liver or protein-losing disease. The 25% solution brings about five times its volume from extravascular water into the vascular space. Thus, patients receiving 25% albumin need to have adequate extravascular water and compensatory mechanisms to deal with the expansion of the blood volume.

Immune Globulin

Immune globulin prepared from pooled plasma is primarily IgG. Although small amounts of IgM and IgA may be present in some preparations, others are free of these contaminating proteins. Products are available for intramuscular or intravenous administration. The intramuscular product must not be given intravenously because severe anaphylactic reactions may occur. The intravenous product must be given slowly to lessen the risk of reaction.

Immune globulin is used for patients with congenital hypogammaglobulinemia[11] and for patients exposed to diseases such as hepatitis A or measles. For hypogammaglobulinemia, monthly injections are usually given because of the 22-day half-life of IgG. The recommended dose is 0.7 mL/kg intramuscularly or 100 mg/kg intravenously. For hepatitis A prophylaxis, 0.02 to 0.04 mL/kg intramuscularly is recommended.

The intravenous preparation of immune globulin is used increasingly in the therapy of autoimmune diseases, such as immune thrombocytopenia[11] and myasthenia gravis. Various mechanisms of action have been postulated. Conceivably, the infused immune globulin blocks the reticuloendothelial system or mononuclear phagocytic system.

Various hyperimmune globulins are available to prevent diseases such as hepatitis B, varicella zoster, rabies, mumps, and others. These are prepared from the plasma of donors who have high antibody titers to the specific virus causing the disease. The dose is recommended in the package insert. It should be noted that preparations such as hepatitis B hyperimmune globulin provide only passive immunity after an exposure. They do not confer permanent immunity and so must be accompanied by active immunization.

Rh immune globulin (RhIG) was developed to protect the Rh-negative female who is pregnant or who delivers an Rh-positive infant (see Chapter 19, "Hemolytic Disease of the Fetus and Newborn [HDFN]"). Much of the IgG in this preparation is directed against the D antigen within the Rh system. Administration of this preparation allows attachment of anti-D to any Rh-positive cells of the infant that have entered the maternal circulation. The antibody-bound cells are subsequently removed by the mother's macrophages, preventing active immunization or sensitization.

Rh immune globulin products, which can be administered intravenously or intramuscularly, are approved for use in idiopathic thrombocytopenic purpura patients who are Rh-positive.[1] The proposed mechanism of action is blockage of the reticuloendothelial system by anti-D–coated RBCs, thereby reducing the destruction of autoantibody-coated platelets.

For RBC transfusion accidents, the number of RhIG vials is calculated by dividing the volume of Rh-positive packed RBCs transfused by 15 mL, the amount of RBCs covered by one vial. The number of vials can be large, so the entire dose is often divided and administered in several injections at separate sites and over 3 days. The intravenous preparation may also be used. Another approach is to perform an exchange transfusion with Rh-negative blood and then calculate the dose based on the number of Rh-positive RBCs remaining in the circulation. For platelets pheresis, one vial is sufficient for 30 or more products, because each unit contains fewer than 0.5 mL RBCs. The dose for leukocyte concentrates can be calculated by obtaining the hematocrit and volume of the product from the supplier.

Immune globulins may cause anaphylactic reactions (flushing, hypotension, dyspnea, nausea, vomiting, diarrhea, and back pain). Caution should be used in patients with known IgA deficiency and previous anaphylactic reactions to blood components.

Special Considerations for Transfusion

Certain categories of patients require the selection of blood products that are leukocyte-reduced, CMV-negative, or irradiated. These special products are detailed here.

Leukocyte-Reduced Cellular Blood Components

Leukocyte-reduction filters are designed to remove more than 99.9% of leukocytes from RBCs and platelet products. The goal is fewer than 5×10^6 (1×10^6 in Europe) leukocytes remaining in the RBC unit. Prestorage filtration in the laboratory or at the time of collection, rather than at the bedside, is more reliable for leukocyte reduction.

Leukocyte-reduced RBCs and platelets can be used to prevent febrile nonhemolytic transfusion reactions, to prevent or delay the development of HLA antibodies, and to reduce the risk of CMV transmission. Controversial effects of leukocyte reduction include decreased mortality and length of hospital stay.[1]

CMV-Negative Cellular Blood Components

CMV is carried, in a latent or infectious form, in neutrophils and monocytes. Transfusion of these virus-infected cells in a cellular product such as RBCs or platelets can transmit infection. CMV infection of the patients can be reduced by using leukocyte-reduction filters[14] or by providing CMV antibody–negative blood. CMV-negative or leukocyte-reduced components are indicated for recipients who are CMV-negative and at risk for severe sequelae of CMV infections.[1] The risk is greatest for CMV-negative pregnant women (mainly for the benefit of the fetus), allogeneic CMV-negative bone marrow and hematopoietic progenitor cell transplant recipients, and premature infants weighing less than 1,200 g.

Irradiated Cellular Blood Components

Blood components are irradiated with gamma radiation to prevent graft-versus-host disease, which requires three conditions to occur:

1. Transfusion or transplantation of immunocompetent T lymphocytes
2. Histocompatibility differences between graft and recipient (major or minor HLA or other histocompatibility antigens)
3. Usually, an immunocompromised recipient[15]

Common after allogeneic bone marrow or hematopoietic progenitor cell transplantation, GVHD is a syndrome affecting mainly skin, liver, and gut (see Chapter 17, "Cellular Therapy").

Transfusion-associated graft-versus-host disease (TA-GVHD), occurring less frequently, is caused by viable T lymphocytes in cellular blood components (e.g., RBCs and platelets). The mortality rate is high;[15] therefore, prevention is key. Prevention centers on irradiating cellular components before administration to significantly immunocompromised individuals. Irradiation doses range from 2,500 to 5,000 cGy, with the higher doses being more effective but more damaging to RBCs. Irradiation decreases or eliminates the mitogenic (blastogenic) capacity of the transfused T cells, rendering the donor T cells immunoincompetent.

At risk for TA-GVHD are transfusion recipients with congenital immunodeficiencies (severe combined immunodeficiency, DiGeorge syndrome, Wiskott-Aldrich syndrome), Hodgkin's lymphoma, bone marrow transplants (allogeneic or autologous), intrauterine transfusion of fetuses, exchange transfusion of neonates, donations from blood relatives, and HLA-matched platelets.[1]

Immunocompetent recipients have experienced TA-GVHD after receiving nonirradiated directed donations primarily from first-degree relatives. The related donor is homozygous for one of the patient's (host's) HLA haplotypes, so the patient is incapable of rejecting the donor's (graft's) T lymphocytes, which then can act against the HLA antigens encoded by the patient's other haplotype. The donor lymphocytes then reject the host. The level of immunosuppression a recipient must have to develop TA-GVHD is unknown, although patients with the severe immunosuppressive conditions listed previously are most at risk. In addition, the dose of lymphocytes needed for TA-GVHD to occur is unknown. For this reason, prevention depends on irradiation and *not* on reduction of lymphocytes by filtration.

Transfusion Therapy in Special Conditions

Some patients require policies and procedures that address particular clinical situations. Patients undergoing elective surgery, autologous collection and transfusion, and emergency and massive transfusion are discussed here. Transfusion of neonatal, pediatric, and oncology patients and those with congenital coagulation deficiencies are detailed here.

Surgical Blood Order Schedule, Type, and Screen

Most surgical procedures do not require blood transfusion. Crossmatching for procedures with a low likelihood of transfusion increases the number of crossmatches performed, increases the amount of blood inventory in reserve and unavailable for transfusion, and contributes to the aging and possible outdating of the blood components. Patients can be better served by performing only a type and antibody screen. If the antibody screen is positive, antibody identification must be completed and compatible units found. However, if the antibody screen is negative, ABO- and Rh-type-specific blood may be released after an immediate spin or electronic crossmatch in those rare instances when transfusion is required. Box 15-2 shows an example of a surgical blood order schedule.

For a patient who is likely to require blood transfusion, the number of crossmatched units should be no more than twice those usually required for that surgical procedure. Thus, the crossmatch-to-transfusion (C/T) ratio will be between 2:1 and 3:1, which has been shown to be optimal practice.

Some transfusion services extend this practice to nonsurgical patients, crossmatching only when the RBCs are requested for issue to the patient. This practice increases the inventory of uncrossmatched units, which can be used for immediate needs.

Autologous Transfusion

Autologous (self) transfusion is the donation of blood by the intended recipient (Fig. 15–1). The infusion of blood

---

BOX 15–2

Surgical Blood Order Schedule

Purpose: Reduce unnecessary crossmatching
Examples:
- Type and screen
  - Exploratory laparotomy
  - Cholecystectomy
- Two units crossmatched
  - CABG
  - Total hip revision

---

from another donor is called **homologous transfusion**. The patient's own blood reduces the possibility of transfusion reaction or transmission of infectious disease.

One type of autologous transfusion is the predeposit of blood by the patient. Collected by regular blood donation procedure, the blood can be stored as liquid or, for longer storage, frozen. Patients may donate several units of blood over a period of weeks, taking iron supplements to stimulate erythropoiesis. Predeposit autologous donation is usually reserved for patients anticipating a need for transfusion, such as for a scheduled surgery. Predeposit autologous transfusion is expensive because about half of the donated units are not used. In addition, patients present for surgery with lower hematocrits, which increases transfusion of homologous units in addition to autologous units. However, patients with multiple RBC antibodies or antibodies to high-incidence antigens may store frozen units for use by themselves or others.

Another type of autologous transfusion, intraoperative hemodilution, is the collection of 1 or 2 units of blood from the patient just before a surgical procedure, replacing the removed blood volume with crystalloid or colloid solution. Then, at the end of surgery, the blood units are infused into the patient. Care must be taken to label and store the blood units properly and to identify the blood units with the patient before infusion.

Meticulous attention to hemostasis and salvage of shed blood has allowed surgical procedures that once required

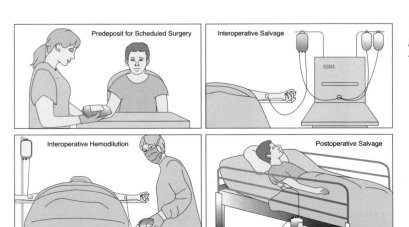

Figure 15–1. Types of autologous transfusions. *(Reprinted with permission from Kennedy, MS (ed): Blood Transfusion Therapy: An Audiovisual Program. AABB, Bethesda, MD, 1985.)*

many units of blood to be performed without the need for homologous blood (see **Fig. 15–1**). Several types of equipment are available for collecting, washing, and filtering shed blood before reinfusion. Washing of intraoperative or postoperative salvaged blood is recommended to remove the cellular debris, fat, and other contaminants. Heparin or citrate solutions may be used for anticoagulation of the shed blood.

Emergency Transfusion

Patients who are rapidly or uncontrollably bleeding may require immediate transfusion. Group O RBCs are selected for patients for whom transfusion cannot wait until their ABO and Rh type can be determined. Group O–negative RBC units should be used if the patient is a female of childbearing potential. An Rh-negative male patient or an older female patient can be switched from Rh-negative to Rh-positive RBCs if few O-negative units are available or if massive transfusion is required. Delaying blood transfusion in emergency situations may be more dangerous than the small risk of transfusing incompatible blood before the antibody screen and crossmatch are completed.

After issuing O blood or type-specific blood, the antibody screen can be completed, and decisions can then be made for the selection of additional units of blood. If the patient has been typed and screened for a surgical procedure and his or her antibody screen is negative, ABO- and Rh-type-specific blood can be given after an immediate spin crossmatch.

Transfusions should be reserved for those patients losing more than 20% of their blood volume. The condition of most patients allows determination of ABO and Rh type and selection of ABO- and Rh-type-specific blood for transfusion.

Massive Transfusion

Massive transfusion is defined as the replacement of one or more blood volumes within 24 hours, or about 10 units of blood in an adult. The strategy for treating massive hemorrhage has changed in recent years, as experience in the military has promoted preventive treatment to avoid coagulopathy. Most medical centers with high-level trauma services have adopted a massive transfusion protocol, one of which is outlined in Table 15–4. Analysis of the patient's clinical status and laboratory tests is essential for guiding appropriate transfusion therapy. The massive transfusion pack can be adjusted for low hemoglobin or platelets or prolonged coagulation tests. For example, platelets are required if the platelet count is less than 50,000/µL, and plasma is needed if the PT ratio is greater than 1.5, or the INR is greater than 1.5, or the activated partial thromboplastin time (PTT) exceeds 60 seconds. Fibrinogen levels should also be monitored because replacement by cryoprecipitate may be indicated when the fibrinogen level is less than 100 mg/dL.

A patient in critical condition and a limited supply of type-specific blood may require a change in ABO or Rh types. An Rh-negative male or postmenopausal female patient may

Table 15–4	**Example of a Massive Transfusion Protocol (MTP)**
INITIAL	**TRANSFUSION STRATEGY**
Draw type and crossmatch	2 units group O RBCs uncrossmatched
Continuing	
Prepare massive transfusion protocol pack by transfusion service	4 to 6 type-specific or crossmatched RBCs 4 plasma 1 platelet pool or plateletpheresis
Monitor CBC, platelet count, PT/INR, PTT, fibrinogen	Add or subtract components based on lab values
Provide additional MTP packs	Continue transfusion until unneeded

be switched from Rh-negative to Rh-positive blood to avoid depleting the inventory of Rh-negative blood. However, an Rh-negative potentially childbearing woman should receive Rh-negative RBC products for as long as possible.

Neonatal Transfusion

Premature infants frequently require transfusion of small amounts of RBCs to replace blood drawn for laboratory tests and to treat the anemia of prematurity (Box 15–3). A dose of 10 mL/kg will increase the hemoglobin by approximately 3 g/dL. Various methods are available for preparing small aliquots for transfusion. Small aliquots of donor blood can be transferred from the collection bag to a satellite bag or transfer bag, or blood can be withdrawn from the collection bag or transfer bag using an injection site coupler and needle and syringe or a sterile docking device and syringe. Red cells in CPD, CPDA-1, or additive solution can be safely used.

The aliquot must be labeled clearly with the name and identifying numbers of the patient and donor. The blood must be fully tested, the same as for adult transfusion. Blood units less than 7 days old are preferred to reduce the risk of hyperkalemia and to maximize the 2,3-diphosphoglycerate levels, although in some institutions CPDA-1 RBCs 14 to 21 days old are used.

BOX 15–3

Neonatal RBC Transfusions

Aliquoted units

- Less than 7 days old, unless infused slowly
- O-negative or compatible with mother and infant
- CMV-negative or leukocyte-reduced
- Hemoglobin S–negative for hypoxic newborns

Dose

- 10 mL/kg over 2 to 3 hours

For very-low-birth-weight infants, the blood should be selected to be CMV-seronegative or leukocyte-reduced to prevent CMV infection, which can be serious in premature infants. Indeed, pregnant women should be given CMV-negative or leukocyte-reduced cellular components if they test negative for CMV.

Irradiation of the blood is recommended to prevent possible TA-GVHD when blood is used for intrauterine transfusion, for an exchange transfusion (see Chapter 19), or for transfusion of a premature (less than 1,200 g) neonate. Transfusions in a full-term newborn infant do not require routine irradiation.

Infants who are hypoxic or acidotic should receive blood tested and negative for hemoglobin S. For more detail on intrauterine and exchange transfusions, see Chapter 19.

Transfusion in Oncology

The bone marrow of oncology patients may be suppressed because of chemotherapy, radiation therapy, or infiltration and replacement of the bone marrow with malignant cells. Repeated RBC and platelet transfusions may lead to the need for rare RBC units or HLA-matched plateletpheresis components because of incompatibility problems. Platelet transfusion requirements may also necessitate a change from Rh-negative to Rh-positive products. RhIG may be given to a woman with childbearing potential to protect against immunization. There is less than 0.5 mL of Rh-positive RBCs present in each Rh-positive plateletpheresis component. A pool of platelets may contain as much as 4 mL of RBCs. One 300-μg dose of RhIg can neutralize the effects of up to 15 mL of Rh-positive cells. Thus, one dose could be used for 30 plateletphereses or 4 platelet pools.

In addition, some malignancies such as chronic lymphocytic leukemia and lymphoma are frequently complicated by autoimmune hemolytic anemia, increased destruction of RBCs, and pretransfusion testing problems.

Oncology patients with hematologic malignancies, such as Hodgkin's disease and lymphoma, are at increased risk of TA-GVHD because of the chemotherapy drugs used for treatment. Therefore, these patients should receive irradiated cellular components.

Coagulation Factor Deficiencies

Factor VIII is normally complexed with another plasma protein, vWF. Both proteins are necessary for normal hemostasis. Patients with hemophilia A, or classic hemophilia, have factor VIII deficiency. Hemophilia A patients have factor VIII levels less than 50%, although clinical disease is generally not apparent unless the factor VIII level is less than 10% (normal is 80% to 120%). Individuals with a level less than 1% have severe and spontaneous bleeding, typically into muscles and joints. The vWF level is usually normal in patients with hemophilia A.

Von Willebrand's disease is defined by a deficiency of vWF. Type I von Willebrand's disease is characterized by a reduced amount of all sizes of vWF multimers and is milder than type III, in which little or no vWF is produced. Type IIA is distinguished by a deficiency of high molecular weight multimers, whereas type IIB is identified by abnormal high molecular weight multimers that have an increased avidity for binding to platelets. Type I patients have the ability to make the full spectrum of vWF multimers but do not produce them in normal amounts. DDAVP, a synthetic vasopressin analog, can stimulate release of the vWF from the vascular endothelium in type I patients. DDAVP, however, is contraindicated in type IIB von Willebrand's disease. Many factor VIII products are assayed for vWF and can be used for type III von Willebrand's disease or in type I or IIA disease when DDAVP treatment has failed.

Hemophilia B is the congenital deficiency of factor IX. Factor IX is activated by factors XIa and VIIa. The activated factor IX (IXa), along with factor VIII, ionized calcium, and phospholipid, activates factor X to Xa. Factor IX deficiency should be treated with recombinant factor IX or prothrombin complex concentrates. Factor IX concentrates are made virus-safe by various sterilization techniques.[10]

All coagulation factors except vWF are made in the liver. With severe liver failure, multiple coagulation factor deficiencies occur. In addition, some of the coagulation factors produced may be abnormal. The liver also produces many of the thrombolytic proteins, leading to imbalance between the coagulation process and the control mechanism. Plasma, having normal amounts of all these proteins, can be used to treat these patients.

Vitamin K aids in the carboxylation of factors II, VII, IX, and X. With the absence of vitamin K or the use of drugs that interfere with vitamin K metabolism, such as warfarin, the inactive coagulation proteins cannot be carboxylated to active forms. Vitamin K administration rather than plasma transfusion is recommended to correct vitamin K deficiency or warfarin overdose. Because several hours are required for vitamin K effectiveness, depending on route of administration, signs of hemorrhage or impending surgery may require transfusion of plasma.

DIC is the uncontrolled activation and consumption of coagulation proteins, causing small thrombi within the vascular system throughout the body. Treatment is aimed at correcting the cause of the DIC: sepsis, disseminated malignancy, certain acute leukemias, obstetric complications, or shock. In some cases, transfusion of plasma, platelets, or cryoprecipitate may be required. Monitoring of the PT, PTT, platelet count, fibrinogen, and hemoglobin and hematocrit levels helps direct the choice of the next component to be used.

Platelet functional disorders may be caused by drugs, uremia, or congenital abnormalities. Platelet transfusions in these patients should be reserved for treating hemorrhage or the impending need for adequate hemostasis (such as a surgical procedure) to decrease development of platelet refractoriness. Drugs that interfere with platelet function, such as clopidogrel (Plavix®), are commonly used in cardiovascular disease and are irreversible for the life of the platelets. Therefore, discontinuing the drug for 5 to 7 days before surgery will minimize hemorrhage and lessen the need for massive transfusion. In uremia, DDAVP may be beneficial as well as dialysis or RBC transfusions. DDAVP releases fresh, functional vWF from endothelial cells. Dialysis removes by-products of protein metabolism that degrade vWF and coat platelets, making both non-functional. RBC transfusion increases viscosity.

General Blood Transfusion Practices

Although blood administration and the hospital transfusion committee are not the responsibility of the transfusion service, nurses, physicians and administrators look to the transfusion specialists to guide policies and practices.

Blood Administration

Blood must be administered carefully for patient safety (Fig. 15–2). The positive identification of the patient, patient's blood specimen, and blood unit for transfusion is essential. Careful identification procedures prevent a major cause of transfusion-related deaths: ABO incompatibility. Clerical errors represent the main cause of transfusion-related deaths and acute hemolytic transfusion reactions.[16] The identification process begins with positive identification of the patient—that is, asking patients to state or spell their name while you read their armband. The patient identification label is compared at the bedside to the patient's

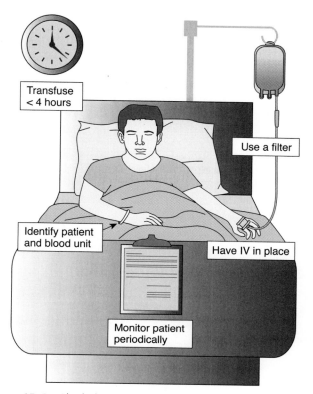

Figure 15–2. Blood administration and patient safety. *(Reprinted with permission from Kennedy, MS (ed): Blood Transfusion Therapy: An Audiovisual Program. AABB, Bethesda, MD, 1985.)*

Transfuse < 4 hours

Use a filter

Identify patient and blood unit

Have IV in place

Monitor patient periodically

hospital armband. This prevents a specimen tube labeled with one patient's name being used for the collection of a specimen from another patient. The labels are applied to the specimen tubes before leaving the bedside to avoid labeling the wrong tube. Electronic systems for patient and label identification are available and should be adopted to reduce clerical errors.

Positive identification is carried out in the laboratory. Clerical check is performed as results are generated and compared to historical results. Another clerical check is done as blood is issued from the blood bank. The final clerical check is performed at the patient bedside as the nurse compares the patient armband with the blood bank tag attached to the component to be transfused.

The patient with difficult veins should have the intravenous infusion device in place before the blood is issued from the transfusion service. All blood components must be filtered (170-μm filter) because clots and cellular debris develop during storage. Blood components are infused slowly for the first 10 to 15 minutes while the patient is observed closely for signs of a transfusion reaction. The blood components should then be infused as quickly as tolerated or, at most, within 4 hours. The patient's vital signs (pulse, respiration, blood pressure, and temperature) should be monitored periodically during the transfusion to detect signs of transfusion reaction (see Chapter 16, "Adverse Effects of Blood Transfusion"). Signs and symptoms are fever with back pain (acute hemolytic transfusion reaction), anaphylaxis, hives or pruritus (urticarial reaction), congestive heart failure (volume overload), and fever alone (febrile non-hemolytic transfusion reaction). A delayed hemolytic transfusion reaction (jaundice, decreasing hematocrit level) may be diagnosed 5 to 10 days after transfusion and thus is not considered an immediate reaction.

In standard blood administration sets, the 170- to 260-μm filter removes gross clots and cellular debris. A standard blood administration filter must be used for transfusion of all blood components.

Rapid transfusion, including exchange transfusion, requires blood warming because the cold blood can cause hypothermia in the patient, which increases the possibility of cardiac arrhythmia and hemorrhage. A patient with paroxysmal cold hemoglobinuria or with potent cold agglutinins may also require blood warming. The blood warmer should have automatic temperature control with an alarm that will sound if the blood is warmed over 42°C. Blood units must not be warmed by immersion in a water-bath or by a domestic microwave oven because uneven heating can cause damage to blood cells and denaturation of blood proteins.

Only isotonic (0.9%) saline or 5% albumin should be used to dilute blood components, because other intravenous solutions may damage the RBCs and cause hemolysis (dextrose solutions such as D_5W) or initiate coagulation in the infusion set (calcium-containing solutions such as lactated Ringer's solution). In addition, some drugs may cause hemolysis if injected through the blood infusion set.

After transfusion, the transfusion set may be flushed with normal saline. The empty blood bag can be discarded or returned to the transfusion service, according to hospital policy. A copy of the blood bag tag is placed in the patient's chart.

Hospital Transfusion Committee

The Joint Commission requires all blood transfusions to be reviewed for appropriate use. A hospital transfusion committee, although not required, may serve as the peer review group for transfusions. Blood usage review may also be performed prospectively if criteria are approved by the transfusion committee and the medical staff.[17] The blood bank director may interact and correspond directly with the chair of individual hospital departments concerning medical staff blood component usage patterns. Appropriate criteria for blood transfusion have been published (Table 15–5), serving as a guide for conducting audits.[3,7,8,18] The results of the audits can be used by the transfusion committee to recommend changes in practice by the hospital staff to improve patient care. The transfusion committee also reviews transfusion reactions to ensure that adverse reactions are unavoidable. In addition, the transfusion committee ensures that appropriate procedures (such as for blood administration) are in place and are followed by hospital personnel.

The transfusion committee is most effective if the various groups who order and administer blood, such as surgeons, anesthesiologists, oncologists, and nurses are represented on the committee. The transfusion committee must have a mechanism for reporting activities and recommendations to the medical staff and hospital administration. Optimally, the transfusion committee ensures that the most appropriate, efficient, and safe use of the blood supply is achieved.

Table 15–5	Criteria for Transfusion Audit
All Blood Components	
Review of patients with transfusion reactions of hemolysis, severe allergic signs or anaphylaxis, circulatory overload, transfusion-related acute lung injury, or infection	
RBCs[18]	
Indications	Decreased oxygen-carrying capacity or acute loss of more than 20% blood volume *or* hemoglobin less than 7 g/dL or hematocrit less than 21%
Exceptions	Patients with hemoglobin less than 8 g/dL and acute coronary syndrome
Outcome	H/H less than 24 hours after transfusion Surgical patients: postoperative hemoglobin less than preoperative hemoglobin
Platelets[7]	
Indications	Platelet count less than 5,000 to 10,000/μL without hemorrhage *or* hemorrhage and platelet count less than 50,000/μL *or* operative procedure and platelet count less than 50,000/μL *or* antiplatelet drugs
Outcome	Platelet count immediately before and 10 minutes to 1 hour post-transfusion except with antiplatelet drugs (e.g., Plavix®)
Plasma	
Indications	Patients with bleeding or invasive procedure PTT greater than 60 sec *or* INR greater than 1.5
Outcome	PT or PTT, less than 4 hours after transfusion
Cryoprecipitate	
Indications	Fibrinogen deficiency or factor XIII deficiency
Outcome	Fibrinogen or factor XIII determination after transfusion

Data from Simon, TL, et al: Practice parameter for the use of red blood cell transfusions. Arch Pathol Lab Med 122:130, 1998; Slichter, SJ: Evidence-based platelet transfusion guidelines. Hematology 127:172–178, 2007; and AuBuchon, JP, et al: Guidelines for blood utilization review, AABB, Bethesda, MD, 2001.
H/H = hemoglobin/hematocrit
PT = prothrombin time
PTT = partial thromboplastin time
INR = international normalized ratio

CASE STUDIES

Case 15-1

A 55-year-old man is contemplating surgery for severe arthritis in the right hip.

1. What should be known to determine how many units of RBCs should be crossmatched?
2. How can it be determined if the patient can donate blood (autologous predeposit) for use during surgery?
3. The patient has a history of bleeding after a tonsillectomy at age 7 years. What tests should be done to further study this potential problem?
4. If the patient is found to have von Willebrand's disease, which blood product might be necessary?

Case 15-2

A 45-year-old woman complains of tiredness and weakness. She appears pale. Laboratory results are as follows: hemoglobin 6.2 g/dL, hematocrit 20%, MCV 75 fL, MCHC 28%. On further questioning, she reports excessive menstrual bleeding, sometimes lasting for several weeks.

1. Does this patient need a transfusion? Justify your answer.
2. If the intern decides to give one unit of RBCs, what would be the resulting hemoglobin and hematocrit levels?

Case 15-3

A 22-year-old woman presents with easy bruising and fatigue. A complete blood count reveals hemoglobin 9 g/dL, hematocrit 27%, WBC 15,000/μL, and platelet count 5,000/μL. The hematologist plans to perform a bone marrow biopsy and aspiration.

1. What blood component(s) is (are) indicated? Why?
2. Describe how the dose is calculated. What laboratory result is desired?
3. The patient receives chemotherapy, and 2 weeks later the hemoglobin is 6.8 g/dL and the hematocrit 20%. The patient complains of shortness of breath when hurrying to the bus stop. The physician decides to order RBC transfusion. What dose of RBCs is indicated? How is this determined?

Case 15-4

A 45-year-old man is admitted to the emergency department vomiting blood. His hemoglobin is 8 g/dL, platelet count 80,000, PT/INR 18/2, fibrinogen 125 mg/dL. The physician orders 4 units of RBCs, 4 units of plasma, and 1 pool of platelets stat.

1. Which blood group(s) should be selected for the RBC transfusions?
2. For FFP and platelets, which blood type(s) should be selected?

His type and screen is B positive with positive antibody screen. The ED nurse calls and informs the blood bank that the massive transfusion protocol has been started.

3. Which components should be prepared?
4. Which blood group and Rh type should be selected?
5. What should be done about the positive antibody screen?

SUMMARY CHART

- ✔ Transfusion therapy is used primarily to treat two conditions: inadequate oxygen-carrying capacity because of anemia or blood loss and insufficient coagulation proteins or platelets to provide adequate hemostasis.
- ✔ A unit of whole blood or RBCs in an adult should increase the hematocrit level 3% or hemoglobin level 1 g/dL.
- ✔ RBCs are indicated for increasing the RBC mass in patients who require increased oxygen-carrying capacity.
- ✔ Platelet transfusions are indicated for patients who are bleeding because of thrombocytopenia. In addition, platelets are indicated prophylactically for patients who have platelet counts under 5,000 to 10,000/μL.
- ✔ Each dose of platelets should increase the platelet count 20,000 to 40,000/μL in a 70-kg human.
- ✔ A plateletpheresis product is collected from one donor and must contain a minimum of 3×10^{11} platelets.
- ✔ Plasma contains all coagulation factors and is indicated for patients with multiple coagulation deficiencies that occur in liver failure, DIC, vitamin K deficiency, warfarin overdose, and massive transfusion.
- ✔ Cryoprecipitate contains at least 80 units of factor VIII and 150 mg of fibrinogen, as well as vWF, and factor XIII.
- ✔ Factor IX is used in the treatment of persons with hemophilia B.
- ✔ Immunoglobulin (IG) is used in the treatment of congenital hypogammaglobulinemia and patients exposed to hepatitis A or measles.
- ✔ Massive transfusion is defined as the replacement of one or more blood volume(s) within 24 hours, or about 10 units of blood in an adult.
- ✔ Emergency transfusion warrants group O RBCs when patient type is not yet known.

Review Questions

1. Leukocyte-reduced filters can do all of the following *except*:
   a. Reduce the risk of CMV infection
   b. Prevent or reduce the risk of HLA alloimmunization
   c. Prevent febrile, nonhemolytic transfusion reactions
   d. Prevent TA-GVHD

2. Albumin should *not* be given for:
   a. Burns
   b. Shock
   c. Nutrition
   d. Plasmapheresis

3. Of the following, which blood type is selected when a patient cannot wait for ABO-matched RBCs?
   a. A
   b. B
   c. O
   d. AB

4. Which patient does *not* need an irradiated component?
   a. Bone marrow transplant recipient
   b. Neonate weighing less than 1,200 g
   c. Adult receiving an RBC transfusion
   d. Adult receiving an RBC transfusion from a blood relative

5. RBC transfusions should be given:
   a. Within 4 hours
   b. With lactated Ringer's solution
   c. With dextrose and water
   d. With cryoprecipitate

6. Which type of transplantation requires all cellular blood components to be irradiated?
   a. Bone marrow
   b. Heart
   c. Liver
   d. Kidney

7. Characteristics of deglycerolized RBCs include the following *except*:
   a. Inexpensive
   b. 24-hour expiration date after thawing
   c. Used for rare antigen-type donor blood
   d. Used for IgA-deficient recipient with history of severe reaction

8. Select the appropriate product for a bone marrow transplant patient with anemia:
   a. RBCs
   b. Irradiated RBCs
   c. Leukoreduced RBCs
   d. Washed RBCs

9. Which blood product should be selected for vitamin K deficiency?
   a. Cryoprecipitate
   b. Factor VIII
   c. Factor IX
   d. Plasma

10. Which fluid should be used to dilute RBCs?
    a. 0.9% saline
    b. 5% dextrose and water
    c. Immune globulin
    d. Lactated Ringers solution

References

1. King, KE (ed): Blood Transfusion Therapy: A Physician's Handbook, 9th ed. AABB, Bethesda, MD, 2008.
2. Circular of Information for the Use of Human Blood and Blood Products. AABB, America's Blood Centers, American Red Cross, Washington, DC, January 2010.
3. Ferraris VA, et al: Perioperative blood transfusion and blood conservation in cardiac surgery: The society of thoracic surgeons and the society of cardiovascular anesthesiologists clinical practice guideline. Ann Thorac Surg 83:S27, 2007.
4. Weiskopf, RB, et al: Oxygen reverses deficits of cognitive function and memory and increased heart rate induced by acute severe isovolemic anemia. Anesthesiology 96:871, 2002.
5. Carson, TH (ed): Standards for Blood Banks and Transfusion Services, 27th ed. AABB, Bethesda, MD, 2011.
6. Quraishy, N, et al: A compendium of transfusion practice guidelines. American National Red Cross, Washington, DC, 2010.
7. Slichter, SJ: Evidence-based platelet transfusion guidelines. Hematology 127:172, 2007.
8. British Committee for Standards in Haematology: Guidelines for the use of fresh-frozen plasma, cryoprecipitate and cryosupernatant. Brit J Haematol 126:11–28, 2004.
9. McVay, PA, and Toy, PTCY: Lack of increased bleeding after liver biopsy in patients with mild hemostatic abnormalities. Am J Clin Pathol 94:747, 1990.
10. Mannucci, PM: Hemophilia: Treatment options in the twenty-first century. J Thrombosis Haemostasis 1:1349–1355, 2003.
11. Knezevic, I, and Kruskall, MS: Intravenous immune globulin: An update for clinicians. Transfusion 43:1460, 2003.
12. Roberts, HR: Recombinant factor VIIa (Novoseven) and the safety of treatment. Semin Hematol 38:48, 2001.
13. Mayer, SA, et al: Efficacy and safety of recombinant factor VII for acute intracerebral hemorrhage. N Eng J Med 358:2127, 2008.
14. Laupacis, A, et al: Prevention of posttransfusion CMV in the era of universal WBC reduction: a consensus statement. Transfusion 41:560, 2001.
15. Shivdasani, RA, et al: Graft-versus-host disease associated with transfusion of blood from unrelated HLA-homozygous donors. N Eng J Med 328:755, 1993.
16. Sazama, K: Reports of 355 transfusion-associated deaths: 1976 through 1985. Transfusion 30:583, 1990.
17. AuBuchon, JP (ed): Guidelines for Blood Utilization Review. AABB, Bethesda, MD, 2001.
18. Simon, TL, et al: Practice parameter for the use of red blood cell transfusions. Arch Pathol Lab Med 122:130, 1998.

Chapter 16

Adverse Effects of Blood Transfusion

Susan Ruediger, MLT, CSMLS, Ileana Lopez-Plaza, MD

OBJECTIVES

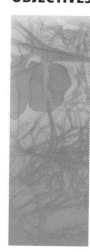

1. Define *transfusion reaction*.

2. Explain the risks of transfusions. Compare and contrast acute transfusion reactions and delayed transfusion reactions.

3. List the types of acute transfusion reactions and delayed transfusion reactions.

4. Differentiate the clinical signs and symptoms of the various types of transfusion reactions.

5. List laboratory findings associated with acute transfusion reactions.

6. Describe the pathophysiology, signs, symptoms, therapy, prevention, and clinical workup of transfusion reactions.

7. Describe the procedures to follow in the event of a suspected transfusion reaction.

8. Explain the importance of the patient's history in relation to medications, transfusion history, and pregnancies.

9. List the logical steps and procedures to follow in a laboratory investigation of transfusion reactions.

10. Describe the appropriate reporting of transfusion reaction workups.

11. List accreditation agencies involved in determining policies regarding transfusion reactions.

12. State the regulatory record requirements and procedures to follow in reporting a fatal transfusion reaction.

Introduction

A transfusion reaction is defined as any transfusion-related adverse event that occurs during or after the transfusion of whole blood, blood components, or human-derived plasma products. Transfusion reactions are also classified according to the time interval between transfusion and the presentation of adverse effects. A transfusion reaction with signs or symptoms presenting during or within 24 hours of transfusion is defined as an **acute transfusion reaction**. A transfusion reaction with signs or symptoms presenting after 24 hours of transfusion is defined as a **delayed transfusion reaction**. Transfusion reactions can further be classified as immune versus nonimmune, and infectious or noninfectious, according to their pathophysiology.

This chapter addresses noninfectious transfusion reactions and transfusion-associated sepsis. Other infection-related transfusion reactions are addressed in Chapter 18, "Transfusion-Transmitted Diseases."

Transfusion Risks

The risks involved with transfusions are variable. Some transfusion-associated adverse events can be prevented, whereas others cannot. Transfusion reactions have different associated outcomes that can be the cause of increased morbidity or even mortality. Therefore, it is of utmost importance that all transfusion decisions be carefully evaluated for their appropriateness. The estimated risks for various transfusion-related adverse events are shown in Table 16–1.[1-9]

Regulations

As with other transfusion service–related activities, the recognition and evaluation of transfusion reactions must follow established regulations. Preventive measurements must be performed when feasible. Transfusion reactions should be promptly recognized and evaluated. Any death that is suspected to be related to a transfusion event must be reported to the federal government and other governmental entities according to the state or jurisdiction.[10] A summary of transfusion reaction–related regulations is provided in Table 16–2.[10-12]

Recognition, Evaluation, and Resolution

The diagnosis and treatment of a transfusion reaction is a multidisciplinary task. It starts with the patient at the bedside and is completed with the interpretation and recommendations by the transfusion service physician.

The initial step occurs at the bedside and involves the patient, the transfusionist, and the physician responsible for the patient at the time of transfusion. The intermediate step and final steps involve the transfusion service technical staff and the transfusion service physician. The execution of each step is critical for the recognition, treatment, evaluation, and recommendations for future transfusions. This underlines the importance of education and competency assessment for

Table 16–1	**Risks for Noninfectious Transfusion Reactions and Transfusion-Associated Sepsis**
ADVERSE EVENT	**INCIDENCE**
Hemolytic, immune	RBC: 1:186,000; PLT: 1:46,000
Hemolytic, nonimmune	Rare
TAS	RBC 1: 250,000; PLT SDP 1:50,000; PLT (PPP) 1:25,000
Febrile non hemolytic	0.1% to 1% (with universal leukocyte reduction)
Allergic, mild	1% to 3%
Severe/anaphylaxis	1:20,000 to 1:50,000
TACO	< 1%
TRALI	RBC 1:143,000; PLT:5.8/million; Plasma: 3.2/million
Massive transfusion related	Dependent on clinical setting
RBC alloimmunization	Adults: 1%, Pediatric incidence is associated to the age at time of initial transfusion exposure
Delayed hemolytic	1:2,500 to 1:11,000
TAGVHD	$< 1 \times 10^6$
Platelet alloimmunization	HLA: 17% (with leukocyte reduction) HPA: 2% to 10% in multiply transfused patients
Post-transfusion purpura	Rare
Iron overload	Any patient with chronic RBC transfusion
Neonatal	1.3% overall
Pediatric	1.6% overall
Autologous	0.43%
Plasma derivatives	Varies among derivatives; severe reactions are rare
Therapeutic apheresis	1.6%

PLT = platelets; PPP = pre-pooled platelets; RBC = red blood cell; SDP = single donor platelet; TACO = transfusion-associated circulatory overload; TA-GVHD = transfusion associated graft versus host disease; TAS = transfusion associated sepsis; TRALI = transfusion-related acute lung injury

nurses, physicians, intermediate-level practitioners, and medical technologists involved in any steps in a transfusion. Figure 16–1 describes the roles for each of the medical personnel involved in the recognition, evaluation, and resolution of a transfusion reaction.

Basic Immunohematology Testing

The initial transfusion reaction workup performed by the technical staff consists of steps to rule out a hemolytic

Table 16–2   Transfusion Reaction Related Regulations

REGULATION	REGULATORY AGENCY		
	CAP	FDA	AABB
Recognition to, immediate response, action to take in event of transfusion reaction	X	X	X
Reporting transfusion reactions to the transfusion service	X		X
Laboratory evaluation of transfusion reaction	X		X
Additional testing during investigation of transfusion reaction	X		X
Transfusion service physician interpretation, reporting of transfusion reaction workup	X		X
Transfusion service physician participation in resolution of system failure (mistransfusions)	X	X	X
Mechanism to notify facility providing blood components of transfusion reactions	X	X	X
Reporting a transfusion reaction–associated fatality	X	X	X
Documentation of investigation of a transfusion reaction	X	X	X
Documentation of annual in-service of criteria for recognition of transfusion reactions	X		X
Evaluation of delayed transfusion reactions	X		X
Instructions for patients that post-transfusion will not be observed by medical personnel	X		X

AABB = American Association of Blood Banks; CAP = College of American Pathologists; FDA = Food and Drug Administration

transfusion reaction.[10] Figure 16–2 describes the basic immunohematology workup performed for the evaluation of any acute transfusion reaction. If the workup suggests the presence of hemolysis, then more specific testing is conducted to confirm the presence of hemolysis and identify its cause. If the workup rules out hemolysis, then other etiologies for the reaction are evaluated according to the patient's signs and symptoms and the evolution of the transfusion reaction. The latter are discussed further in the sections for specific types of transfusion reactions.

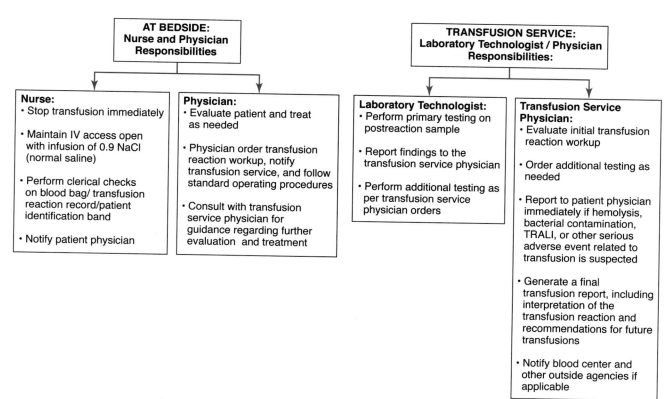

Figure 16–1.   Roles in recognition, evaluation, and resolution of a transfusion reaction. IV = intravenous; TRALI = transfusion-related acute lung injury

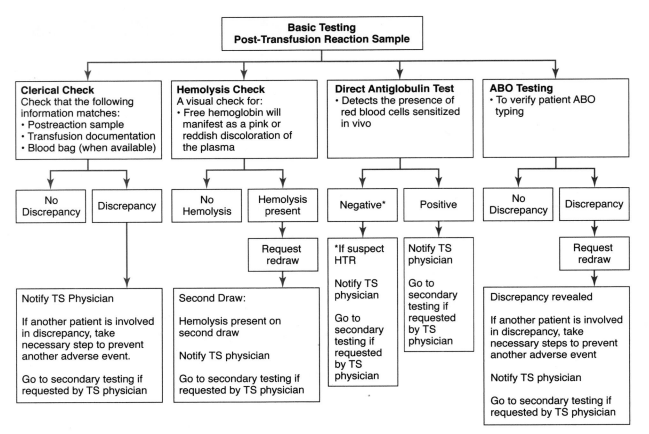

Figure 16–2. Basic immunohematology workup for the evaluation of a transfusion reaction. The purpose of basic immunohematology testing during the evaluation of an acute transfusion reaction is to identify the presence of hemolysis. TS = transfusion service

Figure 16–3 describes the secondary testing performed according to the presenting signs and symptoms and the evolution of the transfusion reaction as requested by the transfusion service physician. Table 16–3 summarizes the medical personnel and their tasks in transfusion reaction recognition, evaluation, and resolution.[13]

Acute Transfusion Reactions

Acute transfusion reaction is defined as a reaction in which signs and symptoms present within 24 hours of a transfusion. Most of the acute reactions can be grouped according to the common etiology that gives similar presenting signs and symptoms, as illustrated in Figure 16–4.[14]

Acute Hemolytic Transfusion Reaction

Acute hemolytic transfusion reaction (AHTR) consists of acute hemolysis with accompanying presenting symptoms within 24 hours of transfusion. Etiology may be of immune or nonimmune origin.

In the immune mediated acute hemolytic transfusion reaction, accompanying signs and symptoms include abdominal, chest, flank, or back pain; pain at infusion site; feeling of impending doom; hemoglobinemia; hemoglobinuria; hypotension; renal failure; shock; and diffuse intravascular coagulopathy. Red or dark urine or diffuse oozing may be the only sign in the anesthetized patient. A small volume of

incompatible blood, as little as 10 mL, can cause rapid hemolysis.[2] The severity of symptoms is closely related to the amount and rate of incompatible blood transfused. The patient's underlying clinical condition can obscure recognition of the reaction. The interaction of preformed antibodies in the recipient with the donor red cell antigens is the basis for the pathophysiology. The most severe reactions are associated with ABO incompatibility.[1]

Figure 16–5 shows the pathophysiology of the transfusion reaction. Previously formed IgM or IgG antibodies in the recipient recognize the corresponding donor red cell antigens, immune complexes are formed, the complement cascade is activated, **vasoactive amines** and **inflammatory mediators** are released into the plasma, and the coagulation cascade is activated.[2] The activated lytic arm (membrane attack complex) of the complement cascade causes hemoglobinemia (Fig. 16–6) and hemoglobinuria, the hallmarks of intravascular hemolysis (Fig. 16–7). The secreted vasoactive amines and inflammatory mediators are responsible for most of the systemic symptoms. The activation of the coagulation cascade causes diffuse intravascular coagulopathy (DIC) and the consequent bleeding. A combination of the vascular collapse and the DIC-initiated end organ microthrombi contribute to renal failure. Without the completion of the complement cascade, the red cell undergoes extravascular hemolysis. This is typical of non-ABO antibodies and delayed hemolytic transfusion reactions.[2]

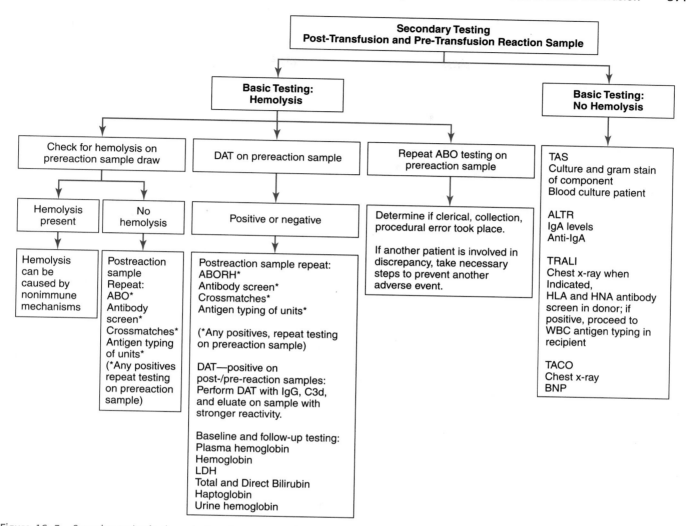

Figure 16–3. Secondary testing for the evaluation of an acute transfusion reaction. A basic immunohematology test indicative of hemolysis will require additional testing in order to investigate the cause of hemolysis. The transfusion service physician may request additional testing as part of the evaluation of suspected nonhemolytic transfusion reactions. ALTR = allergic transfusion reaction; BNP = B-type natriuretic peptide; C3d = complement fragment 3d; DAT = direct antiglobulin test; HLA = human leukocyte antigens; HNA = human neutrophil antigens; IgG = immunoglobulin G; LDH = lactic dehydrogenase; TACO = transfusion-associated circulatory overload; TAS = transfusion-associated sepsis; TRALI = transfusion-related acute lung injury; WBC = white blood cells

Table 16–3	Tasks of Medical Personnel in Recognition, Evaluation, and Resolution of Transfusion Reactions
MEDICAL PERSONNEL	**TASK**
Patient's nurse	Recognize and report to physician any adverse event in relation to a transfusion event
Patient's physician	Evaluate the patient, make recommendations for immediate intervention, and request transfusion reaction workup
TS technologist	Perform basic testing to identify hemolysis and perform secondary additional testing to identify the etiology of hemolysis
TS physician	Order supplemental testing to identify etiologies of hemolysis or other testing to assist in the diagnosis of nonhemolytic transfusion reactions
Quality management (transfusion service, transfusion committee, Biovigilance)	Track and trend transfusion reaction occurrences; perform root cause analysis; recommend corrective and preventive measures

TS = transfusion service

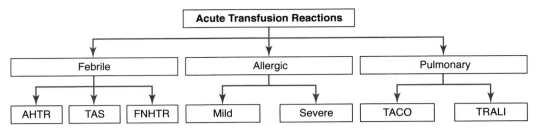

Figure 16–4. Acute transfusion reactions. Acute transfusion reactions are divided according to one of three key presenting symptoms: fever, allergic, or pulmonary. AHTR = acute hemolytic transfusion reaction; FNHTR = febrile nonhemolytic transfusion reaction; TACO = transfusion-associated circulatory overload; TAS = transfusion-associated sepsis; TRALI = transfusion-related acute lung injury

Less frequently, ABO-incompatibility-related acute hemolytic transfusion reaction may be observed with the transfusion of plasma containing sufficient quantities of isohemagglutinins (by volume or antibody titers) against the recipient ABO antigens.[15] This syndrome has been observed with the transfusion of platelets, mainly group O single donor platelets transfused to a non-O recipient.[16] Recent studies have shown that whole blood–derived pooled platelets may contain similar levels of isohemagglutinins.[17]

Nonimmune hemolysis most frequently presents as asymptomatic hemoglobinuria, although it has been occasionally associated with renal dysfunction, and rare related death has been reported.[18] Its pathophysiology is independent of the presence of antibodies. It can be caused by chemical damage or mechanical damage such as improper shipping or storage temperatures; incomplete deglycerolization of frozen red blood cells; needles used for transfusion with an inappropriately small bore size; rapid pressure infuser or roller pumps; improper use of blood warmers; concurrent infusion of unapproved fluids via the transfusion line; and bacterial contamination.

When an immune AHTR is suspected, the transfusion must be discontinued immediately, a clerical verification performed,

and the patient's physician notified. The intravenous access is maintained and used for supportive therapy. Any additional therapeutic intervention at this time should be appropriate to the patient's clinical course with emphasis on maintaining adequate blood pressure and urine output. As soon as possible, the patient's nurse should notify the transfusion service, complete the transfusion reaction documentation, draw the post-transfusion reaction samples, and collect a urine sample, if possible. Once the transfusion service receives the documents, samples, and blood component bag, the technologist should begin the basic reaction evaluation (see **Fig. 16–2**) and notify the transfusion service physician. If a discrepancy is identified during clerical verification, the transfusion service technologist should take any steps necessary to determine whether another patient is involved in order to prevent another adverse event.

If the postreaction blood sample appears hemolyzed upon inspection, the technologist should request a second sample to verify that the hemolysis is not secondary to a difficult blood draw. Perform a direct antiglobulin test (DAT) on the postreaction sample. A negative DAT does not exclude immune hemolysis. If an immune hemolysis is suspected, all prereaction testing is to be repeated using the postreaction

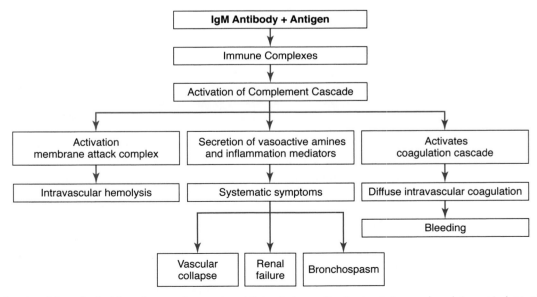

Figure 16–5. Overview of the pathophysiology of an acute immune hemolytic transfusion reaction. In an acute immune hemolytic anemia due to ABO incompatibility, the full complement cascade is activated by the immune complexes formed by the interaction between the incompatible IgM isohemagglutinin and the ABO antigen. The activation of the membrane attack complex damages the red cells. The release of inflammatory mediators, and the activation of the coagulation cascade cause the signs and symptoms associated with the reaction. IgM = immunoglobulin M

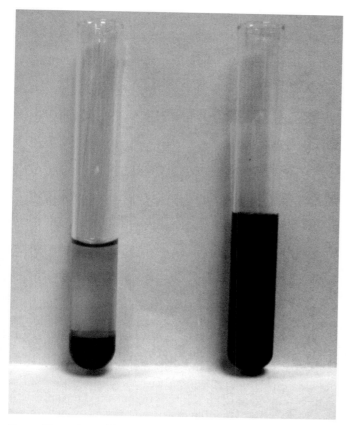

Figure 16–6.   Hemoglobinemia. The sample on the right illustrates the appearance of hemolyzed plasma due to ABO incompatibility. The separation between the plasma layer and the red cell layer is barely discernible. The sample on the left illustrates the appearance of nonhemolyzed plasma.

specimen, including antibody screen, crossmatches, and any antigen typing of the units crossmatched. If any of the repeated testing with the postreaction sample has a positive result, then testing is to be repeated with the prereaction sample (see **Fig. 16–3**).

If the DAT performed in the postreaction sample shows a "new" or stronger positivity than the prereaction sample DAT, then further workup should be performed with the postreaction sample, as this may indicate the presence of incompatible transfused red blood cells. Circulating incompatible red blood cells may give a "mixed-field" appearance when the DAT is read microscopically. The workup should include repeating the DAT with IgG and C3d reagents and performing an eluate. Incompatible red blood cells may absorb sufficient quantities of antibody to make them undetectable in plasma, resulting in a negative antibody screen.[13] If the prereaction DAT shows a stronger positivity when compared with the postreaction sample, then further DAT workup should be performed with the prereaction sample. Tests on baseline and follow-up samples to assess ongoing hemolysis in the patient should also be performed (e.g., free plasma hemoglobin, hemoglobin; LDH; total and direct bilirubin; haptoglobin, free urine hemoglobin, hemosiderin in urine). Figure 16–8 illustrates time frames for the indicators affected by intravascular hemolysis.

INTRAVASCULAR HEMOLYSIS

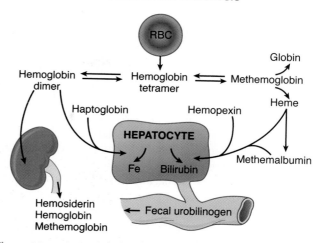

Figure 16–7.   Intravascular hemolysis. This figure illustrates the clearance of hemoglobin associated with intravascular red cell lysis. (*From Hillman, RF, and Finch, CA: Red Cell Manual, 7th ed. F.A. Davis, Philadelphia, 1996, with permission.*)

Promptly recognizing a reaction, discontinuing the transfusion, and maintaining venous access are key interventions for limiting damage for all types of acute hemolytic transfusion reactions. Pharmacological intervention can help maintain hemodynamic stability, treat hypotension, and ensure adequate renal blood flow. Urine output should carefully be monitored. Disseminated intravascular coagulation (DIC), although rare, is extremely difficult to treat. Patients experiencing minimal symptoms may be managed best by careful observation.[13] Due to the association between the volume of incompatible red blood cells transfused and the severity of the symptoms associated with AHTR, a red cell exchange should be considered for symptomatic patients with a strongly reacting DAT. Antigen-negative units should be used once the implicated antibody specificity has been identified.

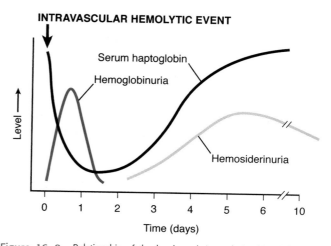

Figure 16–8.   Relationship of the levels and time-relationship of laboratory indicators of hemolysis in relation to an acute hemolytic event. Within a few hours of an acute hemolytic event, free hemoglobin is cleared from plasma and the serum haptoglobin falls to undetectable levels. Hemoglobinuria ceases soon after. If no further hemolysis occurs, the serum haptoglobin level recovers. The urinary hemosiderin can provide more lasting evidence of the hemolytic event. (*From Harmening, DM: Clinical Hematology and Fundamentals of Hemostasis, 5th ed. F.A. Davis, Philadelphia, 2009, with permission.*)

Consultation with appropriate medical specialists early in the course is also recommended. In acute nonimmune hemolytic transfusion reactions in which asymptomatic hemoglobinuria is the only sign observed, adequate hydration is recommended.

Improper patient identification at the time of sample collection or transfusion is the most common cause of an acute immune hemolytic transfusion reaction.[1] Therefore, it is imperative that the patient be properly identified at the bedside. To increase overall transfusion safety, implementation of new technology such as handheld bar-code scanners and radio-frequency chips for patient identification, and a similar system for refrigerators in pharmacy for the release of medication may further reduce misidentification due to human error.[2]

The incidence of hemolytic reactions associated with the transfusion of platelets containing incompatible isoagglutinins has been reduced by 83% overall.[15] This has been done by limiting the volume of incompatible plasma transfused with platelet transfusions or by measuring the isohemagglutinin titers of group O platelets[16,17] to decide if such platelets may be used for transfusion to a non-O recipient. The use of platelet additive solutions as a substitute for plasma to store platelets may further limit the risk of a hemolytic transfusion reaction associated with the transfusion of ABO-incompatible platelets.[19]

Transfusion-Associated Sepsis

Transfusion-associated sepsis (TAS) is an acute nonimmune transfusion reaction presenting with body temperatures usually 2°C or more above normal and rigors that can be accompanied by hypotension. The symptoms usually present shortly after the transfusion begins. TAS occurs when a bacteria-contaminated blood component is transfused. Abruptness of presentation may be similar to AHTR; milder cases may mimic a febrile nonhemolytic transfusion reaction (FNHTR). The number of organisms transfused may influence the clinical presentation and outcome. Mortality risks include contamination by a gram-negative rod, patient's age, volume transfused, and platelet storage time.[13]

Skin flora and, less frequently, gut flora associated with transient bacteremia in an asymptomatic donor are considered the sources of bacterial contamination. Bacterial **endotoxins** generated during storage may contribute to TAS-related morbidity and mortality. Table 16–4 outlines bacterial organisms commonly implicated in TAS. Not surprisingly, bacterially contaminated platelets are considered the most frequent component causing TAS, due to room temperature storage requirements. The contamination rate in association with red blood cell transfusions is related to the inhibition of the growth and viability of most bacteria at the component storage required temperatures (1°C to 6°C) and thus the lower risk for TAS.

Laboratory workup for the diagnosis of TAS consists of ruling out hemolysis and performing a gram stain and culture of the implicated component, as well as getting a blood culture from the patient. The sample from the implicated container must be obtained from within the container and not a segment attached to the component. Blood cultures from the patient should be drawn from a venous site different from the transfusion site. The returned component should be inspected for color changes, presence of bubbles, hemolysis in a red blood cell component, absence of swirling, or presence of clumping in a platelet component. A positive blood culture from the patient without confirmation of the same organism in the transfused component is not sufficient for the diagnosis. Isolation of the same organism in both the implicated blood bag and the patient's blood is key for the diagnosis of TAS. It is important to remember that a colonized or infected central venous catheter used for transfusion may be the source of the bacteria causing the signs and symptoms observed during transfusion.

Treatment consists of discontinuing the transfusion immediately upon suspecting a TAS, providing supportive treatment, and possibly initiating antibiotic therapy. Antibiotic therapy can be initially started with a broad-spectrum coverage and then adjusted to more specific coverage based on the organism identified and its antimicrobial susceptibility.

TAS prevention is directed toward decreasing the risk of bacterial contamination at the time of collection and detecting contamination prior to transfusion. Interventions

Table 16–4	**Bacterial Organisms Associated with Transfusion-Associated Sepsis (TAS)**		
GRAM STAIN	**BACTERIA IDENTIFICATION**	**TAS RISK**	**SOURCE**
Gram-positive	• *Staphylococcus* species • *Streptococcus* species • *Bacillus* species	Red Blood Cells • Risk: 1:500,000 • Mortality: 1:10,000,000 Platelets • Risk: 1:75,000 • Mortality: 1:500,000	• Skin flora • Natural environment
Gram-negative	• *Serratia* species • *Yersinia* species • *Acinetobacter* species • *Escherichia* species • *Pseudomonas* species • *Providencia* species	Red Blood Cells • Risk: 1:500,000 • Mortality: 1:10,000,000 Platelets • Risk: 1:75,000 • Mortality: 1:500,000	• Bloodstream • Natural environment

to prevent the transfusion of a contaminated component are focused only on platelet components. Box 16–1 lists interventions currently in use to decrease the risk of TAS associated with platelet transfusions. The interventions used to detect bacterial growth prior to storage are more sensitive but delay the distribution of platelets for clinical use. The interventions used to detect bacterial contamination at the time of transfusion are more rapid but less sensitive. A donor who has given blood more than 20 times may be at increased risk due to scarring on the antecubital fossa, which makes skin preparation less effective.[13]

A 50% reduction in reported TAS and related fatalities has been observed after the introduction of mandatory testing for the detection of bacterial growth in single donor platelets before distribution, with one institution showing a 69.7% reduction after implementing an automated microbial detection system.[3] A similar standard now applies to pre-pooled and leukoreduced whole blood–derived platelets. Nevertheless, because of the existing risk of contamination at the time of collection, single donor platelets carry a lower risk of contamination when compared to pre-pooled and leukoreduced whole blood–derived platelets, due to the single venipuncture used in the collection of the former and the multiple venipunctures required with the latter.[20]

Febrile Nonhemolytic Transfusion Reaction

Febrile nonhemolytic transfusion reaction (FNHTR) is an acute complication of transfusion presenting with at least a 1°C increase in body temperature that can be accompanied by chills, nausea or vomiting, tachycardia, increase in blood pressure, and tachypnea. Occasionally, shaking chills is the only initial presenting symptom, followed by an increase in body temperature up to 30 minutes after discontinuing the transfusion.[13] An asymptomatic rise in body temperature in

a hypothermic patient to normal body temperature should not be considered to be a FNHTR.[13]

The etiology of FNHTR has been attributed to two different white cell–related mechanisms. The first one is immune mediated and is due to the presence of preformed antibodies[13] reacting against white cells in the blood component for which antigen–antibody specificity is shared, which causes the release of endogenous **pyrogens**. The second mechanism is closely related to platelet storage changes, which involve the production and release of biologically active **cytokines**[21,22] by the white cells present in the component during storage. FNHTR is considered a diagnosis by exclusion. It tends to be self-limited, so treatment may not be required, as fever will resolve within 2 to 3 hours. However, the presence of rigors increases the metabolic rate and many patients express great discomfort. Rigors will not respond to antipyretic therapy, but treatment with **meperidine** may quickly resolve them. However, because of its respiratory-depressant effect, meperidine must be used with extreme caution.

There are several approaches to prevent the FNHTR. The use of prestorage leukocyte reduction has shown to reduce the number of white blood cells present in packed red blood cells and platelet concentrates before their release of cytokines, thus making this intervention the most effective in preventing and reducing the incidence of FNHTR.[23]

Allergic Transfusion Reactions

Allergic transfusion reactions (ALTR) are acute, immune complications of transfusion presenting with a variety of symptoms that can vary according to the reaction's degree of severity. ALTR occurs as a response of recipient antibodies to an allergen present in the blood component. ALTR can range from minor urticarial effects to fulminant anaphylactic shock and death. The more common, milder reactions consist of weals, hives, erythema, or **pruritus**. Severe reactions (anaphylactoid or anaphylactic) are rare and can present with bronchoconstriction (wheezes), angioedema (periorbital edema, tongue swelling), gastrointestinal symptoms (diarrhea), and cardiovascular instability (hypotension, cardiac arrhythmia, loss of consciousness, shock, cardiac arrest).

Symptoms associated with milder reactions can present any time during or after the transfusion. However, symptoms associated with more severe reactions will generally appear shortly after the transfusion has been started and minimal volume has been transfused. The pathophysiology of ALTR is due to the activation of mast cells in the recipient triggered most frequently by an allergen present in the plasma of the blood component. Patient preformed IgE antibodies interact with the donor-derived allergen. The binding of the allergen to the IgE bound to the mast cell results in the release of histamine and other granule contents (type I hypersensitivity reaction).[24] ALTR resulting from non-IgE-mediated release of mast cell mediators are termed *anaphylactoid*.[2]

The triggering factor for most severe ALTR is almost never identified, but the most classic example of such a reaction is the IgA-deficiency-related anaphylactic reaction.

BOX 16–1

Interventions to Prevent Transfusion-Associated Sepsis

At Collection
- Donor history
- Proper phlebotomy technique
- Single arm collection technique
- Diversion pouch

Prior to Storage
- Prestorage leukoreduction
- Pathogen inactivation
- Automated culture

At Time of Transfusion
- Visual inspection
- Biochemical markers
- Microscopy/stains
- Immunoassays

The classic presentation in this population is the development of anaphylaxis shortly after starting a transfusion in a patient who has never been previously transfused. Absolute IgA deficiency (IgA levels less than 0.05 mg/dL) is found in 1:700 individuals of European descent, with only 40% or less forming class-specific anti-IgA antibodies.[25] A similar type of reaction, associated with haptoglobin deficiency, has been described in the Japanese population.[26]

Mild ALTR involving isolated symptoms or signs of urticaria or hives are the only type of transfusion reactions in which discontinuation and restart of the transfusion is allowed if administration of antihistamines improves symptoms. A transfusion reaction report to the transfusion service should still be initiated; however, laboratory workup to rule out hemolysis is not required.[2] In the event that symptoms do not subside with the administration of antihistamines or when other symptoms accompany the hives or urticaria, the transfusion must not be restarted. In general, milder reactions are treated with antihistamines. More severe reactions may require treatment with corticosteroids.

In the presence of anaphylactic symptoms, prompt intervention to maintain oxygenation and stabilize blood pressure must be initiated, including the administration of subcutaneous **epinephrine**.[2] In patients with proven absolute IgA deficiency, anti-IgA testing should be performed. Patients with known anti-IgA antibodies or a reliable history of anaphylactic transfusions must receive blood components and intravenous immunoglobulins deficient in IgA. These patients may receive washed red blood cells and platelets. However, plasma and cryoprecipitate must be obtained from IgA deficient donors.[2] Anti-IgA antibodies are naturally occurring antibodies, so their presence cannot be predicted. Therefore, it is recommended that similar precautions be taken for all patients proven deficient and who are unknown and known to have anti-IgA antibodies.

Transfusion-Related Acute Lung Injury

Transfusion-related acute lung injury (TRALI) consists of an acute transfusion reaction presenting with respiratory distress and severe hypoxemia during or within 6 hours of transfusion in the absence of other causes of acute lung injury (e.g., aspiration, pneumonia, toxic inhalation, lung contusion, near drowning, severe sepsis, shock, multiple trauma, burn injury, acute pancreatitis, cardiopulmonary bypass, drug overdose).[27,28] It can be accompanied by fever or hypotension. This syndrome is now considered the leading cause of transfusion-associated fatalities, surpassing ABO incompatibility and bacterial contamination.[5] Patients with specific clinical diagnoses (i.e., infection, surgery, trauma) have an increased risk of developing TRALI with a significant impact on morbidity and outcome.[29]

Although the pathogenesis of TRALI is not fully understood, two different hypothetical pathways have been postulated.[30,31] One of the pathways ("immune TRALI")[32] consists of an antibody-mediated, one-hit event. Antibodies against the human leukocyte antigen (HLA) or human neutrophil antigens (HNA) in the transfused blood component (up to 89% of cases)[32] react with recipient leukocytes, causing aggregates that occlude the pulmonary circulation. Implicated leukocyte antibodies include HLAI (4% to 23%), HLAII (34% to 47%), both (18% to 21%), and HNA (8% to 28%). Antibodies against class II human leukocyte antigens (HLA), anti-HLA-A2 (antibody against a class I HLA), and HNA-3a (antibody against human neutrophil antigens) are frequently associated with severe (ventilatory support required) and fatal cases.[32]

Blood components implicated are usually donated by multiparous females and are mostly associated with large volumes of plasma; however, blood components with less than 20 mL of plasma and the presence of anti-HNA-3a have also been associated with immune TRALI cases.[32] In rare instances (6%), the antibodies will be present in the recipient, reacting with the transfused donor leukocytes.[32] Immune TRALI may occur in patients with no underlying lung injury or even in healthy individuals.

The other pathway (nonimmune TRALI) consists of a two-hit event. The risk of developing nonimmune TRALI depends on the patient's predisposition to this disorder. The first hit (i.e., lung trauma or an infectious or inflammatory disease in the patient) may result in priming of the patient's neutrophils. Therefore, a proinflammatory priming event of the patient's endothelium, which primes the patient's neutrophils, is a basic requirement for nonimmune TRALI. The second hit (i.e., transfused biologically active substances accumulated during storage or antileukocyte antibodies) causes the activation of the primed neutrophils. Both the immune and nonimmune TRALI lead to a final common pathway that causes damage to the endothelium, leading to pulmonary capillary permeability and resulting in noncardiogenic pulmonary edema.

TRALI is a clinical diagnosis based on clinical (Box 16–2) and radiological parameters (Figs. 16–9 and 16–10). There is a growing appreciation that milder forms of respiratory distress

---

BOX 16–2

Criteria for the Diagnosis of TRALI

Onset

Within 6 hours of transfusion

Oxygenation

PAO2/FiO2 ≤ 300 mm Hg regardless of positive end-expiratory pressure level
or
Oxygenation saturation of ≤ 90% on room air.

Chest X-ray

Bilateral infiltrates on frontal chest radiography

Blood Pressure

Pulmonary artery occlusion pressure ≤ 18 mm Hg when measured
or
No evidence of left atrial hypertension

FiO2 = fraction of inspired oxygen; mm Hg = millimeters of mercury; PAO2 = partial pressure of arterial oxygen; TRALI = transfusion-related acute lung injury
Data from Popovsky, MA: Transfusion associated circulatory overload: The plot thickens. Transfusion 49:2–4, 2009.

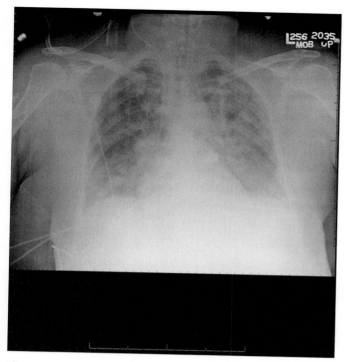

Figure 16–9. Transfusion-related acute lung injury (TRALI) chest radiograph showing pulmonary edema, obtained 4 hours after initial presentation of severe respiratory distress during transfusion of packed red blood cells. *(Courtesy of Spizarny, David, MD, Department of Radiology, Henry Ford Health System.)*

(transient **dyspnea**) may still represent this syndrome. TRALI may be difficult to differentiate from a transfusion-associated circulatory overload (TACO)[33] or from a "possible TRALI" (a transfusion unrelated acute lung injury that is temporally related to a transfusion but that also has at least one other temporally related risk factor for acute lung injury). It is important that the physician treating the patient suspected of TRALI communicate promptly with the transfusion service physician.

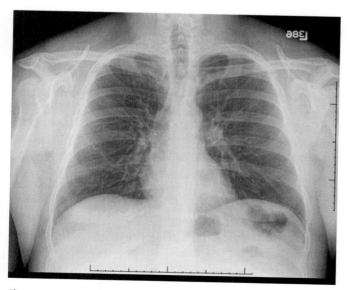

Figure 16–10. Normal chest radiography showing adequately aerated lungs. *(Courtesy of Spizarny, David, MD, Department of Radiology, Henry Ford Health System.)*

Clinical features manifested at the time of presentation of the respiratory failure, and follow-up clinical evaluation necessary to include or exclude the diagnosis of TRALI may include questions such as, Has the patient been evaluated by a critical care specialist? Does the patient have any signs or symptoms of increased left atrial pressure? When was the chest radiography performed or repeated? Was diuresis initiated, and what was the patient response? Was a B-natriuretic peptide level measured, and was it suggestive of congestive heart failure?

The patient with TRALI is managed with supporting therapy similar to other patients with permeability **edema**; both require additional oxygen support, and 72% require mechanical ventilatory support.[2] Typical TRALI cases improve within 48 hours, although in some cases it can persist for up to a week. There seems to be no sustained pulmonary injury. Fatality is observed in 6% to 20% of cases. In contrast to the patient with TACO, the patient with TRALI does not respond to diuresis. A TRALI suspected case should be reported to the blood center for serologic workup of the recipient and the implicated donors for the presence of HLA/HNA antibodies. If such antibodies are present, evidence of leukocyte incompatibility between the donor and the recipient should be documented. A donor implicated in a case of TRALI and found to have antibodies incompatible with the recipient is excluded from any further donations. Because TRALI is based on clinical diagnosis, the absence of demonstrable immune incompatibility between donor and recipient does not preclude the diagnosis of TRALI.

Blood components that contain large plasma volumes donated by alloimmunized donors would be at high risk of causing immune-mediated TRALI. Therefore, preventive efforts are directed toward the donor population. Leukocyte antibodies are found with highest frequency in multiparous female donors, with the incidence increasing with the increased number of pregnancies, from 8% in nonparous to 26% in multiparous females.[20] Blood components with a large volume of plasma include plasma and platelets. Starting in 2003, many countries started adopting a preventive intervention called *predominantly male plasma policy"*; this plasma policy resulted in a significant decrease in the incidence of reported TRALI cases.[5] The predominantly male plasma policy may consist of obtaining plasma from male donors, nulliparous female donors, or multiparous but leukocyte antibody–negative female donors both for the collection and manufacture of plasma, or obtaining platelets from male donors only; testing female donors for the presence of HLA antibodies; testing female-derived platelet products for the presence of HLA antibodies; removing the plasma contents from the platelets; and/or resuspending the platelets in platelet additive solution.[5]

A recent multicenter study conducted in blood centers in the United States evaluated the impact on the different female donor deferrals.[34] The impact of the policy "that would not allow plasma from female whole blood donors to be prepared into transfusable plasma components would result in nearly a 50% reduction in the units of whole blood available for plasma manufacturing."[34] In addition, a loss of 37.1% of all apheresis PLT donations would be lost from deferral of all female apheresis PLT donors; a loss of 22.5% from deferral of parous female apheresis PLT donors; and a loss of 5.4% from deferral of parous female apheresis PLT donors with a positive screening test result for antibodies to HLAs, as reported in this study.[34] Thus far, implementation of the different preventive interventions has been successful in decreasing the risk of immune TRALI and the mortality associated with large plasma volume blood components. Judicious application of the best preventable option, taking into consideration the effect on female donor availability, will facilitate such implementation.

Transfusion-Associated Circulatory Overload

Transfusion-associated circulatory overload (TACO) is an acute, nonimmune complication of transfusion presenting with respiratory distress and hypoxemia that can be accompanied by cough, headache, chest tightness, hypertension, jugular vein distention, elevated central venous pressure, and elevated **pulmonary wedge pressure** during or after transfusion. TACO occurs when the patient's cardiovascular system's ability to handle additional workload is exceeded, manifesting as congestive heart failure. The chest radiography is characterized by the presence of pulmonary edema, cardiomegaly, and distended pulmonary artery (see Figs. 16–10 and 16–11).

The laboratory assay of brain natriuretic peptide (BNP), consisting of the measurement of a peptide secreted from the ventricles in response to increased filling pressures and a marker of congestive heart failure, may be used to aid in the diagnosis of TACO. A post-transfusion to pretransfusion BNP ratio of 1.5, with a post-transfusion level equal or greater than 100 picograms per milliliter as a cutoff point, provides a sensitivity of 81% and a specificity of 89% for diagnosis of TACO.[35] TACO is also associated with increased morbidity and mortality.[33]

Treatment consists of putting the patient in a sitting position, administering supplemental oxygenation, and starting diuresis. Patients with diminished cardiac reserves or with chronic anemia and those who are very young or very old are considered at risk of developing TACO, even with a small transfusion volume. Other patients at risk include those who receive rapid or massive transfusion of blood. For patients at risk of developing TACO, the transfusion rate should be slowed when feasible. Dividing the blood component into smaller aliquots to be transfused over a longer period of time should be considered.

Adverse Events Associated with Massive Transfusions

Massive transfusion is defined as the replacement of one total blood volume in 24 hours or the replacement of 50% of the blood volume in 3 hours.[36] Massive blood replacement may be accompanied by metabolic and coagulation abnormalities related to transfusion volume and infusion rate. Patient-related comorbid factors such as resuscitation maneuvers, underlying disease, severity and duration of hypotensive shock, and hypothermia may further contribute to the metabolic complications and coagulation abnormalities.

Hypothermia can incite metabolic and hemostatic derangements. Studies have shown that the transfusion of one unit of red blood cells with a temperature of 4°C can drop the core body temperature 0.25°C in an average-sized patient.[36] During massive transfusion, the rate of citrate delivery may exceed the liver's capacity for its clearance. Metabolic alkalosis can develop secondarily to the accumulation of bicarbonate, the metabolic by-product of citrate. Citrate toxicity will result in hypocalcemia and cause symptoms such as tingling, shivering, light-headedness, tetany, and hyperventilation. Rarely, hypomagnesemia-associated myocardial depression can be observed with severe citrate toxicity. These complications are mostly observed in patients with liver failure. Citrate-induced hypocalcemia is rarely associated with clinical consequences in other massively transfused patients.

Packed red blood cells leak potassium into the plasma or additive solution of the blood component during storage. Rapid infusion of a large volume of packed red blood cells may put patient populations such as neonates and patients with cardiac, hepatic, or renal dysfunction at risk of developing hyperkalemia.[36] The transient hyperkalemia related to massive transfusion appear to be related to the patient's acid-base balance, ionized calcium levels, and rate of infusion of the packed red blood cells. Extreme hyperkalemia or hypokalemia can compromise the myocardial function.

Coagulation abnormalities can develop secondarily to hemodilution or diffuse intravascular coagulopathy. Use

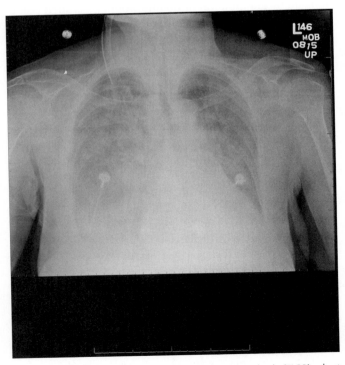

Figure 16–11. Transfusion-associated circulatory overload (TACO) chest radiograph showing pulmonary edema, obtained 2 hours after initial presentation of respiratory distress and significant increase in systemic blood pressure during the transfusion of packed red blood cells. *(Courtesy of Spizarny, David, MD, Department of Radiology, Henry Ford Health System.)*

of large volumes of asanguineous fluids and packed red blood cells during resuscitation in hemorrhagic shock will create platelet and coagulation factor deficiencies. Thrombocytopenia with platelet counts below 50,000/mm^3, hypofibrinogenemia, and coagulation factor levels below 25% generally occur after the replacement of two blood volumes.[37] Tissue injury may disrupt the procoagulant-anticoagulant balance, leading to diffuse intravascular coagulopathy and putting the massively transfused patient at risk of bleeding secondary to a combination of platelet and coagulation factor consumption and secondary fibrinolysis.

Transfusion-related adverse events during massive transfusion can be avoided through careful patient monitoring for the development of sign and symptoms, changes in laboratory values, and the appropriate use of medications and blood components. The infusion of prewarmed resuscitation fluids and refrigerated blood components will help prevent exacerbation of hypothermia. Hyperkalemia can be reversed by slowing the transfusion rate and by maintaining the acid-base balance in the patient. Treatment strategies for the correction of bleeding should be guided by baseline and serial assessment of laboratory parameters. Table 16–5 summarizes the types of acute transfusion reactions.

Table 16–5   Summary: Acute Transfusion Reactions

	SYMPTOMS	DIAGNOSIS	TREATMENT	PREVENTION
AIHTR	Fever/chills Back pain Hemoglobinemia Hemoglobinuria Hypotension, renal failure Shock DIC	DAT positive ↓ Hemoglobin ↑ LDH ↑ Bilirubin ↓ Haptoglobin	Discontinue transfusion Maintain vascular access Maintain blood pressure Maintain renal blood flow Treat DIC if present	Follow standard operating procedures for identification of the patient
ANIHTR	Asymptomatic Hemoglobinuria	DAT negative	Discontinue transfusion Maintain vascular access Maintain renal blood flow	Follow standard operating procedures for equipment operation
TAS	Fever/chills Hypotension Shock	DAT negative Gram stain blood bag Culture blood bag Culture patient	Discontinue transfusion Maintain vascular access Consider initial broad-spectrum antibiotic coverage	Follow standard operating procedures for collection Implement bacterial detection intervention prior to transfusion
FNHTR	Fever/chills Nausea/vomiting Tachycardia Tachypnea ↑ Blood pressure	DAT negative	Treat with antipyretics For rigors, treat with meperidine	Prestorage leukoreduction of PRBC and platelets
Allergic Mild	Erythema Pruritus	Clinical diagnosis DAT not required	Temporary discontinue transfusion Treat with antihistamines If symptoms improve restart transfusion	For repeated reactions, consider premedication with antihistamines
Allergic Severe	Angioedema Wheezing Hypotension Anaphylaxis	DAT negative IgA deficiency workup when indicated	Discontinue transfusion Maintain vascular access Treat with subcutaneous epinephrine Maintain blood pressure Provide respiratory support	For IgA absolute deficient patients provide IgA deficient blood components
TRALI	Severe hypoxemia No evidence of left atrial hypertension	CXR: bilateral infiltrates Donor test for HLA/HNA antibodies Recipient test for HLA/HNA antigens	Discontinue transfusion Maintain vascular access Supplemental oxygen Mechanical ventilation	Use male only plasma Exclude or screen female platelet donors
TACO	Severe hypoxemia ↑ Blood pressure Jugular vein distension ↑ Central venous pressure	CXR: pulmonary edema, cardiomegaly, distended pulmonary artery BNP	Upright posture Supplemental oxygen Diuresis	Slower transfusion rate Transfuse in smaller volumes

AIHTR = acute immune hemolytic transfusion reaction; ANIHTR = acute nonimmune hemolytic transfusion reaction; DAT = direct antiglobulin test; DIC = diffuse intravascular coagulopathy; FNHTR = febrile nonhemolytic transfusion reaction; LDH = lactic dehydrogenase; PRBC = packed red blood cell; TAS = transfusion-associated sepsis

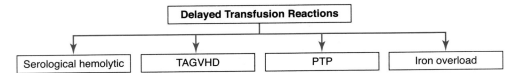

Delayed Transfusion Reactions

Delayed transfusion reactions are defined as reactions in which signs and symptoms present after 24 hours of a transfusion and represent a diverse etiology (Fig. 16–12).

Delayed Serologic/Hemolytic Transfusion Reaction

Delayed serologic/hemolytic transfusion reaction (DSHTR) is defined as the detection of "new" red cell antibodies after 24 hours of transfusion. It usually occurs secondarily to an amnestic response but can also occur during a primary immune response and may (delayed hemolytic) or may not (delayed serologic) be associated with shortened survival of the transfused cells.[38] The DSHTR may be discovered when a new sample is tested during a request for a type and crossmatch and the hemoglobin levels are lower than expected for the transfusion interval, or when a patient returns to see the physician and complains of flulike symptoms, with or without **jaundice**. Most often the only presenting sign is an unexplained or unexpected drop in hemoglobin or hematocrit with increased requirement in the transfusion frequency in the absence of active bleeding.

During pregnancy or transfusion, exposure to non-ABO antigens may stimulate the development of antibodies in the recipient. Primary immune response stimulates IgM antibody production, followed by a switch to IgG production. The primary immune response is usually asymptomatic and becomes apparent by immunohematology testing within weeks to months after transfusion. With time, these antibodies may diminish to undetectable levels when repeat immunohematology testing is performed. In such cases, a subsequent exposure to incompatible red cells elicits a secondary immune response with rapid production of IgG becoming detectable between 2 days to 2 weeks after the reexposure.[1] The degree of accelerated red cell destruction will depend on the characteristics of the implicated antibody such as antibody specificity (usually antibodies directed against the Rh, Kidd, Duffy, and anti-Kell antigens), thermal activity range, and the ability to fix complement. Most frequently, the red cell destruction occurs as extravascular hemolysis (Fig. 16–13).

Transfusion of incompatible blood during emergency or massive transfusion may occasionally be the cause of a delayed hemolytic reaction. Less frequently, after transplantation of a solid organ or hematopoietic progenitor cells, the donor lymphocytes transplanted with the graft may initiate active antibody production, destroying the

recipient's red cells independent of a transfusion event. The resorption of a large hematoma can have manifestations very similar to a DSHTR. Delayed hemolytic transfusion reactions (DHTR), although generally mild, may be severe in chronically transfused patients such as patients with sickle cell disease. Bystander hemolysis (sickle cell HTR syndrome) of autologous red cells and transfused cells may occur in the absence of identifiable red cell alloantibodies.[39]

In addition to the standard basic immunohematology testing (of ABO/Rh, antibody screen and when indicated antibody identification), the immunohematology evaluation (Fig. 16–14) will include a DAT and, when indicated, elution and antigen typing of the units recently transfused and suspected to be implicated in the immune response. An eluate may be necessary to demonstrate the presence of the implicated antibody. If samples from previous immunohematology testing are available, repeat testing should be performed. Antigen typing on the units will be able to provide information regarding the number of antigen-positive transfused units and thus an estimate

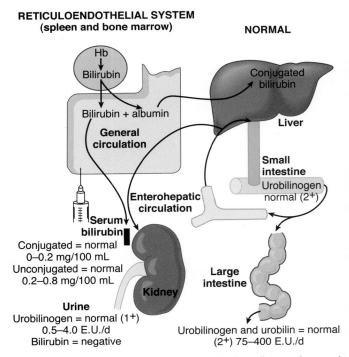

Figure 16–13. Normal extravascular hemolysis. This figure illustrates the normal (extravascular) clearance pathway of red cells. *(From Tietz, MW: Textbook of Clinical Chemistry, W.B. Saunders, Philadelphia, 1986, with permission.)*

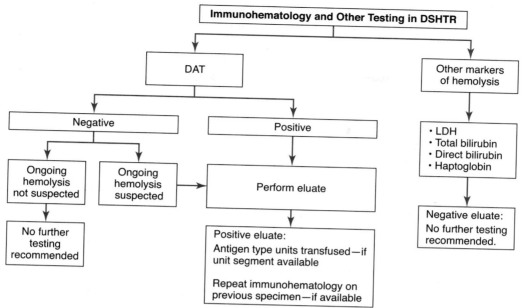

Figure 16–14.   Immunohematology and other testing in delayed serologic/hemolytic transfusion reactions. The evaluation of a suspected delayed serologic/hemolytic delayed transfusion reaction may consist of one or more of the basic and secondary tests performed during the evaluation of an acute immune hemolytic transfusion reaction. DAT = direct antiglobulin test; LDH = lactic dehydrogenase

of the amount of transfused red cells that may have a shortened survival.

Baseline and follow-up samples to assess ongoing hemolysis in the patient should also be performed (hemoglobin; total and direct bilirubin; LDH, haptoglobin). DSHTR in general are mild and may require only careful monitoring of the patient.[18] Treatment, if necessary, should be based on the patient symptomatology. When antigen typing suggests a large burden of antigen-positive cells and other laboratory results are consistent with ongoing hemolysis, a red cell exchange should be considered. The prompt identification and accurate record-keeping of clinically significant red cell alloantibodies are required blood bank practices. Whenever a transfusion is being considered with any patient new to an institution, it is important to inquire about his or her transfusion history. The use of partially or fully phenotypically matched red cell units for some patient populations such as those with sickle cell disease[1] may decrease the risk of alloimmunization and thus the risk of DSHTR. If a sickle cell HTR syndrome is suspected, withholding further transfusions may be required.[39]

Transfusion-Associated Graft-Versus-Host Disease

Transfusion-associated graft-versus-host disease (TA-GVHD) is defined as a delayed immune transfusion reaction due to an immunologic attack by viable donor lymphocytes contained in the transfused blood component against the transfusion recipient. The presenting reaction with a **maculopapular** rash (often pruritic, typically starting centrally and extending to the extremities), fever, watery diarrhea (accompanied by bloody stools and abdominal pain), elevated liver function tests, and pancytopenia occurs between 3 and 30 days

post-transfusion of a nonirradiated cellular blood component. Unlike the hematopoietic progenitor transplant, TA-GVHD leads to profound marrow aplasia with a mortality rate greater than 90%.[2] Death occurs 1 to 3 weeks after first symptoms appear. Three conditions must exist for TA-GVHD to develop in a recipient: HLA antigen difference between donor and recipient, presence of donor immunocompetent cells in the blood component, and a recipient incapable of rejecting the donor immunocompetent cells.[40] The number of lymphocytes in a bag is determined by the age of the blood component and the irradiation status. Fresher blood components contain more viable T lymphocytes.

At-risk immunodeficient patient populations include infants and patients with cancer or compromised immune systems. In patients with an intact immune system, the TA-GVHD can occur when the patient is transfused with a cellular blood component from a donor homozygous for an HLA haplotype that is shared with the heterozygous recipient (Fig. 16–15). In such settings, the recipient's immune system does not recognize the homozygous HLA haplotype of the transfused donor lymphocytes as foreign and therefore will not eliminate them. In contrast, the transfused lymphocytes are able to recognize the recipient nonshared haplotype as foreign and will mount an immune attack on the recipient.

At-risk immunocompetent patient populations include individuals receiving cellular blood components from blood relatives and patients receiving HLA matched or crossmatched platelets or granulocytes. The degree of population genetic diversity influences the TA-GVHD risk of a transfusion from a random donor. For example, in Japan the TA-GVHD risk from a random donor transfusion is as high as 1 in 874 transfusions because of the

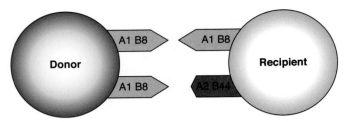

Figure 16–15. Transfusion-associated graft-versus-host disease (TA-GVHD) in an immunocompetent patient. The triggering event involves the transfusion of a cellular blood component from a donor (graft) with a homozygous HLA haplotype to a recipient (host) with a heterozygous HLA type of which a haplotype is shared with the donor. In this figure, the HLA haplotype shared is A1,B8. There is no foreign haplotype to be recognized by the recipient. However, the recognition of the foreign HLA haplotype (A2, B44) by the donor triggers an "unopposed" immune attack against the recipient.

population HLA genetic homogeneity, as compared with France where more HLA genetic heterogeneity exists and the TA-GVHD risk from a random donor transfusion is 1 in 16,835 transfusions.[41]

In cases of TA-GVHD, diagnostic testing includes:

- Skin biopsy for superficial perivascular lymphocyte infiltrate, necrotic **keratinocytes**, and bullae formation.
- Bone marrow examination for hypocellular or aplastic marrow, with only the presence of macrophages.
- Liver biopsy for degeneration and eosinophilic necrosis of small bile ducts, intense periportal inflammation, and lymphocytic infiltration.
- Molecular studies from the patient's buccal swabs or skin fibroblasts, or otherwise from those of first-degree relatives to distinguish between the recipient and donor cells.

Definitive diagnosis requires the identification of donor-derived lymphocytes in the recipient circulation or tissues.[42] On the contrary, the presence of donor-derived lymphocytes alone in the absence of clinical symptoms is not diagnostic for TA-GVHD.[42] Stem cell transplantation may represent the only curative option for TA-GVHD. However, the urgent need for intervention makes the treatment's success very unlikely.

As treatment options are almost nonexistent and because of the condition's high mortality, emphasis is put on recognizing the patient population at risk of TA-GVHD and providing the interventions that prevent it from occurring. Current leukoreduction techniques do not reduce the risk of TA-GVHD. However, exposing the cellular blood component to gamma irradiation reduces the number of viable lymphocytes that prevents TA-GVHD. AABB *Standards* requires a minimum dose of 25 Gy (2,500 cGy) delivered to the central portion of the container and a minimum of 15 Gy (1,500 cGy) dose elsewhere in the container to the products given to at-risk patient populations.[10]

Quality control of irradiation procedures is essential to ensure that the correct dose is administered. Box 16–3 lists the types of patients for whom irradiated blood components are indicated.[39,42] In the United States, gamma irradiation is the only method utilized in the prevention of TA-GVHD.

BOX 16–3

Indications for the Transfusion of Irradiated Cellular Blood Components

Immunocompromised State (Indicated by Patient Condition)

- Intrauterine transfusions
- Low birth weight infants
- Neonates receiving a whole blood exchange
- Neonates undergoing extracorporeal membrane oxygenation
- Congenital immunodeficiencies
- Hematopoietic progenitor cell transplantation
- Solid organ transplantation
- Acute leukemia
- Hodgkin's disease
- Patients with B-cell malignancies
- Patients receiving fludarabine

Immunocompetent State (Indicated by Origin of Blood Component to Be Transfused)

- Directed donations from blood relatives
- HLA-matched platelets or granulocytes
- Crossmatched platelets or granulocytes
- Granulocyte components

HLA = human leukocyte antigen

However, in Europe newer techniques for lymphocyte inactivation such as photochemical treatment of platelets and plasma have been established and used as an alternative to gamma irradiation.[43]

Post-Transfusion Purpura

Post-transfusion purpura (PTP) is a delayed immune complication of transfusion that presents with profound thrombocytopenia, frequently accompanied by bleeding, 1 to 24 days after a blood transfusion.[41] Febrile reactions have been reported retrospectively with the implicated transfusion. PTP occurs when a patient who is previously sensitized to human platelet antigens by pregnancy or transfusion is reexposed via a transfusion. This is characteristically a red blood cell or whole blood transfusion, expressing that human platelet antigen specificity and causing an anamnestic immune response, destroying not only transfused but also the autologous platelets. The mechanism of the autologous platelet destruction and its association with the alloantibody remain unclear, although possible causes include binding of immune complexes to the patient's platelets,[44] coating of the patient platelets by soluble antigens derived from donor plasma,[45] or having an autoimmune response secondary to reexposure to the antigen via the transfused product where the patient's platelets are attacked.[46]

The antigen most commonly implicated in this condition is the human platelet antigen (HPA)1a. HPA antibody specificities detected in one study included HPA-1a (60%) and, less frequently, HPA-1b, HPA-2b, HPA-3a, HPA-5a, HPA-5b, and glycoprotein (GP) IV.[41] The diagnosis is confirmed by demonstrating the presence of antibodies in the patient's plasma against human platelet antigens and the absence of the implicated antigen specificity in the patient's platelets.

PTP is a self-limiting syndrome with the platelet count usually returning to normal within 2 weeks. However, up to a 13% mortality related to intracranial hemorrhage has been reported.[41] The standard of treatment consists of the infusion of intravenous immunoglobulin, 0.5 to 1 grams per kilogram per day over a period of 2 to 10 days, with an average response time of 4 days after initiating therapy.[41] Patients with a documented history of PTP should receive, if possible, antigen-negative blood products for subsequent transfusions.

Iron Overload

Iron overload is a delayed, nonimmune complication of transfusion, presenting with multiorgan (i.e., liver, heart, endocrine organs) damage secondary to excessive iron accumulation. Each unit of red blood cells contains approximately 250 mg of iron. After 10 to 15 red cell transfusions, excess iron is present in the liver, heart, and endocrine organs.[4] Chronic red cell transfusion recipients have the greatest risk for developing iron overload, with a cumulative 50 to 100 red blood cell unit transfusions causing greater morbidity than the underlying anemia. Therefore, preventing the accumulation of iron stores by chelation is extremely important for this patient population. The chelating agents bind to iron in the tissues, helping its removal through the urine and feces. Currently, there are three chelating agents available: parenteral deferoxamine, oral deferiprone, and oral deferasirox.[2] In certain chronic red cell transfusion patient populations, red cell exchange transfusion may be used as an alternative to transfusion therapy and may help delay transfusion-related iron accumulation, preventing

associated organ damage.[47] Table 16–6 summarizes the categories of delayed transfusion reactions.

"Silent" Transfusion-Related Adverse Events

There are some incidents or errors associated with transfusions that do not necessarily present with transfusion-associated symptoms. Therefore, the authors assign the term *silent* to these adverse events. However, any of these have the potential to cause an adverse event if gone unnoticed. Such events include transfusion sample collection errors, red blood cell alloimmunization, platelet alloimmunization, and transfusion over- or underdosing.

Sample Collection Errors

Transfusion sample collection errors consist of those samples that have the wrong blood in the tube (major, risk 1:1,200 to 1:2,800) or those samples that are provided with missing required information (minor, risk 1:71 to 1:165).[48] Surveys have shown an associated risk between the number of minor collection errors occurring at an institution and the risk for the occurrence of a major collection error.[49] Major collection errors are often associated with a properly labeled tube containing all the required information but drawn from the wrong patient. In the absence of a previous historic blood type in the institution for that individual, a great risk occurs for a mistransfusion of incompatible blood. Thus, it is important to track and trend the major and minor collection error rates to provide the appropriate intervention or corrective or preventive action. Current preventive efforts for collection errors include improved patient identification mechanisms such as improved computer technology and barrier systems to prevent transfusion without precise recipient identification.

Table 16–6   Summary of Delayed Transfusion Reactions

	SYMPTOMS	DIAGNOSIS	TREATMENT	PREVENTION
DSHTR	Asymptomatic Fatigue	+ Antibody screen/DAT ↓ Hemoglobin	As needed Transfuse antigen negative, AHG crossmatched compatible PRBC	Accurate record-keeping Obtain transfusion history Limit transfusions
DHTR	Flulike symptoms Pallor Jaundice	↓ Hemoglobin ↑ Total bilirubin	As needed Transfuse antigen negative, AHG crossmatched compatible PRBC	Accurate record-keeping Obtain transfusion history Limit transfusions
TA-GVHD	Rash Fever Diarrhea	Pancytopenia Identify donor engraftment	Not available	Gamma irradiation of cellular blood components as indicated
PTP	Bleeding	Thrombocytopenia HPA antibodies	Intravenous immunoglobulin	Limit transfusions
Iron overload	Multiorgan failure	High ferritin levels	Use of iron-chelating agents	Prophylactic use of iron-chelating agents Red cell exchange

AHG = antihuman globulin; DAT = direct antiglobulin test; DHTR = delayed hemolytic transfusion reaction; DSHTR = delayed serologic/hemolytic transfusion reaction; HPA = human platelet antigen; PRBC = packed red blood cells; PTP = post-transfusion purpura; TA-GVHD = transfusion-associated graft-versus-host disease

Red Blood Cell Alloimmunization

In chronically transfused patients, the risk for them developing antibodies against the red cell antigens (RBC alloimmunization) increases by 2% to 8%; in the sickle cell patient population, this is as high as 40%.[4] Factors influencing the rate of alloimmunization are antigenic differences, dose, frequency of transfusion, recipient immune status, and immunogenicity of the donor HLA antigens.[4] The presence of red cell antibodies not only makes allocation of compatible, antigen-negative units difficult but it also may increase the risk of DSHTR/DHTR.

Platelet Alloimmunization

The presence of antibodies against class I HLA antigens is the most common immune cause of platelet transfusion refractoriness.[4] These antibodies form after exposure to corresponding antigen expressed on contaminating WBCs in transfused blood components and can interfere with adequate platelet count increments to platelet transfusions (platelet transfusion refractoriness). The Trial to Reduce Alloimmunization to Platelets (TRAP) study[50] showed that HLA alloimmunization developed in 45% of the recipients of nonleukoreduced platelets. The rate of HLA alloimmunization decreased to 17% when an intervention to decrease the number of WBCs present by leukoreduction was used. Antibodies against the human platelet antigen system are a less common cause of platelet transfusion refractoriness (rate of 2% to 10% in multiply transfused patients).[4] The leukoreduction of cellular platelets does not seem to decrease the latter risk. Another adverse effect of the development of antibodies against the HPA is post-transfusion purpura.

Transfusion Overdosing and Underdosing

For many years, transfusion practices have been providing blood components in standardized dosing that do not necessarily take into account the component contents, patient blood volume, or the baseline laboratory parameters initiating the request for transfusion. For pediatric transfusions, the volume to be transfused is mostly based on the patient's weight. However, in adults, for the transfusion of RBCs, 2 units have been the standard of practice despite evidence that, in many scenarios, a 1-unit transfusion may suffice.[4] Similarly a 2-unit transfusion practice has been adopted when transfusing plasma despite recommendations of calculating the dose in a way similar to pediatric transfusion practice, which is based on body weight.[51] This persistent practice can lead to overtransfusion, as demonstrated with red cell transfusions,[4] or to undertransfusion of plasma, as has been observed during the correction of coagulopathy.[51]

Transfusion-Related Adverse Events in Special Patient Scenarios

A transfusion-related adverse event study is usually focused on recipients (mainly adults and older children) of allogeneic blood components. However, there are special patient populations and transfusion circumstances that warrant some additional discussion: infusion of plasma derivatives, therapeutic apheresis procedures using blood components as fluid replacement, neonatal transfusions, and transfusion of autologous blood components.

Infusion of Plasma Derivatives

Today, nonviral transfusion reactions are the most common risks seen in association with the transfusion of plasma derivatives such as albumin and intravenous immunoglobulin (IVIg), and human-derived coagulation factor concentrates.[8] These adverse events can be acute or delayed. Most are transient and do not appear to have clinical sequelae. Nevertheless, on rare occasions, these plasma derivatives have the potential for life-threatening adverse reactions. Albumin infusion has been associated with hypotensive reactions when used as the sole replacement fluid during plasmapheresis in patients taking **ACE inhibitors** as treatment for hypertension. IVIg infusion has been associated with numerous adverse effects such as renal dysfunction, related to the use of sucrose as a stabilizing agent; dose-related aseptic meningitis; positive direct antiglobulin test with or without hemolysis; anaphylaxis; TRALI; and thromboembolic events. Infusion of human-derived coagulation factor concentrates may be associated with allergic reactions and, depending on the coagulation protein being replaced, with thrombosis.

Therapeutic Apheresis

During therapeutic apheresis, transfusion reactions can occur, or inherent symptoms to the procedure may be aggravated when the replacement fluids used consist of blood components.[9] Adverse effects most frequently reported include perioral or acral **paresthesias**, seen more frequently when citrated plasma rather than albumin solution is used as the replacement fluid. Anaphylactoid reactions have been reported with the use of albumin as the replacement fluid in patients receiving ACE inhibitors. There are also reported cases of bacterial contamination of albumin solutions.

Neonatal Transfusions

Recognizing transfusion adverse events in neonates may be difficult in the presence of other concomitant clinical factors. The more frequently acute immune-mediated transfusion reactions observed in adults and older children are rarely seen in neonates due to the latter's underdeveloped immune system at birth.[52] More importantly, neonates may be more vulnerable to metabolic complications as a result of their brittle physiological balance.[52] Some symptoms may be associated with the composition of the blood component anticoagulant or preservative solutions, or the temporary discontinuation of fluid replacement during transfusion.

Neonates may be at risk of developing hyperglycemia or hypoglycemia, hypocalcemia, or hyperkalemia in association with transfusion. These metabolic symptoms often present with similar symptoms that may include jitteriness, tremors, convulsions, **hypotonia**, lethargy, **apnea**, and **cyanosis**. The treatment for the transfusion-associated metabolic changes will depend on their expected duration and the infant's underlying condition. Careful planning for replacement balance between transfusion and other fluids will minimize such adverse events.

Development of antibodies is extremely rare in infants due to the inability of the neonatal lymphocytes to recognize foreign antigens.[52] On the rare occasions when an acute immune-mediated transfusion reaction occurs, the reaction is the result of passively transfused antibodies. Rarely, infants with **necrotizing enterocolitis** or sepsis may develop intravascular hemolysis due the exposure of cryptogenic antigens in the autologous red cells that react with antibodies present in the donor plasma that share a similar specificity (**T-antigen activation, polyagglutination syndrome**).[52] Some neonatal patients are also at risk of developing graft-versus-host disease. Finally, the infant is at risk of developing TAS or mistransfusion in a similar fashion to the adult or older children population.

Autologous Blood Transfusions

There are several methods used to collect autologous blood: preoperative autologous donation (PAD; planned collection and storage of patient's own blood until the time of surgery), intraoperative hemodilution (IOH; collection of a patient's own blood at the beginning of the surgery that is then returned to the patient at the end of surgery), and perioperative blood recovery (POBR; the recovery of a patient's blood from the surgical field or postoperative drainage that is washed and returned to the patient).

Autologous transfusions are perceived to be risk-free by many, including patients and their physicians. However, with the exception of transfusion-transmitted diseases and a slight difference in incidence, all other adverse events associated with allogeneic transfusions (FNHTR, TAS, TACO, mistransfusion, AHTR) may also occur in association with the transfusion of autologous blood. These adverse events may be associated with increased morbidity and even death. The most efficient way to avoid adverse events associated with the transfusion of autologous blood is to follow the same rules and regulations that apply to the use of allogeneic blood, as well as the manufacturer's instructions when utilizing perioperative blood recovery.

CASE STUDIES

Case Study 16-1

A 47-year-old male with a history of intravenous drug abuse presented to the emergency department with a 1-week history of back pain, fever, shaking chills, and red urine.

Blood Test Results (Initial)
Hgb: 7 g/L (reference range: 14 to 17.4 g/dL)
Total Bilirubin: 1 mg/dL (reference range: 0.2 to 1.2 mg/dL)
Urinalysis: Blood: large; microscopy: many WBCs and granular casts

Blood Typing: B-positive
Antibody Screen: Negative
Immediate Spin Crossmatching: Compatible

Upon medical evaluation, the patient was diagnosed with acute pyelonephritis and anemia. He was promptly started on antibiotics. Shortly after admission, the patient was transfused with 2 units of packed red blood cells. The patient's clinical course was significant for persistent hypotension despite hydration, requiring the addition of blood pressure support medication. Due to persistent anemia, he received five additional units of packed red blood cells. On day 3 after admission, a new sample was sent to the transfusion service with a request for two additional units of packed red blood cells.

Transfusion Service Evaluation:
Day 3 Sample 1
Blood type: O-positive
Antibody Screen: Neg
Hemolysis: Yes

The day 3 sample revealed a blood type discrepancy. The patient's medical staff was immediately notified and a day 3 second sample was requested. The laboratory technologist examined both pre- and postsamples for clerical errors. Upon initial review, no name discrepancy or other identifying information was identified among the different blood bank samples and transfusion records. Both day 3 samples were noticed to have "orange" appearing plasma when compared to the admission sample. Repeat testing was performed on the pre- and post-transfusion samples with the following results.

Day 3 Sample 1	Day 3 Sample 2	Admission Sample:
Blood type: O-positive	**Blood type:** O-positive	**Blood type:** B-positive
Antibody Screen: Neg	**Antibody Screen:** Neg	**Antibody Screen:** Neg
Hemolysis: Yes	**Hemolysis:** Yes	**Hemolysis:** No

ABO discrepancy and hemolysis were identified.

Transfusion service records indicated that the patient had been transfused with seven B-positive packed red blood cells. **No discrepancies were identified.**

Additional testing was performed with the following results:

Day 3 Sample 2
Direct AHG: Positive (PS 3+, IgG 3+, and C3d 1+)
Eluate: ABS cell I: Neg
ABS cell II: Neg
A cells: Neg
B cells: 3+

Transfusion Service Physician Follow-up

The transfusion service physician promptly notified the patient's physician regarding the ABO incompatibility and the likelihood of an acute hemolytic transfusion reaction. The patient was evaluated for ongoing signs and symptoms of acute hemolysis and was found to be unchanged

Continued

from baseline with the exception of a temporary decrease in urine output that was treated with hydration.

Additional laboratory assays were performed and results are shown below:

LDH	813 (reference range: 100 to 190 IU/L)
Total Bilirubin	3.7 (reference range: 0.2 to 1.2 mg/dL)
Direct Bilirubin	0.3 (reference range: 0.1 to 0.4 mg/dL)
Haptoglobin	Undetectable (reference range: 30 to 200 mg/dL)
Urinalysis	Blood 3 +; many WBC, RBC, granular and red cell casts

During a retrospective review of the patient's clinical course, an increase in body temperature, a decrease in blood pressure, an increase in heart rate and respiratory rate, and shaking chills and back pain were associated with each of the transfusion episodes. These were thought to be related to the patient's underlying condition and therefore not recognized as transfusion-related signs and symptoms. A more detailed examination of the initial sample sent to the transfusion service the day of admission revealed that the tube's original label had a different name and medical record number than the "typenex label" placed on top. Transfusion records of the second name were reviewed, showing that a type and antibody screen had been performed but no crossmatches were requested. The emergency department initiated an investigation to find the cause of the major collection error, revealing that the patients involved in the sample collection error were in the same room when samples were drawn and that the samples were labeled at the nurses' station where addressographs are kept.

Upon follow-up, the patient was found to be improving and was discharged home 10 days after reaction.

Interpretation

This case represents an **acute immune hemolytic transfusion reaction** due to a major collection error with failure to recognize transfusion reaction–related signs and symptoms.

1. Define *acute transfusion reactions*.
2. What does the orange-appearing plasma or hemoglobinemia indicate?
3. The severity of symptoms with acute hemolytic reactions are most likely related to what major factor?
4. What are the key clerical checks to be performed by the laboratory technologist?

Case Study 16-2

A 62-year-old female with spinal stenosis required back surgery. During surgery, 2 units of allogenic red cells and 500 mL of salvaged blood were transfused. Once the patient was in the recovery room, the anesthesiologist became concerned because her urine was "more pink" than usual. The anesthesiologist notified the transfusion service physician, and a transfusion reaction workup was initiated. A postreaction sample was drawn, properly

labeled, and sent to the transfusion service with a copy of the transfusion record listing the reaction. The transfused autologous salvaged units had been discarded and therefore were not available for evaluation.

Transfusion Service Evaluation

The laboratory technologist examined both pre- and postreaction samples for clerical errors. The historic patient records were checked and verified. **No defects were revealed.** Additional testing was performed with the following results:

Postreaction sample:

Blood type:	O-positive; no discrepancies identified
Antibody Screen:	Neg
DAT:	Neg
Hemolysis:	No hemolysis
AHG Crossmatch:	Both units, previously electronic crossmatched, compatible

Repeat ABO confirmatory testing on allogenic unit segments:
O-positive (both units)

Transfusion Service Physician Follow-up

The transfusion service physician notified the anesthesiologist that the transfusion reaction showed no discrepancies or evidence of hemolysis based on the evaluation of the 2 units of allogenic blood issued by the transfusion service and transfused during surgery. The anesthesiologist contacted the hospital's cell saver charge personnel to determine if the cause of the hemoglobinuria could have been caused by the improper use of the cell saver. It was revealed that the proper washing solution (0.9% NaCl) was used and there was no malfunction of the cell saver. However, the surgeon had requested the use of a more potent suction because he stated that the one that came with the cell saver kit was too slow. It was determined that the hemoglobinuria was caused by the use of an inappropriate suction during blood salvage, causing hemolysis of the harvested blood that was then transfused to the patient. The patient's urine cleared overnight and the postoperative course was unremarkable.

Interpretation

This case represents a **nonimmune acute hemolytic transfusion reaction** due to failure to follow the manufacturer's guidelines for the cell saver's use. Communication with other health professionals served as the key to resolving this incident.

1. What is the key to resolving this case?
2. What are the key reasons for nonimmune hemolytic transfusion reactions?

Case Study 16-3

A 57-year-old female bone marrow transplant (BMT) patient with non-Hodgkin's lymphoma required transfusions on a regular basis due to her chronic anemia. During one of her transfusion visits to the clinic, the patient developed a 1.8°C increase in temperature with rigors.

The transfusion was stopped two-thirds of the way through. The nursing personnel performed a clerical check by verifying the patient identification band to the transfusion record and the unit crossmatch tag to confirm that the blood component was given to the correct patient. The patient's physician was notified. The nurse, who had monitored the patient during past transfusions, expressed her concern to the physician regarding the severity of the reaction when compared to previous reactions observed. The physician requested a transfusion reaction workup. A properly labeled postreaction sample was drawn and sent along with the unit of blood, attached tubing, and solutions to the transfusion service for a transfusion reaction workup. The patient was treated with Tylenol and discharged with instructions to continue monitoring her temperature.

Transfusion Service Evaluation

The laboratory technologist examined both pre- and postreaction samples, the blood bag, and the tubing for clerical errors. The attached solution was verified to be 0.9% normal saline, and historic patient records were checked and verified. **No defects were revealed**. Repeat testing was performed on the postreaction sample with the following results:

Postreaction Sample:
Blood type: O-negative
DAT: Neg
Hemolysis: No hemolysis

Three hours later, the patient returned to the emergency department with an increase in temperature and a decrease in blood pressure. The transfusion service physician was consulted, and further testing of the unit of blood was ordered. Immediately, a gram stain and blood culture were performed on the unit of blood implicated with the reaction, and two sets of blood cultures were drawn from the patient.

Gram stain-unit of blood: Gram-positive cocci in clusters

Transfusion Service Physician Follow-up:

The transfusion service physician was immediately notified of the gram-stain results. The results were relayed to the patient's physician, who started the patient on broad-spectrum antibiotic treatment until identification and sensitivity of the cultures were complete. Shortly after, the blood center was notified of the transfusion service physician's preliminary findings, and all available donor products were discarded. The following day, culture results revealed positive growth in both the patient and the unit of blood, and the organism was identified as *Staphylococcus aureus*. A follow-up written notification prepared by the transfusion service physician was sent to the blood center for donor evaluation. Further investigation by the blood center revealed that the donor arm was not cleaned per standard operating procedures, which led to contamination of the unit. The blood center phlebotomist was retrained on proper cleansing techniques.

Interpretation

This case represents a **transfusion-associated sepsis** due to a failure to follow standard operating procedures for the arm preparation prior to donation, most likely resulting in contamination of the unit from the skin flora of the donor.

1. What laboratory workup is performed to diagnose transfusion-associated sepsis?
2. What symptoms usually present with transfusion-associated sepsis?

SUMMARY CHART

- ✓ Transfusion reactions are classified according to symptom time interval. Less than 24 hours: acute transfusion reactions; greater than 24 hours: delayed transfusion reactions. Both further classify into immune or nonimmune.
- ✓ The transfusion reaction workup is designed to rule in or rule out hemolysis.
- ✓ Acute transfusion reaction evaluation or testing includes clerical check, examination for visual hemolysis, DAT, and patient ABO group confirmation.
- ✓ Acute transfusion reactions include acute hemolytic reactions, transfusion-associated sepsis, febrile non-hemolytic reactions, allergic reactions, TRALI, and TACO.
- ✓ Immune hemolysis occurs when previously formed IgM (ABO) or IgG (non-ABO) antibodies in the recipient recognize the corresponding donor RBC antigen and result in complement-mediated intravascular hemolysis. Evidence of immune hemolysis in the postreaction sample from the acute transfusion reaction evaluation or test will need to be followed with comparison to the pretransfusion testing results. If necessary, additional testing in duplicate (pre- and postreaction samples) could include repeat basic immunohematology testing, eluate, and antigen typing to identify the cause of the immune hemolysis.
- ✓ Non-immune hemolysis occurs when the RBC suffers mechanical or chemical damage and is manifested as an asymptomatic hemoglobinuria
- ✓ Transfusion-associated sepsis occurs when bacteria are introduced to the patient via a contaminated blood product, manifested by an increase in body temperature or more than 2°C, rigors, and hypotension. When this condition is suspected, additional testing includes gram staining and cultures of the blood component and the patient. Isolation of the same organism is key for the diagnosis.

Continued

SUMMARY CHART—cont'd

- ✔ Febrile nonhemolytic reactions occur when the recipient is exposed to the donor cytokines present in the WBC or plasma and is manifested by an increase in body temperature of more than 1°C with or without chills. Workup must exclude hemolytic (transfusion reaction workup testing) and septic reactions (symptoms and patient evaluation).

- ✔ Allergic reactions can be mild (hives or itching) or severe (anaphylaxis) and are mainly caused by the release of histamine from the interaction between the allergen present in the donor plasma and the recipient preformed IgE antibodies. A classic example of a severe allergic reaction is the one seen due to the presence of anti-IgA antibodies in a patient with absolute IgA deficiency.

- ✔ TRALI occurs most frequently when donor leukocyte antibodies react with the WBCs in the recipient's lung vasculature, damaging the endothelium and causing noncardiogenic pulmonary edema. High plasma volume blood components from parous female donors are the most commonly associated blood components. Therefore, focus is on prevention achieved by using only male plasma components or plasma components collected from WBC antibody–negative female donors.

- ✔ TACO occurs when the patient's cardiovascular system is unable to handle the transfused volume, resulting in congestive heart failure. This is an underreported complication of transfusion, often responsive to patient diuresis.

- ✔ Delayed transfusion reactions include delayed serologic/hemolytic reactions, transfusion-associated graft-versus-host disease, post-transfusion purpura, and iron overload.

- ✔ Delayed serologic/hemolytic reactions occurs secondary to an anamnestic or primary immune response directed to red cell antibodies that may (delayed hemolytic transfusion reaction) or may not (delayed serologic transfusion reaction) be associated with clinical evidence of shortened red cell survival of the transfused RBCs. Besides standard basic immunohematology testing (ABO/Rh, antibody screen and when indicated antibody identification), additional testing will include DAT and, when indicated, an eluate and antigen typing of the units recently transfused.

- ✔ Transfusion-associated graft-versus-host disease occurs when the transfusion-derived donor lymphocytes attack and destroy the recipient immune system, causing pancytopenia and death. It is prevented by the gamma irradiation of blood components for transfusion to patient populations at risk.

- ✔ Post-transfusion purpura is an acquired profound thrombocytopenia that occurs when a patient with preformed platelet antibodies is transfused with a blood component containing the platelet antigen and sharing specificity with the preformed antibodies, leading to the destruction of the donor and recipient platelets. Anti-HPA-1a is the most common implicated antibody specificity.

- ✔ Iron overload occurs due to long-term accumulation of iron in the body tissues from multiple RBC transfusions. This causes organ damage.

Review Questions

1. What component is most frequently involved with transfusion-associated sepsis?
   a. Plasma
   b. Packed red blood cells
   c. Platelets
   d. Whole blood

2. Fatal transfusion reactions are mostly caused by?
   a. Serologic errors
   b. Improper storage of blood
   c. Clerical errors
   d. Improper handling of the product

3. Early manifestation of an acute hemolytic transfusion reaction can be confused with?
   a. Allergic reaction
   b. Febrile nonhemolytic reaction
   c. Anaphylactic shock
   d. Sepsis

4. Pain at infusion site and hypotension are observed with what type of reaction?
   a. Delayed hemolytic transfusion reaction
   b. Acute hemolytic transfusion reaction
   c. Allergic reaction
   d. Febrile nonhemolytic reaction

5. Irradiation of blood is performed to prevent?
   a. Febrile nonhemolytic transfusion reaction
   b. Delayed hemolytic transfusion reaction
   c. Transfusion-associated graft-versus-host disease
   d. Transfusion-associated circulatory overload

6. The only presenting sign most often accompanying a delayed hemolytic transfusion reaction is?
   a. Renal failure
   b. Unexplained decrease in hemoglobin
   c. Active bleeding
   d. Hives

7. Which transfusion reaction presents with fever, maculopapular rash, watery diarrhea, abnormal liver function, and pancytopenia?

   a. Transfusion-associated sepsis
   b. Transfusion-related acute lung injury
   c. Transfusion-associated graft-versus-host disease
   d. Transfusion-associated allergic reaction

8. A suspected transfusion-related death must be reported to?

   a. AABB
   b. Federal and Drug Administration (FDA)
   c. College of American Pathologists (CAP)
   d. The Joint Commission (TJC)

9. Nonimmune hemolysis can be caused during transfusion by:

   a. Use of small bore size needle.
   b. Use of an infusion pump.
   c. Improper use of a blood warmer.
   d. All of the above

10. Transfusion reactions are classified according to:

   a. Signs or symptoms presenting during or after 24 hours.
   b. Immune or nonimmune.
   c. Infectious or noninfectious.
   d. All of the above

11. With febrile nonhemolytic transfusion reactions:

   a. They are self-limited.
   b. Fever resolves within 2 to 3 hours.
   c. Treatment is required.
   d. A and B are correct
   e. All of the above

12. Absolute IgA deficiency is a classic example of a severe allergic reaction. Results indicating an absolute IgA deficiency:

   a. < 0.05 mg/dL
   b. < 0.50 mg/dL
   c. < 0.50 gm/dL
   d. < 5 mg/dL

13. How are mild allergic transfusion reactions with isolated symptoms or hives and urticaria treated?

   a. Transfusion is stopped and transfusion reaction workup is initiated.
   b. Transfusion is stopped and antihistamines administrated; when symptoms improve, transfusion is restarted.
   c. Stop transfusion and prepare washed red cells.
   d. Continue transfusion with a slower infusion rate.

14. TRALI presents with the following symptoms:

   a. Respiratory distress
   b. Severe hypoxemia and hypotension
   c. Fever
   d. All of the above

15. Which of the following is characteristic of iron overload?

   a. Delayed, nonimmune complication
   b. Chelating agents are used
   c. Multiorgan damage may occur
   d. All of the above

References

1. Eder, AF, and Chambers, LA: Noninfectious complications of blood transfusion. Arch Pathol Lab Med 131:708–718, 2007.
2. Mazzei, CA, Popovsky, MA, and Kopko, PM: Noninfectious complications of blood transfusion. In Roback, JD (ed): Technical Manual, 16th ed. AABB Press, Bethesda, MD, 2009, pp 715–749.
3. Fuller, AK, Uglik, KM, Savage, WJ, et al: Bacterial culture reduces but does not eliminate the risk of septic transfusion reactions to single-donor platelets. Transfusion 49:2588–2593, 2009.
4. Hendrickson, JE, and Hillyer, CD: Noninfectious serious hazards of transfusion. Anesth Analg 108:759–769, 2009.
5. Chapman, CE, Stainsby, D, Jones, H, et al: Ten years of hemovigilance reports of transfusion-related acute lung injury in the United Kingdom and the impact of preferential use of male donor plasma. Transfusion 49:440–452, 2009.
6. Gauvin, F, Lacroix, J, Robillard, P, et al: Acute transfusion reactions in the pediatric intensive care unit. Transfusion 46:1899–1908, 2006.
7. Domen, RE: Adverse reactions associated with autologous blood transfusion: Evaluation and incidence at a large academic hospital. Transfusion 38:296–300, 1998.
8. Callum, J, and Nahirniak, S: Adverse effects of human-derived plasma derivatives. In Popovsky, MA (ed): Transfusion Reactions, 3rd ed. AABB Press, Bethesda, MD, 2007, pp 501–523.
9. McLeod, BC, Sniecinski, I, Ciaravella, D, et al: Frequency of immediate adverse effects associated with therapeutic apheresis. Transfusion 39:282–289, 1999.
10. Price, TH (ed): Standard for Blood Banks and Transfusion Service, 26th ed. AABB, Bethesda, MD, 2009.
11. College of American Pathologists Laboratory Accreditation Program checklists. Northfield, IL: College of American Pathologists, 2009.
12. Code of Federal Regulation. Title 21 CFR Part 606-660. Washington, D.C.: U.S. Government Printing Office, 2008.
13. Davenport, RD: Management of transfusion reactions. In Mintz, PD (ed): Transfusion Therapy Clinical Principles and Practice, 2nd ed. AABB Press, Bethesda, MD, 2005, pp 515–539.
14. Ramirez-Arcos, S, Goldman, M, and Blajchman, MA: Bacterial contamination. In Popovsky, MA (ed): Transfusion Reactions, 3rd ed. AABB Press, Bethesda, MD, 2007, pp 163–206.
15. Fung, MK, Downes, KA, and Shulman, IA: Transfusion of platelets containing ABO incompatible plasma: A survey of 3156 North American Laboratories. Arch Pathol Lab Med 131:909–916, 2007.
16. Josephson, CD, Mullis, NC, Van Demark, C, et al: Significant number of apheresis-derived group O platelet units have a "high titer" anti-A/A,B: Implications for transfusion policy. Transfusion 44:805–808, 2004.
17. Cooling, LL, Downs, TA, Butch, SH, et al: Anti-A and anti-B titers in pooled group O platelets are comparable to apheresis platelets. Transfusion 48:1206–1213, 2008.
18. Davenport, RD: Hemolytic transfusion reactions. In Simon, TL, Dzik, WH, Snyder, EL, Stowell, CP, and Strauss, RG (eds): Rossi's Principles of Transfusion Medicine, 3rd ed. Lippincott, Williams & Wilkins, Philadelphia, 2002, pp 815–828.
19. Sweeney, J: Additive solutions for platelets: Is it time for North America to go with the flow? Transfusion 49;199–201, 2009.

20. Vamvakas, EC: Relative safety of pooled whole blood-derived versus single donor (apheresis) platelets in the United States: A systematic review of disparate risks. Transfusion 49: 2743–2758, 2009.

21. Muylle, L, Joos, M, Wouters, E, et al: Increased tumor necrosis factor alpha (TNFα), interleukin 1, and interleukin 6 (IL-6) levels in the plasma of stored platelet concentrates: Relationship between TNFα and IL-6 levels and febrile transfusion reactions. Transfusion 33:195–199, 1993.

22. Heddle, NM, Klama, L, Singer, J, et al: The Role of the plasma from platelet concentrates in transfusion reactions. N Engl J Med 331:625–628, 1994.

23. King, KE, Shirey, RS, Thoman, SK, et al: Universal leukoreduction decreases the incidence of febrile nonhemolytic transfusion reactions to RBCs. Transfusion 44:25–29, 2004.

24. Hennino, A, Berard, F, Guillot, I, et al: Pathophysiology of Urticaria. Clin Rev Allergy Immunol 30:3–11, 2006.

25. Sadler, G, Malllory, D, Malmaut, D, et al: IgA anaphylactic transfusion reactions. Transfusion Med Rev 9:1–8, 1995.

26. Koda, Y, Watanabe, Y, Soejima, M, et al: Simple PCR detection of haptoglobin gene deletion in anhaptoglobinemic patients with antihaptoglobin antibody that causes anaphylactic transfusion reactions. Blood 95:1138–1143, 2000.

27. Popovsky, MA: Transfusion associated circulatory overload: The plot thickens. Transfusion 49:2–4, 2009.

28. Goldman, M, Webert, KE, Arnold, DM, et al: Proceedings of a consensus conference: Towards an understanding of TRALI. Transfus Med Rev 19:2–31, 2005.

29. Gajic, O, Rana, R, Winters, JL, et al: Transfusion-related acute lung injury in the critically Ill: Prospective nested case-control study. Am J Respir Crit Care Med 176:886–891, 2007.

30. Curtis, BR, and McFarland, JG: Mechanisms of transfused-related acute lung injury (TRALI): Anti-leukocyte antibodies. Crit Care Med 34 (suppl.):S118–123, 2006.

31. Bux, J, and Scahs, UJH: The pathogenesis of transfusion-related acute lung injury (TRALI). Br J Haematol 136:788–799, 2007.

32. Bux, J: Antibody-mediated (immune) transfusion-related acute lung injury. Vox Sanguinis 100:122–128, 2011.

33. Gajic, O, Grooper, MA, and Hubmayr, RD: Pulmonary edema after transfusion: How to differentiate transfusion-associated circulatory overload from transfusion-related acute lung injury. Crit Care Med 34:S109–113, 2006.

34. Rios, JA, Schlumph, KS, Kakaiya, RM, et al: Blood donations from previously transfused or pregnant donors: A multicenter study to determine the frequency of alloexposure. NHLBI Retrovirus Epidemiology Donor Study-II. Transfusion 51: 1197–1206.

35. Zhou, L, Giacherio, D, Cooling, L, et al: Use of B-natriuretic peptide as a diagnostic marker in the differential diagnosis of transfusion-associated circulatory overload. Transfusion 45:1056–1063, 2005.

36. Uhl, L: Complications of massive transfusion. In Popovsky, MA (ed): Transfusion Reactions, 3rd ed. AABB Press, Bethesda, MD, 435–457, 2007.

37. Hippala, ST, Myllyla, GJ, and Vahtera, EM: Hemostatic factors and replacement of major blood loss with plasma-poor red-cell concentrates. Anesth Analg 81:360–365, 1995.

38. Ness, PM, Shirey, RS, Thoman, SK, et al: The differentiation of delayed serologic and delayed hemolytic transfusion reactions: Incidence, long-term serologic findings, and clinical significance. Transfusion 30:688–693, 1990.

39. Petz, LD, Cahoun, L, Shulman, IA, et al: The sickle cell hemolytic transfusion reaction syndrome. Transfusion 37:382–392, 1997.

40. Billingham, R: The biology of graft-versus-host reactions. In The Harvey Lecture series, 1966–1967. Academic Press, Orlando, FL, 1968, pp 62:21–78.

41. McFarland, JG: Posttransfusion purpura. In Popovsky, MA (ed): Transfusion Reactions, 3rd ed. AABB Press, Bethesda, MD, 2007, pp 275–299.

42. Alyea, EP, and Anderson, KC: Transfusion-associated graft-versus-host disease. In Popovsky, MA (ed): Transfusion Reactions, 3rd ed. AABB Press, Bethesda, MD, 2007, pp 229–249.

43. Dwyre, DM, and Holland, PV: Transfusion-associated graft-versus-host disease. Vox Sanguinis 95:85–93, 2008.

44. Shulman, NR, Aster, RH, Leitner, A, et al: Immunoreactivity involving platelets. V. Post-transfusion purpura due to a complement fixing antibody against a genetically controlled platelet antigen. A proposed mechanism for thrombocytopenia and its relevance in autoimmunity. J Clin Invest 40:1597–1620, 1961.

45. Kickler, TS, Ness, PM, Herman, JH, et al: Studies on the pathophysiology of post-transfusion purpura. Blood 68:347–350, 1986.

46. Strickler, RB, Lewis, BH, Corash, L, et al: Post-transfusion purpura associated with an autoantibody directed against a previously undefined platelet antigen. Blood 69:1458–1463, 1987.

47. Kim, HC, Dugan, NP, Silber, JH, et al: Erythrocytapheresis therapy to reduce iron overload in chronically transfused patients with sickle cell disease. Blood 83:1136–1142, 1994.

48. Dzik, WH, Murphy, MF, Andreu, G, et al: An international study of the performance of sample collection from patients. Vox Sanguinis 85:40–47, 2003.

49. Lamadue, JA, Boyd, JS, and Ness, PM: Adherence to a strict specimen-labeling policy decreases the incidence of erroneous blood grouping of blood bank specimens. Transfusion 37:1169–1172, 1997.

50. The Trial to Reduce Alloimmunization to Platelets Study Group: Leukocyte reduction and ultraviolet B irradiation of platelets to prevent alloimmunization and refractorines to platelet transfusions. N Engl J Med 337:1861–1869, 1997.

51. Dzik, WH: Component therapy before bedside procedures. In Mintz, PD (ed): Transfusion Therapy Clinical Principles and Practice, 2nd ed. AABB Press, Bethesda, MD, 2005, pp 1–26.

52. Pisciotto, PT, and Luban, NLC: Complications of neonatal transfusion. In Popovsky, MA (ed): Transfusion Reactions, 3rd ed. AABB Press, Bethesda, MD, 2007, pp 459–499.

Chapter 17

Cellular Therapy

Melanie S. Kennedy, MD, and Scott Scrape, MD

OBJECTIVES

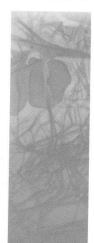

1. List and define the categories of hematopoietic progenitor cell (HPC) donors.
2. List five assessments of an HPC donor.
3. Name a registry for HPC unrelated donors.
4. State the chance of an HLA match between siblings.
5. Describe the differences in health screening of cord blood donors compared with other HPC donors.
6. Compare and contrast the collection of HPC-M and HPC-A.
7. Name the antigen that defines HPCs.
8. Identify three diseases treated with HPC transplantation.
9. Explain the reason few HPC transplants are performed for nonmalignant diseases.
10. List five tests performed on all HPC products.
11. Explain when cultures are necessary during processing of HPCs.
12. State the temperature for frozen storage of HPCs.
13. Identify the cryoprotectant generally used for HPCs.
14. List two methods of determining HPC viability.
15. Describe the freezing process of HPCs.

Continued

OBJECTIVES—cont'd

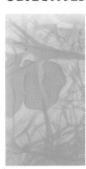

16. Contrast myeloablative with nonmyeloablative recipient conditioning.
17. Compare major, minor, and bidirectional ABO incompatibility between HPC donor and recipient.
18. Define engraftment for neutrophils, platelets, and all cell lines.
19. Define graft-versus-host disease (GVHD).
20. Define acute versus chronic GVHD.
21. State the purpose of donor lymphocyte infusion.
22. List three important conditions to prevent when transfusing blood products.
23. Select the correct ABO type(s) when transfusing RBCs and plasma to a B recipient with an O donor.

Introduction

Cellular therapy encompasses a wide variety of cells for transplantation. This chapter will focus on the cells used for blood and bone marrow transplantation. The bone marrow contains the **hematopoietic stem cells** (HSC) from which all the cells of the blood are formed. These stem cells differentiate into hematopoietic progenitor cells (HPC), which are committed to specific cell lines. The myeloid line differentiates into erythrocytes, platelets, neutrophils, basophils, eosinophils, monocytes, and macrophages. The lymphoid line forms dendritic cells and lymphocytes, including T cells, B cells, and **NK cells**. Therefore, a bone marrow transplant repopulates not only myeloid cells (erythrocytes, platelets, and granulocytes), but also lymphocytes and **dendritic cells**.

The population of hematopoietic stem cells in the bone marrow is small, about 0.01%. These cells are not a uniform population but are in varying states of development. As they mature, the daughter cells commit to specific cell lines and are known as **hematopoietic progenitor cells** (HPC).

Purpose and Goals of HPC Transplantation

HPCs are collected and transplanted for three main reasons: (1) to serve as bone marrow replacement following total-body irradiation or chemotherapy given to treat primary marrow and nonmarrow disorders, (2) to provide a graft-versus-leukemia (or tumor) reaction, or (3) to replenish diseased or destroyed bone marrow.

Categories of Transplantation

HPC transplants fall into three general categories: autologous, allogeneic, and syngeneic (Box 17–1). **Autologous** means the source of HPCs is the patient, who donates the cells for transplantation. **Allogeneic** includes both related and unrelated donors. **Syngeneic** is when the donor and recipient are identical twins. The type of transplantation used is dependent on, among other things, the type of disease being treated and the availability of the donor.

Autologous bone marrow or peripheral blood HPCs are selected for most patients, especially those with marrow

---

> **BOX 17–1**
>
> ### Categories of HPCs for Transplantation
>
> Autologous
> - From self
>
> Allogeneic
> - From one human to another
> - Related or unrelated
>
> Syngeneic
> - Identical twin or triplet

malignancies or metastatic solid tumors. These individuals are generally in disease remission, so the blood or bone marrow is less likely to be contaminated with malignant cells.

Allogeneic HPC transplantation is used for patients who cannot donate their own cells because of multiple cycles of chemotherapy, irradiation of bone marrow, disease in marrow (e.g., aplastic anemia), or genetic disease. There is a one in four chance of an HLA match with siblings for a related transplant, so many patients must receive HPCs from an unrelated, HLA-matched, or mismatched donor (Box 17–2). These donors are often registered with the National Marrow Donor Program (NMDP) or are part of other registries.

Syngeneic HPC transplantation is performed infrequently because of the relative rarity of identical twins or triplets. Identical twins or triplets do not have minor histocompatibility differences, which means graft rejection, graft-versus-host disease, or graft versus leukemia does not

---

> **BOX 17–2**
>
> ### HLA Matching for Related Transplantation
>
> Sibling—HLA
> - 25% identical
> - 50% one haplotype
> - 25% mismatch
>
> Parents—HLA
> - 100% one haplotype

occur. In contrast, HLA-matched siblings have minor incompatibilities, which can cause graft-versus-host disease.

Donor/Patient Selection

The FDA regulates transplantation similar to that of blood donors, except that the HPC donors undergo greater scrutiny because of the increased risks associated with the HPC donation process.[1] Each donor's workup includes a complete history and physical, lab tests, EKG, chest x-ray, donor health history, and extensive informed consent. Infectious disease marker tests are required for HBsAg, anti-HBc, HCV NAT, anti-HCV; HIV-1,-2 NAT, anti-HIV-1,-2; HTLV-I,-II NAT; and syphilis. Other tests that may be performed are WNV NAT, HBV NAT, anti-CMV, and others, as indicated.

Autologous Donors/Patients

Autologous donors are usually patients who have a hematologic malignancy. The patient should be in clinical remission to decrease the risk of collecting malignant cells with the HPCs. Pulmonary function tests and cardiac stress tests are performed, as are the tests listed above. Infectious disease testing is important for the autologous donor because of possible reactivation after the transplant. Also, if positive, the HPC product is stored to prevent cross-contamination of other products.

Unrelated Donors and National Marrow Donor Program

Allogeneic unrelated donors are selected from a registry, such as the National Marrow Donor Program (NMDP), which is the largest registry in the world (Box 17–3). These donors previously agreed to join the registry and have basic information, such as ABO, Rh, and HLA type recorded. The NMDP's goal is to match 90% of requests, although the percentage is less for ethnic and racial minorities. The NMDP has targeted these underrepresented groups for recruiting drives to increase the HLA diversity of the registry.

The recipient's institution initiates the search for the best matched donor. After the search, the selected donor is contacted for initial screening and more testing, including high-resolution (DNA) HLA typing (see Chapter 21, "The HLA System"). After the donor's workup, the recipient's institution accepts the match and selects dates for the transplant.

The donor selects the most convenient date for the donation. After HPCs are collected, the fresh product is shipped to the recipient's institution. The recipient may be anywhere in the world that has an HPC transplant program.

Related Donors

Siblings or other related donors are screened and tested as outlined above for unrelated donors. Health history and infectious disease testing may reveal sensitive information, such as high-risk sexual behavior. The donor must agree for the information to be shared with the recipient, so the recipient can give informed consent for the transplant. If the related donor does not agree, the donor cannot proceed to HPC collection.

Umbilical Cord Blood

The NMDP also coordinates umbilical cord blood transplants, locating the appropriate cord blood bank that has the best matched cord blood. Cord blood is most appropriate for children needing transplantation because of their smaller size. Cord blood is immunologically naïve, so there is less risk of graft-versus-host disease than with adult HPCs. In addition, HLA mismatches are better tolerated by the recipient.

Before delivery, the mother must consent to the collection of umbilical cord blood. The mother is screened for health issues, infectious disease risks, and family history for genetic diseases. The cord blood is collected at or after delivery, with no risk to the mother or infant.

HPC Collection

HPCs intended for transplantation are collected in one of three ways: bone marrow collection, known as HPC-marrow (HPC-M); peripheral blood progenitor cell (leukapheresis) collection, called HPC-apheresis (HPC-A); and umbilical cord blood collection, referred to as HPC-cord (HPC-C).

Bone Marrow Collection (HPC-M)

Bone marrow is harvested similar to a diagnostic bone marrow aspiration, except with a stronger and longer needle. The procedure must be done using general or epidural anesthesia. The posterior iliac crest is the most frequently used. Multiple aspirations are performed, moving the needle within the skin puncture to various points within the marrow and making additional bone marrow punctures. The marrow aspirates are transferred within a sterile system. The usual volume goal for marrow is 10 to 15 mL/kg, using the weight of the donor or recipient, whoever is smaller, with 1,500 mL or more collected.

Because of the volume collected, some donors may need RBC transfusion. Many donors donate their own blood days to weeks before the HPC-M collection to be transfused during or after the collection.

The risks of HPC-M collection include anesthesia, pain (acute and chronic), bruising, allogeneic blood transfusion, and, in rare cases, nerve damage.

BOX 17–3

National Marrow Donor Program (NMDP)

- Contains the largest registry of recruited donors
- Coordinates searches for HLA-matched adult donors and cord blood
- Recruits donors to provide match for 90% of recipients
- Emphasizes recruitment of racial and ethnic minorities for HLA diversity
- Provides for collection and transport of the HPC product

Leukapheresis (HPC-A)

HPCs are more frequently harvested from peripheral blood by **leukapheresis** (see Chapter 14, "Apheresis"). Because few HPCs are in circulating blood (0.05%), numerous days would be required to collect sufficient quantities for a successful transplant. However, if the HPCs are "mobilized" from the marrow to the peripheral blood with cytokines, the number of leukapheresis procedures can usually be reduced to one or two. The leukapheresis procedure generally processes 3 to 4 blood volumes to collect a product of 150 to 500 mL. The higher volumes are the result of the difficulty in stabilizing the white cell layer during the collection.

Autologous donors (patients) also may be given chemotherapy to take advantage of the rebound of the bone marrow and the increase in circulating HPCs (Box 17–4). The donors receive the cytokine analog, **granulocyte colony-stimulating factor** (G-CSF) filgrastim to stimulate the release of more HPCs into the peripheral blood. Less commonly, **granulocyte-macrophage colony-stimulating factor** (GM-CSF) is used. The usual dose of either cytokine analog is 10 μg per kilogram of body weight per day (10 μg/kg/day).

Allogeneic donors, mobilized by G-CSF, are collected on day 5 and, if needed, day 6. These donors do not receive chemotherapy. Autologous donors may be slower to mobilize and need more time to achieve a high enough HPC level to be collected. A few may require plerixafor, an antagonist to the chemokine receptor 4 on CD34+ cells, to aid in mobilization.

As a side effect of these cytokines, the donor may have bone pain from the marrow expansion. Other side effects may include headache, myalgia (muscle pain), nausea and vomiting, fatigue, and insomnia. These signs and symptoms quickly resolve when the collection meets the goal and the G-CSF (and plerixafor) is discontinued. Commonly, the platelet count decreases with cytokine stimulation and HPC collection. A few donors need platelet transfusions. Rare side effects are chronic thrombocytopenia and splenic bleeding.

Umbilical Cord Blood (HPC-C)

Umbilical cord blood is rich in HPCs and is another donor source for transplantation. Although umbilical cord blood is used less frequently than HPC-A products for transplantation, the rate of cord blood transplant is increasing as the availability increases.[2]

Cord blood is collected after the baby's delivery and clamping of the cord and either before or after delivery of the placenta (Box 17–5). Most collections are performed soon after delivery of the placenta either in the sterile delivery room or a separate sterile room. The HPC-C is collected by gravity into a FDA-approved collection bag containing CPD anticoagulant, using a needle or cannula in the cord blood vessel. Only 100 to 150 ml are usually collected.[3] The collection is of no risk to the mother or infant.

Detection and Measurement of HPCs

HPCs can be identified by, among other things, the presence of the surface CD34 antigen and the absence of lineage-specific antigens. The **CD34 antigen** is a cell surface transmembrane protein expressed on hematopoietic progenitor cells and vascular endothelium throughout the body. The CD34 antigen is used routinely to determine when a patient or donor should be collected by leukapheresis. Cellular therapy labs measure CD34+ cells to determine the quantity of HPCs harvested by bone marrow, apheresis, or cord blood collection. The HPCs in a sample can be quantified by flow cytometry using antibody to the CD34 antigen. HPCs also express HLA, but not ABO blood group antigens.

The CD34 antigen is measured in autologous and allogeneic donors who are to be collected by leukapheresis. The donor should have a minimum of 10 CD34+ cells/μL in the peripheral blood for collection to begin. The collection goal for an adult is 2 to 6 × 10⁶ CD34 positive cells per kilogram of recipient body weight ($2–6 \times 10^6$/kg). Generally, the yield of CD34+ cells is less for autologous than for allogeneic donors, so more days of collection are required.

Indications for Transplantation

The most common indication for HPC transplantation is to treat malignant diseases, such as acute leukemia, chronic myelogenous leukemia, multiple myeloma, Hodgkin's disease and non-Hodgkin's lymphoma, and solid childhood tumors (Box 17–6). HPC transplantation can extend survival and cure disease.[4,5] However, the risks must be weighed against the chance of recurrence of the malignancy and expected survival.

BOX 17–4

Leukapheresis (HPC-A) Mobilization

Autologous
- Granulocyte colony-stimulating factor (G-CSF)
- Chemotherapy
- Plerixafor

Allogeneic
- G-CSF

BOX 17–5

Umbilical Cord Blood (HPC-C) Collection

- Mother delivered infant and cord clamped
- Collect from placenta through cord blood vessel
- 100 to 150 mL volume
- No risk for mother or infant

HPC transplants are also performed for nonmalignant diseases, such as aplastic anemia, severe combined immunodeficiency disease (SCID), and Wiskott-Aldrich syndrome.[6] Inborn metabolic disorders such as adrenoleukodystrophy, mucopolysaccharidoses, and lysosomal disorders have also been treated with HPC transplants.

Multiple clinical trials are assessing the success of HPC transplants in other disorders such as multiple sclerosis, paroxysmal nocturnal hemoglobinuria, and sickle cell disease. Even though thousands of HPC transplantations are performed each year, it remains a risky procedure with multiple possible complications. Currently, the risk of fatal complications of allogeneic transplantation ranges from 20% to 60%, which is too high for HPC transplantation to gain wide acceptance in the treatment of nonmalignant and nonhematologic conditions.[6] Some studies have also reported the use of HPCs to regenerate muscle, liver, bone, blood vessels, and brain tissue.[7–9]

Processing HPC Products

The cellular therapy laboratory receives the HPC products from the collection facilities for further processing, storage, and transportation. The lab is essential to assure the quality and quantity of the product before storage, transportation, and dispensing. Careful labeling and preventing mix-ups during processing and storage are fundamental. Processing must meet the regulations of the FDA[1] and should meet the requirements of the AABB *Standards for Cellular Therapy Product Services*.[10]

Initial Testing

Upon receipt, the product is examined for proper labeling, clumps of platelets, hemolysis, and integrity of the collection container. A sample from the product is tested for CBC, platelets, WBC differential, CD34+ cells (HPCs), and viability. Sampling is performed in a laminar flow hood, with the use of a sterile connecting device or integral sampling tubes attached to the collection set.

Cell counts are usually performed on automated instruments, with the differential confirmed manually to confirm mononuclear cells, which contain the HPCs. CD34+ cells are determined by flow cytometry, and viability can also be determined by flow, using markers for **apoptosis**. Viability is traditionally determined by dye exclusion, as dead cells cannot exclude the dye from their cytoplasm.

Bacterial and fungal cultures may be performed at several steps of processing. Culture is required after product is prepared for infusion to the recipient. If a culture is positive, antibiotic sensitivity is determined so the appropriate antibiotic(s) can be given to the recipient when the product is infused.[11]

Initial Processing

Bone marrow products are filtered to remove bone spicules, fat, and debris. An automated cell separator device can be used to separate the buffy coat (nucleated WBC) from the RBCs and plasma. Another way to concentrate the buffy coat is to use a sedimenting agent such as Ficoll, dextran, or hydroxyethyl starch (HES). These agents form a density gradient using centrifugation, with the plasma or supernatant on top, the RBCs on the bottom, and the **buffy coat** (containing WBC, HPCs, and platelets) in between. The buffy coat is resuspended in autologous plasma or a balanced salt solution and dextrose. This process is used to deplete RBCs and plasma for major and minor ABO incompatibility and to reduce volume for frozen storage.[12]

Allogeneic and syngeneic HPCs collected from bone marrow or peripheral blood are usually transplanted fresh or are stored 24 to 72 hours at 20°C to 24°C or at 4°C. The product is labeled with standard ISBT bar codes, and a tag with the patient's name, medical record number, and other identifying information is attached before release from the laboratory. The product is then infused into the recipient.

Preparation for Freezing HPCs

Autologous HPCs are frozen while the donor or recipient is prepared for the transplant. The volume of the collected product is reduced to limit the aliquots for freezing, and RBCs are removed from bone marrow products, because the freezing and thawing process causes the cells to lyse and release **nephrotoxic** hemoglobin and RBC stroma. HPC-A products have a smaller RBC volume, with hematocrit of 3% to 10% in a volume from 150 to 500 ml. The larger products need to be volume reduced before freezing. Contaminating granulocytes, which are higher in HPC-A products, can cause febrile reactions with chills in the recipient because of lysing during thawing.

After processing, the products are transferred to freezing bags in small aliquots of about 45 to 70 ml. The cryoprotective chemicals—dimethyl sulfoxide (DMSO) or DMSO and hydroxyethyl starch (HES)—are slowly added to a final concentration of 5% to 10% DMSO.[13] DMSO and HES cross the cell membrane and protect the cells from ice damage and cell dehydration during the freezing and thawing process. The amount of DMSO needs to be limited because of its toxicity. For that reason, many labs concentrate the buffy coat as much as possible and thus reduce the DMSO required.

Umbilical Cord Blood Processing

Umbilical cord blood requires special processing. Both the mother's blood sample and the cord blood are tested for ABO, Rh, and, for the mother's sample, antibodies (Box 17–7). The product is tested for the total nucleated cell (TNC) count and the CD34 content. Testing for **hemoglobinopathies** is performed. Serologic and DNA testing for HLA A, B, and DRB1 is performed on both mother and cord to assure no mix-ups occurred. It is wise to store samples of viable cells and DNA of both the cord and the mother.

The maternal sample is tested for HIV-1,-2; HBV; HCV; and HTLV-I,-II. Also, HBsAg, anti-HBc, and syphilis status is determined. The cord blood is cultured for cytomegalovirus (CMV). In some cases, WNV by nucleic acid tests (NAT) is performed.

Several ways of processing the cord blood product exist; one method is described. The cord blood is diluted with dextran and albumin or hetastarch, which improves the viability of the HPCs. The cells are allowed to sediment, and the buffy coat and plasma are transferred to another bag. Centrifugation is used to separate and then remove plasma. The final volume is about 20 ml. Then 5 mL of 50% DMSO is slowly added for a final content of 10%. At the end of processing, a sample from the product is tested for viability and cell count. Bacterial and fungal cultures are performed.

To prevent mix-ups, one national cord blood bank uses a master bar code label that can be scanned to generate additional labels for transfer bags and the final aliquots.

Cell Enrichment

CD34+ cells can be separated from the other cells by a device using antibodies and magnetic beads with attached antibodies. Mouse anti-CD34 is incubated with the product, magnetic beads with sheep antimouse are added, and the cells are separated by magnetic force, giving an enriched product of CD34+ cells. Another method of enrichment is fluorescent cell sorting.

Cell Purging and Reduction

Unfortunately, leukemic cells also are mobilized from the marrow by **cytokine** therapy and are collected by HPC-A. Bone marrow can also contain leukemic precursors. The cellular laboratory can use a process called *cell purging* to remove the malignant cells from the HPCs. Antibodies specific for the malignant cell antigen can be used to bind and then remove (purge) the malignant cells.

T, B, and NK cells can be reduced by using antibodies to specific antigens that define these cells. The risk of graft-versus-host disease is reduced, but the rate of relapse is increased.

Product Storage and Shipping

Factors involved with product storage and shipping include shipping fresh products, freezing for long-term frozen storage, shipping frozen products, and thawing and preparing products for transplant.

Shipping Fresh Products

Fresh products can be shipped by air for long distances at room temperature or at 4°C. An insulated container with cooling packs at appropriate temperature should be used to ship the product. Complete paperwork must accompany the product for security checks and customs. A courier hand-carrying the product, as practiced by the NMDP, can avoid irradiation of the product by airport security x-ray, which would damage the HPCs.

Long-Term Frozen Storage

The HPCs are best preserved in liquid nitrogen below −196°C or in the vapor phase (just above the liquid nitrogen). A disadvantage of the vapor phase is that as the level of liquid nitrogen lowers, the temperature at the top of the vapor phase is warmer and further increases when the freezer is opened. However, the cells need steady temperature, as warming damages them. A problem with the liquid phase is that it can harbor viruses and can cross-contaminate the products. Careful processing so that the bags are clean externally and the canisters are cleaned after breakage lessens the chance of cross-contamination. Some cellular therapy labs use an overwrap to quarantine products.

The freezing rate must be controlled, as either too slow or too fast freezing can damage the cells and reduce viability. The best rate is 1°C to 3°C per minute. Automatic controlled rate freezers are available for this purpose.

Mechanical −80°C freezers are also used for short-term storage of weeks to 2 years. This method does not require controlled-rate freezing.

Freezers must have alarms that are monitored 24 hours a day, 7 days a week to prevent loss of products. Backup freezers must be readily available in case a freezer fails.

Shipping Frozen Products

Frozen HPC products can be shipped short distances in liquid nitrogen; however, the shipping container must be kept upright. The canister has a large mouth opening to accommodate the bags, leading to dangerous situations for the shipping company and loss of the HPC product. Available are "dry shippers," which are packed with absorbent material

---

BOX 17–7

Cord Blood Testing

- ABO and Rh
- CD34 cells and TNC
- Hemoglobinopathies
- HLA A, B, DRB1
- Infectious diseases
- Antibody screen—mother

for the liquid nitrogen. Dry shippers are much safer and can be shipped longer distances.

Thawing and Preparing Products for Transplant

Thawing and preparing the HPCs for transplant includes testing the product for TNC count, CD34 count, and viability and culturing for contamination. Each product bag must be thawed quickly at 37°C and infused through the recipient's IV within 1 to 2 hours. Significant loss of HPCs has been found when the product is kept at room temperature for a short time. Some transplant units thaw each bag at the bedside to minimize delay in starting the infusion.

The thawed products can be washed, especially if DMSO toxicity is a problem for the recipient. Based on recipient body weight, no more than 10 ml/kg of a product having 10% DMSO should be given during one infusion.

Transplanting the Recipient

The conditioning of the recipient includes gamma irradiation, high-dose chemotherapy, or both to ablate (eliminate) the recipient's marrow and immune system. In this way, the recipient can accept the HPC transplant. Most conditioning regimens completely ablate the bone marrow and immune system. Once this conditioning has occurred, the recipient must receive a transplant or he or she will die. The transplant is thus "rescue."

More recently, some recipients have received nonmyeloablative conditioning, which allows part of their bone marrow and immune system to survive. The theory is to establish a stable **chimerism** (two cell populations) so that donor cells recognize malignant cells as foreign and destroy them. Potential recipients who are not suitable for **myeloablative** conditioning may be candidates for **nonmyeloablative** transplantation. These recipients include those who have serious comorbidity or are elderly.

Infusion of HPCs

Fresh products (allogeneic) are infused slowly to minimize volume overload and adverse reactions. Leukapheresis products can be infused over an hour or two, and bone marrow, because of the larger volume, can be infused over 2 to 4 hours. The tradition was not to use a filter, although a regular blood transfusion filter has been recommended more recently. A

Table 17–1	ABO Incompatibility		
	RECIPIENT	**DONOR**	**POSSIBLE OUTCOME**
Major	O	A	Hemolysis of donor RBCs Delayed RBC engraftment
Minor	A	O	Hemolysis of recipient RBCs Passenger lymphocyte syndrome

leukocyte-reduction filter must never be used because many of the HPCs would be removed.

ABO Incompatibility

ABO-incompatible products require special care. Major incompatibility occurs when the recipient has ABO antibody against the donor; for example, the recipient is group O and the donor is A (Table 17–1). The recipient's plasma contains anti-A, which can hemolyze the donor RBCs in the product. Because HPC-A and HPC-C products have only a few milliliters of RBCs, a serious hemolytic reaction is less likely. However, bone marrow contains a much higher portion of RBCs, requiring the cellular therapy laboratory to remove most of the RBCs and thus prevent a serious acute hemolytic reaction. The recipient may also have delayed RBC engraftment if group O RBCs containing anti-A are selected for transfusion.[14]

Minor ABO incompatibility is less likely to cause adverse reaction. In **Table 17–1**, the first recipient is A and the donor is O. The donor may have high-titered anti-A or anti-A,B, which may cause hemolysis of the recipient's group A cells. In addition, the donor's T lymphocytes are primed to make anti-A and may cause ongoing hemolysis of the recipient's RBCs and may attack other cells bearing the A antigen. This is called **passenger lymphocyte syndrome**.

Bidirectional mismatches have both major and minor ABO incompatibility (Table 17–2). Thus, both the recipient and the graft may have adverse effects following the transplant.

More than one donor cord blood may be selected for transplant to an adult or teenager. The two or three cords are selected for HLA match, so as many as three different ABO types may be infused. However, cord blood products are RBC and plasma reduced, so ABO reactions are less frequent than when bone marrow is used.

Table 17–2	Major, Minor, and Bidirectional ABO Incompatibility for Donors and Recipients			
	RECIPIENT			
ABO Type (Antibody Produced)	**A (anti-B)**	**B (anti-A)**	**AB**	**O (anti-A, anti-B)**
Donor				
A (anti-B)	Matched	Bidirectional mismatch	Minor mismatch	Major mismatch
B (anti-A)	Bidirectional mismatch	Matched	Minor mismatch	Major mismatch
AB	Major mismatch	Major mismatch	Matched	Major mismatch

Adverse Recipient Reactions

The recipient may receive premedication to lessen or avoid reactions, similar to the process for blood transfusion.[15] DMSO has an odor like the sulfur in garlic or rotten eggs, so the recipient may have this odor. The most common adverse reactions are flushing and nausea. In addition, vomiting and changes in heart rate and blood pressure may occur.

Contamination with granulocytes may lead to fever and chills because of the release of cytoplasmic granules and their content by freezing and thawing.[16] Red blood cells are not preserved by DMSO, so the free hemoglobin and red blood cell stroma may lead to renal damage.

Other transplant-related complications include liver or lung toxicity caused by myeloablative chemotherapy, which, in the autologous recipient, may mimic graft-versus-host disease.

Engraftment

After the HPC products are infused, engraftment should occur. Early engraftment is generally defined as the interval from transplant to the absolute neutrophil count greater than 500/μL. This occurs in 9 to 30 days. Platelet engraftment is defined as platelet count greater than 20,000/μL without transfusion and requires 15 or more days. RBC engraftment and immune reconstitution occurs 90 days or longer. The standard measurement of success is engraftment of all three cell lines at 100 days. The rate of engraftment varies by the source of the HPCs, the number and viability of CD34+ cells, cellular processing, the conditioning regimen of the recipient, and other variables.[17] For example, engraftment of neutrophils and platelets occur earlier with higher CD34 counts in the HPC product. Cord blood and leukapheresis products generally engraft earlier than bone marrow products. However, because of the smaller CD34+ cell dose in cord blood, engraftment can be delayed or, in about 20%, never occur. Cord blood transplantation is most successful in children weighing less than 45 kg. Transplanting two or three HPC-C products may be used successfully in children weighing more than 45 kg and in adults. The longer the engraftment takes, the higher the risk of severe viral or fungal infection. Major ABO mismatch can also delay RBC engraftment.

Graft Rejection

Graft rejection can occur in the nonmyeloablative transplant, in which host cells can mount an immunological response to the graft. Graft rejection is mediated by T cells or NK cells. Also, a graft mismatched for HLA and sex has a higher risk of graft rejection.

Graft-Versus-Host Disease

Graft-versus-host disease (GVHD) is mediated by the T cells that are transplanted with allogeneic HPC products. Cord blood transplants, even with HLA mismatch, are less likely to cause severe GVHD than other sources of HPCs.

Acute GVHD is defined as occurring within the first 100 days and **chronic GVHD** after 100 days.[18] About 25% to 50% of allogeneic recipients develop chronic GVHD.[19] The most affected body sites are the skin, gastrointestinal tract, liver, lung, and eyes (Table 17–3). **Immunosuppressive** drugs are required to treat GVHD, which increases the risk of infection.

Relapse of Disease and Donor Lymphocyte Infusion

Leukemia and lymphoma can reoccur because of inadequate conditioning or contamination of the autologous graft. The incidence of relapse is lower in recipients with chronic GVHD. With allogeneic transplants, the donor can be asked to donate another leukapheresis with the goal to collect T cells to attack the malignancy. The process is called *donor leukocyte infusion* (DLI). For DLI collection, the donor is not stimulated with cytokines, such as G-CSF or plerixafor.

The purpose of DLI is to induce graft versus leukemia, which can aid in controlling the leukemia or lymphoma relapse. DLI works best for CML and less well for other hematologic malignancies.

Outcomes

Following myeloablative therapy, autologous HPC transplantation has proved to provide an improved quality of life and increased disease-free survival for patients with multiple myeloma, acute myelogenous leukemia (AML), non-Hodgkin's lymphoma, and Hodgkin's disease. Several cancer centers have also proven the benefits of two sequential autologous transplants for patients with multiple myeloma.

Allogeneic transplants have had less success, mainly because of acute GVHD and infections caused by immunosuppressive therapy.

Transfusion Therapy for HPC Transplantation

Once a patient is recognized as an HPC transplant candidate, the blood bank personnel should be vigilant to provide blood products which prevent alloimmunization to HLA antigens, CMV infection, or graft-versus-host disease. This can be accomplished with cellular products that have been leukocyte

Table 17–3	Graft-Versus-Host Disease
BODY SITES	**SIGNS AND SYMPTOMS**
Skin	Rash, scarring
Liver	Jaundice, elevated enzymes, cirrhosis
Lung	Dyspnea, decreased oxygen
Gastrointestinal system	Ulcers, nausea, vomiting, diarrhea
Eyes	Dryness, photophobia

reduced, gamma-irradiated, and, in special circumstances, CMV seronegative.

HLA Alloimmunization

Leukocyte-reduced cellular products help to minimize the incidence of **alloimmunization** to HLA antigens. HLA alloimmunization can interfere with platelet transfusion support in the critical pre- and post-transplantation periods. Platelet engraftment may be delayed weeks, leading to increased risk of hemorrhage if the patient is refractory to platelet transfusion.

In the multi-institutional Trial to Reduce Alloimmunization to Platelets (TRAP) study,[20] a significant number of patients (17% to 20%) developed HLA antibodies, even though all of their RBC and platelet components had been leukocyte reduced. However, leukocyte reduction decreases the incidence of HLA antibodies and is believed to benefit patients on platelet therapy.

Some studies have shown that minimizing the HLA alloimmunization may reduce the incidence of complement fixing HLA antibodies, which may result in a positive serological HLA crossmatch with the donor before HPC transplantation.[21] These recipients are at increased risk of graft rejection with an HLA-mismatched related donor and perhaps with an unrelated HLA-matched donor.

CMV Transmission

Leukocyte-reduced products benefit HPC transplantation candidates and recipients by decreasing the risk of transfusion-transmitted CMV infections. CMV-seropositive rates among whole blood donors in different areas of the United States range from 40% to 80%.[22,23] However, very few CMV-seropositive donors have active CMV infections.

Allogeneic recipients are immunosuppressed because of drugs used to treat acute and chronic GVHD. Thus, these recipients are at risk for acquiring a life-threatening CMV infection from a CMV-infective blood component.[24] The use of CMV-seronegative or leukocyte-reduced cellular components decreases the risk of CMV transmission.

The supporting data for leukocyte-reduced or CMV seronegative products were obtained from studies of neonatal and hematologic malignancy patients and anecdotally applied to HPC transplantation recipients. Although no formal recommendations exist for how long CMV-seronegative patients should use CMV-seronegative blood, a prudent course may be to continue use until immunosuppression is withdrawn.

For CMV-seropositive recipients, the most common cause of CMV disease is reactivation of latent CMV from prior exposure. Therefore, CMV seronegative blood products are not recommended for seropositive recipients.

Transfusion-Associated Graft-Versus-Host Disease

Transfusion-associated graft versus disease (TA-GVHD) is caused by donor T lymphocytes engrafting in a susceptible immunosuppressed host. Donor lymphocytes can cause a type of **microchimerism**, surviving for months to years in the recipient's circulation.[25] Although TA-GVHD is uncommon, the mortality rate is over 90%. The clinical symptoms may include fever, **maculopapular** rash, bloody diarrhea, or **pancytopenia** and may begin 1 to 4 weeks after transfusion.

Gamma irradiation for all cellular blood components is recommended in the pre-HPC transplantation period and when a patient is considered a potential HPC transplant candidate. Irradiation is required, beginning at conditioning. The recommended dose of radiation is 2,500 cGy to the center of a freestanding irradiation canister, with a minimum of 1,500 cGy at any other area of the canister. Usually, the patient receives irradiated blood products for life, but no studies are available to support this practice.

Transfusion in ABO-Mismatched Transplant

ABO-mismatched transplants present interesting transfusion problems. RBCs and platelets or plasma will have separate preferred ABO blood groups in most cases (Table 17–4). The table is based on the selection of the ABO blood groups that are compatible with both the recipient and the donor.

In the first line of Table 17–4, both the donor and the recipient can receive group O RBCs, so group O is selected for RBCs. For plasma and platelets, anti-A must be avoided, so A or AB products are selected. If group A or AB platelets are unavailable, the next choice would be group O. In the second line of the table, the recipient is A and the donor is B (bidirectional). Group O is the only choice for RBCs. To avoid anti-A- or anti-B-containing plasma or platelets, AB is preferred, with B as the second choice and A the third choice. An important point is that group O plasma or platelets should be avoided except in unusual circumstances, such as when HLA-matched platelets are required and the preferred ABO group is not available.

As the HPC cells engraft, the recipient will slowly become the donor's ABO group. In the first line of the table, the A RBCs of the recipient will become fewer over several weeks, eventually becoming undetectable. During that time, small proportions of donor group O cells will be detected as mixed-field reactions. Eventually, the recipient will type as group O, generally at the same time as RBC engraftment is achieved.

In the second line of the table, the group A recipient has anti-B, so the group B donor RBCs may be hemolyzed during the infusion. In addition, the engraftment of RBCs may be delayed because of the circulating anti-B. Only group O RBCs or AB plasma and platelets should be transfused. Eventually, the donor's B cells will engraft in the recipient, with the loss of the recipient's anti-B. Generally, the donor's lymphocytes will not make anti-A because of the A antigens on the recipient's endothelial tissue.

In all ABO-incompatible transplants, transfusing the blood groups of choice for RBCs, plasma, and platelets is extremely important to prevent hemolysis and delayed RBC engraftment.

Table 17–4 Selection of ABO Blood Products

ABO Recipient	ABO Donor	ABO OF BLOOD COMPONENT			
		Red Cells	FFP	Platelets	
				1st choice	2nd, 3rd choice
A	O	O	A, AB	A, AB	O
A	B	O	AB	AB	B, A
A	AB	A	AB	AB	A, B
B	O	O	B, AB	B, AB	O
B	A	O	AB	AB	A, B
B	AB	B	AB	AB	B, A
AB	O	O	AB	AB	A, B
AB	A	A	AB	AB	A, B
AB	B	B	AB	AB	B, A
O	A	O	A, AB	A, AB	B, O
O	B	O	B, AB	B, AB	A, O
O	AB	O	AB	AB	A, B

CASE STUDIES

Case Study 17-1

A 45-year-old man is diagnosed with non-Hodgkin's lymphoma. He types as B, Rh-positive. His brother is found to be HLA matched but is A, Rh-positive. The brother donates HPC-A, which is transplanted in the patient on January 25, 2010. The patient requires long-term transfusion support and receives 47 RBCs, 56 platelets apheresis, 16 FFP, and 6 cryoprecipitate.

1. Which blood group(s) should be selected for the RBC transfusions?
2. For FFP and platelets, which blood type(s) should be selected?

The patient's ABO testing for specific days post-transplant is shown below.

DAY POST-TRANSPLANTATION	ANTI-A	ANTI-B	A CELLS	B CELLS
Day 117	0	1+ (mf)	1+	0
Day 147	0	wk (mf)	2+	0
Day 156	0	0	1+	0
Day 200	wk (mf)	0	0	0

mf = mixed field

3. What is the interpretation of his ABO group on day 147?
4. What is the blood group interpretation on day 200? On day 156?

SUMMARY CHART

- ✔ The categories of HPC donors are autologous (self), allogeneic (another person, related or unrelated), and syngeneic (twin or triplet).
- ✔ HPC donors are assessed by history and physical, lab tests, EKG, chest x-ray, and donor health history.
- ✔ The National Marrow Donor Program (NMDP) recruits donors, stores data, and searches for donors requested by recipient institutions.
- ✔ A recipient has a 25% chance of an HLA match with a sibling.
- ✔ Umbilical cord blood donation requires the consent, history, and lab testing of the mother.
- ✔ HPC-M is the collection of bone marrow by aspiration. The donor undergoes general or epidural anesthesia and may need RBC transfusion.
- ✔ HPC-A is the collection of HPCs from the peripheral blood by leukapheresis. The HPCs are mobilized by cytokine.
- ✔ Transplantation is used to treat leukemia, lymphoma, and multiple myeloma.
- ✔ Allogeneic transplantation is not routinely used for nonmalignant diseases because of the serious risks.
- ✔ HPC products are tested for CBC, WBC differential, CD34+ cells, and viability.
- ✔ Bacterial and fungal cultures are required after thawing.
- ✔ HPCs are stored at 20°C to 25°C or 4°C and −196°C.
- ✔ DMSO is used as a cryoprotectant.
- ✔ Viability can be determined by dye exclusion or by flow cytometry.

- ✔ Freezing of HPCs requires the slow addition of DMSO and freezing in a controlled-rate freezer at 1°C to 3°C/min.
- ✔ Myeloablative conditioning completely destroys the bone marrow and the immune system. Nonmyeloablative conditioning partially destroys bone marrow and the immune system.
- ✔ Major ABO incompatibility in HPC transplantation is when the donor's RBCs are incompatible with the recipient's antibody.
- ✔ Minor ABO incompatibility is when the donor's plasma is incompatible with the recipient's RBCs.
- ✔ Engraftment is defined as PMNs greater than 500/μL (about 10 days) and platelets greater than 20,000/ μL (about 15 days), and recipient is no longer RBC transfusion dependent (90 to 100 days).
- ✔ Graft-versus-host disease is defined as donor T cells attacking the recipient's cells and tissues.
- ✔ Acute GVHD occurs during the first 100 days after transplant; chronic occurs after 100 days.
- ✔ Donor lymphocyte infusion is used to treat relapse of chronic myelogenous leukemia.
- ✔ In HPC transplant recipients, leukocyte-reduced and irradiated cellular products are selected to reduce the risk of HLA alloimmunization, CMV transmission, and GVHD. CMV seronegative cellular blood products may also be selected.
- ✔ The blood type selected for blood transfusion must be compatible with both the donor and the recipient.

Review Questions

1. Which of the following terms describe an HPC transplant where the donor and recipient may be unrelated?
   a. Allogeneic
   b. Autologous
   c. Syngeneic
   d. Hematopoietic

2. Stem cells from HPC donors may be mobilized with:
   a. Plerixafor.
   b. Granulocyte colony-stimulating factor (G-CSF).
   c. Chemotherapy.
   d. All of the above

3. Which choice is an advantage of an HPC transplant using umbilical cord blood?
   a. Recipient weight of no concern
   b. Donor screening and testing abbreviated
   c. Higher risk of GVHD
   d. No significant risk to the donor or mother

4. Graft-versus-host disease (GVHD) is primarily caused by:
   a. Neutrophils.
   b. T lymphocytes.
   c. B lymphocytes.
   d. Monocytes.

5. The minimum number of CD34+ cells required in an HPC-apheresis collection to ensure timely engraftment is:
   a. 2×10^2 CD34+ cells/kg.
   b. 2×10^4 CD34+ cells/kg.
   c. 2×10^6 CD34+ cells/kg.
   d. 2×10^8 CD34+ cells/kg.

6. The mother of a cord blood donor is tested for:
   a. ABO.
   b. HIV.
   c. Antibody screen.
   d. All of the above

7. The cellular marker used to quantify the collection of HPCs is:
   a. CD4.
   b. CD33.
   c. CD34.
   d. CD59.

8. The recommended dose of gamma radiation administered to a blood product to reduce the risk of graft-versus-host disease is:
   a. 1,500 cGy to any point within the canister.
   b. 1,500 cGy to the midplane of the canister.
   c. 2,500 cGy to the midplane of the canister.
   d. 2,500 cGy to any point within the canister.

9. During HPC processing, cultures must be performed:
   a. At initial testing.
   b. Before freezing.
   c. After thawing.
   d. After infusion.

10. HPC products are required to be tested for:
    a. Hepatitis C.
    b. Epstein-Barr virus.
    c. Variant CJD.
    d. Herpes simplex virus.

11. Which of the following terms describe an HPC transplant where donor and recipient are the same person?
    a. Allogeneic
    b. Autologous
    c. Syngeneic
    d. Hematopoietic

12. Which of the following terms describe an HPC transplant where donor and recipient are identical twins?
    a. Allogeneic
    b. Autologous
    c. Syngeneic
    d. Hematopoietic

References

1. Code of Federal Regulations, CFR—Title 21 Part 1271. Human cells, tissues, and cellular and tissue-based products. Washington, DC, U.S. Government Printing Office, 2010.
2. Grewal, SS, Barker JN, Davies SM, et al: Unrelated donor hematopoietic cell transplantation: Marrow or umbilical cord blood? Blood 101:4233–4244, 2003.
3. Wagner, JE, Barker, JN, Defor, TE, et al: Transplantation of unrelated donor umbilical cord blood in 102 patients with malignant and nonmalignant diseases: Influence of CD34 cell dose and HLA disparity on treatment related mortality and survival. Blood 100:1611–1618, 2002.
4. Attal, M, Harrousseau, JL, Facon, T, et al: Single versus double autologous stem cell transplantation for multiple myeloma. N Engl J Med 349:2495–2502, 2003.
5. Lenhoff, S, Hjorth, M, Holmberg, E, et al: Impact on survival of high dose therapy with autologous stem cell support in patients younger than 60 years with newly diagnosed multiple myeloma: A population based study. Nordic Myeloma Study Group. Blood 95:7–11, 2000.
6. Burt, RK, Loh, Y, Pearce, W, et al: Clinical applications of blood-derived and marrow-derived stem cells for nonmalignant diseases. JAMA 299:925–936, 2008.
7. Bitter, RE, Schofer, C, Weipoltshammer, K, et al: Recruitment of bone marrow derived cells by skeletal and cardiac muscle in adult dystrophic mdx mice. Anat Embryol 199:391–396, 1999.
8. Petersen, BE, Bowen, WC, Patrene, KD, et al: Bone marrow as a potential source of hepatic oval cells. Science 284:1168–1170, 1999.
9. Cogle, CR, Yachnis, AT, Laywell, ED, et al: Bone marrow transdifferentiation in brain after transplantation: A retrospective study. Lancet 363:1432–1437, 2004.
10. Padley, D (ed): Standards for Cellular Therapy Product Services, 4th ed. AABB, Bethesda, 2009.
11. Klein, MA, Kadidlo, McCollough, J, et al: Microbial contamination of hematopoietic stem cell products: Incidence and clinical sequelae. Biol Blood Marrow Transplant 12:1143–1149, 2006.
12. Larghero, J, Rea, D, Esperou, H, et al: ABO-mismatched marrow processing for transplantation: Results of 114 procedures and analysis of immediate adverse events and hematopoietic recovery. Transfusion 46:309–402, 2006.
13. Berz, D, McCormack, EM, Winer, ES, et al: Cryopreservation of hematopoietic stem cells. Am J Hematol 82:463–472, 2007.
14. Worel, N, Greinix, HT, Schneider, B, et al: Regeneration of erythropoiesis after related and unrelated donor BMT or peripheral blood HPC transplantation: A major ABO mismatch means problems. Transfusion 40:543–560, 2000.
15. Sauer-Heilborn, A, Kadidlo, D, and McCullough, J: Patient care during infusion of hematopoietic progenitor cells. Transfusion 44:507–516, 2004.
16. Camels, B, Lemarie, C, Esterni, B, et al: Occurrence and severity of adverse events after autologous hematopoietic cell infusion are related to the amount of granulocytes in the apheresis product. Transfusion 47:1268–1273, 2007.
17. Bittencourt, H, Rocha, V, Chevret, S, et al: Association of CD34 cell dose with hematopoietic recovery, infections, and other outcomes after HLA-identical sibling bone marrow transplantation. Blood 99:2726–2733, 2002.
18. Goker, H, Haznedaroglu, IC, and Chao, NJ: Acute graft-versus-host disease: Pathobiology and management. Exp Hematol 29:259–277, 2001.
19. Lee, SJ, Vogelsang, G, and Flowers, MED: Chronic graft-versus-host disease. Biol Blood Marrow Transplant 9:215–233, 2003.
20. Slichter, SJ: Leukocyte reduction and ultraviolet B irradiation of platelets to prevent alloimmunization and refractoriness to platelet transfusions: The trial to reduce alloimmunization to platelets study group. N Engl J Med 337:1861–1869, 1997.
21. Kaminski, ER, Hows, JM, Goldman, JM, and Batchelor, JR: Pretransfused patients with severe aplastic anaemia exhibit high numbers of cytotoxic T lymphocyte precursors probably directed at non-HLA antigens. Br J Haematol 76:401–405, 1990.
22. Goodrich, JM, Bowden, RA, Fisher, L, Keller C, Schoch, G, and Meyers, JD: Ganciclovir prophylaxis to prevent cytomegalovirus disease after allogeneic bone marrow transplant. Ann Intern Med. 118:173–178, 1993.
23. Winston, DJ, Ho, WG, Bartoni, K, et al: Ganciclovir prophylaxis of cytomegalovirus infection and disease in allogeneic bone marrow transplant recipients: Results of a placebo-controlled, double-blind trial. Ann Intern Med 118:179–184, 1993.
24. Broeckh, M, Nichols, WG, Papanicolaou, G, et al: Cytomegalovirus in hematopoietic stem cell transplants: Current status, known challenges, and future strategies. Biol Blood Marrow Transplant 9:543–558, 2003.
25. Lee, TH, Paglieroni, T, Ohto, H, et al: Survival of donor leukocyte subpopulations in immunocompetent transfusion recipients: Frequent long-term microchimerism in severe trauma patients. Blood 93:3127–3139, 1999.

Chapter 18

Transfusion-Transmitted Diseases

Elizabeth F. Williams, MHS, CLS(NCA), MT(ASCP)SBB; Patsy C. Jarreau, MHS, CLS(NCA), MT(ASCP); Michele B. Zitzmann, MHS, CLS(NCA), MT(ASCP); and Christine Pitocco, MS, MT(ASCP)BB

OBJECTIVES

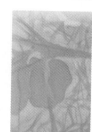

1. Describe the pathology, epidemiology, laboratory testing, and prophylaxis/treatment of the following diseases: hepatitis A through G, HIV 1 and 2, human T-cell lymphotropic viruses I and II, and West Nile virus (WNV).

2. Explain the implications of the following diseases for blood transfusions: Epstein-Barr virus, cytomegalovirus (CMV), parvovirus B19, herpesvirus 6 and 8, general bacterial contamination, syphilis, *Babesia microti*, *Trypanosoma cruzi*, malaria (*Plasmodium* species), and Creutzfeldt-Jakob disease and variant Creutzfeldt-Jakob disease.

3. Describe procedures for look-back and recipient follow-up.

4. Describe pathogen inactivation for plasma and cellular components.

Introduction

Blood is a lifesaving resource. In the United States, blood components are subjected to rigorous testing that makes them extremely safe and renders the likelihood of a transfusion-transmitted disease (TTD) very small. However, bacterial, viral, parasitic, and prion pathogens constantly evolve and, if not detected in the testing process, can cause harm and even death.

Donor Testing

Once a donor passes the medical screen and donor questionnaire, required serologic testing is performed for hepatitis B surface antigen (HBsAg), antibody to hepatitis B core antigen (anti-HBc), antibody to hepatitis C virus (anti-HCV), antibodies to human immunodeficiency virus (anti-HIV 1/2), antibody to human T-cell lymphotropic virus types I and II (anti-HTLV-I/II), syphilis, HCV RNA, and WNV RNA (Table 18–1).[1,2]

Table 18–1	**Disease Transmission Prevention—Required Tests**
DISEASES	**REQUIRED TESTS**
Hepatitis B	HBsAg anti-HBc
Hepatitis C	Anti-HCV HCV RNA
HIV	Anti-HIV-1/2 HIV-1 RNA
HTLV	Anti-HTLV-I/II
Syphilis	STS
West Nile Virus	WNV RNA

As current test methods are extremely sensitive, confirmatory tests are used to detect false-positives. These tests, which vary by the disease, include polymerase chain reaction (PCR), Western blot (WB), radioimmunoprecipitation assay (RIPA), and recombinant immunoblot assay (RIBA).

Surrogate markers (alanine aminotransferase [ALT] and anti-HBc) were used in the past to detect non-A, non-B hepatitis. Due to the sensitivity of the current testing for HCV, ALT is no longer required. However, most blood centers are continuing to perform both tests. ALT testing has continued because the European Union requires it for recovered plasma. The FDA recommends performance of anti-HBc in part because of cases of liver donors who were HBsAg-negative but anti-HBc-reactive and transmitted HBV to the recipients.[3]

Many other organisms may be transfusion-transmitted; however, tests for them are not routinely performed in the blood screening process. These include other viruses such as Epstein-Barr virus (EBV), CMV, parvovirus B19 (B19), bacteria (now considered to be the leading cause of death from transfusion),[4] parasites such as *Babesia microti* and *Trypanosoma cruzi*, malaria, and prion diseases.

Transfusion-Associated Hepatitis

Hepatitis is a generic term describing inflammation of the liver. Symptoms typically include jaundice, dark urine, hepatomegaly, anorexia, malaise, fever, nausea, abdominal pain, and vomiting. The clinical symptoms of hepatitis range from being asymptomatic to death.

It can be caused by many things, including viruses, bacteria, noninfectious agents such as chemicals (including drugs and alcohol), ionizing radiation, and autoimmune processes.[4] EBV, CMV, parvovirus, and herpes simplex virus (HSV) can cause hepatitis as a complication, but because it is not the primary disease, these viruses are not considered hepatitis viruses.[4] The hepatitis viruses affect the liver as the primary clinical manifestation. Hepatitis viruses can be transmitted through the fecal-oral route or parenterally (through contact with blood and other body fluids).

Hepatitis A (HAV) and hepatitis E (HEV) are mainly transmitted through the fecal/oral route. Hepatitis B (HBV), hepatitis C (HCV), hepatitis D (HDV), and hepatitis G (HB-C/HGV) are primarily transmitted parenterally.[4]

Hepatitis A

Hepatitis A (HAV) belongs to the *Picornaviridae* family of viruses and is a small, nonenveloped, single-stranded enterovirus RNA virus. Of all the forms of hepatitis viruses, it is the most common.[4]

Clinical Manifestations and Pathology

Symptoms, if they occur at all, generally appear abruptly and last fewer than 2 months but may persist for as long as 6 months in some individuals. They may include nausea, vomiting, anorexia, fatigue, fever, jaundice, dark urine, and abdominal discomfort. Less than 10% of children under 6 years will develop jaundice. Jaundice is more common in older children and adults, occurring in 40% to 50% of children between 6 to 14 years and 70% to 80% of individuals older than 14 years.[5] The disease is rarely fatal. Fulminant, cholestatic, or relapsing hepatitis may occur. Symptoms usually resolve within 3 weeks and are generally self-limiting.[6] In rare cases, a patient may develop fulminant liver failure.

Epidemiology and Transmission

Transmission is primarily through the fecal-oral route—spread through water, food, and person-to-person contact. Poor hygiene and poor sanitation contribute to the spread of HAV. Because young children are generally asymptomatic, the disease is predominantly spread from person to person within the household. Other individuals at risk are those who are exposed in day-care centers, neonatal intensive care units, and institutions for the mentally handicapped or who have sexual contact with infected individuals or illegal-drug users.[6] A risk factor cannot be identified in 46% of cases.[7]

The incubation period for HAV is 28 days on average, and the peak viremic period occurs 2 weeks before the onset of the elevation of liver enzymes or the appearance of jaundice.[1] Transmission of HAV by clotting factor concentrates treated with solvent or detergent pathogen process has been reported.[8] Rates in the United States have been dropping and are the lowest in the last 40 years (Table 18–2). This may be due to the introduction of the Hep A vaccine in 1995.[9] Acute viral hepatitis has declined 92% since 1995, from 12 cases per 100,000 population to 1 per 100,000 population in 2007.[9] This number may be low due to underreporting of asymptomatic or unrecognized cases.[7]

Laboratory Diagnosis

Most of the virus is shed in the feces during the incubation period and declines to low levels by the onset of symptoms (Fig. 18–1). The presence of IgM anti-HAV antibody is required for diagnosis of hepatitis A. IgM antibodies are detectable at or prior to the onset of clinical illness and decline in 3 to 6 months.[6] IgG antibodies to HAV appear soon after IgM and may persist for years after the infection.[7]

Prophylaxis and Treatment

A vaccine to HAV was licensed in the United States in 1995 for anyone older than 2 years. The number of cases has been decreasing since then, especially in areas and populations where the vaccine has been routinely given to all

Table 18–2   Disease Burden From Hepatitis A, B, and C in the United States

	HEPATITIS A		HEPATITIS B		HEPATITIS C	
	2007	2000	2007	2000	2007	2000
Number of acute cases reported	2979	13,397	4519	8036	849	No data
Estimated number of acute clinical cases	45,000	57,000	22,000	22,000	4,000	5,700
Estimated number of new infections	25,000	143,000	43,000	81,000	25,000	35,000
Number of persons with chronic infections	No chronic infection		1.25 million		2.7 million	
Estimated annual number of chronic liver disease deaths	No chronic infection		5,000		8,000–10,000	
Percent ever infected	31.3%		4.9%		1.8%	

Data from Centers for Disease Control (www.cdc.gov/hepatitis/Statistics/)

children. By 1998, the levels had dropped to historic lows. Health professionals now routinely vaccinate children, travelers to certain countries, and other persons who may be at risk.[9] The vaccine is produced from inactivated HAV. It is believed that the risk is low for pregnant women and that no special precautions should be taken for immunocompromised persons.[7] Other prevention methods include improvement in water purification, good hygiene, and improved sanitation.

Immune globulin can be used pre-exposure to protect those traveling to high HAV–endemic areas or postexposure to prevent infection in those exposed within a family, after an outbreak at a day-care center, or from a common source of exposure such as a restaurant. Immune globulin should be used postexposure within 2 weeks for maximum protection.[8]

Hepatitis B

Hepatitis B (HBV) is a partially double-stranded circular DNA virus of the *Hepadnaviridae* family.[5]

Clinical Manifestations and Pathology

Acute viral hepatitis has declined 82%, from 8.5 cases per 100,000 in 1990 to 1.5 cases per 100,000 population in 2007

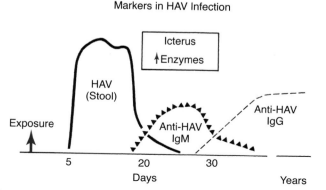

Figure 18–1.   Markers in acute HAV infection. The typical pattern of HAV infection includes early shedding of virus in the stool, appearance of IgM anti-HAV, and immunity on recovery.

(see **Table 18–2**).[10] The clinical picture of HBV infection is highly variable. Most people with acute illness will recover with no liver damage, 15% to 25% of chronically infected persons develop liver disease, and an estimated 3,000 persons in the United States die from HBV-related illness per year.[10] The individual may be completely asymptomatic or may present with typical signs of disease, including jaundice, dark urine, hepatomegaly, anorexia, malaise, fever, nausea, abdominal pain, and vomiting. For children younger than 5 years, fewer than 10% show signs of jaundice and clinical illness. However, infections acquired at birth or between ages 1 to 5 years result in a chronic infection 90% and 30% of the time, respectively. For those older than 5 years, up to 50% will have clinical illness, but only 2% to 10% will develop a chronic infection. Mortality rates in acute HBV are approximately 0.55% to 1% as compared with a 15% to 25% death rate following chronic HBV infection.[9]

Epidemiology and Transmission

HBV is transmitted through exposure to bodily fluids containing the virus from an infected individual. Concentrations of the virus are at high levels in blood, serum, and wound exudates; at moderate levels in semen, vaginal fluids, and saliva; and at low levels in urine, feces, sweat, tears, and breast milk. Transmission may be sexual, parenteral, or perinatal.[4] Percutaneous transmission may occur through needle stick (drug use, occupational hazard, acupuncture, tattooing, or body piercing), hemodialysis, human bite, transfusion of unscreened blood or blood products, or sharing razors. Permucosal transmission can occur through sexual intercourse or vertically from mother to infant (transplacental or through breast milk).[4] According to the Surveillance for Viral Hepatitis Report of 2007, higher rates of hepatitis B continue among adults, especially among males between the ages of 30 to 44 years.[10]

Laboratory Diagnosis

HBV consists of several proteins or antigens to which the body can make antibodies (Fig. 18–2). A surface antigen protein, HBsAg, is on the outer envelope of the virus. It can also be found floating free in the plasma. Antibodies can be

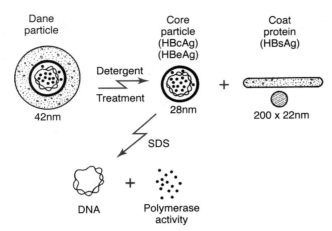

Figure 18–2. Diagram of the intact Dane particle (HB virion) as seen by electron microscopy. Detergent treatment disrupts the particle into a core particle and outer coat protein, releasing DNA (double- and single-stranded) and DNA polymerase activity.

produced to two proteins within the core: hepatitis B core antigen (HBcAg) and hepatitis Be antigen (HBeAg). Viral replication levels of these markers along with the host's production of IgM or IgG antibodies are all used to make an initial diagnosis and follow the course of infection (Table 18–3).[6]

HBV DNA is the first marker to appear and can be detected by polymerase chain reaction (PCR) testing before HBsAg reaches detectable levels.[3] There have been only incremental benefits of HBV minipool NAT over a sensitive HBsAg assay.[3] HBsAg is detectable 2 to 12 weeks postexposure during the acute stage and becomes undetectable in 12 to 20 weeks after development of anti-HBsAg (Fig. 18–3). If the patient develops chronic HBV, the level of HBsAg remains high. HBsAg can be used to monitor the stages of HBV from the acute, active infection to recovery or a chronic infection. It is also used to screen donor blood.[7]

HBeAg appears after the HBsAg and, in recovering patients, disappears before HBsAg. In chronic patients, it remains elevated. HBeAg is present during the time of active replication of the virus and is considered a marker of high infectivity.[7]

HBcAg is present in the serum but is undetectable. However, IgM anti-HBc is the first antibody to appear, and it persists for about 6 months. Appearance of this antibody indicates current or recent acute infection.[7]

ALT testing is no longer required in the United States. However, it continues to be performed because the European Union requires it for recovered plasma.[3]

Prophylaxis and Treatment

The donor questionnaire is used to identify individuals at risk for HBV infection. For those who are not eliminated by that process, testing for HBsAg and anti-HBc can be performed.

An HBV vaccine was licensed in 1981 and introduced in 1982. Hepatitis vaccination programs will eliminate domestic HBV transmission, and the increased vaccination of adults with risk factors will help accelerate the progress toward elimination.[10]

Hepatitis B immune globulin injections (HBIG) and the vaccine given soon after exposure or within 12 hours of birth, if the mother is infected, may prevent infection. Three other treatments licensed by the FDA are interferon (IFN)-α-2b,[11] lamivudine, and adefovir dipivoxil.[12] Once a patient has been diagnosed, family members should be tested. If uninfected, they should be vaccinated. If infected, they should be treated.

Hepatitis C

Hepatitis C (HCV) is a member of the *Flaviviridae* virus family and is caused by a virus with an RNA genome.[4] Hepatitis C is transmitted parenterally, although the sexual and fecal-oral routes as modes of transmission have been documented.[4] In 2007, a total of 849 confirmed cases of HCV were reported with an overall national rate of 0.3 cases per 100,000 population.[10] Blood transfusions were a major source of infection before 1992, before routine screening was implemented. Testing has reduced the incidence of transmission.[7]

Clinical Manifestations and Pathology

The incubation period of HCV is 2 to 26 weeks. The average incubation period is 7 to 8 weeks, followed by seroconversion occurring in 8 to 9 weeks.[7] Of all HCV cases, 60% to 70% are asymptomatic, with an additional 10% to 20% having nonspecific symptoms such as anorexia, malaise, fatigue, or abdominal pain. Most symptomatic cases are very mild. Of HCV-infected individuals, 75% to 85% become chronic carriers, 60% to 70% develop chronic liver disease, 5% to 20% develop cirrhosis over a period of 20 to 30 years, 1% to 5% will die from cirrhosis or liver cancer, and an estimated 12,000 persons in the United States die from HCV-related illness per year.[9]

Epidemiology and Transmission

Because most HCV cases are asymptomatic, the worldwide incidence is unknown (see **Table 18–2**). It is estimated that there are over 4 million people in the United States and 170 million chronic carriers worldwide.[7] The risk of posttransfusion HCV has declined dramatically since the introduction of testing.

HCV can be transmitted percutaneously through needle stick, hemodialysis, human bite, transplant, or transfusion, or by acupuncture, tattooing, or body piercing. It can also be transmitted permucosally through sexual intercourse, contact with infected toothbrush or razor, or perinatally. Hepatitis C is transmitted mainly by exposure to contaminated blood, with IV drug use being the main source of infection.[7]

Laboratory Diagnosis

Diagnosis of HCV is difficult. Not only are symptoms so mild in acute cases as to make separation of acute HCV from chronic HCV difficult, but also separating HCV from other forms of liver disease is not easy. Diagnosis depends on biochemical changes suggestive of HCV, detection of HCV RNA or anti-HCV in serum, or a known exposure to the virus.

Table 18–3 Molecular and Serologic Tests in the Diagnosis of Viral Hepatitis

VIRUS			TEST REACTIVITY					INTERPRETATION
HBV	**DNA**	**HBsAg**	**Anti-HBc Total**	**IgM**	**Anti-HBs**	**HBeAg**	**Anti-HBe**	
	+	+	+/−	+/−	−	+/−	−	Early acute HBV infection/chronic carrier
	+	+	+	+	−	+	−	Acute infection
	+/−	−	+	+	−	+/−	+/−	Early convalescent infection/possible early chronic carrier
	+/_	+	+	−	−	+/−	+/−	Chronic carrier
	−	−	+	−	+	−	+/−	Recovered infection
	−	−	−	−	+	−	−	Vaccination or recovered infection
	−	−	+	−	−	−	−	Recovered infection? False-positive?
	+	−	−	−	−	−	−	Window period

HDV	**RNA**	**HBsAG**	**anti-HBc**		**Anti-HBs**	**anti-HDV**		
	+	+	+		−	+		Acute or chronic HDV infection
	−	−	+		+	+		Recovered infection

		Anti-HCV		Recombinant Antigens				
HCV	**RNA**	**Screening EIA**	**5-1-1**	**c100-3**	**c33c**	**c22-3**		
	+/−	+		Not available				Possible acute or chronic HCV infection
	−	+	−	−	−	−		False-positive
	+/−	+	+	+	−	−		Possible false-positive (if RNA is negative); possible acute infection (if RNA is positive)†
	+/−	+	−		+	+		Early acute or chronic infection (if RNA is positive); false-positive or late recovery (if RNA is negative)†
	+	+	+	+	+	+		Acute or chronic infection
	−	+	+/−	+/−	+	+		Recovered HCV†

HAV	**RNA**	**anti-HAV**						
		Total	IgM					
	+	+	+					Acute HAV
	−	+	−					Recovered HAV/vaccinated

HEV	**RNA**	**anti-HEV**						
		Total	IgM					
	+	+	+					Acute HEV
	+	+	−					Recovered HEV

Taken from *AABB Technical Manual*, 15th ed., pp. 670–671. Bethesda, Maryland, 2005 with permission.

HBsAg = hepatitis B surface antigen; anti-HBc = antibody to hepatitis B core antigen; anti-HBs = antibody to HBsAg; HBeAg = hepatitis Be antigen; anti-HDV = antibody to hepatitis D virus; anti-HAV = antibody to hepatitis A virus; anti-HCV = antibody to hepatitis C virus; anti-HEV = antibody to hepatitis E virus.

*Those with HBeAg are more infectious and likely to transmit vertically.

†Anti-5-1-1 and anti-c100-3 generally appear later than anti-c22-3 and anti-c33c during seroconversion and may disappear spontaneously, during immunosuppression or after successful antiviral therapy.

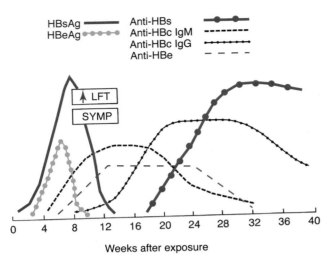

HBsAg ——   Anti-HBs ●—●—●
HBeAg ●●●●   Anti-HBc IgM ------
          Anti-HBc IgG ·-·-·-·
          Anti-HBe – – –

↑ LFT
SYMP

Weeks after exposure

Figure 18–3.   Markers in HBV infection.

Today, anti-HCV testing via EIA or ChLIA methodology is performed on all donor units.[3] Currently licensed confirmatory tests such as recombinant blot immunoassay (RIRA) or HCV RNA are performed on all positive tests[3] (see **Table 18–3**).

Recombinant immunoblot assays (RIBA), licensed by the FDA, can be used to confirm anti-HCV tests. Seventy to 90% of all RIBA-positive tests are also positive for HCV by NAT methods. Those units that are positive for HCV RNA approach 100% infectivity. The repeatedly reactive EIA tests that are RIBA-negative or indeterminate (approximately 37% of EIA repeatedly reactive donors) are rarely infectious.[3]

Prophylaxis and Treatment

Currently there is no HCV vaccine. Prevention consists of worldwide screening of blood and blood products; destruction or sterilization of needles and surgical or dental instruments; universal precautions; and education about the risks.

Patients with chronic HCV infection are usually treated with pegylated interferon and ribavirin.[4] Optimal therapy is now considered to be pegylated IFN and ribavirin combination for chronic HCV.[13] In a small study by Gerlach and colleagues,[13] 50% of patients with acute HCV spontaneously and permanently cleared the virus within the first 3 to 4 months. Patients who were still viremic at 3 months and were treated at that point had an 80% clearance rate. However, most cases were not symptomatic and therefore were not noticed and treated until the patient was in the chronic phase. Treatment with INF-α and ribavirin in these chronic cases achieved only a 30% to 54% sustained viral clearance.[13]

Hepatitis D

Hepatitis D (HDV) is a defective, single-stranded RNA virus that is found only in patients with HBV infection. It requires HBsAg in order to synthesize an envelope protein and replicate. It was previously called the delta antigen. If HBV and HDV are contracted concurrently, this coinfection, as compared with HBV alone, appears to cause a more severe acute disease, with a higher risk of fulminant hepatitis (2% to 20%) but a lesser risk of developing chronic hepatitis.

Those at highest risk of infection are IV drug users. This infection can also be transmitted sexually. It is believed that 20 million people are infected worldwide, but the number of new infections appears to be declining, most likely due to the implementation of the Hep B vaccine.[4]

HDV is detected by testing for IgM or IgG anti-HDV or HDAg and HDV RNA in the serum. Tests for HDV are not required for blood donations. If a donor has HBV, the unit will not be used for transfusion. As HDV cannot exist without HBV, testing for HBV will eliminate any infections with HDV.

Hepatitis E

Hepatitis E (HEV) is a member of the *Caliciviridae* family of nonenveloped RNA viruses. It is rare in the United States, and there are no recorded cases of transfusion transmission.[5] As in HAV, HEV is spread through the fecal-oral route, usually through contaminated drinking water in developing countries. A carrier state does not develop after the acute, usually self-limiting, illness.[7]

Clinical Manifestations and Pathology

Symptoms are the same as for any hepatitis. Generally, these cases are short-lived but can be prolonged. HEV causes an acute, self-limiting hepatitis that may last from 1 to 4 weeks in most people.[14]

Epidemiology and Transmission

HEV usually occurs in developing countries and is responsible for acute, sporadic cases of infection that can be short-lived or prolonged. The fecal-oral route is the most common form of transmission. Most cases in the United States are found in travelers returning from an endemic country.[14] HEV does not progress to a chronic state. Rare cases have been reported among persons with no history of travel.[14]

Laboratory Diagnosis

Both IgM and IgG antibody to HEV (anti-HEV) may occur following HEV infection. The titer of IgM anti-HEV declines rapidly during early convalescence; IgG anti-HEV persists and appears to provide at least short-term protection against disease (see **Table 18–3**). Antibodies are usually identified using highly sensitive enzyme immunoassays that are recombinant and synthetic HEV antigens.[7]

Prophylaxis and Treatment

Water supplies must be cleaned and sewage disposal handled properly to prevent the spread of HEV. Currently, no commercially available vaccines exist for the prevention of hepatitis E.

Hepatitis G Virus

GB virus C (GBV-C) and hepatitis G virus (HGV) are two genotypes of the same enveloped RNA virus that belongs to the *Flaviviridae* family. Approximately 1% to 2% of U.S.

donors have tested positive for HGV, making this virus more common than HCV.[15] However, recent reports do not implicate GBV-C/HGV as a cause of hepatitis.

Clinical Manifestations and Pathology

Although acute, chronic, and fulminant hepatic failure cases have been associated with GBV-C/HGV, there are other studies that do not implicate GBV-C/HGV. One article showing a strong association with fulminant hepatitis dealt with a certain mutated strain of GBV-C/HGV.[16] In another article by Halasz,[17] 33 GBV-C/HGV individuals were identified who had no coinfection with other known hepatitis viruses. No evidence of liver disease, clinical or biochemical, was found. In fact, there is some evidence that patients with HIV who have a coinfection with HGV have a slower progression to AIDS.[15] Overall data do not support GBV-C/HGV as a major cause of liver failure.

Epidemiology and Transmission

HGV is transmitted by the blood-borne route. Parental transmission through contaminated blood and the presence of the virus in bile, stool, and saliva suggest transmission through the fecal-oral and respiratory routes.[7] It has been found in 20% to 24% of intravenous drug users and in higher rates among people with HIV.[18] Vertical or perinatal transmission from mother to child has been documented.[19]

Most adult infections appear to be transient, with viral clearance followed by antibody to the viral envelope (E2) production. Vertical or perinatal infections and other infections established early in life can last for years but do not cause liver disease.[17,19]

Laboratory Diagnosis

Reverse transcription polymerase chain reaction (RT-PCR) for GBV-C/HGV-RNA is used to diagnose a current, ongoing infection. Anti-E2 along with a negative PCR for GBV-C/HGV-RNA indicates a past infection and recovery. Individuals who never develop the GBV-C/HGV E2 antibody are still infected.[20] These assays are first generation, and the evaluation has not been completed on the sensitivity and specificity of these assays.[17]

Prophylaxis and Treatment

Interferon-α treatment has been used with conflicting results. In most cases, the level of the GBV-C/HGV-RNA returned to normal levels once therapy was discontinued. Only a small percentage of cases with low pretreatment viral loads had a predictable sustained response.[21]

HIV Types 1 and 2

HIV-1 and HIV-2 are well recognized as the etiologic agents of AIDS. AIDS was first diagnosed in 1981, but the causative agent was not identified until 1984.

HIV is a retrovirus that is spherical in shape, with an approximate diameter of 100 nm. It consists of an envelope of glycoproteins, core proteins, and an inner core of viral RNA and reverse transcriptase. Infection with the virus

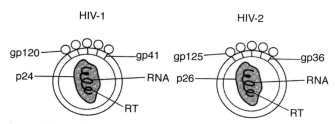

Figure 18–4. Schematic representation of human immunodeficiency virus genomes, HIV-1, and HIV-2. RT = reverse transcriptase.

causes a slowly progressing immune disorder. The causative viruses, HIV-1 and HIV-2, are similar in structure, varying primarily in the envelope proteins (Fig. 18–4 and Table 18–4). Almost all cases in the United States result from infection with the HIV-1 virus. HIV-2 is prevalent in West Africa but very rarely diagnosed in the United States; when it is diagnosed in the States, it is usually linked to an association with West Africa.

Profile

Clinical Manifestations and Pathology

Primary infection with HIV may be asymptomatic or may result in a mild, chronic lymphadenopathy with symptoms similar to those seen in infectious mononucleosis. Symptoms may occur within 6 to 12 weeks of infection and persist for a few days to 2 weeks. HIV enters the cell by the binding of the virus glycoprotein 120 with cell surface receptors. Cells possessing these receptors include CD4+ lymphocytes, macrophages, and other antigen-presenting cells. The disease may have a long, clinical latency period with the absence of clinical symptoms. During this period, antibody concentration and viral load reach equilibrium. As the viral load increases and the CD4 count decreases, the patient progresses toward clinical AIDS. When the CD4 count is less than 200/μL, the patient is classified as having clinical AIDS. The resultant immunodeficiency allows the onset of opportunistic infections such as *Pneumocystis carinii* pneumonia, Kaposi's sarcoma, fungal infections, and a host of others. About 50% of patients do not progress to clinical AIDS for 10 years or more.[22]

Table 18–4	**Components of the HIV Virus**		
	BANDS OBSERVED		
Gene	**HIV-1**	**HIV-2**	**Protein**
Gag	p18, p24, p15	p16, p26, p55	Core
Pol	p31		Endonuclease
	p51, p65	p68	Reverse transcriptase
Env	gp41	gp36	Transmembrane protein
	gp120, gp160	gp140, gp125	Envelope unit

gp = glycoprotein (number indicates molecular weight); p = protein

Epidemiology and Transmission

The number of cases of HIV infection rose rapidly in the 1980s after identification of the disease. After the incorporation of combination retroviral drug therapy in treatment protocols in the late 1990s, there was a significant reduction in the reported numbers of new AIDS cases and deaths. Reduction of death rates has resulted in an increased number of persons living with AIDS. The CDC estimates that 1.1 million adults and adolescents were living with diagnosed and undiagnosed HIV infection at the end of 2006 in the United States.[23]

HIV is transmitted through sexual contact with an infected person, use of contaminated needles during drug use, and very rarely through transfusion of blood or blood components. Congenital transmission may also occur. High-risk populations include men who have sex with men and IV drug users. The blood supply is most at risk from those individuals who have been recently infected with the virus but have not yet produced antibodies.

It was recognized over a decade ago that transfusion of blood and components from HIV-infected individuals may result in HIV infection in the recipient and development of transfusion-associated AIDS. HIV infection may occur after receiving a single contaminated unit of whole blood or its components. Albumin and immune globulins have not been reported to transmit HIV. Blood donor screening practices have dramatically reduced the incidence of transfusion-related transmission, but the possibility of transmitting HIV remains when the donor has not yet seroconverted and the level of virus in the blood is low. This subpopulation of HIV-infected persons who are unaware of their positive serostatus may pose the greatest risk to the blood supply.

Laboratory Diagnosis

The use of very sensitive serologic testing in screening the blood supply has resulted in an extremely low risk of HIV transmission. The pattern of serologic markers detected in HIV infection is shown in Figure 18–5. The window period is that time after infection but before antibody or antigen is detectable by currently available testing procedures. Only a very small number of donors donate in the window period, about 1 in 4 million.[24] It is possible for a donation to be infectious but to test negative for HIV-1/HIV-2 antibodies when the donor is in the window period. Antibodies are detectable at about 22 days after infection.

In 1985, using an EIA to screen all blood donations for antibodies to HIV-1 was instituted. Testing for HIV-2 was initiated in 1992. EIA is used for the qualitative detection of HIV-1 and HIV-2 in a ChLIA test. Positive screening tests are repeated in duplicate, and if at least one of the duplicates also tests positive, a confirmatory test is performed. The confirmation of HIV-1 and HIV-2 is performed using one or a combination of tests. These include HIV-1 indirect immunofluorescence assay (IFA) and HIV-2 EIA, which is a rapid diagnostic test used for HIV-1 and HIV-2 differentiation.[24] HIV RNA detection by NAT closes the window

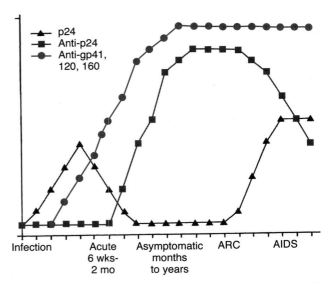

Figure 18–5. Pattern of serologic markers detected in HIV infection. ARC = AIDS-related complex.

period between time of infection and the detection of antibody by approximately 4 to 7 days. Interpretation of HIV antibody results related to blood donations is described in Figure 18–6.[3]

In 1996, donor screening protocols were expanded to include p24 core antigen testing, which reduced the window period from an estimated 22 days to 16 days. Using HIV antigen and antibody screening, the estimated risk of transmission of HIV through a single antibody negative component is 1 in 2,000,000.[24]

The FDA approved the use of NAT HIV-1 RNA testing under its investigational new drug exemptions policy in 1999. Screening of donations using NAT testing was implemented nationwide. NAT testing has reduced the window period. The first NAT test procedure was licensed in February 2002. Blood donations may be tested for HIV-1 RNA by single donor or minipool using NAT. Minipool testing involves pooling 16 donations and testing for evidence of HIV infection. As automated procedures are not available, pooling allows implementation of NAT testing by reducing costs and time involved for required testing. This procedure is limited due to the dilution effect of HIV-negative donations in the pool. It is possible to obtain a negative NAT test on a pool that includes a positive donor.

Prophylaxis and Treatment

In 2005, the CDC revised recommendations for routine testing and has implemented an initiative aimed at reducing barriers to early diagnosis of HIV infection entitled *Advancing HIV Prevention: New Strategies for a Changing Epidemic*. This initiative also aims to increase access to medical care, treatment, and prevention for those persons living with HIV.[25] To reduce perinatal transmission, the CDC recommends routine HIV testing of all pregnant women and screening of all neonates whose mothers have not been tested.

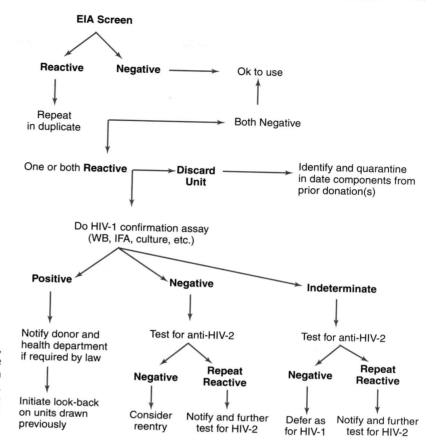

EIA Screen

Reactive → Repeat in duplicate

Negative → Ok to use

Both Negative → Ok to use

One or both **Reactive** → **Discard Unit** → Identify and quarantine in date components from prior donation(s)

Do HIV-1 confirmation assay (WB, IFA, culture, etc.)

Positive → Notify donor and health department if required by law → Initiate look-back on units drawn previously

Negative → Test for anti-HIV-2

Negative → Consider reentry

Repeat Reactive → Notify and further test for HIV-2

Indeterminate → Test for anti-HIV-2

Negative → Defer as for HIV-1

Repeat Reactive → Notify and further test for HIV-2

Figure 18–6.   Decision tree for human immunodeficiency virus, types 1 and 2 (anti-HIV-1, -2) testing of blood donors. If enzyme immunoassay (EIA) testing is nonreactive, nucleic acid amplification testing must also be nonreactive before release of a donation. IFA = immunofluorescence assay; WB = Western blot. *(From American Association of Blood Banks: Technical Manual, 16th ed, 2008, p 270, with permission.)*

Treatment with highly active antiretroviral therapy has lengthened life and improved quality of life for those infected with HIV. Use of this therapy has resulted in the most stable HIV morbidity and mortality rates since 1998.[22]

Human T-Cell Lymphotropic Viruses Types I/II (HTLV-I/II)

HTLV-I and HTLV-II are RNA retroviruses. HTLV-I causes a T-cell proliferation with persistent infection.[26] Once the RNA has been transcribed into DNA, it is integrated randomly into the host cell's genome.[27] Once integrated into the DNA, the provirus can either complete its replication cycle or remain latent for many years.

Profile

Clinical Manifestations and Pathology

HTLV-I was the first retrovirus to be associated with a human disease. That association was with adult T-cell lymphoma/leukemia (ATL), a highly aggressive, mature T-cell non-Hodgkin's lymphoma with a leukemic phase.[3] ATL does not respond well to chemotherapy, and mean survival time with acute ATL is less than 1 year. Immunodeficiency similar to that of patients with AIDS develops, making the ATL patient susceptible to other hematologic malignancies.[27] HTLV-I is also associated with the progressive neurological disorder known as HTLV-I-associated myelopathy or tropical spastic

paraparesis (HAM/TSP). A few case reports in the literature suggest that HTLV-II may impact the development of neurological diseases, including HAM, but subsequent studies have failed to support this with convincing evidence.[28]

Epidemiological data suggest blood donors infected with HTLV-I or HTLV-II have an excess of infectious syndromes, such as pneumonia, bronchitis, and urinary infections.[29] HTLV-I is associated with uveitis and infective dermatitis of children, Sjögren's syndrome, polymyositis, and facial nerve palsy.[7]

Epidemiology and Transmission

HTLV-I is transmitted vertically (breastfeeding), sexually (transmission from male to female more common), and parenterally (blood transfusion or IV drug abuse).[7] Because recipients of RBCs, platelets, and whole blood, but not fresh frozen plasma, have seroconverted, it is believed that transmission requires introduction of infected living white blood cells (WBCs).[26,27] This theory is supported by the fact that units stored for at least 7 days before transfusion are less likely to transmit the virus.

There appears to be a strong correlation between disease development and host factors such as cytotoxic T lymphocytes and HLA types. Susceptibility to ATL seems to correlate with polymorphisms of the tumor necrosis factor α (TNF-α) that result in an increased production of TNF-α.[27] In individuals with HAM/TSP, both cellular and humoral immune responses are increased as compared with those of asymptomatic carriers and seronegative controls.[28] However, ATL seems to occur in persons who were infected as infants, with a latent period of approximately 67 years, whereas HAM/TSP is generally seen in individuals who are infected in childhood or as an adult, with a variable latency as short as weeks to months. There is a 40% to 60% probability of seroconversion within 51 days following an infected blood transfusion.[26] For both diseases, the host's ability to keep the proviral load low correlates with asymptomatic carriers.[27,28]

Worldwide, it is estimated that 10 to 20 million people are infected with HTLV-I and HTLV-II.[27,28] It is endemic in parts of southern Japan, central and West Africa, the Caribbean, the Middle East, Melanesia, Papua New Guinea, the Solomon Islands, and in Australian aborigines. In the United States, HTLV-I and HTLV-II are seen primarily in IV drug users. HTLV-I is also seen in immigrants from endemic areas, whereas HTLV-II is seen in some Native American populations.[26,28] Indications from the high numbers of carriers and low numbers of individuals diagnosed with actual disease are that most carriers are asymptomatic their entire lives.[26,27]

The risk of transmitting HTLV through infected blood is estimated to be between 10% to 30%.[3] Leukocyte reduction and serologic testing greatly reduces the risk of HTLV transmission.[3]

Laboratory Diagnosis

Because the majority of carriers are asymptomatic, diagnosis is based on seroconversion after exposure. In the United States, FDA-licensed EIA using whole virus lysates from both viruses is used to detect both anti-HTLV-I and anti-HTLV-II. With 60% homology between HTLV-I and HTLV-II, antibody cross-reactivity makes it difficult to distinguish between the two viruses. Results are reported as reactive or negative for HTLV-I/II. No licensed confirmatory test is currently available, but most blood centers perform a confirmatory test under the Investigational New Drug (IND) protocol. Confirmatory tests are not performed until the test is repeatedly reactive and retested by EIA from a different manufacturer (Fig. 18–7).[30] All donated blood is currently screened by EIA to remove units positive for HTLV-I or HTLV-II from the donor pool.

The AABB[30] and FDA have published guidelines on the use of the unit for transfusion and donor notification as shown in Figure 18–7. The guidelines state that if the donor is repeatedly reactive by the test of record (original EIA) but negative by the second licensed EIA of a different type (different manufacturer), the donor is still eligible for donation. The donor can continue to donate as long as the test-of-record EIA is negative on the next donation. If the donor is repeatedly reactive by test of record on two separate occasions or on the same donation by the test-of-record assay and the different manufacturer's EIA, the donor is indefinitely deferred.

Prophylaxis and Treatment

ATL does not respond well to treatment. However, early treatment with corticosteroids appears to have some effect on HAM/TSP. There is no treatment for chronic or advanced disease.[26] The best prophylaxis is to prevent exposure. However, as the majority of infected individuals are asymptomatic, it is difficult to prevent spread to an uninfected individual vertically or sexually. Infected mothers should not breastfeed.

West Nile Virus

West Nile Virus (WNV) is a member of the *Flavivirus* family and is a human, avian, and equine neuropathogen. It is a single-stranded RNA lipid-enveloped virion[31] that is common in Africa, West Asia, and the Middle East. WNV is a member of the Japanese encephalitis virus antigenic complex that includes St. Louis encephalitis virus prevalent in the Americas, Japanese encephalitis virus prevalent in East Asia, and Murray Valley encephalitis virus and Kunjin virus prevalent in Australia.[32] WNV was first documented in the Western Hemisphere when 149 cases were reported in New York in 1999. In the United States in 2009, a total of 720 human cases of WNV-associated illness with 32 fatalities were reported in 44 states and the District of Columbia.[33]

Profile

Clinical Manifestations and Pathology

WNV is usually subclinical but may cause a mild flulike disease. However, the strain in the United States is often associated with more severe disease. In 2002, outbreaks determined by antibody screening found that 20% to 30% of infected individuals exhibited symptoms ranging from mild fever and headache to extensive rash, eye pain, vomiting, inflamed lymph nodes, prolonged lymphocytopenia, muscle weakness, disorientation, and even acute flaccid paralysis and poliomyelitis.[31] The association of paralysis and poliomyelitis with WNV is recent. It is a peripheral demyelinating process similar to Guillain-Barré syndrome.[34] WNV is capable of crossing the blood-brain barrier and can cause what is known as *West Nile encephalitis*, *West Nile meningitis*, or *West Nile meningoencephalitis*.[35] Approximately 1 in 150 infections results in severe neurological disease that may cause permanent neurological impairment, with encephalitis reported more often than meningitis. The risk of severe neurological disease increases markedly for anyone over the age of 50 years.[35]

Epidemiology and Transmission

Birds are the primary amplifying hosts in a mosquito-bird-mosquito cycle. Incidentally, mosquitoes feed off infected birds and then bite humans. Although at least 16 species of mosquitoes have been found to carry WNV, the genus *Culex* is the chief vector.[30–32] The infection in humans has an incubation period of approximately 3 to 14 days following the mosquito bite, with symptoms lasting 3 to 6 days. Other animals can become infected, including horses, cats, dogs, bats, chipmunks, skunks, squirrels, and domestic birds and rabbits. Although mosquito bites are the most common route of infection, there is a slight risk of contracting WNV from

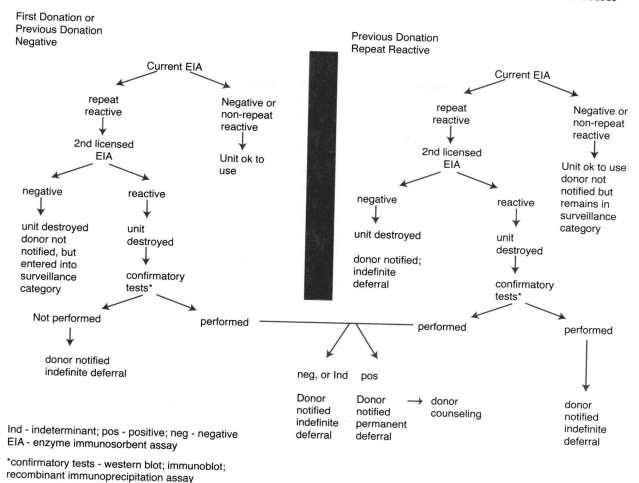

First Donation or
Previous Donation
Negative

Current EIA

repeat reactive → 2nd licensed EIA

Negative or non-repeat reactive → Unit ok to use

negative → unit destroyed donor not notified, but entered into surveillance category

reactive → unit destroyed → confirmatory tests*

Not performed → donor notified indefinite deferral

performed

Previous Donation
Repeat Reactive

Current EIA

repeat reactive → 2nd licensed EIA

Negative or non-repeat reactive → Unit ok to use donor not notified but remains in surveillance category

negative → unit destroyed donor notified; indefinite deferral

reactive → unit destroyed → confirmatory tests*

performed

neg, or Ind → Donor notified indefinite deferral

pos → Donor notified permanent deferral → donor counseling

performed → donor notified indefinite deferral

Ind - indeterminant; pos - positive; neg - negative
EIA - enzyme immunosorbent assay

*confirmatory tests - western blot; immunoblot; recombinant immunoprecipitation assay

Figure 18–7.   Flowchart for HTLV-I/II testing.

blood components, organ transplants, pregnancy, and breast milk. During the epidemic outbreak of 2002, 23 persons were reported to have been infected through transfusion.[2]

Laboratory Diagnosis

Viremia usually lasts approximately 6 days and peaks around the onset of symptoms. Once clinical symptoms occur, the IgM WNV-specific antibody titer increases, and the virus concentration in the blood stream decreases. Until July 2003, diagnosis depended on the clinical findings and specific laboratory tests. IgM antibody-capture enzyme-linked immunosorbent assay (ELISA) was the method used to detect IgM antibody to the WNV in serum and cerebrospinal fluid (CSF). In the 1999 and 2000 outbreak in New York, 95% of all infected patients for whom CSF was tested had a demonstrable IgM antibody. However, because all *Flaviviruses* are antigenically similar, cross-reactivity has been observed in testing persons who have been vaccinated for a *Flavivirus,* such as yellow fever or Japanese encephalitis, or who have been recently infected with another *Flavivirus,* such as St. Louis encephalitis or dengue fever. The plaque reduction neutralization test is the most specific test for arthropod-borne *Flaviviruses* and helps to distinguish false-positive IgM antibody-capture ELISA from cross-reactivity.[36] In fatal cases,

immunohistochemistry can be used by testing brain tissue with virus-specific monoclonal antibodies.[37]

Clinically, the serologic tests for IgM antibodies to WNV using ELISA can be used for testing symptomatic patients. Because the virus is in the bloodstream before either symptoms or antibodies develop, blood screening tests for WNV that identify the virus itself were needed. In June 2003, two commercial WNV-screening NATs were distributed, and implementation of donor blood testing began "under phase III investigational new drug (IND) FDA approval."[2] As of July 14, 2003, all civilian blood donations were being screened by NAT. Units are initially screened individually or in pools of 6 or 16, depending on the kit manufacturer. Individual samples are tested only if the pool is positive with NAT.[2] The implementation of NAT testing for West Nile virus resulted in the detection of 183 confirmed cases, with an additional 47 cases of infected units being detected by testing targeted individual units.[38]

If an individual donor tested NAT-positive, all current blood components were discarded, and any unused components donated within the last 14 to 28 days by that individual were retrieved. Additional NAT tests were performed by another laboratory for confirmation, using a different amplification technique or different primers. The original sample collected from the donor was assayed for WNV-specific IgM antibody. The donor was questioned again about "recent travel history, other exposure history, and review of symptoms compatible with WNV illness before or after illness."[39] Donors were classified as viremic if the initial donor sample was NAT-positive by pool and by individual testing, and the individual sample was repeatedly reactive using alternate NAT protocols.[2] With the implementation of NAT testing, approximately 2.5 million units were screened for WNV from June to mid-September 2003. Only 1,285 (0.50%) were WNV-positive by NAT. Of the positive units, 601 (0.02%) were considered viremic, and results are pending for an additional 209.[2]

WNV has become a major area of focus for transfusion safety, especially since there have been large outbreaks in the United States when comparing WNV with other transmissible diseases tested by NAT testing. There is a similar interval in which it is detected, but when comparing testing by minipool method, WNV has a much shorter duration of viremia.[38]

Prophylaxis and Treatment

Individuals should avoid mosquitoes and wear mosquito repellant and appropriate clothing if they are going to be in a mosquito-infested area. Once infected, there is no licensed treatment, only supportive therapy. Research is ongoing for the use of ribavirin, interferon-α,[31] and West Nile immune globulin to treat WNV. Having survived the illness, a person is immune for life.

Other Viruses

Cytomegalovirus

Cytomegalovirus (CMV) is a member of the herpesvirus group[40] and is found in all geographic locations and socioeconomic groups, with a higher prevalence in developing countries. In areas with lower socioeconomic conditions, the prevalence approaches 100%. Of adults in the United States, 50% to 85% have been exposed to CMV by the age of 40 years.

Clinical Manifestations and Pathology

When exposure occurs after birth to an individual with a competent immune system, there are generally few symptoms. Rarely, mononucleosis-like symptoms with fever and mild hepatitis occur. Once an individual is exposed, CMV can remain latent in the tissues and leukocytes for years, with reactivation occurring from a severe immune system impairment.[40]

Those at the highest risk of a CMV infection are fetuses and individuals receiving allogeneic marrow transplants. CMV-seronegative recipients transplanted with CMV-seronegative allogeneic marrow are at risk if they receive untested and non-WBC-reduced blood components. The risk of seroconversion and serious disease is 20% to 50%. CMV-seronegative women who become infected in the first two trimesters have a 35% to 55% chance of delivering an affected infant, many of which will have clinically apparent disease. Intrauterine transfusions with CMV-positive components is also a high risk to the fetus.[41]

Individuals at moderate risk are recipients of solid organ transplants, persons with HIV, and individuals who may require an allogeneic marrow transplant in the future. When the individual becomes immunosuppressed, a reactivation of a latent infection is possible, resulting in a clinically apparent infection.[41]

Low-birth-weight neonates and autologous marrow recipients are considered to be at low risk. Preterm, multitransfused neonates weighing less than 1,200 grams are currently considered to be at a lower risk than once considered, as a result of better transfusion techniques and management of their condition. However, leukocyte-reduced or CMV-negative units reduce the risk of CMV infection in these low birth-weight neonates.[3] The neonate may be exposed at the time of delivery, through breastfeeding or contact with seropositive individuals. Approximately 1% of all newborns are infected with CMV, but most are asymptomatic at birth.[42] The fetus that is exposed to the mother's reactivation of the virus during pregnancy rather than a primary exposure rarely has any damage.[42] The autologous marrow recipient is not as immunosuppressed as the allogeneic marrow recipient, and therefore CMV infection does not present a problem.[41] CMV infection from transfusion is between 1% to 3%.[3]

Epidemiology and Transmission

Transmission occurs from person to person through contact with infected body fluids, which may include urine, semen, saliva, blood, cervical secretions, and breast milk. CMV is the most frequently transmitted virus from mother to fetus.[42]

Seronegative individuals who have received organ transplants or hematopoietic progenitor cells from a seronegative donor and AIDS patients who are not currently infected with CMV are also at risk.[3] The rate of transmission of CMV to bone marrow recipients or to neonates has been documented at 13% to 38%.[43]

Laboratory Diagnosis

Antibodies formed to CMV last a lifetime and can be detected by ELISA. Other laboratory tests include fluorescence assays, indirect hemagglutination, and latex agglutination. If the patient is symptomatic, active infection can be detected by viral culture of urine, throat swabs, and tissue samples.[40]

CMV DNA tests are currently being investigated for use in detecting blood donors who have been exposed but have not yet seroconverted. Tests for anti-CMV would be negative for these individuals when, in fact, their blood might be capable of transmitting the disease. In one study by Roback and colleagues, previously described CMV PCR assays were compared.[43] The performances of the seven assays varied greatly in sensitivity, specificity, and reproducibility.[43]

Prophylaxis and Treatment

Currently, there is no treatment for CMV for a healthy individual; vaccines are still in the research and development stage. Infants are being evaluated using antiviral drug therapy, and ganciclovir is being used for patients with depressed immunity.

Blood and blood components are not universally screened for CMV because of the generally benign course of this disease and the high percentage of virus carriers. To prevent CMV transmission, leukocyte-reduced blood or blood from seronegative donors may be used. Leukoreduction using high-efficiency filters such that the final level of leukocytes is less than or equal to 5×10^6 leukocytes per component appears to work well with high-risk neonates (weighing less than 1,200 grams) and transplant recipients.[3] In an AABB bulletin, prestorage leukoreduction was encouraged rather than bedside leukoreduction.

Epstein-Barr Virus

Epstein-Barr virus EBV is a ubiquitous member of the herpesvirus family. As many as 95% of the adult population in the United States have been exposed to the virus by the age of 40 years and maintain an asymptomatic latent infection in B lymphocytes for life. Infections occurring in infants or young children are usually asymptomatic. In adolescence and young adulthood, EBV causes infectious mononucleosis in 30% to 50% of patients.[44]

Although transfusion transmission is rarely an individual's first exposure to the virus and reactivation usually occurs only in immunocompromised individuals, there are a few cases in the literature of transfusion-associated EBV. EBV is not detected by current practices and could cause severe consequences in immunocompromised patients, particularly organ transplant patients.[45]

EBV has been called the "kissing disease" because the virus usually replicates in the cells of the oropharynx, possibly in infected B cells. The virus is shed in the saliva and is most frequently associated with infectious mononucleosis.

EBV was first discovered in 1964 in Burkitt's lymphoma cells.[46] Since then it has been associated with many illnesses besides infectious mononucleosis and cancers such as nasopharyngeal carcinoma, non-Hodgkin's lymphoma, oral hairy leukoplakia in AIDS patients, T-cell lymphomas, and Hodgkin's disease.[7]

Parvovirus B19

Human B19 parvovirus (B19) is a small, single-stranded DNA nonenveloped virus.[3] It causes a common childhood illness called "fifth disease" and is usually transmitted through respiratory secretions. Fifth disease presents with a mild rash described as "slapped cheek" when occurring on the face and a lacy red rash when occurring on the trunk and limbs. Approximately 50% of adults have been exposed as children or adolescents and have protective antibodies. Primary infection in an adult is usually asymptomatic, but a rash or joint pain and swelling may occur transiently.[47,48]

As in all viral infections, the virus must enter the cell through a specific cell receptor. B19 parvovirus enters the red blood cell (RBC) via the P antigen and replicates in the erythroid progenitor cells.[49] The cytotoxicity of erythroid precursors can lead to serious illness in individuals with chronic hemolytic anemia, such as sickle cell disease and thalassemia, who may have a transient aplastic crisis. Severe RBC aplasia or chronic anemia may manifest in patients with chronic or acquired immunodeficiency or malignancies or in organ transplant recipients. Hydrops fetalis and fetal death can occur when the virus is transmitted during pregnancy.

The viremic stage occurs shortly after infection. A donor would be asymptomatic but capable of transmitting the virus during this period. This is a concern for donor centers because the rate of seroconversion is high after exposure. In one study, B19 DNA was found in approximately 1 out of 800 donations. B19 is very resistant to heat and detergent and has been found through PCR to be present in plasma components. Because of the lack of inactivation in the manufacturing process, B19 has been implicated in several studies, with transmission through factor concentrates and, in one study, through an antithrombin III concentrate.[50]

There has been ongoing regulatory concern about the safety of plasma derivatives that has led some manufacturers and regulatory authorities to require B19 DNA qualification testing of plasma and release testing of manufactured lots.[51] The FDA recommends manufacturers of plasma-derived products to engage in practices that will reduce the time between product collection and process testing in order for the collection establishments to be notified of positive test results within the in-date period of any blood components that are intended for transfusion.[52]

In a study by Weimer and colleagues,[50] plasmas were tested for B19 DNA levels by PCR, and those with high titers were eliminated from the pool used in the manufacture of antithrombin III (ATIII). After the manufacturing process, PCR was used to compare ATIII concentrates made from a pool in which high titers were excluded and ATIII concentrates that were made from a pool that had not been tested for B19 DNA. None of the concentrates manufactured with high-titer plasma eliminated from the pool were PCR-positive, whereas 66% of the concentrates that were not tested prior to manufacturing were PCR-positive. This indicates the effectiveness of eliminating high-titer plasmas in reducing the B19 DNA to undetectable levels.

Disease transmission of parvovirus B19 is rare. Very high levels of parvovirus B19 (up to 10^{12} IU/ml) in plasma of acutely infected asymptomatic donors may pose a greater risk for plasma derivatives. This is due to the pooling of larger plasma units by manufacturers when processing these products.[52] There have been no confirmed reports that immunoglobulin and albumin products have transmitted parvovirus B19 infection.[52]

Human Herpesvirus 6 and Human Herpesvirus 8

Human herpesvirus 6 (HHV-6) is a very common virus that causes a lifelong infection. Seroprevalence approaches 100% in some populations. The virus replicates in the salivary gland and then remains latent in lymphocytes, monocytes, and perhaps other tissues.

In childhood, HHV-6 causes roseola infantum, also known as *exanthem subitum* or *sixth disease*. Symptoms are those of a mild, acute febrile disease. In immunocompetent adults, it is very rare to find infection or reaction from sites other than the salivary gland where secretions from saliva are a known source of transmission. Side effects are not common but can include lymphadenopathy and fulminant hepatitis.

HHV-6 has been associated with a number of diseases other than roseola infantum, such as multiple sclerosis and lymphoproliferative and neoplastic disorders. There is no evidence to support a TTD association; with the high level of seropositivity in the population, blood components are not being tested for HHV-6.[3]

HHV-8 is another human herpesvirus. Unlike HHV-6, it is not common in the population but has been seen in Africa.[53] Only 3% of donors are seropositive in the United States.[54] It is associated with several diseases that generally affect the immunosuppressed patient. These include Kaposi's sarcoma (KS), primary effusion lymphoma, and multicentric Castleman's disease. Spread is generally through sexual contact. However, in KS patients, 30% to 50% have circulating lymphocytes harboring HHV-8, which lends support to the premise that exposure to HHV-8 could be transfusion-associated. There has been no evidence to support this to date.[54] In post-transplant patients who develop KS, it appears to be due to reactivation. The transmission of HHV-8 has been associated with organ transplants and injection drug use.[53]

Bacterial Contamination

Overview

As the infection risk for other diseases has decreased due to better donor testing, bacterial contamination has come to the forefront and has become a great concern as a transfusion-transmitted disease.[55] Although the incidence of transfusion-associated bacterial sepsis is low, the morbidity and mortality rates are high. Common sources of bacterial contamination include donor skin and blood. Less common sources are the environment and disposables.[3] Platelets have been the most frequent source of septic transfusion reactions, due to the fact that room temperature storage promotes bacterial growth.[3] In 2004, implementation of bacterial contamination screening methods has lowered the rate of contamination.

Clinical Manifestations and Pathology

The most common signs and symptoms of transfusion-associated sepsis are rigors, fever, and tachycardia.[56] Other symptoms may include shock, low back pain, disseminated intravascular coagulation (DIC), and an increase or decrease in systolic blood pressure.[3] The mortality rate from sepsis and toxemia due to bacterially contaminated RBC units is greater than 60%.[3] Although the number of contaminated platelet units is much greater, the mortality rate is not as high as it is for RBCs. However, platelet contamination is considered to be underreported. Sepsis due to platelets can occur hours after the transfusion, and the connection may be unrecognized. This may be because many patients who receive platelets are already immunosuppressed because of their condition or treatment, and the sepsis may be attributed to the immunosuppression.[3]

Epidemiology and Transmission

Bacterial contamination usually originates with the donor, either through skin contamination at the phlebotomy site or an asymptomatic bacteremia. It may also occur through contamination during processing.[3] Contamination rates in the United States have been estimated to be 0.2% for RBCs and as high as 10% for platelets. It is estimated that a febrile transfusion reaction caused by contaminated blood occurs once for every 10 to 20,000 units and that a death occurs once for every 6 million units.[56]

According to the CDC,[57] *Yersinia enterocolitica* is the most common isolate found in RBC units, followed by the *Pseudomonas* species. Together, these two account for more than 80% of all bacterial infections transmitted by RBCs. In a study by Kunishima,[58] *Propionibacterium acnes*, a common isolate of human skin, was the most common bacterial contaminant in RBCs. It is a slow-growing anaerobic bacteria that can go unrecognized if tested in aerobic conditions or by using short-term bacterial cultural methods. Although *P. acnes* has been implicated in only a few cases of transfusion-related sepsis, studies are needed to confirm long-term safety, as it has been associated with sarcoidosis.

Staphylococcus epidermidis, and *Bacillus cereus* (both gram-positive) are the organisms most frequently recovered from donated blood and contamination of platelets.[55]

Laboratory Diagnosis

Before the unit of RBCs or platelets is issued, the unit should be inspected for discoloration (dark purple or black), which strongly indicates contamination. The unit may have no visible evidence of contamination at the time of issue. However, clots in the unit and hemolysis may also indicate contamination. Because the bacteria in the unit consume the oxygen, the cells may lyse, resulting in discoloration in the unit as compared with the segments that remain normal in color.[3]

To detect bacterial contamination, both the donor blood component and the recipient's blood should be tested. It is better to test the component itself and not the segments, as they may be negative.[3] The FDA has cleared two culture methods for quality-control monitoring of bacterial contamination in platelets. Both methods can be used for leukocyte-reduced apheresis platelets, whereas only one can be used for leukocyte-reduced whole blood–derived platelets.

Bacterial screening of platelets was implemented in the United States from 2003 to 2004. This has reduced the risk of transfusing contaminated platelets to patients. Between 2004 and 2006, the American Red Cross documented a residual risk of clinically relevant septic shock reactions of 1 in 74,807, and a fatality rate of at least 1 in 498,711, with platelets that were distributed (to outside facilities) after routine bacteria detection by culture techniques.[59] This shows a 50% reduction in reported reactions and fatalities in a 10-month period after bacteria screening was implemented.

The FDA has allowed individual blood collection facilities to apply for extension of platelet storage from 5 to 7 days. This extension is based on the track record and successful implementation of a bacterial-detection system.[3]

Prophylaxis and Treatment

The 26th edition of the AABB *Standards* states that "the blood bank or transfusion service shall have methods to detect or inactivate bacterial contamination in all platelet components."[1] Use of apheresis platelets, careful phlebotomy technique, and phlebotomy diversion are listed by the AABB as methods to limit bacterial contamination of platelets.

Use of apheresis platelets rather than pooled whole blood–derived platelets from multiple donors reduces the incidence of contamination occurring during phlebotomy. However, apheresis platelets cannot meet all platelet transfusion needs, and whole blood–derived platelets are still needed. Therefore, proper arm preparation for phlebotomy is of paramount importance. Standard 5.6.2 in the 26th edition of *Standards* states that the use of green soap will no longer be allowed.[1] Improved bacterial disinfection has been correlated with the use of an iodine-based scrub. In donors allergic to iodine, chlorhexidine or double isopropyl alcohol skin disinfectant may be used.[55]

Phlebotomy diversion consists of collecting the first 20 to 30 mL of blood in a separate container to be used for testing. This reduces the quantity of skin contaminants entering the unit during phlebotomy and appears to be very effective in reducing *Staphylococcus* species contamination.[60] Several blood bag manufacturers have developed systems with a diversion pouch.

Leukodepletion of units can be helpful in removing phagocytized bacteria along with the leukocytes. Some advocate this for RBCs to reduce *Yersinia* contamination. Other methods under consideration listed in the AABB *Technical Manual* include endotoxin assays, detection of by-products of bacterial metabolism, NAT, and pathogen inactivation methods.[3]

Water baths used in a blood bank can have high bacterial counts unless disinfected frequently. An overwrap is recommended for any components placed in the water bath, with inspection of the outlet ports before use.

If transfusion-associated sepsis is suspected, treatment should begin immediately without waiting for laboratory confirmation. Treatment should include IV antibiotics and necessary therapy for whatever symptoms are present, such as shock, renal failure, and DIC.[3]

Syphilis

Treponema pallidum, the causative agent of syphilis, is a spirochete. It is usually spread through sexual contact but can be transmitted through blood transfusions. In 2006 in the United States, 36,000 cases of syphilis was reported.[61]

Between 2005 and 2006, the number of reported cases of primary and secondary syphilis increased 11.8%.[62]

The standard serologic tests for syphilis (STS) usually do not detect a donor in the spirochetemia phase who has not yet seroconverted. Spirochetemia is short, and seroconversion usually occurs after this phase.[3] However, the STS is still required for blood donors despite the fact that in 1978 a federal advisory panel recommended that this requirement be eliminated. The FDA withheld the proposed rule to drop STS from donor testing. The 26th edition of the AABB *Standards* continues to require the STS.[1]

Polymerase chain reaction followed by Southern blotting and a labeled probe have been used to confirm the presence of treponemal antigen. The test is capable of detecting as few as one treponeme in CSF.[61] Nontreponemal EIAs, fluorescent treponemal antibody absorption (FTA-ABS), treponema pallidum immobilization (TPI), and treponema pallidum hemagglutination (TPHA) are the methodologies utilized. Blood donations that are reactive may not be used unless a confirmatory test such as FTA is determined to be nonreactive.[3] Donors that have confirmed positive results can be reinstated for donation after 12 months with documentation of treatment.[3]

Tick-Borne Bacterial Agents

Lyme disease, Rocky Mountain spotted fever (RMSF), and ehrlichiosis are all bacterial diseases spread by a tick bite. Lyme disease is caused by the spirochete *Borrelia burgdorferi* and RMSF (*Rickettsia rickettsii*) and ehrlichiosis (*Ehrlichia* species) are caused by bacteria that are obligate intracellular pathogens.

Transfusion-Associated Parasites

At least three parasites have been associated with transfusion-associated infections: *Babesia microti*, *Trypanosoma cruzi*, and malaria (*Plasmodium* species). Several additional parasites have been identified in association with transfusion-associated disease. These include *Leishmania* species, other *Trypanosoma* species, *Toxoplasma gondii*, and the microfilarial parasites. Most of these infections occur on rare occasions and typically involve patients who are severely immunocompromised. The risk for acquiring a blood transfusion containing these parasites may be underreported in endemic areas but has always been very low in the United States. However, in October 2003, the AABB put forth a recommendation to blood collection facilities that all individuals who had been in Iraq should be deferred for 1 year from the last date of departure. This was done after cases of leishmaniasis were reported in personnel stationed in Iraq.

Babesia Microti

Babesiosis, a zoonotic disease, is usually transmitted by the bite of an infected deer tick. Infection is caused by the protozoan parasite, *Babesia*, which infects the RBCs. Most human cases of *Babesia* infection that occur in the United States are caused by the *Babesia microti* parasite.[63] There have been reported cases of simultaneous transmission of *B. microti* and *Borrelia burgdorferi*, the causative agent of Lyme disease, because the tick vectors are the same for the two organisms.[64] Other reported species are *B. duncani*, formally called WA1-type *Babesia*, CA1-type *Babesia*, and *B. divergens*–like agents such as the MO1-type *Babesia*.[65] *Babesia* infection may also be acquired by blood transfusion and solid organ transplant. Estimates between 70 and 100 cases of transfusion-transmitted *Babesia* (TTB) have occurred over the last 30 years in the United States, with at least 12 fatalities in transfusion recipients diagnosed with babesiosis.[66,67]

Clinical Manifestations and Pathology

Most cases of babesiosis are asymptomatic. Symptomatic patients usually develop a malaria-type illness characterized by fever, chills, lethargy, and hemolytic anemia. The risk for developing severe complications, which include renal failure, DIC, and respiratory distress syndrome, increases for elderly, asplenic, or immunocompromised patients. Reported incubation periods for symptomatic patients range from 1 to 8 weeks after transfusion; therefore it is important that physicians consider babesiosis when diagnosing a febrile illness following a transfusion.[3]

Epidemiology and Transmission

Areas of the United States, such as the northeast, mid-Atlantic, upper Midwestern states are said to have endemic transmission.[65] The incidence is higher during the spring and summer months, which corresponds to the increase in tick activity and outdoor recreation of humans. Persons infected with *Babesia* may not have clinical signs of illness for an extended time. Infected persons who donate blood during the asymptomatic period pose the greatest risk to the blood supply, as they probably have infectious organisms circulating in their bloodstreams. Units of packed RBCs (liquid stored and frozen deglycerolized) and platelet units, which contain RBCs, have been associated with transmission.[66,68] *B. microti* can survive in refrigerated, uncoagulated blood for 21 to 35 days.[3] There have been 63 transfusion-transmitted babesiosis cases in the United States between 2004 and 2008.[65]

Laboratory Diagnosis

Prompt diagnosis is essential, as *Babesia* responds well to antibiotic therapy but can be fatal in certain risk groups if not properly treated. There is no specific test to diagnose an infection with *B. microti*. Thick and thin blood smears stained with Giemsa or Wright stain can be examined for intraerythrocytic organisms. A single negative smear does not rule out an infection. Serologic studies such as immunofluorescence assays can be used to detect circulating antibody.[65] Currently there is no screening test for blood donors.

Prophylaxis and Treatment

Babesiosis can be effectively treated with antibiotic therapy. There is no specific drug of choice, but quinine and clindamycin are very effective. In addition, the combination of atovaquone and azithromycin can be as effective in patients without a life-threatening illness.[69] Apheresis has also been successful in patients who fail to respond to antibiotic therapy.[70,71]

There is no test currently available to screen for asymptomatic carriers of *Babesia*. Many blood banks have added questions to their donor questionnaire that address topics such as living in an endemic area and previous *Babesia* infection. Some blood banks have chosen to defer individuals who reside in areas that are heavily tick-infested in the summer months.[72] This practice may have little value, as donors may remain asymptomatic for months after exposure to the organism. Donors with a history of babesiosis should be deferred from donating blood for an indefinite period of time.[3] Because *B. microti* can be transmitted by blood donated from asymptomatic donors, effective measures for preventing transmission are needed. The AABB Transfusion Transmitted Disease Committee (TTD) has described Babesiosis as a red category agent.[52] These agents are given a low to high scientific or epidemiological risk regarding blood safety with a potential for severe outcomes.[51]

Trypanosoma Cruzi

Trypanosoma cruzi is a flagellate protozoan that is the etiologic agent of Chagas' disease (American trypanosomiasis). It is estimated that 300,000 people are infected within the United States.[73] The disease is naturally acquired by the bite of a reduviid bug, thus making it a zoonotic infection. Insect transmission is the most common mode of infection but the organism has also been transmitted by blood transfusion and organ transplants.

Clinical Manifestations and Pathology

The acute phase of Chagas' disease is initiated when the organism enters the host. The reduviid bug bite produces a localized nodule, referred to as a *chagoma*. The chagoma is usually painful and may take up to 3 months to heal. Clinical symptoms may be mild or absent; therefore, many cases are not diagnosed until the chronic phase of the disease. Symptoms include anemia, weakness, chills, intermittent fever, edema, lymphadenopathy, myocarditis, and gastrointestinal symptoms. Death may occur within a few weeks or months after initial infection.

Following the acute phase, the disease may enter a latent phase, which can last up to 40 years.[73] During this phase, the patient is usually asymptomatic but has parasites circulating in the bloodstream. Transfusion-associated Chagas' disease is most likely to occur during this phase.

Chagas' disease usually progresses to the chronic phase years or decades after the acute phase.[73] In the chronic phase, the organism begins to cause damage to cardiac tissue, thus causing cardiomyopathy. Since Chagas' disease is not very common in the United States, it can be easily misdiagnosed. One study revealed that 72% of Chagas' disease patients in the United States had been treated for other cardiomyopathies for as long as 9 years before Chagas' disease was diagnosed.[73]

Epidemiology and Transmission

Chagas' disease is endemic in Central and South America and some areas of Mexico.[3,73] Infected individuals pose a risk of infecting recipients of their donated blood. There have been four reported cases of *T. cruzi* infection acquired by blood transfusion in North America.[3,73] All cases occurred in immunocompromised patients. This number could be higher if we consider there may be other cases not detected in immunocompetent patients receiving blood. *T. cruzi* can survive in platelets stored at room temperature, RBC units at 4°C, and during cryopreservation and thawing.[73] In addition to blood transfusions, Chagas' disease can be transmitted congenitally or transplacentally or through solid organ transplantation.[73]

Screening for Chagas' disease was implemented in January 2007, shortly after licensing of the screening test in the United States confirmed 1 in 121,000 positive blood donors after 3 months of screening.[3] By January of 2008, there were 1,112 repeat antibody-positive blood donors identified.[3]

Laboratory Diagnosis

Acute Chagas' disease is diagnosed by detecting the organism in the patient's blood. Blood smears stained with Giemsa or Wright stain may be examined for the characteristic C- or U-shaped trypomastigote (Fig. 18–8). Anticoagulated blood or the buffy coat may also be evaluated for motile organisms.

Chronic Chagas' disease is diagnosed serologically. Such testing includes complement fixation, immunofluorescence, and ELISA. False-positive reactions are common; therefore it is recommended that patient specimens be analyzed using more than one assay. Trypomastigotes are rare or absent in the peripheral blood during the chronic phase, so examination of blood smears is not useful.

Prophylaxis and Treatment

National screening of the blood supply was initiated in 2007. Since that time, more than 1,000 donors with *T. cruzi* infection have been identified.[74] The FDA approved a second test to screen blood, tissue, and organ donors in April 2010. The

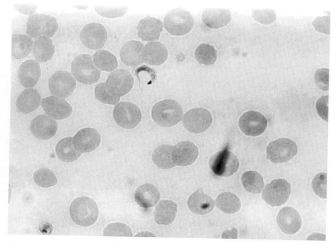

Figure 18–8. *T. cruzi* trypomastigote.

test, called the Abbott Prism Chagas, is highly sensitive and specific for the detection of antibodies to *T. cruzi*.[74]

The AABB TTD committee has given *T. cruzi* an orange category rating.[51] An orange category agent is considered a low scientific or epidemiological risk regarding blood saftey.[51] *T. cruzi* was assigned a moderate rating by the TTD committee based on public and regulatory attention to introducing blood donor screening.[51]

In the United States, medication for Chagas' disease may only be obtained by contacting the CDC.

Malaria (*Plasmodium* Species)

Malaria, another intraerythrocytic protozoan infection, may be caused by several species of the genus *Plasmodium* (*P. malaria*, *P. falciparum*, *P. vivax*, and *P. ovale*). Natural transmission occurs through the bite of a female *Anopheles* mosquito, but infection may also occur following transfusion of infected blood. Malaria is very rare in the United States, but it is the most common parasitic complication of transfusion.[3] There are approximately 1,500 cases of malaria diagnosed in the United States each year.[75] Between 1963 and 2009, there have been 96 reported cases of transfusion-transmitted malaria in the United States.[75]

Clinical Manifestations and Pathology

Symptoms include fever, chills, headache, anemia, hemolysis, and splenomegaly. There may be variations in symptoms among the different species of *Plasmodium*. Malaria often mimics other diseases, and its diagnosis is often delayed due to lack of suspicion in nonendemic areas.

Epidemiology and Transmission

Malaria is endemic in tropical and subtropical areas and in West Africa. The World Health Organization (WHO) estimated that in 2008, malaria caused 190 to 311 million clinical episodes and 708,000 to 1,003,000 deaths.[75] Many people associate malaria with a history of traveling to an endemic area. However, other transmission modes are possible, including blood transfusions and congenital infection.

Transfusion-associated malaria is acquired by receiving blood products from an asymptomatic carrier. *Plasmodium* can survive in blood components stored at room temperature or 4°C for at least a week, and deglycerolized RBCs can transmit disease.[3]

Laboratory Diagnosis

Examination of thick and thin blood smears is performed to diagnose infection with malaria. Although each species of *Plasmodium* varies morphologically, diagnosis can be quite difficult. Depending on the species of *Plasmodium* and the stage of the parasite's life cycle, timing is crucial when evaluating the blood smear. A single negative smear does not rule out a diagnosis of malaria.

Prophylaxis and Treatment

A practical or cost-effective serologic test to screen asymptomatic donors does not exist. According to AABB *Standards*, persons who have traveled to an endemic area are deferred for 1 year, and those who have had malaria or who have immigrated from or lived in an endemic area are deferred for 3 years.[1,3]

Chloroquine is generally effective for chemoprophylaxis and treatment of all four species of *Plasmodium*, except *P. vivax* acquired in Indonesia or Papua New Guinea, which is best treated with atovaquone-proguanil, with mefloquine or quinine plus tetracycline or doxycycline as alternatives.[76] Therapy has become more complicated due to the increase in resistance of *P. falciparum* and, more recently, *P. vivax* to chloroquine. It is important for the physician to carefully evaluate the species of *Plasmodium* causing the illness, the estimated parasitemia, and the patient's travel history. This information is necessary to prescribe appropriate therapy and decrease the chance of resistance by the organism.

Some individuals have a natural immunity to certain species of malaria, caused by a genetic alteration in their RBCs. These include persons who have sickle cell anemia or trait, G6PD deficiency, or RBCs that lack the Duffy blood group antigen.

Prion Disease

Creutzfeldt-Jakob Disease

Creutzfeldt-Jakob disease (CJD) is one of the transmissible spongiform encephalopathies (TSE). These are rare diseases characterized by fatal neurodegeneration that results in spongelike lesions in the brain. Although a definitive diagnosis can be made only at autopsy, neurological signs and symptoms and disease progression are used to make a preliminary diagnosis. Animals, such as sheep, goats, cattle, cats, minks, deer, and elk, and humans can be affected by TSE. In humans, sporadic CJD is the most common form, representing 85% to 90% of all cases, generally occurring in late middle age (average age 60 years). An inherited form due to a gene mutation accounts for another 5% to 10% of cases, and iatrogenic CJD acquired through contaminated neurosurgical equipment, cornea or dura mater transplants, or human-derived pituitary growth hormones accounts for less than 5% of cases. The sporadic, inherited, and iatrogenic CJD are considered the classic CJD.[76,77] In 1996, a variant form of CJD (vCJD) affecting younger individuals was noted, and epidemiological evidence linked vCJD to bovine spongiform encephalopathy, possibly from eating contaminated beef. Of the 129 cases reported from 1996 to 2002, most were in the United Kingdom.[76]

The causative agent of all TSEs is believed to be a "prion," which is described as a self-replicating protein. It does not contain nucleic acid but is formed when the confirmation of the normal cell surface glycoprotein, the prion protein, is changed to an abnormal form. This abnormal form accumulates in the brain and makes the brain tissue highly infectious. It is resistant to inactivation by heat, radiation, and formalin.[78]

The median duration of illness for vCJD is 13 to 14 months.[77] However, the incubation period in humans varies from 4 to 20 years and may eventually prove to be longer in some cases.

There is no epidemiological evidence linking classic CJD to TTD. However, in vCJD cases, prion particles have been found in lymphoreticular tissues, including the tonsils, spleen, and lymph nodes. As blood is intimately involved with the lymphoreticular system, concerns arose regarding the ability of vCJD individuals to transmit the prion to recipients of blood or blood products.[77]

Currently, there is no reliable diagnostic test that can detect asymptomatic individuals. Therefore, deferral of donors with connection to the United Kingdom and parts of Europe is used to prevent transmission.[3]

Pathogen Inactivation

The safety of the blood supply in the United States has improved greatly over the years, with improved screening of donors and testing of the blood product. However, pathogen inactivation methods have been developed to account for residual risks associated with serologic window periods, virus variants, and laboratory errors and for organisms for which testing is not performed routinely.[79] The possibility of newly emerging pathogens also exists as evidenced by WNV that can be transmitted by blood.

Plasma Derivatives

Heat inactivation, the first pathogen inactivation intervention, has been used since 1948 to treat albumin.[3] Even before the introduction of third-generation testing for HBsAg, heat inactivation prevented the transmission of HBV. The transmission of viruses or bacteria has been prevented due to albumin's pasteurization method (60°C for 10 hours).[3]

In 1973, third-generation assays for HBsAg were licensed. Only one case of HBV transmission by immune globulin was ever documented before then. Intramuscular immune globulin has never transmitted HIV or HCV. All immunoglobulin plasma pools were screened for HBsAg, and only those that were negative were used. Viral inactivation included cold-ethanol (Cohn-Oncley) fractionation and anion-exchange chromatography (for one IV immunoglobulin). However, in 1994, the FDA required viral clearance processing or proof of absence of HCV by NAT testing because of outbreaks of HCV from anion-exchange chromatography in Ireland and Germany that did not use a viral clearance procedure. NAT is now used in the processing of all source plasmas.[3]

Coagulation factors had a high rate of viral transmission until the early 1980s. Chronic hepatitis was the biggest problem until HIV emerged. More than 50% of all hemophiliacs receiving concentrates became infected with HIV. Since 1987, these clotting factors have become very safe with implementation of a variety of virus inactivation steps, and there have been no cases of HIV transmission. Today, all manufacturers use methods that either remove the virus or inactivate it. The lipid-enveloped viruses—HIV, HBV, HCV, HTLV, EBV, CMV, HHV-6 and HHV-8—are all inactivated by use of organic solvents and detergents. This process is not effective with non-lipid-enveloped viruses such as HAV and parvovirus B-19.[3,80]

The current risk of enveloped virus transmission is very low because of the combination of treatments such as heat treatment, solvent and detergent treatment, and nanofiltration.[81] These methods are often used in combination during the manufacturing process. With the exception of one case of HCV transmission in IV immune globulin in 1994, there have been no cases of HBV, HCV, or HIV since 1985 by any U.S. licensed plasma derivative.[80]

Cellular Components

Pathogen inactivation using psoralen activated by ultraviolet light has been tested with platelet concentrates. It has been shown to inactivate cell-associated viruses, cell-free viruses, and selected prokaryotic organisms. Whether this process will work against intracellular bacterial organisms has not been established. There are three licensed platelet pathogen reduction systems that are currently in use in the United States and Canada: the Cerus Corporation INTERCEPT Blood System, CaridianBCT Biotechnologies Mirasol PRT, and the MacoPharma's Theraflex UV.[51] These companies also have processes for pathogen reduction in plasma.[51]

CaridianBCT Biotechnologies is currently using a photochemical process for red cell pathogen reduction. This system incorporates riboflavin and UV light.[51] A process for RBCs that uses a chemical cross-linker specific for nucleic acid is being designed by Cerus Corporation.[51]

Limitations of pathogen reduction systems include agents with intrinsic resistance, such as prions, some bacterial spores, and nonenveloped viruses.[51] Some viruses may not be inactivated if they are of high titer, including B19V and HBV.[51]

Quarantine and Recipient Tracing (Look-Back)

All blood banks and transfusion services are required to have a process to detect, report, and evaluate any complication of transfusion, including recipient development of HBV, HCV, HIV, or HTLV. There must be an established method to notify donors of any abnormality with the predonation evaluation, laboratory testing, or recipient follow-up. A report should be submitted to the collecting agency when the recipient of a blood component develops a TTD.[1]

Current donations that test positive for HBV, HCV, HIV, or HTLV cannot be used for transfusion.[1] All prior donations from these donors become suspect. The timeline and standards using the look-back procedure to identify recipients of a component from the implicated donation or other donations by the same donor differ depending on the disease. Any prior components still in date must be quarantined, and the disposition depends on results of licensed supplemental tests.[3]

If on recipient follow-up it is noted that a patient developed HBV, HCV, HIV, or HTLV after receiving a single unit from one donor, that donor is permanently deferred. If the recipient received donations from several donors, all donors do not have to be excluded. These implicated donors may be called in for retesting. If a donor has been implicated in more than one case of TTD, this donor should be retested and possibly permanently deferred.[3] Once a donor has been implicated in a TTD, other recipients of a component from the suspected donor should be contacted. The donor must be placed on the appropriate donor deferral list if subsequent tests are positive.[3] Donors who have been permanently deferred due to positive test results must be notified of the fact. Notification and a thorough explanation of the positive tests results and their implications must be given to the donor.[3] Follow-up testing should be performed by the donor's own physician.[3]

Autologous donations positive for HBV, HCV, HIV, HTLV, or syphilis can be used. If they are not transfused at the collecting facility, the collecting facility must notify the transfusion service. Testing must be repeated every 30 days on at least the first unit to be shipped. Information about abnormalities must be transmitted to the patient and the patient's physician.[1]

Any fatalities due to a TTD must be reported to the director of the Center for Biologics Evaluation and Research within 1 working day, followed by a written report within 7 days.[81] Table 18–5 summarizes the laboratory tests for transfusion-transmitted diseases.

Table 18–5   Summary of Laboratory Tests for Transfusion-Transmitted Diseases

DISEASE	TESTING	DATE IMPLEMENTED	TEST METHOD	CONFIRMATORY TEST METHOD	RISK OF TRANSMISSION
Hepatitis B Virus (HBV)	B surface antigen (HB$_s$A$_q$)	1971	ChLIA	Antigen neutralization	1 in 200,000 and 1 in 500,000[1,2]
	Hepatitis B core antibody (HB$_c$)	1986	ChLIA	Ultrasensitive HBV DNA detection by PCR	1 in 200,000 and 1 in 500,000[1,2]
	Confirmatory testing	2009	NAT	All TMA-reactive donations confirmed by PCR	

Continued

Table 18–5 Summary of Laboratory Tests for Transfusion-Transmitted Diseases—cont'd

DISEASE	TESTING	DATE IMPLEMENTED	TEST METHOD	CONFIRMATORY TEST METHOD	RISK OF TRANSMISSION
Human T-Lymphotropic Virus (HTLV-I/II)	Qualitative antibody detection for both HTLV-I and HTLV-II in a combined test	1998	ChLIA		(HTLV-I) less than 1 in 2 million[3] (HTLV-II is not yet proven unequivocally to be of significant clinical concern).
Hepatitis C Virus (HCV)	Antibody testing	1990	ELISA	RIBA	1 in 1,390,000[1]
	Nucleic Acid Testing (NAT)	1999	NAT (using TMA in minipools of 16...)	NAT	
Human Immunodeficiency Viruses, Types 1 and 2 (HIV 1, 2)	Antibody Testing	1985	EIA	One or a combination of: HIV-1 IFA and HIV-2 EIA ("A rapid diagnostic test is used for HIV-1 and HIV-2 differentiation)	1 in 2 million[1]
	NAT	1999	NAT (using TMA in minipools of 16...)		
Chagas' Disease (*T. cruzi*)	Antibody testing—qualitative detection of antibodies to *T. cruzi*	2007	ELISA	RIPA	At least 7 reported in the U.S. and Canada[4]
Syphilis (*Treponema pallidum*)	Antibody testing—qualitative screening test detects presence of antibodies to *Treponema pallidum*	1950s	*NAT	EIA, as well as a test for regain (a protein-like substance that is present during acute infection and for several months following resolution of infection).	0* (No cases of transfusion-transmitted syphilis have been recorded for more than 30 years).
West Nile Virus (WNV)	WNV RNA detection	2003	*NAT (same type of assay as used for HBV, HIV-1, and HCV).		9 documented cases (since the introduction of blood donor screening).

ChLIA = Chemiluminescent immunoassay; ***NAT** = Nucleic Acid Testing (Polymerase chain reaction (PCR) for anti-HBc; Transcription mediated amplification (TMA) for HBV DNA); **ELISA** = Enzyme-Linked, Immunosorbent Assay Test System; **RIBA** = Recombinant Immunoblot Assay; **EIA** = Enzyme Immunoassay; **IFA** = Indirect Immunofluorescence Assay; **RIPA** = Radioimmunoprecipitation Assay.

References: Cited in American Red Cross, Infectious Disease Testing, on: http://www.redcrossblood.org/learn-about-blood/what-happens-donated-blood/blood-testing

1. Stramer S. Current risks of transfusion-transmitted agents—A Review. Arch Pathol Lab Med. 2007; 131: 702-707.
2. Zou S, et al. Current Incidence and residual risk of hepatitis B infection among blood donors in the United States. Transfusion 2009; 49:1609-1620.
3. Dodd RY, et al. Current prevalence and incidence of infectious disease markers and estimated window-period risk in the American Red Cross blood donor population. Transfusion 2002; 42: 975-97.
4. Young C, Losikoff P, Chawla A, Glasser L, Forman E. Transfusion-acquired *Trypanosoma cruzi* infection. Transfusion 2007;47:540-4. in Perkins HA and Busch MP, Transfusion-associated infections: 50 years of relentless challenges and remarkable progress. Transfusion 2010; 8-9. doi: 10.1111/j.1537-2995.2010.02851.x

SUMMARY CHART

- ✔ The first and most important step in ensuring that transfused blood will not transmit a pathogenic virus is careful selection of the donor.
- ✔ HAV is usually spread by the fecal-oral route in communities where hygiene is compromised.
- ✔ On infection with HBV, the first serologic marker to appear is HBsAg, followed by HBeAg and IgM anti-HBc within the first few weeks of exposure.
- ✔ HBIG is an immune globulin prepared from persons with a high titer of anti-HBs and is used to provide passive immunity to health-care workers and others who are exposed to patients with HBV infection.
- ✔ A combined vaccine for HAV and HBV is available to provide immunity.
- ✔ HDV infection is common among drug addicts and can occur simultaneously with HBV infection; diagnosis depends on finding anti-HDV or HDV RNA in the serum.
- ✔ Of all HCV infections, 60% to 70% are asymptomatic. With the implementation of NAT testing for HCV, the window period has been reduced to 10 to 30 days.
- ✔ HCV is the leading cause of liver transplants in the United States.
- ✔ Diagnosis of HIV-1 and HIV-2 infection is dependent on the presence of antibodies to both envelope and core proteins; HIV-positive persons with fewer than 200 CD4+ T cells per μL are considered to have AIDS in the absence of symptoms.

- ✔ Transfusion-associated CMV infection is a concern for seronegative allogeneic organ transplant recipients and fetuses. Reactivation of a latent infection can occur when an individual becomes severely immunocompromised.
- ✔ The risk of CMV infection for low-birth-weight neonates is not as great as it was in the past due to better transfusion techniques and management of their conditions.
- ✔ The WB confirmation test detects the presence of anti-HIV and determines with which viral proteins the antibodies react.
- ✔ The window period for HIV can be shortened by using the polymerase chain reaction, which detects HIV infection before tests for antigen or antibody are positive.
- ✔ Bacterial contamination is the most frequent cause of transfusion-transmitted infection.
- ✔ Because routine screening for parasitic infections is not currently available, many blood banks have added questions to their donor questionnaire that address topics associated with risk for parasitic infection.
- ✔ Pathogen inactivation methods are under development to remove the residual risk of transfusion-associated disease due to the window period, virus variants, laboratory mistakes, and new, emerging diseases.
- ✔ Look-back is a process mandated by the FDA that directs collection facilities to notify donors who test positive for viral markers, to notify prior recipients of the possibility of infection, and to quarantine or discard implicated components currently in inventory.

Review Questions

1. The fecal-oral route is common in transmitting which of these hepatitis viruses?
   a. HAV
   b. HBV
   c. HDV
   d. HCV

2. Which of the following is the component of choice for a low-birth-weight infant with a hemoglobin of 8 g/dL if the mother is anti-CMV negative?
   a. Whole blood from a donor with anti-CMV
   b. RBCs from a donor who is anti-CMV negative
   c. Leukoreduced platelets
   d. Solvent detergent–treated plasma

3. Which of the following tests is useful to confirm that a patient or donor is infected with HCV?
   a. ALT + anti-HBc
   b. Anti-HIV 1/2
   c. Lymph node biopsy
   d. RIBA

4. Currently, which of the following does the AABB consider to be the most significant infectious threat from transfusion?
   a. Bacterial contamination
   b. CMV
   c. Hepatitis
   d. HIV

5. Which of the following is the most frequently transmitted virus from mother to fetus?
   a. HIV
   b. Hepatitis
   c. CMV
   d. EBV

6. Jaundice due to HAV is seen most often in the:
   a. Adolescent.
   b. Adult.
   c. Child younger than 6 years old.
   d. Newborn.

7. Currently, steps taken to reduce transfusion-transmitted CMV include:
   a. Plaque reduction neutralization test.
   b. NAT testing.
   c. Leukoreduction.
   d. Minipool screening.

8. HBV remains infectious on environmental surfaces for 1:
   a. Day.
   b. Week.
   c. Month.
   d. Year.

9. HBV is transmitted most frequently:
   a. By needle sharing among IV drug users.
   b. Through blood transfusions.
   c. By unknown methods
   d. By sexual activity

10. Which of the following is the most common cause of chronic hepatitis, cirrhosis, and hepatocellular carcinoma in the United States?
    a. HAV
    b. HBV
    c. HCV
    d. HDV

11. The first retrovirus to be associated with human disease was:
    a. HCV
    b. HIV
    c. HTLV-I
    d. WNV

12. All of the following statements are true concerning WNV except:
    a. 1 in 150 infections results in severe neurologic disease.
    b. Severe disease occurs most frequently in the over-50 age group.
    c. Deaths occur more often in those over 65 years who present with encephalitis.
    d. Fatalities occur in approximately 38% of infected individuals.

13. The primary host for WNV is:
    a. Birds.
    b. Horses.
    c. Humans.
    d. Bats.

14. Tests for WNV include all of the following except:
    a. ELISA.
    b. NAT.
    c. Plaque reduction neutralization test.
    d. Immunofluorescent antibody assay.

15. Individuals exposed to EBV maintain an asymptomatic latent infection in:
    a. B cells.
    b. T cells.
    c. All lymphocytes.
    d. Monocytes.

16. Fifth disease is caused by:
    a. CMV.
    b. EBV.
    c. Parvovirus B19.
    d. HTLV-II.

17. Transient aplastic crisis can occur with:
    a. Parvovirus B19.
    b. WNV.
    c. CMV.
    d. EBV.

18. Reasons why syphilis is so rare in the United States blood supply include all of the following except:
    a. 4°C storage conditions.
    b. Donor questionnaire.
    c. Short spirochetemia.
    d. NAT testing.

19. Nucleic acid amplification testing for HIV was instituted in donor testing protocols to:
    a. Identify donors with late-stage HIV who lack antibodies.
    b. Confirm the presence of anti-HIV in asymptomatic HIV-infected donors.
    c. Reduce the window period by detecting the virus earlier than other available tests.
    d. Detect antibodies to specific HIV viral proteins, including anti-p24, anti-gp41, and anti-gp120.

20. Screening for HIV is performed using the following technique:
    a. Radio immunoassay
    b. WB
    c. Immunofluorescent antibody assay
    d. NAT

21. The first form of pathogen inactivation was:
    a. Chemical.
    b. Heat.
    c. Cold-ethanol fractionation.
    d. Anion-exchange chromatography.

22. What is the most common parasitic complication of transfusion?
    a. *Babesia microti*
    b. *Trypanosoma cruzi*
    c. *Plasmodium* species
    d. *Toxoplasma gondii*

23. Which organism has a characteristic C- or U-shape on stained blood smears?

   a. *Trypanosoma cruzi*
   b. *Plasmodium vivax*
   c. *Plasmodium falciparum*
   d. *Babesia microti*

24. Which transfusion-associated parasite may have asymptomatic carriers?

   a. *Babesia microti*
   b. *Trypanosoma cruzi*
   c. *Plasmodium* species
   d. All of the above

25. Which disease is naturally caused by the bite of a deer tick?

   a. Chagas' disease
   b. Babesiosis
   c. Malaria
   d. Leishmaniasis

References

1. American Association of Blood Banks: Standards for blood banks and transfusion services, 26th ed. AABB, 2009.
2. Centers for Disease Control and Prevention: Detection of West Nile virus in blood donations—United States, 2003. MMWR 59:25, 2010.
3. Roback, JD (ed): Technical Manual, 16th ed. American Association of Blood Banks, Bethesda, MD, 2008.
4. Bishop, ML, et al: Clinical Chemistry Techniques, Principles and Correlations, 6th ed. Lippincott, Williams & Wilkins, Baltimore, MD, 2010.
5. Lemon, SM: Type A viral hepatitis: Epidemiology, diagnosis, and prevention. Clin Chem 43;8:1494, 1994.
6. Soucie, JM, et al: Hepatitis A virus infections associated with clotting factor concentrates in the United States. Transfusion 38:573, 1998.
7. Miller, LE: Serology of viral infections. In Stevens, CD (ed): Clinical Immunology and Serology: A Laboratory Perspective, 2nd ed. FA Davis Company, Philadelphia, 2003, p 324.
8. Centers for Disease Control and Prevention: Hepatitis A Information for the Public. Available at www.cdc.gov/hepatitis/A/afap.htm#transmission. Accessed July 30, 2010.
9. Centers for Disease Control and Prevention: Hepatitis B virus. Available at www.cdc.gov/hepatitis/resources/professionals/pdfs/ABCTable_BW.pdf. Accessed August 9, 2010.
10. Centers for Disease Control and Prevention: Surveillance for Acute Viral Hepatitis—United States, 2007. Available at www.cdc.gov/mmwr/PDF/ss/ss5803.pdf. Accessed August 9, 2010.
11. Lox, ASF, and McMahon, BF: AASLD practice guidelines: Chronic hepatitis B. Hepatology 34:1225, 2001.
12. Marcellin, P, et al: Adefovir dipivoxil for treatment of hepatitis B antigen-positive chronic hepatitis B. N Engl J Med. 348:808, 2003.
13. Gerlach, JT: Acute hepatitis C: High rate of both spontaneous and treatment-induced viral clearance. Gastroenterology 125:80, 2003.
14. Centers for Disease Control and Prevention: Hepatitis E virus. Available at www.cdc.gov//hepatitis/HEV?HEVfaq.htm#section1. Accessed August 9,2010.
15. Alter, H, et al: The incidence of transfusion associated hepatitis G virus infection and its relation to liver disease. N Engl J Med 336:747, 1997.
16. Heringlake, S, et al: Association between fulminant hepatic failure and a strain of GB virus C. Lancet 348:1626, 1996.
17. Halasz, R, et al: GB virus C/hepatitis G virus. Scand J Infect Dis 33:572, 2001.
18. Nunnari, G, et al: Slower progression of HIV-1 infection in persons with GB virus C coinfection correlates with an intact T-helper 1 cytokine profile. Ann Intern Med 139:26, 2003.
19. Zanetti, AR, et al: Multicenter trial on mother-infant transmission of GBV-virus. J Med Virol 54:107, 1998.
20. Sathar, MA, et al: GB virus C/hepatitis G virus (GBV-C/HGV): Still looking for a disease. Int J Exper Pathol 81:305, 2000.
21. Jarvis, LM, et al: The effect of treatment with alpha-interferon on hepatitis G/GBV-C viraemia. The CONSTRUCT Group. Scand J Gastroenterol 33:195, 1999.
22. Centers for Disease Control and Prevention: HIV/AIDS Prevalence Estimates, United States, 2006. Available at www.cdc.gov/mmwr/preview/mmurhtm/mm5739a2.htm. Accessed August 11, 2010.
23. Centers for Disease Control and Prevention: HIV and AIDs in the United States. Available at www.cdc.gov/hiv/resources/factsheets/us.htm. Accessed August 11, 2010.
24. American Red Cross: Blood Testing. Available at www.redcross/blood.org/learn-about-blood/what-happens=donated-blood/blood-testing. Accessed August 11, 2010.
25. Centers for Disease Control: Advancing HIV prevention: New strategies for a changing epidemic—United States, 2005. Available at www.cdc.gov/hiv/topics/prev_prog/AHP/default.htm. Accessed August 11, 2010.
26. Manns, A, Hisada, M, and La Grenade, L: Human T-lymphotropic virus type I infection. Lancet 353:1951, 1999.
27. Matsuoka, M: Human T-cell leukemia virus type I and adult T-cell leukemia. Oncogene 22:5131, 2003.
28. Nagai, M, and Osame, M: Human T-cell lymphotropic virus type I and neurological diseases. J Neurovirol 9:228, 2003.
29. Murphy, EL, et al: Increased prevalence of infectious diseases and other adverse outcomes in human T lymphotropic virus types I- and II-infected blood donors. J Infect Dis 176:1468, 1997.
30. American Association of Blood Banks: Dual enzyme immuno assay (EIA) approach for deferral and notification of anti-HTLV-I/II EIA reactive donors. Association Bulletin #99–9. Available at www.aabb.org/members_only/archives/association_bulletins/ab99–9.htm. Accessed on August 11, 2010.
31. Prowse, CV: An ABC for West Nile virus. Transfus Med 13:1, 2003.
32. Petersen, LR, Marfin, AA, and Gubler, DJ: West Nile virus. JAMA 290:524, 2003.
33. Centers for Disease Control and Prevention: West Nile virus statistics, surveillance and control archive. Available at www.cdc.gov/ncidod/dvbid/westnile/surv&control.htm. Accessed August 13, 2010.
34. Centers for Disease Control and Prevention: Acute flaccid paralysis syndrome associated with West Nile virus infection—Mississippi and Louisiana, July–August 2002. MMWR 51:825, 2002.
35. Centers for Disease Control and Prevention: West Nile virus: Overview of West Nile virus. Available at www.cdc.gov/ncidod/dvbid/westnile/qa/overview.htm. Accessed August 13, 2010.
36. Petersen, LR, and Marfin, AA: West Nile virus: A primer for clinicians. Ann Intern Med 137:173, 2002.
37. Centers for Disease Control and Prevention: Epidemic/Epizootic West Nile virus in the United States: Guidelines for surveillance, prevention, and control. Available at www.cdc.gov/ncidod/dvbid/westnile/lab_DiagnosticTesting.htm. Accessed August 16, 2010.
38. Busch, MP, et al: Screening the blood supply for West Nile virus RNA by nucleic acid amplification testing. N Engl J Med 353:460–467, 2005.
39. Centers for Disease Control and Prevention: Dispatch: Update: Detection of West Nile virus in blood donations—United States, 2003. MMWR 52:2003. Available at www.cdc.gov/mmwr/preview/mmwrhtm/mm5232a3.htm. Accessed August 16, 2010.

40. Centers for Disease Control and Prevention: Cytomegalovirus (CMV) infection. Available at www.cdc.gov/cmv/overview.html. Accessed August 17, 2010.

41. Laupacis, A, et al: Conference report: Prevention of posttransfusion CMV in the era of universal WBC reduction: A consensus statement. Transfusion 41:560, 2001.

42. Ely, JW, Yankowitz, J, and Bowdler, NC: Evaluation of pregnant women exposed to respiratory viruses. Available at http://aafp.org/afp/20000515/3065.html. Accessed August 17, 2010.

43. Roback, JD, et al: Multicenter evaluation of PCR methods for detecting CMV DNA in blood donors. Transfusion 41:1249, 2001.

44. Centers for Disease Control and Prevention: Epstein-Barr virus and infectious mononucleosis. May 16, 2006. Available at www.cdc.gov/ncidod/diseases/ebv.htm. Accessed August 17, 2010.

45. Tattevin, P, et al: Transfusion-related infectious mononucleosis. J Infect Dis 34:777, 2002.

46. Epstein, MA, Achong, BG, and Barr, YM: Virus particles in cultured lymphoblasts from Burkitts's lymphoma. Lancet 1:702, 1964.

47. Centers for Disease Control and Prevention: Parvovirus B19 (fifth disease). Available at www.cdc.gov/ncidod/dvrd/revb/respiratory/paro_b19/.htm. Accessed August 17, 2010.

48. Centers for Disease Control and Prevention: Parvovirus B19 infection and pregnancy. Available at www.cdc.gov/ncidod/dvrd/revb/respiratorys/B19&preg.htm. Accessed August 17, 2010.

49. Brown, KE, et al: Resistance to parvovirus B19 infection due to lack of virus receptor (erythrocyte P antigen). New Engl J Med 330:1192, 1994.

50. Weimer, T, et al: High-titer screening PCR: A successful strategy for reducing the parvovirus B19 load in plasma pools for fractionation. Transfusion 41:1500, 2001.

51. Stramer, SL, et al: Emerging infectious disease agent supplement and their potential threat to transfusion safety. Transfusion 49:2009.

52. FDA Guidance for Industry: Nucleic acid testing (NAT) to reduce the possible risk of parvovirus B19 transmission by plasma-derived products. Available at www.FDA.gov/BiologicsBlood Vaccines/Guidance Compliance Regulatory Information/Guidance/Blood/ucm071592.htm.

53. Hladik, W, et al: Transmission of human herpesvirus-8 by blood transfusion. N Engl J Med 355:1331–1338, 2006.

54. Pellett, PE, et al: Multicenter comparison of serologic assays and estimation of human herpesvirus 8 seroprevalence among US donors. Transfusion 43:1260, 2003.

55. Brecher, ME, and Hay, SN: Bacterial contamination of blood products. Clin Microbiol Rev 18(1): 195–204, 2005.

56. Kuehnert, MJ, et al: Transfusion-transmitted bacterial infection in the United States, 1998 through 2000. Transfusion 41;1493, 2001.

57. Centers for Disease Control: Red blood cell transfusions contaminated with *Yersinia enterocolitica*—United States, 1991–1996, and initiation of a national study to detect bacteria-associated transfusion reactions. MMWR 46:553, 1997.

58. Kunishima, S, et al: Presence of *Propionibacterium acnes* in blood components. Transfusion 41:1126, 2001.

59. Eder, A, Kennedy, J, Dy, B, et al: Bacterial screening of apheresis platelets and the residual risk of septic transfusion. The American Red Cross Experience (2004–2006). Transfusion 47:1134–1142, 2007.

60. de Korte, D, et al: Diversion of first blood volume results in a reduction of bacterial contamination for whole blood collections. Vox Sang 83:13, 2002.

61. Stevens, CD: Spirochete diseases. In Clinical Immunology and Aerology: A Laboratory Perspective, 2nd ed. FA Davis Company, Philadelphia, 2003, p 294.

62. Centers for Disease Control: Sexually Transmitted Diseases—Syphilis Fact Sheet. Available at www.cdc.gov/std/syphillis/stdfact-Syphillis.htm. Accessed August 23, 2010.

63. Centers for Disease Control: Babesiosis Fact Sheet. Available at www.cdc.gov/babesiosis/factsheet.htm/#intro. Accessed August 24, 2010.

64. Machon, CR, et al: Textbook of Diagnostic Microbiology. Saunders Elsevier, St., Louis, MO, 2007.

65. U.S. Food and Drug Administration: July 26–27, 2010: Blood Products Advisory Committee Meeting Presentations. Available at www.FDA.gov/advisory/committees/committeesmeeting-materials/BloodVaccines and other Biologics/BloodProducts AdvisoryCommittee/UCM221857.htm. Accessed August 24, 2010.

66. Leiby, DA: Transfusion-transmitted Babesia spp.: Bull's-eye on Babesia microti. Clin Microbiol Rev Jan:24(1):14–28, 2011.

67. Stramer, SL, Hollinger, FB, Katz, LM, et al: Emerging infectious disease agents and their potential threat to transfusion safety. Transfusion 49 Suppl 2:1S–29S, 2009.

68. Lettau, LA: Nosocomial transmission and infection control aspects of parasitic and ectoparasitic diseases part II. Infect Control Hosp Epidemiol 12:111, 1991.

69. Lux, JZ, et al: Transfusion-associated babesiosis after heart transplant. Emerg Infect Dis 9:116, 2003.

70. Jocoby, GA, et al: Treatment of transfusion-transmitted babesiosis by exchange transfusion. New Engl J Med 303:1098, 1980.

71. Evenson, DA, et al: Therapeutic apheresis for babesiosis. J Clin Apher 13:32, 1998.

72. McCullogh, J: Transfusion Medicine. McGraw-Hill, New York, 1998, p 377.

73. Pan, AA, and Winkler, MA: The threat of Chagas' disease in transfusion medicine. Lab Med 28:269, 1997.

74. U.S. Food and Drug Administration: FDA approves Chagas Disease Screening Test for Blood Tissue & Organ Donors. Available at www.FDA.gov/newsevents/newsroom/PressAnnouncements/ucm210429.htm.

75. Griffith, KS, et al: Treatment of malaria in the United States: A systemic review. JAMA 297(20):2007.

76. World Health Organization: Variant Creutzfeldt-Jakob disease. Fact Sheet No. 180. Revised November 2002. Available at www.who.int/mediacentre/factsheets/fs180/en/print.html. Accessed August 26, 2010.

77. Centers for Disease Control and Prevention: Bovine spongiform encephalopathy and Creutzfeldt-Jakob disease. Questions and answers regarding Creutzfeldt-Jakob disease infection-control practices. Available at www. cdc.gov/ncidod/dvrd/vcjd/indexhtm. Accessed August 26, 2010.

78. McKnight, C: Clinical implications of bovine spongiform encephalopathy. Clin Infect Dis 32:1726, 2001.

79. Purmal, A, et al: Process for the preparation of pathogen-inactivated RBC concentrates by using PEN110 chemistry: Preclinical studies. Transfusion 42:139, 2002.

80. Tabor, E: The epidemiology of virus transmission by plasma derivatives: Clinical studies verifying the lack of transmission of hepatitis B and C viruses and HIV type 1. Transfusion 39:1160, 1999.

81. Food and Drug Administration: Transfusion/Donation Fatalities. Available at www.fda.gov/BiologicsBloodVaccines/SafetyAvailability/ReportaProblem/transfusiondonationFatalities/default.htm. Accessed September 3, 2010.

Hemolytic Disease of the Fetus and Newborn (HDFN)

Melanie S. Kennedy, MD

OBJECTIVES

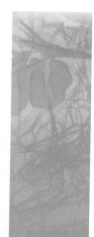

1. State the definition and characteristics of hemolytic disease of the fetus and newborn (HDFN).
2. Describe the role of the technologist in the diagnosis and clinical management of HDFN.
3. Compare and contrast ABO versus Rh HDFN in terms of:
   - Pathogenesis
   - Incidence
   - Blood types of mother and baby
   - Severity of disease
   - Laboratory data: anemia, direct antiglobulin test (DAT), and bilirubin
   - Prevention and treatment
4. Define Rh-immune globulin and describe its function.
5. Identify the indications and contraindications for administration of Rh-immune globulin.
6. List the tests used for detecting fetomaternal hemorrhage.
7. Outline the protocol for testing maternal and cord blood in cases of suspected HDFN.
8. Given maternal and infant ABO blood group phenotypes, state the possible ABO donor blood group(s) that would be selected for an exchange transfusion. Be specific as to donor blood groups for both the plasma and the red blood cells (RBCs).
9. State the blood components and the maximum age of the donor unit preferred for intrauterine or exchange transfusions.
10. State the source of cells and plasma (serum) to crossmatch an RBC unit for a newborn.

Introduction

Hemolytic disease of the fetus and newborn (HDFN) is the destruction of the red blood cells (RBCs) of a fetus and neonate by antibodies produced by the mother. The mother can be stimulated to form the antibodies by previous pregnancy or transfusion and sometimes during the second and third trimester of pregnancy. Previously, about 95% of the cases of HDFN were caused by antibodies in the mother directed against the **Rh antigen D, or Rh(D)**. The incidence of the disease caused by anti-D has steadily decreased since 1968 with the introduction of **Rh-immune globulin** (RhIG). Rh(D) incompatibility is common, although other RBC incompatibilities have surpassed D in frequency at referral centers.[1] Because Rh(D) incompatibility was a major concern for many years, the diagnosis and treatment of HDFN caused by anti-D has been the emphasis of much investigation. These findings can be applied to other clinically significant RBC antibodies that cause HDFN, with the exception of ABO antibodies, which are described separately.

In addition to the use of RhIG, many other advances have been made in the diagnosis and treatment of HDFN. Ultrasonography, Doppler assessment of middle cerebral artery peak systolic velocity, cordocentesis, allele-specific gene amplification studies on fetal cells in amniotic fluid, fetal DNA analysis in maternal plasma, and intravascular intrauterine transfusion have greatly increased the success of accurately diagnosing and adequately treating this disease.

This chapter will discuss the disease process, diagnosis, therapy, and outcomes of HDFN.

Etiology

Although the clinical findings in the fetus and newborn were noted as early as the 17th century, it was not until 1939 that Levine and Stetson reported a transfusion reaction from transfusing a husband's blood to a postpartum woman. They postulated that the mother had been immunized to the father's antigen through **fetomaternal hemorrhage**. The antigen was later identified as Rh(D).

HDFN is caused by the destruction of the RBCs of a fetus by antibodies produced by the mother. Only antibodies of the immunoglobulin G (IgG) class are actively transported across the placenta; other immunoglobulin classes, such as IgA and IgM, are not. Most IgG antibodies are directed against bacterial, fungal, and viral antigens, so the transfer of IgG from the mother to the fetus is beneficial. However, in HDFN, the antibodies are directed against those antigens on the fetal RBCs that were inherited from the father.

Rh HDFN

In Rh(D) HDFN, the Rh-positive firstborn infant of an Rh-negative mother usually is unaffected because the mother has not yet been immunized. During gestation and particularly at delivery, when the placenta separates from the uterus, variable numbers of fetal RBCs enter the maternal circulation. When D antigen is inherited from the father, these fetal cells immunize the mother and stimulate the production of anti-D. Once the mother is immunized to D antigen, all subsequent offspring who inherit the D antigen will be affected. The maternal anti-D crosses the placenta and binds to the fetal Rh-positive cells (Fig. 19–1). The sensitized RBCs are destroyed (hemolyzed) by the fetal monocyte-macrophage system, resulting in anemia.

There are several factors that affect immunization and severity of HDFN, including antigenic exposure, host factors, immunoglobulin class, antibody specificity, and influence of the ABO group.

Antigenic Exposure

Fetomaternal hemorrhage during pregnancy can cause significant increases in maternal antibody titers, leading to increasing severity of HDFN. Transplacental hemorrhage of fetal RBCs into the maternal circulation occurs in up to 7% of women during gestation, as determined by the acid-elution method for detecting fetal hemoglobin.[2] In addition, interventions such as amniocentesis and chorionic

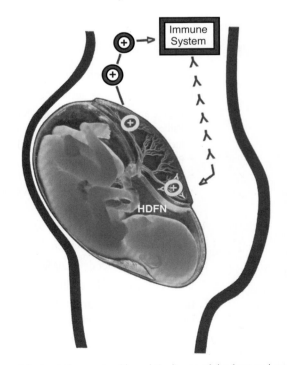

Hemorrhage of D-positive fetal RBCs into D-negative mother
↓
Maternal antibody formed against paternally inherited D antigen
↓
Next D-positive pregnancy
↓
Placental passage of maternal IgG anti-D
↓
Maternal antibody attaches to fetal RBCs
↓
Hemolysis of fetal RBCs

Figure 19–1. Pathogenesis of hemolytic disease of the fetus and newborn caused by D incompatibility between the fetus and mother. The pathogenesis of other blood group incompatibilities (except ABO) follows the same pattern.

villus sampling and trauma to the abdomen can increase the risk of fetomaternal hemorrhage. At delivery, the incidence is more than 50%. In the majority of cases, the volume of fetomaternal hemorrhage is small; however, as little as 1 mL of fetal RBCs can immunize the mother.[3]

The number of **antigens** on the fetal RBCs corresponds to heterozygous RBCs, because all fetal antigens incompatible with the mother have been inherited from the father, who can give only one set of genes to the fetus.

Host Factors

The ability of individuals to produce antibodies in response to antigenic exposure varies, depending on complex genetic factors. In Rh-negative individuals who are transfused with 200 mL of Rh-positive RBCs, approximately 85% respond and form anti-D.[4] Nearly all of the nonresponders will fail to produce anti-D even with repeated exposure to Rh-positive blood. On the other hand, if RhIG is not administered, the risk of immunization is only about 16% for an Rh-negative mother after an Rh-positive pregnancy.

Immunoglobulin Class

Immunoglobulin class and subclass of the maternal antibody affects the severity of the HDFN. Of the immunoglobulin classes (i.e., IgG, IgM, IgA, IgE, and IgD), only IgG is transported across the placenta. The active transport of IgG begins in the second trimester and continues until birth. The IgG molecules are transported via the FC portion of the antibodies (see Chapter 3, "Fundamentals of Immunology").

Of the four subclasses of IgG antibody, IgG_1 and IgG_3 are more efficient in RBC hemolysis than are IgG_2 and IgG_4. Therefore, the subclass(es) in the mother can affect the severity of the hemolytic disease. All subclasses of IgG are transported across the placenta.

Antibody Specificity

Of all the RBC antigens, D is the most antigenic. For this reason, only Rh-negative blood is transfused to Rh-negative females of childbearing potential. Other antigens in the Rh system, such as C, E, and c, are also potent immunogens (although less than D; Table 19–1). These other Rh antibodies have been associated with moderate to severe cases of HDFN. Anti-E and anti-c have caused severe HDFN that required intervention and treatment.

Of the non–Rh system antibodies, anti-Kell is considered the most clinically significant in its ability to cause HDFN. **Kell antigens** are present on immature erythroid cells in the bone marrow, so severe anemia occurs not only by destruction of circulating RBCs but also by precursors.[5] Almost any IgG RBC antibody is capable of causing HDFN, although the disease caused by these antibodies is usually mild to moderate in severity. Nevertheless, all pregnant women with IgG RBC antibodies should be followed closely for HDFN. Vengelen-Tyler lists and discusses 64 different RBC antibody specificities reported to cause HDFN.[6]

Table 19–1	Antibodies Identified in Prenatal Specimens as a Cause of HDFN	
COMMON	**RARE**	**NEVER**
Anti-D	Anti-Fy^a	Anti-Le^a
Anti-D + C	Anti-s	Anti-Le^b
Anti-D + E	Anti-M	Anti-I
Anti-C	Anti-N	Anti-IH
Anti-E	Anti-S	Anti-P$_1$
Anti-c	Anti-Jk^a	
Anti-e		
Anti-K		

Influence of ABO Group

When the mother is ABO incompatible with the fetus (major incompatibility), the incidence of detectable fetomaternal hemorrhage is decreased. Investigators noted many years ago that the incidence of D immunization is less in mothers with major ABO incompatibility with the fetus. The ABO incompatibility protects somewhat against Rh immunization, apparently by the hemolysis of ABO-incompatible D-positive fetal RBCs in the mother's circulation before the D antigen can be recognized by her immune system.

Pathogenesis

Pathogenesis is the effect of the maternal antibody on the fetus, the reasons for the effects, and the ensuing signs and symptoms.

Hemolysis, Anemia, and Erythropoiesis

Hemolysis occurs when maternal IgG attaches to specific antigens of the fetal RBCs (see **Fig. 19–1**). The antibody-coated cells are removed from the circulation by the macrophages of the spleen. The rate of RBC destruction depends on antibody titer and specificity and on the number of antigenic sites on the fetal RBCs. Destruction of fetal RBCs and the resulting anemia stimulate the fetal bone marrow to produce RBCs at an accelerated rate, even to the point that immature RBCs (erythroblasts) are released into the circulation. The term *erythroblastosis fetalis* was used to describe this finding. When the bone marrow fails to produce enough RBCs to keep up with the rate of RBC destruction, erythropoiesis outside the bone marrow is increased in the hematopoietic tissues of the spleen and liver. These organs become enlarged (hepatosplenomegaly), resulting in portal hypertension and hepatocellular damage.

Severe anemia and hypoproteinemia (caused by decreased hepatic production of plasma proteins) lead to the development of high-output cardiac failure with generalized edema, effusions, and ascites, a condition known as *hydrops fetalis*.

In severe cases, hydrops fetalis can develop by 18 to 20 weeks' gestation. In the past, hydrops fetalis was almost uniformly fatal; today, most fetuses with this condition can be treated successfully.

The process of RBC destruction continues even after such an infant is delivered alive—in fact, it continues as long as maternal antibody persists in the newborn infant's circulation. The rate of RBC destruction after birth decreases because no additional maternal antibody is entering the infant's circulation through the placenta. However, IgG is distributed both extravascularly and intravascularly and has a half-life of 25 days, so antibody binding and hemolysis of RBCs continue for several days to weeks after delivery.

Bilirubin

RBC destruction releases hemoglobin, which is metabolized to **bilirubin** (Table 19–2). This bilirubin is called *indirect* because indirect methods are required to measure the bilirubin in the laboratory. The indirect bilirubin is transported across the placenta and conjugated in the maternal liver to "direct" bilirubin. The **conjugated** bilirubin is then excreted by the mother. Although levels of total bilirubin in the fetal circulation and amniotic fluid may be elevated, they do not cause clinical disease in the fetus. However, after birth, accumulation of metabolic by-products of RBC destruction can become a severe problem for the newborn infant. The newborn liver is unable to conjugate bilirubin efficiently, especially in premature infants. With moderate to severe hemolysis, the unconjugated, or indirect, bilirubin can reach levels toxic to the infant's brain (generally, more than 18 to 20 mg/dL) and if left untreated can cause **kernicterus** or permanent damage to parts of the brain.

Diagnosis and Management

The diagnosis and management of HDFN requires close cooperation among the pregnant patient, her obstetrician, her spouse or partner, and the personnel of the clinical laboratory performing the serologic testing. Serologic and clinical tests performed at appropriate times during the pregnancy can accurately determine the level of antibody in the maternal circulation, the potential of the antibody to cause HDFN, and the severity of RBC destruction during gestation (Fig. 19–2).[7] If clinical and serologic data indicate that the fetus is becoming

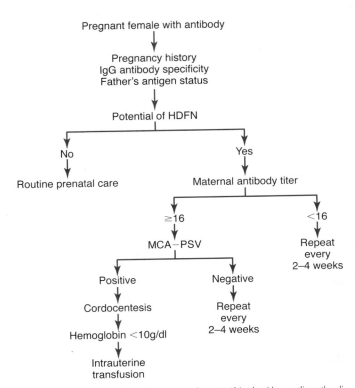

Figure 19–2. Diagnosis and Treatment of HDFN. This algorithm outlines the diagnostic tests and transfusion therapy indicated when antibody that can cause HDFN is identified. The history of previous pregnancies and the antigen typing of the father contribute to the expected severity of the HDFN. Titers of the mother's plasma guide decisions for more testing. When the MCA-PSV indicates anemia, cordocentesis will determine whether intrauterine transfusion is indicated.

severely anemic, interventions such as intrauterine transfusion can be used to treat the anemia and prevent the development of severe disease.

Serologic Testing of the Mother

The recommended obstetric practice is to perform the type and antibody screen at the first prenatal visit, preferably during the first trimester.[8] At that time, the pregnant woman can be asked about previous pregnancies and their outcomes and prior transfusions. Previous severe disease and poor outcome predict similar findings in the current pregnancy. Although antibody titers are useful in assessing the extent of intrauterine fetal anemia during the first affected pregnancy, antibody titers are less predictive in subsequent pregnancies.

ABO, Rh, and Antibody Screen

The prenatal specimen must be typed for ABO and Rh. The antibody screening method must be able to detect clinically significant IgG alloantibodies that are reactive at 37°C and in the antiglobulin phase. At least two separate reagent screening cells, covering all common blood group antigens (preferably homozygous), should be used. For tube testing, an antibody-enhancing medium such as polyethylene glycol (PeG) or low ionic strength solution (LISS) can increase sensitivity of the assay.

Prenatal patients may produce clinically insignificant antibodies, such as anti-Le[a] or anti-Le[b]. Therefore, immediate

Table 19–2	**Bilirubin Metabolism in the Fetus and Newborn**

DURING GESTATION	
Fetus	**Mother**
Indirect bilirubin (unconjugated)	Direct bilirubin (conjugated)

POSTDELIVERY	
Neonate	**Phototherapy**
Indirect bilirubin (kernicterus)	Bilirubin isomers (nontoxic)

spin and room temperature incubation phases are omitted, and anti-IgG rather than polyspecific antiglobulin reagent is used. These steps reduce detection of IgM antibodies, which cannot cross the placenta. Other antibody screening methods, such as solid phase or gel column, may be used.

If the antibody screen is nonreactive, repeat testing is recommended before RhIG therapy in Rh-negative prenatal patients and in the third trimester if the patient has been transfused or has a history of unexpected antibodies.[8]

Antibody Identification

If the antibody screen is reactive, the antibody identity must be determined. Follow-up testing will depend on the antibody specificity. Cold reactive IgM antibodies such as anti-I, anti-IH, anti-Le[a], anti-Le[b], and anti-P[1] can be ignored. Lewis system antibodies are rather common in pregnant women but have not been reported to cause HDFN.

Antibodies such as anti-M and anti-N can be IgM or IgG or a combination of both. Both anti-M and anti-N can cause mild to moderate HDFN, although rarely. To establish the immunoglobulin class, the serum can be treated with a sulfhydryl reagent, such as dithiothreitol or 2-mercaptoethanol, and then retested with appropriate controls. The J-chain of IgM antibodies will be destroyed by this treatment; IgG antibodies will remain reactive.

Many Rh-negative pregnant women have weakly reactive anti-D, particularly during the third trimester. Most of these women have received RhIG, either after an event with increased risk of fetomaternal hemorrhage or at 28 weeks' gestation (antenatal). The passively administered anti-D will be weakly reactive in testing and will remain demonstrable for 2 months or longer. This must be distinguished from active immunization. A titer higher than 4 almost always indicates active immunization; with a titer under 4, active immunization cannot be ruled out, but it is less likely.

If the antibody specificity is determined to be clinically significant and the antibody is IgG, further testing is required. Other than anti-D, the most common and most significant antibodies are anti-K, anti-E, anti-c, anti-C, and anti-Fy[a] (see Table 19–1).

Paternal Phenotype and Genotype

A specimen of the father's blood should be obtained and tested for the presence and zygosity of the corresponding antigen. If the mother has anti-D and the father is D-positive, a complete Rh phenotype can help determine his chance of being homozygous or heterozygous for the D antigen. A more sensitive and precise genotype can be determined by DNA methods. The information is helpful in determining further testing of the mother and in counseling her about potential treatment plans and complications of HDFN.

In cases of antibody specificity other than D, testing the father can save a great deal of time, expense, and worry if he is shown to lack the corresponding antigen. For example, only 9% of the random population is positive for the Kell antigen. The mother must be counseled in private as to the paternity of the fetus to ensure accurate paternal phenotyping.

Fetal DNA Testing

If the mother has anti-D and the father is likely to be heterozygous for the D antigen, amniocentesis or chorionic villous sampling can be performed as early as 10 to 12 weeks' gestation to determine whether the fetus has the gene for the D antigen. During the second trimester, maternal plasma can be tested for fetal DNA to determine genotype.[9] Testing can be performed for the genes coding c, e, C, E, K, Fy[a], Fy[b], Jk[a], Jk[b], M and others.

Antibody Titers

The relative concentration of all antibodies capable of crossing the placenta and causing HDFN is determined by **antibody titration**. The patient serum or plasma is serially diluted and tested against appropriate RBCs to determine the highest dilution at which a reaction occurs.[9] The method must include the indirect antiglobulin phase using anti-IgG reagent. The result is expressed as either the reciprocal of the titration endpoint or as a titer score.

The titration must be performed exactly the same way each time the patient's serum is tested. The recommended method is the saline antiglobulin tube test, with 60-minute incubation at 37°C and the use of anti-IgG reagent.[8] The RBCs used for each titration should have the same genotype (preferably homozygous for the antigen of interest), approximately the same storage time, and the same concentration. The first serum or plasma specimen should be frozen and run in parallel with later specimens. Only a difference of greater than 2 dilutions, or a score change of more than 10, is considered a significant change in titer.

The method chosen is critical for the appropriate clinical correlation. Methods using enhancing media or gel column result in higher titers, as shown by comparative proficiency testing. Therefore, the critical titer level for these other methods must be determined by reviewing the outcome of several pregnancies complicated by HDFN.

For the recommended method, 16 is considered the critical titer. If the initial titer is 16 or higher, a second titer should be done at about 18 to 20 weeks' gestation. A titer reproducibly and repeatedly at 32 or above is an indication for color Doppler imaging to assess middle cerebral artery peak systolic velocity (MCA-PSV) after 16 weeks' gestation.[10]

When the titer is less than 32, it should be repeated at 4-week intervals, beginning at 16 to 20 weeks' gestation and then every 2 to 4 weeks during the third trimester.

Antibody titer alone cannot predict severity of HDFN.[8] In some sensitized women, the antibody titer can remain moderately high throughout pregnancy while the fetus is becoming more severely affected. Similarly, a previously sensitized woman can have consistently high antibody titer whether pregnant or not, and whether the fetus is Rh-positive or Rh-negative. In others, the titer can rise rapidly, which portends increasing severity of HDFN. However, antibody titers consistently below the laboratory's critical titer throughout the pregnancy reliably predict an unaffected or mild-to-moderately affected fetus, with the exception of anti-K with a K-positive fetus.

Titration studies at time of delivery are not recommended, because they provide no clinically useful information.

Color Doppler Middle Cerebral Artery Peak Systolic Velocity

At about 16 to 20 weeks' gestation, further diagnosis and treatment are begun. Patients with a history of a severely affected fetus or early fetal death may require earlier intervention. The measurement of the fetal **middle cerebral artery peak systolic velocity** (MCA-PSV) with color Doppler ultrasonography can reliably predict anemia in the fetus.[10] Color Doppler indicates the direction of blood flow, using red for arterial flow and blue for venous. The middle cerebral artery is used because of its easy accessibility. The measurement is based on the reduced blood viscosity at low hematocrit and the resulting faster velocity. The peak systolic (arterial) velocity is plotted on a standardized graph to determine the critical point for cordocentesis. MCA-PSV is noninvasive and poses no adverse effects for the fetus.

Cordocentesis

Advanced sonography allows clinicians to obtain a sample of fetal blood through a procedure called **cordocentesis**. Using high-resolution ultrasound with color Doppler enhancement of blood flow, the umbilical vein is visualized at the level of the cord insertion into the placenta. A spinal needle is inserted into the umbilical vein, and a sample of the fetal blood is obtained. The fetal blood sample can then be tested for hemoglobin, hematocrit, bilirubin, blood type, direct antiglobulin test (DAT), and antigen phenotype and genotype.

Amniocentesis

For management of HDFN, amniocentesis is uncommonly used, because MCA-PSV is noninvasive and gives the same information.[11] The concentration of bilirubin pigment in the amniotic fluid estimates the extent of fetal hemolysis. The amniotic fluid is tested by a spectrophotometric scan at steadily increasing wavelengths, so the change in the optical density (ΔOD) at 450 nm (the absorbance of bilirubin) can be calculated. The measurement is plotted on a graph according to gestational age. An increasing or unchanging ΔOD 450 nm as pregnancy proceeds predicts worsening of the fetal hemolytic disease and the need for frequent monitoring and intervention if indicated. High values indicate severe and often life-threatening hemolysis (fetal hemoglobin less than 8 g/dL) and require urgent intervention.

Intrauterine Transfusion

Intervention in the form of intrauterine transfusion becomes necessary when one or more of the following conditions exists:

- MCA-PSV indicates anemia.
- Fetal hydrops is noted on ultrasound examination.
- Cordocentesis blood sample has hemoglobin level less than 10 g/dL.
- Amniotic fluid ΔOD 450 nm results are high.

Intrauterine transfusion is performed by accessing the fetal umbilical vein (cordocentesis) and injecting donor RBCs directly into the vein.[12] The goal of intrauterine transfusion is to maintain fetal hemoglobin above 10 g/dL. Once intrauterine transfusion is initiated, the procedure is repeated every 2 to 4 weeks until delivery. The initial intrauterine transfusion is rarely performed after 36 weeks' gestation. Intrauterine transfusion apparently suppresses the fetal bone marrow RBC production. During the first weeks after birth, the infant may require additional RBC transfusion.

Cordocentesis, intrauterine transfusion, and amniocentesis have several risks, including infection, premature labor, and trauma to the placenta, which may cause increased antibody titers because of antigenic challenge to the mother through fetomaternal hemorrhage.

Phototherapy

After delivery, the neonate can develop hyperbilirubinemia of unconjugated bilirubin. Phototherapy at 460 to 490 nm is used to change the unconjugated bilirubin to isomers, which are less lipophilic and less toxic to the brain.[13] Relatively high doses are given by using two banks of lights to surround the infant's body. In infants with mild-to-moderate hemolysis or history of intrauterine transfusion, phototherapy is generally sufficient.

Intravenous Immune Globulin

Intravenous immune globulin (IVIG) is increasingly used to treat hyperbilirubinemia of the newborn caused by HDFN. The IVIG competes with the mother's antibodies for the FC receptors on the macrophages in the infant's spleen, reducing the amount of hemolysis.

Exchange Transfusion

Exchange transfusion is the use of whole blood or equivalent to replace the neonate's circulating blood. Exchange transfusion is rarely required because of advances in phototherapy and the use of IVIG. In addition, less than one-half of the cases of HDFN are caused by anti-D, so the majority is generally less severe. Exchange transfusions are used primarily to remove high levels of unconjugated bilirubin and thus prevent kernicterus. Premature newborns are more likely than full-term infants to require exchange transfusions for elevated bilirubin because their livers are less able to conjugate bilirubin. Other advantages of exchange transfusion include the removal of part of the circulating maternal antibody, removal of sensitized RBCs, and replacement of incompatible RBCs with compatible RBCs; all of these help interrupt the bilirubin production caused by hemolysis.

Serologic Testing of the Newborn Infant

Serologic testing of the cord blood is used to confirm HDFN and prepare for possible transfusion.

ABO Grouping

ABO antigens are not fully developed in newborn infants, so newborns may show weaker reactions than older children and adults. In addition, infants do not have their own isoagglutinins but may have those of the mother, so reverse grouping cannot be used to confirm the ABO group.

Rh Typing

Rarely, the infant's RBCs can be heavily antibody-bound with maternal anti-D, causing a false-negative Rh type, or what has been called *blocked Rh.* An eluate from these RBCs will reveal anti-D, and typing of the eluted RBCs will show reaction with anti-D.

Direct Antiglobulin Test

The most important serologic test for diagnosing HDFN is the DAT with anti-IgG reagent. A positive test result indicates that the antibody is coating the infant's RBCs; however, the strength of the reaction does not correlate well with the severity of the HDFN. A positive test result may be found in infants without clinical or other laboratory evidence of hemolysis (e.g., mother received RhIG).

Elution

The routine preparation of an eluate of all infants with a positive DAT result is unnecessary. Elution in cases of known HDFN and postnatal ABO incompatibility is not needed, because eluate results do not change therapy. The preparation of an eluate may be helpful when the cause of HDFN is in question. As noted earlier, the resolution of a case of blocked Rh requires an eluate.

Newborn Transfusions

The newborn may receive small aliquot transfusions, which can be used to correct anemia when the bilirubin is successfully treated with phototherapy or IVIG. The suppression of erythropoiesis by small aliquot or exchange transfusions may cause anemia to occur after the immediate neonatal period.

Although full-term newborn infants normally have rather high hemoglobin levels (14 to 20 g/dL), a level below 10 g/dL may require transfusion, especially if the neonate has hypoxia needing oxygen supplementation. A hemoglobin level lower than 7 g/dL is considered severe anemia. A cord blood sample closely correlates with the levels during gestation.

Selection of Blood for Intrauterine and Neonatal Transfusion

Most centers treating HDFN use group O RBCs for intrauterine and neonatal transfusions. The RBCs must be antigen-negative for the mother's respective antibodies. Donors are usually cytomegalovirus (CMV)-negative as well. Physicians in these centers are transfusing neonates for other indications, such as RBC replacement for blood samples taken for laboratory tests. This allows a small inventory of group O CMV-negative donor units to be set aside for intrauterine and neonatal transfusions. Rh-negative units are selected for fetuses and neonates whose blood types are unknown or are Rh-negative.

For intrauterine transfusion, the hematocrit level of the RBCs should be greater than 70% because of the small volume transfused and the need to correct severe anemia.

For the rare exchange transfusions, one practice is to prepare RBCs from whole blood units and then replace the plasma with group AB plasma to reduce the amount of blood group antibodies transfused. This procedure is not necessary if both the neonate and the mother are the same ABO group.

Blood transfused to the fetus and premature infant should also be irradiated to prevent graft-versus-host disease (see Chapter 15, "Transfusion Therapy"). Blood for exchange transfusion should be irradiated and should not contain hemoglobin S, because the decreased oxygen tension that may occur early in the neonatal period may cause hemoglobin S trait blood to sickle. Traditionally, blood units less than 7 days from collection from the donor are selected. Special circumstances, such as the need for units of the mother's blood when high-incidence antibodies are involved, have shown that older blood units can be safe and effective for the newborn when infused slowly.

RhIG

Active immunization induced by RBC antigen can be prevented by the concurrent administration of the corresponding RBC antibody. This principle has been used to prevent immunization to D antigen by the use of high-titered RhIG.

During pregnancy and delivery, fetal and maternal blood are mixed. If the mother is Rh-negative and the fetus is Rh-positive, the mother has up to a 16% chance of being stimulated to form anti-D.[2] As little as 1 mL of fetal RBCs can elicit a response. Before delivery, the risk of sensitization is 1.5% to 1.9% in susceptible women, indicating that a significant amount of fetal RBCs can enter the maternal circulation during pregnancy.[2] However, the greatest risk of immunization to Rh is at delivery.

Mechanism of Action

The administered RhIG attaches to the fetal Rh-positive RBCs in the maternal circulation. The antibody-coated RBCs are removed by the macrophages in the maternal spleen. The amount of antibody necessary to prevent alloimmunization has been determined experimentally and is known to be less than that required to saturate all D-antigen sites. The mechanism of action of RhIG is uncertain. Evidence indicates it interferes with B-cell priming to make anti-D, although other modes of action may occur.[14]

Indications

This section describes the clinical indications for administering RhIG to the mother during pregnancy and after delivery.

Antenatal

Because of the known risk of Rh immunization during pregnancy, RhIG should be given early in the third trimester, or

Other Indications for RhIG

- Amniocentesis
- Chorionic villus sampling
- Abortion (spontaneous and induced)
- Ectopic pregnancy
- Abdominal trauma
- Greater than 40 weeks' gestation
- Accidental or inadvertent transfusion

at about 28 weeks' gestation. The dose does not pose a risk to the fetus, as this amount will cause a titer of only 1 or 2 in the mother.[2] However, a positive DAT result may be observed in the newborn. Box 19–1 lists antenatal, postpartum, and transfusion indications for RhIG administration.

Postpartum

The Rh-negative nonimmunized mother should receive RhIG soon after delivery of an Rh-positive infant. Based on experiments conducted many years ago, the recommended interval is within 72 hours after delivery. Even if more than 72 hours have elapsed, RhIG should still be given, as it may be effective and is not contraindicated.

Figure 19–3 outlines a decision tree for the indications and dose of postpartum RhIG administration. The mother

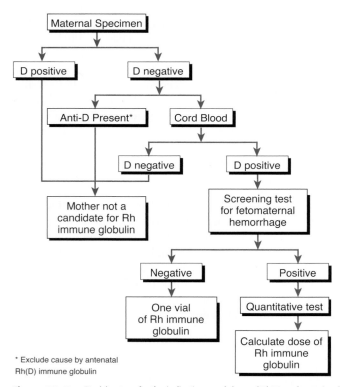

* Exclude cause by antenatal
Rh(D) immune globulin

Figure 19–3. Decision tree for the indications and dose of RhIG as determined by laboratory test results. If the cord or neonatal blood specimen is unavailable, assume the fetus is D-positive. *(Modified with permission from Kennedy MS: Rho(D) immune globulin. In Rayburn, W, and Zuspan, FP (eds): Drug Therapy in Gynecology and Obstetrics, 3rd ed. CV Mosby, St. Louis, 1991, p 235.)*

should be D-negative, and the infant should be D-positive or D-variant. If the type of the infant is unknown (e.g., if the infant is stillborn), RhIG should also be administered. Antibody titers are not recommended because the amount of circulating RhIG does not correlate with effectiveness of the immune suppression or with the amount of fetomaternal hemorrhage.

The half-life of IgG is about 25 days, so only about 10% of the antenatal dose will be present at 40 weeks' gestation. It is essential that the anti-D from antenatal RhIG present at delivery not be interpreted erroneously as active rather than passive immunization. Omission of the indicated dose after delivery may lead to active immunization.

Dose and Administration

The regular-dose vial of RhIG in the United States contains sufficient anti-D to protect against 15 mL of packed RBCs or 30 mL of whole blood. This is equal to 300 μg of the World Health Organization (WHO) reference material. In the United Kingdom, the regular-dose vial contains about 100 μg, which appears to be adequate for postpartum prophylaxis. The microdose (United States) can be used for abortions and ectopic pregnancies before the 12th week of gestation. The total fetal blood volume is estimated to be less than 5 mL at 12 weeks.

IV preparations of RhIG are approved for use in the United States. These products also contain 300 μg in each vial and can be administered either intramuscularly or intravenously. Additional manufacturing steps are required to allow IV use, so the products are more expensive.

Massive fetomaternal hemorrhages of more than 30 mL of whole blood occur in less than 1% of deliveries.[3] These massive hemorrhages can lead to immunization if adequate RhIG is not administered. A maternal sample should be obtained within 1 hour of delivery and screened—using a test such as the rosette technique—for massive fetomaternal hemorrhage. If positive, quantitation of the hemorrhage must be done by Kleihauer-Betke or by flow cytometry.

In the **Kleihauer-Betke test**, a maternal blood smear is treated with acid and then stained with counterstain. Fetal cells contain fetal hemoglobin (Hgb F), which is resistant to acid and will remain pink. The maternal cells will appear as ghosts. After 2,000 cells are counted, the percentage of fetal cells is determined, and the volume of fetal hemorrhage is calculated using this formula:

$$\frac{\text{Number of fetal cells} \times \text{Maternal blood volume}}{\text{Number of maternal cells}} = \text{Volume of fetomaternal hemorrhage}$$

The calculated volume of fetomaternal hemorrhage is then divided by 30 to determine the number of required vials of RhIG. A simpler way to calculate the dose is to multiply the fetal cell percentage by 50, which gives the volume of fetomaternal hemorrhage in milliliters. Because the Kleihauer-Betke is an estimate, one vial is added to the calculated answer.[15] If needed, additional vials of RhIG should be administered within 72 hours of delivery or as soon as possible.

The RhIG must be injected according to the product label. The IV product can also be given intramuscularly. The intramuscular form must be given intramuscularly only. IV injections of intramuscular preparations can cause severe anaphylactic reactions because of the anticomplementary activity of these products. RhIG also contains IgA and may be contraindicated in patients with anti-IgA and IgA deficiency who have had anaphylactic reactions to blood products.

Other Considerations

RhIG is of no benefit once a person has been actively immunized and has formed anti-D. However, care must be taken to distinguish women who have been passively immunized by antenatal administration of RhIG from those who have been actively immunized by exposure to Rh-positive RBCs.

Care must also be taken that fetal Rh-positive RBCs in the maternal circulation are not interpreted as maternal, because then the mother would be erroneously assumed to be weak D-positive. The difference is distinguished by a quantitative test such as the Kleihauer-Betke or by flow cytometry using antibody to hemoglobin F.

RhIG is not indicated for the mother if the infant is found to be D-negative. The blood type of fetuses in abortions, stillbirths, and ectopic pregnancies usually cannot be determined; therefore, RhIG should be administered in these circumstances. RhIG must not be given to the newborn infant.

There is no risk of transmission of the viral diseases hepatitis A and B and HIV with the administration of RhIG.

ABO HDFN

ABO incompatibility between the mother and newborn infant can cause HDFN. Maternal ABO antibodies that are IgG can cross the placenta and attach to the ABO-incompatible antigens of the fetal RBCs. However, destruction of fetal RBCs leading to severe anemia is extremely rare. More commonly, the disease is manifested by the onset of hyperbilirubinemia and jaundice within 12 to 48 hours of birth. The increasing levels of bilirubin can be treated with phototherapy. Severe cases requiring exchange transfusion are extremely rare. A comparison of ABO versus Rh HDFN is shown in Table 19–3.

As the incidence of HDFN caused by Rh(D) has declined, ABO incompatibility has become the most common cause of HDFN. Statistically, mother and infant are ABO-incompatible in one in every five pregnancies.

Factors Affecting Incidence and Severity

ABO antibodies are present in the plasma of all individuals whose RBCs lack the corresponding antigen. These antibodies, the result of environmental stimulus, occur more frequently as high-titered IgG antibodies in group O individuals than in group A or B individuals. Hence, ABO HDFN is nearly always limited to A or B infants of group O

Table 19–3	**Comparison of ABO Versus Rh HDFN**	
CHARACTERISTIC	**ABO**	**Rh**
First pregnancy	Yes	Rare
Disease predicted by titers	No	Yes
Antibody IgG	Yes (anti-A,B)	Yes (anti-D, etc.)
Bilirubin at birth	Normal range	Elevated
Anemia at birth	No	Yes
Phototherapy	Yes	Yes
Exchange transfusion	Rare	Uncommon
Intrauterine transfusion	None	Sometimes

mothers with potent anti-A,B. Most occur in group A infants in white populations. In the black population, however, group B infants are more often affected, and the overall incidence of ABO HDFN is several times greater than in other groups.

The mother's history of prior transfusions or pregnancies seems unrelated to the occurrence and severity of the disease. Thus, ABO HDFN can occur in the first pregnancy and in any, but not necessarily all, subsequent pregnancies. However, tetanus toxoid administration and helminth parasite infection during pregnancy have been linked to the production of high-titered IgG ABO antibodies and severe HDFN.

Even high-titered IgG antibodies that are transported across the placenta seem incapable of causing significant RBC destruction in an ABO-incompatible fetus. These infants are delivered with mild anemia or normal hemoglobin levels. The mild course of ABO HDFN is related more to the poor development of ABO antigens on fetal RBCs than the characteristics of the maternal antibody. ABO antigens are not fully developed until after the first year of life. Group A infant RBCs are serologically more similar to A_2 adult cells, with group A_2 infant RBCs much weaker. The weakened A antigen on fetal and neonatal RBCs is more readily demonstrable with human than with monoclonal anti-A reagents. As expected, group A_2 infants are less likely to have ABO HDFN.

The laboratory findings in ABO HDFN differ from those shown in Table 19–3 for Rh disease. Microspherocytes and increased RBC fragility in the infant are characteristic of ABO HDFN, but not of Rh HDFN. The severity of the disease is independent of the presence of a positive DAT result or demonstrable anti-A, anti-B, or anti-A,B in the eluate of the infant's RBCs.

The bilirubin peak is later, at 1 to 3 days. Phototherapy is usually sufficient for slowly rising bilirubin levels. With rapidly increasing bilirubin levels, IVIG or exchange transfusion with group O RBCs may be required. The serious consequences of Rh and other blood groups causing HDFN, such as stillbirth, hydrops fetalis, and kernicterus, are extremely rare in ABO HDFN.

Prenatal Screening

Many investigators have tried to use the immunoglobulin class and titer of maternal ABO antibodies to predict ABO HDFN. These tests are laborious and at best demonstrate the presence of IgG maternal antibody, but they do not correlate well with the extent of fetal RBC destruction. Consequently, detection of ABO HDFN is best done after birth.

Postnatal Diagnosis

No single serologic test is diagnostic for ABO HDFN. When a newborn develops jaundice within 12 to 48 hours after birth, various causes of jaundice need to be investigated, and ABO HDFN is only one. The DAT on the cord or neonatal RBCs is the most important diagnostic test. In all cases of ABO HDFN requiring transfusion therapy, the DAT result has been positive.[16] On the other hand, the DAT result can be positive even in the absence of signs and symptoms of clinical anemia in the newborn infant. However, these infants may have compensated anemia, or the RBCs are not destroyed by the reticuloendothelial system.

Collecting cord blood samples on all delivered infants is highly recommended. The sample should be collected by venipuncture to avoid contamination with maternal blood and Wharton's jelly (the material surrounding the blood vessels) and should be anticoagulated for storage. If the neonatal infant develops jaundice, ABO, Rh, and DAT results can be assessed. The DAT result is neither strongly nor consistently positive, although 90% of the cases complicated by jaundice are positive.[16] When the DAT result is negative but the infant is jaundiced, other causes of jaundice should be investigated. In the rare cases in which ABO incompatibility can be the only cause of neonatal jaundice, but the DAT result is negative, the eluate of the cord RBCs always reveals ABO antibodies. The eluate can also be helpful when the mother's blood specimen is not available.

CASE STUDIES

Case 19-1

Mother: gravida 1 para 0
Current pregnancy:
ABO/Rh(D) typing: O-negative
Today's antibody screen: Positive
Antibody identification: Anti-D
4 weeks ago antibody screen: Negative
6 months ago antibody screen: Negative
Gestational age: 32 weeks

1. What is the most probable cause of anti-D in this mother?
2. After delivery, is this mother an Rh immune globulin candidate?

Case 19-2

Mother: gravida 4 para 2
History:
Firstborn child unaffected
Second-born child mildly affected, positive DAT at birth and required no treatment
Third child stillborn
Mother had anti-D during second and third pregnancies
Current pregnancy:
ABO/Rh(D) typing: O-positive
Antibody screen: Positive
Antibody identification: Anti-D
Antibody titer:
Saline: negative
AHG: 128 (1:128)
Gestational age: 8 weeks

Same father as the three previous pregnancies (he is homozygous for the D antigen)

1. What is the most likely Rh(D) type of the fetus?
2. When should the titer be repeated?
3. Is there any intervention that should be done now? Why?
4. When should MCA-PSV be performed?

Case 19-3

Mother: gravida 3 para 2
History:
Firstborn child unaffected, mother's antibody screen negative
Second-born child mildly affected, ABO/Rh(D) typing A-positive, positive DAT, jaundice
Mother O-positive, antibody screen negative
Current pregnancy:
ABO/Rh(D) typing: O-positive
Antibody screen: Positive
Antibody identification: Anti-Le[a]
Gestational age: 32 weeks

1. What is the most probable cause of the second-born child being mildly affected?
2. Is the antibody identified in the current pregnancy clinically significant? Why?

Case 19-4

At a rural hospital near a migrant farm camp, a 32-year-old Hispanic woman just delivered a severely anemic infant. At 6 weeks' gestation, the mother had been typed as A-negative, with positive antibody screen. The antibody was identified as anti-D, titer 256. A report states that she had an intrauterine transfusion 3 weeks earlier at a university hospital in another state. The cord blood collected at delivery is typed as A-negative. On a heel-stick specimen, the infant's hemoglobin is reported as 4.3 g/dL and bilirubin as 3.9 mg/dL. Typing results of this specimen are as follows:

Anti-A	Anti-B	Anti-D	DAT
0	0	0	+/−

1. What is the infant's blood type? Why is the infant so anemic? What further testing is indicated?

Further testing shows the following:

	Cord Blood	Heel-stick
Anti-I	4 +	3 +
Kleihauer-Betke	0/1,000	23/1,000

The results indicate the cord blood specimen is all adult blood and the heel-stick specimen is nearly all adult blood.

2. How could that happen?

Further testing is done on the heel-stick specimen:

Anti-A	Anti-B	RBC Eluate
4°C0	+	Anti-D

These results indicate that the infant is B-positive and has HDFN caused by anti-D.

SUMMARY CHART

✔ HDFN is the destruction of the RBCs of the fetus and neonate by IgG antibodies produced by the mother.

✔ Only antibodies of the IgG class are actively transported across the placenta.

✔ In Rh HDFN, the Rh-positive firstborn infant of an Rh-negative mother is unaffected because the mother has not yet been immunized; in subsequent pregnancies, fetal cells carrying the Rh antigen immunize the Rh-negative mother and stimulate production of anti-D.

✔ In ABO HDFN, the firstborn infant may be affected as well as subsequent pregnancies in which the mother is group O and the newborn is group A, B, or AB; the IgG antibody, anti-A,B in the mother's circulation, crosses the placenta and attaches to the ABO-incompatible antigens of the fetal RBCs.

✔ Erythroblastosis fetalis describes the presence of immature RBCs or erythroblasts in the fetal circulation because the splenic removal of the IgG-coated RBCs causes anemia; the term commonly used now is *HDFN*.

✔ Although anti-D is the most antigenic of the Rh antibodies, anti-Kell is considered the most clinically significant of the non-Rh-system antibodies in the ability to cause HDFN.

✔ Prenatal serologic tests for obstetric patients include an ABO, Rh, and antibody screen during the first trimester of pregnancy.

✔ A cord blood workup includes tests for ABO and Rh as well as DAT; the most important serologic test for diagnosis of HDFN is the DAT with anti-IgG reagent.

✔ RhIG administered to the mother within 72 hours following delivery is used to prevent active immunization by the Rh(D) antigen on fetal cells; RhIG attaches to fetal Rh-positive RBCs in maternal circulation, blocking immunization and subsequent production of anti-D.

✔ A Kleihauer-Betke test or flow cytometry is used to quantitate the number of fetal Rh-positive cells in the mother's circulation as a result of a fetomaternal hemorrhage.

Review Questions

1. HDFN is characterized by:
   a. IgM antibody.
   b. Nearly always anti-D.
   c. Different RBC antigens between mother and father.
   d. Antibody titer less than 32.

2. The main difference between the fetus and the newborn is:
   a. Bilirubin metabolism.
   b. Maternal antibody level.
   c. Presence of anemia.
   d. Size of RBCs.

3. Kernicterus is caused by the effects of:
   a. Anemia.
   b. Unconjugated bilirubin.
   c. Antibody specificity.
   d. Antibody titer.

4. The advantages of cordocentesis include all of the following except:
   a. Allows measurement of fetal hemoglobin and hematocrit levels
   b. Allows antigen typing of fetal blood
   c. Allows direct transfusion of fetal circulation
   d. Decreases risk of trauma to the placenta

5. Middle cerebral artery-peak systolic velocity is used to:
   a. Measure bilirubin.
   b. Determine fetal blood type.
   c. Determine change in optical density.
   d. Assess for anemia.

6. Blood for intrauterine transfusion should be all of the following except:
   a. More than 7 days old.
   b. Screened for CMV.
   c. Gamma-irradiated.
   d. Compatible with maternal serum.

7. RhIG is indicated for:
   a. Mothers who have anti-D.
   b. Infants who are Rh-negative.
   c. Infants who have anti-D.
   d. Mothers who are Rh-negative.

8. RhIG is given without regard for fetal Rh type in all of the following conditions except:
   a. Ectopic pregnancy rupture.
   b. Amniocentesis.
   c. Induced abortion.
   d. Full-term delivery.

9. A Kleihauer-Betke test or flow cytometry indicates 10 fetal cells per 1,000 adult cells. For a woman with 5,000 mL blood volume, the proper dose of RhIG is:
   a. One regular-dose vial.
   b. Two regular-dose vials, plus one.
   c. One regular-dose vial, plus one.
   d. Two microdose vials.

10. RhIG is indicated in which of the following circumstances?
    a. Mother D-positive, infant D-positive
    b. Mother D-negative, infant D-positive
    c. Mother D-positive, infant D-negative
    d. Mother D-negative, infant D-negative

11. ABO HDFN is usually mild because:
    a. ABO antigens are poorly developed in the fetus.
    b. ABO antibodies prevent the disease.
    c. ABO antibodies readily cross the placenta.
    d. ABO incompatibility is rare.

12. A woman without prenatal care delivers a healthy term infant. A cord blood sample shows the infant is A-positive with a positive DAT. The workup of the unexpected finding should include:
    a. Anti-C3 antiglobulin test.
    b. ABO testing of the mother.
    c. Direct antiglobulin testing of the mother's specimen.
    d. ABO and Rh typing of the father.

References

1. Geifman-Holtzman, O, et al: Female alloimmunization with antibodies known to cause hemolytic disease. Obstet Gynecol 89:272–275, 1997.
2. Klein, HG, and Anstee, DJ: Mollison's Blood Transfusion in Clinical Medicine, 11th ed. Blackwell Scientific, London, 2005, pp 496–545.
3. Bowman, JM: The prevention of Rh immunization. Transfus Med Rev 2:129–150, 1988.
4. Klein, HG, and Anstee, DJ: Mollison's Blood Transfusion in Clinical Medicine, 11th ed. Blackwell Scientific, London, 2005, pp 163–208.
5. Vaughan, JI, et al: Inhibition of erythroid progenitor cells by anti-Kell antibodies in fetal alloimmune anemia. N Engl J Med 338:798–803, 1998.
6. Vengelen-Tyler, V: The serological investigation of hemolytic disease of the newborn caused by antibodies other than anti-D. In Garratty, G (ed): Hemolytic Disease of the Newborn. American Association of Blood Banks, Arlington, VA, 1984, pp 145–172.
7. Moise, KJ: Management of Rhesus alloimmunization in pregnancy. Obstet Gynecol 100:600–611, 2002.
8. Judd, WJ, Johnson, ST, and Storry, JR: Judd's Methods in Immunohematology, 3rd ed. AABB, Bethesda, MD, 2008.
9. Finning, K, et al: Fetal genotyping for the K (Kell) and Rh C, E, c, and E blood groups on cell-free DNA in maternal plasma. Transfusion 47:2126–2133, 2007.
10. Mari, G, et al: Noninvasive diagnosis by Doppler ultrasonography of fetal anemia due to maternal red-cell alloimmunization. Collaborative group for Doppler assessment of the blood velocity in anemic fetuses. N Eng J Med 342:9–14, 2000.
11. Oepkes, D, et al: Doppler ultrasonography versus amniocentesis to predict fetal anemia. N Engl J Med 354:156–164, 2006.
12. Schumacher, B, and Moise, KJ: Fetal transfusion for red blood cell alloimmunization in pregnancy. Obstet Gynecol 88:137–150, 1996.
13. Maisels, MJ, and McDonagh, AF: Phototherapy for neonatal jaundice. N Engl J Med 358:920–928, 2008.
14. Brinc, D, et al: Immunoglobulin G-mediated regulation of the murine response to transfused red blood cells occurs in the absence of active immunosuppression: Implications for the mechanism of action of anti-D in the prevention of haemolytic disease of the fetus and newborn? Immunology 124:141–146, 2008.
15. Kennedy, MS: Perinatal issues in transfusion practice. In Roback, JD (ed): Technical Manual, 16th ed. AABB, Bethesda, 2008, pp 625–637.
16. Herschel, M, et al: Isoimmunization is unlikely to be the cause of hemolysis in ABO-incompatible but direct antiglobulin test-negative neonates. Pediatrics 110:127–130, 2002.
17. Kennedy, MS: Rho(D) immune globulin. In Rayburn, W, and Zuspan, FP (eds): Drug Therapy in Gynecology and Obstetrics, 3rd ed. CV Mosby, St. Louis, 1991, p 297.

Chapter 20

Autoimmune Hemolytic Anemias

Denise M. Harmening, PhD, MT(ASCP), CLS(NCA); Karen Rodberg, MBA, MT(ASCP)SBB; and Ralph E. B. Green, B. App. Sci, FAIMS, MACE

OBJECTIVES

1. Define *autoantibody* and compare the types of immune hemolytic anemias with respect to thermal amplitude, method of red blood cell (RBC) destruction, and the type of immunoglobulin that characteristically coats the RBCs.

2. Characterize autoantibodies that react at temperatures below 37°C and identify the common specificities of benign cold autoagglutinins.

3. Describe problems encountered in the laboratory testing of specimens containing cold autoagglutinins.

4. Explain the techniques used to investigate serologic findings and detect underlying clinically significant alloantibodies in the presence of cold autoantibodies.

5. Describe pathological cold autoagglutinins, including laboratory testing and treatment.

6. Differentiate between idiopathic warm autoimmune hemolytic anemia (WAIHA) and drug-induced immune hemolytic anemia.

7. Describe the clinical and laboratory findings in WAIHA, including indicators of RBC hemolysis, difficulties in serologic testing, and selection of blood for transfusion.

8. Explain procedures used to investigate serologic findings and detect underlying clinically significant alloantibodies in the presence of warm autoantibodies.

9. Compare the mechanisms for drug-induced hemolysis and give examples of medications causing each type.

10. Describe the Donath-Landsteiner test.

Introduction

Immune hemolytic anemia is defined as shortened RBC survival mediated through the immune response, specifically by humoral antibody. Immune hemolysis is destruction of RBCs as a result of antibody production and is an acquired characteristic of the RBC membrane associated with demonstrable antibodies, as opposed to intracorpuscular defects such as enzyme deficiencies and hemoglobinopathies, which represent intrinsic abnormalities of the patient's RBCs.

The three broad categories of immune hemolytic anemias are:

1. Alloimmune
2. Autoimmune
3. Drug-induced

In an **alloimmune response**, the patient produces antibodies to foreign or non-self RBC antigens introduced into the circulation through transfusion, transplant, or pregnancy. In cases in which an alloantibody clears the antigen-positive RBCs from circulation, intravascularly or extravascularly, a transient hemolytic process may result (e.g., a hemolytic transfusion reaction), sometimes causing anemia in the transfusion recipient or the affected fetus. For a discussion of alloantibody production, refer to Chapter 9, "Detection and Identification of Antibodies"; Chapter 16, "Adverse Effects of Blood Transfusion"; and Chapter 19, "Hemolytic Disease of the Fetus and Newborn (HDFN)."

This chapter focuses on the latter two categories of immune hemolytic anemias: **autoimmune hemolytic anemia** (AIHA) and **drug-induced immune hemolytic anemia** (DIIHA). An autoimmune response occurs when a patient produces antibodies against his or her own RBC antigens. A drug-induced hemolytic anemia is the result of a patient's production of antibody to a particular drug or drug complex, with ensuing damage to the patient's RBCs.

Autoantibodies

A serologist who is able to recognize and investigate both alloantibodies and autoantibodies can assist the clinician in both the diagnosis of immune hemolytic anemia and the proper selection of blood components for transfusion.

Definition

Antibodies that are directed against the individual's own RBCs are termed **autoantibodies** or **autoagglutinins**. Most autoantibodies react with high-incidence RBC antigens. They typically agglutinate, sensitize, or lyse RBCs of most random donors as well as their own. RBC survival may be shortened by this circulating humoral antibody. Some individuals will produce an autoantibody that readily attaches to their own RBCs but does not cause RBC destruction. Approximately 1 in 1,000 healthy blood donors will have a positive **direct antiglobulin test** (DAT) but will have a normal hematocrit and be asymptomatic. In these individuals, the presence of autoantibody alone does not necessarily cause decreased RBC survival.[1]

Studies in animal models suggest that production of antibodies against the self occurs because the immune regulatory responses fail.[2,3] According to this model, under normal circumstances, immunoglobulins made by B lymphocytes are regulated by T lymphocytes. Helper T cells assist these immunocompetent B cells in making antibody against foreign antigens. Another population of T lymphocytes, suppressor T cells, has the opposite effect on B-cell activity; they prevent excessive proliferation of B cells and overproduction of antibodies. Suppressor T cells are thought to act through a feedback mechanism. An increasing concentration of antibody activates these T cells and suppresses further antibody production.[4]

In a normal individual, it is theorized that autoantibody production is prevented through a similar mechanism. Suppressor T cells induce tolerance to self-antigens by inhibiting B-cell activity. Conversely, loss of suppressor T-cell function could result in autoantibody production. Support for this concept comes from animal studies[3] and patients taking the drug alpha-methyldopa.[5] The cause of the regulatory system's dysfunction is not understood, but microbial agents and drugs have been suggested.[6] For further discussion of the immune response, see Chapter 3, "Fundamentals of Immunology."

Recognition of autoantibodies in routine serologic investigations is extremely important. Identifying an autoantibody may explain decreased RBC survival in vivo to offer an explanation for an otherwise unexplained anemia. In serologic investigations, the presence of an autoantibody may complicate some aspects of routine testing, including ABO/Rh typing, antibody screening, and compatibility testing. If a patient's RBCs are coated with autoantibody, the patient may present with a serologic ABO discrepancy, a positive Rh control, or a positive DAT. If the patient's serum contains autoantibody, RBC antibody screening procedures, compatibility testing, and serum (reverse) ABO typing of the individual may present difficulty. It is likely that the patient's serum will be incompatible with all random donors. Techniques that can be used to resolve these difficulties are discussed in greater detail below. Serologic and clinical problems can be found separately or together.

Characterization

In individuals who have not been recently transfused, the presence of a positive DAT, a positive autocontrol, or serum autoantibody does not necessarily confer the diagnosis of autoimmune hemolytic anemia (AIHA). In themselves, these findings merely indicate the presence of autoantibody. It has been reported that approximately 0.1% of normal blood donors and up to 15% of hospitalized patients have positive DATs with no evidence of hemolytic anemia.[7] Before the presence of an AIHA is established, it is important to verify the presence of immune-mediated RBC destruction. Evidence of increased RBC destruction is not always accompanied by decreased hemoglobin and hematocrit levels. These may become evident only when the individual is no longer able to compensate for increased RBC destruction. In many instances, even before decreases in hemoglobin and hematocrit are obvious, there will be evidence of compensation for increased RBC destruction, including increases in reticulocyte count, unconjugated (indirect) bilirubin levels, and lactate dehydrogenase (LDH) levels, and a decrease in haptoglobin.

The individual who has immune RBC destruction may experience either compensated or uncompensated anemia. In compensated anemia, the rate of RBC production will nearly equal the rate of RBC destruction. These individuals will demonstrate an increased reticulocyte count but may have only a mild decrease in hemoglobin and hematocrit levels, depending on the rate of RBC production. Those individuals with uncompensated anemia demonstrate a rate of RBC destruction that exceeds the rate of RBC production. Hemolytic anemia is often demonstrated in a blood smear by macrocytosis (evidence of a young cell population) or spherocytosis (evidence of cell membrane damage). The reticulocyte count of these individuals is generally greater than 3%,[8] and the unconjugated bilirubin levels and LDH levels are also increased due to accelerated RBC destruction; however, haptoglobin levels are markedly decreased due to its role of clearing hemoglobin from the plasma. With intravascular RBC destruction, hemoglobinemia and hemoglobinuria may occur.

Because there are other causes of hemolysis (e.g., hereditary spherocytosis, hemoglobinopathies, and RBC enzyme defects), AIHA must be confirmed by additional serologic testing. Diagnostic tests in a symptomatic patient include:

1. Direct antiglobulin test (DAT) using **polyspecific** and **monospecific antiglobulin reagents** (refer to Chapter 5, "The Antiglobulin Test")
2. Characterization of the autoantibody in the serum or eluate using standard antibody detection and identification procedures (refer to Chapter 9)

Based on these results and the clinical evaluation of the patient, AIHA may be diagnosed and classified as cold reactive, warm reactive, or drug-induced. The expected laboratory findings for each type are discussed in the following sections. In their book *Immune Hemolytic Anemias*, Petz and Garratty devote several chapters to the differential diagnosis of the hemolytic anemias and another chapter to drug-induced immune hemolytic anemia. The reader is referred to their text for a complete discussion.[7]

As previously stated, some individuals may have autoantibodies in their sera and on their RBCs but display no evidence of decreased RBC survival. All normal RBCs have a small amount of IgG and complement on their surfaces. Studies have shown that there may be 5 to 90 molecules of IgG/RBC and 5 to 500 molecules of complement/RBC in the average healthy individual.[7] Because conventional tube testing will normally detect 100 to 500 molecules of IgG/RBC and 400 to 1,100 molecules of complement/RBC, these individuals are not routinely identified as DAT-positive.[9]

It should be noted that column agglutination (gel) or solid phase methodologies may have an increased sensitivity in the detection of IgG-coated RBCs. Therefore, with the increase in the use of methods other than conventional test tube technique, it is possible that a greater number of individuals may be found to be DAT-positive, with or without detectable evidence of RBC destruction. As mentioned above, the incidence of positive DATs in normal blood donor populations has been reported to be as high as 1 in 1,000 in the U.S. population,[1] whereas the incidence in hospitalized patients ranges from 0.3 to 1%, using anti-IgG antiglobulin reagent[10,11] and as high as 15% using polyspecific antiglobulin reagent.[12] Many of the latter group have only complement bound to the RBCs. The differences between individuals who are affected (i.e., those who have AIHA) and those who are unaffected by autoantibodies are not clearly understood. Among the possibly significant factors are:

- Thermal amplitude of antibody reactivity[13]
- IgG subclass of the antibody[14]
- Amount of antibody bound to the RBCs[14]
- Ability of the antibody to fix complement in vivo[15]
- Activity of the individual's macrophages[7]
- Quantitative or qualitative change in band 3 and proteins 4.1 and 4.2 in the RBC membrane structure[16]

The opposite situation also occurs; in some patients with hemolytic anemia, autoantibodies cannot be demonstrated by routine techniques. Some patients have more IgG than normal on their RBCs but less than the amount detectable by the routine antiglobulin test.[17] In other cases, the patient's RBCs are sensitized with anti-IgA or anti-IgM, not routinely demonstrable using commercial antiglobulin reagents.[18–20] Because polyspecific antihuman globulin (AHG) reagents are required by the FDA to contain anti-IgG and anti-C3d,[21,22] antibodies to other immunoglobulins (e.g., IgA and IgM) are not consistently present in the reagent, and cells sensitized with IgA or IgM may not give a positive direct antiglobulin test.

Autoantibodies can be characterized by their optimal temperature of reactivity. About 70% of the reported cases of AIHA are those that react best at warm temperatures (30°C to 37°C), whereas cold reactive (4°C to 30°C) autoagglutinins account for about 18%. Drug-induced autoagglutinins are present in about 12% of the reported cases of AIHA. Characterization of autoantibodies is important because treatment of the patient and resolution of the serologic problems will differ according to the optimal temperature of reactivity and the immunoglobulin responsible; treatment of the patient will depend on the nature of the autoantibody. The remainder of this chapter details the clinical and laboratory aspects of cold reactive, warm reactive, and drug-induced autoantibodies.

Cold Reactive Autoantibodies

Cold reactive autoantibodies are frequently encountered in serologic testing. Most of the time, the antibodies detected are not clinically significant but nevertheless can present challenges for the blood banker. Occasionally, cold autoantibodies are clinically significant and cause immune hemolytic anemia. The antibody specificity may be of interest to the technologist or may be a clue to the disease process, but the important distinction between clinically significant and benign cold autoantibodies is their thermal range. Any antibody that reacts at or near body temperature (30°C to 37°C), regardless of specificity, is potentially clinically significant; this includes "cold" autoantibodies.

Benign Cold Autoantibodies

When testing is performed at 4°C, the most commonly encountered autoantibody is a benign cold agglutinin that may be found in the serum of most normal, healthy individuals. Normally these antibodies present no serologic problem because routine antibody detection tests are not performed at this temperature. The typical cold agglutinin has a relatively low **titer** (less than 64 at 4°C). Occasionally, these benign cold autoantibodies may agglutinate cells at room temperature (20°C to 24°C); however, even in this situation, strongest reactivity is found at 4°C. **Table 20–1** compares the characteristics of benign (normal) cold autoantibodies with those of pathological cold autoantibodies, which are discussed later in this chapter. Most cold agglutinins react strongly with enzyme-treated cells; therefore, cold agglutinins are quite likely to be detected when ficin-treated cells are tested. Cold autoantibodies are IgM immunoglobulins and therefore can activate complement in vitro. In serum testing, reactivity may be seen in the antiglobulin phase if polyspecific antihuman serum (i.e., containing anticomplement) is used in antiglobulin testing. **Table 20–2** contrasts titers and thermal amplitudes typical of benign versus pathologic cold autoagglutinins.

Laboratory Tests Affected by Cold Autoagglutinins

Cold agglutinins sometimes interfere with routine serum and cell testing performed at room temperature (RT). The extent to which they cause problems depends on whether antibody detection tests are performed at room temperature and how strongly the antibody reacts at this temperature (i.e., the concentration and **thermal amplitude** of the antibody). Although the cold autoantibodies found in the serum

of normal people do not typically interfere with testing, they are one of the more common causes of serologic problems; therefore, one should be able to recognize these circumstances and employ methods to resolve problems associated with these antibodies. If a cold agglutinin is strong enough to interfere with ABO typing, it may also interfere with indirect antiglobulin testing even if the antibody detection method does not intentionally include an RT incubation step. In these cases, troubleshooting a positive antibody screening should include RT testing to prove the existence of a cold reacting antibody.

ABO Typing

If an individual's RBCs are heavily coated with cold agglutinins, they may directly agglutinate, causing false-positive reactions with routine ABO reagents. In most cases, valid results can be obtained by using patient's cells that have been washed once or twice with normal saline warmed to 37°C. The cold autoantibody is eluted from the cells during warm washing. For example, group O cells coated with cold autoantibody might show the following reactions before and after warm washing:

	ANTI-A	ANTI-B
Serum-suspended RBCs	1+	1+
Warm-washed, saline-suspended RBCs	0	0

If more potent autoagglutinins are present, it may be necessary to incubate the patient's whole blood sample at 37°C prior to warm washing.[23] In some cases, it may be inconvenient to adhere closely to a protocol of maintaining the sample at 37°C from the point of collection; similar success has been found with warming the sample in a waterbath or heat block to 37°C for 15 to 30 minutes and then warm washing the RBCs. The warm incubation elutes the cold agglutinin from the patient's RBCs, and the warm washes remove it to prevent it from reattaching in vitro. In the rare situation in which washing with warm saline is not effective, thiol reagents (e.g., dithiothreitol) can be used to disperse the autoagglutination.[24]

Table 20–1   Characteristics of Normal (Benign) Cold and Pathological Cold Autoantibodies

CHARACTERISTIC	NORMAL (BENIGN)	PATHOLOGICAL
Thermal range	Reactive ≤ 20°C–24°C	Reactive ≥ 30°C
Titer at 4C	≤ 64	≥ 1,000
Reactivity	Marginally enhanced with albumin	Strongly enhanced with albumin
Common specificity	Anti-I or anti-IH	Anti-I
Capable of binding complement	Yes (in vitro) DAT: 0 – 1+ due to C3	Yes (in vivo) DAT: 2 – 4+ due to C3
Clinically significant	No	Yes
Associated with disease	No	Yes—may be secondary to viral infections or *M. pneumonia.*

Table 20–2 Benign Cold Agglutinin Compared With Pathological Cold Agglutinin: Titers and Thermal Amplitudes*

Benign Cold Agglutinin

Tube #	1	2	3	4	5	6	7	8	9	10	11	12	Titer
Dilution →	N	2	4	8	16	32	64	128	256	512	1,024	2,048	
Temp ↓													
37°C	0	0	0	0	0	0	0	0	0	0	0	0	0
30°C	0	0	0	0	0	0	0	0	0	0	0	0	0
20°C	3+	2+	1+	0	0	0	0	0	0	0	0	0	4
4°C	4+	4+	3+	2+	1+	0	0	0	0	0	0	0	16

Pathological Cold Agglutinin

Tube #	1	2	3	4	5	6	7	8	9	10	11	12	Titer
Dilution →	N	2	4	8	16	32	64	128	256	512	1,024	2,048	
Temp ↓													
37°C	1+	±	0	0	0	0	0	0	0	0	0	0	1
30°C	2+	1+	0	0	0	0	0	0	0	0	0	0	2
20°C	4+	4+	3+	3+	2+	1+	0	0	0	0	0	0	32
4°C	4+	4+	4+	4+	4+	3+	3+	3+	2+	2+	1+	1+	>2,048

*Titrations performed using normal group O RBCs.

 See Procedure 20-1 on the textbook's companion website.

Because serum ABO grouping is performed at room temperature, cold autoagglutinins frequently cause discrepancies in the serum ABO (reverse) typing also. In the following example, the cell typing results suggest the cells are group AB. In a group AB individual, one does not expect the serum to agglutinate either the A₁ or B cells, as seen in this example. Although a number of explanations for this discrepancy exist, a cold agglutinin is the most likely cause. Group O and autologous cells should also be tested in the investigation of a serologic ABO discrepancy. If a cold autoagglutinin is present, the autologous and group O cells (the negative controls) will most likely be positive as well:

	ANTI-A	ANTI-B
RBCs	4+	4+

	A₁ RBCs	B RBCs	O RBCs	AUTOLOGOUS RBCs
Serum (or Plasma)	1+	1+	2+	1+

Such a discrepancy is easily resolved if the cold reactive autoantibody is removed by an **autoadsorption** technique,

and the tests with the A₁, B, O and autologous cells are repeated with autoadsorbed serum.

 See Procedure 20-2 on the textbook's companion website.

Although it may be possible to resolve this discrepancy with prewarmed testing, one must remember that not all ABO isoagglutinins are reactive at 37°C, and erroneous test results may be obtained; therefore, autoadsorption procedures are preferred.

	A₁ RBCs	B RBCs	O RBCs	AUTOLOGOUS RBCs
Autoadsorbed Serum	0	0	0	0

Rh(D) Typing

As in ABO cell grouping, false-positive reactions can be seen with Rh reagents when RBCs coated with cold autoagglutinins are tested. This was previously a common problem encountered in typing with **polyclonal** high-protein anti-D reagent where the anti-D and the Rh control were both positive, rendering the test invalid. Today, the Rh reagents in common use are **monoclonal** or a blend of monoclonal and low-protein anti-D reagents, which normally yield valid results. When a monoclonal reagent is used, many manufacturers consider a negative reaction with any of the ABO reagents as a control for the D typing; however, an Rh control reagent is available from some manufacturers. As stated above, if a discrepancy exists in the ABO typing, washing the cells with warm saline usually gives acceptable results. This also holds true when testing with low-protein anti-D. Thiol reagents may be required when washing with warm saline is ineffective.

Cold reactive IgM autoagglutinins can activate the complement cascade in vitro, causing complement components to be bound to the RBC surface, which can lead to false-positive reactions in the weak D (antiglobulin) test if cells from a clotted sample and polyspecific antihuman serum are used. In this instance, the Rh control test will also be positive. The use of monospecific anti-IgG for weak D testing or RBCs collected into ethylenediaminetetraacetic acid (EDTA) can eliminate the problem of complement-binding cold agglutinins in D typing. The following examples illustrate these results:

	ANTI-D	Rh CONTROL
Immediate spin phase	0	0
Indirect antiglobulin phase (poly AHG)	1+	1+
Indirect antiglobulin phase (anti-IgG)	0	0
RBCs collected in EDTA	0	0

Similar problems can be encountered with other antisera used in **RBC phenotyping** (e.g., anti-K, anti-S, anti-Fy^a) that require the use of an indirect antiglobulin test. The use of anti-IgG antiglobulin reagent or a sample collected in EDTA is recommended when cold autoagglutinins are present. Fortunately, most samples collected for the blood bank today are collected in EDTA.

Direct Antiglobulin Test

When a properly collected specimen is used (EDTA-anticoagulated RBCs), the DAT of a patient with benign cold autoagglutinins is negative; however, one frequently obtains a positive result using polyspecific antihuman serum if a clotted specimen is used, because complement can be activated in vitro. This in vitro sensitization is usually weak—less than or equal to 1+. If monospecific reagents are used, these cells are reactive with anti-C3d but not with anti-IgG. A negative control of 6% albumin or saline, used in parallel with the antiglobulin reagents, is recommended for direct antiglobulin testing, particularly when there has been difficulty obtaining valid ABO or Rh typing.

Antibody Detection and Identification

The frequency with which cold autoagglutinins interfere with detection and identification of RBC alloantibodies depends to a large extent on the routine procedures used in patient testing. As shown in **Table 20–2**, cold agglutinins react best at 4°C but are generally not detected because routine antibody screening is no longer performed at this temperature. Antibodies reactive only at room temperature are usually considered to be of no clinical significance. Benign cold autoagglutinins do not react at 37°C, but they may interfere with testing at the antiglobulin phase if polyspecific antihuman reagent is used, inasmuch as they may bind to cells at lower temperatures when the serum and cells are mixed together initially or during centrifugation following the 37°C incubation, and complement may be activated. Although the antibody elutes from the cell surface during the incubation or washing phases, the complement remains bound. Polyspecific antihuman serum will agglutinate the cells coated with complement. When enzyme-treated cells are used, reactions in all phases may be stronger. Often, omitting room temperature incubation and the use of anti-IgG for the indirect antiglobulin test (IAT) are all that is needed to avoid detecting cold agglutinins at the IAT.

Because most clinically significant antibodies capable of causing accelerated RBC destruction are detected by the antiglobulin test, reactions in this phase must be investigated. Reactivity caused by cold autoagglutinins can mask the presence of clinically significant alloantibodies. Although the use of anti-IgG antiglobulin reagents will eliminate most problems with cold autoagglutinin reactivity in the IAT phase, it may be necessary to remove the cold reacting autoantibody by cold adsorption procedures to thoroughly investigate the reactivity observed in antiglobulin testing. Rabbit erythrocyte stroma is known to be rich in I antigen and is commercially available and easy to use. There have been some reports that clinically significant antibodies have been adsorbed using rabbit erythrocyte stroma, so caution is advised.[25]

Other techniques useful in differentiating between cold autoantibodies and alloantibodies are prewarm technique or testing with cold autoadsorbed serum.[23] Cold autoadsorption technique is preferred because the prewarm test has become quite controversial. There have been reports of clinically significant alloantibodies being unintentionally "prewarmed away," either due to poor technique or because the antibodies were partially IgM, yet this technique persists in practice and does have value in investigating an identified antibody's thermal amplitude.

The principle of the prewarm test is that by first warming the cell suspension and serum prior to mixing, avoiding room temperature centrifugation after 37°C incubation, and washing with saline warmed to 37°C, any reaction between the cold autoagglutinin and RBC antigens can be prevented, thus avoiding complement activation. While cold reacting antibodies should not react by this method, alloantibodies that are reactive at 37°C (i.e., potentially clinically significant) would still bind to the cells and be detectable at the antiglobulin phase.

 See Procedure 20-3 on the textbook's companion website.

An example of the results of testing a serum that contains a cold autoagglutinin and anti-Fy^a using routine antiglobulin testing with polyspecific antiglobulin and testing with the

Table 20–3	**Typical Reactivity Observed With Patient Serum Containing a Clinically Significant Alloantibody (anti-Fyᵃ) and Cold Autoagglutinin**		

RBCs TESTED	STANDARD ANTIGLOBULIN TESTING WITH POLYSPECIFIC AHG	PREWARMED ANTIGLOBULIN TESTING WITH POLYSPECIFIC AHG	STANDARD ANTIGLOBULIN TESTING WITH ANTI-IgG
Fy(a+b−)	2+	2+	2+
Fy(a+b+)	2+	2+	2+
Fy(a−b+)	1+ᵂ	0	0
Auto control	1+ᵂ	0	0

prewarmed technique is shown in Table 20–3. Reactions are present in routine antiglobulin tests with both Fy(a+) and Fy(a−) cells. In a prewarmed test, only the reactions expected of the anti-Fyᵃ are evident. The weak reactions of the cold autoagglutinin are eliminated by prewarm technique. The prewarm technique is simple and successful in most cases; however, if the cold autoantibody is very potent, it may be difficult to maintain the cells and serum at 37°C to avoid the antigen-antibody interaction and complement activation.

Although prewarm technique may appear to be very helpful in resolving problems caused by cold autoagglutinins, this technique should not be used indiscriminately. Cases have been reported in which clinically significant alloantibodies have been missed after prewarming.[26] Prewarming should be used only when the reactions obtained indicate the likely presence of a cold autoagglutinin (i.e., positive autocontrol and reactivity noted below 37°C). Because there is no immediate spin reading or room temperature incubation in the prewarmed procedure, IgM immunoglobulin components of a newly forming alloantibody may not be detected in this testing. Therefore, this testing must not be performed with patients transfused within the previous 3 months or patients without an accurate transfusion history. A cold autoagglutinin is not apt to be the answer if weak reactions are present only in the antiglobulin phase with anti-IgG (i.e., there is no evidence of reactivity at immediate spin or room temperature).

When strong cold autoantibodies are present or if one wishes to identify a room temperature–reactive alloantibody, autologous adsorption must be performed to remove the autoantibody. Cold autologous adsorption, described in Procedure 20-2 on the companion website, may be performed if the patient has *not* been transfused within 3 months. In autoadsorption procedures, an aliquot of patient cells is incubated with an equal volume of the patient's serum at 4°C. Autoantibody is adsorbed onto the cells, and alloantibody remains in the serum. It may be necessary to repeat the adsorption several times if the autoantibody is of high titer. In order to enhance the adsorption process, the patient's RBCs may be treated with enzymes before adsorption to increase the amount of autoantibody removed by the adsorption; however, enzyme pretreatment should not be performed without confirming that the serum antibody is reactive with enzyme-treated cells. Autologous

adsorption should not be performed if a patient has been recently transfused, because donor RBCs will be present in the patient's circulation. Alloantibodies and autoantibodies will be adsorbed if an "auto" adsorption is performed on a recently transfused patient. In this situation, it is best to use allogeneic adsorption or cold adsorption using rabbit erythrocyte stroma.

 See Procedure 20-4 on the textbook's companion website.

If anti-IgG antiglobulin reagent is used, the problems caused by most cold agglutinins can be avoided. The use of anti-IgG reagents is an attractive alternative when prewarming is not effective and there is not enough time to adsorb the serum.

Compatibility Testing

The difficulties encountered in antibody detection and identification tests are also found in **compatibility tests**, because the most commonly encountered cold autoantibody (autoanti-I) is directed against an antigen that is found on the RBCs of most random donors and on most reagent RBCs. Compatibility tests, like antibody identification tests, can be performed using prewarmed or autoadsorbed serum or allogeneic adsorbed serum or using anti-IgG antiglobulin reagent.

Two other common cold agglutinins, anti-IH and anti-H, distinguish between group O reagent RBCs and group A, B, or AB donor cells. Because these antibodies react with the H antigen that is only weakly expressed on the RBCs of group A, B, or AB individuals, they are not always obvious as autoantibodies when encountered. As discussed in the following section on specificity, anti-IH and anti-H react best with group O cells; they react least with group A_1 and A_1B cells, perhaps only at 4°C. Anti-IH and anti-H are found most often in the serum of group A_1 and A_1B persons; therefore, the units selected for compatibility testing (group A or AB) are those that give the weakest, if any, reactivity. On the other hand, group O cells (e.g., antibody screening cells) give the strongest reactions.

Specificity of Cold Autoagglutinins

The specificity of the cold autoantibody is often associated with the patient's diagnosis. It is important to be familiar

Table 20–4   Typical Reactivity Observed at 4°C With Serum Containing Autoanti-I with I_{adult} and i_{cord} Cells

SERUM	SERUM DILUTION	I_{adult} CELLS	I_{cord} CELLS
Benign cold	Neat	3+	$1+^W$
	1:2	1+	0
	1:4	$1+^W$	0
	1:8	0	0
Pathological cold	Neat	4+	3+
	1:2	4+	2+
	1:4	4+	1+
	1:8	3+	0

with the properties and characteristics of these types of autoantibodies.

Anti-I, Anti-i. Most cold reactive autoantibodies have anti-I specificity. The I antigen is fully expressed on the RBCs of virtually all adults, whereas it is only weakly expressed on cord RBCs. At birth, an infant's RBCs express the i antigen. As an infant matures, the antigen expressed is converted from the i antigen to the I antigen; the amount of I antigen increases until the adult levels are reached at about 2 years of age.[23] Very rarely do adult RBCs lack the I antigen; if they do, they are termed i *adults* and may produce alloanti-I, which is a potentially clinically significant alloantibody because it is typically an IgG antibody that reacts at 37°C.

The reactivities of several examples of anti-I are given in Table 20–4. As shown, anti-I specificity may be apparent when a serum is tested with adult and cord RBCs. Benign cold autoantibodies, for example, react with adult RBCs but not with cord RBCs. Pathological cold autoantibodies react with both adult and cord cells, but the preference for the adult cells is still obvious. Alloanti-I is frequently present in the serum of i adults.[27]

Anti-i is a relatively uncommon autoantibody. As shown in Table 20–5, this antibody reacts in a manner antithetical to anti-I. Cord cells and i adult cells have the strongest expression of the i antigen; adult $_I$ cells have the least.

Anti-H, Anti-IH. Cold agglutinins found in the sera of group A_1 and A_1B individuals (and occasionally group B) may have anti-H specificity. This antibody distinguishes between cells of various ABO groups. Group O and A_2 cells react best because they have the largest amounts of H antigen. Group A_1 and A_1B cells have the least H antigen, so they react weakly. Because the A_1 and A_1B individual's own cells demonstrate a very weak expression of the H antigen, anti-H and anti-IH are actually autoantibodies that may react only with autologous RBCs at 4°C, but that can be easily managed by the selection of type-specific RBCs. The pattern of reactivity seen

Table 20–5   Reactivity of Cold Autoagglutinins at 4°C With ABO-Compatible RBCs

RBC PHENOTYPE	ANTI-I	ANTI-i	ANTI-H	ANTI-IH	ANTI-Pr*
Group O I_{adult}	4+	0 to 1+	4+	4+	4+
Group A_1 I_{adult}	4+	0 to 1+	0 to 1+	0 to 1+	4+
Group A_2 I_{adult}	4+	0 to 1+	2+	2+	4+
Bombay O_h I_{adult}	4+	0 to 1+	0	0 to 2+	4+
Group O i_{adult}	0 to 1+	4+	4+	0 to 1+	4+
Group O i_{cord}	0 to 1+	4+	4+	0 to 1+	4+
Group A_1 i_{adult}	0 to 1+	4+	0 to 1+	0	4+
Group A_2 i_{adult}	0 to 1+	4+	2+	0 to 2+	4+
Bombay O_h i_{adult}	0 to 1+	4+	0	0	4+
Group O I_{adult} ficin-treated	4+	1+ to 2+	4+	4+	0

*Anti-Pr is a less commonly encountered cold autoagglutinin that frequently mimics autoanti-I.

with anti-H is shown in **Table 20–5**. See Chapter 6, "The ABO Blood Group System," for a discussion of the ABO system and H substance.

It is very important not to confuse cold reactive anti-H with the anti-H found in the serum of O_h (Bombay) individuals who lack the H antigen. Cold reactive anti-H may be found in A_1 or A_1B individuals as an autoantibody even though the cells of the antibody maker (A_1 or A_1B) may give considerably weaker reactions. The anti-H in the O_h person is a potent alloantibody, which reacts at 4°C to 37°C with all cells except the rare O_h cell, and is capable of causing rapid intravascular RBC destruction.

Anti-IH, another of the usually harmless cold autoagglutinins, is also found more commonly in the serum of A_1 and A_1B individuals. This antibody agglutinates only RBCs that have both the I and the H antigens. As with anti-H, group O and group A_2 cells react best. The difference between these two antibodies is that group O i_{cord} cells and group O i_{adult} cells react as strongly as group O I_{adult} cells with anti-H but not with anti-IH (see **Table 20–5**).

Other Cold Reactive Autoagglutinins

A number of other less commonly encountered cold autoagglutinins have been described, such as anti-Pr, anti-Gd, and anti-Sd^x (anti-R$_x$).[28] Cold autoantibodies with the specificity of anti-M have also been described.[29] Most researchers agree that specificity of cold reactive autoantibodies is primarily of academic interest and usually not clinically important; however, development of autoantibodies with specificities for integral components of the RBC membrane, such as the glycophorins or band 3, may be precursors for developing other autoimmune disorders such as systemic lupus erythematosus or rheumatoid arthritis.[30]

Pathological Cold Autoagglutinins

Differentiating the serologic characteristics of a benign cold autoagglutinin from a pathological cold agglutinin may aid the clinician in making a diagnosis. This is very important in terms of the treatment that is required for pathological cold autoantibodies as opposed to no treatment required for benign cold autoantibodies.

Cold Hemagglutinin Disease (Idiopathic Cold AIHA)

Most cold autoagglutinins do not cause RBC destruction, but in some patients they can cause hemolytic anemia that varies in severity from mild to life-threatening intravascular lysis. Cold reactive immune hemolytic anemia may be a chronic, idiopathic (no identifiable cause) condition or an acute, transient disorder often associated with an infectious disease such as *Mycoplasma pneumoniae* pneumonia or infectious mononucleosis. Cold agglutinin syndrome, also called **cold hemagglutinin disease** (CHD) or idiopathic cold AIHA, represents approximately 18% of the cases of AIHA. A moderate chronic hemolytic anemia is produced by a cold autoantibody that optimally reacts at 4°C but also reacts at temperatures between 25°C and 30°C. The antibody is usually an IgM immunoglobulin that quite efficiently activates complement.

Clinical Picture. CHD occurs predominantly in older individuals, with a peak incidence in those over 50 years of age. Antibody specificity in this disorder is almost always anti-I, less commonly anti-i, and rarely anti-Pr. It is rarely severe and is usually seasonal because the winter months often precipitate the signs and symptoms of this chronic hemolytic anemia. Acrocyanosis of the hands, feet, ears, and nose is frequently the patient's main complaint along with a sense of numbness in the extremities. Changes take place when the person is exposed to the cold, because the cold autoantibody agglutinates the patient's RBCs as they pass through the skin capillaries, resulting in localized blood stasis. During cold winter weather, the temperature of an individual's blood falls to as low as 28°C in the extremities, activating his or her cold autoantibody. The antibody then agglutinates the RBCs and fixes complement as the cells flow through the capillaries of the skin, causing signs of acrocyanosis. These patients may also experience hemoglobinuria, because the complement fixation may result in intravascular hemolysis. **Figure 20–1** illustrates the relationship between ambient temperatures and LDH concentration (a reflection of the severity of hemolysis) over a period of 18 months.[31] However, this intravascular hemolytic episode is not associated with fever, chills, or acute renal insufficiency, any one of which is characteristic of patients with paroxysmal cold hemoglobinuria (PCH) or severe WAIHA.

Patients usually display weakness, pallor, and weight loss, which are characteristic symptoms of a chronic anemia. CHD usually remains quite stable; however, if it does progress in severity, it is insidious in intensity. Physical findings such as hepatosplenomegaly are infrequent because of the mechanism of hemolysis. Other clinical features of CHD include jaundice and Raynaud's disease (symptoms of cold intolerance, such as pain and bluish tinge in the fingertips and toes as a result of vasospasm). Patients with severe CHD usually live more comfortably in warmer climates.

Laboratory Findings. Laboratory findings in CHD include reticulocytosis and a positive DAT due to complement only. It is suggested that a simple serum screening procedure be performed initially to test the ability of the patient's serum to agglutinate autologous saline-suspended RBCs at 18°C to 20°C. If this test result is positive, further steps may be taken to determine the titer and thermal amplitude of the patient's cold autoantibody, which typically reacts as pathological cold autoagglutinins as described in **Table 20–2**. If it is negative, the diagnosis of CHD is unlikely. The peripheral smear of a patient with CHD may show agglutinated RBCs, polychromasia, mild to moderate anisocytosis, and poikilocytosis (**Fig. 20–2**). Autoagglutination of anticoagulated whole blood samples is characteristic of CHD and occurs quickly as the blood cools to room temperature, causing the binding of cold autoantibodies to the patient's RBCs in vitro. As a result of this autoagglutination, it is extremely difficult to perform automated blood counts and preparation of blood smears with these patients' samples.

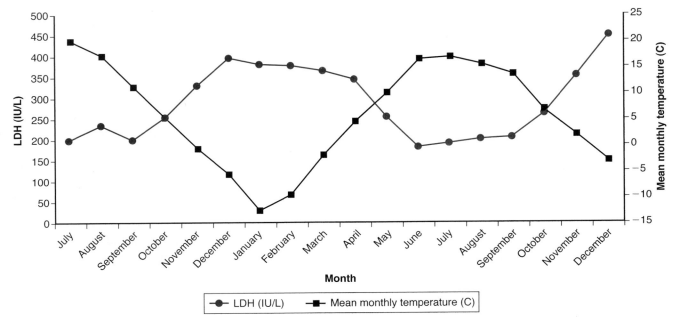

Figure 20–1. Seasonal hemolysis in cold agglutinin disease. As the ambient temperature decreases, the amount of hemolysis (reflected in serum lactate dehydrogenase levels) increases. During warmer months, LDH levels return to normal. *(Adapted with permission from Lyckholm, LJ, and Edmond, MB: Seasonal hemolysis due to cold-agglutinin syndrome. N Engl J Med 334:437, 1996.)*

Leukocyte and platelet counts are usually normal. Box 20–1 lists the clinical criteria for diagnosis of CHD.

Selection of Blood for Transfusion. Most patients with CHD do not require transfusion; however, when they do, it is sometimes challenging to perform the pretransfusion testing. As previously described, potent cold autoantibodies interfere with most routine tests. Perhaps the most difficult problem is detecting and identifying alloantibodies. Procedures to manage these problems were described earlier in this chapter, but cold autoadsorption of the serum should be the method of choice, if possible. It is important to provide RBCs compatible with any clinically significant alloantibodies. Most patients tolerate transfusion of blood that is incompatible with the autoantibody. Units of i_{adult} RBCs are extremely rare and should be reserved for the rare i_{adult} patient with alloanti-I.

The issue of transfusion in CHD patients is most relevant in those undergoing surgical procedures that use hypothermia (lowering of the body temperature to 22°C to 30°C), such as cardiac procedures. For patients with CHD, blood for transfusion can be warmed by an approved blood warmer, or the operative procedures can be performed without subjecting the patient to hypothermia.[32] Patients with benign cold autoagglutinins do not require these special arrangements.

Cold Autoantibodies Related to Infection (Secondary Cold AIHA)

CHD can also occur as a transient disorder secondary to infection. Episodes of cold AIHA often occur after upper respiratory infections. Approximately 50% of patients suffering from pneumonia caused by *M. pneumoniae* have cold

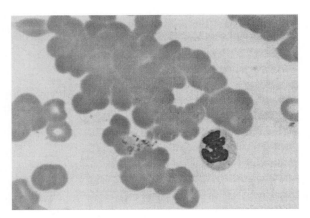

Figure 20–2. Cold agglutinin disease (peripheral blood).

BOX 20–1

Clinical Criteria for the Diagnosis of CHD

- Clinical signs of an acquired hemolytic anemia, with a history (which may or may not be present) of acrocyanosis and hemoglobinuria on exposure to cold
- Positive DAT result using polyspecific antihuman sera
- Positive DAT result using monospecific anti-C3 antisera
- Negative DAT result using monospecific anti-IgG antisera
- Presence of reactivity in the patient's serum due to a cold autoantibody
- Cold agglutinin titer of 1,000 or greater in saline at 4°C with visible agglutination of anticoagulated blood at room temperature

Adapted from Harmening, DM: Clinical Hematology and Fundamentals of Hemostasis, 4th ed. FA Davis, Philadelphia, 2002, p 210, with permission.

agglutinin titer levels higher than 64. In the second or third week of the patient's illness, CHD may occur in association with the infection, and a rapid onset of hemolysis is observed. Pallor and jaundice are characteristically present. Acrocyanosis and hemoglobinuria are uncommon and not consistently present. Usually, resolution of the episode occurs within 2 to 3 weeks because the hemolysis is self-limiting, resolving when the infection subsides. The offending cold autoantibody is an IgM immunoglobulin with a characteristic anti-I specificity. Very high titers of cold autoagglutinins are seen almost exclusively in patients with *M. pneumoniae*. It has been theorized that the cold agglutinin produced in this infection is an immunologic response to the mycoplasma antigens and that this antibody cross-reacts with the I antigen on RBCs.

The antibodies produced in primary CHD and in this disorder secondary to *M. pneumoniae* both have anti-I specificity, and the RBCs are sensitized with complement components. If the complement cascade does not proceed to C9 (cell death by lysis), the macrophages of the reticuloendothelial system can still clear the sensitized RBCs through their receptors for C3b fragments, thereby causing hemolysis.

Infectious mononucleosis also may be associated with a hemolytic anemia resulting from a cold autoantibody. Although infrequent, it has been well documented that a high-titered IgM anti-i with a wide thermal range plays a major role in hemolytic anemia associated with this viral infection. Acute illness with a sore throat and a high fever, followed by weakness, anemia, and jaundice, are characteristic features of infectious mononucleosis. Lymphadenopathy and hepatosplenomegaly are common findings. A larger percentage of patients with infectious mononucleosis has been reported to develop anti-i, but only a small number of these patients develops the antibody of sufficient titer and thermal amplitude to induce in vivo hemolysis.

Treatment for CHD. Therapy for CHD is generally unnecessary. Most patients require no treatment and are instructed to avoid the cold, keep warm, or move to a milder climate. Patients with moderate anemia are given the same instructions and are urged to tolerate the symptoms rather than to use drugs on a therapeutic trial basis. There is some advantage to the use of plasma exchange in more severe cases, inasmuch as IgM antibodies have a predominantly intravascular distribution; however, response to plasma exchange is still variable in this patient population, and repeated plasma exchanges are often required on a frequent basis to maintain low plasma levels of autoagglutinating antibodies.

Corticosteroids also have been used but generally have a poor response. In some patients whose RBCs are strongly coated with C3, successful results have been reported with corticosteroids. Some favorable responses also have been reported with the alkylating drug chlorambucil. Splenectomy is generally considered ineffective.

Paroxysmal Cold Hemoglobinuria. **Paroxysmal cold hemoglobinuria** (PCH) is the least common type of AIHA, with an incidence between 1% and 2%. It is most often seen in children who have had viral illnesses such as measles, mumps, chickenpox, infectious mononucleosis, and the ill-defined flu syndrome. Originally, PCH was described in association with syphilis, with an autoantibody formed in response to *Treponema pallidum* infection; however, with the effective treatment of syphilis with antibiotics, PCH is no longer commonly reported in relation to syphilis.

In PCH, RBC destruction is caused by a cold autoantibody referred to as a biphasic autohemolysin, which binds to the patient's RBCs at lower temperatures and fixes complement. Hemolysis occurs when the sensitized RBCs circulate and are exposed to 37°C and the sensitized cells undergo complement-mediated intravascular lysis. In contrast to the other cold reactive autoagglutinins, the antibody in PCH is an IgG immunoglobulin with biphasic activity. The classic antibody produced in PCH is called the Donath-Landsteiner antibody and is an autoantibody with anti-P specificity. Other specificities have been reported, including anti-i[33] and anti-Pr-like.[34] These antibodies are not identifiable using regular serologic techniques. The antibody specificity is only demonstrated in the **Donath-Landsteiner test**, which is the test used to confirm the diagnosis of PCH.

The Donath-Landsteiner test involves the collection of a fresh blood sample from the patient. The sample is maintained at 37°C after collection and the serum is then separated. Three sets of three test tubes, labeled A1–A2–A3, B1–B2–B3, and C1–C2–C3, containing the patient's serum are incubated at various temperatures with group O RBCs that express the P antigen (i.e., RBCs of common phenotype). In this test, tubes 1 and 2 of each set contain 10 drops of patient's serum, and tubes 2 and 3 of each set contain 10 drops of fresh normal serum as a complement source. One volume of 50% suspension of washed P+ RBCs is added to each tube, and all tubes are mixed. After mixing, the three A tubes are then placed in a melting ice bath for 30 minutes and subsequently for 1 hour at 37°C (biphasic incubation). The three B tubes are placed in a melted ice bath for 90 minutes. The three C tubes are kept at 37°C for 90 minutes. After the appropriate time has passed, the tubes are centrifuged, and supernatant fluids are examined for hemolysis. Table 20–6 summarizes the reactions of a positive Donath-Landsteiner test.

As the name PCH implies, paroxysmal or intermittent episodes of hemoglobinuria occur upon exposure to cold. These acute attacks are characterized by sudden onset of fever, shaking chills, malaise, abdominal cramps, and back pain. All the signs of intravascular hemolysis are evident, along with hemoglobinemia, hemoglobinuria, and bilirubinemia, depending on the severity and frequency of the attack (Fig. 20–3). This results in a severe and rapidly progressive anemia with hemoglobin levels frequently as low as 4 or 5 g/dL. Polychromasia, nucleated RBCs, and poikilocytosis are demonstrated in the peripheral smear, findings that are consistent with hemolytic anemia. These signs and symptoms, as well as hemoglobinuria, may resolve in a few hours or persist for days. Splenomegaly, hyperbilirubinemia, and renal insufficiency may also develop.

Table 20–6   Reactions of a Positive Donath-Landsteiner Test

INCUBATION PHASES	TUBES 1 PATIENT SERUM (TUBES A1, B1, C1)	TUBES 2 PATIENT SERUM PLUS NORMAL SERUM* (TUBES A2, B2, C2)	TUBES 3 NORMAL SERUM* (TUBES A3, B3, C3)
Ice bath followed by 37°C (all A tubes)	+	+	0
Ice bath only (all B tubes)	0	0	0
37°C only (all C tubes)	0	0	0

+ = with hemolysis
0 = without hemolysis
* Tubes with normal serum are used as control
Note: The patient's blood should be clotted at 37°C and the serum separated at this temperature to avoid the loss of the autoantibody by cold autoadsorption prior to testing. Fresh normal serum should be included in the reaction medium as a source of complement, as PCH patients may have low levels of serum complement. Omit the patient serum-only tubes (A1, B1, C1) if a limited amount of blood is available (e.g., a young child).

PCH is an acute hemolytic anemia occurring almost exclusively in children and young adults and almost always represents a transient disorder. Table 20–7 compares and contrasts PCH with CHD.

Treatment for PCH. For chronic forms of PCH, protection from cold exposure is the only useful therapy. Acute postinfection forms of PCH are transient and usually terminate spontaneously after the infection resolves. Steroids and transfusion may be required, depending on the severity of the attacks.

Note: Paroxysmal nocturnal hemoglobinuria (PNH) is often confused with PCH because of the similarity of the names and acronyms. Autoantibody has not been implicated in PNH; a membrane defect is thought to be involved. RBC destruction in PNH is complement-mediated because of the absence or reduced amounts of some complement regulatory proteins.[35]

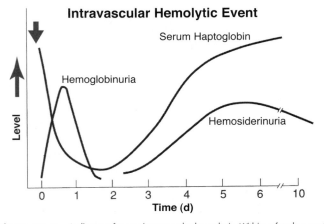

Figure 20–3. Indicator of acute intravascular hemolysis. Within a few hours of an acute hemolytic event, free hemoglobin is cleared from plasma, and the serum haptoglobin falls to undetectable levels. Hemoglobinuria ceases soon after this. If no further hemolysis occurs, the serum haptoglobin level recovers and methemalbumin disappears within several days. The urinary hemosiderin can provide more lasting evidence of the hemolytic event. *(From Hillman, RS, and Finch, CA: Red Cell Manual, 7th ed. FA Davis, Philadelphia, 1996, p 112, with permission.)*

Warm Autoantibodies

Autoantibodies that react best at 37°C are not found as often in the random population as the almost universal cold autoanti-I. However, many more of the true AIHAs are of the warm type (70%) than of the cold reactive type (18%).[7] As with the cold reactive autoantibodies, some individuals have apparently harmless warm autoantibodies; however, unlike their cold counterparts, the harmless autoantibodies are serologically indistinguishable from the harmful ones. There are no diagnostic tests to predetermine which autoantibodies will cause RBC destruction. When a warm autoantibody is encountered, it should be characterized as such and reported to the patient's physician. The presence of the antibody may alert the physician to an underlying autoimmune process.

Clinical Findings

Patients with warm autoimmune hemolytic anemia (WAIHA) present a different problem to the blood bank than those with cold AIHA. A significant percentage of cases suffer from an anemia of sufficient severity to require transfusion. The extent of anemia is variable; however, hemoglobins less than 7 g/dL are not uncommon. The onset of WAIHA may be insidious and may be precipitated by a variety of factors such as infection,[36] trauma, surgery, pregnancy,[37] or underlying disease. In other patients, the onset is sudden and unexplained. WAIHA may be idiopathic with no underlying disease process or may be secondary to a pathological disorder. Box 20–2 lists the disorders most commonly associated with WAIHA.

Signs and symptoms appear when a significant anemia has developed. Pallor, weakness, dizziness, dyspnea, jaundice, and unexplained fever are occasionally presenting complaints. Hemolysis is usually acute at onset and may stabilize or may continue to accelerate at a variable rate. The peripheral blood smear usually exhibits polychromasia and macrocytosis, reflecting reticulocytosis, or even the presence of nucleated RBCs, which is evidence of a hyperactive bone

Table 20–7 Comparison of Paroxysmal Cold Hemoglobinuria (PCH) and Cold Hemagglutinin Disease (CHD)

FACTORS	PCH	CHD
Patient population	Children and young adults	Elderly or middle-aged adults
Pathogenesis	Following viral infection	Idiopathic, lymphoproliferative disorder; following *M. pneumoniae* infection
Clinical features	Hemoglobinuria, acute attacks upon exposure to cold (symptoms resolve in hours to days)	Acrocyanosis; autoagglutination of blood at room temperature
Severity of hemolysis	Acute and rapid	Chronic and rarely severe
Site of hemolysis	Intravascular	Extravascular/intravascular
Autoantibody class	IgG (anti-P specificity; biphasic hemolysin)	IgM (anti-I/i) monophasic
DAT	3–4+ monospecific C3 only	3–4+ monospecific C3 only
Thermal range	Moderate (< 20°C)	High (up to 30°C–31°C)
Titer	Moderate (< 64)	High (> 1,000)
Donath-Landsteiner test result	Positive	Negative
Treatment	Supportive (disorder terminates when underlying illness resolves)	Avoid cold

Harmening DM: Clinical Hematology and Fundamentals of Hemostasis, 4th ed. FA Davis, Philadelphia, 2002, p 212, with permission.

marrow (Fig. 20–4). Spherocytosis and occasionally RBC fragmentation, indicating extravascular hemolysis, may also be demonstrated in a blood smear from a patient with immune hemolytic anemia. An uncommon manifestation of WAIHA is reticulocytopenia. This may be associated with a hypoplastic marrow that is secondary to an underlying disease state. Because antigenic determinants on erythrocyte precursors can also react with the patient's RBC autoantibodies, reticulocytes may be destroyed as they are released from the bone marrow. Therefore, reticulocytopenia at a

time of intense hemolysis is associated with a high mortality rate. Products of hemolysis, such as bilirubin (particularly the unconjugated indirect fraction) and urinary urobilinogen, are increased. In severe cases, depleted serum haptoglobin, hemoglobinemia, hemoglobinuria, and increases in LDH may be laboratory markers that help confirm the diagnosis.

RBC Hemolysis

Most patients with WAIHA have both IgG and complement on their RBCs (67%). A minority have either IgG only (20%) or complement only (13%). Fewer still are patients with WAIHA with IgA (2% to 3%) or IgM (less than 2%) coating their RBCs.[7] The IgG subclass of coating antibody has been studied in hopes of finding a correlation with severity of

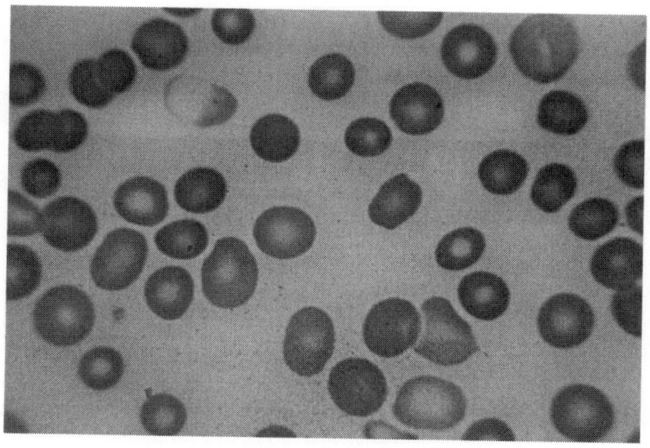

BOX 20–2

Diseases Frequently Associated With WAIHA Hemolytic Anemia

- Reticuloendothelial neoplasms, such as chronic lymphocytic leukemia, Hodgkin's disease, non-Hodgkin's lymphomas, myelofibrosis, and myelodysplastic syndromes
- Collagen disease, such as systemic lupus erythematosus and rheumatoid arthritis
- Infectious diseases, such as viral syndromes in childhood and adults
- Immunologic diseases, such as hypogammaglobulinemia, dysglobulinemia, and other immune-deficiency syndromes
- Gastrointestinal diseases, such as ulcerative colitis
- Carcinoma (nonovarian)
- Pregnancy
- Chronic renal failure

Adapted from Sokol, RJ, Booker, DJ, and Stamps, R: The pathology of autoimmune haemolytic anaemia. J Clin Path 45:1047–1052, 1992, with permission

Figure 20–4. Autoimmune hemolytic anemia (peripheral blood).

hemolysis, with IgG1 predominating (87%). Unexpectedly, approximately the same percentages of patients with a positive DAT but no evidence of hemolysis and normal blood donors with a positive DAT had IgG1 on their RBCs. Nance and Garratty reported that, in general, the strength of the DAT correlated with the presence of multiple IgG subclasses on the RBCs, which in turn correlated with the severity of the hemolysis.[38]

In general, IgG3 antibodies are the most destructive to RBCs, followed by IgG1. IgG2 antibodies are less destructive, and IgG4 shows little or no RBC destruction. The subclasses, or isotypes, of IgG are distinguished by the number of disulfide bonds present in the hinge region of the molecule, accounting for their different electrophoretic mobility and biological properties. Refer to Chapter 3 for a complete discussion of the properties of the IgG subclasses. All IgG subclasses, except IgG4, possess the ability to bind complement via the classic pathway of activation, with IgG3 being more efficient than IgG1, which in turn is more efficient than IgG2.

Immune RBC destruction resulting from sensitization with IgG antibody is primarily extravascular, taking place in the fixed reticuloendothelial system (RES) cells of the liver and spleen. The spleen is 100 times more efficient than the liver in removing IgG-sensitized RBCs. Macrophages are equipped with two important biological receptors on their membranes:

1. Receptors for the FC fragments of IgG1 and IgG3 immunoglobulins
2. Receptors for the C3b fragment of complement

Sensitized RBCs are phagocytized by interaction with RES mononuclear phagocytes, depending on which protein coats the erythrocytes. If only IgG coats the RBCs, gradual phagocytosis of the erythrocytes occurs. If both IgG and C3b coat the RBCs, there is a rapid phagocytosis, because the C3b fragment augments the action of IgG, enhancing sequestration and phagocytosis of the coated erythrocytes. If only C3b coats the RBCs, transient immune adherence occurs. It has been estimated that more than 100,000 molecules of the complement fragment would be required to induce phagocytosis; therefore, the activity of the macrophages and the severity of hemolysis via phagocytosis of sensitized RBCs depend on various factors, summarized in Box 20–3.

BOX 20–3

Factors Affecting Activity of Macrophages

- Subclass of IgG, especially IgG1 and IgG3
- Presence of complement (C3b) fragments
- Quantity of immunoglobulin or complement
- Number and activity of helper T cells (CD4)
- Number and activity of suppressor T cells (CD8)

Adapted from Pittiglio, D, and Sacher, RA: Clinical Hematology and Fundamentals of Hemostasis. FA Davis, Philadelphia, 1987, p 153, with permission.

Serologic Characteristics and Laboratory Tests Affected

Because warm reactive autoantibodies are typically IgG immunoglobulins, they react best by the indirect antiglobulin technique. As a rule, they do not directly agglutinate saline-suspended RBCs after 37°C incubation. The antibodies may activate complement and are usually enhanced by enzyme techniques. Most of these autoantibodies react with a high-incidence RBC antigen, often with a general specificity within the Rh blood group system, but there are reports of autoantibodies associated with most of the other blood group systems. Identification of autoantibodies is discussed later in this chapter.

Warm autoantibodies can interfere with most routine blood bank tests, and they may present more of a serologic dilemma than cold autoagglutinins. While most cold autoantibodies can be avoided if room temperature incubation is omitted, if testing is performed at 37°C, or if anti-IgG antiglobulin is used, with WAIHAs, both clinically significant alloantibodies and the autoantibodies themselves react best at the indirect antiglobulin phase; therefore, more complicated and time-consuming procedures for resolving the problems may have to be used.

ABO Typing

Since most warm autoantibodies are not direct agglutinins, ABO grouping is usually not affected. Even though the patient's cells may be heavily coated with antibody, the antibodies typically do not cause spontaneous agglutination of RBCs at room temperature when reagent anti-A and anti-B are added. Similarly, warm autoantibodies in the serum usually do not directly agglutinate saline-suspended A_1 and B cells.

Rh(D) Typing

False-positive Rh typing can occur when the patient's cells are coated with immunoglobulins. The high-protein Rh antisera, previously the mainstay of Rh typing, demonstrated numerous testing problems. Potentiators were added to many high-protein Rh typing reagents that caused direct agglutination of RBCs strongly coated with IgG. For this reason, a negative control consisting of patient cells and the matching Rh diluent had to be tested in parallel with the D typing. The results of the D antigen typing were valid only when the control test result was negative.

The current reagents available for D typing are predominantly monoclonal antisera containing no more than 7% protein additive. Monoclonal antisera have a low incidence of false-positive test results, but false positive results still may occur if the RBCs are heavily coated with IgG.[39] Some manufacturers offer an Rh control reagent designed to be tested in parallel with the anti-D serum. Other manufacturers recommend that a negative test with an antiserum of a similar protein concentration (e.g., ABO antisera) is sufficient to detect a false-positive reaction. If a patient types group AB Rh positive (i.e., all tubes in the ABO cell typing and the D typing are positive), a separate Rh control (commercial matched diluent or 6% albumin) must be tested alongside to ensure that the ABO/Rh typing is valid. If the diluent or 6% albumin control is positive, it may be necessary to pretreat the cells using EDTA/glycine acid (EGA) or choloroquine diphosphate (CDP) to remove coating IgG immunoglobulins from the RBCs to obtain a valid ABO/Rh test.[40]

 See Procedures 20-5 or 20-10 on the textbook's companion website.

If the DAT of the EGA-treated or CDP-treated RBCs is negative, it is then possible to use these cells for weak D testing; however, an Rh control serum or 6% albumin should again be tested in parallel to detect false-positive reactivity. *Note*: Even if some IgG remains on the RBCs after EGA or CDP treatment, they are usually suitable for testing with directly agglutinating monoclonal reagents, including anti-D, anti-C, anti-E, anti-c, anti-e, anti-K, anti-Jk^a, anti-Jk^b and others, as long as the negative control is valid.

Another technique to detect a weak D type is the rosette test (see Chapter 19), which is commonly used in the detection of fetal-maternal hemorrhage. This screening test, used to detect fetal D+ cells in the circulation of the D– mother, will also detect D+ cells in any cell population. If the patient's cells are D+, the rosette test will be strongly positive. Because the rosette test does not incorporate an antiglobulin phase, a patient with a positive DAT can be accurately typed for the D antigen by this method. It is not absolutely necessary to determine the correct weak D typing of a patient with WAIHA, because D– (Rh negative) RBCs can be transfused if necessary.

DAT

A positive DAT is expected in association with warm autoantibodies. As autoantibody is produced, it adsorbs onto the antigen of that defined specificity present on the patient's own RBCs. The RBCs may then be coated with IgG alone (20%), IgG and complement (67%), or complement alone (13%).[7] In rare cases, the DAT may be negative or cells may be coated only with IgA or IgM.[18–20]

Antibody Detection and Identification

The serum of a patient with warm autoantibodies may contain only autoantibody or, if the patient has been previously transfused or pregnant, a mixture of autoantibody and alloantibody. When smaller amounts of autoantibody have been produced, the autoantibody may be detected only on the patient's cells, adsorbed in vivo, with no free autoantibody detectable in the serum. If the amount of antibody produced exceeds the number of RBC antigen sites available, when the antigen-antibody equilibrium is reached, serum antibody will be detected in the indirect antiglobulin phase of testing. When warm autoantibodies are present in the serum or on the patient's cells, the extent of further testing could be based on the patient's history, but reliable transfusion histories are notoriously difficult to obtain. It must be confirmed that the antibody coating the patient's cells is an autoantibody, and limited effort should be expended

determining its specificity. The main goal of additional testing should be to detect and identify all clinically significant alloantibodies that might be masked by the autoantibody. If the patient has had a previous transfusion or has been pregnant, there is an inherent risk of previous alloimmunization.

Evaluation of Autoantibody

A positive DAT can result from RBC alloantibodies coating recently transfused donor cells or drug-induced antibodies and RBC autoantibodies. IgG immunoglobulins will most likely be present on the cells in each case. It is important to differentiate the causes of a positive DAT because selection of RBCs for transfusion and treatment protocols differ. To make the distinction between these causes, one must have the patient's medical history, including an accurate history of previous transfusions and pregnancies, diagnoses, and medications.

If a patient has had a recent transfusion, the possibility that alloantibodies and not autoantibodies are coating the circulating transfused donor cells must be considered. In most cases, by examining the DAT microscopically for **mixed-field agglutination** (which indicates a mixed-cell population of DAT+ and DAT– RBCs) and by determining the specificity of the antibody in the eluate, it is possible to establish alloantibodies as the cause (see Chapter 16). Because warm autoantibodies are frequently associated with certain diseases, such as systemic lupus erythematosus, and with medications, such as Aldomet, the patient's diagnosis and drug history are informative tools in helping establish autoantibodies as the cause of the positive DAT. The specificity of the antibody compared to the patient's RBC phenotype is also helpful in differentiating between autoantibody and alloantibody.

To identify the specificity of a warm reactive autoantibody, an eluate prepared from the patient's RBCs must be tested, in addition to the patient's serum, with a panel of reagent RBCs.

 See Procedure 20-6 on the textbook's companion website for instructions in preparing a digitonin acid eluate. *Note*: A commercial kit is also available for the preparation of acid eluates.

If the patient has a well-documented history showing that he or she has not been transfused within the past 3 months, and there is no evidence of a mixed-cell population in any phenotyping results, it is reasonably safe to assume that antibody activity in the eluate is autoantibody. But if the patient has a history of recent transfusion or pregnancy, the serum may contain alloantibody in addition to autoantibody.

The specificity of an autoantibody may be different in the serum and in the eluate. Warm autoantibodies in the serum may show a relative anti-e specificity, reacting weakest with e– RBCs, while the eluate may show pan-agglutination of all RBCs tested. This apparent difference in antibody specificity may be qualitative or quantitative. The concentration of antibody removed from the cells in the elution process may be greater than the quantity of antibody in the serum. **Table 20–8** illustrates an example of such reactivity. It should also be noted that elution procedures vary in their ability to remove coating immunoglobulins (i.e., a heat or freeze/thaw eluate generally reacts less strongly than an acid eluate or one of the chemical eluates, such as dichloromethane or ether).

A majority of the IgG antibodies detected in eluates prepared from the WAIHA patient's RBCs or in the patient's serum have a complex Rh-like specificity, similar to those shown in **Table 20–9**. Occasionally, an autoantibody may have what is termed "simple" anti-e specificity that reacts with all red cells except R_2R_2 (D+C–E+c+e–) cells. Much more frequently, reactivity is observed with all RBCs of normal Rh phenotype. In order to identify the specificity of a complex Rh-like autoantibody, one must have an extensive library of rare cells, which includes Rh_{null} and D-- cells. Testing of these cells should allow one to categorize the antibody as anti-nl (normal), which reacts with all cells of common/normal Rh phenotypes but not those that are partially deleted or Rh_{null}; anti-pdl (partially deleted), which reacts with all cells except Rh_{null}; or anti-dl (deleted), which reacts with all cells.[41] This information is of historic value because of early work done by Weiner, Vos, and Race. Fortunately, this level of antibody identification is of academic interest, since few laboratories have access to these rare RBCs for testing purposes, let alone have them available for transfusion.

There are numerous reports of autoantibodies with specificities other than Rh, many of which appear to be directed against RBC antigens of high incidence or a null phenotype. Among the other specificities are autoanti-U, autoanti-Wr[b], autoanti-En[a], autoanti-Kp[b], autoanti-Vel, and autoanti-Ge.[42–44] The reader is referred to Petz and Garratty[7] for a detailed discussion of autoantibody specificity. Apparent specificities such as these can cause confusion, especially when the patient has had a recent transfusion. Determining the patient's phenotype is one of the most valuable tools used to classify the antibody as "auto" or "allo." As previously discussed, monoclonal antisera and commercially available IgG removal agents have made this challenge easier. In recently transfused patients, molecular genotyping of the patient's white blood cells may be helpful in predicting the patient's phenotype. Most researchers agree that it is not necessary to do extensive studies to identify the specificity of the autoantibody, but testing of at least one example of RBCs that is phenotypically similar to those of the patient is important to help distinguish between autoantibody (the phenotypically similar RBCs will be reactive) and multiple alloantibodies (the phenotypically similar RBCs will be nonreactive).

Specificity of the autoantibody, if obvious, may influence selection of blood for transfusion. Some practitioners prefer to transfuse RBCs that are compatible with the autoantibody if simple specificity can be assigned, such as anti-e, and if there are no preexisting circumstances that would prevent this transfusion (e.g., one would not select Rh-positive

Table 20–8 Warm Autoantibody With Relative Anti-e Specificity Noted in Serum Testing, but Broad Reactivity Noted in Eluate

Cell		D	C	E	c	e	Cell	SERUM			ELUATE	
								RT	LISS 37° C	IAT	Eluate IAT	LAST WASH IAT
R_1R_1 - 44	1	+	+	0	0	+	1	0	0	3+	4+	0✓
R_1R_1 - 39	2	+	+	0	0	+	2	0	0	3+	4+	0✓
R_2R_2 - 23	3	+	0	+	+	0	3	0	0	±	4+	0✓
r r - 33	4	0	0	0	+	+	4	0	0	3+	4+	0✓
r r - 26	5	0	0	0	+	+	5	0	0	3+	4+	0✓
r′ r - 4	6	0	+	0	+	+	6	0	0	3+	4+	0✓
r″ r - 17	7	0	0	+	+	+	7	0	0	3+	4+	0✓
R_0 r – 13	8	+	0	0	+	+	8	0	0	3+	4+	0✓
R_1 r – 14	9	+	+	0	+	+	9	0	0	3+	4+	0✓
R_1R_2 - 8	10	+	+	+	+	+	10	0	0	2+	4+	0✓
Auto Control (untt'd RBCs)	11						11	0	0	3+	4+	3+
Auto Control (EGA-tt'd)	12						12	0	0	3+	4+	0✓

0✓ = negative IAT reading with check cells added and reactive, as expected; untt'd = untreated; EGA-tt'd = EDTA glycine acid treated.

Table 20–9	Typical Serologic Reactions of Warm Autoantibodies With RBCs of Selected Rh Phenotypes			
Rh PHENOTYPE	**AUTOANTI-e**	**ANTI-nl**	**ANTI-pdl**	**ANTI-dl**
R_1R_1 (normal)	+	+	+	+
R_2R_2 (normal)	0	+	+	+
rr (normal)	+	+	+	+
D– – (partially deleted)	0	0	+	+
Rh_{null} (fully deleted)	0	0	0	+

dl = fully deleted; nl = normal; pdl = partially deleted

e– RBCs for an Rh-negative patient with autoanti-e). Selecting donor units that are compatible with the patient's autoantibody, however, cannot guarantee normal RBC survival. Unfortunately, the transfused cells will probably be destroyed as rapidly as the patient's own cells, regardless of phenotype.

Detection and Identification of Alloantibodies

All researchers agree that detection and identification of all alloantibodies is of primary concern when one must transfuse a patient with WAIHA, especially when the patient has had a previous transfusion or pregnancy. When autoantibody is found in the serum, it will typically mask any alloantibodies present. In this situation, one can use several techniques:

1. If the autoantibody demonstrates a simple specificity, such as anti-e, test a panel of cells negative for the corresponding antigen (e– in this case) and positive for all common clinically significant RBC antigens (Rh, Kell, Duffy, Kidd, S, and s) to exclude or identify the presence of underlying alloantibodies.

2. If the patient has not had a recent transfusion (within the past 3 months), determine the patient's RBC phenotype using either monoclonal antisera, which does not require antiglobulin testing, or using the patient's RBCs treated with an agent known to remove coating IgG immunoglobulins. The cells may be treated with chloroquine diphosphate (CDP) solution or EGA prior to phenotyping. (The EGA procedure will denature all Kell system antigens, among others.) If there is a sufficient quantity of patient RBCs available, prepare autologous cells to be used for autoadsorption procedures. Pretreat the cells to remove coating autoantibody, using either of the methods described above or a chemical such as ficin or ZZAP (a combination of ficin and DTT).

 See Procedure 20-7B on the textbook's companion website. This treatment will free antigen sites for adsorption of autoantibody.

3. If autoadsorption studies are not possible because the patient was recently transfused, and there is evidence of reticulocyte production, it may be possible to determine the patient's phenotype using a reticulocyte harvesting

procedure. This phenotyping information can be used to select RBCs that are phenotypically similar to those of the patient by matching the common RBC antigens: Rh, Kell, Kidd, Duffy, S, and s. Allogeneic adsorptions performed using this method to select phenotypically similar donor or reagent RBCs will remove autoantibody, but it will also adsorb an alloantibody to any high incidence RBC antigen, if present.

 See Procedure 20-11 on the textbook's companion website.

4. If it is not possible to determine the patient's RBC phenotyping, differential allogeneic adsorptions may be performed by selecting three donor units that are known to lack common RBC antigens and are of complimentary Rh antigen combinations. Typically, these cells include each of the following Rh types: R_1R_1 (D+C+E–c–e+), R_2R_2 (D+C–E+c+e–), and rr (D–C–E–c+e+). Allogeneic adsorptions performed using this method will remove autoantibody but will also adsorb an alloantibody to any high-incidence RBC antigen, if present. Ficin or ZZAP treatment of the allogeneic adsorbing cells is recommended because it increases antibody uptake but also alters the phenotype of the adsorbing cells—for example, ficin will render the RBCs M–N–S– Fy(a–b–) and ZZAP will render them K–k–s–. Keep in mind the cell treatment used when interpreting the pattern of results in the adsorbed sera.

In typical warm adsorption procedures, the patient's serum and the prepared adsorbing cells are incubated at 37°C, allowing the autoantibody to bind to antigen sites on the prepared cells, leaving unadsorbed alloantibody in the serum. The number of adsorptions needed to remove all autoantibody depends on the amount of autoantibody present in the patient's serum and the test procedure used. Usually the strength of reactivity in the indirect antiglobulin phase of the antibody screen or panel is a good indicator of how many adsorptions will be necessary. If there is strong reactivity (3+ to 4+) of autoantibody in the serum and gel or polyethylene glycol (PEG) enhancement is used in testing, then more than one adsorption will be necessary. Testing the adsorbed serum with the DAT– (e.g., EGA or CDP-treated) autologous RBCs or allogeneic adsorbing cells used is a useful way of determining if autoantibody has been adsorbed and the adsorbed serum is ready to test with additional selected cells. Table 20–10 shows an example of a patient with a warm autoantibody demonstrable by LISS indirect antiglobulin test (IAT) and alloanti-E detected in the autoadsorbed serum.

 See **Procedure 20-7** on the textbook's companion website.

When performing adsorption procedures, the following circumstances must be considered:

- Autoadsorption procedures are never recommended in patients who have been transfused within the previous 3 months. In vitro studies have determined that as few as 10% of antigen-positive RBCs are sufficient to adsorb the alloantibody.[45] This small amount of antigen-positive cells may not be obvious in phenotyping.
- If the patient is severely anemic, it may not be possible to obtain sufficient autologous cells for multiple adsorptions.
- Whenever an adsorption is performed, whether with autologous or allogeneic cells, the serum is diluted to some extent. Some saline remains in "packed" RBCs. A weakly reactive alloantibody could be diluted and missed if multiple adsorptions are performed.
- If allogeneic adsorptions are performed, it is possible to adsorb an alloantibody to a high-incidence RBC antigen that is present on the allogeneic cells that is not present on the patient's own cells.

When the patient has had a recent transfusion or is severely anemic, cells of selected phenotypes for adsorption can be used. If the patient's phenotype is unknown and cannot be determined, adsorptions can be performed using a trio of selected cells (R_1R_1, R_2R_2, and rr). These cells should also lack one or more antigens for the more commonly encountered clinically significant alloantibodies (i.e., anti-D, anti-C, anti-E, anti-c, anti-e, anti-S, anti-s, anti-K, anti-Fy^a, anti-Fy^b, anti-Jk^a, anti-Jk^b). As shown in Table 20–11, if the patient's serum is adsorbed with cells from donors of selected phenotypes and then the adsorbed sera are tested, alloantibodies to the common antigens can be detected.

Alternatively, if a pretransfusion phenotype is available for the patient, phenotypically matched RBCs can be used for adsorption. (See discussion of antigen typing the patient with a positive DAT in this chapter.) With the exception of possible adsorption of an antibody to a high-incidence antigen, adsorption with donor RBCs of similar phenotype to the patient's is a useful alternative to autologous adsorption. The patient should not form alloantibodies to RBC antigens that he or she possesses; therefore, it is advised to focus mainly on the antigens the patient lacks. For example, if the patient's RBCs phenotype is E–c–S–K–Fy(a–)Jk(b–) and donor RBCs are available that are E–c–K–Jk(b–), ficin treatment of the donor RBCs would render them also S– and Fy(a–), a phenotype-similar to the patient's.

It is impossible to detect all clinically significant alloantibodies using allogeneic adsorptions, like those directed against high-incidence antigens. For example, an anti-k would be adsorbed onto virtually all random donor cells, because the k antigen is present on the cells of more than 99% of the population (including the R_1R_1, R_2R_2, and rr adsorption cells) unless ZZAP treatment of the adsorbing cells is used. An antibody such as this would be differentiated from the autoantibody only if a cell negative for the high-incidence antigen happened to be present among the cells used for adsorption. Nevertheless, allogeneic (differential) adsorption technique is valuable when there is no alternative.

Table 20–12 shows an example of a warm autoantibody with underlying anti-K and anti-Jk^a. The allogeneic adsorptions were performed using phenotyped donor RBCs that are of phenotypes complimentary to each other as a "set." Note that the phenotype of the donor RBCs is unknown for P_1, M, N, Le^a, and Le^b. Because antibodies to these antigens would not be expected to be clinically significant unless they were reactive at 37°C, they can be ignored. If interpretation of the reactivity pattern in the adsorbed sera suggested one of these antibodies was present, the adsorbing cells could be phenotyped at that point for the antigen of interest.

When alloantibodies are detected in the serum of a patient with WAIHA, it is desirable to test the patient's untransfused RBCs for the absence of the corresponding antigen, if not already done. If no pretransfusion sample is available, underlying antibodies must be assumed to be alloantibody in nature.

Selection of Blood for Transfusion

Many patients with WAIHA never require transfusion; they can be managed with medical treatment. Occasionally, however, the anemia is so severe that transfusion cannot be avoided. In addition, patients who have a nonhemolytic WAIHA pose problems when blood is needed for a surgical procedure. In these cases, after thorough serologic investigation, the primary concern is to ensure compatibility with any alloantibodies in the patient's serum. Compatibility with the autoantibody is controversial. If the autoantibody shows a simple specificity, such as anti-e, local practice may be to select donor units that are negative for the corresponding antigen, when practical.

As previously mentioned, this may be difficult if the donor RBCs selected precipitated alloantibody formation that would bring bigger challenges. For example, because virtually all Rh-negative (D–) cells are e+, an Rh-negative (D–) patient with autoanti-e specificity should not receive a transfusion of Rh-positive (D+) RBCs that lack the e antigen.[46] Singh and colleagues report hemoglobin increments in patients with AIHA comparable to the expected increment even when e+ units were transfused to patients with an apparent autoanti-e.[47] Finding compatible units for patients with a broad specificity warm autoagglutinin is virtually impossible. Even if the units are nonreactive with the adsorbed serum, these units will be "least incompatible" when crossmatched with unadsorbed serum. Also, the selection of in vitro least incompatible RBCs may not translate to in vivo

Table 20–10 Warm Autoantibody With Underlying Alloanti-E

Cell		D	C	E	c	e	P₁	M	N	S	s	Leᵃ	Leᵇ	K	k	Fyᵃ	Fyᵇ	Jkᵃ	Jkᵇ	OTHER	CELL	RT	LISS 37°C	IAT	FICIN AUTO-ADS SERUM IAT
R₁R₁ - 44	1	+	+	0	0	+	+	+	+	0	+	0	+	0	+	+	0	+	+	Cw+	1	0	0	3+	0✓
R₁R₁ - 39	2	+	+	0	0	+	+	+	+	0	+	0	+	0	+	+	+	+	0	Co(b+)	2	0	0	3+	0✓
R₂R₂ - 23	3	+	0	+	+	0	+	0	+	0	+	0	+	0	+	0	+	+	0		3	0	2+	4+	3+
r r - 33	4	0	0	0	+	+	0	+	0	+	+	+	0	0	+	0	+	0	+		4	0	0	3+	0✓
r r - 26	5	0	0	0	+	+	+	+	+	+	+	0	+	+	+	+	+	+	0		5	0	0	3+	0✓
r' r - 4	6	0	+	0	+	+	0	+	0	+	+	0	0	+	+	0	+	0	+		6	0	0	3+	0✓
r'' r - 17	7	0	0	+	+	+	+	+	+	+	0	0	+	0	+	+	0	0	+		7	0	1+	4+	2+
R₀ r - 13	8	+	0	0	+	+	+	+	+	+	0	0	0	0	+	0	0	+	+	V+ VS+	8	0	0	3+	0✓
R₁ r - 14	9	+	+	0	+	+	+	0	+	+	+	+	0	0	+	+	0	+	+		9	0	0	3+	0✓
R₁R₂ - 8	10	+	+	+	+	+	0	+	0	+	+	0	+	0	+	0	+	+	+	Kp(a+)	10	0	1+	4+	2+
Auto Control (untt'd RBCs)	11																				11	0	0	3+	3+
Auto Control (EGA-tt'd)	12																				12	0	0	3+	0✓

Anti-E is also detectable at 37°C as a directly agglutinating antibody, which is not uncommon with many examples of Rh antibodies. Adsorption x3 with ficin-treated autologous RBCs removed the warm autoantibody and left alloanti-E detectable in the autoadsorbed serum. EGA-treated autologous RBCs react with the unadsorbed serum but are nonreactive with the autoadsorbed serum. ADS = Adsorbed.

0✓ denotes negative IAT reading with check cells added and reactive as expected.

Table 20–11	Differential Adsorption Technique for Detecting Alloantibodies in the Serum of a Patient With Warm-Reacting Autoantibodies		
RBC	**EXAMPLE OF PHENOTYPE OF ADSORBING RBCs**	**ANTIBODY REMOVED BY ADSORPTION**	**ANTIBODY REMAINING IN ADSORBED SERUM**
R_1R_1 (D+C+E–c–e+)	K–k+ Fy(a+b–) Jk (a–b+) S+s+	D, C, e, k, Fy^a, Jk^b, S, s	E, c, K, Fy^b, Jk^a
R_2R_2 (D+C–E+c+e–)	K–k+ Fy(a–b+) Jk (a+b–) S–s+	D, E, c, k, Fy^b, Jk^a, s	C, e, K, Fy^a, Jk^b, S
rr (D–C–E–c+e+)	K+k– Fy(a–b+) Jk(a+b+) S+s–	c, e, K, Fy^b, Jk^a, Jk^b, S	D, C, E, k, Fy^a, s

most compatible RBCs. The transfused donor cells are likely to be destroyed as rapidly as the patient's own RBCs. It is much more important that donor units be selected that are compatible with any alloantibodies identified.

Treatment of WAIHA

Therapy is generally aimed at first treating the underlying disease, if one is present. General measures to support cardiovascular function are important for patients who are severely anemic. Transfusion should be avoided, if possible, because it may only accelerate the hemolysis; however, transfusion should not be avoided if the anemia is life-threatening. The volume of red blood cells transfused should be conservative, aiming for a relief in symptoms, not restoring a normal hematocrit. In many cases, even small amounts of transfused RBCs (even ½ to 1 unit of packed RBCs) are sufficient to relieve the symptoms of the anemia.[48] Forms of treatment other than transfusion are described in the following section.

Corticosteroid Administration and Use of IV Immunoglobulin

One form of therapy involves the use of corticosteroids, such as prednisone. Initially, high doses (100 to 200 mg) of prednisone are maintained until the patient's hematocrit level stabilizes. Patients who have not had transfusions seem to respond to steroid therapy more rapidly than those who are transfused.

Several mechanisms have been proposed for the action of prednisone,[49] including:

- Reduction of antibody synthesis
- Altered antibody activity
- Alteration of macrophage receptors for IgG and C3, which reduces the clearance of antibody-coated RBCs

The dosage of prednisone should be reduced when the hematocrit begins to rise and the reticulocyte count drops. The steroids are withdrawn slowly over 2 to 4 months. A beneficial response to the administration of prednisone is demonstrated in 50% to 65 % of all cases of WAIHA. An androgenic steroid, danazol, has also been beneficial in prednisone-resistant cases.[49]

Intravenous immunoglobulin (IVIG) has also been used in patients who do not respond to prednisone therapy.

Its mechanism for effectiveness is not understood and appears to be most effective when used in conjunction with corticosteroid therapy.[7] The use of intravenous immune globulin in patients unresponsive to corticosteroid treatment is controversial and appears to have limited efficacy.[50]

Splenectomy

If steroid therapy fails, or if a patient requires large doses of steroids to control hemolysis, splenectomy is usually recommended. The decision to perform a splenectomy requires clinical evaluation and judgment. There are three reasons for performing a splenectomy:

1. Failure of steroid therapy
2. Need for continuous high-dose steroid maintenance
3. Complications of steroid therapy

Splenectomy results in decreased production of antibody and removes a potent site of RBC damage and destruction. Patients who had a good initial response to steroids respond better with splenectomy than do those who failed initial steroid therapy. It has been reported that as many as 60% of patients with WAIHA benefit from splenectomy if steroid dosages greater than 15 mg per day are also used to maintain remission.

Immunosuppressive Drugs

The use of immunosuppressive drugs is usually the last approach for managing WAIHA. The field of organ transplantation has seen advances in development of immunosuppressive drugs, some of which have been used effectively in the treatment of WAIHA that has failed other forms of therapy. Azathioprine (Imuran) and cyclophosphamide are examples of immunosuppressive drugs that interfere with antibody synthesis by destroying dividing cells. Detrimental side effects of these drugs are infection, infertility, risk of birth defects, and development of malignancies. Cyclosporin has also been used, but the risk of renal damage is high. One of the most promising drugs is Rituximab, a monoclonal antibody that targets antibody-producing B lymphocytes, but it also has adverse effects, especially when used long-term.

Mixed-Type Autoantibodies

Individuals demonstrating antibody activity that appears to have both "warm" and "cold" components are considered to

Table 20–12 Warm Autoantibody With Underlying Alloanti-K and -Jkᵃ

CELL	D	C	E	c	e	P₁	M	N	S	s	Leᵃ	Leᵇ	K	k	Fyᵃ	Fyᵇ	Jkᵃ	Jkᵇ	CELL	UNADS. LISS RT	UNADS. 37°C	UNADS. IAT	R1R1 ALLO-ADS IAT	R2R2 ALLO-ADS IAT	r r ALLO-ADS IAT
R₁R₁ - 10	+	+	0	0	+	?	?	?	0	+	?	?	0	+	+	0	+	+					0✓		
R₂R₂ - 18	+	0	+	+	0	?	?	?	+	+	?	?	0	+	+	+	0	0						0✓	
r r - 14	0	0	0	+	+	?	?	?	+	0	?	?	+	+	0	+	0	+							0✓
R₁R₁ - 16	+	+	0	0	+	+	+	0	0	+	0	+	0	+	+	+	+	0	1	0	0	3+	0✓	0✓	3+
R₂R₂ - 25	+	0	+	+	0	+	0	+	+	+	+	0	0	+	+	+	0	+	2	0	0	3+	3+	0✓	0✓
r r - 9	0	0	0	+	+	0	+	+	0	+	0	+	0	+	0	+	+	+	3	0	0	3+	0✓	3+	2+
r r - 17	0	0	0	+	+	+	+	+	+	0	0	+	+	+	0	0	0	+	4				0✓	0✓	0✓
R₀r - 13	+	0	0	+	+	+	+	+	0	+	0	0	0	+	0	0	0	+	5				3+	3+	0✓
R₁r - 17	+	+	0	+	+	0	+	0	+	+	+	0	0	+	+	0	+	0	6				0✓	0✓	3+
R₁R₂ - 12	+	+	+	+	+	+	0	+	0	+	0	+	0	+	+	0	+	+	7				0✓	0✓	0✓
Auto Control (untt'd RBCs)																			8	0	0	3+	NT	NT	NT
Auto Control (EGA-tt'd)																			9	0	0	3+	0✓	0✓	0✓

Adsorbing cells chosen by phenotype (R₁R₁-10, R₂R₂-18, r r-14). Set of 3 antibody detection cells (1, 2, 3). Selected RBCs to confirm and exclude common alloabys (4, 5, 6, 7).

Each column in the adsorbed sera columns must be interpreted separately for purposes of antibody identification, keeping in mind the phenotype of the adsorbing cells after ficin treatment; for example, the R₁R₁, R₂R₂, and rr adsorbing cells would all become Fy(a–b–). This means that if anti-Fyᵃ or –Fyᵇ were present in the adsorbed sera, they would be present in all three aliquots.

Differential adsorption x3 with ficin-treated allogeneic RBCs removed the warm autoantibody and left alloanti-K and alloanti-Jkᵃ detectable in the alloadsorbed serum. EGA-treated autologous RBCs react with the unadsorbed serum but are nonreactive with the autoadsorbed serum.

? = phenotype of adsorbing cell is unknown

0✓ = negative IAT reading with check cells added and reactive as expected

NT = cell not tested

have a mixed-type AIHA. Serologic testing will show autoantibody components typical of both warm and cold AIHA. The mere presence of a warm and cold autoantibody in a patient does not define "mixed-type" AIHA. Although the cold autoagglutinin in these individuals will demonstrate strongest reactivity at 4°C, it is usually reactive at 30°C or above. It is the thermal amplitude of the cold autoantibody that is key to its pathogenicity. The cold agglutinin is an IgM hemagglutinin capable of binding complement. The warm component is an IgG antibody; therefore, the patient will typically demonstrate a positive DAT with both IgG and complement on the RBCs. This type of AIHA is rare.

Patients with mixed-type AIHA often present with extremely acute hemolysis and frequently require transfusion. Because there are two separate autoantibodies present, adsorption procedures must include both cold and warm adsorptions to completely remove autoagglutinins. In routine adsorption procedures, the patient's serum or plasma may first be adsorbed at 4°C with one or more aliquots of selected cells and then adsorbed at 37°C with additional aliquots of selected cells, using the procedures previously described; however, the procedures may be performed on the same aliquot of adsorbing cells if the order is reversed. Warm adsorption followed by cold adsorption in the same tube saves time and adsorbing cells. The warm antibody will remain bound at 4°C while the cold antibody is secondarily adsorbed. It has been found that corticosteroid treatment is most often effective in treating individuals with mixed-type AIHA.[51]

IgM Warm Autoantibodies

An unusual type of WAIHA is one associated with IgM warm autoantibodies. The serologic characteristics are often unimpressive when compared to the clinical havoc these antibodies wreak. Usually the patient's RBCs are strongly coated with complement and frequently cause difficulty in obtaining valid ABO/Rh typing and DAT because the cells spontaneously agglutinate. This **spontaneous agglutination** is not prevented by warm washing because the antibody is a warm agglutinin. Treatment of the RBCs with 0.01M DTT is necessary to remove enough IgM from the RBCs to allow for valid ABO/Rh and DAT results. IgM can sometimes be detected on the RBCs, if suitable anti-IgM is available, but flow cytometry is the most reliable technique in detecting the IgM. In antibody detection tests, there is usually no reactivity of the serum at room temperature, a weak agglutinin at 37°C, and very weak or no reactivity at the antiglobulin phase. If enzyme-treated RBCs are tested, many examples react strongly or are lysed by these antibodies. If antibody specificity is done, these antibodies may show a specificity for antigens on glycophorins (e.g., anti-En^a, anti-Pr, anti-Ge, anti-Wr^b).[51] If the IgM warm autoantibodies detected are associated with a severe clinical anemia (hgb less than 5 g/dL), the prognosis is poor. Some patients have been treated with plasma exchange, IVIG, steroids, or transfusion, but treatment is not always successful and the disease may be fatal.[7]

DAT Negative Autoimmune Hemolytic Anemia

Although the vast majority of patients presenting with signs and symptoms of autoimmune hemolytic anemia will have a positive DAT and other serologic evidence to support their diagnoses, there is a minority of affected patients who appear to have a negative DAT when tested with commercial reagents (polyspecific AHG, anti-IgG, and anti-C3). Sometimes, the amount of IgG coating the RBCs is lower than the detectable limit of commercial IgG reagents. However, if the hematologist has a laboratory value to confirm his diagnosis, he may order a "super Coombs'" test. Few laboratories have the reagents and experience to perform this test, more accurately called a "DAT hemolytic anemia workup," but the laboratories that do this sort of testing have found the following tests to be most productive: cold saline/cold LISS wash prior to DAT testing (to detect low-affinity IgG that is lost if washing is done at RT), direct polybrene DAT, DAT testing with anti-IgA and anti-IgM (noncommercial reagents standardized for RBC agglutination), and DAT by solid phase or column agglutination method. Researchers have also used flow cytometry, enzyme-linked antiglobulin assays, monocyte monolayer assays (MMAs), and concentrated eluates. Even with these esoteric methods, immunoglobulins are only detected on the patient's RBCs about half of the time.[7] Table 20–13 shows a summary contrasting the main characteristics of warm and cold autoantibodies.

Drug-Induced Immune Hemolytic Anemia

Therapeutic drugs may have unintended consequences, including immune destruction of RBCs, white blood cells (WBCs), and platelets, although the incidence is rare. Hemolytic anemia, leukopenia, and thrombocytopenia can occur separately, but in some patients more than one cell line is affected. The cells may be coated with antibody, antibody and complement, or complement alone. The discussion in this section is limited to RBC problems, but many of the same principles also apply to platelets and leukocytes.

Drug-mediated problems may come to the attention of the blood bank technologist in one of two ways:

1. A request for diagnostic testing on a patient with suspected hemolytic anemia
2. Unexpected results in routine testing; for example, a positive autologous control in the antiglobulin phase of antibody screening or compatibility testing, or a positive DAT

Drugs should be suspected as a possible explanation for immune hemolysis or a positive DAT when there is no other reason for the serologic and hematologic findings and if the patient has a recent history of taking high doses of antibiotics or other drugs associated with drug-induced immune hemolytic anemia (DIIHA). Drug-induced positive DATs and hemolytic anemia are relatively rare (estimated at 1 in 1 million), so other potential causes should be considered and investigated first.[52]

Table 20–13	Comparison of Warm and Cold AIHA	
FACTORS	**WARM AIHA**	**COLD AIHA**
Optimal reaction temperature	> 32°C	< 30°C
Immunoglobulin classification	IgG	IgM
Complement activation	May bind complement	Binds complement
Site of hemolysis	Usually extravascular (no cell lysis)	Extravascular/intravascular (cell lysis)
Frequency	70%–75% of cases	16% of cases (PCH 1%–2%)
Specificity	Frequently broad Rh specificity	Ii system (PCH autoanti-P)

Adapted from Harmening, DM: Clinical Hematology and Fundamentals of Hemostasis, 4th ed. FA Davis, Philadelphia, 2002, p 213, with permission.

Drug-induced hemolytic anemias were first reported in the 1950s, but most of these reports were limited to association of the onset of hemolytic anemia with the onset of drug therapy and resolution of the anemia when the drug was stopped.[53,54] Since these events could just be coincidental, proving drug-inducement would have required reinstigating the drug therapy to prove that hemolytic anemia would again ensue. This practice could certainly endanger the patient, so was not usually done, nor is it recommended. However, this approach was used to associate methyldopa (Aldomet) with DIIHA in the 1960s. Few early studies demonstrated the presence of antibody serologically, which is the approach used today.

In their first volume, Petz and Garratty[7] reviewed the four classic mechanisms then proposed to account for drug-induced problems: immune complexes, drug adsorption, membrane modification/nonspecific protein adsorption, and autoantibody formation. Specific drugs have often been associated with one particular mechanism, but not all drugs associated with hemolytic anemia neatly fit one model.[55,56] The lines are often blurred. Other theories postulate combining aspects of these earlier proposed mechanisms.[41] Current thinking on these mechanisms is termed a *unifying hypothesis* where more than one drug-associated antibody specificity is present. Figure 20–5 depicts the three mechanisms proposed to support the unifying hypothesis:

1. Drug binds to the RBC membrane and antibody formed is directed at the drug (test methodology involves testing drug-coated RBCs)
2. Drug does not bind covalently to RBCs but rather complexes with drug antibody (test methodology involves testing in the presence of the drug)
3. Drug induces an autoimmune response but the antibody is directed at the RBC membrane (testing cannot differentiate between drug-induced or idiopathic autoantibody)

Drug-related positive DATs may be additionally classified as "drug-dependent" or "drug-independent." Drug-dependent antibodies are those that require the presence of the drug in order to react; drug-independent antibodies are those that mimic warm autoantibodies serologically but where the formation of autoantibody was stimulated by the drug.

Drug-Adsorption (Hapten) Mechanism

Drugs operating through the drug-adsorption mechanism bind firmly to proteins, including the proteins of the RBC membrane (Fig. 20–6). Presumably because of their ability to bind to proteins, these drugs are good immunogens. Antibodies to penicillin, the drug most commonly associated with this mechanism, are found in about 3% of hospitalized patients receiving large doses of penicillin; of these, fewer than 5% develop a hemolytic anemia.[23] Even with the relatively high incidence of antipenicillin antibodies and the drug's ability to bind to the RBC membrane, penicillin-induced positive DATs are rare.[12] The low incidence may reflect the fact that the patient must receive massive doses (10 million units per day) of penicillin for the cells to be coated adequately. Also, most penicillin antibodies are IgM and therefore not detected by the antiglobulin test. The penicillin antibody responsible for a positive DAT is most often IgG, less often IgM, IgA, or IgD, and rarely binds complement.[41]

Laboratory test results are consistent with this description of the mechanism. Cells from patients with a positive DAT due to drug adsorption are usually coated with IgG alone; however, sometimes both IgG and complement are present on the cells. The patient's serum and eluate are nonreactive

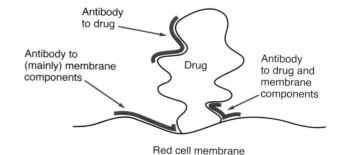

Antibody to drug

Antibody to (mainly) membrane components

Drug

Antibody to drug and membrane components

Red cell membrane

Figure 20–5. Unifying hypothesis. The drug binds loosely or firmly to the RBC membrane and antibody reacts with the drug itself (drug adsorption), mostly with the RBC membrane altered by the drug (mimics typical warm autoantibody) or with a combination of drug and RBC membrane (so-called immune complex). *(From Garratty, G: Target antigens for red-cell-bound autoantibodies. In Nance, SJ (ed): Clinical and Basic Science Aspects of Immunohematology, American Association of Blood Banks, Arlington, VA, 1991, p 55.)*

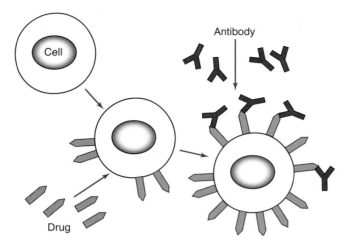

Antibody

Cell

Drug

Figure 20–6.   Drug adsorption mechanism.

with reagent RBCs and random donor cells. Therefore, the antibody screen is negative, and crossmatches are compatible in all phases. In order to demonstrate the antibody, the serum and eluate must be tested with penicillin-coated cells; reactivity occurs in the antiglobulin phase.[57] Because many patients have low-titered antipenicillin antibodies, Garratty emphasizes that when tested with drug-coated cells, the serum antibody must be high titered and the eluate must also contain antipenicillin antibodies before the findings are definitive.[7] Interpretation of the confirmatory tests to demonstrate antidrug antibody reactive by the drug adsorption method is outlined in Table 20–14.

 The procedure for preparing the penicillin-coated cells is given in Procedure 20-9 on the companion website.

Only a small percentage of those patients with penicillin-induced positive DATs exhibit hematologic complications. The clinical features of such a hemolytic episode differ from those of immune complex–mediated problems in several ways. Because the complement cascade is usually not activated, cell destruction is predominantly extravascular rather than intravascular; therefore, the anemia develops more slowly and is not life-threatening unless the cause for the hemolysis is not recognized and the penicillin therapy is

continued. Penicillin-induced hemolysis occurs only when the patient receives massive doses of the antibiotic, in contrast to the small amounts of drug that are necessary for hemolysis due to immune complexes. The patient improves once the drug is withdrawn, but hemolysis continues at a decreasing rate until cells heavily coated with penicillin are removed. The DAT may remain positive for several weeks. Mixed-field agglutination in the DAT can be expected because some cells are penicillin-coated while others are not.

Antipenicillin antibody may cross-react with ampicillin and methicillin. Antipenicillin reacts with Keflin-treated cells and anti-Keflin with penicillin-coated cells. Garratty suggests that comparing the strength of the reactivity of the serum or eluate (titer or score) with penicillin-coated and Keflin-coated cells may be of value.[58]

Other drugs that cause a positive DAT and hemolytic anemia by this mechanism are most notably the cephalosporins. Distinguishing between cephalosporin-induced problems and penicillin-induced problems is technically difficult because the drugs have antigenic determinants in common, and antipenicillin is frequently in the serum. Reports of severe hemolytic episodes associated with the second- and third-generation cephalosporins appear to be increasing.[41,59–61] Several of these cases appear to involve aspects of both the immune complex and the drug-adsorption mechanisms. Immune-mediated hemolysis has occurred rapidly after administering only a small amount of the drug. Because these antibiotics are routinely used in both adult and pediatric populations, any evidence of intravascular hemolysis should be noted and evaluated.

Cefotetan-induced hemolysis has been the most frequently encountered DIIHA (greater than 50%) by Garratty in the last 40 years.[62] It causes intravascular lysis of RBCs. Cefotetan is often given prophylactically for surgeries such as Caesarian sections and appendectomies and is often given during surgery. Even without additional doses, the patient may present with profound anemia 7 to 10 days after the procedure. This previously healthy patient may present with a very low hemoglobin (e.g., 4 g/dL). DIIHA is not suspected because the patient is unaware of receiving the drug. Finding documentation of the drug may involve searching through the surgical notes. If a second dose is given, the results can be fatal.

Table 20–14	**Test Results Observed in the Presence of Anti-Drug Antibody Reactive by the Drug Adsorption Mechanism**			
TEST	**PATIENT SERUM OR ELUATE**	**DRUG-COATED RBCs**	**UNCOATED RBCs**	**RESULTS**
Patient's serum control	X	–	X	If negative, indicates no alloantibody to RBC present.
Drug/RBC control	–	X	–	If negative, indicates drug-coated cells did not spontaneously agglutinate.
Patient's serum test	X	X	–	If agglutination is present and controls are all negative, indicates the presence of antidrug antibody. If negative, no antidrug present.

X = sample added to tube; – = no sample added to tube

Drug-Dependent or Immune Complex ("Innocent Bystander") Mechanism

Although the occurrence is rare, many drugs have been implicated in causing immune-mediated problems by the so-called immune complex mechanism. This mechanism was first described in the early 1960s, and it was thought that drugs operating through this mechanism combine with plasma proteins to form immunogens.[63] The antibody produced (often IgM, but IgG antibodies may also be present) recognizes determinants on the drug. If the patient ingests the same drug (or a drug bearing the same haptenic group) after immunization, the formation of a drug-antidrug complex may occur. The complement cascade may be activated because of this antigen-antibody interaction. RBCs are thought to be involved in this process only as "innocent bystanders."[64] The soluble drug-antidrug complex nonspecifically adsorbs loosely to the RBC surface. Complement, when activated, sensitizes the cell and may proceed to lysis (Fig. 20–7).

More recently, the concept of "neoantigen" formation has been proposed. In this model, the drug interacts in a noncovalent manner with a specific membrane component and forms a new antigen ("neoantigen") determinant consisting of both drug and membrane components. This explanation is the basis of the unifying hypothesis discussed above.

Because complement activation is involved in the immune complex, clinically affected patients frequently present with acute intravascular hemolysis. Up to half of the patients affected also have renal failure. When other causes for hemoglobinemia and hemoglobinuria have been excluded, a drug-antidrug reaction should be considered. When obtaining the medication history, it is important to realize that this group of patients needs to take only small doses of the drug to be affected. The patient recovers rapidly once the drug is withdrawn.

If polyspecific antihuman serum is used in DAT testing, the patient's DAT will usually be positive. If monospecific reagents are used, the DAT may be positive due to complement alone. Tests with anti-IgG are usually negative, even when the antibody is of the IgG class, because the drug-antidrug complex is thought to elute from the cells during the washing procedure before the antiglobulin test.[58,65] Other routine blood bank tests are negative in all phases; the antibody is directed against a drug or the drug-RBC membrane "neoantigen," not a true RBC antigen. Therefore, the antibody screening procedures and compatibility tests are negative, unless an alloantibody is also present. An eluate tested with reagent RBCs will also be nonreactive. A summary of typical serologic results is given in Table 20–15.

To confirm that a positive DAT is caused by a drug-antidrug reaction through the immune-complex mechanism, it must be demonstrated that the antibody in the patient's serum reacts only if the drug is added to the test system. The patient's serum is incubated with a solution of the drug in question and ABO-compatible (and antigen-negative if there is alloantibody present) RBCs. Complement activation is the usual indicator of an antigen-antibody reaction; therefore, one should observe for hemolysis after incubation and use reagents containing anti-C3 for the antiglobulin test.

 A general procedure for demonstrating antibodies reacting by the immune complex mechanism, suggested by Garratty,[57] is given in Procedure 20-8 on the companion website.

For the test results to be interpreted correctly, adequate controls must be performed. The patient's serum must not react with the cells when saline or the diluent used to dissolve the drug is substituted for the drug solution, and the drug solution must not hemolyze the suspension of cells nonspecifically. Examples of typical reactions with the patient's serum and control are given in Table 20–16. An eluate from the patient's cells is usually nonreactive even if the drug and a source of complement are added. Very little antibody, if any, remains on the cells after washing.

In most blood banks, confirmatory testing is done only when the patient has hematologic complications and not when he or she simply has a history of taking the drug and a positive DAT. Some of the drugs known to cause immune complex–mediated problems are in frequent use, and there are large numbers of patients with positive DATs but no evidence of hemolysis. A full workup may only be of academic interest and is not required before release of RBCs for transfusion. Treatment involves discontinuing the use of the drug. Although hemolysis by this mechanism is rare, the onset is usually sudden and may be characterized by intravascular hemolysis and renal failure. Therefore, immediate cessation of the drug is essential. Steroid treatment may also be given.

Membrane Modification (Nonimmunologic Protein Adsorption)

It is hypothesized that the cephalosporins, especially cephalothin (Keflin), both operate through the drug-adsorption mechanism and are able to modify RBCs so that plasma

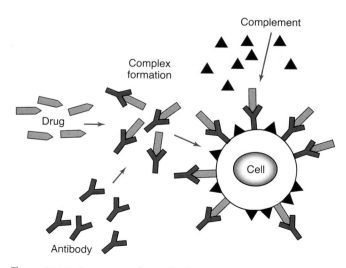

Figure 20–7. Immune complex mechanism.

Table 20–15   Serologic Reactions Observed With Drug-Induced Positive DATs

MECHANISM	IMMUNOGLOBULIN ON RBC	SERUM AND ELUATE REACT WITH:
Immune complex	C3 and occasionally IgG and IgM	Cells, only if serum was incubated with the drug prior to testing. Routine testing with reagent RBCs is negative.
Drug adsorption	IgG—rarely C3 may be present	Cells only if they are coated with the specific drug prior to testing. Routine testing with reagent RBCs is negative.
Drug-independent	IgG	All "normal" RBCs. Routine testing with reagent RBCs is positive
Membrane modification	IgG, IgM, IgA, C3	No cells tested. The mechanism is nonimmunologic protein adsorption.

proteins (e.g., IgG, IgM, IgA, and complement) can bind to the membrane (Fig. 20–8).[66] Consequently, RBCs from approximately 3% of patients receiving Keflin may exhibit a positive DAT with polyspecific and monospecific reagents. The uptake of immunoglobulins or complement components is not the result of a specific antigen-antibody reaction, so this mechanism is nonimmunologic. Because antibodies with blood group specificities are not involved, tests with the patient's serum and eluate are negative (see **Table 20–15**). Numerous cases of cephalosporin-associated hemolytic anemia have been reported, but, as stated earlier, RBC destruction seems to have been mediated through the drug adsorption or immune complex mechanism rather than the membrane modification mechanism. There is no treatment approach because hemolytic anemia associated with the ingestion of these drugs has not been described in relation to membrane modification.

Autoantibody Formation

Unlike the drugs acting through the previously described mechanisms that induce production of an alloantibody against a determinant on a drug or on a combination of the drug and RBC membrane, alpha-methyldopa (Aldomet) induces the production of an autoantibody that recognizes RBC antigens.[67,68] Although Aldomet is used rarely to treat hypertension in current practice, a review of its history is important

because it has been so well studied. The antibodies produced are serologically indistinguishable from those seen in patients with WAIHA. Presence of the drug is not required to obtain positive reactions. Positive DATs are encountered in approximately 10% to 20% of patients receiving Aldomet as an antihypertensive; however, very few (0.5% to 1%) of this group of patients subsequently develop significant immune hemolytic anemia,[7,69] and this occurs only after patients have been taking Aldomet for approximately 6 months. If the drug is stopped, the hemolytic anemia gradually resolves. Other drugs that also cause autoantibody production are L-dopa, mefenamic acid (Ponstel), procainamide, and diclofenac.[69,70] The second- and third-generation cephalosporins, fludarabine, and cladribine, have also been associated with autoantibody formation.

Several mechanisms by which Aldomet causes the production of autoantibodies have been proposed.[4,62,68] Kirtland, Horwitz, and Mohler[5] propose that methyldopa alters the function of T-suppressor cells and suggest that this upset in the immune system would allow production of antibody against self. Worlledge and associates[68] suggest that the drug alters RBC membrane components, similar to the theory of "neoantigen" formation.

The serologic features of this type of drug-induced problem are very different from those of the other drug-related immune hemolytic anemias. As shown in Table 20–17, the antibody in the eluate *does* react with normal RBCs in the absence of the

Table 20–16   Test Results Observed in the Presence of Anti-Drug Antibody Reactive by the Immune Complex Mechanism

TEST	PATIENT	FRESH SERUM*	DRUG	RBCs	RESULTS
Patient's serum control	X	–	–	X	If negative, indicates no alloantibody to RBC present.
Fresh serum control	–	X	X	X	If negative, indicates no alloantibody to RBC or drug present.
Drug/RBC control	–	–	X	X	If negative, indicates drug solution will not cause agglutination alone.
Patient's serum test	X	X	X	X	If agglutination is present and controls are all negative, indicates the presence of antidrug antibody. If negative, no antidrug present.

*Fresh serum is the source of complement in this test.
X = sample added to tube; – = no sample added to tube

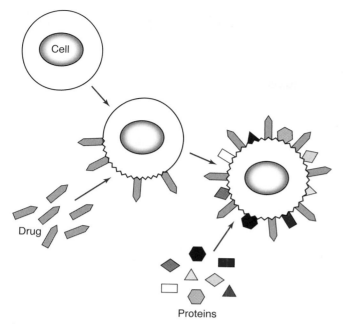

Figure 20–8. Nonimmunological adsorption of proteins onto RBCs.

drug. Antibodies of similar specificity and reactivity may be found in the serum. The patient's RBCs are usually coated with IgG and rarely with complement components.

Because the serology of Aldomet-induced positive DAT/immune hemolytic anemia is identical to that of the idiopathic WAIHA, one cannot establish in the laboratory that Aldomet is the instigating factor; however, if the patient is receiving the drug, one should be highly suspicious. If Aldomet is withdrawn, autoantibody production will eventually stop, but it may be several months before the DAT is negative.

Treatment of Drug-Induced Immune Hemolytic Anemia

Discontinuation of the drug is the treatment of choice for patients with a drug-induced hemolytic anemia. The presence of a positive DAT result does not necessarily imply that the drug must be discontinued if its effects are of therapeutic benefit and significant hemolysis is not present. In general, other drugs should be substituted, and the patient should be observed for resolution of the anemia to confirm a drug-induced hemolytic process. If the patient has a positive DAT without hemolysis, continued administration of the drug is optional. Generally, the prognosis for patients with drug-induced hemolytic anemia is excellent, as long as the cause is recognized and the drug is stopped. Table 20–17 compares the four recognized mechanisms leading to the development of drug-related antibodies.[71] Table 20–18 contrasts the antibody characteristics of the various types of AIHAs.[71]

By understanding the mechanisms by which drugs can cause a positive DAT or immune hemolytic anemia, it can quickly be decided which laboratory tests are most likely to be informative. Many other drugs have been cited as a cause for hemolytic anemia; however, the majority of these have only one reported case, and the association between the hemolytic anemia and the drug may be unclear. Before any special testing is done, proceed in the following manner:

1. Obtain the patient's medical history, including transfusions, pregnancies, medications, and diagnosis.
2. Perform a DAT using RBCs collected in EDTA. Test the cells with a polyspecific antihuman serum and monospecific reagents.
3. Screen the patient's serum for RBC alloantibodies.
4. Prepare and test an eluate for RBC alloantibodies if the patient has been recently transfused.

Table 20–17 Mechanisms Leading to Development of Drug-Related Antibodies

MECHANISM	PROTOTYPE DRUGS	Ig CLASS	DAT RESULTS	ELUATE	FREQUENCY OF HEMOLYSIS
Immune complex	Quinidine Phenacetin	IgM or IgG	Positive—often C3 only, but IgG may be present	Often negative	Small doses of drugs may cause acute intravascular hemolysis with hemoglobinemia/hemoglobulinuria; renal failure common.
Drug adsorption	Penicillins Streptomycin Cephalosporin	IgG	Strongly positive	Often negative	3%–4% of patient on large doses (10,000,000 U) of penicillin, which is one of the most common causes of immune hemolysis, usually extravascular.
Membrane modification	Cephalosporins	Many plasma proteins	Positive because of variety of serum proteins	Negative	No hemolysis; however, 3% of patients receiving the drug develop a positive DAT.
Methyldopa induced	Methyldopa (Aldomet)	IgG	Strongly positive	Positive—warm autoantibody identical to that found in WAIHA	0.8% develop a hemolytic anemia that mimics a warm AIHA; 15% of patients receiving methyldopa develop a positive DAT.

Adapted from Harmening, DM: Clinical Hematology and Fundamentals of Hemostasis, 4th ed. FA Davis, Philadelphia, 2002, p 215, with permission.

Table 20–18　Summary of Antibody Characteristics in AIHA

CHARACTERISTICS	WARM REACTIVE AUTOANTIBODY	COLD REACTIVE AUTOANTIBODY	PAROXYSMAL COLD HEMOGLOBINURIA	DRUG-RELATED AUTOANTIBODY
Immunoglobulin characteristics	Polyclonal IgG—occasionally IgM and IgA may be present	Polyclonal IgM in infection monoclonal kappa chain IgM in cold agglutinin disease	Polyclonal IgG	Polyclonal IgG
Complement activity	Variable	Always	Always	Depends on the mechanism of drug, antibody, and RBC interaction
Thermal reactivity	20°–37°C (optimum 37°C)	4°C–32°C, rarely to 37°C (optimum 4°C)	4°C–20°C biphasic hemolysin	20°C–37°C (optimum 37°C)
Titer of free antibody	Low to moderate (< 32) may be detectable only with enzyme-treated cells	High (>1,000 at 4°C)	Moderate to low (< 64)	Depends on the mechanism of drug, antibody, and RBC interaction
Reactivity of eluate with antibody screening cells	Usually pan-reactive	Nonreactive	Nonreactive	Pan-reactive with methyldopa type; nonreactive in all other cases
Most common specificity	Anti-Rh precursor; anti-common Rh; anti-LW; anti-U	Anti-I, anti-i, anti-Pr	Anti-P	Anti-e-like, methyldopa antidrug
Site of RBC destruction	Predominantly spleen with some liver involvement	Predominantly liver, rarely intravascular	Intravascular	Intravascular and spleen

Adapted from Harmening DM: Clinical Hematology and Fundamentals of Hemostasis, 4th ed. FA Davis, Philadelphia, 2002, p 217, with permission.

After evaluating this information, one can decide whether drugs are a possible cause of the problem and which of the mechanisms may be involved. It is wise to also note that many drugs cause an immunologic reaction by both drug-dependent and drug-independent mechanisms. When other causes (e.g., transfusion reaction) have been excluded and the clinical situation warrants additional testing, drug-coated cells or solutions of the drug can be prepared for confirmatory tests. Testing procedures for the investigation of drug-induced AHIA require a library of control sera and cells and expertise in this testing. Without appropriate controls, it is possible to misinterpret test results and report either false-positive or false-negative results.

CASE STUDIES

Case 20-1

A 71-year-old man from northern Minnesota is admitted to the hospital with complaints of severe fatigue, shortness of breath, "pounding heart," and numbness in his fingers. He first noticed the symptoms when setting up his lake shelter for ice fishing as he does every year. Although he was mostly annoyed, his wife was concerned and made him go to the doctor. An automated CBC done at the doctor's office showed a hemoglobin value of 7.8 g/dL and hematocrit of 23.5%. His doctor has ordered a bone marrow biopsy, a type and crossmatch for 3 units of packed red blood cells, and a "direct Coombs" test. A sample of his blood is drawn and sent to the blood bank for the crossmatch and DAT.

The type and screen results are:

		RBC (Forward) Typing				Serum (Reverse) Typing	
	Anti-A	Anti-B	Anti-D	6% alb		A₁ RBCs	B RBCs
Pt's RBCs	4+	2+	4+	2+	Pt's Serum	4+	4+

Note: The technologist also commented that the EDTA tube appeared "clotted" when it was first received in the blood bank.

Antibody Screening	Immediate Spin	LISS 37°C	IAT Anti-IgG
S I	4+	1+	0✓
S II	4+	1+	0✓
S III	4+	1+	0✓
Auto Control	2+	1+	0✓

Note: 0✓ indicates negative IAT reading with check cells added and reactive as expected.

		Direct Antiglobulin Test		
	Polyspecific	Anti-IgG	Anti-C3	6% alb
Pt's RBCs	3+	0✓	3+	0

1. What is the patient's ABO/Rh type?
2. How do the results of the antibody screening help explain the ABO discrepancy?
3. What immunoglobulin is coating the patient's RBCs?
4. What is the most likely cause of this combination of results? What is the most logical next step?

The results of additional testing is below:

	RBC (Forward) Typing					Serum (Reverse) Typing	
	Anti-A	Anti-B	Anti-D	6% alb		A_1 RBCs	B RBCs
Pt's warm washed RBCs	4+	0	4+	0	Pt's cold adsorbed serum	0	4+

Antibody Screening Using Cold Autoadsorbed Serum	Immediate Spin	LISS 37°C	IAT ANTI-IgG
S I	0	0	0✓
S II	0	0	0✓
S III	0	0	0✓
Auto Control (with warm washed RBCs)	0	0	0✓

5. What is the patient's ABO/Rh type?
6. What sample should be used to perform crossmatching?
7. What other diagnostic testing might be useful?

Case 20-2

A 52-year-old female high school band teacher nearly fainted one afternoon while demonstrating some trombone-playing techniques to one of her students. She went to her physician complaining of shortness of breath, mild depression, irritability, and a loss of appetite (which was uncharacteristic). Her physician noted signs of anemia and had some hematology tests done. Most notable was her hemoglobin of 5.2 g/dL, hematocrit of 14.8%, and reticulocyte count of 10.5%. He sent blood samples to the hospital blood bank for type and crossmatch for 4 units of red blood cells for outpatient transfusion ASAP. The patient was not thrilled at the prospect of a transfusion since she'd had a bad experience one time previously when transfused for multiple fractures incurred in a motorcycle accident in her wilder days.

The blood bank tested her samples and got the following results:

| | RBC (Forward) Typing | | | | | Serum (Reverse) Typing | |
	Anti-A	Anti-B	Anti-D	6% alb		A₁ RBCs	B RBCs
Pt's RBCs	0	0	3+	0	Pt's Serum	4+	4+

Antibody Screening	Immediate Spin	LISS 37°C	IAT ANTI-IgG
S I	0	0	2+
S II	0	0	2+
S III	0	0	4+
Auto Control	0	0	3+
Unit 1	0	0	4+
Unit 2	0	0	2+
Unit 3	0	0	2+
Unit 4	0	0	4+

1. What is the patient's ABO/Rh type?
2. What do the results of the antibody screening and crossmatches suggest?
3. What is the next logical step in investigating these preliminary results?

The results of additional testing is below:

| | Direct Antiglobulin Test | | | |
	Polyspecific	Anti-IgG	Anti-C3	6% alb
Pt's RBCs	3+	3+	1+	0

The patient's serum was warm autoadsorbed x3 with ficin-treated aliquots of her RBCs. An antibody identification panel with the autoadsorbed serum gave the following results:

Cell	D	C	E	c	E	P₁	M	N	S	s	Leᵃ	Leᵇ	K	k	Fyᵃ	Fyᵇ	Jkᵃ	Jkᵇ	LISS IAT
1	+	+	0	0	+	+	+	+	0	+	0	+	0	+	+	0	+	+	2+
2	+	+	0	0	+	+	+	+	0	+	0	+	+	+	+	+	+	0	3+
3	+	0	+	+	0	+	0	+	0	+	0	+	0	+	0	+	0	+	0✓
4	0	0	0	+	+	0	+	0	+	+	+	0	0	+	0	+	0	+	0✓
5	0	0	0	+	+	+	+	+	+	+	0	+	0	+	+	+	+	+	2+
6	0	+	0	+	+	0	+	0	+	+	0	0	+	+	0	+	0	+	0✓
7	0	0	+	+	+	+	+	+	+	0	0	+	0	+	+	0	+	+	2+
8	+	0	0	+	+	+	+	+	+	0	0	0	0	+	0	0	0	+	0✓
9	+	+	0	+	+	+	0	+	+	+	+	0	0	+	0	+	0	+	0	3+
10	+	+	+	+	+	0	+	0	+	+	0	+	0	+	0	+	+	+	2+
11	+	+	0	0	+	+	+	+	0	+	0	+	0	+	+	0	0	+	0✓
12	0	0	0	+	+	+	0	+	+	+	0	0	0	+	+	+	+	+	2+

4. What do the results of the DAT suggest?
5. What alloantibody is identified in the warm autoadsorbed serum?
6. What is the appropriate blood selection for this patient?
7. What other treatment is she likely to receive?

Case 20-3

A 32-year-old female is admitted to the hospital in active labor at term with her first baby. After 8 hours of labor with not much progress, there are signs of fetal distress and she is taken for an emergency Caesarian section. The baby is soon delivered and is healthy. After 3 days of care, mother and baby are discharged. A week later, the mother returns to the emergency room of the hospital with complaints of extreme weakness, mild jaundice, and some back pain. An automated CBC reveals a hemoglobin of 6.9 g/dL and hematocrit of 21.3%. The ER physician orders 3 units for transfusion STAT. A sample is drawn and sent to the blood bank.

The type and screen results are:

| | RBC (Forward) Typing | | | | | Serum (Reverse) Typing | |
	Anti-A	Anti-B	Anti-D	6% alb		A_1 RBCs	B RBCs
Pt's RBCs	0	4+	4+	0	Pt's Serum	4+	0

Note: The technologist performing the testing commented that the EDTA plasma and serum were dark red, but the phlebotomist denied having difficulty drawing the samples.

Antibody Screening	Immediate Spin	LISS 37°C	IAT ANTI-IgG
S I	0	0	0✓
S II	0	0	0✓
S III	0	0	0✓
Auto Control	0	0	3+

1. What is the patient's ABO/Rh?
2. What are the results of the antibody screening?
3. Are there any atypical results worth pursuing before setting up the crossmatch?

Further testing reveals:

| | | Direct Antiglobulin Test | | |
	Polyspecific	Anti-IgG	Anti-C3	6% alb
Pt's RBCs	3+	3+	2+	0

Eluate prepared from the DAT+ RBCs:

Antibody Screening	Eluate IAT Anti-IgG	Last Wash IAT Anti-IgG
S I	0✓	0✓
S II	0✓	0✓
S III	0✓	0✓
Auto Control	3+	0✓

(EGA-ttd = EDTA glycine acid treated)

4. What do the results of the DAT suggest?
5. What do the results of the eluate suggest?
6. Should additional testing be done?

Cefotetan-coated RBCs were tested with the patient's serum and eluate in parallel with the same donor RBCs not treated with cefotetan. Patients with DIIHA have high-titered antibodies (e.g., greater than 10,000), so dilutions of the serum and eluate are tested. Also, many normal individuals have "naturally occurring" anticefotetan antibodies (cephalosporins are added to cattle food) that agglutinate cefotetan-coated RBCs, but naturally occurring antibodies are of low titer, so testing for DIIHA employs the use of diluted serum and eluate:

	Cefotetan-Treated RBCs		Untreated RBCs	
	37°C	IAT	37°C	IAT
Patient's serum 1:100	4+	4+	0	0✓
Patient's eluate 1:20	0	3+	0	0✓
Last wash 1:20	0	0✓	0	0✓
Positive control	3+	3+	0	0✓
Negative control	0	0✓	0	0✓

Anticefotetan was identified in the patient's serum and eluate. The patient must be warned that she should never receive cefotetan again. Renal failure and fatality were seen in 19% of such cases in one study.[7]

SUMMARY CHART

✔ Immune hemolytic anemia is defined as shortened RBC survival mediated through the immune response, specifically by humoral antibody.

✔ In alloimmune hemolytic anemia, patients produce alloantibodies to foreign RBC antigens introduced into their circulation, most often through transfusion or pregnancy.

✔ Alloimmune hemolytic anemia is self-limiting; when the foreign RBCs are cleared from circulation, RBC destruction stops.

✔ In autoimmune hemolytic anemia (AIHA), patients produce antibodies against their own RBC antigens.

✔ In AIHA, the autoantibody is directed against the patient's own RBCs; therefore, there is a consistent source of antibody and antigen present for continuous RBC destruction.

✔ In drug-induced immune hemolytic anemia, patients produce antibody to a particular drug or drug complex, with subsequent damage to RBCs.

✔ AIHA may be classified as cold reactive (18%), warm reactive (70%), or drug-induced (12%); diagnostic tests include the DAT and characterization of the autoantibody in the serum or eluate.

✔ In AIHA, serum antibody will not be detected until the amount of antibody produced exceeds the number of RBC antigen sites available on the patient's own RBCs.

✔ The common antibody specificity in both benign and pathological cold autoagglutinins is anti-I.

✔ In CHD, the DAT will be positive because of complement coating of the RBCs; an antibody titer greater than 1,000 may cause visible agglutination of anticoagulated blood at room temperature.

✔ The classic antibody produced in PCH is called the Donath-Landsteiner antibody, and it has the specificity of autoanti-P. This biphasic antibody binds to patient RBCs at low temperatures and fixes complement. Hemolysis occurs when coated cells are warmed to 37°C and complement-mediated intravascular lysis occurs.

✔ In WAIHA, most patients (67%) have both IgG and complement on their RBCs, but 20% have only IgG and 13% have only complement.

✔ Warm reactive autoantibodies are generally enhanced by enzyme techniques and often have a broad specificity within the Rh blood group system.

✔ When transfusing a patient with WAIHA, the primary concern is detection and identification of all alloantibodies that are masked by the warm autoantibody.

✔ In the immune complex drug mechanism, the soluble drug-antidrug complex nonspecifically adsorbs loosely to the RBC surface, yielding a positive DAT with anti-C3 and sometimes with anti-IgG.

✔ In the drug-adsorption (hapten) mechanism, drugs such as penicillin or cefotetan bind firmly to proteins of the RBC membrane. The DAT will show reactivity with anti-IgG and often with anti-C3.

✔ In the membrane modification drug mechanism, drugs such as the cephalosporins modify the RBCs so that plasma proteins can bind to the membrane nonimmunologically. The DAT will often demonstrate reactivity with both anti-IgG and anti-C3.

✔ In the autoantibody drug mechanism, the drug (e.g., alpha-methyldopa/Aldomet) induces production of an autoantibody that recognizes RBC antigens. Both the autoantibody and eluate are reactive with normal RBCs. The DAT is reactive with anti-IgG.

Review Questions

1. Immune hemolytic anemias may be classified in which of the following categories?
   a. Alloimmune
   b. Autoimmune
   c. Drug-induced
   d. All of the above

2. When preparing cells for a cold autoadsorption procedure, it is helpful to pretreat the cells with which of the following?
   a. Dithiothreitol
   b. Ficin
   c. Phosphate-buffered saline at pH 9
   d. Bovine albumin

3. The blood group involved in the autoantibody specificity in PCH is:
   a. P
   b. ABO
   c. Rh
   d. Lewis

4. Which of the following blood groups reacts best with an anti-H or anti-IH?
   a. O
   b. B
   c. A_2
   d. A_1

5. With cold reactive autoantibodies, the protein coating the patient's cells and detected in the DAT is:
   a. C3
   b. IgG
   c. C4
   d. IgM

6. Problems in routine testing caused by cold reactive autoantibodies can usually be resolved by all of the following except:
   a. Prewarming
   b. Washing with warm saline
   c. Using anti-IgG antiglobulin serum
   d. Testing clotted blood specimens

7. Pathological cold autoagglutinins differ from common cold autoagglutinins in:
   a. Immunoglobulin class
   b. Thermal amplitude
   c. Antibody specificity
   d. DAT results on EDTA specimen

8. Cold AIHA is sometimes associated with infection by:
   a. *Staphylococcus aureus*
   b. *Mycoplasma pneumoniae*
   c. *Escherichia coli*
   d. Group A *Streptococcus*

9. Many warm reactive autoantibodies have a broad specificity within which of the following blood groups?
   a. Kell
   b. Duffy
   c. Rh
   d. Kidd

10. Valid Rh typing can usually be obtained on a patient with WAIHA using all of the following reagents or techniques *except*:
    a. Slide and modified tube anti-D
    b. Chloroquine-treated RBCs
    c. Rosette test
    d. Monoclonal anti-D

11. In pretransfusion testing for a patient with WAIHA, the primary concern is:
    a. Treating the patient's cells with chloroquine for reliable antigen typing
    b. Adsorbing out all antibodies in the patient's serum to be able to provide compatible RBCs
    c. Determining the exact specificity of the autoantibody so that compatible RBCs can be found
    d. Discovering any existing significant alloantibodies in the patient's circulation

12. Penicillin given in massive doses has been associated with RBC hemolysis. Which of the classic mechanisms is typically involved in the hemolytic process?
    a. Immune complex
    b. Drug adsorption
    c. Membrane modification
    d. Autoantibody formation

13. Which of the following drugs has been associated with complement activation and rapid intravascular hemolysis?
    a. Penicillins
    b. Quinidine
    c. Alpha-methyldopa
    d. Cephalosporins

14. A patient is admitted with a hemoglobin of 5.6 g/dL. Initial pretransfusion workup appears to indicate the presence of a warm autoantibody in the serum and coating his RBCs. His transfusion history indicates that he received 6 units of RBCs 2 years ago after an automobile accident. Which of the following would be most helpful in performing antibody detection and compatibility testing procedures?
    a. Adsorb the autoantibody using the patient's enzyme-treated cells.
    b. Perform an elution and use the eluate for compatibility testing.
    c. Crossmatch random units until compatible units are found.
    d. Collect blood from relatives who are more likely to be compatible.

15. A patient who is taking Aldomet has a positive DAT. An eluate prepared from his RBCs would be expected to:
    a. React only with Aldomet-coated cells
    b. Be neutralized by a suspension of Aldomet
    c. React with all normal cells
    d. React only with Rh$_{null}$ cells

16. One method that can be used to separate a patient's RBCs from recently transfused donor RBCs is:
    a. Chloroquine diphosphate treatment of the RBCs
    b. Reticulocyte harvesting
    c. EGA treatment
    d. Donath-Landsteiner testing

17. Monoclonal antisera is valuable in phenotyping RBCs with positive DATs because:
    a. Both polyspecific and monospecific antihuman serum can be used in antiglobulin testing
    b. Anti-C3 serum can be used in antiglobulin testing
    c. It usually does not require antiglobulin testing
    d. It does not require enzyme treatment of the cells prior to antiglobulin testing

18. Autoadsorption procedures to remove either warm or cold autoantibodies should not be used with a recently transfused patient. Recently means:
    a. 3 days
    b. 3 weeks
    c. 6 weeks
    d. 3 months

References

1. Allan, J, and Garratty, G: Positive direct antiglobulin tests in normal blood donors (abstract). Proceedings of the International Society of Blood Transfusion, Montreal, 1980.
2. Izui, S: Autoimmune hemolytic anemia. Curr Opin Immunol 6:926, 1994.
3. Barthold, DR, Kysela, S, and Steinberg, AD: Decline in suppressor T cell function with age in female NZB mice. J Immunol 112:9, 1974.
4. Banacerraf, B, and Unanue, ER: Textbook of Immunology. Williams & Wilkins, Baltimore, 1979.
5. Kirtland, HH, Horwitz, DA, and Mohler, DN: Inhibition of suppressor T cell function by methyldopa: A proposed cause of autoimmune hemolytic anemia. N Engl J Med 302:825, 1980.
6. van Loghem, JJ: Concepts on the origin of autoimmune diseases: The possible role of viral infection in the etiology of idiopathic autoimmune diseases. Semin Hematol 9:17, 1965.
7. Petz, LD, and Garratty, G: Immune Hemolytic Anemias, 2nd ed. Churchill Livingstone, Philadelphia, 2004.
8. Hillman, RS, and Finch, GA: Red Cell Manual, 7th ed. FA Davis, Philadelphia, 1996.
9. Roback, JD (ed): Technical Manual, 16th ed. American Association of Blood Banks, Bethesda, MD, 2008.
10. Okuno, T, Germino, F, and Newman, B: Clinical significance of autologous control (abstract). American Society Clinical Pathologists 16, 1984.
11. Lau, P, Haesler, WE, and Wurzel, HA: Positive direct antiglobulin reaction in a patient population. Am J Clin Pathol 65:368, 1976.
12. Judd, WJ, et al: The evaluation of a positive direct antiglobulin test in pretransfusion testing. Transfusion 20:17, 1980.
13. Garratty, G, Petz, LD, and Hoops, JK: The correlation of cold agglutinin titrations in saline and albumin with haemolytic anaemia. Br J Haematol 35:587, 1977.
14. Engelfriet, CP, et al: Autoimmune hemolytic anemias: Serological studies with pure anti-immunoglobulin reagents. Clin Exp Immunol 3:605, 1968.
15. Rosse, WF: Quantitative immunology of immune hemolytic anemia: The relationship of cell-bound antibody to hemolysis and the effect of treatment. J Clin Invest 50:734, 1971.
16. De Angelis, V, et al: Abnormalities of membrane protein composition in patients with autoimmune haemolytic anaemia. Br J Hematol 95:273, 1996.
17. Gilliland, BC, Baxter, E, and Evans, RS: Red cell antibodies in acquired hemolytic anemia with negative antiglobulin serum tests. N Engl J Med 285:252, 1971.
18. Garratty, G: Autoimmune hemolytic anemia. In Garratty, G (ed): Immunobiology of Transfusion Medicine. Marcel Dekker, New York, 1994, p 493.
19. Stratton, F, et al: Acquired hemolytic anemia associated with IgA anti-e. Transfusion 12:197, 1972.
20. Sturgeon, P, et al: Autoimmune hemolytic anemia associated exclusively with IgA of Rh specificity. Transfusion 19:324, 1979.
21. Hoppe, PA: The role of the Bureau of Biologics in assuring reagent reliability. In Considerations in the Selection of Reagents. American Association of Blood Banks, Washington, DC, 1979, p 1.
22. Garratty, G, and Petz, LD: An evaluation of commercial antiglobulin sera with particular reference to their anticomplement properties. Transfusion 11:79, 1971.
23. Roback, JD (ed): Technical Manual, 16th ed. American Association of Blood Banks, Bethesda, MD, 2008.
24. Reid, ME: Autoagglutination dispersal utilizing sulfhydryl compounds. Transfusion 18:353, 1978.
25. Storry, JR, Olsson, MI, and Moulds, JJ: Rabbit red blood cell stroma bind immunoglobulin M antibodies regardless of blood group specificity (letter). Transfusion 46:1260, 2006.
26. Judd, WJ: Controversies in transfusion medicine: Prewarmed tests: Con Transfusion 35:271, 1995.
27. Chaplin, H, et al: Clinically significant allo-anti-I in an I-negative patient with massive hemorrhage. Transfusion 26:57, 1986.
28. Marsh, WL: Aspects of cold-reactive autoantibodies. In Bell, CA (ed): A Seminar on Laboratory Management of Hemolysis. American Association of Blood Banks, Washington, DC, 1979, p 79.
29. Combs, MR, et al: An auto-anti M causing hemolysis in vitro. Transfusion 31:756, 1991.
30. Garratty, G: Target antigens for red-cell-bound autoantibodies. In Nance, ST (ed): Clinical and Basic Science Aspects of Immunohematology. American Association of Blood Banks, Arlington, VA, 1991, p 33.
31. Lyckholm, LJ, and Edmond, MB: Seasonal hemolysis due to cold-agglutinin syndrome. N Engl J Med 334:437, 1996.
32. Aoki, A, et al: Cardiac operation without hypothermia for the patient with cold agglutinin. Chest 104:1627, 1993.
33. Shirey, RS, et al: An anti-i biphasic hemolysin in chronic paroxysmal cold hemoglobinuria. Transfusion 26:62, 1986.
34. Judd, WJ, et al: Donath-Landsteiner hemolytic anemia due to an anti-Pr-like biphasic hemolysin. Transfusion 26:423, 1986.
35. Reid, M: Association of red blood cell membrane abnormalities with blood group phenotype. In Garratty, G (ed): Immunobiology of Transfusion Medicine. Marcel Dekker, New York, 1994, p 257.
36. Salloum, E, and Lundberg, WB: Hemolytic anemia with positive direct antiglobulin test secondary to spontaneous cytomegalovirus infection in healthy adults. Acta Hematol 92:39, 1994.
37. Benraad, CEM, Scheerder, HAJM, and Overbeeke, MAM: Autoimmune haemolytic anaemia during pregnancy. Eur J Obstet Gynecol Reprod Biol 55:209, 1994.

38. Nance, S, and Garratty, G: Subclass of IgG on red cells of donors and patients with positive direct antiglobulin tests (abstract). Transfusion 23:413, 1983.

39. Rodberg, K, Tsuneta, R, and Garratty, G: Discrepant Rh phenotyping results when testing IgG-sensitized RBCs with monoclonal Rh reagents (abstract). Transfusion 35(Suppl):67S, 1995.

40. Edwards, JM, Moulds, JJ, and Judd, WJ: Chloroquine dissociation of antigen-antibody complexes: A new technique for typing red blood cells with a positive direct antiglobulin test. Transfusion 22:59, 1982.

41. Issitt, P, and Anstee, D: Applied Blood Group Serology, 4th ed. Montgomery Scientific Publications, Durham, NC, 1998, p 1021.

42. Win, N, et al: Autoimmune haemolytic anaemia in infancy with anti-Kp^b specificity. Vox Sang 71:187, 1994.

43. Becton, DL, and Kinney, TR: An infant girl with severe autoimmune hemolytic anemia: Apparent anti-Vel specificity. Vox Sang 51:108, 1986.

44. Reynolds, MV, Vengelen-Tyler, V, and Morel, PA: Autoimmune hemolytic anemia associated with auto anti-Ge. Vox Sang 41:61, 1981.

45. Laine, EP, Leger, RM, Arndt, PA, et al: In vitro studies of the impact of transfusion on the detection of alloantibodies after autoadsorption. Transfusion 40:1384–1387, 2000.

46. Wilkinson, SL: Serological approaches to transfusion of patients with allo- or autoantibodies. In Nance, ST (ed): Immune Destruction of Red Blood Cells. American Association of Blood Banks, Arlington, VA, 1989, p 227.

47. Singh, M, Thompson, H, and Pallas, C: Response to transfusions in autoimmune hemolytic anemia. Abstracts of South Central Association of Blood Banks Annual Meeting, Tucson, AZ, 1997.

48. Jeffries, LC: Transfusion therapy in autoimmune hemolytic anemia. Hematol Oncol Clin North Am 8:1087, 1994.

49. Anderson, DR, and Kelton, JG: Mechanisms in intravascular and extravascular cell destruction. In Nance, ST (ed): Immune Destruction of Red Blood Cells. American Association of Blood Banks, Arlington, VA, 1989, p 39.

50. Flores, G, et al: Efficacy of intravenous immunoglobulin in the treatment of autoimmune hemolytic anemia: Results in 73 patients. Am J Hematol 44:237, 1993.

51. Garratty, G, Arendt, P, and Domen, R: Severe autoimmune hemolytic anemia associated with IgM warm autoantibodies directed against determinants on or associated with glycophorin A. Vox Sang 72:124–130, 1997.

52. Arndt, PA, and Garratty, G: The changing spectrum of drug-induced immune hemolytic anemia. Semin Hematol 42:137–144, 2005.

53. Snapper, I, Marks, D, Schwarta, L, et al: Hemolytic anemia secondary to mesantoin. Ann Intern Med 39:619, 1953.

54. Harris, JW: Studies on the mechanism of a drug-induced hemolytic anemia. J Lab Clin Med 47:760, 1956.

55. Kerr, RO, et al: Two mechanisms of erythrocyte destruction in penicillin-induced hemolytic anemia. N Engl J Med 298:1322, 1972.

56. Ries, CA, et al: Penicillin-induced immune hemolytic anemia. JAMA 233:432, 1975.

57. Garratty, G: Laboratory Investigation of Drug-Induced Immune Hemolytic Anemia and/or Positive Direct Antiglobulin Tests. American Association of Blood Banks, Washington, DC, 1979.

58. Garratty, G: Drug-induced immune hemolytic anemia. In Garratty, G (ed): Immunobiology of Transfusion Medicine. Marcel Dekker, New York, 1994, p 523.

59. Eckrich, RJ, Fox, S, and Mallory, D: Cefotetan-induced immune hemolytic anemia due to the drug-adsorption mechanism. Immunohematology 10:51, 1994.

60. Bernini, JC, et al: Fatal hemolysis induced by ceftriaxone in a child with sickle cell anemia. J Pediatr 126:813, 1995.

61. Lascari, AD, and Amyot, K: Fatal hemolysis caused by ceftriaxone. J Pediatr 126:816, 1995.

62. Garratty, G: Drug-induced immune hemolytic anemia. Hematology Am Soc Hematol Educ Program 73–79:2009.

63. Shulman, NR: Mechanism of blood cell destruction in individuals sensitized to foreign antigens. Trans Assoc Am Physicians 76:72, 1963.

64. Dameshek, W: Autoimmunity: Theoretical aspects. Ann N Y Acad Sci 124:6, 1965.

65. Petz, LD, and Mueller-Eckhardt, C: Drug-induced immune hemolytic anemia. Transfusion 32:02, 1992.

66. Spath, P, Garratty, G, and Petz, LD: Studies on the immune response to penicillin and cephalothin in humans: Immunohematologic reactions to cephalothin administration. J Immunol 107:860, 1971.

67. Carstairs, KC, et al: Incidence of a positive direct Coombs' test in patients on alpha-methyldopa. Lancet 2:33, 1966.

68. Worlledge, SM, Carstairs, KC, and Dacie, JV: Autoimmune hemolytic anemia associated with methyldopa therapy. Lancet 2:135, 1966.

69. Petz, LD: Drug-induced hemolytic anemia. Transfus Med Rev 7:242, 1993.

70. Lopez, A, et al: Autoimmune hemolytic anemia induced by diclofenac. Ann Pharmacother 29:787, 1995.

71. Harmening, DM: Clinical Hematology and Fundamentals of Hemostasis, 5th ed. FA Davis, Philadelphia, 2009, pp 252–265.

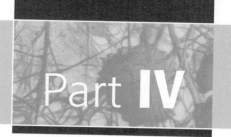

Leukocyte Antigens and Relationship Testing

Part IV

Chapter 21

The HLA System

Donna L. Phelan, BA, CHS(ABHI), MT(HEW) and Gerald P. Morris, MD, PhD

OBJECTIVES

1. Define the abbreviations HLA, MLR, SSO, SSP, SBT, TRALI, and MHC.

2. Describe the three regions of the HLA complex located on the short arm of chromosome 6.

3. List the characteristics of HLA genes.

4. List the three exceptions to the practice of naming all serologic specificities on the basis of correlation with an identified sequence that eliminates the need for a provisional w designation.

5. Describe the current nomenclature for HLA genes.

6. Define the term *haplotype*.

7. Describe the difference between HLA phenotype and HLA genotype.

8. List the characteristics, importance, and clinical relevance of HLA class I and class II gene products.

9. Describe the characteristics of HLA antibodies.

10. Define *linkage disequilibrium*, a characteristic of HLA antigens.

11. Describe the techniques used for HLA antigen and allele detection.

12. Describe the techniques for HLA antibody detection.

13. Describe crossmatch technology to evaluate tissue compatibility.

14. Describe the role of HLA typing in paternity testing, disease association, platelet transfusion, TRALI, and transplantation.

15. Explain the role of virtual crossmatches with single antigen antibody testing.

Introduction

Human leukocyte antigen (HLA) testing is a specialized branch or division of immunology for human histocompatibility testing. HLA testing supports a number of clinical specialties in transplantation, transfusion, and immunogenetics. Because of its specialized nature, however, HLA is given relatively little attention in training programs such as nursing and medical technology.

This chapter is intended to serve as an introduction to the basic concepts of HLA and clinical applications of HLA testing. It is written for the reader with some training in the biomedical sciences and familiarity with general immunology concepts.

The emphasis of the chapter is on the principles and concepts of HLA structure and function, HLA procedures, and the clinical application of HLA testing to immunogenetics (e.g., paternity and disease association), transfusion practices, and transplantation. Although HLA testing is a technologically complex area, this chapter provides a general overview of the topic.

Historical Perspective

Evidence for human leukocyte blood groups was first advanced in 1954 by Jean Dausset,[1] with the observation that patients whose sera contained leukoagglutinins had received a larger number of blood transfusions than other patients. He determined that these agglutinins were not autoantibodies as had been thought previously but rather were alloantibodies produced by the infusion of cells bearing alloantigens not present in the recipient. Dausset[2] determined that patients with alloantibodies segregated into two groups, based upon their reactivity; antibodies from group 1 specifically recognized antigens on group 2. Through this method, Dausset identified HLA-A2, the first known HLA molecule.

Nomenclature

The **HLA genetic region** is a series of closely linked genes that determine major histocompatibility factors—that is, surface antigens or receptors responsible for the recognition and elimination of foreign tissues. The region is also referred to as the **major histocompatibility complex** (MHC). The HLA complex contains an estimated 35 to 40 genes physically grouped into three regions located on the short arm of chromosome 6: class I, class II, and class III regions (Fig. 21–1).

The class I region encodes genes for the classic transplantation molecules HLA-A, HLA-B, and HLA-C. It also encodes for additional nonclassic genes, including HLA-E, HLA-F, and HLA-G. The class II region encodes genes for the molecules HLA-DR, HLA-DP, and HLA-DQ composed of both α and β chains. DP molecules are the product of DPA1 and DPB1 alleles (Fig. 21–2); DPB2 and DPA2 are pseudogenes, genes with mutations that prevent gene activation or transcription. DQ molecules are the product of DQA1 and DQB1

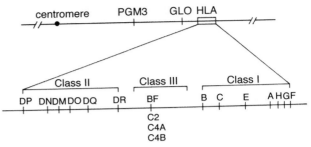

Human Chromosome 6

Figure 21–1. The HLA complex on the short arm of chromosome 6.

alleles. DR molecules use DRA but can use alleles coded by DRB1 (the classic DR specificities), DRB3 (DR52 molecules), DRB4 (DR53), and DRB5 (DR51).

The class III region encodes structurally and functionally diverse molecules, including C2, C4, Bf (the complement factors), 21-hydroxylase, and tumor necrosis factor. In addition, two other genes, glyoxalase-1 (GLO) and phosphoglucomutase-3 (PGM-3) are linked with the HLA complex.

One very important characteristic of HLA genes is that they are highly polymorphic, and several alleles exist at each locus. The antigenic specificities, defined by serologic reactivity, are designated by numbers following the locus symbol (e.g., HLA-A1, HLA-A2, HLA-B5, HLA-B7, and so on). Table 21–1 lists the current specificities of the HLA system recognized by the WHO Nomenclature Committee for Factors of the HLA System.[3] Several HLA alleles demonstrate serologic cross reactivity due to structural similarity. For example, HLA-A9, HLA-A23, and HLA-A24 all react with antibodies specific for HLA-A9, but HLA-A23 and HLA-A24 can be "split" from A9 by unique reactivity with antibodies specific for each. Two exceptions to HLA nomenclature are the Bw4 and Bw6 epitopes, where the "w" is present to distinguish them as significant serologic epitopes found on multiple HLA-A and HLA-B alleles, rather than independent HLA specificities (Table 21–2).

Continued investigation into HLA using molecular techniques of DNA sequence analysis revealed many HLA allelic variants that were not detectable by traditional serologic

Class II

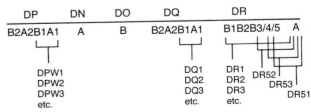

Figure 21–2. The loci that code for the major categories of HLA class II gene products. *(From Rodey, GE: HLA Beyond Tears. De Novo, Atlanta, GA, 1991, p 12, with permission.)*

Table 21–1	**Recognized HLA Serologic and Cellular Specificities**				
A	**B**	**C**	**DR**	**DQ**	**DP**
A1	B5	Cw1	DR1	DQ1	DPw1
A2	B7	Cw2	DR103	DQ2	DPw2
A3	B703	Cw3	DR2	DQ3	DPw3
A9	B8	Cw4	DR3	DQ4	DPw4
A10	B12	Cw5	DR4	DQ5 (1)	DPw5
A11	B13	Cw6	DR5	DQ6 (1)	DPw6
A19	B14	Cw7	DR6	DQ7 (3)	
A23 (9)	B15	Cw8	DR7	DQ8 (3)	
A24 (9)	B16	Cw9 (w3)	DR8	DQ9 (3)	
A2403	B17	Cw10 (w3)	DR9		
A25 (10)	B18		DR10		
A26 (10)	B21		DR11 (5)		
A28	B22		DR12 (5)		
A29 (19)	B27		DR13 (6)		
A30 (19)	B2708		DR14 (6)		
A31 (19)	B35		DR1403		
A32 (19)	B37		DR1404		
A33 (19)	B38 (16)		DR15 (2)		
A34 (10)	B39 (16)		DR16 (2)		
A36	B3901		DR17 (3)		
A43	B3902		DR18 (3)		
A66 (10)	B40		DR51		
A68 (28)	B4005		DR52		
A69 (28)	B41		DR53		
A74 (19)	B42				
A80	B44 (12)				
	B45 (12)				
	B46				
	B47				
	B48				
	B49 (21)				
	B50 (21)				
	B51 (5)				
	B5102				
	B5103				
	B52 (5)				

Table 21–1   Recognized HLA Serologic and Cellular Specificities—cont'd

A	B	C	DR	DQ	DP
	B53				
	B54 (22)				
	B55 (22)				
	B56 (22)				
	B57 (17)				
	B58 (17)				
	B59				
	B60 (40)				
	B61 (40)				
	B62 (15)				
	B63 (15)				
	B64 (14)				
	B65 (14)				
	B67				
	B70				
	B71 (70)				
	B72 (70)				
	B73				
	B75 (15)				
	B76 (15)				
	B77 (15)				
	B78				
	B81				
	B82				
	Bw4				
	Bw6				

Data from Marsh, SGE, et al: Nomenclature for factors of the HLA system. Tissue Antigens 75:291, 2010.

Table 21–2   Bw4 and Bw6 Associated Specificities

Bw4	B5, B5102, B5103, B13, B17, B27, B37, B38 (16), B44 (12), B47, B49(21), B51(5), B52 (5), B53, B57 (17), B58(17), B59, B63(15), B77 (15) and A9, A23(9), A24(9), A2403, A25 (10), A32 (19)
Bw6	B7, B703, B8, B14, B18, B22, B2708, B35, B39(16), B3901, B3902, B40, B4005, B41, B42, B45(12), B46, B48, B50 (21), B54 (22), B55 (22), B56 (22), B60(40), B61(40), B62 (15), B64 (14), B65 (14), B67, B70, B71 (70), B72 (70), B73, B75 (15), B76 (15), B78, B81, B82

techniques. This complexity has necessitated the development of the following nomenclature for HLA genes:

1. HLA-prefix designates the MHC gene complex.
2. A capital letter indicates a specific locus (A, B, C, D, etc.) or region. All genes in the D region (class II genes) are prefixed by the letter D and followed by a second capital letter indicating the subregion (DR, DQ, DP, DO, DN, etc.).
3. Loci coding for the specific class II alpha and beta peptide chains are identified at this point (i.e., DRA1, DRA2, DRB1, DRB2).
4. The broad allele family, or serologic reactivity, is designated by a two-digit numeral that defines the serologic

group reactivity (i.e., A2 reactivity is described as HLA-A*02).

5. Following the allele family, separated by a colon (:), is a two digit numeral that defines the specific allele. For example, the serologically defined HLA-B27 specificity is actually made up of 43 distinct allelic variations. These alleles are defined as HLA-B *27:01 through *27:36. It is mandatory to include the leading zeros that are part of the defined alleles.

6. The following two-digit series, separated by a colon, convey other, less clinically relevant but scientifically important information. Alleles that differ only by synonymous nucleotide substitutions within the coding sequence are distinguished by the use of the fifth and sixth digits (i.e., noncoding silent substitutions).

7. Lastly, alleles that only differ by sequence polymorphisms in the introns are distinguished by the use of the seventh and eighth digits. See Table 21–3 for examples of all loci with the new nomenclature changes.[3]

Antigens and Antibodies

It is necessary to evaluate the HLA antigen composition in prospective donor-recipient pairs before organ transplantation and in candidates for platelet therapy refractory to random donor platelets. Even more important is the evaluation and identification of HLA antibodies in the serum of recipients before transplantation and transfusion. Evidence clearly indicates that presensitization to HLA antigens may cause rapid rejection of transplanted tissue or poor platelet survival following transfusion.[4] HLA-antigen testing is also used in disease correlation, relationship testing, and anthropologic studies.

Each person has two alleles for each locus. Both alleles of a locus are expressed co-dominantly—that is, there is equal expression of both alleles. The presence of one allele does not suppress the expression of the other. If there are two different alleles on one locus, the person is heterozygous. If both alleles on that locus are the same, the person is homozygous.

Inheritance

The physical linkage of the HLA genes on chromosome 6 results in all of the genes on a single chromosome typically being inherited together. The entire set of A, B, C, DR, DQ, and DP genes located on one chromosome is called a *haplotype*. Genetic crossovers and recombination in the HLA region are uncommon (less than 1%), and thus a complete set of alleles located on a chromosome is usually inherited by children as a unit (haplotype). **Figure 21–3** illustrates the segregation of HLA haplotypes in a family. The two haplotypes of the father are labeled a and b, and the mother's haplotypes are c and d. Each offspring inherits two haplotypes, one from each parent. Thus, only four possible haplotypes—ac, ad, bc, and bd—can be found in the offspring. It can be calculated that 25% of the offspring will have identical HLA haplotypes, 50% will share one HLA haplotype, and 25% will share no HLA haplotypes. An important corollary is that a parent and child can share only one haplotype, making an identical match between the two unlikely. It should also be apparent that uncles, grandparents, and cousins are very unlikely to have identical haplotypes with any given child. These are important factors when looking for a well-matched organ or blood donor.

The HLA phenotype, then, represents the surface markers or antigens detected in histocompatibility testing of a single individual. The HLA genotype represents the association of the alleles on the two chromosomes as determined by family studies, and the term *haplotype* refers to the allelic makeup of a single chromosome, illustrated in Figure 21–4.

Crossing Over

An event that infrequently complicates HLA-typing interpretation and haplotype determination is **crossing over**, or

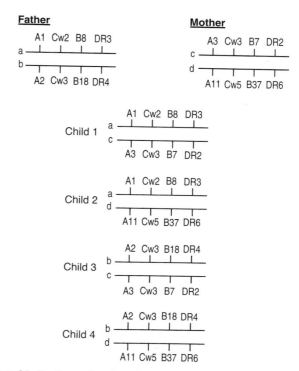

Figure 21–3. Segregation of HLA haplotypes in a pedigree. *(From Tiwari, JL, and Terasaki, PI: HLA and Disease. Springer-Verlag, New York, 1985, p 8, with permission.)*

Table 21–3 HLA Nomenclature	
EXISTING NOMENCLATURE	**NEW NOMENCLATURE**
A*01010101	A*01:01:01:01
B*150102	B*15:01:02
Cw*020201	C*02:02:01
DRB1*03010101	DRB1*03:01:01:01
DQB1*0202	DQB1*02:02
DPB1*0403	DPB1*04:03

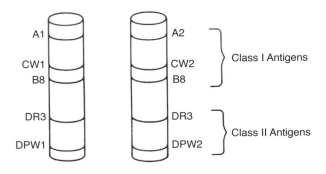

Phenotype: A1,2; B8,-; CW1, W2; DR3,-; DPW1, W2

Genotype: A1,2; B8,8; CW1, W2; DR3, 3; DPW1, W2

Haplotype: A1, B8, CW1, DR3, DPW1/A2, B8, CW2, DR3, DPW2

Figure 21–4. Schematic representation of the HLA loci on the short arm of chromosome 6. *(From Miller, WV, and Rodey, G: HLA Without Tears. American Society of Clinical Pathologists, Chicago, 1981, p 10, with permission.)*

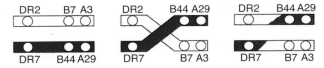

Figure 21–5. Schematic of a recombination event between HLA-B and HLA-DR.

recombination. During meiosis, exchange of material between the paired chromosomes can occur. During chromosomal replication, replicated chromosomes often overlay each other, forming x-shaped chiasmata (**Fig. 21–5**). When the chromosomes are pulled apart during meiotic division, breaks can occur at the crossover site, resulting in complementary exchange of genetic material. The farther apart two loci are on a given chromosome, the more likely it is that genetic exchanges will take place. For example, recombination between HLA-A and HLA-DP occurs commonly, whereas recombination between HLA-DQ and HLA-DR is a rare event. Crossing over has the effect of rearranging the genes on the chromosome to produce new haplotypes in the general population.

Linkage Disequilibrium

An important characteristic of HLA antigens is the existence of linkage disequilibrium between the alleles of the loci. **Linkage disequilibrium** is when HLA genes occur more frequently in the same haplotype than would be expected by chance alone. In the Rh system, the blood groups C, D, and e are found together more often than would be expected based on their individual gene frequencies. This is commonly found within the HLA system.[4] In a random mating population at Hardy-Weinberg equilibrium, the occurrence of two alleles from closely linked genes will be the product of their individual gene frequencies. If the observed value of the joint frequency is significantly different from the expected frequency (the product of the individual allele frequencies), the alleles are said to be in linkage disequilibrium.

For example, if HLA-A1 and HLA-B8 gene frequencies are 0.16 and 0.1, respectively, in a population, the expected occurrence of an HLA haplotype bearing both A1 and B8 should be 0.16 × 0.1 × 100, or 1.6%. In certain white populations, however, the actual occurrence of this haplotype is as high as 8%, far in excess of the expected frequency. The HLA alleles frequently associated through disequilibrium are listed in **Table 21–4**. Disequilibrium between the B and DR loci alleles may account for problems in correlating B locus

serotyping with allograft survival and disease associations, inasmuch as matching or typing for B locus alleles would, by disequilibrium, often result in matching or typing for DR locus alleles, which have been found to be clinically significant to allograft survival.

HLA Gene Products

HLA gene products are globular glycoproteins, each composed of two non-covalently linked chains.

Structure

Class I (HLA-A, HLA-B, and HLA-C) molecules consist of a heavy chain with a molecular weight of 45,000 daltons associated non-covalently with β_2-microglobulin, a non-polymorphic protein of 12,000 dalton molecular weight found in serum and urine. The heavy chain folds into three domains and is inserted through the cell membrane via a hydrophobic sequence.[5]

Class II (HLA-DR, HLA-DQ, and HLA-DP) molecules consist of two similar-sized chains of a molecular weight of 33,000 (α) and 28,000 (β) daltons associated noncovalently throughout their extracellular portions. In these molecules, both chains are inserted through the membrane via hydrophobic regions. The extracellular portions of these chains fold into two domains.[6]

Class I molecules are present on all nucleated cells, dendritic cells, and platelets, whereas class II molecules have a much more restricted distribution. They are found only on B lymphocytes, activated T lymphocytes, macrophages, monocytes, and endothelial cells. Although class I and class II molecules have some obvious structural differences, they are thought to be very similar in overall three-dimensional configuration (**Fig. 21–6**). The folding of class I and class II molecules forms a pocket that is used to present short linear peptides to T cells for immune recognition.[7,8]

Early structural models of class I molecules indicated that the α-1 and α-2 domains consisted of stretches of amino acids that were arranged into helical structures rather than sheets typical of globular proteins. The crystallography studies of Bjorkman and colleagues[5] elucidated the three-dimensional structure of the class I, HLA-A2 molecule. The α_1 and α_2 domains form a platform overlaid by two helical structures to form the peptide-binding site (**Fig. 21–7**). This groove holds processed peptides for presentation to T cells. Class I and class II molecules are also alike in that most of the polymorphism is expressed in the portion of the molecule farthest from the cell membrane involved in presenting peptide antigens to T cells.[9]

Table 21–4	**HLA Alleles Frequently Associated Through Disequilibrium**		
HLA-A, HLA-C, HLA-B	**POPULATION**		**HLA-A, HLA-B, HLA-DR**
	White		
A1, Cw7, B8			A1, B8, DR3
A3, Cw7, B7			A3, B7, DR2
A2, Cw5, B44			A29, B44, DR7
A1, Cw6, B57			A3, B35, DR1
A11, Cw4, B35			A1, B17, DR7
A30, Cw6, B13			A30, B13, DR7
	Black		
A36, Cw4, B53			A1, B8, DR3
A1, Cw7, B8			A30, B42, DR3
A11, Cw2, B35			A28, B64, DR7
A24, Cw4, B35			A2, B58, DR11
A2, Cw2, B72			A28, B58, DR14
A2, Cw7, B58			A3, B7, DR3
	Asian		
A30, Cw6, B13			A24, B52, DR2
A2, Cw1, B46			A33, B44, DR14
A24, Cw1, B54			A24, B7, DR1
A33, Cw3, B58			A33, B44, DR13
A24, Cw7, B7			A30, B13, DR7
A11, Cw4, B62			A24, B54, DR4

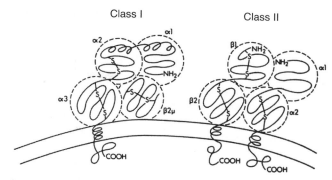

Figure 21–6. Three-dimensional configurations of class I and II molecules. β2μ = B₂-microglobulin. *(From Rodey, GE: HLA Beyond Tears. DeNovo, Atlanta, 1991, p 17, with permission.)*

mapped, very numerous, and distinct from the serologically defined ones.

Function

The primary role of the adaptive arm of the immune system is to recognize and eliminate foreign antigens. An essential feature of this function is the ability to discriminate between self and nonself, or foreign antigens. HLA class I and II molecules play a crucial role in the process of discrimination at the molecular, cellular, and species levels between self and nonself elements by presenting foreign protein antigens to T cells. The large degree of polymorphism seen in MHC is directly related to this function, as it is thought to have evolved to present a large range of foreign peptide antigens.[9]

Antibodies to HLA

The majority of HLA alloantibodies are IgG. Antibodies to HLA molecules can be divided into two groups:

1. Those that detect a single HLA gene product ("private" antibodies binding to an epitope unique to one HLA gene product)
2. Those that detect more than one HLA gene product

The surface topography, created by the folding of globular proteins into three-dimensional configurations, is large and irregular, containing multiple, nonrepeating sites (antigenic determinants or epitopes) that are potentially immunogenic. It is possible that the entire surface of the HLA molecule consists of these multiple, overlapping epitopes. An epitope is estimated to involve a minimum of five to six amino acid residues, but larger sequences are often necessary to construct the appropriate conformation. Serologic epitopes are formed by the three-dimensional protein structure and can be determined by discontinuous amino acids.

Epitopes that differ among individual members of the same species are alloepitopes. HLA alloepitopes are defined with well-characterized alloantibodies and cloned T lymphocytes. Serologically defined epitopes are located primarily in and around the peptide groove and are finite in number. The epitopes recognized by T lymphocytes are less precisely

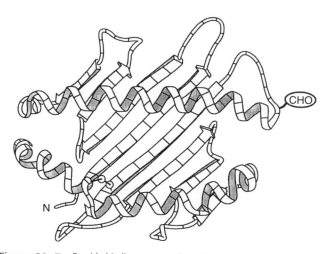

Figure 21–7. Peptide-binding groove of an HLA class I molecule. CHO = attached carbohydrate unit; N = amino terminus. *(Courtesy of Dr. Peter Parham.)*

These may be "public" (binding to epitopes shared by more than one HLA gene product) or cross-reactive (binding to structurally similar HLA epitopes).[4]

The monoclonal HLA antibody (MoAb) is produced by fusing HLA antibody-producing B cells with plasmacytoma lines.[10] Plasmacytoma cells arise from the malignant transformation of plasma cells or differentiated B cells. These cells continue to secrete antibody after transformation. MoAbs detect a broader range of epitopes because they are derived through xenoimmunization—immunization across different species. Monoclonal antibodies are still used for serologic typing, especially class II; however, they are more currently used as capture antibodies in newer-generation immunoassays.

Cross Reactivity

Cross reactivity is a phenomenon in which an antiserum directed against one HLA antigenic determinant reacts with other HLA antigenic determinants as well. Cross-reactive antigens share important structural elements with one another but retain unique, specific elements. HLA serologists recognized very quickly that many of the HLA alloantibodies were serologically cross-reactive with HLA specificities.[11–13] Dausset and colleagues[14] suggested that these antibodies might detect public specificities shared by multiple HLA gene products. The broadly reactive antibodies used in van Rood and von Leeuwen's original computer-derived HLA clusters also defined many of the current major cross-reactive groups (CREGs).

The majority of cross-reactive alloantibodies detect HLA specificities of allelic molecules coded by the same locus. On the basis of these reactions, most specificities can be grouped into major CREGs (Figs. 21–8 and 21–9).[15,16] For example, the HLA-A locus antigens A2, A23, A24, and A28 share a common determinant and therefore make up the A2 CREG, or A2C. HLA-A28 also shares a common determinant with A26, A33, and A34, defining the A28 CREG. There are also at least three interlocus cross reactions detected by alloantisera and MoAbs that occur between the HLA-A and HLA-B loci: HLA-A23, HLA-A24, HLA-A25, and HLA-A32 with HLA-Bw4;[14,17–19] HLA-A11 with HLA-Bw6;[20] and HLA-A2 with HLA-B17.[21–23] Recently, cross-reactive groups have been defined molecularly using amino acid residues. CREGs are used predominantly in the definition of antibodies present in recipient antisera and in the definition of antigens to avoid in potential organ donors when performing virtual crossmatches.

Techniques of Histocompatibility Testing

The principles used in histocompatibility testing are conceptually similar to those used for red blood cell (RBC) testing. HLA antigens are identified using sera with known anti-HLA antibodies and DNA-based molecular typing, recipient serum is screened for the presence of HLA antibodies using immunoassays, and compatibility is directly determined by crossmatching of donor cells and recipient sera.

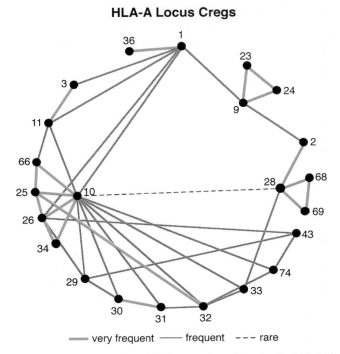

Figure 21–8. Cross reactions within the HLA-A locus. *(From Bender, K: The HLA System. Biotest Diagnostics, 1991, p 21, with permission.)*

HLA Antigen Detection

The agglutination methods initially used to define HLA antigens have been succeeded by a precise microlymphocytotoxicity test.[24] Cytotoxicity techniques require only 1 to 2 µL of serum and are sensitive and reproducible. For this purpose, acid-citrated dextrose or phenol-free heparinized blood

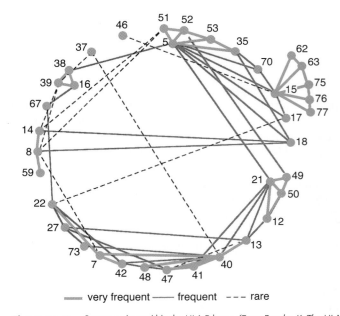

Figure 21–9. Cross-reactions within the HLA-B locus. *(From Bender, K: The HLA System. Biotest Diagnostics, 1991, p 22, with permission.)*

is used for testing. A purified lymphocyte suspension is prepared by layering whole blood on a Ficoll-Hypaque gradient and centrifuging. Residual RBCs and granulocytes are forced to the bottom of the gradient, and platelets remain in the supernatant. Lymphocytes collect at the gradient's interface and can be harvested, washed, and adjusted to appropriate test concentrations (Fig. 21–10). HLA-A, HLA-B, and HLA-C typing is performed on this lymphocyte suspension. HLA-DR typing requires identification of B lymphocytes.

Purified B-lymphocyte suspensions can be prepared by nylon wool separation,[25,26] where B cells adhere preferentially to nylon wool, from which they can be eluted. An additional technique currently used is immunomagnetic beads to positively select (target cells rosetted on beads) lymphocyte subpopulations for use in HLA typing, both for class I and II antigens. The technique for isolating either T or B cells is based on the capture monoclonal antibody coated on the bead's surface.[27] These techniques provide rapid isolation of cells with a high degree of purity and use immunofluorescence lymphocytotoxicity. Alternatively, B cells can be identified by fluorescent labeling.[28] Fluorescent labeling involves incubating lymphocytes with fluorescein isothiocyanate (FITC)–labeled anti-immunoglobulin. B lymphocytes develop distinct fluorescent caps because of the binding of the labeled anti-immunoglobulin to the cell surface immunoglobulin found on B cells and not on T cells. A major advantage of the fluorescent labeling technique is that it does not involve the physical separation of T and B cells.

Serologic HLA testing uses a form of **complement-dependent microlymphocytotoxicity** (CDC) performed in 60-well or 72-well microtiter trays (Fig. 21–11). Antiserum test trays are prepared by dispensing 1 μL of serum with known HLA reactivity into the bottom of each well, which contains mineral oil. Mineral oil is used to prevent evaporation of antisera during test incubations. Antiserum trays are frozen at –70°C until just before use. Upon use, they are removed from the freezer and thawed for 3 to 5 minutes. For CDC HLA typing, 1 μL of antisera is mixed with 1 μL of cells and incubated at room temperature for 30 minutes. Rabbit serum (5 μL) is added as a source of complement, and the cells are further incubated at room temperature for 60 minutes. Complement-mediated cell membrane injury that is induced in cells binding HLA antibody is visualized by the uptake or release of eosin-Y or trypan blue dye. The test is a tertiary binding assay that depends heavily on many factors—time, temperature, antibody strength—that influence the efficiency with which the antibodies will activate the complement cascade.

Trays are usually read on inverted phase contrast microscopes. In the properly adjusted phase, cells that have not been injured appear small, bright, and refractile. Injured cells that have taken up eosin-Y or trypan blue owing to antibody and complement-mediated damage will flatten and appear large, dark, and nonrefractile. The percent of cell death is coded numerically: the number 8 is used for a strong positive with essentially all cells killed; the number 1 is used for a negative reaction in which cell viability is the same as in the negative control. By scoring the reaction

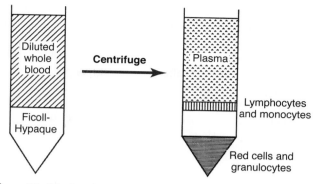

Figure 21–10. Lymphocyte separation.

of each known serum with test cells, a phenotype can be assigned. Antigen assignment is made by looking at the specificity of the defined HLA antibody in the positive wells. For example, if all wells containing HLA-A3 antibody are positive (eight reactions), the A3 antigen is assigned to the phenotype.

HLA Molecular Techniques

HLA class I (HLA-A, HLA-B, HLA-C) and class II (HLA-DR, HLA-DQ, HLA-DP) typing is performed in most laboratories by DNA analysis techniques.[29] These procedures have replaced serologic typing in many laboratories. Molecular typing for class I and II alleles is required in hematopoietic stem cell transplantation, as serologic typing does not adequately determine HLA compatibility. The three most common molecular assays employed in the clinical laboratory are **sequence-specific oligonucleotides** (SSO), **sequence-specific primers** (SSP), and **sequence-based typing** (SBT).

Sequence-Specific Oligonucleotides

Sequence-specific oligonucleotides (SSO) typing involves PCR amplification of a chosen sequence using primers flanking that sequence. The amplified DNA is immobilized on a membrane and hybridized with selected, labeled oligonucleotide probes. The reverse of this technique is utilized in

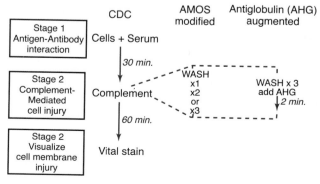

Figure 21–11. Complement-dependent microlymphocytotoxicity assay with two variations: three-wash AMOS and antiglobulin.

laboratories with low throughput, where oligonucleotide probes are immobilized on membranes and hybridized with amplified DNA.

All known HLA alleles can be identified with one or a combination of allele-specific oligonucleotide probes. Different strategies are used, depending on the extent of resolution required. Figure 21–12 illustrates a basic strategy for oligonucleotide typing. Although SSO is a powerfully reliable and accurate technology, it has been superseded by the more rapid technique of PCR-SSP.

Sequence-Specific Primers

In the sequence-specific primers (SSP) technique, oligonucleotide primers are designed to obtain amplification of specific alleles or groups of alleles. The typing method is based on the principle that a completely matched primer will be more efficiently used in the PCR reaction than a primer with one or more mismatches. The specificity of the typing system is part of the PCR reaction. Assignment of alleles is based on the presence or absence of amplified product normally detected by agarose gel electrophoresis and transillumination.

Sequence-Based Typing

Direct nucleotide sequencing of HLA genes is utilized for high-resolution typing and is required in the definition of a new allele. Most commonly, sequence-based typing (SBT) is performed by terminal-end incorporation of fluorescently labeled nucleotides during PCR reactions amplifying the most polymorphic regions of the HLA genes: exons 2, 3, and 4 of class I genes, and exon 2 of the class II β chain genes. The fluorescently tagged DNA fragments are sorted by capillary electrophoresis and interpreted by computer software to provide a DNA sequence. Generated DNA sequences are then compared to the known DNA sequences of HLA alleles to find a match, identifying the HLA allele. Detection is not based on the use of sequence-specific oligonucleotide probe, and prior knowledge of the nucleotide sequences is not required.[30,31] Therefore, previously undefined alleles can be detected.

SBT has become the preferred method of high-resolution typing for hematopoietic stem cell transplantation.

HLA Antibody Detection Techniques

Preformed antibodies to the tissue of the donor and recipient may cause significant complications in transplantation or transfusion. Recipient lymphocytotoxic HLA antibodies to donor antigens have been associated with accelerated graft rejection and with poor response to platelet transfusion. Antibody in donor plasma to recipient leukocytes has been associated with severe pulmonary infiltrates and respiratory distress following transfusion, known as **transfusion-related acute lung injury** (TRALI). Thus, the clinical management of patients, pre- and post-transplant, includes screening for and determining the specificity of anti-HLA class I and II antibodies that may be present.

Crossmatching involves serologic and cellular procedures. Serologic crossmatching is performed by cytotoxicity and flow cytometric techniques.[24] **Enzyme-linked immunosorbent crossmatch assays** (ELISA) are in development. Detection and identification techniques of HLA antibodies are similar to those for RBC antibodies. The unknown serum is tested against a panel of cells or soluble antigen of known HLA phenotype. Targets from a large panel of donors must be selected if antibodies to all HLA specificities are to be detected. A panel of at least 30 carefully selected targets is required for initial screening in the determination of panel reactive antibody (PRA), and a panel of at least 60 cells is required for accurate antibody identification.

Microlymphocytotoxicity

The **microlymphocytotoxicity** method depends on the purpose of the screen. When seeking alloantisera as typing reagents, it is essential to screen using the method for the typing procedure, the standard CDC being the most common. When screening recipient serum samples, a more sensitive technique—Amos-modified, extended incubation, or antihuman globulin—should be employed. The Amos-modified technique introduces a wash step after the initial serum-cell incubation. The wash step removes anticomplementary activity: aggregated immunoglobulin in the serum that can activate complement, making it unavailable for binding on the cell membranes. Standard CDC tests rarely detect 100% of the antigen-binding specificities of cross-reactive antibodies.[32,33]

Sensitivity of the CDC test can be greatly enhanced by adding an anti-human globulin reagent following serum and cell incubation.[32] Addition of goat anti-human kappa chain increases the likelihood of complement binding and subsequent cell injury, especially in circumstances in which the amount of HLA-antibody binding is below the threshold of detection in the standard technique. The anti-human globulin test functions like a complement-independent technique with respect to HLA alloantibodies. It is also similar to the addition of Coombs in testing for antibodies to red blood cell antigens. If antibodies to class II molecules (DR and DQ) are to be identified, then separated or labeled B-lymphocyte suspensions of known phenotype must be used. Serum can be screened

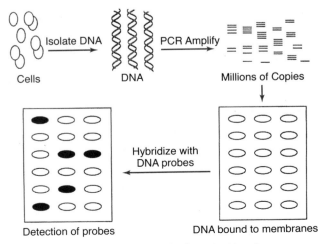

Figure 21–12. Strategy for allele-specific oligonucleotide typing.

using freshly prepared lymphocytes or lymphocytes frozen in bulk or in trays. Lymphocytes frozen in trays have the advantage of rapid preparation, enabling serum to be screened in just a few hours.

The lymphocytotoxicity assay has several disadvantages. First, viable T and B lymphocytes are essential for an accurate assessment of the presence of antibody. Many laboratories routinely use frozen cells to maintain a consistent, representative panel of antigens. The process of freezing renders lymphocytes more fragile and susceptible to cell lysis, resulting in false positives. A second problem is the necessity to maintain a reliable and consistent antigen panel that reflects the ethnic composition of the patient population; HLA antigen frequencies are known to vary among different races. The requirement for activating complement in the cytotoxicity assay results in a third disadvantage: the inability to detect non-complement-fixing antibodies. Differentiation between HLA-specific and non-HLA-specific antibodies and between IgG and IgM antibodies is not possible with the standard cytotoxicity assays. Three techniques have been introduced as alternatives to the lymphocytotoxicity assay for the detection of anti-HLA antibodies. They employ ELISA, flow cytometry, and Luminex technologies, and overcome many of the pitfalls of the standard cytotoxicity assays.

Enzyme-Linked Immunosorbent Crossmatch Assays

The enzyme-linked immunosorbent crossmatch assays (ELISA) test uses purified HLA antigens instead of lymphocytes or cells as targets for antibodies that may be present in the patient's sera. The increased specificity of the assay, due to the use of purified HLA antigens, offers the advantage of recognizing false-positive non-HLA reactions and distinguishing class I and II specificities. In addition, this method also differentiates between IgG and IgM antibody isotypes by the use of appropriate secondary detection antibody. ELISA can be used as a screening assay for the detection of anti-HLA antibodies and as a method to determine antibody specificity. The screening assay utilizes a pool of purified HLA antigens. Results are interpreted as either positive or negative. The specificity determination assay utilizes a panel of purified antigens, rather than a pool, permitting the evaluation of PRA and HLA antibody specificity.

HLA class I and II antigens are purified from either transformed cell lines or from platelets with known HLA phenotypes. The affinity-purified HLA antigens, either pooled or specific, are bound directly to wells of microtiter plates. The specific binding of antibody from the test serum sample with any of the antigens is detected by subsequent incubation with alkaline phosphatase-conjugated antibody that recognizes human IgG. A quantitative measure of the reaction is obtained by spectrophotometry after the appropriate enzyme substrate is added.

Flow Cytometry

The **flow cytometric antibody screen** detects antibody binding directly. Therefore, complement activation is not necessary as in the case of the lymphocytotoxicity assay. As with

ELISA, flow screening can distinguish between IgG and IgM antibodies with the use of either anti-IgG or anti-IgM secondary antibodies. Flow screening can also detect noncomplement-fixing antibodies, because binding of the antibodies rather than complement fixation is measured. Flow cytometric antibody screens utilize T and B lymphocytes as targets or, in a newer technique, employ purified HLA antigens coated onto microparticles 2 to 4 μm in diameter.

Flow cytometry may be used to screen for the presence of HLA antibodies and determine antibody specificity in the same manner as the ELISA assays by utilizing either pooled or specific HLA antigen-coated microparticles as targets. Lymphocytes as targets have two problems:

1. Difficulty in distinguishing between HLA-specific and non-HLA antigens on lymphocytes
2. Inability to distinguish class I or II antibody specificity, as B lymphocytes express both class I and II markers

The use of microparticles/beads coated with purified class I or II antigens circumvents these problems. HLA antibodies present in patient sera react specifically with the beads. After incubation of serum with beads, followed by staining with a fluorescently labeled antihuman IgG antibody, the anti-HLA IgG-positive serum shows a fluorescent channel shift as compared with the negative serum. Percent PRA is represented by the percentage of pooled beads that react positively with the serum.

Multiplex Immunoassay (Luminex)

The highly polymorphic nature of HLA requires testing a large number of cell types to accurately screen for alloantibodies by either serologic, lymphocytotoxicity crossmatching or by ELISA with cell lysate techniques. The development of the **multiplex flow assay** using recombinant individual HLA proteins, the **Luminex single antigen**, improved upon ELISA, increasing assay throughput, sensitivity, and simplified determination of anti-HLA specificity.[34–38] The Luminex assay involves testing patient sera against a panel of recombinant soluble HLA antigens, each bound to specific microbeads. Each microbead is labeled with a distinct set of fluorophores, enabling direct evaluation of antibody binding specificity. Anti-HLA antibody binding is detected by labeling with PE-conjugated anti-Ig and measured on a specialized flow cytometer. Positive reactions are described as the mean fluorescence intensity (MFI) of positive beads.

The increased sensitivity of the Luminex assay is clinically relevant, as detection of **donor-specific antibody (DSA)** by immunoassay is a strong predictor of antibody-mediated rejection, particularly in patients with negative or equivocal serologic crossmatch results.[39–41] However, several studies have demonstrated that not all DSA detected by Luminex are correlated with positive crossmatch and that these antibodies may not preclude transplantation.[42–44] There is currently much interest in defining DSA concentrations that preclude tissue compatibility, though no clear cutoffs between clinically relevant and irrelevant antibodies have been agreed upon.

Panel Reactive Antibody

Prior to development of single antigen assays, determining the specificities of anti-HLA antibodies detected by screening serum was problematic. Therefore, it was useful to describe the overall degree of reactivity of the serum as a predictor of immunologic compatibility. This was described as **panel-reactive antibody** (PRA), which denoted the percentage of cells in the panel that the serum was capable of binding. The advent of single antigen immunoassays enabled the specificities of detected anti-HLA antibodies to be determined, though it is still useful to consider the overall degree of HLA sensitization. For this purpose, percent PRA is represented by the percentage of pooled beads that react positively with the serum. However, the single antigen screen does not reflect a true PRA, as it is falsely low. If single donor antibody screens are available, PRAs should be calculated (cPRA) based on antigen frequency in the population. The United Network for Organ Sharing (UNOS) utilizes an algorithm based on frequency tables to calculate PRAs in listed patients when antibody specificities are entered.

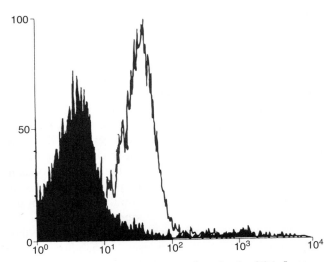

Figure 21–13. Flow cytometry histogram illustrating the shift in fluorescence light intensity emitted by a cell population coated with fluorescein-labeled antibody. The horizontal abscissa represents increasing cell numbers and the y-axis represents increasing fluorescence. *(From Rodey, GE: HLA Beyond Tears. DeNovo, Atlanta, 1991, p 17, with permission.)*

HLA Crossmatch Techniques

Lymphocytotoxicity

Numerous techniques have been described and applied as crossmatch procedures for transplantation and transfusion. **Lymphocytotoxicity** is the most widely used technique because the assays are rapid and reproducible, and they use small volumes of recipient antisera and small numbers of donor cells. The primary purpose of crossmatching before transplantation or transfusion is to identify antibodies in the serum of the potential recipient to antigens present on donor tissues.

Flow Cytometry

To facilitate detection of low levels of antibodies in potential recipients, sensitive techniques must be used, as in recipient serum screens. The correlation between hyperacute rejection and the presence of serum antibody against donor tissue is well established.[4] Cases of irreversible rejection during the first days after transplantation may be a result of low levels of antibody undetected by less sensitive techniques.[45,46] Bray[47] observed that crossmatches performed with an immunofluorescence **flow cytometric technique** are highly sensitive in detecting donor HLA antibodies in potential allograft recipients, which were undetected by standard serologic techniques (Amos and antihuman globulin). The **flow cytometry** crossmatch is performed by incubating donor cells with recipient sera, followed by a fluoresceinated goat antihuman immunoglobulin. A phycoerythrin-labeled antibody to detect either T or B cells is used to discriminate between the two subpopulations of lymphocytes. Cells are analyzed, and results are expressed as positive or negative, based on the shift in fluorescence intensity of the test serum with respect to negative serum (**Fig. 21–13**). To achieve good graft survival rates, centers are investigating more sensitive crossmatch techniques to detect donor-specific HLA alloantibodies.

The three newer detection methods for the presence of anti-HLA antibodies, ELISA, flow cytometry, and Luminex were developed to overcome disadvantages inherent in the traditional lymphocytotoxicity assay. All three assays are more sensitive than lymphocytotoxicity and can differentiate between antibodies to HLA and non-HLA antigens. Furthermore, these assays can discriminate between IgG and IgM isotypes, making them the preferred choice for detecting anti-HLA antibodies in screening a patient serum. However, clinical correlation between the presence of antibodies detected by these sensitive assays and graft survival is not yet established. For this reason, PRA and antibody specificity determined by the newer methods are considered only as initial tests and are not used as the sole basis for clinical decision-making. A final crossmatch with specific donor targets is required prior to transplant because not all HLA antigens are represented in the pools or panels of targets utilized in either of the assays.

Virtual Crossmatch

Significant evidence demonstrates the importance of clinical testing for DSA in solid organ transplantation. Since the first description of anti-HLA antibodies detected by CDC as a defining risk factor for graft rejection, improvements in the detection of DSA have nearly eliminated hyperacute rejection. Serologic crossmatch remains the gold standard assay for determining immunologic compatibility, though the labor-intensive nature, complex interpretation, and limited donor and recipient samples preclude performing crossmatching for all potential donor and recipient pairs. The strategy of **virtual crossmatching**, or selecting donor-recipient pairs based upon knowledge of donor HLA type and recipient alloantibody profile, has led to improved organ allocation, directing shared organs to centers with the most likely compatible matches.[48–50]

Virtual crossmatching is not infallible, however, as it is critically limited by the information used to determine compatibility: Accurate evaluation of immunologic compatibility requires full knowledge for donor HLA type and recent alloantibody profile of the recipient. Knowledge of the donor organ HLA type is often limited to HLA-A, HLA-B, and HLA-DR antigens, while multiplex alloantibody testing is most commonly limited to anti-HLA antibodies, ignoring the contribution of allotypic antibodies against MICA and other alloantigens. This reinforces the necessity of serologic or flow crossmatch with donor cells being performed prior to any solid organ transplantation to minimize the risk of hyperacute rejection.

Clinical Significance of the HLA System

The identification of HLA antigens was driven by their potential clinical application to transplantation. The HLA system is still of primary clinical importance in transplantation, but it has recently become of great interest to individuals in the field of human genetics and to investigators of disease associations. HLAs are associated with disease susceptibility to a greater extent than any other known genetic marker in humans, and the HLA system has the highest exclusion probability of any single system in resolving cases of disputed paternity.[51]

Paternity

Relationship testing involves analyzing genetic markers from the mother, child, and alleged father to determine whether the tested man could be the biological father of a child. To accomplish this, the laboratory uses several techniques to accurately identify the polymorphic genetic markers in a paternity trio. Combinations of various genetic markers are used, including RBC markers and enzymes, serum proteins, HLA typing, and DNA testing.[51] Previously, the most common combination of testing included RBC markers together with HLA typing. Owing to increased costs of HLA typing reagents and the significantly high power of exclusion when testing multiple DNA loci, DNA methodologies are used increasingly more than HLA typing (see Chapter 22, "Parentage Testing").

Disease Association

It has been determined that HLA antigens are associated with disease susceptibility to a greater extent than any other known genetic marker.[52] Many genetic markers have been suspected to be associated with disease, the most extensively studied being blood groups, enzymes, and serum proteins. Relative risk indicates how many times more frequently the disease occurs in individuals positive for the marker than in individuals negative for the marker. In contrast, the association between HLA-B27 and ankylosing spondylitis has a relative risk ranging from 60 to 100, depending on the population studied. To date, over 500 diseases have been studied.[53] A list of the most significant HLA and disease associations is given in Table 21–5.

The exact cause for the association of HLA to disease is unclear. There is no question that genetic factors coded within or near the HLA complex confer susceptibility for a variety of diseases. This susceptibility may somehow be related to altered immunologic responsiveness in many cases. It is also probable that the diseases in question may be a result of both multiple gene interactions and environmental factors. In some cases, it has been documented to result from presentation of unique pathogenic epitopes to T cells. Although the study of HLA and disease associations is very important in understanding disease susceptibility and manifestation, HLA alone is not clinically useful as a diagnostic tool.

Platelet Transfusion

Hematopoietic stem cell transplantation and more aggressive use of chemotherapy in the treatment of malignancies have led to a dramatic increase in platelet transfusions in the past decade. Human leukocyte class I antigens are expressed variably on platelets.[54–58] Alloimmunization to the HLA results in refractoriness to random donor platelet transfusions. Refractoriness is manifested by the failure to achieve a rise in the circulating platelet count 1 hour after infusion of adequate numbers of platelets. The refractory state is often associated with lymphocytotoxic HLA antibodies.

Considering the highly polymorphic nature of the HLA system, it is impossible to obtain sufficient numbers of HLA-typed donors to provide HLA-matched platelets for all alloimmunized patients. Duquesnoy and associates[60] demonstrated that platelet transfusions from donors mismatched only for cross-reactive antigens can effectively provide hemostasis for refractory patients. For example, an HLA-A1,B7; HLA-A11,B22 recipient might benefit from the platelets of an A1,B7; A3,B27 donor because A3 and A11 and B27 and B22 are cross-reactive. Table 21–6 lists the major cross-reactive groups and the private specificities associated with each. As a result of these observations, the donor pool necessary to sustain an HLA-matched platelet program can be reduced from 8,000 to 10,000 to manageable numbers of 2,000 to 5,000.

Good platelet survival and HLA matching are not absolute. For example, poor transfusion results are sometimes obtained despite a perfect HLA match. Poor recovery may be a result of sensitization to non-HLA antigens, such as platelet-specific antigens. In contrast, excellent transfusion results are at other times obtained in the presence of complete HLA mismatch. Good recovery may be a function of:

- A restricted pattern of alloimmunization—private versus public antibodies
- Variable expression of HLA antigens on the platelet surface

Leukocytes are more immunogenic than platelets, and refractoriness is probably initiated by HLA antigens on the

Table 21–5 Significant HLA Disease Associations

DISEASE	HLA	RELATIVE RISK*
Narcolepsy	DR2	129.8
Ankylosing spondylitis	B27	87.4
Reiter's syndrome	B27	37.1
Dermatitis herpetiformis	DR3	17.3
	B8	9.8
Pemphigus vulgaris	DR4	14.6
	A26	4.8
	B38	4.6
Goodpasture's syndrome	DRB1*1501	7.4
Celiac disease	DQA1*0501/DQB1*0201	24.9
	DQA1*0301/DQB1*0302	2
Acute anterior uveitis	B27	8.2
Psoriasis vulgaris	Cw6	7.5
	B17	5.3
	B13	4.1
Idiopathic hemochromatosis	A3	6.7
	B7	2.9
Systemic lupus erythematosus	DR3	5.8
Sjögren's syndrome	Dw3	5.7
	B8	3.3
Hashimoto's disease	DR3	2.2
Behçet's disease	B51	3.8
Rheumatoid arthritis	DR4	4.2
Grave's disease	DR3	3.7
Type 1 diabetes	DRB1*0301/DQB1*0201	2.4
	DRB1*0401/DQB1*0302	9.5
Myasthenia gravis	B8	3.4
	DRB1*03	2.5
Multiple sclerosis	DR2	4.1

*Relative risk of the disease in the white population. Frequencies for other races can be found in Tiwari, JL, and Terasaki, PI: HLA and Disease. Springer-Verlag, New York, 1995, p 33.

contaminating leukocytes. Evidence for this is based on a study by Brand and others,[60] in which they demonstrated a decreased rate of alloimmunization to random donor platelets when contaminating leukocytes were removed before transfusion. Herzig and colleagues[61] were also able to improve the transfusion response to HLA-matched platelets by removing the leukocytes. This type of approach might be useful for those patients who are unable to produce a response to HLA-matched platelets.

Transfusion-Related Acute Lung Injury

Transfusion-related acute lung injury (TRALI) is the clinical syndrome of new **acute lung injury** (ALI) that develops with

Table 21–6 Major CREGs

MAJOR CREG	ASSOCIATED SEROLOGIC ALLELES
A1 CREG	A1, 36, 3, 9 (23, 34), 10 (25, 26, 34, 66), 11, 19 (29, 30, 31, 32, 33), 28 (68, 69), 43, 74, 80
A2 CREG	A2, 9 (23, 24), 28 (68, 69), B17
B5 CREG	B5 (51, 52), 15 (62, 63, 75, 76, 77), 17 (57, 58), 18, 35, 12 (49, 50), 53, 70 (71, 72), 78, 37
B7 CREG	B7, 42, 22 (54, 55, 56), 27, 40 (60, 61), 13, 41, 46, 47, 48, 81, 37, 73
B8 CREG	B8, 14 (64, 65), 16 (38, 39), 18, 59, 67
B12 CREG	B12 (44, 45), 21 (49, 50), 13, 40 (60, 61), 41, 48, 82
4c CREG	A9 (23, 24), A25, A32, Bw4
6c CREG	Bw6, Cw1, Cw3, Cw7

a clear temporal relationship to transfusion, in patients with or without alternate risk factors for ALI.[62] TRALI manifests as fever, hypoxemia, and pulmonary edema occurring acutely (within 6 hours) following transfusion of blood components. The phenomenon of respiratory distress following transfusion has been observed for 60 years, though TRALI has only been recognized as a distinct clinical entity since 1985.[63] TRALI is the most severe adverse outcome from transfusion, with estimates of prevalence ranging from 0.02% to 0.16% of patients receiving transfusions.[63,64] Treatment is supportive, with supplemental oxygen and respiratory support if necessary. Most cases resolve within 96 hours, though a mortality rate of 5% to 10% is reported.[65]

The exact pathophysiology of TRALI is unclear, though TRALI is strongly associated with the presence of allotypic antibodies present in donor blood products. Antibodies against HLA class I and class II molecules have been found in 50% to 89% of products associated with TRALI.[63,66,67] Additionally, antibodies to HNA-1a, HNA-1b, HNA-2a, and HNA-3a, alloantigens found specifically on neutrophils, have been described in as many as 72% of blood products associated with TRALI.[63] The current model of TRALI suggests that these allotypic antibodies activate neutrophils in the lung, which release cytokine and chemokine mediators that cause pulmonary edema.[63] In rare cases, TRALI has been described to be mediated by allotypic antibodies in the recipient that react with donor granulocytes. However, no causative antibody can be found in over 15% of reported cases, demonstrating the limitations of current testing.[68]

Suspected cases of TRALI are typically evaluated by analyzing the donor blood product for anti-HLA and anti-HNA antibodies. This can be performed by immunoassay or by serologic techniques. However, the diagnosis of TRALI is primarily upon clinical symptoms correlated with a recent transfusion event. While laboratory evaluation is not required to make a diagnosis of TRALI or begin treatment, it is important for confirmation, particularly to evaluate the potential risks of transfusing blood products from donors associated with TRALI. Demonstration of anti-HLA or anti-HNA antibodies will likely not affect treatment decisions regarding a patient with symptoms of TRALI, but they are important to determine whether the donor associated with the suspected causative blood product should be removed from the donor pool.

Transplantation

Clinical transplant immunology is a difficult field. Unlike animal experimentation, in which studies are performed under controlled conditions in selected inbred strains, transplant immunology deals with actual patients with different medical histories and backgrounds. Individuals working in transplant immunology must determine how best to select recipients and donors, when to increase or decrease immunosuppressive treatment, and how to precondition potential recipients so that their immune systems will accept a graft. Decisions are based on the relative merits of laboratory findings viewed against complex medical histories. Differences of opinion exist from center to center about the significance of immunologic test results and their considerations in clinical treatment protocols.

Hematopoietic Stem Cell Transplantation

Hematopoietic stem cell transplantation (HSCT) is the term used for the transplantation of multipotent hematopoietic stem cells (HSC). Under normal conditions, HSC in the bone marrow continuously generates red blood cells, leukocytes, and platelets. However, under certain conditions, including hematologic malignancies, congenital and acquired aplasias, and after intense radiation and chemotherapy, the bone marrow's hematopoietic capability is compromised. In these instances it is beneficial to transplant HSC, either collected from the patient prior to bone marrow ablation (autologous HSCT) or from a healthy donor (allogeneic HSCT) to reconstitute normal hematopoietic function. Allogeneic HSCT enables reconstitution with fully functioning, healthy HSC, replacing those compromised by malignancy or metabolic defects, with demonstrated benefit in immune-mediated antitumor function (graft versus leukemia, GVL). However, it has adverse consequences, most notably the development of graft-versus-host disease (GVHD). Both GVHD and GVL are directly related to the degree of alloantigenic mismatch. This has led to the development of several donor-recipient matching strategies, each with distinct trade-offs between GVHD and GVL.

Because of the continuous difficulty of finding well-matched related (approximately 33% of patients) and unrelated (less than 50%) donors for HSCT, umbilical cord blood transplantation (UCBT) has increased over the past 15 years. UCBT is an accepted alternative to HSCT, because the functional and phenotypic immaturity of UCB lymphocytes or the reduced T-cell dose contribute to UCB reduced alloreactivity. Therefore, limited HLA mismatches are better tolerated, and there is a decreased incidence of GVHD. The most limiting factor of UCBT is cell dosage in that quite frequently there are insufficient hematopoietic stem or progenitor cells in one UCB unit. UCB dose is of paramount importance in engraftment and survival after unrelated UCBT. The single most important factor for the potential increase of HSCT is expanding the donor pool to include both related and unrelated individuals. To meet the needs of patients who do not have a matched, related donor, the U.S. Congress authorized a federal contract in 1986 to establish a national marrow donor registry.

In response to a request for proposal, the National Marrow Donor Program (NMDP) was formed with cosponsorship of the American Association of Blood Banks, American Red Cross, and the Council of Community Blood Centers. The goals were to recruit a large number of informed HLA-typed volunteers to be listed as potential marrow donors, to combine all available donor HLA data into a centralized registry, and to establish a national coordinating center for facilitating donor searches and communication between donor and transplant centers. The NMDP currently operates the Be The Match registry of volunteer donors and umbilical cord blood units in the United States. It is the world's largest hematopoietic cell registry, listing more than 8 million individuals and 160,000 cord blood units. As of January 2010, the NMDP had facilitated more than 38,000 unrelated transplants worldwide.

Kidney Transplantation

Kidney transplantation is used to treat end-stage renal disease. Transplantation is preferred over dialysis in treating patients with chronic renal failure because it is more cost-effective, and it usually returns patients to a state of relatively normal health. The best graft survival rates occur when kidneys are obtained from HLA-identical, ABO-compatible siblings, but such donors are available for relatively few patients.[69,70] Three general strategies are used by transplantation surgeons and immunologists to minimize graft rejection:

1. Immunosuppressive agents
2. Reduction of graft "foreignness"
3. Induction of tolerance

Immunosuppressive agents such as azathioprine, prednisone, thymoglobulin, cyclosporine, and tacrolimus are used to diminish the destructive immunologic responses to the graft. These agents are nonselective and carry risks of serious side effects, especially life-threatening infection.[72] Extensive efforts are used to minimize graft "foreignness" through matching of donor and recipient antigens. Antigen disparities that most influence graft rejection include the ABO blood group antigens and the HLA antigens. Although it is still not clear what combinations of HLA gene products promote optimal graft survival rates, it is evident that 0 and 1 antigen mismatches result in increased graft survival.[72] In highly sensitized recipients, it is necessary to match for HLA-A and HLA-B because of the presence of class I HLA antibodies. Sanfilippo

and colleagues[73] found that matching based on public cross-reactive antigens can provide the same association with graft outcome as private antigens. Matching for public antigens also promotes and increases the transplantation of minority patients. When matching for highly sensitized recipients, by either private or public antigens, identification of HLA serum antibodies is important. Oldfather and others[74] observed that crossmatch results can be predicted in highly sensitized recipients based on careful analysis of serum HLA-antibody specificities. Thus, single antigen antibody testing plays an enormous role in the detection of antibodies and, ultimately, the prediction of crossmatch results.

The third strategy is based on the induction of tolerance to donor-specific antigens. The evidence that transfusion of blood products before transplantation promotes graft acceptance suggests that tolerance induction may be feasible. In 1973, Opelz and coworkers[75] reported that blood transfusion might promote renal allograft survival in patients receiving kidneys from crossmatch-negative donors. In their retrospective study, graft survival rates at 1 year were significantly improved in patients who had received more than 10 transfusions (66%), compared with patients who had received 1 to 10 units (43%) or no transfusions (29%). Salvatierra and colleagues[76] applied this observation to the potential benefits of donor-specific blood transfusions and transplants between living related individuals. The effects of blood transfusion on the success of renal transplantation are complex and paradoxical. Transfusion of blood usually leads to HLA alloimmunization, and when this leads to HLA antibody production, it is difficult to find compatible donors. Yet graft survival rates are improved when pretransplant blood is given to the recipient with no resulting sensitization. However, with new drug therapies, transfusion protocols have not been utilized due to the risk of recipient sensitization to potential organ donors.

Two modalities—plasmapheresis and intravenous immune globulin (IVIG)—are used in the treatment of rejection post-transplant and in the pretransplant desensitization of the patient.[77] Plasmapheresis has been demonstrated to remove HLA-specific antibody in many different clinical settings.[78,79] IVIG has been used to modulate immune responses and suppress alloantibody. Several groups have had success using IVIG to decrease levels of anti-HLA antibody and to lower panel-reactive antibody among highly sensitized patients awaiting transplantation.[80,81] Most recently, rituximab has been added to antirejection and desensitization treatments to destroy antibody producing B cells.

Heart Transplantation

Heart transplantation is used to treat cardiomyopathies and end-stage ischemic heart disease. Because of the organ's extremely short total ischemic time (3 hours for hearts, compared with 72 hours for kidneys), HLA matching and prospective crossmatching is not feasible. Total ischemic time is the amount of time there is no blood flow through the organ. The single most important HLA pretransplant test is the HLA-antibody screen. Recipients with no preformed HLA antibodies receive transplants without crossmatching. Those with preformed HLA antibodies require either pretransplant crossmatches to determine recipient-donor compatibility or donor HLA phenotype to perform virtual crossmatching.

Liver Transplantation

Orthotopic liver transplantation has become an established and successful therapeutic modality for patients with end-stage liver disease. Immunologic factors in recipient/donor matching for liver transplantation and recipient presensitization have largely been ignored in the past because of the liver's unique abilities to act as a sink for anti-HLA antibodies and to regenerate itself if destroyed by antibody. The consequences of HLA presensitization and ABO incompatibility were recently underlined in three reports.[82–84] In the first, a retrospective analysis of preformed HLA antibodies demonstrated 1-year graft survival rate of 40% in the presensitized individuals as compared with 83% in the nonsensitized individuals. In the second, survival of patients with emergency ABO-incompatible transplants was 30% compared with 76% in patients with emergency ABO-compatible grafts and 80% in patients with elective ABO-compatible grafts.

Lung Transplantation

An overall review of the indications for lung transplantation during the past several years reveals that emphysema and cystic fibrosis account for the majority of double-lung transplants. The major indications for single-lung transplantation include pulmonary fibrosis (33%) and emphysema (41%). In addition, single-lung transplants for primary hypertension are being performed instead of heart-lung transplantation. As with hearts, short cold ischemic times for lungs preclude prospective histocompatibility testing. However, the HLA matching between donor and recipient may play an important role in live-donor lung transplantation (2% to 3%) in an attempt to improve post-transplant conditions and graft survival rates.[85] Virtual crossmatching also plays an important role in those sensitized patients awaiting lung transplantation.

Pancreas and Islet Cell Transplantation

The primary indication for pancreas transplantation is diabetes. The majority of pancreas transplants performed are simultaneous pancreas and kidney transplants (81%), with pancreas following kidney (12%) and pancreas alone (5%). HLA matching, as reported by one of the largest pancreas transplant centers, has a major effect on graft survival,[86] particularly in the pancreas after kidney and pancreas alone transplants. Because of increased risks of myocardial complications with pancreas transplantation, islet cell transplantation has been actively pursued. Although islet cell transplantation is technically simple, difficulty has been encountered in achieving sustained engraftment in humans due to insufficient cell numbers. To overcome this, sufficient islet mass is attained by transplanting islets from two donor pancreases when cell numbers are low. To date, the effect of HLA matching has not been studied, but data are being stored for future analyses.

United Network for Organ Sharing

In an effort to provide solid organs (a rare commodity) equitably, the United Network for Organ Sharing (UNOS) was established in 1986. This organization received the federal contract to operate the national Organ Procurement and Transplantation Network (OPTN) and to develop an equitable scientific and medically sound organ allocation system. The OPTN is charged with developing policies that maximize use of organs donated for transplantation, ensuring quality of care for transplant patients, and addressing medical and ethical issues related to organ transplantation in the United States.

SUMMARY CHART

✔ The HLA genetic region is a series of closely linked genes located on the short arm of chromosome 6 that determine major histocompatibility factors—that is, surface antigens or receptors that are responsible for recognizing and eliminating foreign tissues.

✔ The HLA class I region encodes genes for the classic transplantation molecules HLA-A, HLA-B, and HLA-C; the class II region encodes genes for the molecules HLA-DR, HLA-DP, and HLA-DQ; the class III region encodes genes for C2, C4, Bf (complement factors), 21-hydroxylase, and tumor necrosis factor.

✔ The HLA genotype represents the association of the alleles on the two C6 chromosomes as determined by family studies, and the term *haplotype* refers to the allelic makeup of a single C6 chromosome.

✔ The majority of HLA alloantibodies are IgG and can be grouped into private antibodies (binding to an epitope unique to one HLA gene product), public antibodies (binding to epitopes shared by more than one HLA gene product), or cross-reactive (binding to structurally similar HLA epitopes) antibodies.

Continued

SUMMARY CHART—cont'd

✔ Techniques of histocompatibility testing include antigen and allele typing; HLA antibody detection and identification, in which recipient serum is tested against a panel of cells or a panel of single antigens; and crossmatching, in which specific donor cells and recipient sera are tested for compatibility. The ability to perform "virtual" crossmatches due to the specific and sensitive single antigen screening assay has refined pretransplant histocompatibility testing and improved organ allocation algorithms. This has led to improved clinical outcomes.

✔ The general strategies employed by transplantation immunologists include use of immunosuppressive drugs, reduction of graft "foreignness," and induction of tolerance.

✔ Platelet refractoriness is manifested by the failure to achieve a rise in circulating platelet count 1 hour after infusion of adequate numbers of platelets.

✔ TRALI is the most severe adverse outcome from transfusion manifested by fever, hypoxemia, and pulmonary edema.

Review Questions

1. The HLA genes are located on which chromosome?
   a. 2
   b. 4
   c. 6
   d. 8

2. The majority of HLA antibodies belongs to what immunoglobulin class?
   a. IgD
   b. IgE
   c. IgG
   d. IgM

3. What is the test of choice for HLA antigen testing?
   a. Agglutination
   b. Molecular
   c. Cytotoxicity
   d. ELISA

4. Of the following diseases, which one has the highest relative risk in association with an HLA antigen?
   a. Ankylosing spondylitis
   b. Juvenile diabetes
   c. Narcolepsy
   d. Rheumatoid arthritis

5. Why is HLA matching not feasible in cardiac transplantation?
   a. No HLAs are present on cardiac cells
   b. No donors ever have HLA antibodies
   c. Total ischemic time is too long
   d. Total ischemic time is too short

6. DR52 molecules are the product of which alleles?
   a. DRA and DRB1
   b. DRA and DRB3
   c. DRA and DRB4
   d. DRA and DRB5

7. What is the molecular technique that detects undefined alleles?
   a. Restriction fragment length polymorphism
   b. Sequence-specific primer typing
   c. Sequence-specific oligonucleotide typing
   d. Direct nucleotide sequencing

8. What represents the association of the alleles on the two C6 chromosomes as determined by family studies?
   a. Haplotype
   b. Genotype
   c. Phenotype
   d. Xenotype

References

1. Dausset, H: Leukoagglutinins: Leukoagglutinins and blood transfusion. J Vox Sang 4:190, 1954.
2. Dausset, J: Iso-leuco-anticorps. Acta Haematol 20:156, 1958.
3. Marsh, SGE, et al: Nomenclature for Factors of the HLA System. Tissue Antigens 75:291, 2010.
4. Kissmeyer-Nielson, F, et al: Hyperacute rejection of kidney allografts associated with preexisting humoral antibodies against donor cells. Lancet 1:662, 1966.
5. Bjorkman, PJ, et al: Structure of the HLA class I histocompatibility antigen, HLA-A2. Nature 329:506, 1987.
6. Brown, JH, et al: Three-dimensional structure of the human class II histocompatibility antigen HLA-DR1. Nature 364:33, 1993.
7. Townsend AR, et al: The epitopes of influenza nucleoprotein recognized by cytotoxic T lymphocytes can be defined with short synthetic peptides. Cell 44:959, 1986.
8. Babbit, BP, et al: Binding of immunogenic peptides to Ia histocompatibility molecules. Nature 317:359, 1985.
9. Little, AM, and Parham, P: Polymorphism and evolution of HLA class I and II genes and molecules. Rev Immunogenet 1:105, 1999.
10. Kohler, G, and Milstein, C: Derivation of specific antibody producing tissue culture and tumor lines by cell fusion. Eur J Immunol 6:611, 1976.
11. Dausset, J, et al: Un nouvel antigene du systeme HL-A (Hu-1), l' antigene 15 allelle possible des antigenes 1, 11, 12. Nouv Rev Fr Hematol 8:398, 1968.
12. Kissmeyer-Nielsen, F, Svejgaard, A, and Hange, M: Genetics of the HL-A transplantation system. Nature 291:1116, 1968.

13. Svejgaard, A, and Kissmeyer-Nielsen, F: Crossreactive human HL-A iso-antibodies. Nature 219:868, 1968.
14. Legrand, L, and Dausset, J: The complexity of the HLA gene product: Possible evidence for a "public" determinant common to the first and second HLA series. Transplantation 19:177, 1975.
15. Rodey, G, et al: ASHI HLA class I public epitope workshop: Phase I report. Transpl Proc 19:872, 1987.
16. Rodey, GE, et al: Public epitopes and the antigenic structure of HLA molecules. Crit Rev Immunol 7:229, 1987.
17. Scalamogne, M, et al: Crossreactivity between the first and second segregant series of the HLA system. Tissue Antigens 7:125, 1976.
18. Kostyu, DD, Cresswell, P, and Amos, DB: A public HLA antigen associated with HLA-A9, Aw32, and Bw4. Immunogenetics 10:433, 1980.
19. Muller, C, et al: Monoclonal antibody (Tu 48) defining alloantigenic class I determinants specific for HLA-Bw4 and HLA-Aw23, -Aw24 as well as -Aw32. Hum Immunol 5:269, 1982.
20. Belvedere, M, Mattiuz, PL, and Curtoni, ES: An antibody cross-reacting with LA and four antigens of the HLA system. Immunogenetics 1:538, 1975.
21. McMichael, AJ, et al: A monoclonal antibody that recognizes an antigenic determinant shared by HLA-A2 and B17. Hum Immunol 1:121, 1980.
22. Ahern, AT, et al: HLA-A2 and HLA-B17 antigens share an alloantigenic determinant. Hum Immunol 5:139, 1982.
23. Claas, F, et al: Alloantibodies to an antigenic determinant shared by HLA-A2 and B17. Tissue Antigens 19:388, 1982.
24. Troup, CM, and Walford, RL: Cytotoxicity test for the typing of human lymphocytes. Am J Clin Pathol 51:529, 1969.
25. Eisen, SA, Wedner, HJ, and Parker, CW: Isolation of pure human peripheral blood T-lymphocytes using nylon wool columns. Immunol Commun 1:571, 1972.
26. Lowry, R, et al: Improved B cell typing for HLA-DR using nylon wool column enriched B lymphocyte preparations. Tissue Antigens 14:325, 1979.
27. Vartdal, F, et al: HLA class I and II typing using cells positively selected from blood by immunomagnetic isolation: A fast and reliable technique. Tissue Antigens 28:301, 1986.
28. van Rood, JJ, van Leeuwen, A, and Ploem, JS: Simultaneous detection of two cell populations by two-color fluorescence and application to the recognition of B cell determinants. Nature 262:795, 1976.
29. Tiercy, JM, Jannet, M, and Mach, B: A new approach for the analysis of HLA class II polymorphism: HLA oligo typing. Blood Rev 4:9, 1990.
30. Zemmour, J, and Parham, P: HLA class I nucleotide sequences. Hum Immunol 31:195, 1991.
31. Marsh, SGE, and Bodmer, J: HLA class II nucleotide sequences. Hum Immunol 31:207, 1991.
32. Fuller, TC, et al: Antigenic specificity of antibody reactive in the antiglobulin-augmented lymphocytotoxicity test. Transplantation 34:24, 1982.
33. Fuller, TC, and Rodey, GE: Specificity of alloantibodies against antigens of the HLA complex. In Theoretical Aspects of HLA: A Technical Workshop. American Association of Blood Banks, Arlington, VA, 1982, p 51.
34. Pei, R, et al: Simultaneous HLA class I and class II antibodies screening with flow cytometry. Hum Immunol 59:313, 1998.
35. Pei, R, et al: Single human leukocyte antigen flow cytometry beads for accurate identification of human leukocyte antibody specificities. Transplantation 75:43, 2003.
36. El-Awar, N, Lee, J, and Terasaki, PI: HLA antibody identification with single antigen beads compared to conventional methods. Hum Immunol 66:989, 2005.
37. Ishida, H, et al: Evaluation of flow cytometric panel reactive antibody in renal transplant recipients—examination of 238 cases of renal transplantation. Transpl Int 18:163, 2005.
38. Patel, AM, et al: Renal transplantation in patients with pretransplant donor-specific antibodies and negative flow cytometry crossmatches. Am J Transplant 7:2371, 2007.
39. Amico, P, et al: Incidence and prediction of early antibody-mediated rejection due to non-human leukocyte antigen-antibodies. Transplantation 85:1557, 2008.
40. Amico, P, et al: Clinical relevance of pretransplant donor-specific HLA antibodies detected by single-antigen flow-beads. Transplantation 87:1681, 2009.
41. Vlad, G, et al: Relevance of different antibody detection methods for the prediction of antibody-mediated rejection and deceased-donor kidney allograft survival. Hum Immunol 70:589, 2009.
42. Reinsmoen, N, et al: Acceptable donor-specific antibody levels allowing for successful deceased and living donor kidney transplantation after desensitization therapy. Transplantation 86:820, 2008.
43. Phelan, D, et al: Living donor renal transplantation in the presence of donor-specific human leukocyte antigen antibody detected by solid phase assay. Hum Immunol 70:584, 2009.
44. Morris, G, et al: Virtual crossmatch by identification of donor-specific anti-human leukocyte antigen antibodies by solid phase immunoassay. A 30-month analysis in living donor kidney transplantation. Hum Immunol 3:268, 2010.
45. Lucas, ZG, et al: Early renal transplant failure associated with subliminal sensitization. Transplantation 10:522, 1970.
46. Patel, R, and Briggs, WA: Limitation of the lymphocyte cytotoxicity crossmatch test in recipients of kidney transplants having preformed anti-leukocyte antibodies. N Engl J Med 284:1016, 1971.
47. Bray, RA: Flow cytometry in the transplant laboratory. Ann NY Acad Sci 677:138, 1993.
48. Bray, RA, et al: Transplanting the highly sensitized patient: The Emory algorithm. AM J Transplant 6:2307, 2006.
49. Vaidya, S, et al: Prediction of crossmatch outcome of highly sensitized patients by single and/or multiple bead luminex assay. Transplantation 82:1524, 2006.
50. Bielmann, D, et al: Pretransplant risk assessment in renal allograft recipients using virtual crossmatching. Am J Transplant 7:626, 2007.
51. Polesky, HF: Impact of molecular (DNA) testing on determination of parentage. Arch Pathol Lab Med. 123:1060, 1999.
52. Tiwari, JL, and Terasaki, PI: HLA and Disease. Springer-Verlag, New York, 1985.
53. Mourant, AE, Kopec, AC, and Domaniewska-Solczak, K: Blood Groups and Diseases. Oxford University Press, New York, 1978.
54. Colombani, J: Blood platelets in HL-A serology. Transpl Proc 3:1078, 1971.
55. Svejgaard, A, Kissemeyer-Nielson, F, and Thorsby, E: HL-A typing of platelets. In Terasaki, PI (ed): Histocompatibility Testing 1970. Munksgaard, Copenhagen, 1970, p 160.
56. Leibert, M, and Aster, RH: Expression of HLA-B12 on platelets, on lymphocytes, and in serum: A quantitative study. Tissue Antigens 9:199, 1977.
57. Aster, RH, Szatkowski, N, and Liebert, M: Expression of HLA-B12, HLA-B8, W4, and W6 on platelets. Transpl Proc 9:1965, 1977.
58. Duquesnoy, RJ, Testin, J, and Aster, RH: Variable expression of W4 and W6 on platelets: Possible relevance to platelet transfusion therapy of alloimmunized thrombocytopenic patients. Transpl Proc 9:1827, 1977.

59. Duquesnoy, RJ, Filip, DJ, and Rody, GE: Successful transfusion of platelet "mismatched" for HLA antigens to alloimmunized thrombocytopenic patients. Am J Hematol 2:219, 1977.

60. Brand, A, van Leeuwen, A, and Eernisse, JG: Platelet immunology with special regard to platelet transfusion therapy. Excerpta Medica International Congress 415:639, 1978.

61. Herzig, RH, Herzig, GP, and Biell, MI: Correction of poor platelet transfusion responses with leukocyte-poor HLA-matched platelet concentrates. Blood 46:743, 1975.

62. Toy, P, et al: Transfusion-related acute lung injury: Definition and review. Crit Care Med 33:721, 2005.

63. Popovski, MA, and Moore, SB: Diagnostic and pathogenic considerations in transfusion-related acute lung injury. Transfusion 25:573, 1985.

64. Sillimann, CC, et al: Transfusion-related acute lung injury: Epidemiology and a prospective analysis of etiologic factors. Blood 101:454, 2003.

65. Popovski, MA, et al: Transfusion-related acute lung injury: A neglected, serious complication of hemotherapy. Transfusion 32:589, 1992.

66. Kopko, PM, et al: HLA class II antibodies in transfusion-related acute lung injury. Transfusion 41:1244, 2001.

67. Eder, AF, et al: Transfusion-related acute lung injury surveillance (2003–2005) and the potential impact of the selective use of plasma from male donors in the American Red Cross. Transfusion 47:599, 2007.

68. Engelfriet, CP, and Reesink, HW: Transfusion-related acute lung injury (TRALI). Vox Sang 81:269, 2001.

69. Siegler, HF, et al: Comparisons of mixed leukocyte skin graft survival in families genotyped for HLA-A. Transpl Proc 3:115, 1971.

70. Hamburger, J, et al: The value of present methods used for the selection of organ donors. Transpl Proc 3:260, 1971.

71. Alexander, JW: Impact of transplantation on microbiology and infectious diseases. Transpl Proc 12:593, 1980.

72. Cecka, JM: The UNOS scientific renal transplant registry 2000. Clin Transpl 1, 2001.

73. Sanfilippo, F, Vaughn, WK, and Spees, EKL: The effect of HLA-A, -B matching on cadaver renal allograft rejection comparing public and private specificities. Transplantation 38:483, 1984.

74. Oldfather, JW, et al: Prediction of crossmatch outcome in highly sensitized dialysis patients based on the identification of serum HLA antibodies. Transplantation 42:267, 1986.

75. Opelz, G, et al: Effect of blood transfusions on subsequent kidney transplants. Transpl Proc 5:253, 1973.

76. Salvatierra, O, Jr, et al: Deliberate donor-specific transfusions prior to living related renal transplantation: A new approach. Ann Surg 192:543, 1980.

77. Montgomery, RA, et al: Plasmapheresis and intravenous immune globulin provides effective rescue therapy for refractory humoral rejection and allows kidneys to be successfully transplanted into cross-match positive patients. Transplantation 70:887, 2000.

78. Ross, CN, et al: Renal transplantation following immunoadsorption in highly sensitized recipients. Transplantation 55:785, 1993.

79. Hodge, EE, et al: Pretransplant removal of anti-HLA antibodies by plasmapheresis and continued suppression on cyclosporine-based therapy after heart-kidney transplant. Transpl Proc 26:2750, 1994.

80. Kickler, T, et al: A randomized, placebo-controlled trial of intravenous gamma globulin in alloimmunized thrombocytopenic patients. Blood 75:313, 1990.

81. Tyan, DB, et al: Intravenous immunoglobulin suppression of HLA alloantibody in highly sensitized transplant candidates and transplantation with a histoincompatible organ. Transplantation 57:553, 1994.

82. Karuppan, S, Ericzon, BG, and Moller, E: Relevance of a positive crossmatch in liver transplantation. Transpl Int 4:18, 1991.

83. Gugenheim, J, Samuel, D, and Reynes, M: Liver transplantation across ABO blood group barriers. Lancet 336:519, 1990.

84. Mathew, J, et al: Biochemical and immunological evaluation of donor-specific soluble HLA in the circulation of liver transplant recipients. Transplantation 62:217, 1996.

85. Shaw, LR, Miller, JD, and Slutsky, AS: Ethics of lung transplantation with live donors. Lancet 338:461, 1991.

86. Gruessner, AC, and Sutherland, DER: Analysis of United States (US) and non-US pancreas transplants reported to UNOS and the International Pancreas Transplant Registry as of October, 2001. Clin Transpl 2001:41, 2002.

Chapter 22

Relationship Testing

Robert W. Allen, PhD, and Chantal Ricaud Harrison, MD

OBJECTIVES

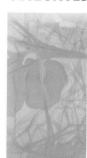

1. State the goals of parentage testing.
2. List the criteria used to select a genetic system for parentage testing.
3. Briefly describe the testing technologies used for the different types of genetic systems.
4. Outline the advantages and disadvantages of the different types of genetic systems.
5. Define and give examples of false direct and indirect exclusions.
6. List at least two causes of false exclusions produced using serologic testing and one cause of false exclusion with DNA typing.
7. Define paternity index, probability of paternity, and power of exclusion.
8. List organizations involved and resources available in quality improvement for parentage testing laboratories.

Introduction

The frequency with which relationship (parentage) testing is performed in the United States has risen to the point that in 2008 the AABB Annual Report Summary for Testing listed approximately 415,000 cases performed. The growth of parentage testing in the United States has its roots in the rapid rise in illegitimacy during the 1960s and 1970s and the government's efforts to identify primarily delinquent fathers and force them to provide financially and emotionally for their children. However, the field of parentage testing, or more appropriately now "relationship testing," has expanded over the past 20 years to include criminal investigations, immigration, and the identification of human remains from disasters, war, or genocide.

Relationship testing also has relevance to the physician or blood banker in the visualization in real life of somewhat abstract concepts learned in genetics in school and perhaps practiced with fruit flies in an undergraduate laboratory. Genetic disease, transplantation, and even transfusion of specialized blood products may call for basic knowledge and ability in predicting the passage of genetic traits from one generation to the next. **Relationship** or **parentage testing** refers to the testing of genetic markers that are inherited to confirm or refute a biological relationship. This test is most commonly applied to determine whether a male is the biological father of a child, but it can also be applied to determining maternity and other kinships.

History

The processes currently used to resolve cases of questioned parentage can be traced back to the statistical analysis published by Bernstein[1] in 1924 demonstrating that the ABO blood group frequency distribution in Austria was most compatible with a three-allele theory. ABO blood group test results were first used to establish nonpaternity in Vienna in 1926. As other blood groups were described and their inheritance established, they were used with the ABO system for paternity studies. In 1955, Smithies[2] described the charge polymorphism of haptoglobin, which could be revealed through gel electrophoresis; this opened the door to a new type of genetic system: enzymes and proteins.

The next step occurred in 1972, when the extreme polymorphism of the human leukocyte antigen (HLA) system was demonstrated at the Evian workshop organized by Dausset.[3] All these genetic systems were expressed on different elements of the blood (red blood cells [RBCs], proteins, and leukocytes), but they had one important aspect in common: The detection of the polymorphisms were all dependent on a complex biochemical expression of the original genes. This group of genetic systems is often termed the **classic systems**.

The molecular genetics technology developed over the next decade laid the foundation for a revolution in parentage testing, heralded by the description by Jeffreys[4] in 1985 of a new type of polymorphism in human DNA: hypervariable minisatellites often referred to as **variable number tandem repeats** (VNTR). New genetic systems, tested by technologies that directly assess the variability of DNA, have now become the norm. These are called **DNA polymorphisms**.

Over the past decade, there has been a rapid evolution of the DNA polymorphism testing technologies used for relationship testing and forensic analysis. Early on, VNTR systems were tested by treating the extracted DNA with restriction enzymes followed by Southern blotting and hybridization to VNTR probe(s). This technology, referred to as **restriction fragment length polymorphism** (RFLP) testing, dominated the field for several years. Figure 22–1 is a schematic representation of RFLP analysis from genomic DNA.

However, RFLP testing ceded precedence to **polymerase chain reaction** (PCR) technology. Originally, PCR was often used to detect polymorphisms caused by point mutations or sequence-specific polymorphisms but soon was used to analyze VNTR-type loci in which the repeated unit was small

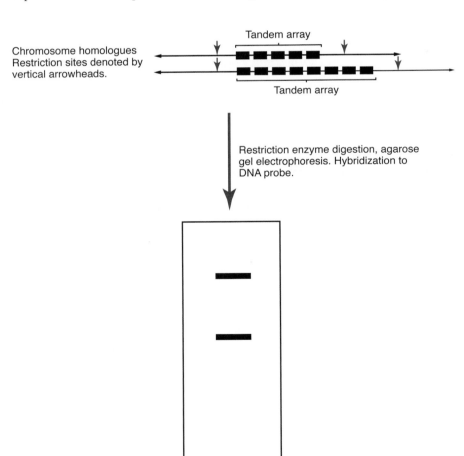

Chromosome homologues Restriction sites denoted by vertical arrowheads.

Tandem array

Tandem array

Restriction enzyme digestion, agarose gel electrophoresis. Hybridization to DNA probe.

Figure 22–1. Schematic representation of RFLP analysis from genomic DNA. Chromosomal DNA extracted from a biological specimen (i.e., blood, buccal swab, or some other tissue) is digested with restriction endonuclease (vertical arrowheads). One pair of homologous chromosomes is shown that contains a VNTR. Among the thousands of restriction fragments produced are the two shown in the figure that harbor the tandemly repeated sequence (five repeats in one chromosome and eight repeats in the other). The restriction digest is electrophoresed in an agarose gel, and the fragments are transferred to a nylon membrane using Southern blotting. The membrane is hybridized to a labeled DNA probe targeting the tandem array, and the specific VNTR alleles are visualized through autoradiography (if the probe is radioactively labeled) or through another visualization method (colorimetric or chemiluminescence).

(i.e., 4 to 5 nucleotides). Such loci are termed *short tandem repeat* or **small tandem repeat** (STR) loci.

Goals of Testing

The ultimate goal of relationship testing is to confirm or refute a specific biological relationship between two or more individuals whose relationship is in question (usually a child and a father or a mother). When applied to the usual trio (mother, child, and alleged father), the goals are to exclude all falsely accused men and to provide compelling inclusionary evidence if a man is not excluded.

Criteria for Selection of Genetic Systems

The following factors are considered when selecting genetic systems to use for parentage testing:

1. The system should be polymorphic—that is, it should have multiple alleles, ideally in Hardy-Weinberg equilibrium.
2. The inheritance pattern should be well established and follow Mendel's rules.
3. The mutation rate should be known and should be low.
4. Possible genotypes should be readily deducible from the phenotype.
5. Testing methodology should be reliable, reproducible, and available in more than one laboratory.
6. Markers tested should be stable and not affected by environmental factors, age, disease, reagents, or methodology employed.
7. Databases of allele frequencies should be available for all ethnic groups that may be tested.
8. Allelic distributions should be able to provide a high probability of excluding a falsely accused man.
9. Each genetic system should be known to be genetically independent (e.g., no linkage disequilibrium) of all other genetic systems used by the laboratory in the test battery.

Types of Genetic Systems and Technology Used

Box 22–1 lists the most common classic genetic systems that were widely used in the past. In the last few years, there has been an almost entire migration of laboratories to rely on DNA polymorphism testing using STR systems and PCR technology. Although literally thousands of STR loci exist in human DNA, 13 core STR loci plus amelogenin (for sex determination) were officially recognized by the FBI as the "core" loci to be used to create and query the database of convicted offender DNA profiles (CODIS). Table 22–1 lists the chromosomal locations of the most common STR loci in current use.

RBC Antigens

Six blood groups have been routinely used in paternity testing: ABO, Rh, MNSs, Kell, Duffy, and Kidd. These systems have been in use for a very long time, and their potential pitfalls in interpretation are well known from the vast, worldwide experience accumulated. Phenotype determination is based on standard RBC agglutination techniques with regulated

---

BOX 22–1

Classic Genetic Systems Used in Parentage Testing

RBC Antigens

- ABO
- Rh
- MNSs
- Kell
- Duffy
- Kidd

RBC Enzymes and Serum Proteins

- PGM1
- ACP
- ESD
- Hp
- Gc

Immunoglobulin Allotypes

- Gm
- Km
- Am

HLA

- A and B locus

Table 22–1	Chromosomal Locations of Most Common STR Genetic Systems in Current Use	
LOCUS	**CHROMOSOMAL LOCATION**
D2S1338	2
D3S1358	3p21
D5S818	5q21–q31
D7S820	7q
D8S1179	8q24.1–24.2
D13S317	13q22–q31
D16S539	16q22–24
D18S51	18q21.3
D19S433	19
D21S11	21p11.1
CSF1PO	5q33.3–34
FGA	4q28
HUMTHO1	11pl5–15.5
TPOX	2p23–2pter
VWA	12p12–pter

reagents and, with some extra built-in quality control steps, is indistinguishable from testing performed daily in most blood banks or transfusion services. This is why, prior to the introduction of DNA testing methods, the majority of laboratories performing relationship testing were associated with a blood bank or a transfusion service. In performing serologic testing, duplicate testing of each specimen was required, and it was also recommended that testing be done by two individuals using two different sources of antisera. Such test redundancy ensured the accuracy of test results traceable to interpretive errors and antiserum reagent variability. There may be only one or two laboratories that still conduct antigen testing for cases of questioned parentage. The College of American Pathology, which administers the only proficiency test for parentage, no longer reports participant responses (because no laboratory submits them) for serologic testing; therefore it is difficult to know the number of laboratories still using this technology as part of their testing.

RBC Enzymes and Serum Proteins

Testing of RBC enzymes and serum proteins is also rarely, if ever, performed. Testing methodology consists of separating the different allelic proteins based upon net charge using electrophoresis, followed by staining. Subtyping of the *PGM1* and *Gc* alleles may be done using isoelectric focusing, which allows separation of molecules with only slightly differing net charge, thereby increasing the extent of polymorphism of the system. When isoelectric focusing is used, it is customary to refer to the system with a subscript letter i (e.g., $PGM1_i$ or Gc_i).

Phenotypes are identified by the number or respective position of the bands detected and comparison with control specimens expressing at least two known allotypes that are tested in parallel with the unknown specimens. Interpretation of the band patterns must be performed independently by two observers. Rare variants exist in most systems, and the laboratories should maintain a file of variants to permit identification of rare phenotypes when they are encountered.

Immunoglobulin Allotypes

Three immunoglobulin chains demonstrate a polymorphism that has been applied to paternity testing. The gamma heavy chain expresses the Gm polymorphism, the kappa light chain expresses Km (also termed Inv), and the alpha heavy chain expresses Am. Determination of the phenotype is done by hemagglutination inhibition using indicator RBCs coated with antibodies of known phenotype and reagent anti-Gm, anti-Km, or anti-Am. Reagents are not widely available, genetic interpretation is complex, and phenotypic interpretation is often not possible in infants younger than 6 months of age because of interference with maternal immunoglobulins. For these reasons, few laboratories in the world now use these genetic systems. They are described here solely for the sake of completion and historical perspective.

HLA

The HLA complex represents the most polymorphic genetic system in the human genome. As discussed in the previous chapter, it comprises multiple linked loci expressed as class I and class II antigens. In relationship testing with classic methodology (non-DNA), only antigens expressed by the A and the B loci are part of the testing performed.

The usual method for revealing the HLA phenotype is termed *microlymphocytotoxicity*. HLA phenotyping depends on the evaluation of the reactions of live lymphocytes with a panel of cytotoxic antibodies of known specificity in the presence of complement. Testing is performed in 60 or 72 microwell trays preloaded with reagent antisera. A sufficient number of antisera should be used so that all HLA-A and HLA-B specificities recognized by the 1980 HLA Nomenclature Committee of the World Health Organization can be reliably identified. Additional antigens should be tested if appropriate antisera can be obtained. The larger the number of antigens that can be defined, the more powerful the system becomes—that is, the better it can exclude falsely accused men. Because of the large number of existing antigens, no single tray can identify all relevant antigens. Some antigens occur more frequently in specific racial groups, and specially designed trays are available for African Americans and Asians. Such trays should be selected when appropriate.

Antisera are of human origin (alloantisera) or are monoclonal (created in the laboratory), and monospecific sera are generally not available for a large number of antigens. It is required that each antigen be defined by at least two different operationally monospecific sera, by one monospecific and two multispecific sera, or by three multispecific sera. Phenotypes must be verified by reading two independent trays or tray sets. Each tray or tray set must be read independently.

In interpreting phenotypes, a certain amount of expertise is needed, requiring knowledge of cross reactivity between antigens and splits of broader reactivity (e.g., A9 splitting into A23 and A24) and familiarity with the unexpected reactivity of the antisera used (false-negative or extra reactions). Because of the variability of HLA antisera, it is recommended that all individuals in a parentage case be tested in the same laboratory, ideally with the same reagents.

DNA Polymorphisms: RFLP

RFLP refers to polymorphisms in DNA that can be revealed by restriction enzyme digestion because of nucleotide sequence differences that either create or destroy restriction sites; this alters their linear arrangement on a chromosome and, hence, the size of DNA fragments produced by the accompanying digestion. Restriction enzymes recognize specific DNA sequences of four to six bases and cut the double-stranded DNA at that site. These enzymes have been isolated from bacteria and are named after the bacteria from which they were isolated (e.g., Eco RI from *Escherichia coli* RY13; Hae III from *Haemophilus aegyptius*).

After DNA is incubated with the restriction enzyme (digestion step), it is electrophoresed in an agarose gel to separate the DNA fragments according to length. DNA present in the gel is then denatured and transferred by blotting (Southern blotting) to a membrane that is then subsequently hybridized with a labeled probe to reveal the DNA fragments corresponding to the locus tested. Phenotypes are defined as the length of the DNA fragments in kilobases (kb), estimated through comparison to a sizing ladder consisting of DNA fragments of known size. Some variability in migration may occur within a gel, depending on the position of the electrophoretic lane (band shifting), and it is recommended that mixtures of DNA of each alleged parent with each child be electrophoresed together in a single lane to maximize resolution and to normalize potential electrophoretic anomalies. Ultimately, the goal of the process is to confirm or refute sharing of alleles between alleged parent and child. **Figure 22–2** illustrates this process.

Although RFLP analysis is a suitable technique to reveal insertion or deletion or single nucleotide substitution–type

polymorphisms, it is VNTR-type polymorphisms that were the target of RFLP analysis by parentage laboratories because of their high discriminatory power characteristics. As shown in **Figure 22–2**, the fragment size of VNTR alleles depends on the number of repeats they contain and the restriction enzyme utilized. This is an important concept: The phenotype of the same individual at the same locus will differ between two laboratories if each uses a different restriction enzyme. This is why, when reporting RFLP results, it is mandatory to identify not only the locus and probe tested but also the restriction enzyme used. In the United States, the most common restriction enzymes used were Hae III and Pst I, whereas in Europe, Hinf I was more popular. **Table 22–2** illustrates the different band sizes obtained on the same individuals at the same locus when using different restriction enzymes.

An important limitation of RFLP analysis of VNTR polymorphisms is that allele identification is based upon an estimate of the size of a restriction fragment that generally consists of thousands of nucleotides. As in any quantitative measurement, there is variability, which is referred to as sigma (σ). One variable is the ability to distinguish two alleles that are similar in size (alleles differing by only a few repeats). Resolution may vary greatly among laboratories, depending on the methodology utilized, especially the technical conditions used during electrophoresis. The limit of resolution is referred to as delta (δ).

Because of these two sources of variability, allele frequency distribution of VNTR alleles using RFLP analysis is continuous as opposed to the discrete distribution of allele frequencies as in the classic genetic systems. For example, in most laboratories, a DNA fragment measured at 1.60 kb cannot be considered different from a fragment measured at 1.57 kb or 1.63 kb. Through the use of validation, each laboratory must identify the limit of resolution for which two closely spaced alleles cannot be distinguished from one another. This range of "matching sizes" is called a *bin*. The allele frequency used in the statistical calculations is actually the frequency of all the alleles falling into the bin for the allele size measured. Since the bin size varies with the technical characteristics of the laboratories, the final statistical result (i.e., likelihood ratio, probability of parentage, or probability of exclusion) may differ between two laboratories for the same locus with the same restriction enzyme, even if their band sizes are identical.

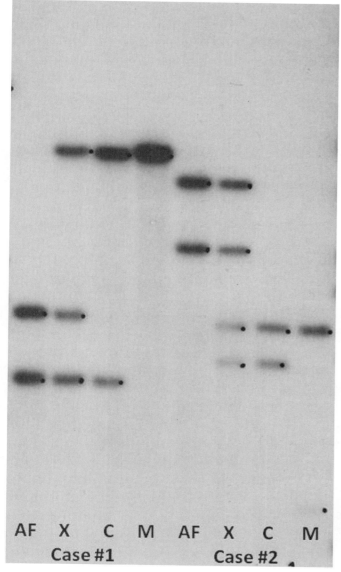

Figure 22–2.   RFLP analysis in two paternity cases. DNA extracted from blood samples of an alleged father (AF), child (C), and mother (M) in two paternity cases were subjected to RFLP analysis using a radioactively labeled DNA probe directed against the D16S85 locus. Profiles visualized in case #1 show the AF to be included because he shares the smaller of his two alleles with the child, and this is the obligate gene in the child's profile. In contrast in case #2, the AF and the child do not share any alleles; this is evidence of nonpaternity for this tested man. The lanes marked "X" represent mixtures of DNA from the AF and the C to maximize resolution of the RFLP process.

Table 22–2	**DNA-RFLP Results in a Parentage Test at the D2S44 Locus**		
RESTRICTION ENZYME USED FOR DIGESTION			
INDIVIDUAL TESTED	**Hae III**	**Hinf I**	**Pst I**
Mother	3.43, 4.25	4.55, 5.36	12.68, 13.53
Child	2.91, 3.43	4.03, 4.55	12.16, 12.68
Alleged father	2.91, 3.13	4.03, 4.25	12.16, 12.46

These VNTR loci are very polymorphic and thus are very powerful for excluding falsely accused men and in providing compelling inclusionary evidence in true biological relationships. However, their mutation rate can be up to 2 per 1,000, which is small but not negligible.[5] In the past 5 years, laboratories have stopped using RFLP to test VNTR genetic systems, moving instead to technologies that involve PCR amplification of VNTR-type polymorphisms.

DNA Polymorphisms: PCR

The transition of relationship testing laboratories from serology and HLA to RFLP analysis was short lived, largely because of the characterization of VNTR loci consisting of tetranucleotide repeats that could be amplified using PCR. **Figure 22–3** shows PCR amplification of STR loci using fluorescent detection. The figure shows STR amplification products separated in one of four capillaries in the array that are labeled with either red or green fluorescent dye (depending on the particular STR locus). Electropherograms are displayed as fluorescent bands (right panel) or as a histogram, the latter of which is the more common method for STR profile presentation. The banding results are correlated with the histogram by capillary number. The lane or histogram panel shown in capillary #2 represents an allelic ladder containing all common alleles in the population for the different STR loci amplified and is used as a reference to identify the alleles in unknowns.

DNA typing using STR loci and PCR amplification eliminated many of the shortcomings associated with RFLP analysis. The amount of DNA required for testing dropped about a thousandfold; this made it possible to use buccal swabs as a source of DNA instead of blood samples, which were often difficult to collect from newborns. The reduced quantity of DNA needed also allowed for direct DNA testing from prenatal samples of amniotic fluid or chorionic villi (CVS).

A second advantage of STR analysis is the increased resolution of alleles associated with **polyacrylamide gel electrophoresis** (PAGE) and **capillary electrophoresis** (CE), which can reliably distinguish two DNA fragments differing by a single base pair. With the enhanced resolution of the electrophoresis systems came the ability to designate STR alleles as discrete alleles, naming each based upon the number of repeats of the tetranucleotide or pentanucleotide contained within the PCR amplicon. Eliminating the use of bins in the matching process and in determining allele frequencies also greatly improved the acceptance of STR typing in court. Third, the technology allows simultaneous testing of several loci by multiplex amplification and very fast allele identification by capillary electrophoresis. This is conducive to automation and a faster turnaround time.

The panels of STR loci currently in use consist mostly of repeats with core sequences of four bases (tetranucleotide repeats), although a few loci based on core sequences of five bases (pentanucleotides) have recently been introduced. A group of 12 loci dominates the field in conjunction with a 13th locus, amelogenin, that identifies the sex of the sample donor and nothing else. This group has been selected by the FBI as the core testing panel for a nationwide databank of crime scene DNA evidence material and reference samples from convicted felons. **Box 22–2** lists the STR loci included in the FBI Combined Offender DNA Index System (CODIS) database.

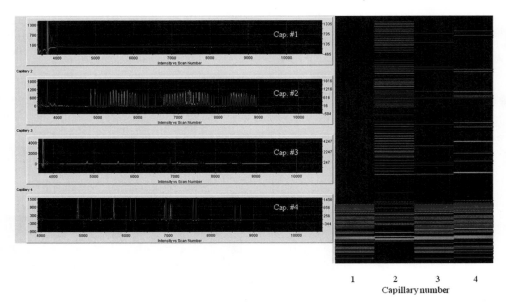

Figure 22–3. PCR amplification of STR loci using fluorescent detection. Genomic DNA recovered from a biological sample is added to a multiplex PCR reaction containing fluorescently labeled primers for multiple STR loci. Following amplification, PCR products are separated by size using polyacrylamide gel or, in this case, capillary electrophoresis. The gel or capillary is then irradiated with a laser, causing the STR alleles to emit light at several wavelengths depending on the particular fluorescent dye coupled to the different primers. In this figure, STR alleles are displayed in one of two formats—horizontal bands in a gel track much like traditional RFLP profiles or in the newer histogram format that is the norm among STR typing laboratories that use capillary electrophoresis platforms to separate STR alleles. In addition, whereas current STR multiplex kits contain PCR primers targeting as many as 16 different loci and labeled with 4 different fluorescent dyes, the allele pattern shown in Figure 22–4 has been simplified to show only the STR loci amplified from primers labeled with green or red fluorescent dyes. Size of the PCR amplicons and the color emitted serve to identify the particular genetic marker visualized and the particular allele present in a sample.

STR Systems Included in the FBI Combined Offender DNA Index System (CODIS) Database

- D3S1358
- D5S818
- D7S820
- D8S1179
- D13S317
- D16S539
- D18S51
- D21S11
- CSF1PO
- FGA
- THO1
- TPOX
- VWA
- Amelogenin

Readily available commercial kits provide convenient multiplex amplification for loci selected to match the CODIS STR core loci plus additional STR markers to further enhance the discriminatory power of the multiplex. A group of STR loci located on the Y chromosome has also become available and has successfully delineated the male lineage within family groups. Y-STR analysis can be especially useful for establishing or refuting a claimed relationship within the male lineage of a pedigree. However, caution must be used in reporting results since all males within the lineage are equally likely to be the parent, brother, grandfather, uncle, and so on, of a male child whose paternity is in question.

Phenotypes for all STR loci should be reported following the recommendations of the International Society for Forensic Genetics, which means that alleles are identified by the repeat number. Variants that have additional bases to an exact repeat number are identified by the repeat number followed by a period and the number of additional bases (e.g., a common allele of TH01 is 9.3, which means that it has 9 tetranucleotide repeats and 3 additional bases).

Mitochondrial DNA

In addition to polymorphism contained within nuclear DNA, **mitochondrial DNA** (mtDNA) exhibits **single nucleotide polymorphisms** (SNPs), which can be useful in kinship testing. To reveal these SNPs, noncoding hypervariable segments (the displacement loop) of mtDNA are amplified by PCR and then sequenced. The sequence is then compared with a published reference mtDNA sequence. Since mitochondria are passed on with the cytoplasm of the oocyte and not by spermatozoa, mitochondrial DNA is passed from mother to child. Therefore, mtDNA typing is especially useful when analyzing a questioned maternal lineage.

Mitochondrial DNA appears to be stable for extremely long periods (thousands of years), probably because the mtDNA genome is small and there are 500 to 1,000 copies present in most cells in the body. These genetic systems have been applied to anthropological studies aimed at solving human evolution questions. Preserved mitochondrial DNA has also been isolated from mummies and fossils.[6] This technique is very useful in demonstrating maternal lineage in long-distance relatives such as grandmother to grandchild, and it was applied to the authentication of the remains of the family of Tsar Nicholas II of Russia, who were assassinated during the Bolshevik uprising.[7]

Terminology and the Interpretation of Results

In interpreting the testing results on a classic trio (mother, child, and alleged father), it is always assumed that the mother is the biological mother. This assumption sets the stage for the analysis of results in that it is expected that the mother and child will share at least one allele. Therefore, the remaining allele in the child's profile is of paternal origin and can be compared with the profile of the alleged father (AF). If the AF lacks the paternally inherited allele in the child, he is excluded as the biological father. If he is not excluded, a statistical analysis is performed to determine his relative probability of being the biological father of the child as compared with a random man unrelated to him or to the mother.

There is terminology associated with relationship testing that deserves some discussion. Two terms that ultimately define the overall result of the testing are **exclusion** and **inclusion**. Although the definitions of these terms may seem obvious, the criteria by which these terms are used to communicate results have evolved along with the technologies used for testing. For example, when serology was widely used for testing, a single inconsistent test result between alleged parent and child could be sufficient to exclude parentage. For example, a type AB child could not be the offspring of a type O alleged parent.

Exclusion Criteria for Classical Systems

In classical systems, inconsistencies have been customarily referred to as *exclusions*, direct or indirect, with the rule that a single direct exclusion was enough to exclude the alleged father as the biological father of the child, while at least two indirect exclusions were necessary to form a final conclusion of exclusion. A **direct exclusion** exists when either the child possesses a marker that is not present in either the mother or the alleged father (e.g., the child is K-positive while both the mother and the alleged father are K-negative) or when the alleged father demonstrates two different markers in the same system and the child does not demonstrate either (e.g., an AB alleged father with an O child).

On the other hand, an **indirect exclusion**, also referred to as **apparent opposite homozygosity**, exists when the child demonstrates only one marker (i.e., appears to be homozygous for the marker) and the alleged father demonstrates a different single marker (i.e., appears to be homozygous for an opposite marker). As this situation requires the assumption of homozygosity, it is considered indirect evidence. The transmission of an alternate allele that is either silent or not routinely tested for can lead to this apparent opposite homozygosity in a true biological parent/child pair. Such alleles exist at a low but significant frequency in most of the classical systems.

Exclusion Criteria for DNA Systems

One consequence of the technology shift to DNA-related methods was the discovery of the rather high mutation rate characteristic of the VNTR systems.[5,8] Such mutation rates were sufficiently high to cause a laboratory to be wary of single DNA mismatches between alleged parent and child as compelling evidence of exclusion. Mutations associated with VNTR loci are generally the result of DNA replication errors that occur during meiosis and alter the number of repeats in the tandem array. Changes in the number of repeats is usually small (i.e., 1% to 3% of allele size for VNTR loci detected with RFLP methods and single repeat changes for STR loci), and repeats can be added to or subtracted from daughter alleles with approximate equal frequency.[5,8] There is a confirmed difference in mutation rate in the male versus female lineages, with males exhibiting a 10- to 20-fold higher rate than females for some loci, possibly due to an increased number of cell divisions that occur during spermatogenesis (Table 22–3).

Although the mechanism underlying alterations in repeat number resulting from mutation in VNTR loci is not certain, current evidence does not support unequal recombination between sister chromosomes during meiosis as the mechanism. Rather, it appears the replicative complex responsible for DNA replication "slips and jumps" as it moves down a chromosome. If the complex "slips" and remains in one spot on the chromosome while replicating, a new repeat may be added to the daughter strand. If the complex "jumps" over a repeat due to a loopout of the DNA template or for some other reason, a repeat may be lost from the daughter chromosome. The net effect of either occurrence will be the production of a gamete harboring a genetic marker distinct from the parent. If this gamete is involved in conception, the offspring will differ from the parent. When an inconsistency in the inheritance pattern is detected in a DNA system, the term *exclusion* is not used; instead, the terms *mismatch* or *inconsistency* are used to indicate that the alleles between the child and the alleged father do not match. The term *exclusion* is reserved for the final interpretation of the entire set of genetic systems tested. A minimum of two mismatches is required before an opinion of nonpaternity (or nonmaternity) is rendered. Interestingly, because of the large number of STR loci tested routinely, some laboratories require three mismatches to conclusively exclude an alleged parent, especially if all three mismatches involve single repeat changes.

Inclusionary Calculations

Three types of statistical evaluations can be calculated when the alleged father is not excluded: the parentage index (PI), the probability of paternity (PP), and the probability of exclusion (PE). The three calculations producing the values defined by these terms are based on the assumption that the "random man" with whom the tested man is compared is biologically unrelated to him or to the mother. The standard calculations are not valid if a brother, father, uncle, or other close biological relative of the tested man is a possible biological father of the child.

Another important aspect of the calculations is the need to have accurate allele frequencies for each genetic system tested, estimated from databases drawn from an adequate sample population of the appropriate ethnic group. When referring to a sample size for a database, the term *adequate* will depend largely upon the degree of polymorphism exhibited by the genetic marker in question. In general, the larger the number of alleles exhibited by the marker, the larger the population sampling needed to create a valid allele frequency database. In contrast, databases created for STR loci may consist of only 200 to 300 individuals because there are far fewer alleles possible.

Paternity Index

The **paternity index** (PI) compares two mutually exclusive hypotheses that are expressed as a likelihood ratio. The numerator generally states the mathematical probability of producing a child genetically identical to the tested child, through a mating of the known parent with the alleged

Table 22–3	Summary of Mutation Rates for STR Loci	
LOCUS	**PATERNAL LINEAGE**	**MATERNAL LINEAGE**
CSF1PO	0.002021	0.000283
D13S317	0.001743	0.000436
D16S539	0.001127	0.000481
D18S51	0.00253	0.000748
D19S453	0.000745	0.000596
D21S11	0.001709	0.001295
D2S1338	0.001526	0.000245
D3S1358	0.001691	0.000211
D5S818	0.001742	0.0003
D7S820	0.001348	0.000073
D8S1179	0.002031	0.000333
FGA	0.003713	0.000522
PENTA D	0.000259	<0.000253
PENTA E	0.00026	<0.000253
THO1	0.00007	0.000043
TPOX	0.00013	0.000081
VWA	0.003258	0.000494

Data from the 2008 AABB Annual Report Summary for Relationship Testing Laboratories. Available at www.aabb.org/sa/facilities/Documents/rtannrpt08.pdf.

parent. The denominator mathematically states the probability of producing the child through a mating of the known parent with a randomly selected, unrelated individual in the same ethnic population. The PI is calculated one genetic system at a time and is sometimes referred to as the *system index* (SI). If all the genetic systems tested are independent from one another, the overall final PI is the product of all the system indices calculated. When the PI is greater than 100, the evidence for paternity is considered very strong. Figure 22–4 shows STR typing in a paternity case involving two alleged fathers, and Table 22–4 outlines the testing results for the case. For the D3S1358 system, the mother and child share the 18 allele, thus the obligatory gene (paternal

allele in the child) is 16. Alleged father #1 (AF1) is heterozygous for this allele; thus, his chance of passing it on to an offspring is 50% (i.e., 0.5). Alleged father #2 (AF2) is homozygous for allele 16 and thus will pass it to 100% of his offspring. The population frequency for allele 16 is 0.232. Therefore, the system index calculation for AF1 takes the following form:

$$SI = [(0.5M \text{ passing } 18)(0.5AF \text{ passing } 16)]/[(0.5M \text{ passing } 18)(0.232RM \text{ passing } 16)]$$
$$SI = 0.5/0.232 = 2.16.$$

Therefore, based upon this test result alone, AF1 is 2.16 times more likely to be the father of the child than is a

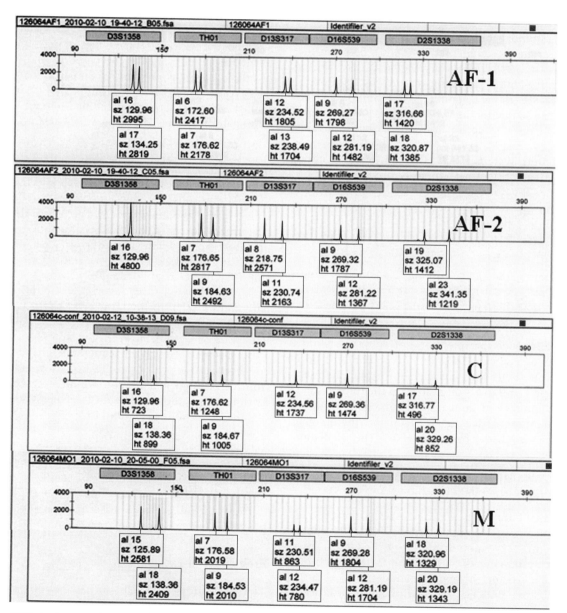

Figure 22–4.   STR typing in a paternity case involving two alleged fathers. DNA was extracted from buccal swabs from two alleged fathers (#1 and #2), a child, and a mother and subjected to STR analysis using the Identifiler STR typing kit (Applied Biosystems, Foster City, CA). Products were separated and analyzed using capillary electrophoresis on an ABI310 Genetic Analyzer (Applied Biosystems, Foster City, CA). Shown in the figure are the results from those loci labeled with the green fluorescent dye known as JOE consisting of 5 of the 15 STR loci co-amplified with the Identifiler kit. Shown under each peak in the histogram are labels containing the allele identification (labeled "al"), the size of the amplicon (labeled "sz"), and the intensity of the fluorescence (labeled "ht"). The results of the analysis are shown in Table 22–4.

Table 22–4	System Indices Produced in a Paternity Case with Two Alleged Fathers					
SYSTEM	**MOTHER**	**CHILD**	**ALLEGED FATHER #1**	**PI (AF#1)**	**ALLEGED FATHER #2**	**PI (AF#2)**
D3S1358	15, 18	16, 18	16, 17	2.1598	16	4.32
TH01	7, 9	7, 9	6, 7	1.4819	7, 9	2.96
D13S317	11, 12	12	12, 13	1.6197	8, 11	0
D16S539	9, 12	9	9, 12	4.8077	9, 12	4.8
D2S1338	18, 20	17, 20	17, 18	2.8835	19, 23	0

PI = Parentage Index

random man of the same ethnic background. Interestingly, AF2 is twice as likely to be the father of the child as is AF1, because he is homozygous in phenotype at the D3S1358 locus. However, he is excluded as the child's father at the D13S317 and D2S1338 loci because he lacks the obligate alleles seen in the child. This is one reason why it is important for a parentage testing laboratory to test multiple genetic markers in a trio so that random coincidences are not overly emphasized in developing an opinion of inclusion and exclusion about a case.

In the second system listed, the mother and child are phenotypically identical, so it is uncertain which allele, 7 or 9, is the obligatory gene. AF1 is heterozygous for allele 7 and thus is included as a possible father. However, the SI calculation must consider both allele 7 and allele 9 as possible obligatory genes and takes the following form:

SI = [(0.5M passing 9)(0.5AF passing 7) + (0.5M passing 7)(0AF passing 9)]/[(0.5M passing 7)(0.0.165RM passing 9) + (0.5M passing 9)(0.172RM passing 7)]
SI = 1.48

Again, AF2 has twice the likelihood of being the child's father, in this case because his phenotype contains both possible obligate alleles seen in the child (i.e., he can transmit either allele 7 or 9 to his offspring). In the third system, the child is homozygous and inherits one copy of allele 12 from the mother. AF1 is heterozygous for the obligate allele and will pass it with a frequency of 0.5. The calculation thus becomes:

SI = [(0.5M passing 12)(0.5AF passing 12)]/[(0.5M passing 12)(0.309RM passing 12)] SI = 1.62

The overall PI for both AF1 and AF2 is the product of the individual system indices for the five STR systems shown in **Figure 22–4** and **Table 22–4**. For AF2, since two of those systems have SI values of 0, the combined paternity index is 0 and the man is excluded. For AF1, the individual system indices are multiplied to produce a combined paternity index of 71.74. This value means that AF1 is about 72 times more likely than is a random man to produce the single sperm that contains all the genetic information this child inherited from his or her biological father.

Probability of Paternity

The **probability of parentage** (PP) is a restatement of the weight of the evidence for parentage, expressed in percentage form. To calculate the PP, the parentage index previously discussed is incorporated into a statistical theory developed by Bayes that allows multiple types of evidence for and against a hypothesis to be combined into a final statement of probability: In the case of parentage testing,

PP = ([(PI)(prior for)]/[(PI)(prior for) + prior against]

In order to calculate the PP, a value for a prior probability favoring a hypothesis must be chosen and included in the formula. The value for the prior essentially reflects the probability of the hypothesis being true before the testing was performed. In the case of a relationship test, the prior probability reflects the evidence favoring parentage of a child before any genetic testing is performed. Typically, Relationship (parentage) testing laboratories assign a neutral prior of 0.5 (i.e., 50%), neither favoring nor refuting the alleged parent/child relationship. However, based upon available information, a judge can change the prior to something other than 0.5. For example, if an alleged father has a sperm count 1% of normal, that could reduce his fertility and a judge could reduce the prior probability to 1% or at least reduce it from 50%. Such a reduction would necessitate a higher PI value to get the same final PP value. When the prior is 0.5, the PP formula is reduced to:

$$PP = PI/(PI + 1)$$

Currently, laboratories target a PP of 99% or greater as the threshold of proof of parentage for an alleged parent. At the 99% level, the burden of proof shifts from the known parent to prove the alleged parent is a true parent to the alleged parent to prove they are not a true parent.

Probability of Exclusion

The **probability of exclusion** (PE) is the probability of excluding a falsely accused man, given the phenotypes of the mother and the child. This probability is entirely dependent on the mother-and-child phenotype combination and does not require knowledge of the alleged father's phenotype. It is evaluated by first calculating the proportion of men who would not be excluded; this number is called *random men not excluded* (RMNE). The probability of exclusion is 1 − RMNE. If p is the sum of all frequencies of the possible paternal alleles, then RMNE = p (2 − p) for each genetic system. The overall RMNE for all the genetic systems tested is the product of the RMNE values for each system, and the overall probability of exclusion is 1 − overall RMNE. In the case shown in **Table 22–4**, the overall RMNE is:

$$0.410 \times 0.560 \times 0.197 \times 0.316 = 0.0075,$$

and the combined probability of exclusion is 0.9925. The probability of exclusion represents the proportion of untested men who would have been excluded by the extent of testing performed (99.25% in this case) and can sometimes be more easily understood by a layperson, such as a jury member or a judge. The PP is a more accurate way to quantify the situation, because it includes all the genetic information available, whereas the probability of exclusion does not take into account the phenotype of the alleged father.

Nonclassic Situations

The majority of parentage testing cases consist of the classic trio of mother, child, and alleged father. However, nonclassic cases are more and more frequently encountered. This is largely because the newer DNA technologies are better able to give reliable answers in these situations. It is not unusual to attempt to establish the presence or absence of a biological relationship between an alleged parent and a child when the known parent is unavailable for testing.[9] Calculations in such situations follow the typical procedure with the exception that a "random known parent" is substituted into the PI equation in place of the known transmission frequency for the allele shared between the known parent and the child, which is generally 0.5 to 1 (depending on the zygosity). When a "random known parent" must be included in the calculation, both alleles in a heterozygous child could have come from the known parent and their respective transmission probabilities are set to equal the population frequency for each.[9]

Occasionally, the alleged parent is deceased, and a reconstruction of his or her possible genetic makeup is attempted by testing all available and known parents, siblings, and other undisputed children of the alleged father. Other biological relationships, such as siblings, may be in question in adoption, immigration, or inheritance cases.

Advantages and Disadvantages of Genetic Systems

The classic systems have the advantage of the vast experience accumulated over the decades during which they have been in place in many countries. Phenotypes are well recognized and consistently reproducible from laboratory to laboratory. Potential pitfalls have been thoroughly studied, gene frequency distributions are available for almost every population in the world, and the mutation rate has been shown to be extremely low (less than one in a million). Statistical analyses in inclusion cases give extremely consistent results between laboratories.

However, they do have some serious drawbacks when compared with the newer technologies that test DNA polymorphisms. In particular, each genetic system, except for the HLA-A and HLA-B antigens, has a relatively low average power of exclusion. The highest power of exclusion for a classical system is achieved by $PGM1_i$ at 0.32, followed by MNSs and Gc_i at 0.31 and Rh 0.27, respectively. Virtually all other systems have a power of exclusion below 0.20. In contrast, the HLA-A and HLA-B antigens, analyzed as a haplotype, have a power of exclusion of 0.87. By testing all the classic systems, a high power of exclusion can be achieved, but it is almost impractical to go beyond 0.99. In addition, to get the full benefit of these systems, one must be competent with a multiplicity of techniques.

Fairly rigid restrictions exist on the type, amount, and quality of samples needed for testing. Because of the small number of alleles existing in each system, often no more than two or three, serologic test batteries lack efficacy in nonclassic cases. Finally, because serologic markers represent the products of genes, mutations in those genes altering expression can complicate the interpretation of parentage test results, producing false direct and false indirect exclusions of alleged parents who are true parents of a child.

The DNA polymorphisms by RFLP are extremely powerful genetic systems with average powers of exclusion almost always above 0.50 and often reaching above 0.90 per genetic system. Thus, testing only four different loci by DNA-RFLP ensures very high levels of PP for nonexcluded men. The sample required is any tissue or body fluid from which sufficient DNA can be extracted. Peripheral blood, buccal smears, amniotic fluid, chorionic villi, and tissue biopsies can be analyzed. Once extracted, DNA can be kept frozen for an indefinite period. However, the technique is time-consuming and labor-intensive, and turnaround times are long. The main drawback, however, may be the lack of precise correlation in the final PI value between laboratories testing the same loci. This is because, as previously discussed, the phenotypes consist of measured band sizes, with the unavoidable difficulties caused by a built-in incertitude in measurement. This can be very confusing when results from a case tested in several different laboratories are compared, and the results may give a false impression of unreliability to someone who is unfamiliar with the limitations of the methodology.

The DNA polymorphisms analyzed using PCR avoid this difficulty because they return to a discrete allele distribution. When identifying alleles of an STR genetic system based on fragment length polymorphisms, one can actually identify the number of repeats and not simply a length of DNA subject to an imprecision in measurement. This technique has the least restriction in the amount and type of sample needed but the highest requirement for environmental controls to prevent sample contamination because it is based on high amplification of a very small amount of DNA.

A great advantage of DNA-PCR technology is the ability to amplify as many as 15 or more loci in a single amplification reaction. Current instrument technology allows the routine resolution of 15 STR loci with analysis within 4 to 5 hours. Individually, these systems are not as powerful as individual DNA-RFLP systems, and so two to three times the number of STR markers need to be analyzed to achieve the same discriminatory power as DNA-RFLP systems. Both types of DNA polymorphisms have in common a significantly higher mutation rate than the classic systems have. As previously discussed, this has resulted in abandoning the concept of direct and indirect exclusion that has been so effective in classic systems. A mismatch observed in a DNA polymorphism system should lead to the calculation of a system index, which takes into account the rate of mutation for that system. A single mismatch should never lead to an interpretation of nonpaternity but rather to the testing of additional systems.

Social and Legal Issues

Currently, more than 400,000 cases of relationship testing are performed every year in the United States (www.aabb.org/sa/facilities/Documents/rtannrpt08.pdf). The majority of these cases are done to establish paternity for children, with the aim of obtaining child support. Child support enforcement agencies in all states actively pursue the identification of the biological father of children who are eligible for their Aid to Families with Dependent Children for the purpose of seeking child support. Contracts with child support agencies account for most of the activity of many relationship testing laboratories. The majority of cases outside the child support enforcement agencies also have a legal implication, such as child support, custody in divorce cases, inheritance rights, immigration, and more recently, the identification of human remains in natural disasters or in cases of murder. Occasionally, cases also have criminal implications relating to incest or statutory rape. STR testing is also widely used in other areas of medicine, including monitoring engraftment in patients who received a bone marrow transplant, assessing the purity of DNA presumably extracted from pregnant mothers that may actually represent a mixture of maternal and fetal DNA, and the identification of pathological specimens thought to perhaps be mislabeled or contaminated with someone else's tissue during processing.

Regardless of the application for the technology, every step in the collecting, storing, processing, and testing of the samples must be carefully documented as to time of occurrence and person performing the task. An unbroken chain of custody must be maintained. The individuals tested must be carefully verified, and procedures must be in place to ensure that unauthorized persons do not have access to the samples or test results. Without careful attention to these aspects, the results may not be valid in court. If called to testify on the validity and significance of the testing results, the laboratory director must be able to re-create from the documented evidence every step in the handling of the case.

Accreditation and Quality Issues

Approximately 30 years ago, the American Association of Blood Banks (AABB) took the lead in promoting the establishment of standardization and quality in the field of paternity testing and created a standing committee on parentage testing. This committee offered educational opportunities such as workshops and publications. With the participation of the American Medical Association, the American Bar Association, and the Office of Child Support Enforcement, the Committee on Parentage Testing organized an international conference in 1982 in Airlie, Virginia, where a group of international experts established a consensus approach for the interpretation of inclusionary evidence. An accreditation program for parentage testing laboratories was implemented, and the first edition of *Standards for Parentage Testing Laboratories* was published in 1990. A complementary *Accreditation Requirements Manual* followed in 1991. The College of American Pathologists, with joint sponsorship by the AABB, initiated a proficiency testing program for parentage testing laboratories in 1993.

Continuing involvement by professional organizations in the promotion of quality improvement and in the provision of opportunities for continuing education in the field of paternity testing is essential to maintain a high level of accuracy and consistency in ascertaining biological relationships (see Chapter 23, "Quality Management").

CASE STUDIES

Case 22-1

An African American trio consisting of a mother, child, and alleged father is tested to establish paternity. The following results are obtained:

Genetic System	Mother	Child	Alleged Father
ABO	O	B	A
D3S1358	15,18	16,18	16,17
THO1	7,9	7,9	6,7
D13S317	11,12	12	8,11
D16S539	9,12	9	9,12
D2S1338	18,20	17,20	17,18

1. Which of the genetic systems tested excludes the AF?
   a. THO1 and D16S539
   b. ABO and D13S317
   c. ABO and THO1
   d. No system excludes the AF
2. Given the test results in question 1, if this was the only testing performed, would you exclude the AF based upon currently accepted standards for parentage testing?
   a. Yes
   b. No

Case 22-2

A white trio consisting of a mother, child, and alleged father is tested to establish paternity. The following results are obtained:

Genetic System	Mother	Child	Alleged Father
ABO	A	O	B
MNSs	MNs	MNs	NSs
D10S28/Hae III	3.34, 2.98	3.34, 4.52	1.95, 4.52
D2S44/Hae III	3.42, 4.24	2.90, 3.42	2.90, 3.11
D3S1358	15, 16	15, 17	14, 18
FGA	21, 22	22, 25	20, 25
TH01	6, 9.3	9, 9.3	7, 9

1. The fourth genetic system tested (D2S44/Hae III) represents a(n):
   a. RBC antigen system tested by agglutination
   b. RBC enzyme system
   c. DNA polymorphism tested by RFLP
   d. STR-DNA polymorphism tested by PCR

2. The fifth genetic system tested (D3S1358) represents a(n):
   a. RBC antigen system tested by agglutination
   b. RBC enzyme system
   c. DNA polymorphism tested by RFLP
   d. STR-DNA polymorphism tested by PCR

3. Among the following statements relating to the interpretation of these results, choose the one that is true:
   a. The alleged father is excluded due to a direct exclusion at D3S1358.
   b. The alleged father may be excluded due to an inconsistency at D3S1358.
   c. A mutation may have occurred at D3S1358.
   d. The alleged father is excluded due to a direct exclusion in the ABO system.

SUMMARY CHART

✔ Relationship (parentage testing) refers to the testing of genetic markers that are inherited to determine the presence or absence of a biological relationship.

✔ The ultimate goal of relationship (parentage testing) is to confirm a specific biological relationship with the individual in question, usually a father or a mother or sometimes a sibling.

✔ The blood group systems used most often in paternity testing are ABO, Rh, MNSs, Kell, Duffy, and Kidd.

✔ The HLA complex represents the most polymorphic genetic system in the human genome; only antigens expressed by the A and B loci are considered for relationship testing with non-DNA-based typing.

✔ RFLP refers to polymorphisms of the DNA that can be detected by restriction enzymes; polymorphisms detected in relationship testing relate to the presence of VNTR.

✔ In PCR, the DNA fragment of interest is amplified in amount thousands of times, and the resulting product is normally identified directly through fluorescence resulting from fluorescently labeled primers incorporated in the PCR reaction.

✔ STRs have repeats that are 4 to 5 bp long.

✔ STR present on the Y chromosome can verify only male lineage.

✔ Mitochondrial DNA can verify only maternal lineage.

✔ The term *mismatch* is used when the bands between the child and the alleged father do not match; a minimum of two mismatches is required before an opinion of nonpaternity (or nonmaternity) is rendered.

✔ A direct exclusion occurs when a marker is detected in the child and is absent in the mother and the alleged father or when the alleged father's phenotype demonstrates two markers and the child has neither one of them.

✔ An indirect exclusion occurs when a single marker is detected in the child and a different single marker is detected in the alleged father.

✔ False direct exclusions can occur as the result of mutations that are significant enough to alter the final product, lack of precursor substance, suppressor activity at a locus unlinked to the one tested, or chimeric state of one of the tested individuals.

✔ False indirect exclusions occur secondary to the presence of silent alleles (e.g., *Fy*).

Review Questions

1. Among the combinations of attributes described below, select the one that would *not* be suitable for a genetic system used in parentage testing analysis.
   a. The system has multiple alleles in Hardy-Weinberg equilibrium.
   b. The system has a high mutation rate.
   c. Databases of allele frequencies are available for all ethnic groups tested by the laboratory.
   d. All systems selected are genetically independent from each other.

2. In which of the following genetic systems is the allele frequency distribution continuous (not discrete)?
   a. DNA polymorphisms by RFLP
   b. DNA polymorphisms by PCR
   c. RBC antigens
   d. RBC enzymes

3. A false direct exclusion in RBC antigen genetic systems can be caused by:
   a. A silent allele
   b. A lack of precursor substance
   c. An alternate untested allele
   d. Weak reagents

4. Among the following organizations, which one offers an accreditation program for parentage testing laboratories?
   a. AABB
   b. ASCP
   c. FDA
   d. HCFA

References

1. Bernstein, F: Ergebnisse einer biostatischen zusammenfassenden Betrachtung über die erblichen Blutstrukturen des Menschen. Klin Wschr 3:1495, 1924.
2. Smithies, O: Zone electrophoresis in starch gels: Group variations in the serum proteins of normal human adults. Biochem J 61:629, 1955.
3. Histocompatibility Testing 1972. Proceedings of the 5th International Conference. Evian. Munksgaard, Copenhagen, 1973.
4. Jeffreys, AJ, Wilson, B, and Thein, SL: Hypervariable "minisatellite" regions in human DNA. Nature 314:67, 1985.
5. Brinkman, B, et al: Mutation rate in human microsatellites: Influence of the mutation and length of the tandem repeat. Am J Hum Genet 62:1408, 1998.
6. Krings, M, et al: Neanderthal DNA sequences and the origin of modern humans. Cell 90:19, 1997.
7. Ivanov, P, et al: Mitochondrial DNA sequence heteroplasmy in the grand duke of Russia: Giorgig Romanov establishes the authenticity of remains of Tsar Nicholas II. Nat Genet 12:417, 1996.
8. Edwards, M, and Allen, RW: Characteristics of mutations at the D5S818 locus studied using a tightly linked marker. Transfusion 44:83–90, 2004.
9. Brenner, CH: A note on paternity computation in cases lacking a mother. Transfusion 33:51, 1993.

Bibliography

AABB: Guidance for Standards for Parentage Testing Laboratories, 5th ed. American Association of Blood Banks, Bethesda, MD, 2002.

AABB: Standards for Parentage Testing Laboratories, 5th ed. American Association of Blood Banks, Bethesda, MD, 2001.

Allen, RW, Wallhermfechtel, M, and Miller, WV: The application of restriction fragment length polymorphism mapping to parentage testing. Transfusion 30:552, 1990.

Annual report summary for relationship testing laboratories. American Association of Blood Banks, 2008. Available at www.aabb.org/sa/facilities/Documents/rtannrpt08.pdf.

Brinkmann, B, Klintschar, M, Neuhuber, F, Huhne, J, and Rolf, B: Mutation rate in human microsatellites: Influence of the structure and length of the tandem repeat. Am J Hum Genet 62:1408–1415, 1998.

Committee on DNA Forensic Science: The Evaluation of Forensic DNA Evidence: An Update. National Academic Press, Washington, DC, 1996, pp 53–54.

Edwards, M, and Allen, RW: Characteristics of mutations at the D5S818 locus studied using a tightly linked marker. Transfusion 44:83–90, 2004.

Polesky, HF: Parentage testing: Use of DNA polymorphisms and other genetic systems. In Henry, JB (ed): Clinical Diagnosis and Management by Laboratory Methods, 20th ed. WB Saunders, Philadelphia, 2001, pp 1390–1401.

Walker, RH: Molecular biology in paternity testing. Lab Med 23:752, 1992.

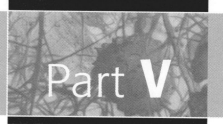

Quality and Compliance Issues · Part V

Chapter 23

Quality Management

Lucia M. Berte, MA, MT(ASCP)SBB, DLM, CQA(ASQ)CMQ/OE

OBJECTIVES

1. Explain the differences between compliance and quality management.
2. List the three building blocks of quality.
3. Describe the framework of a quality system for a blood bank and a medical laboratory.
4. List 12 quality management system (QMS) essentials and the blood bank operations to which they are applied.
5. Describe a process using a flowchart.
6. Explain the role of validation in introducing a new process.
7. Name at least five blood bank process controls.
8. Describe the differences between a form and a record.
9. Explain the importance of document control for procedures.
10. State the differences between remedial and corrective action.
11. Describe the role of auditing in a QMS.
12. Identify at least six sources of input that can be used to improve processes.
13. Define the activities in a problem-solving process.
14. Describe the four types of quality costs.
15. Explain how to transition the QMS of a blood bank into that for a whole laboratory.

Introduction

Several dictionaries define *quality* as "the degree to which a product or service meets requirements." Blood banks must provide quality to their customers in many forms, including:

- Safe, satisfying donation experiences for blood donors.
- Accurately labeled and tested blood components provided to transfusion services.
- Timely, accurate transfusion services provided to physicians and other health-care personnel.
- Safe and efficacious blood transfusions to patients.

Blood centers, hospital blood banks, and transfusion services need to embrace the following quality philosophy to ensure a high degree of safe blood donation and transfusion practices to regulatory agencies, accrediting agencies, blood donors, physicians, patients, and patients' families:

> Quality, safety, and effectiveness are built into a product; quality cannot be inspected or tested into a product. Each step in the process must be controlled to meet quality standards.[1]

The method for bringing this quality philosophy into all operations involves each facility developing the building blocks of quality: quality control (QC), quality assurance (QA), and quality management system (QMS). When the building blocks are assembled, and the facility's management and staff are actively involved in monitoring and maintaining the QMS, quality management (QM) has been achieved.

Compliance Versus Quality Management

Blood bank compliance with federal regulations and accreditation standards is required by the following organizations:

- United States Food and Drug Administration (FDA)[2,3]
- The Joint Commission[4,5]
- College of American Pathologists (CAP)[6]
- American Association of Blood Banks (AABB)[7]

Compliance programs evaluate how effectively the facility meets the requirements by detecting errors, deficiencies, and deviations. **Compliance inspections** (also called *surveys* or *assessments*) measure the state of the facility's program with respect to the applicable requirements at a single point in time and are usually conducted every 1 to 2 years. Although this process may seem logical, compliance programs alone are inadequate to identify and prioritize a facility's problems.

Compliance simply requires the correction of identified deviations and deficiencies and usually leaves the facility with the false sense that it has solved its problems and has been brought into compliance. However, subsequent inspections often reveal the same deviations and deficiencies because the facility's current QC and QA programs do not identify the fundamental quality problems. Remember that quality cannot be inspected into a process; regulatory and accreditation inspections only find deviations and deficiencies *after* they occurred. Facilities need to design work processes in a way that *prevents* deficiencies and errors from occurring in the first place.

Quality management (QM) is actively and continuously practiced by the blood bank's leaders, managers, and staff throughout all blood bank operations. With QM, the blood bank is always ready for an inspection because it validates its processes, monitors process performance, knows where the problems are, continuously takes action to determine root causes of problems and removes them, and documents its actions. In QM organizations, quality is everyone's job all the time. Quality is not something we do in addition to our jobs—it's built *into* our jobs!

Quality Building Blocks

The building blocks of quality are **quality control** (QC), **quality assurance** (QA), and **quality management systems** (QMS). **Figure 23–1** demonstrates these building blocks and their internationally accepted definitions.[8]

Quality Control

Most blood bank technologists are familiar with routine blood bank QC procedures, such as daily testing of the reactivity of blood typing reagents; calibrating serologic centrifuges; and monitoring temperatures of refrigerators, freezers, and thawing devices. Requirements for the type and frequency of QC are determined in regulations and accreditation standards, manufacturers' operator manuals and package inserts, and state and local requirements. Regular performance of QC reveals when a method, piece of equipment, or procedure is not working as expected.

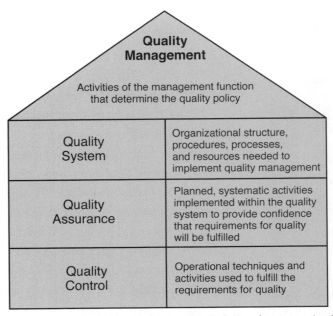

Figure 23–1. The building blocks of quality. *(Definitions from International Organization for Standardization: ISO 9000:2005 Quality management systems—Fundamentals and vocabulary. International Organization for Standardization, Geneva, 2005.)*

Quality Assurance

QA is a set of planned actions that ensure that systems and elements that influence the quality of the product or service are working as expected, individually and collectively.[8] QA looks beyond the performance of a test method or piece of equipment; it addresses how well an entire process, which is a sequence of activities, is functioning. This is particularly important in those processes that cross functional or departmental lines. For example, a blood center could monitor the number of times and reasons why a set of collected whole blood units transported from the collection site to the component processing site did not arrive in time or was not in an acceptable condition to make blood components. In the transfusion service, it is important to monitor the source, the number of times, and the reason why specimens collected for compatibility testing do not meet predetermined acceptance criteria. Box 23–1 lists common QC and QA activities and indicators practiced by most blood banks.[9]

Quality Management Systems

A quality guideline published by the FDA[10] set the meaning, emphasis, and organization of quality activities for blood banks. Accrediting agencies such as the Joint Commission and AABB have established their quality requirements to be more comprehensive and more coordinated than either QC or QA. A QMS provides a framework for applying quality principles and practices uniformly across all blood bank operations, starting with donor selection and proceeding through transfusion outcomes.

In its *Standards for Blood Banks and Transfusion Services*,[8] the AABB defined **quality system essentials** (QSEs) for blood collection and transfusion service facilities and the blood bank operations to which they are applied. Box 23–2 lists the QSEs and blood bank operations on which the AABB assesses blood banks in its accreditation program.

The next sections of this chapter describe the blood bank's role and responsibilities in fulfilling QMS essentials, which extend far beyond historic QC and QA practices. Figure 23–2 demonstrates that the QMS essentials are the building blocks that support blood bank operations in the path of workflow for both donor centers and transfusion services.

Quality Management System Essentials

The QMS essentials are in a logical order that can be explained as follows for any new or changed product or service. The blood center or transfusion service organization develops its mission, vision, values, goals, and objectives around the products and services it plans to offer. The facility should have a customer focus by determining the needs and expectations of its customers and designing its processes and procedures to meet those needs and all regulatory and accreditation requirements. The blood center or transfusion service should have the physical facilities to support the products and services offered and ensure that safety

---

BOX 23–1

Common Blood Bank QC Activities and QA Indicators

QC Activities

Collection Equipment
- Microhematocrit instrument
- Hemoglobin instrument
- Apheresis equipment
- Blood-weighing scales

Blood Components
- Red blood cell hematocrit
- Cryoprecipitated antihemophilic factor
- Platelet counts in platelet units
- Residual leukocyte counts in leukocyte-reduced components
- Bacterial contamination of platelet units

Reagents
- Copper sulfate
- Reagent red blood cells
- Reagent antisera
- Test kits for infectious disease testing

Laboratory Equipment
- Heating instruments
- Water baths
- Thawing devices for blood components
- pH meters
- Cell counters
- Centrifuges, refrigerated and serologic
- Cell washers
- Blood irradiators
- Refrigerators
- Freezers
- Platelet incubators
- Blood warmers
- Shipping containers

QA Indicators
- Number of donor forms with incomplete or incorrect information
- Number and types of unusable units and blood components
- Number of blood typing discrepancies in donors and patients
- Number of and reasons for invalid tests
- Number of and reasons for labeling check failures
- Number and source of improper and incomplete requests for blood components
- Number and location of patients without proper identification at time of specimen collection or transfusion
- Number of, source of, and reasons for unacceptable specimens
- Number of times wrong component or ABO was selected for crossmatch or use
- Number and type of transfusion complications
- Number of and reasons for turnaround time failures

---

requirements are met. The facility determines the qualifications needed for each job and hires qualified personnel who are trained and who maintain competence in their assigned duties.

Before products and services can be provided to customers, equipment and materials need to be purchased and maintained in inventory. Equipment needs to be managed according to manufacturer, regulatory, and accreditation requirements. Before any work can commence, the facility needs to design, document, and validate work processes with appropriate management to ensure their correct performance. Documents provide instructions for how the work generates records of work performance. Patient and donor information is managed in a way to ensure that requirements

---

BOX 23–2

QMS Essentials and Blood Bank Operations

QMS Essentials[8]

- Organization
- Facilities and safety
- Personnel
- Purchasing and inventory
- Equipment
- Process management
- Documents and records
- Nonconformance management
- Assessments
- Continual improvement

Blood Bank Operations[8]

- Donor qualification
- Autologous donor qualification
- Apheresis donor qualification
- Blood collection
- Cytapheresis collection
- Preparation of components
- Testing of donor blood
- Final labeling
- Final inspection before distribution
- Patient samples and requests
- Serologic confirmation of donor blood ABO/D
- Pretransfusion testing of patient blood
- Selection of compatible blood and components for transfusion
- Crossmatch
- Special considerations for neonates
- Selection in special circumstances
- Issue for transfusion
- Blood administration
- Rh-immune globulin

---

resources, and receives reports and information from all hospital departments. The hospital-based blood bank or transfusion service must participate in blood bank quality-related activities, laboratory-wide quality initiatives, and the hospital's continual improvement program. The blood bank should state in writing its policies, goals, and objectives for each of the QMS essentials and relate them to the bigger laboratory and hospital quality goals. There should be an organizational chart showing the following:

- Relationships among blood bank personnel by job title
- The blood bank's link to the laboratory
- The blood bank's link to the hospital
- How the blood bank links to the hospital's quality function

A freestanding blood center must develop and manage the entirety of its QMS. There may be a quality council represented by top-level management from the various departments. The council develops the blood center's QMS policies, goals, and objectives and its strategies for QMS implementation; provides resource support; prioritizes identified improvement projects; and provides support for cross-functional process improvements. There may also be a quality steering committee composed of senior managers and department staff who operationalize the quality strategies and implement process improvements.

for confidentiality and information integrity are met. The process of capturing information on nonconformances is managed to identify recurring process problems that can affect patient safety, laboratory credibility, and the operating budget. Internal and external assessments measure and monitor the facility's performance to identify opportunities for improvement. The facility should constantly strive for continual improvement.

Organization

The type and size of the organization determine the configuration of the blood bank's QMS. In hospitals, there is usually an organization-wide quality function or department that prioritizes and coordinates quality projects, approves

Customer Focus

Although both blood centers and transfusion services toil on behalf of patients, the real customers of these facilities is the entity or person who receives and must be satisfied with a product or service.[8] For blood centers, the customers are the donors, who want a safe and satisfying donation experience, and the transfusion services served by the blood center, which want properly tested and labeled blood components of the appropriate types on demand. For transfusion services, customers are the physicians, who want the blood transfusions they order to occur in a timely manner, and the nurses, who want the correctly issued blood components in a timely manner for administration to patients. For all types of facilities, internal customers are the employees.

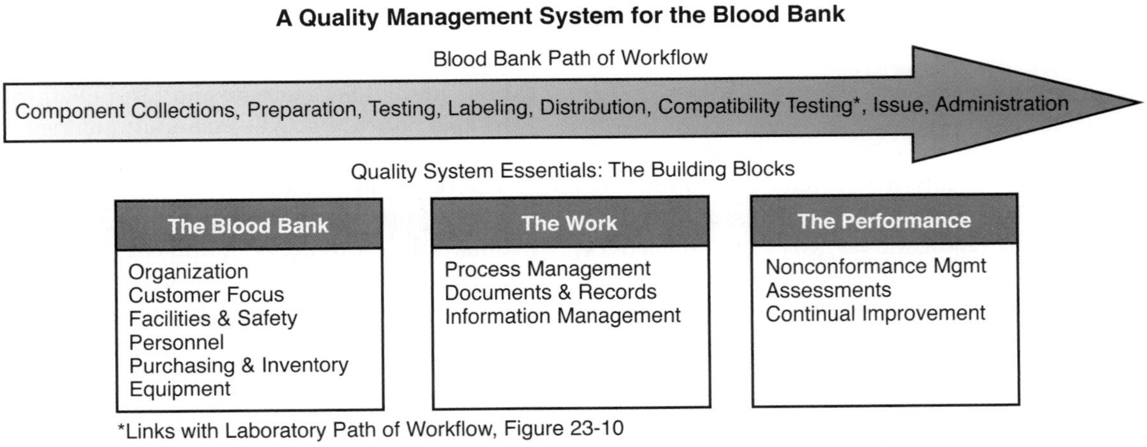

A Quality Management System for the Blood Bank

Blood Bank Path of Workflow

Component Collections, Preparation, Testing, Labeling, Distribution, Compatibility Testing*, Issue, Administration

Quality System Essentials: The Building Blocks

The Blood Bank	The Work	The Performance
Organization	Process Management	Nonconformance Mgmt
Customer Focus	Documents & Records	Assessments
Facilities & Safety	Information Management	Continual Improvement
Personnel		
Purchasing & Inventory		
Equipment		

*Links with Laboratory Path of Workflow, Figure 23-10

Figure 23–2. A quality system for the blood bank, showing the relationship of quality management system essentials to blood bank operations.

The important issue about having a customer focus is to understand the customer's needs and design the work processes and procedures to meet those needs. In addition to fulfilling customer needs, the processes and procedures must also meet regulatory and accreditation requirements.

Facilities and Safety

In hospitals, the Joint Commission mandates an environmental control program that addresses all significant environmental issues for facility management and maintenance such as temperature control, electrical safety, fire protection, and so forth.[4] The Joint Commission also requires that hospital laboratories have training programs for all laboratory personnel on emergency preparedness, chemical hygiene, and infection control.[4] Therefore, hospital-based blood banks and transfusion services are already participating in facilities management and safety training. In addition, any blood bank that performs irradiation of blood components must also have a radiation safety program and document appropriate training.

A freestanding blood center must develop its own facility management program. All regulations and accreditation requirements for emergency preparedness, chemical hygiene, infection control, and radiation safety training and documentation also apply.

Personnel

Quality begins and ends with people. However, a quality problem is seldom an individual employee's fault. Rather, a quality problem is almost always due to a faulty work process. All the quality policies, goals, and objectives in the world do not ensure safe and effective blood components and transfusions unless the people involved in blood banking know how their job fits into the organization, are trained to know the work processes and procedures, and demonstrate ongoing competence by doing it right the first time, every time. Blood bank management needs to work with the blood center's or hospital's human resources departments to define qualifications for all blood bank jobs and to write job descriptions that include educational qualifications, experience, and federal, state, and local licensing requirements, where applicable, so that qualified persons can be hired. Box 23–3 lists the major types of training that personnel need to receive once they are hired. This training extends significantly beyond only the task specifics of a particular job. Periodic evaluation and documentation of the continuing competence of personnel to perform their assigned job functions and tasks is also required. Competence assessment challenges can include direct observation of job task performance, review of records, and written, verbal, or practical tests.

Purchasing and Inventory

In hospital-based blood banks and transfusion services, contract and purchasing issues are usually handled by the hospital's purchasing department. Blood bank personnel may or may not have control over the specific vendors with

---

BOX 23–3

Training for New Employees

Orientation
- Organization
- Department
- Section

Quality Training
- Current good manufacturing practice (cGMP)
- QMS
- Team skills
- Problem-solving skills

Computer Training
- Facility information system (hospital, blood center)
- Department information system (e.g., laboratory)
- Personal computers
- E-mail
- Scheduling
- Online documentation

Safety Training
- Emergency preparedness
- Accident reporting

- Chemical hygiene program
- Hazardous waste disposal program
- Infection control (including universal precautions, bioterrorism)
- Radiation safety, where applicable

Work Processes and Procedures Training
- Work processes performed on the job
- Procedures performed
- New work processes and procedures
- Revised work processes and procedures

Compliance Training
- Medicare necessity requirements
- Fraud and abuse reporting
- Concerns about quality and safety

---

which the organization has agreements to purchase blood components, reagents and kits for testing, equipment, and other important supplies and materials. At a minimum, hospital-based blood banks and transfusion services need to have a process by which incoming blood components and critical supplies are inspected and tested, where required. In addition, blood banks and transfusion services need to have effective processes for managing inventories of reagents, supplies, and blood components.

Blood centers need to have specified processes for selecting vendors of equipment, supplies, and services, and for entering into and amending agreements. In addition, blood centers must also have processes for receipt, inspection, and testing (where required) of incoming critical materials (such as blood bags and infectious disease testing kits), blood components (such as leukocyte-reduced platelets), and blood products (such as albumin, clotting factor concentrates, and immune globulins).

Equipment

The blood bank needs to have a process for installing new equipment and ensuring its proper functioning before it is used in daily operations. Schedules for calibration, preventive maintenance, and QC are required, with frequencies determined by regulations, accreditation requirements, manufacturers' written instructions, usage, testing volume, and equipment reliability. In addition to temperature-controlled equipment (e.g., refrigerators, freezers, incubators), instruments such as automated analyzers, readers, pipettors, and washers must also be installed and functioning properly before routine use. Defective equipment and instruments must be identified and repaired when necessary. Records must be kept of all installation, calibration, maintenance, and repair activities.

Process Management

A **process** can be defined as a set of interrelated resources and activities that transforms inputs into outputs. **Process control** is a set of activities that ensures a given work process will keep operating in a state that is continuously able to meet process goals without compromising the process itself. **Total process control** is the evaluation of the performance of a process, comparison of actual performance to a goal, and action taken on any significant difference. Process control is a means to build quality, safety, and effectiveness into the product or service from the beginning. It is important to understand and document the sequence of activities in a process, develop and write procedures for the individual activities, validate the entire process to ensure that it works as expected before actual use, measure process parameters to see that they stay in control, and understand when and why the process has variations.

The FDA has published its requirements for process control as the current *Good Manufacturing Practices* (cGMP) that are cited in the Code of Federal Regulations.[2,3] The cGMP requires that facilities design their processes and procedures to ensure that blood components are manufactured consistently to meet the quality standards appropriate for their intended use.

Flowcharts

Figure 23–3 is a sequential flow of the elements of total process control. An effective tool for understanding a process is the flowchart. **Flowcharts** graphically represent the sequence of activities in a process and show how the inputs are converted into outputs. Flowcharts help to develop a common understanding of a process. Mapping a facility's current work processes reveals bottlenecks; missing actions; decision points; dead ends; and choices that can lead to errors, delays, and unnecessary work. Mapping a new process facilitates understanding of where human and other resources will be needed for successful accomplishment. Flowcharts can be created on paper or with commercially available software programs. Figure 23–4 is a sample flowchart for the activities in the pretransfusion testing process. It illustrates different decision points and test method choices.

Standard Operating Procedures

A **work process** involves one or more persons who perform a sequence of activities over a period of time. A process flowchart describes "who does what and when" in a visual manner and provides a big picture of "how it happens." The boxes in the flowchart represent activities performed by one person; these activities need instructions that answer the question, "How do I do this activity?"

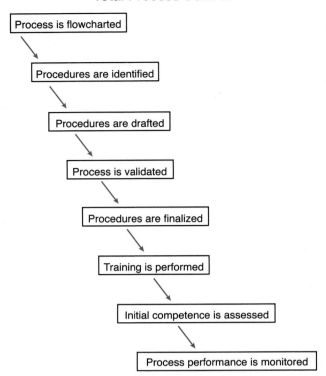

Total Process Control

Figure 23–3. The sequential activities in total process control.

Standard operating procedures provide instructions for each activity in the larger process. For example, the process to provide a physician with a patient's ABO and Rh type involves ordering the test, collecting an appropriate specimen, delivering it to the laboratory, performing the test, and reporting the results. Different people order the test, collect the specimen, perform the ABO/Rh test, and deliver the results. In this process, there needs to be specific written procedures for ordering tests manually or on the computer system, collecting and labeling the blood specimen, delivering the specimen to the laboratory, performing and recording the ABO/Rh testing, and reporting the results.

Validation

To ensure that new processes will work as intended, they must be validated before being put into use. **Validation** tests all activities in a new process to ensure that the process will work in the live environment. For example, when a new test for a transfusion-transmitted disease is added to those performed on donated blood units, the new test method—with its associated instruments, test kits, computer functions, and procedures—must be validated in each blood bank that will perform the new test. The validation ensures that the new test will perform as expected with that blood bank's instrumentation, written procedures, personnel, and computer systems. The culmination of this activity is a validated process and set of new procedures on which all personnel who will perform the new test must be trained. Training must be documented and personnel determined to be competent in the new process and procedures before they are implemented in the live environment.

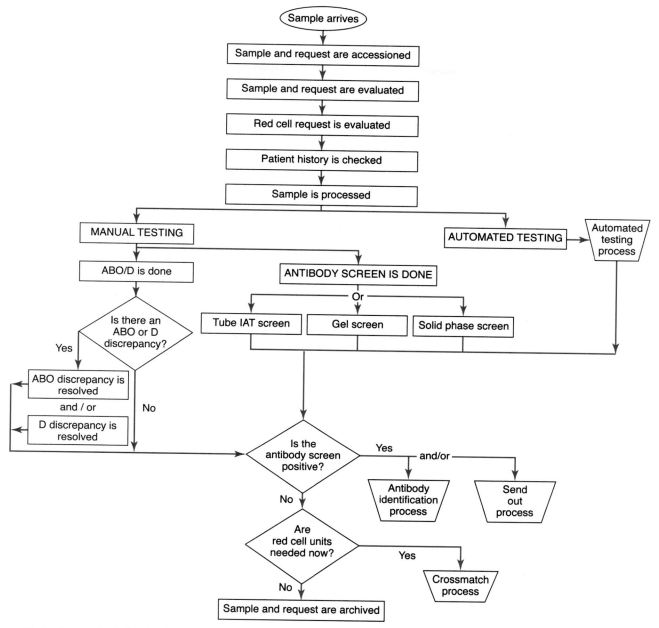

Figure 23–4. An example of a flowchart for the pretransfusion testing process. (*Adapted from Berte, LM (ed): Transfusion Service Manual of SOPs, Training Guides and Competence Assessment Tools, 2nd ed. American Association of Blood Banks, Bethesda, MD, 2007.*)

Process Controls

It is essential to monitor processes to ensure that they are performing as required, to correct process problems before they affect output, and to improve processes to meet changing needs and technology. Routine process controls include:

- QC of test methods and reagents
- Review of work and QC records
- Capture of occurrences when the process did not perform as expected

These routine process controls monitor whether a process is functioning as needed.

Proficiency testing is another example of a process control. In proficiency testing, one laboratory's methods and procedures are compared with those of other laboratories for the ability to get the same result on a set of unknown specimens. Regulations require that all laboratories participate in proficiency testing for diagnostic laboratory testing. Blood bank proficiency test challenges include serologic testing for blood types, detecting and identifying unexpected antibodies, checking compatibility of crossmatched blood, testing for diseases transmitted through blood transfusion, and checking for contamination of prepared blood components.

Other process controls include manual and automated steps to prevent the occurrence of errors. One common process control in serologic testing is the use of green-colored antiglobulin serum to ensure that the antiglobulin serum was indeed added at the antiglobulin phase of testing. Another common process control is the addition of IgG-coated reagent red blood cells after the antiglobulin phase reading to ensure that the antiglobulin serum was working. Computer process controls include automatic comparison of current blood type interpretation with the previous computer records on the same donor or patient to prevent ABO errors and warning signals when ABO-incompatible units are issued for transfusion.

Documents and Records

Documents are approved information contained in a written or electronic format. Documents define the QMS for external inspectors and internal staff. Examples of documents include written policies, process flowcharts, procedures and instructions, forms, manufacturers' package inserts, computer software and instrument operator manuals, and copies of regulations and standards. **Records** capture the results or outcomes of performing procedures and testing on written forms or electronic media, such as manual worksheets, instrument printouts, tags, or labels. Both documents and records must be controlled to provide evidence that regulations and standards are being met.

Document Control

A structured **document control system** links a facility's policies, processes, and procedures and ensures that only the latest approved copies of documents are available for use. A typical document control system is structured as a pyramid, as shown in Figure 23–5. The following example best illustrates how a blood bank should link its policies, processes, and procedures.

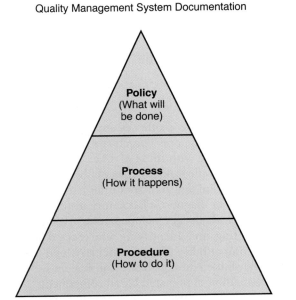

Quality Management System Documentation

Figure 23–5. A simple structure for organizing QMS documents.

The blood bank should have a written policy document stating that the blood bank maintains a process and relevant procedures for correcting erroneous entries or results on a paper record or in the computer. A second document (such as a process flowchart) should describe the sequence of activities in identifying the need for a correction, obtaining any necessary approvals for the changed information, making the correction in the computer or on paper (or both), and notifying all appropriate parties of the correction. Procedure documents instruct staff members how to record the need for a correction, how to obtain any necessary approvals for making the change, how to properly record a change to an entry on a paper record, how to properly record a change to an entry in a computer record, and how to notify appropriate parties of the change and document the notification. The process and procedures should be written in a way that ensures that all regulatory and accreditation requirements are met. Recording the actions taken throughout the process provides a tracking record to provide evidence that the requirements were met.

The blood bank needs a system to control identification, approval, revision, and archiving of its policies, process descriptions, procedures, and related forms. The document control system includes instructions for creating documents in approved formats, assigning document identification and version designation, approving new and revised documents, preparing a master document list, and maintaining document history files. This "change control" process usually requires the completion and routing of a form that contains information about the reason for a new document or a change to an existing one. Other important change information includes when the change was requested; who wants the change; what other documents, if any, are affected by this change; and dates for approval, training, and in-use.

A master copy of the new, approved version is added to the master document history file, which contains copies of all previous versions of that same document. The hard copies within this master file capture the original signatures and provide a paper backup when electronic files cannot be accessed. The master document list is updated with the new version number. When a revised version of a document is ready for release, the distribution process needs to be controlled to ensure that copies of the obsolete document (e.g., procedures in a working manual) are replaced with the new version and the obsolete copies destroyed. Employees should not keep and refer to copies of procedures and forms stashed in lockers, drawers, and personal files. Use of unapproved, outdated documents could lead to errors or omissions that could cause harm to patients.

Records Management

Forms are specially designed documents—either paper or electronic—on which are recorded the results or outcomes of performing a given procedure. Forms are subject to the document control activities described in the previous paragraph. The document identification system should link the form to its respective procedure. Instructions for completion of forms, when needed, can be conveniently placed on the front or back side of the form. When a form (either paper or electronic) is filled out, it becomes a record. Regulations and accreditation requirements mandate the review of records by authorized personnel and specify the type of records and length of time they are stored for possible future reference. State, local, and facility requirements for record retention periods may also apply.

Information Management

Whereas documents provide information about what to do, records tell what happened, who did it, and when it was done. **Information management** activities include using and manipulating the donor or patient information and test results in the facility's paper and electronic information systems. For example, maintaining the confidentiality of privileged donor and patient information is mandated by government regulations,[11] and the facility needs to ensure its processes preserve that confidentiality. The facility must also ensure the integrity of any data or information sent inside or outside the facility, whether the medium used is paper or electronic. For example, the facility needs to verify that information faxed, e-mailed, or sent across instrument and computer interfaces is identical to the original information.

Nonconformance Management

FDA regulations require that blood banks report any error or accident in the manufacture of blood components that may affect the safety, purity, potency, identity, or effectiveness of the component or that compromises the safety of the blood donor or recipient. Each blood bank must have a process for detecting, reporting, evaluating, and correcting deviations and any nonconformance with its own procedures, products, or services. **Nonconformance management** is one name for such a process. Other commonly used names include occurrence, incident, or variation management. Table 23–1 provides definitions of terms used to further classify occurrences of nonconformance in blood banks.

Nonconformance Reporting

Information about events involving the blood bank that deviate from accepted policy, process, or procedure need to be captured and acted upon. Hospitals usually have a risk management program in place; this program type typically captures information about events involving patients and visitors that could result in financial loss to the facility. An internal blood bank nonconformance management system captures and analyzes information about events that occurred across the entire path of workflow for blood collection and transfusion service activities whether or not a patient was involved.

All employees need to participate in nonconformance reporting. It is essential that staff not perceive nonconformance reporting as a tool for finger-pointing or disciplinary action. Instead, all staff needs to understand that nonconformances represent blood bank processes that do not work as they should, so knowledge of these problems provides opportunities for improvement. Nonconformances may be identified

Table 23–1	**Common Classifications of Various Types of Nonconformances**
NONCONFORMANCE TYPE	**DEFINITION**
Accident	Nonconformance generally not attributable to a person's mistake, such as a power outage or an aged instrument's malfunction
Adverse reaction	Complications that occurred to the donor during or after the donation process or to the recipient of transfused blood components
Complaint	Expression of dissatisfaction from internal customers (physicians, employees) or external customers (donors, patients)
Discrepancy	Difference or inconsistency in the outcomes of a process, procedure, or test results
Error	Nonconformance attributable to a human or system problem, such as a problem from failure to follow established procedure or a part of a process that did not work as expected
Postdonation	The receipt of information (call or information letter) from a donor with additional details regarding his or her donation, such as subsequent illness or neglecting to mention an illness or medication

either by staff in the course of routine activities or by supervisors during review of records. Complaints received in the blood bank are also considered nonconformances. The facility needs to capture information about all nonconformances, including those identified before blood components are distributed or issued. In the reporting process, employees describe the who, where, and when and then briefly describe what happened and what they did at the time to remediate the problem. A standard report form can be used to capture information on all occurrences of nonconformance (Fig. 23–6).

Investigation and Corrective Action

Supervisors and quality function personnel record the nonconformances in a spreadsheet or database so that the resolution process can be tracked. The nonconformances are reviewed, investigated, and further classified as errors, accidents, complaints, or another definition.

The immediate action, which is the initial quick-fix solution, is known as **remedial action**. Such remedial actions do not address the real cause of the problem, which can be determined only through investigation. Investigation of complaints or errors provides an opportunity to identify underlying factors that contributed to the problem. Process improvement tools (discussed later in this chapter) are

NONCONFORMANCE REPORT FORM

Database number: ____________________

ORIGINATOR: Reported by: ______________________________
Date and time occurred: ______________________________ Date and time discovered: ____________
Date and time reported: ______________________________

Explain the error / complaint / incident / nonconformance. Attach copies of any relevant records, as needed.

How was the error / complaint / incident / nonconformance discovered?

Describe what you did to take care of the immediate problem (remedial action):

INVESTIGATOR: Name: ______________________________
Findings of investigation: Attach copies of any related paperwork, as needed.

Will remedial action be effective in eliminating future nonconformances of this same type?
Circle one: Yes No

If no, what further action should be taken?

QUALITY DEPARTMENT: Name:______________________________ Date: ____________

Is this nonconformance FDA reportable? Circle one: Yes No
If yes, initiate FDA-CBER report – see procedure.

What further action needs to be taken?

System, process, procedure, form change needed to reduce or eliminate recurrence:

DATABASE ADMINISTRATOR
Entered into database by: ______________________________ Date: ____________

Figure 23–6. An example of a nonconformance report form.

used to identify these contributing factors and to determine the best way to remove them through implementing corrective action.

Most corrective action involves making changes in the process. All employees performing that process must then be informed of the changes and retrained when necessary. Sometimes the corrective action involves retraining only specific individuals who may not have been adequately trained initially or who have been taking unapproved deviations from the established processes or procedures.

The nonconformance reporting process needs to be clearly defined so that information is tracked and acted upon and feedback is provided. The person responsible for the quality function in the blood bank (usually called the QA officer or quality manager) reviews all nonconformance reports, assigns an accession number, and forwards the report form to the sections or departments that will be involved in the investigation. The completed report is returned to the quality officer, who reviews it for completeness and appropriateness of remedial and corrective action. If an identified error or accident needs to be reported to the FDA, the corresponding process is initiated.

In a good nonconformance management program, the nonconformances are also mapped to the specific involved processes in the blood bank's workflow path. This information is trended to determine which processes have the most problems. Identifying problematic processes provides significant support for defending when a process needs to be changed. Facility staff must make a conscious decision not simply to respond with remedial actions but also to use nonconformance information for removing the underlying root causes of the problem and to make improvements that truly contribute to the safety and efficacy of transfusion medicine.

Assessments

Assessments measure the state of a facility's quality program with respect to the applicable requirements at a single point in time. There are internal and external assessments for measuring and monitoring a facility's performance to identify opportunities for improvement.

Internal Assessments

Blood banks need to have processes in place to continuously monitor the effectiveness of its QMS (see **Fig. 23–2** for a review of the QSEs supporting the blood bank's workflow path). Both the quality essentials and the facility's specific operations need to be assessed. Compliance inspection and other checklists[4–8] can be used as assessment tools; however, these assess the adequacy of only the listed items. The quality indicators monitored by hospital-based blood banks and transfusion services as part of the laboratory's QA program are also helpful but do not usually cover all important aspects of each operation.

Each blood bank should review all its processes and ask the question, "What can we monitor on a scheduled basis to ensure that this process is working as needed?" Quantitative indicators can then be derived for which the numerator is the number of times the process did or did not work, and the denominator is the total number of times the process was performed. Common transfusion service examples include the percentage of specimens received in the compatibility testing laboratory not acceptable for testing and the number of times the transfusion service met its established turnaround time for emergency release of uncrossmatched blood to the emergency department (see **Table 23–1** for additional examples of quality indicators).

A very effective assessment tool is the **internal audit**. Unlike compliance inspections, audits review a specific facility process and determine—by examining documents and records, interviews, and observations—whether the facility is meeting the applicable requirements. For example, in a retrospective audit of transfusion service records, an auditor could randomly select a unit number for a red blood cell component and track through each activity involved in how the component was received, tested, issued, and transfused. The training and competence assessment records of each employee involved in handling the component are reviewed, as are the QC records for the storage refrigerator and the reagents, centrifuges, and other instruments used in compatibility testing for that unit. The performance on the proficiency test most recent to the unit's testing is reviewed. Copies of procedures and forms used at the workstations for all testing and QC are examined to determine whether they are the most current version, according to the master list. Samples of records are reviewed for inclusion of all required information, interpretations, and required supervisory reviews.

For blood collection operations, a donor name or number could be randomly selected and the same process repeated for the donation record, computer files, all related procedures, training and competence records, component production records, serologic and infectious disease testing records, and related QC, labeling, storage, and shipping records.

When prospective audits are conducted, the auditor watches the staff performing activities in the selected process. The auditor may ask questions of staff members such as, "How were you trained to perform this procedure and when?" or "Where in the procedure are the instructions for what you just did?"

Audits should be conducted by personnel who have been trained to perform audits and to identify system problems. Auditors should not audit the procedures they perform in their jobs. In a hospital-based blood bank or transfusion service, there may be insufficient personnel to have a separate quality function, and the supervisor or senior personnel or staff from another laboratory area may have to perform some auditing activities. A freestanding blood center should have sufficient personnel to designate a quality officer and to separate the quality function from routine operations.

The auditor presents his or her findings to the appropriate management and operations personnel at the closing meeting on a form similar to that in Figure 23–7. The auditor may request corrective action for each finding. A process should be in place for management personnel to evaluate and review the audit to ensure that corrective actions were implemented. Follow-up audits may be necessary to ensure that the corrective action was successful in removing the causes of the findings. Facilities must prepare an annual summary of their audit findings and the corrective actions taken.

External Assessments

There are two types of **external assessments**—proficiency testing and external inspections. Proficiency testing is a means to demonstrate that the facility's testing processes provide results comparable to those of other facilities with the same instruments and methods. In proficiency testing, the facility receives samples for testing from a designated provider and performs the testing using its routine processes, procedures, and staff. Results are compared to those of the provider and the other laboratories and the facility gets a report of its performance. Successful performance on proficiency testing challenges is a requirement for laboratory licensure and accreditation.[12]

The second type of external assessment is the **external inspection**, performed by regulatory and accreditation organizations for the purposes of obtaining and maintaining the facility's license or accreditation. External assessments are periodically conducted by the FDA, the Joint Commission, the CAP, and the AABB to determine the facility's compliance with the respective requirements.[2–7,12]

Continual Improvement

Information gathered from quality management activities provides the facility's leadership with a "report card" of how well laboratory processes are functioning so that action can be taken to improve any problematic processes.

QUALITY ASSURANCE INTERNAL AUDIT

Area/Function Assessed

Subject Area: _____ Date: _____

Key Positive Findings:

Key Opportunity Areas:

Recommendations for Improvements:

Auditors: _____ Date: _____

Response: Planned Actions and Completion Dates

Area Mgmt.: _____ Date: _____

Approved by: _____ Date: _____

Figure 23–7. An example of an internal audit form.

Identifying Opportunities for Improvement

Opportunities for improvement for both blood collection facilities and transfusion services can be identified from several main sources:

- The nonconformance trending process pointing to operational areas that are not functioning as well as intended
- Customer feedback such as complaints, solicited feedback, or suggestions from external customers the facility serves and from internal customers (employees)
- Information derived from monitoring quality indicators of operations, particularly when it is compared with that of peer groups in other institutions
- Internal audit feedback, whereby objective evidence collected by the auditor should support the facility's understanding of why corrective action is needed and should be taken
- Feedback from periodic external compliance inspections (however, if the blood bank is already seriously involved in the previous four activities, there should be little new information learned of which the facility is not already aware)
- Reports from other departments in the hospital's organization-wide quality committee function, such as nursing or emergency department problems in dealing with the blood bank

Using Teams

The hospital blood bank or laboratory's quality committee, or the blood center's quality council, should set priorities for the problems that need the most immediate attention. Many organizations have successfully used teams to solve problems or to design process improvements. Names such as *process improvement teams*, *quality action teams*, *continuous improvement teams*, and *corrective action teams* have all been used to refer to groups of people representing different parts of a given process who have been brought together to identify and implement ways to remove the causes of the problem and thereby improve the process. Teams need good team skills to perform their assignments successfully. Team members should receive team-building and problem-resolution training to ensure the most effective outcome for the time and resources expended.[13] Common team dos and don'ts are listed in Box 23–4.

Resolving Problems

Many approaches to the problem-solving process have been published. All the published problem-solving approaches contain essentially the same activities of identifying problems, prioritizing, selecting the top-priority problem, collecting data, analyzing the data, identifying possible solutions, implementing the chosen solution, monitoring the performance of the revised process, evaluating the effectiveness of the implemented solution, and sustaining the gains. Figure 23–8 depicts one common approach to managing the problem-solving process that includes these main activities:[14]

- Developing a customer-oriented action plan
- Putting the plan into action
- Measuring and monitoring to determine effectiveness of the action
- Determining what to do based on the measurements

BOX 23–4

Appropriate Focus Points for Process Improvement Teams

Teams Should Improve Processes That Affect:

- Quality of product
- Quality and reliability of service to internal and external customers
- Efficiency and accuracy of job performance
- Waste reduction, scrap, rework, and operating costs
- Equipment performance, up-time, and reliability
- Interdepartmental and intradepartmental communications
- Improved process controls
- Safety, hygiene, and work environment
- Processes, procedures, training, and competence
- Learning new skills, upgrading knowledge of the business, developing personal capabilities, team process

Teams Should *Not* Work on These Issues:

- Problems governed by or directly related to union contracts
- Grievances and grievance procedures
- Seniority
- Job classifications
- Job assignments
- Pay rates or benefits

Plan-Do-Check-Act Process

Step1: Plan

A mission-consistent, customer-oriented action plan
- Identify opportunities for improvement from data sources
- Prioritize improvement activities
- Develop an action plan for the selected activity, either
  - initiating a new process, or
  - improving an existing process
- Identify
  - customer needs
  - participants
  - timeframes
  - outcome measurements
  - success criteria

Step 2: Do

Put the plan into action
- Implement the action plan
  - do a pilot project first
  - broaden only after success
- Collect performance data

Step 3: Check

Has the planned and implemented change created intended improvement?
- Analyze collected data
- Compare performance data to established success targets and original performance data to determine if improvement was achieved
- Identify any unexpected peripheral benefits
- Identify unanticipated problems in other areas

Step 4: Act

Decide what to do next
- Determine if customer needs were met
- Take action based on the results:
  - Success:
    - revise the processes for further improvements (optional), and
    - assess again to determine if improvement is maintained, and
    - if a pilot project, standardize to the bigger group
  - Lack of success—re-do the action plan and repeat

Figure 23–8.   Plan-Do-Check-Act Process. A common quality improvement process.

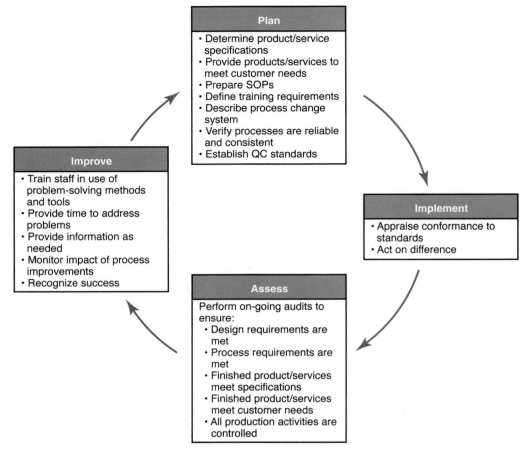

Figure 23–9. The cycle of organization-wide quality management.

A formalized problem-resolution process is just one piece of continual improvement. **Figure 23–9** illustrates the whole cycle that encourages continual improvement.

A Quality Management System for Medical Laboratories

A laboratory-wide QMS can be derived by simply replacing the blood bank path of workflow (see **Fig. 23–2**) with the medical laboratory's path of workflow, as shown in **Figure 23–10**. All the quality system essentials (QSEs) supporting the path of workflow remain the same because these quality elements are universal. In fact, at the point of compatibility testing in the blood bank path of workflow, the laboratory's (and transfusion service's) path of workflow is entered for all transfusion service testing.

A review of the International Organization for Standardization quality standards demonstrates that blood bank and laboratory QSEs are included in the international standards.[15,16] Therefore, all the discussion in the section on

A Quality Management System for the Laboratory

Laboratory Path of Workflow

← ————— Preanalytic ————— **Analytic** **Postanalytic** →

Test Order, Sample Collection, Transport, Receipt and Process, Testing, Reporting,Sample Archiving

Quality System Essentials: The Building Blocks

The Blood Bank	**The Work**	**The Performance**
Organization Customer Focus Facilities & Safety Personnel Purchasing & Inventory Equipment	Process Management Documents & Records Information Management	Nonconformance Mgmt Assessments Continual Improvement

Figure 23–10. A QMS for the medical laboratory.

QSEs applies equally to hospital laboratories. It is not only possible but also highly desirable to expand the blood bank's QMS building efforts so that the entire laboratory benefits from improved organization, coordination, and effectiveness of its many processes.[17]

The Cost of Quality

Although it may sound like much work and expense to implement a QMS in a blood bank, transfusion service, or medical laboratory, the costs involved are significantly lower than the expenses the facility experiences when there are major and minor nonconformances that need correction. Expenses are multiplied when the same nonconformance recurs and needs to be "fixed" again. A basic understanding of the four different types of quality costs is vital to comprehending the value of quality management to the customers and patients served by the facility.[18]

Prevention Costs

The cost of implementing processes and controls to prevent the occurrence of nonconformances is considered a "good" quality cost. In the blood bank, transfusion service, and medical laboratory, **prevention costs** include validation activities, preventive maintenance, work process training, and quality management activities such as improvement teams and quality system training. A small amount of money spent in these activities greatly reduces the chance of process problems in the path of workflow that could compromise the quality of the services provided or patient safety. Every budget should contain funds for prevention activities.

Appraisal Costs

The cost of implementing processes and controls to appraise or evaluate the blood bank, transfusion service, or medical laboratory's performance is also considered a "good" quality cost. There are internal and external **appraisal costs**. Internal evaluation costs include those for calibration materials and reagents, equipment calibration, quality control materials and reagents, any interim inspections of blood products or records, and the internal audit program. External evaluation costs include those for proficiency testing and periodic licensure or accreditation inspections. The budget usually always contains funds for these activities because they are mandated by regulatory and accreditation agencies. Appraisal helps ensure that problems are caught and corrected so as to minimize any negative impact on customers and patients.

Internal Failure Costs

Internal failure costs are one of two costs considered to be "bad" quality costs (the other is external failure costs). Examples include discarded donated blood units, samples unacceptable for compatibility testing that need recollection, retesting when controls don't give the proper results, instrument failures, and downtime. Internal failures are those caught and corrected before they adversely affect customers or patients. However, operating funds have been expended and wasted because the activity was not performed correctly the first time. Additional operating funds are then expended to correct the failure, thus eroding the operating budget.

External Failure Costs

External failure costs are "bad" quality costs that are expensive and hard to measure because they include both actual and intangible costs incurred to correct a nonconformance that has reached the customer. Examples of external failure costs include customer complaint resolution, misdiagnoses, recalls, and lawsuits. Consider the time, effort, and expense involved in investigating nonconformances related to issuing an erroneous report or blood component. The cost to correct these and other "never" events greatly erodes the facility's operating budget and definitely erodes customer confidence in the facility's quality and credibility.

Reports have shown that some businesses waste up to 40% of their operating budgets correcting internal and external failures! Whereas there are no published data for blood banks, transfusion services, and medical laboratories, there is little reason to believe that the expenditures for internal and external are significantly less. The important issue is for a facility to identify its prevention, appraisal, and internal and external failure costs and to use prevention and appraisal activities to reduce failure costs wherever possible. The old adage "An ounce of prevention is worth a pound of cure" was never more appropriate!

Importance of a Facility Quality Management System

Today, working in a QMS environment is needed to achieve the standards of excellence necessary for surviving the changes facing the nation's health-care industry and providing the level of patient safety that our donors and patients both expect and deserve. Purchasers of health-care services want evidence that health-care providers such as hospitals and blood centers are involved in organization-wide quality improvement programs that increase the safety of donors and patients. Only those organizations demonstrating measurable quality improvements are approved for agreements for products and services. The cultural change needed to create a QMS takes time, and organizations that have not started must begin immediately to keep pace. Consumers of blood center, hospital, and transfusion services accept no less than total quality. Organizations that provide less will not survive.

SUMMARY CHART

✔ Blood bank compliance with federal regulations and accreditation requirements is mandated by the FDA, the Joint Commission, the AABB, and the CAP.

✔ Compliance inspections measure the state of the facility's program with respect to the applicable requirements at a single point in time and are usually conducted every 1 to 2 years.

✔ Quality control procedures in blood banking may include daily testing of the reactivity of blood typing reagents, positive and negative controls in infectious disease testing, calibration of serologic centrifuges, and temperature monitoring of refrigerators, freezers, and thawing devices.

✔ Quality assurance is a set of planned actions to provide confidence that processes and activities that influence the quality of the product or service are working as expected individually and collectively.

✔ A QMS provides a framework for uniformly applying quality principles and practices across all blood bank operations, starting with donor selection and proceeding through transfusion outcomes.

✔ Process control is a set of activities that ensures a given process will keep operating in a state that is continuously able to meet process goals without compromising the process itself.

✔ cGMP requires that facilities design their processes and procedures to ensure that blood components are manufactured consistently to meet the quality standards appropriate for their intended use.

✔ Process validation challenges all activities in a new process before implementation to provide a high degree of assurance that the process will work as intended.

✔ Routine QC procedures, review of records, and capture of nonconformances when the process did not perform as expected are routine process control measures that monitor whether a process is functioning as needed.

✔ Nonconformance management is a name for processes that detect, report, evaluate, and correct events in blood bank operations that do not meet the facility's or other requirements.

✔ An internal audit reviews a specific facility process and determines—by examining documents and records, interviews, and observations—whether the facility is meeting applicable requirements and its own policies, processes, and procedures.

✔ A process improvement team is a group of people who represent different activities in a given process and who have been brought together to identify and implement ways to solve process problems.

Review Questions

1. A QMS is:
   a. Synonymous with compliance.
   b. Active and continuous.
   c. Part of quality control.
   d. An evaluation of efficiency.

2. QSEs are applied to:
   a. Just the blood bank's management staff.
   b. Blood bank quality control activities.
   c. Only blood component manufacturing.
   d. The blood bank's path of workflow.

3. cGMP refers to:
   a. Regulations pertaining to laboratory safety.
   b. Validation of testing.
   c. Nonconformance reporting.
   d. Manufacturing blood components.

4. Internal and external failure costs are:
   a. Readily identifiable in facility reports.
   b. Controlled through prevention and appraisal.
   c. Built into the facility's operating budget.
   d. Part of prevention and appraisal.

5. Which *one* statement below is correct?
   a. A process describes how to perform a task.
   b. A procedure simply states what the facility will do.
   c. A procedure informs the reader how to perform a task.
   d. A policy can be flowcharted.

6. A blank form is a:
   a. Record.
   b. Procedure.
   c. Flowchart.
   d. Document.

7. An example of a remedial action is:
   a. Applying the problem-solving process.
   b. Starting a process improvement team.
   c. Resolving the immediate problem.
   d. Performing an internal audit.

8. The PDCA cycle is used for:
   a. Problem resolution.
   b. Process control.
   c. Validation.
   d. Auditing.

9. The difference between the blood bank and laboratory QMSs is that:

   a. The laboratory has a different path of workflow.

   b. The blood bank does not include computer systems.

   c. The QSEs are different.

   d. The blood bank excludes testing.

10. The QSEs for the blood bank QMS can be used for the laboratory because:

   a. The paths of workflow are identical.

   b. Both the laboratory and blood bank experience accreditation inspections.

   c. The QSEs are universal.

   d. The QSEs are required by international standards.

References

1. Food and Drug Administration, Center for Biologics Evaluation and Research: Guideline on General Principles of Process Validation. Food and Drug Administration, Rockville, MD, 2011.

2. Food and Drug Administration, Department of Health and Human Services: Code of Federal Regulations, Title 21, Parts 200–299. U.S. Government Printing Office, Washington, DC, revised annually.

3. Food and Drug Administration, Department of Health and Human Services: Code of Federal Regulations, Title 21, Parts 600–799. U.S. Government Printing Office, Washington, DC, revised annually.

4. The Joint Commission: Comprehensive Accreditation Manual for Hospitals. Joint Commission Resources, Oakbrook Terrace, IL, 2010.

5. The Joint Commission: Comprehensive Accreditation Manual for Laboratories and Point-of-care Testing. Joint Commission Resources, Oakbrook Terrace, IL, 2010.

6. College of American Pathologists: Inspection Checklists for Laboratory Accreditation. College of American Pathologists, Northfield, IL, 2010.

7. American Association of Blood Banks: Standards for Blood Banks and Transfusion Services, 27th ed. American Association of Blood Banks, Bethesda, MD, 2011.

8. International Organization for Standardization: ISO 9000:2005 Quality management systems—Fundamentals and vocabulary. International Organization for Standardization, Geneva, 2005.

9. American Association of Blood Banks: Technical Manual, 16th ed. Bethesda, MD, 2008.

10. Food and Drug Administration, Center for Biologics Evaluation and Research: Guideline on Quality Assurance in Blood Establishments (Docket No. 91N-0450). Food and Drug Administration, Rockville, MD, 1995.

11. Department of Health and Human Services: Code of Federal Regulations, Title 45, Parts 160 and 164. U.S. Government Printing Office, Washington DC, revised annually.

12. Centers for Medicare and Medicaid Services: Code of Federal Regulations, Title 42, Parts 430 to end. U.S. Government Printing Office, Washington, DC, revised annually.

13. Scholtes, PR, et al: The Team Handbook, 3rd ed. Goal-QPC, Salem, MA, 2003.

14. McCloskey, LA, and Collet, DN: TQM: A Primer Guide to Total Quality Management. GOAL/QPC, Methuen, MA, 1993.

15. International Organization for Standardization: ISO 9001:2008 Quality management systems—Requirements. International Organization for Standardization, Geneva, 2008.

16. International Organization for Standardization: ISO 15189:2007 Medical laboratories—Particular requirements for quality and competence. International Organization for Standardization, Geneva, 2007.

17. Clinical and Laboratory Standards Institute: A Quality Management System Model for Laboratory Services; Approved Guideline, GP26, 4th ed. Wayne, PA, 2011.

18. Campanella, J (ed): Principles of Quality Costs: Principles, Implementation, and Use, 3rd ed. American Society for Quality Press, Milwaukee, WI, 1999.

Bibliography

Berte, LM (ed): Transfusion Service Manual of SOPs, Training Guides and Competence Assessment Tools, 2nd ed. American Association of Blood Banks, Bethesda, MD, 2007.

Clinical and Laboratory Standards Institute: Training and Competence Assessment, 3rd ed. Approved guideline GP21-A3. Clinical and Laboratory Standards Institute, Wayne, PA, 2009.

Laboratory Documents: Development and Control. Approved guideline GP2A-5. CLSI, Wayne, PA, 2006.

Tague, NR: The Quality Toolbox, 2nd ed. ASQC Press, Milwaukee, 2005.

Chapter 24

Utilization Management

Julie L. Cruz, MD, and Steven F. Gregurek, MD

OBJECTIVES

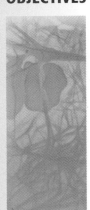

1. Distinguish the differences between blood utilization review and blood utilization management.
2. Describe the purpose and goals of a blood utilization management program.
3. Explain the principles and limitations of the Lean approach within the context of blood utilization management.
4. Describe how to perform a value stream assessment within the blood bank environment.
5. Develop a strategy for creating standardization and metrics used in blood utilization management.
6. Explain how adoption of transfusion guidelines can improve the value stream and help to develop utilization review criteria.
7. Explain how to assess the current and future state of blood utilization within a hospital system.
8. Identify the differences among the prospective, concurrent, and retrospective blood utilization reviews.
9. List intervention strategies and describe how they may be employed with the various blood utilization review models.
10. Explain the importance of a well-planned policy deployment and the need for continuous improvement within the context of blood utilization management.

Introduction

Since 1965, utilization review and management programs have been required in U.S. hospitals that participate in Medicare and Medicaid programs. By definition, they assess the appropriateness of the delivery of health care to patients using evidence-based guidelines and predetermined criteria. The terms *utilization review* and *utilization management* are similar, although the former emphasizes the actual review methodology and the latter emphasizes the entire process, including improvement strategies and aggressive interventions such as denial of service. Both concepts are well incorporated in pharmacy services and managed care.[1,2] This chapter defines **blood utilization review** as a focused review or audit of a particular population of transfused patients. **Blood utilization management** is the *process* that unites blood utilization review with particular intervention strategies to reduce inappropriate transfusion and improve patient safety.

The overarching goal of a blood utilization management program is to better manage limited blood resources and eliminate waste while providing maximum benefit to the patient. Benefits may be realized in terms of increased safety, component availability, reduced total expenditure, and more responsible stewardship of what is ultimately the voluntary gift of willing donors. There are many parallels with the application of Lean strategies in manufacturing. **Lean** manufacturing (aka "the Toyota Production System") is a production practice focusing on eliminating waste to generate efficiencies and ultimately deliver exactly what the customer wants precisely when it is needed. In fact, hospital systems and medical laboratories are increasingly training personnel and modifying their systems to adopt Lean strategies, and it has been noted that transfusion services already apply some Lean concepts such as standardization.[3] This chapter outlines one approach to designing a blood utilization management program utilizing Lean tools and concepts. Each individual institution should develop a blood utilization management strategy best suited to the unique challenges within its own system.[4]

Approval and Support

Blood utilization programs cannot exist in isolation within the hospital. Guidelines for transfusion and phone calls to clinicians regarding appropriateness of transfusion orders have the potential to lead to animosity and accusations of intrusiveness by clinicians accustomed to ordering autonomy. These physicians may perceive a loss of control over their medical decisions.[5] Hospital leadership must support the inception of the blood utilization management program and continue to empower the program once a credible plan is designed and approved. It is extremely important to obtain this commitment from hospital leadership before proceeding with a program of even low complexity.

Blood utilization programs may have multiple dedicated personnel for auditing, educational activities, and reporting and can require significant resources. However, most improper ordering is related to overtransfusion. If properly executed, blood utilization management can produce significant indirect and direct cost savings.[6] These potential savings should be summarized and presented to the administrative staff and should not be limited to projected savings related simply to decreased purchasing of blood components. Assessment of the potential cost savings by preventing severe transfusion reactions associated with significant morbidity and mortality such as TRALI (transfusion-related acute lung injury), circulatory overload, bacterial contamination, and hemolytic transfusion reactions should also be discussed.[7] Although demonstrable cost savings are often a priority for administrative support of the program, it is important to remember that other key benefits, including enhanced safety and greater stewardship of a limited resource, can be achieved. These things often cannot be easily quantified in dollars but should be considered just as critical in terms of rationale for development and continued support of the program.[8]

Like hospital administration, senior medical and nursing leadership must also be actively engaged, educated, and recruited to devise and support a successful program. In particular, consensus regarding transfusion guidelines and utilization program objectives should be achieved between the blood bank and physician leadership. Education, commitment, and compromise are necessary to create a cooperative environment and promote system-wide acceptance rather than a combative "blood bank versus the hospital" mentality. All must share a vision that existing processes must be changed in order to improve service to patients and to lower costs. It is critical that the change leaders reach every stakeholder in the process to *repetitively communicate* the importance of focusing on patients while also addressing the concerns and needs of employees who will inevitably be required to change work habits. The physician groups with the greatest blood use should be selectively targeted for policy agreement and educational activities. Armed with a thorough understanding of appropriate indications, risks, and the blood utilization process, nurses can be instrumental in achieving success and compliance. Once the program is launched, they can help ensure that the blood order indication and dose are appropriate, that the necessary interval laboratory data are obtained, and that essential clinical information is relayed.[9] Continued approval and support from these areas of hospital culture leadership are necessary to drive acceptance and provide the motivation and awareness to achieve the long-term goals of the blood utilization program.

Lean Approach to Blood Utilization Management

When selecting a strategy for blood utilization management, it is important to consider a systems-based approach that is compatible with the unique challenges of the safe and effective administration of blood components. The authors find Lean to be a particularly useful blood utilization management strategy, although other quality management systems may also be employed. Tools for identifying and eliminating waste while improving quality and ensuring customer satisfaction are key components of any utilization strategy.

Overview

Simply put, Lean is a systematic approach to identifying actions within a process that create value, then optimizing the alignment of these actions to deliver to customers exactly what is desired, in the quantity desired, precisely when it is required. It is based upon an approach first developed by the Toyota Corporation following World War II to better manage operations, including customer relations, supply chain management, development, and production.[10] Central to accomplishing this goal is the elimination of waste (also described by the Japanese term *muda*).

Waste is any action that does not create value as defined by the customer. DOWNTIME is a useful acronym utilized in Lean for identifying types of waste: Defects, Overproduction, Waiting, Nonvalue Added Processing, Transportation, Inventory Excess, Motion, Employee/People waste. Table 24–1 delineates types of waste identified in Lean and gives examples found in transfusion medicine.[10] Although some transfusion services may consider the ordering clinician to be the customer, the patient is the true customer, and value is ultimately determined by the therapeutic benefit (or harm) the patient receives from blood component transfusion. The system strives for "just in time" delivery as determined by

Table 24–1   Types of Waste and Corollaries to Transfusion Medicine

TYPES OF WASTE	TRANSFUSION MEDICINE COROLLARY
Inventory waste • Misallocation of resources	• Available units diverted from patients with greater need • Unused issued components improperly returned
Overproduction "just in case"	• Not trusting of timely delivery if ordered as needed (pull not met) • FFP thawed for the OR that expires unused • Unused washed units allowed to expire on floor
People	• Personnel diverted to perform unnecessary tasks
Motion	• Inappropriate "STAT" order
Transport	• Delivered components that were not transfused
Processing waste • Lack of communication • Customer need not clearly defined	• Failure to discontinue standing order for HLA-matched platelets • CMV seronegative transfused when leukoreduced appropriate

Adapted from Womack, JP, and Jones DT: Lean Thinking: Banish Waste and Create Wealth in Your Corporation. Free Press, New York, 2003.

customer need (also known as *pull*). Laboratorians are most familiar with this concept as turnaround time.

Lean utilization is not a one-time strategy that is deployed and delivers a fixed benefit. Rather, it relies upon a monitoring of metrics carefully chosen to reflect value and a process of continuous improvement (*kaizen*). It is designed to move the system ever closer to pure value (perfection) with minimal waste.[11] Perfect value with zero waste is unattainable in a blood utilization program, as some actions fitting the strict Lean definition of waste are necessary to enhance safety. Infectious disease testing is an example. However, significant improvement opportunities can still be identified. Blood utilization management attempts to optimize value (safety and therapeutic benefit) while minimizing waste. Here, the discussion and applications of Lean concepts are by no means representative of Lean in its entirety but merely illustrate the possibilities for application in blood utilization management. Those interested in applying Lean concepts are referred to the literature, and a number of professional organizations and consultancies offer resources.[12]

The traditional Lean model focuses on the elimination of waste (*muda*) to drive production toward value (as defined by the customer). However, in transfusion medicine, there is an additional facet to be considered—peril. All transfusions (even optimally selected, fully tested, appropriately stored and matched components produced under good manufacturing practices and properly administered by skilled personnel) pose an inherent baseline risk of adverse events. For example, despite intense mitigation strategies that have reduced the risk of TRALI, residual risk remains.[13]

Improper blood utilization and management practices decrease value and drive the result toward peril and waste. Thus, there are not only financial, labor, and resource losses but also human losses in terms of the patient's health and well-being. For example, the transfusion of a blood component to a healthy person creates no value but increases waste and peril. The Cruz-Gregurek model, shown in Figure 24–1, demonstrates this concept. Optimal value is the penultimate goal and is accomplished by developing standardized methods targeted to reduce waste and peril. As noted in the figure, some inappropriate practices create waste and peril. These practices represent high-yield opportunities for intervention. In addition to financial and safety benefits, such interventions are expected to reduce variability in practice and

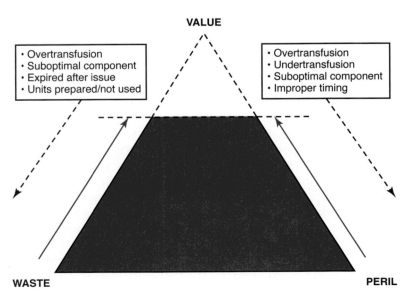

VALUE

• Overtransfusion
• Suboptimal component
• Expired after issue
• Units prepared/not used

• Overtransfusion
• Undertransfusion
• Suboptimal component
• Improper timing

WASTE   **PERIL**

Figure 24–1. The Cruz-Gregurek model of optimization. Inappropriate utilization practices result in both waste and peril. Measures to improve utilization drive transfusion practice toward optimal value, ultimately defined as the patient's clinical response to safe and effective transfusion. Interventions addressing some inappropriate practices will reduce both waste and peril and are therefore high yield.

provide better stewardship through optimization of a limited resource.

Value Stream Assessment

Application of the Lean paradigm begins with iteration of the **value stream** and assessment of the current state. The value stream mapping team identifies all subprocesses necessary to bring the finished product to the customer (in our case, the patient). Value stream mapping (VSM) is a strategy development tool to aid in identifying opportunities throughout the process for waste elimination. After identifying problems with the current state, the strategy development team creates an improved "future state" that will be translated into a "Lean transformation plan" and subsequent improvement (*kaizen*) projects. When considering the value stream, it becomes apparent that "improvements" in one area can cause downstream impacts with the potential to increase waste over the total system.[14] For this reason, it is critical that executive management be involved in the VSM process, or at least endorse the VSM team's future state value stream.

As applied to transfusion medicine, the traditional, or "current state," map of the value stream reveals two disjointed processes, as shown in Figure 24–2. One process is under tight quality control within the purview of the transfusion service, but the portion of the value stream involving the patient, the clinician, and the nursing staff is disconnected with respect to the assessment of the patient and the decision to transfuse. Here, the blood bank serves merely as a dispensary, and what happens after the component is issued (and before it is ordered) occurs out of the blood bank's control. As the figure demonstrates, all the processes are considered under the penumbra of the utilization program. This maximizes opportunity for the identification and elimination of waste, which can be generated along the stream at any point.

Considered another way, traditional methods to mitigate peril focus on interventions designed to increase the safety of the individual blood component, such as donor deferral questions, infectious disease testing, the crossmatch, and the second label check. Quality assurance processes ensure that safe, pure, and potent components are manufactured in the blood center and released for transfusion by the blood bank. The transfusion service mantra is "the right blood, right patient, right time."[9] The "right patient" in this context refers to identity (e.g., John A. Smith in bed A vs. John J. Smith in bed B). In contrast, the utilization program ensures the patient actually requires each transfusion. Figure 24–3 demonstrates the paradigm shift, illustrating that greater risk reduction can be achieved by considering both individual component safety measures and utilization optimization strategies.

To receive benefits from transfusion, the patient must have a deficiency or pathological lesion that can be remedied by functioning stored components. This process can be perfected by ensuring optimal timing and administering the optimal dose for correction without exposing the patient to increased transfusion risk. In this case, "the right patient" refers to his or her suitability to receive the requested transfusion, taking into account both individual clinical factors and established guidelines. In this context, blood utilization management is the complement to the crossmatch. The

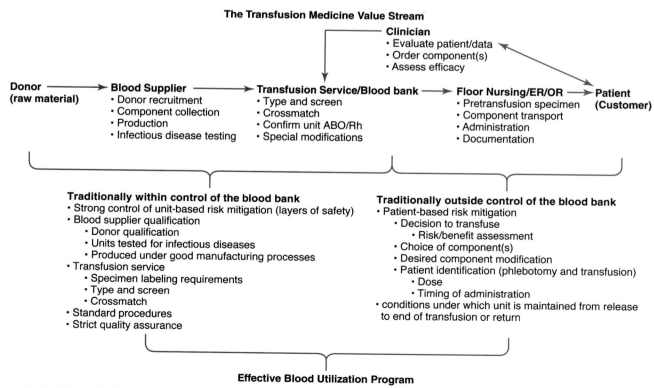

Figure 24–2.   Effective blood utilization management places the *entire* value stream under the penumbra of evidence-based practice and risk management to maximize benefit and optimally reduce peril.

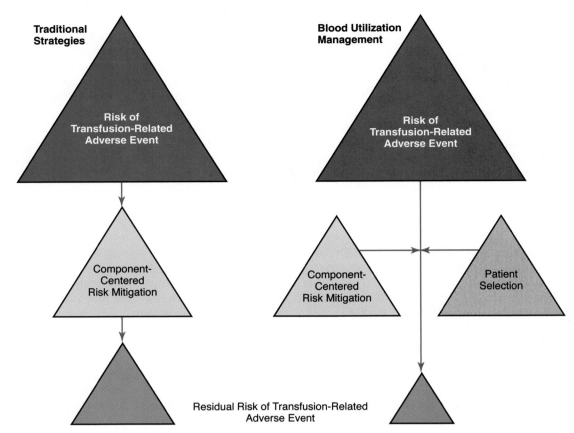

Figure 24–3.   Traditional transfusion service risk mitigation strategies are focused on increasing the safety of the individual component, yet inherent residual risk remains. Blood utilization management confers additional safety by incorporating consideration of patient-based factors to ensure transfusion is appropriate and optimally selected, hence a greater safety benefit is achieved.

crossmatch assesses the safety of a particular component for the patient, while utilization management ensures that the patient is appropriate for the transfusion.

Although cost savings are often emphasized, the safety of blood transfusion is the single most important aspect of effective blood utilization. According to Dzik, "the 'decision to transfuse' is perhaps the most critical step in patient transfusion safety."[15] Despite the layers of safety designed to reduce risk associated with blood components, inherent risk remains, thus zero risk is equivalent to no transfusion.[7]

Appropriate blood utilization and management also recognizes the risk of undertransfusion (i.e., failure to transfuse when benefits outweigh risk) and inappropriate or suboptimal component selection. From this perspective, the safest transfusion is the one that is given appropriately. Although many transfusion risks are preventable, rare errors account for a significant number of fatal transfusion-related events. Fortunately, rigorous attention to procedure and good manufacturing practice has decreased the incidence of these untoward events. However, it is important to recognize that despite our best efforts, total elimination of all transfusion risk (peril) is impossible.

Certainly there are many interventions the blood supplier or transfusion service may implement to improve transfusion safety (e.g., manufacturing plasma exclusively from male donors to prevent HLA antibody-associated TRALI, bacterial detection in platelet components), but residual risk remains.

For instance, yet unrecognized blood-borne pathogens and noninfectious complications whose mechanisms are not yet well understood. This is well understood from the immunohematological model of red blood cell antigen-antibody interaction. Unfortunately, the sickest and most physiologically vulnerable patients are also the most frequently transfused.[16] Examples of such individuals include cardiac, gastrointestinal, critical care, massive trauma, and oncology patients.

Standardization and Metrics

Having introduced the concept of utilization and discussed its importance in transfusion medicine, we can now turn to the basic elements important in any utilization program. Metrics must be chosen to allow an assessment of the current state and scope of the problem. Evidence-based **transfusion guidelines** must then be written and deployed. Finally, review criteria must be established to monitor physician compliance with guidelines.

Metrics

Assessment of the current state is an important initial step in Lean utilization. A baseline status must be established by selecting metrics that will both adequately reflect the system as is and serve as indicators of success (or failure) in execution of the future state. Those chosen should be meaningful within the system, readily evaluable, and widely disseminated.

This will allow for individuals, cross-functional kaizen teams, and departments at all levels of the system to continuously monitor their own subprocess performance and progress toward improvement targets and to benchmark themselves against other components of the value stream.

Many of these may already be trended and tracked by the blood bank or quality assurance personnel, such as crossmatch-to-transfusion ratio and number of mislabeled or unlabeled specimens. However, instead of automatically including existing metrics, one should consider their potential impact across the entire value stream. Consider not only what is measured and reported, but also how. For example, the number of mislabeled or unlabeled specimens in a particular time period is often tracked and reported to the transfusion committee and to individual nursing units. Yet might this information have greater impact if reported not just as the number of "defects" or opportunities for sentinel events, but also communicated as extension of turnaround time?

Waste begets waste within a system, and in this example the interval between the blood order and the availability of the component for transfusion is significantly prolonged while a subsequent properly labeled specimen is obtained and delivered to the blood bank. Such delays may contribute to the perception that blood bank turnaround time is too long and may be partially responsible for the overproduction issues previously noted in **Table 24–1**. Would selecting metrics that both include the absolute numbers of such specimens and quantify the delay in the system caused by them (in minutes or hours) increase the ability to drive behavior? Would it better demonstrate that as waste is removed, flow improves, thus decreasing strain on blood bank resources and resulting in more timely provision of appropriate units? These types of questions must be considered, and ultimately the metrics chosen will reflect the individual institution's goals, priorities, and beginning state.

Transfusion Guidelines

Once metrics are chosen, facility guidelines must be drafted, approved, and disseminated. The involvement of a multidisciplinary team is critical. A well-written transfusion guideline will contain the indications for transfusion and thresholds used in screening and auditing of transfusion records.[17] If the existing guidelines are not current, then current evidence-based medicine should be reviewed and the guidelines amended to reflect best practices. Evidence-based guidelines should be carefully scrutinized and included only if they fit within the scope of the hospital's practice and patient population. In cases where the evidence is limited, adoption of expert consensus panels should be considered in conjunction with local practices.

New guidelines should not be adopted until input is obtained from physician and nurse champions. Physician groups with high utilization should also be offered the opportunity to review and comment upon the proposed guidelines. Emphasis should be placed on the hazards of transfusion, therapeutic indications, and conservative transfusion practices. It is critical to obtain input from clinical staff and support of guidelines to improve compliance by ensuring they are broad and flexible enough to meet the majority of clinical situations. If guidelines are too restrictive or ignore significant clinical literature consensus opinions or guidelines in favor of more stringent recommendations from the transfusion medicine literature, compliance will be poor. Published evidence-based guidelines and consensus opinions are widely available and should be referenced.[18–24]

Current State and Scope of Problem

The next step is to assess the scope of inappropriate transfusion. A retrospective and representative sample of records from transfused patients should be reviewed to identify existing issues and patterns of misuse. The review should compare the indications used for actual transfusions against the transfusion guidelines. Specific areas and physician practice groups should be ranked by total utilization and appropriateness. Next, specific goals should be determined by the members of the planning committee who are considering the available resources and the desired monetary and safety outcomes.

Program complexity should be determined, including type, frequency, and scope of audit. Special attention should be given to each type of blood component. Will all components be reviewed equally? Will there be disproportionate representation of more frequently ordered components? Consideration must also be given to which patient populations will be audited, such as pediatric, neonatal, high-complexity surgery, hematology-oncology, and so on. Particular populations may require tailored auditing and intervention methods. To ensure the program moves forward expeditiously, a timetable should be created. Hospital leadership will often request this, along with early projections of the expected costs and benefits of the program.

After the determination of metrics and the assessment of the current state, it is important to ask the following questions regarding the future desired state: Is the current state adequate without any intervention? How will the program increase safety or eliminate waste? Are there enough resources available for successful implementation and continuance of the program? Will our program become too restrictive and potentially cause undertransfusion or prohibit compliance? The answers should be used to alter the design as indicated.

Review Criteria

After the transfusion guidelines are updated and the scope of the program is defined, criteria should be generated for use in the audit process. If the transfusion service is small and sufficient personnel are available, 100% manual review of records could be considered. However, as the number of transfusions increases, this method can quickly exhaust available resources. Screening criteria can be selected to flag cases with a high probability of inappropriate use and unflag those with low probability. This maximizes the efficiency of the review process. Algorithms can be developed that include laboratory data and information from **blood order sets**. Screening criteria that are too specific will fail to identify many inappropriate transfusions, while overly sensitive criteria will result in detailed review of many appropriate transfusions, making the program inefficient. In most cases, screening thresholds using fixed lab values or excluding certain conditions or indications are used.[18]

Blood Utilization Review

As previously discussed, blood utilization review attempts to optimize transfusion utilization by minimizing inappropriate transfusion. Most programs emphasize overutilization of blood products; only a few institutions monitor for underutilization of blood. The rare studies that have addressed underutilization have failed to show significant practice deviations. However, with continued efforts to lower transfusion thresholds and reduce overutilization, the risk may increase.[25,26] This may be especially true if educational efforts to improve utilization are strongly focused on potential transfusion-associated adverse events.

Blood utilization review is comprised of three broad categories of audits: **retrospective**, **concurrent**, and **prospective**. These strategies have direct corollaries from managed care.[2] Two subtypes of prospective review—**targeted** and **discontinuous**—are particularly useful when there are resource constraints.

The feature common to all methods is the requirement for comparison of transfusion records from individual patients to criteria developed from standardized guidelines. Each transfused component is assessed for medical necessity, adherence to indication guidelines, component dosing, and timing of administration. It is then categorized as either appropriate or inappropriate. Results of the audit are often submitted for further review and possible intervention strategies. Some methods are better suited for particular end goals.

Reviews can be manual, semiautomated, or automated. Manual reviews are often time-consuming, involve detailed medical record review of the entire selected audit population, and require the involvement of clinical health-care professionals such as nurses or physicians. Semiautomated reviews include computerized screening criteria that flag particular records for manual review. A screening process may add efficiency to the process by removing records for review that are below a predetermined screening threshold and by flagging the remaining records for review.[27] It is important to note that the screening threshold is different from the review criteria threshold. Screening thresholds must be carefully selected to prevent missing inappropriate transfusions, yet not be so strict as to compromise efficiency and speed. They are usually delineated in terms of a specific algorithm.

Automated review is carried out completely by algorithm and can be very quick and expeditious. Such reviews lack the detail of a manual system but can be an excellent method to display trending. Most common utilization benchmarks in the blood bank are examples of automated review. Many times the screening process or automated review can be performed entirely electronically.[15] The automated screening process is particularly effective when a transfusion indication must be linked to a decision support function when computerized physician order entry is available. This process has led to significant cost savings.[28]

Retrospective Review

Retrospective blood utilization review can be performed after the transfusion event has taken place and can occur when convenient without interrupting other staff duties. Detailed chart reviews can be performed by nursing or physician staff to determine appropriateness. Large numbers of transfusions can be reviewed and compared to previous data if medical records are readily available. Hence, this method is often used to generate trending reports on a large scale, including utilization within the hospital, particular physician practice group, or diagnosis and billing code.

In retrospective reviews, the feedback communication usually consists of letters, focused educational efforts, or both. The goal of either method is to educate clinicians and raise their awareness of current guidelines, thereby improving future transfusion decisions.[29] The major disadvantage of this methodology is that transfusion events occur in the past and the inappropriate transfusion is not prevented, merely identified later. Another drawback is feedback and clinician education occur remotely from the event, decreasing the likelihood that the clinician will remember the specifics of the transfusion decision. Of note, a longitudinal study of the impact of retrospective review alone in the sister field of drug utilization review failed to demonstrate significant improvement.[30]

Concurrent Review

Managed care audit models define **concurrent review** as a type of retrospective utilization review that occurs shortly after delivery of service, usually during the hospital stay.[31] Concurrent review is a type of retrospective review that occurs shortly after the transfusion while case details are still fresh in the mind of the ordering practitioner. It provides the blood bank with the opportunity to obtain further information to facilitate review.[21] In blood utilization models, it allows review of the relevant guidelines with the ordering physician to encourage future compliance. This type of review process is more labor-intensive than retrospective reviews because of the additional requirement to contact the ordering physician. Also like the retrospective audit, interventions occur after transfusion and focus on preventing future occurrence.

Prospective Review

Prospective blood utilization review is the most complex method and requires the interaction of many of the key players discussed below. This type of audit methodology uses manual or semiautomated methods and requires real-time evaluation of component requests. If prospective review is performed, the blood bank staff will be intimately involved in the audit process. Blood bank personnel are responsible for correctly screening transfusion orders in a timely manner that does not delay preparation of the component. The clinician's order is reviewed in real time in light of available patient laboratory data and clinical information. It is compared to evidence-based criteria and the facility's established transfusion guidelines. The component is issued as ordered if transfusion is indicated, within guidelines, and the component optimally selected. If the order appears to deviate from facility-approved transfusion guidelines, or if the requested component is suboptimal, blood bank personnel can communicate with the clinician to obtain more information or offer guidance and education. Mechanisms must be in place for notifying the on-call physician evaluator. Possible outcomes include approval of the order after additional information is provided, consultation and agreement upon a more appropriate component, or a more informed decision resulting in cancellation of the transfusion order.

If the prospective review process is used, the corresponding blood bank standard operating procedure should address four issues:

1. The type of screening method must be incorporated into the procedure, including required computer data entry or algorithm. Validation of the screening algorithm should be specifically addressed to prevent errors.
2. There must be specific instructions for handling flagged blood orders detailing the circumstances under which products are issued, denied, or the physician consulted.
3. There must be a process that describes what action to take in unusual circumstances or if the physician evaluator cannot be reached.
4. An efficient method of recording details of the event, including the pertinent discussion, disposition of the component order, and the name of the approving physician evaluator, is needed.

This process should not cause unnecessary delay in issuing components for patients in urgent need.[15] However, the majority of transfusions are not performed urgently, and there is ample time for consultation to make the best therapeutic choice for the patient. A well-written standard operating procedure with adequate training time is essential to ensure a robust, consistent process. Obstacles to performing prospective review are the considerable time and resources required and the potential for conflict between the transfusion service and clinician.[29]

Targeted Prospective Review

Targeted prospective review is a subtype of prospective review used during drug utilization review to pinpoint a high-priority, expensive, or potentially hazardous medication.[32] When this concept is applied to the blood bank, targeted prospective review involves ongoing prospective monitoring of one or a few specifically selected products or indications. These should be chosen from areas where intervention and behavior modification are expected to have high-yield results. This process is most useful when resources are limited and specific inappropriate utilization "targets" are readily

identifiable. However, there is evidence that this strategy fails to provide long-term improvements, likely because it is a "point" intervention rather than one that concentrates on overall transfusion practice.[33]

Discontinuous Prospective Review

Discontinuous prospective review is a process that can be employed by facilities with limited transfusion medicine resources or by facilities with only occasional deviations from transfusion utilization benchmarks. It is a method to conserve resources when intervention that is more aggressive is not expected to yield a significantly better response. Typically, it is combined with retrospective or concurrent review strategies and is selectively triggered when significant deviations are identified. It may be limited to a particular product type, DRG (diagnosis related group—a categorization system utilized for medical billing, based on diagnosis) clinical service, or individual clinician. In fact, a multi-institutional study revealed that less than 30 diagnostic categories accounted for more than 75% of the cost of transfusion.[34] Once improvement has been demonstrated and a steady state achieved, intense review may be discontinued until significant deviations are again identified. The risk in employing this strategy is that during periods of "relaxation," appropriate monitoring does not occur, and the review process is not reactivated in a timely manner.

Intervention Strategies

Each particular hospital and situation may require different interventions or perhaps a combination of strategies to mitigate inappropriate practices.[35] Interventions may be categorized as educational, punitive, or confrontational. They may be employed individually or collectively, depending on the culture of the institution. Tinmouth and colleagues conducted a comparative study and reported that "no particular intervention or combination of interventions appeared more effective in reducing utilization" of blood components.[36]

Educational strategies may require a hospital-wide focus if inappropriate utilization occurs in multiple departments or in groupings that are not easily categorized. Lectures, grand rounds, and job aids are all useful resources. If greater inappropriate usage is found among specific physician practice groups or in patients with a particular disease, classification-focused educational interventions are useful. Small group lectures or discussions ("lunch and learn") and phone conversations are excellent vehicles to relay current practice guidelines.

Punitive strategies involve reporting aberrant ordering practices to certain peer groups or hospital administrative groups relevant to the ordering physician. These groups must agree with the mission of the blood utilization program and endorse the metrics and guidelines or such reports will be ignored. Transfusion utilization may be included in annual "physician report cards." Practitioners may then be required to complete annual training that emphasizes evidence-based practice and the facility guidelines criteria.

Confrontational methods involve preventing or obstructing certain physician orders. With institutional approval, system-wide constraints can be placed on transfusion orders. Restrictions prevent the release of specific blood components for indications that are blatantly ineffective or better remedied by other lower risk or more cost-effective strategies. An example would be restricting all "fresh" blood to certain age populations. **Gatekeeping** is another confrontational method that requires approval of any transfusion order that does not meet predefined criteria. Decision support logic added to blood order sets is an example of a gatekeeping role that has been shown to reduce inappropriate blood utilization.[37] This intervention can also be used to deny release of components for transfusion order requests when indications are clearly inappropriate. If product release is denied or delayed, it must follow specific direction from the transfusion medicine physician or must follow strict adherence to explicit instructions for denial within the standard procedures.

Although the preceding strategies focus on correcting aberrant ordering behavior, positive feedback should occur as well. The development of physician champions has been successful in improving quality in other areas of health care.[38] Physicians who practice consistently within established guidelines should be recognized and, where possible, asked to share their practice philosophy with peers. These individuals may make excellent "utilization ambassadors," assisting in shifting the institutional culture toward the desired goal. As practicing physicians, they will also have an additional level of credibility with other clinicians who are absent in communications with laboratory personnel or transfusion service medical directors.

Behavioral Influences

There are three types of behavioral influences that can impact program success and should be considered in the planning process: direct, local, and external. Direct influences are the communications and actions between the physician or nursing staff involved in ordering a blood product and the blood bank staff involved in manipulation and dispensation of the product. Local influences include directing forces particular to the institution or locality, including habitual ordering practices, administrative expectations, blood bank resources, and physician group demands. External influences include standard of care issues and obstacles outside the immediate control of the hospital, such as conflicts between current evidence-based studies or consensus agreements. Blood supplier resources are also an external influence. With a common goal to improve safe and effective blood utilization practices, all three of these must be addressed to ensure quality and uniformity of care while avoiding unnecessary conflict and confusion.

If planned interventions include component denial or administrative actions, then it is of great importance to have transfusion committee endorsement before implementing such actions. Consideration should be given to methods of creating official hospital policy and seeking administrative support. In addition, consensus and support should be obtained from physician practice groups that frequently order components or have expected utilization issues. Groups with poor utilization should be notified and educated before any stricter policies are enforced. Mechanisms must be included for bypassing any potential for delay in a truly emergent situation such as massive hemorrhage.

Blood Order Sets

In Lean manufacturing, visual control is important as a means of standardization.[10] A utilization management equivalent is the use of blood order sets. This is a standardized method to clarify indications and enforce guidelines during physician order entry. This process may be paper or electronic. Such tools should be simple, intuitive to use, and not cluttered or overwhelming. They must also be readily available, whether electronic or paper-based. It is important to keep in mind that blood order sets are not foolproof methods for preventing inappropriate orders. Order sets that are too complex, difficult to access, or too restrictive will result in the development of "workarounds" to bypass the screening process. Those who had employed this tactic reported they were directed to do so by a more superior physician. Such "solutions" on the part of clinical staff impede flow in the blood bank, increase waste, and inhibit the ability to provide "just in time" service according to customer pull.[28,37]

Generally, any blood utilization program will use a screening tool such as the blood order set. Care should be taken to address issues such as massive and emergent transfusion. It may be necessary to address special populations such as neonates and pediatric patients with separate specifically tailored order sets. Blood should not be denied simply because a specific clinical indication was not included among the choices on the blood order form. These rare instances require consultation with the blood bank physician before issuing or denying product and may provide opportunities for continuous improvement of the form through updated versions.

Education

Numerous studies suggest that educational efforts alone may impart a substantial improvement to blood utilization.[17,29,39] Physician training in transfusion medicine is variable and often limited to behavior learned "on the floor." Pressure from specialists or more senior medical staff may influence transfusion-related decisions made by medical residents. Educational activities can be focused on a single practitioner or group. A direct phone call may be made to a physician who appears to order inappropriately. Another example is a small group discussion with a physician group about current guidelines for plasma transfusion. Formal lectures at grand rounds are also excellent methods for relaying transfusion guidelines to the community. Resident education is an ideal way to instill proper transfusion practice. If educational efforts are burdensome on available resources and time, consideration should be given to participation in hospital grand rounds or sponsorship of invited expert speakers.

Brief prepackaged computer-based training modules can be included annually to reinforce guidelines.

Sufficient lead time must be allocated for training and competency of technical staff. Staffing responsibilities and limitations should be addressed. Even a small retrospective program should develop consistent methods for auditing, recording, and reporting of data, thereby creating transparency and improving training efficiency. Complex programs involving real-time prospective audits require a team approach with readily available call schedules, written expectations for physician evaluators, and consistent documentation of outcomes. Transfusion service personnel should help validate the implementation or adjustment of the program. The blood bank staff can be crucial in identifying and reporting any unexpected delays in issuing or preparing product.

Policy Deployment

Just as a utilization management program needs careful assessment and thoughtful development of policies and guidelines, initiating such a program requires planning. Enacting sweeping changes at the launch of the program may overwhelm participants, leading to poor compliance and unforeseen risks. Employing the total quality management principle of **hoshin kanri**, the program should prioritize the elimination of waste as outlined in the future state VSM, via policy deployment and control. Hoshin kanri is a strategy of examining all of the desired goals and ordering projects based on balancing priority with ease of accomplishment to ensure progress. Change is thereby enacted in smaller pieces rather than through broad instantaneous reform. For example, the program may first take actions to address inappropriate red blood cell use. Once improvement is noted, measures to address plasma use can be instituted, and so on. An institution may first address the largest amount of waste, the greatest opportunity for expense reduction, the area of greatest peril, or any other area according to institutional priorities. Stepwise or phased deployment also provides an opportunity to incorporate lessons learned into the design of subsequent phases.[40]

Personnel

Once the scope and nature of the blood management program is agreed upon, attention focuses on allocation of resources and identification of personnel for planning, approval, and implementation. Although the planning stage involves many steps, a well-designed program begets a smooth implementation. Since blood management programs involve the interaction of multiple departments throughout the institution, the planning team must develop specific policies, guidelines, and procedures that fall within the constraints and expectations of the entire hospital system. Planners will lay the foundation for a successful utilization program, and once the program is implemented, they may continue in other leadership roles. Continued involvement allows them to serve as a resource for continuous improvement and to provide motivation and inspiration.

As the planning committee is established, team leadership should include personnel well versed in blood bank operations and others with a thorough understanding of blood use, including knowing appropriate indications and risk. The team must be skilled in communication and negotiation since multiple interdepartmental actions are required. Effective negotiation in the planning stage ensures a smooth implementation and favors acceptance, and it provides a buffer to administrative problems that may arise later. At a minimum, planning must include the medical director and supervisor of the blood bank. Even with limited-scope utilization programs, the medical director is responsible for maintaining guidelines and approving blood bank procedures. The medical director is also ultimately responsible for the safety and efficacy of transfused blood components. This individual has the authority to appoint appropriate surrogates to these duties, including screening procedures, denying product in prospective programs, and providing feedback regarding inappropriate transfusion in retrospective audit.

A thorough understanding of current evidence and guidelines is necessary for key players and should be promoted throughout the hospital system. As complexity of the utilization program increases, additional input and advice should be sought from such sources as the transfusion committee, blood utilization champions, and transfusion safety officers. Blood utilization champions are the physicians, practitioners, and nurses who order and administer blood components. They are useful in bridging the gap between the blood bank and clinicians and can be recruited through newsletters, e-mails, or directly at hospital lectures and presentations. Current publications and local and national organizations provide resources for implementation of blood management and utilization programs and can be very useful for planning teams unfamiliar with this process. Dedicated blood management personnel are essential to the success of the utilization program, and the duties and assignments should be described in detail in a standard operating procedure. The utilization program should be conducted with the same level of rigor as other functions within the blood bank. Each facility will have staffing needs determined based on its particular goals.

The skill and training required of an evaluator is based upon the complexity of the blood utilization program. The initial screening is usually accomplished by blood bank staff, sometimes in conjunction with automated screening algorithms. With a retrospective review at a small institution, the transfusion safety officer (TSO) may be able to accomplish retrospective auditing. However, a large prospective review with potential denial of product will require control by a dedicated on-call physician or designee. Prospective audits may require the interaction of several physician evaluators. Review benchmarks should be developed and the goals of the utilization program should be clearly and carefully defined.

Transfusion Safety Officer

The **transfusion safety officer** (TSO) is a unique career role that developed in Canadian and European blood banks. TSOs are typically medical laboratory scientists or nurses (BSN). Essentially, they coordinate and participate in most functions within the blood utilization program, including but not limited to audits of transfusion records, quality assurance, and educational functions. This role requires excellent communication skills, clinical knowledge, and ability to manipulate database software. This allows the TSO to perform audits, educate physicians and nurses, and assist with the development of other transfusion safety programs.[41] Coordinating auditing functions and educational activities and ensuring that resources and personnel are correctly tasked is essential during implementation. In addition to prospective or retrospective auditing, meticulous records should be kept for trending purposes. The coordinator must have sufficient knowledge of blood banking if no TSO is appointed.

Information Technology

For most programs, the inclusion of a team member from information technology will be important. Data mining and analysis will be critical in assessing the current state and designing reports for continuous monitoring. A great deal of information can be gleaned and processed by well-constructed queries to the Library Information System (LIS), electronic medical record, billing system, and other databases. Often these systems do not readily interface, and in-house design of well-tailored validated programs may provide the best solution. However, before any such design is undertaken, there must be agreement upon and clear communication of the precise data and metrics that will be desired. Redesign and rework of such programs is resource intensive. Additional waste is generated if the ultimate result does not serve the purpose for which it was intended.

Design Considerations

At first glance, the apparent increased complexity of the blood management model versus simple component dispensation (order filling) may seem prohibitive. However, delays can be prevented by well-designed, properly implemented standard operating procedures. Intervention strategy styles should be paired with an appropriate audit type, since not all are complementary to each other. Figure 24–4 shows a schematic of the interactions between blood utilization review and intervention strategies and the potential impact on the ordering clinician. It is important to remember that even in facilities where there are significant improvement opportunities, many of the

transfusions are appropriate and have a therapeutic effect.[35] The program should not be structured in such a way as to limit the capabilities of the primary clinician, especially in emergencies.

Figure 24–5 illustrates one model of process flow for a utilization management program. Most important is recognizing that the program design requires a cyclic model to ensure continuous improvement and maintain currency. Members of the utilization team may be responsible for specific phases of the cycle or may follow a particular component or issue through the entire cycle. Regular updates and communications among team members are essential for monitoring progress and ensuring that learning experiences are shared. Important key players are listed in Table 24–2.

Continuous Improvement

Continuous improvement (also known as *kaizen*) through Lean or another quality process is required for long-term success of a blood utilization management program.[12] Within the strategy established in the future state map, improvement teams should be deployed at all organizational levels. For example, blood bank technologists, nursing staff, and ordering practitioners should be included in the strategy. One study has demonstrated that without such measures, improvements in utilization tend to decrease after as little as 3 years.[33] It follows that the long-term success of the program should be considered a safety and cost-saving investment, which is dependent on the adequate allocation of resources. While teams may be empowered to make recommendations for improvements, implementation of process changes must be endorsed by management to ensure safety and total value stream optimization. Monitoring and continuous improvement may include most of the same players involved in the planning stages. The medical director must be aware of trending patterns and anticipate changes to the screening criteria. A significant reduction in usage may require changes in staffing and ordering components from vendors. An increase in inappropriate utilization or a failure to improve may require reallocation of resources and more intense auditing procedures. Additional personnel resources for chart review and clinician interaction may be required.

The transfusion committee is an ideal forum for the review and assessment of the program's success. Because of its multidisciplinary nature, feedback can be shared between the blood bank and clinicians, preventing the development

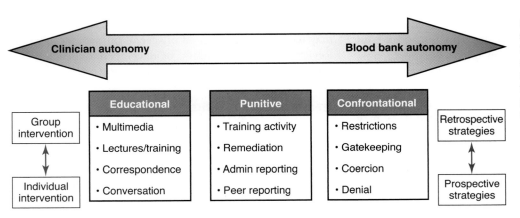

Figure 24–4. Common intervention strategies in blood utilization management. Strategies on the left encourage clinician autonomy while those on the right encourage blood bank autonomy. Strategies near the top of the figure are designed for large groups, and those near the bottom are designed for individuals.

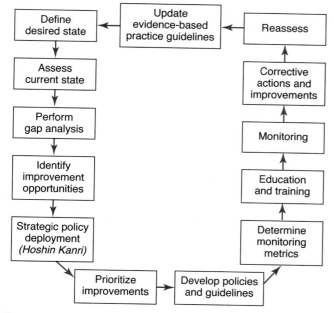

Figure 24–5. Sample utilization management process flow: The cyclic nature is critical to continuous improvement and program currency.

Table 24–2	Key Players in a Utilization Management Program
ROLE	**EXAMPLES**
Planners	• Medical director of blood bank • Transfusion committee • Supervisor of blood bank • Transfusion safety officer • Delegated clinical leadership • Quality assurance • Information technology
Approvers Policy approval, resource provision, program support, and awareness	• Executive staff for physicians • Physician groups with high blood utilization • Nursing leadership • Hospital administration
Implementers Day-to-day operations	• Coordinator (transfusion safety officer) • Evaluators (auditors, controller, screeners) • Educators (consultant, lecturer) • Physician ambassadors • Nursing ambassadors • Suppliers (blood bank staff following utilization procedure)
Reviewers Reassessment and refinement of existing program	• Medical director of blood bank • Transfusion committee • Supervisor of blood bank • Transfusion safety officer • Hospital leadership and administration (for policy changes)

of an adversarial relationship. This forum also allows for the review of flagged occurrences of misuse and determination of appropriate actions. However, in the philosophy of continuous improvement, it is critical that metrics are shared across the entire system, and reporting is not confined to the transfusion committee or hospital administration. This recognizes all participants as stakeholders and opens the door for improvement suggestions to be generated by personnel at all levels across the entire value stream. Organizational newsletters or intranet home pages are ideal forums for this and for disseminating evidence-based literature. To maintain support for the transformation and build the foundation for a continuous improvement culture, it is absolutely critical that management maintains personal two-way communication with every kaizen team. Likewise, insightful feedback should be provided to kaizen teams and individuals when their recommendations cannot be adopted. Without such personal interaction, employees will perceive that they are not truly empowered and participation will decline.

CASE STUDIES

Case Study 24-1

You are the blood bank supervisor at a medium-sized hospital. Administration has been impressed by reported cost-reduction realized in other facilities with active blood utilization and management programs. You have been directed to begin such a program in your facility.

1. What will you tell administration about cost reduction as the goal for a blood utilization and management program?
2. What will your first steps be?
3. Who will be included on the blood utilization management team?
4. How will you establish appropriate utilization criteria?
5. What type(s) of review might you consider?

Case Study 24-2

You are the transfusion safety officer of a large, growing tertiary-care hospital facility. Your facility's blood utilization management program consists of monthly retrospective analysis of blood usage by diagnosis and procedure codes. Your results are reported at the quarterly transfusion committee, where review determines whether placement of a letter in the physician's file is warranted. You notice an increasing trend in both plasma usage and plasma wastage. You must report your findings and analysis at the next transfusion committee meeting.

1. How will you assess the source of the problem?
2. How will you assess the decrease in value as a result of the problem?
3. What strategies should be used to develop possible improvements?
4. How will the corrective action be monitored?

SUMMARY CHART

✔ Cost savings and risk reduction can be realized from a well-designed blood utilization management program. The program should be multidisciplinary, tailored to the needs of the institution, rely upon evidence-based criteria, and employ mechanisms for continuous monitoring and improvement. Lean or another quality process can be utilized to organize the system and provide consistency and value.

✔ Blood utilization management is a process designed to ensure that blood transfusions are administered in accordance with evidence-based guidelines and predetermined criteria. Effective program design and good compliance ensure that patients receive transfusions only when necessary and medically appropriate.

✔ Concepts derived from Lean manufacturing or from other quality systems may be employed in the design and organization of an effective blood utilization management program.

✔ Standardization is achieved through thoughtfully prepared transfusion guidelines and carefully selected evidence-based criteria. Blood order sets may also be employed to promote uniformity and complete documentation.

✔ Meaningful metrics are chosen to reflect the progress of the system toward facility-defined goals. Trending and tracking these metrics allows monitoring of program effectiveness and indicates opportunities for continuous improvement.

✔ Blood utilization review consists of retrospective, concurrent, and prospective methods. Based on current and future needs, a facility may choose a single method or may use them in combination.

✔ When review processes identify deviations, interventions are triggered. Like review processes, there are multiple interventions, and selected types are determined based on institutional culture and needs. However, not all review processes and interventions are mutually compatible.

✔ Key personnel in the blood utilization management include the transfusion service medical director, blood bank supervisory personnel, and representatives from nursing and the facility's practicing physicians. Some institutions may employ a transfusion safety officer. A representative from information technology may also prove invaluable to the team.

✔ Support and approval by hospital administration is crucial to the survival and success of the program.

Review Questions

1. Which type of review does not require direct discussion between the ordering clinician and transfusion service personnel?
   a. Discontinuous prospective
   b. Targeted prospective
   c. Concurrent
   d. Retrospective

2. Improper specimen labeling contributes to waste (muda) within the system by requiring rework and prolonging turnaround time.
   a. True
   b. False

3. There is no value in a transfusion if the patient suffers any transfusion-related adverse event.
   a. True
   b. False

4. To receive benefit from a transfusion the patient must have:
   a. A hemoglobin level less than 8 g/dL.
   b. An invasive procedure planned.
   c. A pathological lesion or deficiency that can be remedied by functioning stored components.
   d. A blood order signed by the attending physician.

5. All of the following regarding the transfusion medicine value stream are true except:
   a. The patient is the customer.
   b. Waste can be generated in any department.
   c. Transfusion guidelines are a form of standardization.
   d. Value is decreased when waste and peril are decreased.

6. Continuous improvement (kaizen) is important only when targeted or discontinuous prospective review is utilized.
   a. True
   b. False

7. All interventions are compatible with all utilization review methods, and they can be utilized in any combination.
   a. True
   b. False

8. The blood utilization management program planning team should include:
   a. Nursing representatives.
   b. Representatives from the facility's practicing clinicians.
   c. The blood bank medical director.
   d. All of the above.

9. Metrics should be:

a. Chosen to indicate progress during the process of continuous improvement.

b. Tracked and disseminated only to members of the blood utilization management team.

c. The same for all institutions.

d. Selected only by the transfusion service leadership.

10. Perfect value with zero risk and no peril is attainable for any facility willing to invest in a blood utilization management program.

a. True

b. False

References

1. Restuccia, JD: The evolution of hospital utilization review methods in the United States. Int J Qual Health Care 7:253, 1995.
2. Assistant Secretary for Planning and Evaluation: Managed Care Terminology. http://aspe.hhs.gov/Progsys/forum/mcobib.htm, 2010. Cited February 4, 2010.
3. Kim, CS, Spahlinger, DA, and Billi, JE: Creating value in health care: The case for Lean thinking. J Clin Outcomes Manage 16:6, 2009.
4. Goodnough, LT, and Shander, A: Blood management. Arch Pathol Lab Med 131:695, 2007.
5. Shea, AM, et al: Use and perceptions of clinical practice guidelines by internal medicine physicians. Am J Med Qual 22:170, 2007.
6. Laird, J, and Soutar, R: Effective transfusion audit can improve and alter clinical practice: Something that is often questioned. Transfus Med 18:141, 2008.
7. Hendrickson, JE, and Hillyer, CD: Noninfectious serious hazards of transfusion. Anesth Analg 108:759, 2009.
8. Shulman, IA, and Saxena, S: The transfusion services committee—responsibilities and response to adverse transfusion events. Hematology Am Soc Hematol Educ Program 483, 2005.
9. Gray, A, et al: Promoting safe transfusion practice: Right blood, right patient, right time. Br J Nurs 17:812, 2008.
10. Womack, JP, and Jones, DT: Lean Thinking: Banish Waste and Create Wealth in Your Corporation. Free Press, New York, 2003.
11. Melanson, SE, et al: Applying Lean/Toyota production system principles to improve phlebotomy patient satisfaction and workflow. Am J Clin Pathol 132:914, 2009.
12. Womack, JP, and Jones, DT: Lean Solutions: How Companies and Customers Can Create Value and Wealth Together. Free Press, New York, 2005.
13. Chapman, CE, et al: Ten years of hemovigilance reports of transfusion-related acute lung injury in the United Kingdom and the impact of preferential use of male donor plasma. Transfusion 49:440, 2009.
14. Dickson, EW, et al: Application of lean manufacturing techniques in the emergency department. J Emerg Med 37:177, 2009.
15. Dzik, S: Use of a computer-assisted system for blood utilization review. Transfusion 47:142S, 2007.
16. Cobain, TJ, et al: A survey of the demographics of blood use. Transfus Med 17:1, 2007.
17. Garrioch, M, et al: Reducing red cell transfusion by audit, education and a new guideline in a large teaching hospital. Transfus Med 14:25, 2004.
18. Goodnough, LT: Transfusion triggers. Surgery 142:S67, 2007.
19. Blajchman, MA, et al: New strategies for the optimal use of platelet transfusions. Hematology Am Soc Hematol Educ Program 198, 2008.
20. Wong, MP: Guidelines for frozen plasma transfusion. BC Med J 49:311, 2007.
21. Spiess, BD: Red cell transfusions and guidelines: A work in progress. Hematol Oncol Clin North Am 21:185, 2007.
22. Slichter, SJ: Evidence-based platelet transfusion guidelines. Hematology Am Soc Hematol Educ Program 172, 2007.
23. American Society of Anesthesiologists Task Force on Perioperative Blood Transfusion and Adjuvant Therapies: Practice guidelines for perioperative blood transfusion and adjuvant therapies: An updated report by the American Society of Anesthesiologists Task Force on Perioperative Blood Transfusion and Adjuvant Therapies. Anesthesiology 105:198, 2006.
24. Hill, SR, et al: Transfusion thresholds and other strategies for guiding allogeneic red blood cell transfusion. Cochrane Database Syst Rev 2002:CD002042, 2002.
25. Saxena, S, et al: Monitoring for underutilization of RBC components and platelets. Transfusion 41:587, 2001.
26. Vincent, JL, and Piagnerelli, M: Transfusion in the intensive care unit. Crit Care Med 34:S96, 2006.
27. So-Osman, C, et al: Triggers and appropriateness of red blood cell transfusions in the postpartum patient—a retrospective audit. Vox Sang 98:65, 2010.
28. Fernandez-Perez, ER, Winters, JL, and Gajic, O: The addition of decision support into computerized physician order entry reduces red blood cell transfusion resource utilization in the intensive care unit. Am J Hematol 82:631, 2007.
29. Tinmouth, A: Reducing the amount of blood transfused by changing clinicians' transfusion practices. Transfusion 47:132S, 2007.
30. Hennessy, S, et al: Retrospective drug utilization review, prescribing errors, and clinical outcomes. JAMA 290:1494, 2003.
31. Murray, ME, and Henriques, JB: An exploratory cost analysis of performing hospital-based concurrent utilization review. Am J Manag Care 9:512, 2003.
32. Navarro, R: Managed Care Pharmacy Practice, 2nd ed. Jones and Bartlett, Sudbury, 2009.
33. Tobin, SN, Campbell, DA, and Boyce, NW: Durability of response to a targeted intervention to modify clinician transfusion practices in a major teaching hospital. Med J Aust 174:445, 2001.
34. Beguin, C, et al: Concentration of transfusion resources on a few pathologies and a few patients: Analysis of the comprehensive in-hospital patient database. Transfusion 47:217, 2007.
35. Damiani, G, et al: Appropriateness of fresh-frozen plasma usage in hospital settings: A meta-analysis of the impact of organizational interventions. Transfusion (epub) August 31, 2009.
36. Tinmouth, A, et al: Reducing the amount of blood transfused: A systematic review of behavioral interventions to change physicians' transfusion practices. Arch Intern Med 165:845, 2005.
37. Scheurer, D, et al: Effectiveness of computerized physician order entry with decision support to reduce inappropriate blood transfusions. J Clin Outcomes Manage 17:10, 2010.
38. Holland, R, et al: Creating champions for health care quality and safety. Am J Med Qual (epub) December 4, 2009.
39. Brandt, MM, et al: Transfusion insurgency: Practice change through education and evidence-based recommendations. Am J Surg 197:279, 2009.
40. Hutchins, DC: Hoshin Kanri: The Strategic Approach to Continuous Improvement. Gower, Burlington, VT, 2008.
41. Dzik, WH: Emily Cooley Lecture 2002: Transfusion safety in the hospital. Transfusion 43:1190, 2003.

Chapter 25

Transfusion Safety and Federal Regulatory Requirements

Judy Ellen Ciaraldi, BS, MT(ASCP)SBB, CQA(ASQ), and Alan E. Williams, PhD

OBJECTIVES

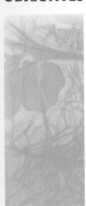

1. Describe why laws governing the regulation of biological products were enacted.
2. Define a biological product manufacturer.
3. Describe the regulatory process.
4. List the requirements for and responsibilities of being registered with the FDA.
5. List the requirements for and responsibilities of FDA licensure.
6. Describe the FDA's inspectional authority of biological product manufacturers.
7. Distinguish between licensed and unlicensed manufacturers and between interstate and intrastate commerce.
8. Describe the role of the FDA current good manufacturing practice (CGMP) in biological product manufacturing.
9. List the possible enforcement actions.
10. List the FDA's five layers of safety for protecting the blood supply.

Introduction

The Department of Health and Human Services (DHHS) is the United States government's principal health agency for protecting the health of all Americans. The Centers for Disease Control and Prevention (CDC), the Centers for Medicare and Medicaid Services (CMS), the National Institutes of Health (NIH), and the Food and Drug Administration (FDA) are the primary agencies of the DHHS with responsibilities directly related to blood. DHHS is part of the executive branch of the U.S. government.

In addition to regulating other products such as food, veterinary medicine, and tobacco, the FDA promulgates and enforces regulations to ensure the safety and efficacy of biological products, drugs, and devices, which include human blood and blood components, blood collection supplies and instruments, blood establishment computer systems, blood bank reagents, and infectious disease tests. Regulations for biological products promulgated under the Public Health Service (PHS) Act and the Federal Food, Drug, and Cosmetic (FD&C) Act are found in Parts 210-211, 600-680, and 800-820 of Title 21, Code of Federal Regulations (CFR).[1] These regulations set forth the regulatory requirements under the statutes, including adherence to current good manufacturing practice (CGMP) requirements. In addition, the regulations address licensing of biological products and establishment registration, as well as product-specific standards for blood and blood components.

This chapter describes the history of biologics regulations, the FDA's regulatory process and requirements, the FDA's inspection and enforcement activities, and the CGMP requirements for blood and blood components. The appropriate citations for specific regulations are provided next to the topic. Common abbreviations used here and throughout the chapter are listed in Box 25-1.

History of Biologics Regulation

Public Health Service Act

The regulation of biological products in the United States began when Congress passed the Biologics Control Act of 1902 (also known as the Virus-Toxin Law).[2]

In 1901, there was a serious epidemic of diphtheria that resulted in a great demand for the diphtheria antitoxin. At that time, there were no requirements for safety testing. A horse from which serum was obtained to produce the diphtheria antitoxin had contracted tetanus, which resulted in tetanus infection in persons who received the diphtheria antitoxin. The Biologics Control Act of 1902 was passed following the deaths of 13 children who received injections of diphtheria antitoxin contaminated with tetanus.[3]

The Biologics Control Act required biological products to be manufactured in a manner that ensured the safety and purity of the product. The Act included provisions for licensing products, suspending or revoking the license for violations,

---

BOX 25–1

Commonly Used Abbreviations

BLA	Biologics License Application
BPDR	Biological Product Deviation Report
DHHS	Department of Health and Human Services
CBER	Center for Biologics Evaluation and Research
CFR	Code of Federal Regulations
CGMP	Current Good Manufacturing Practice(s)
CMS	Center for Medicare and Medicaid Services
CSO	Consumer Safety Officer
FDA	Food and Drug Administration
FD&C Act	Federal Food, Drug, and Cosmetic Act
FR	Federal Register
FY 2008	Fiscal Year 2008 (October 1, 2007 to September 31, 2008)
OBRR	Office of Blood Research and Review
OCBQ	Office of Compliance and Biologics Quality
ORA	Office of Regulatory Affairs
PHS Act	Public Health Service Act

---

labeling requirements, and authorizing entry of federal officials into manufacturing facilities to conduct inspections.

The Biologics Control Act was incorporated into the Public Health Service (PHS) Act in 1944 as Section 351. The new PHS Act required a biologics license to be in effect before a biological product enters into interstate commerce.[4] A biologics license application can be approved only after the manufacturer demonstrates that both the product and the manufacturing facility meet standards to ensure the continued safety, purity, and potency of the products.

The 1902 Act did not include all biological products; specifically, it did not address the regulation of blood and blood components. In 1970, the definition of a biological product within the PHS Act was expanded to include blood and blood components and derivatives.

Federal Food, Drug, and Cosmetic Act

The Federal Food, Drug, and Cosmetic (FD&C) Act was passed in 1938 to further define the government's regulatory authority. This act requires manufacturers to demonstrate that a drug is safe and effective before marketing it. In addition, it authorizes facility inspections of drug manufacturers and requires drug manufacturers to register. The FD&C Act prohibits the introduction or delivery for introduction into interstate commerce any food, drug, device, or cosmetic that is adulterated or misbranded.[5] A drug or device is misbranded if its labeling is false or misleading. A drug is adulterated if the methods used in its manufacture do not conform with CGMP to ensure the drug is safe, and has the identity and strength, and meets the quality and purity characteristics which it is represented to possess.

The FD&C Act has been amended many times to incorporate new provisions. For example, in 1976 the FD&C Act was amended to strengthen the FDA's authority to regulate medical devices. In 1992, the Prescription Drug User Fee Act (PDUFA) was passed to expand the FDA's capability to hire reviewers using industry application and supplement submission processing fees in exchange for FDA's agreement to complete drug reviews within specified time frames. Device user fees were first enacted in 2002. In 1997, the Food and Drug Administration Modernization Act (FDAMA) was enacted to implement many changes, including those to bring the regulation of biological products in closer harmony with the regulations for drugs. Some of the provisions in FDAMA include eliminating the need for establishment licenses, streamlining the approval process for manufacturing changes, and incorporating risk-based regulation of medical devices. In 2007, the FDA Amendments Act (FDAAA) renewed the Prescription Drug and Device User Fee programs, increased the public transparency of current regulatory actions, and provided the FDA with numerous new authorities to assess and act on safety issues that may only be recognized after a drug is marketed.

Food and Drug Administration

Originally, the Laboratory of Hygiene of the Marine Hospital Service was charged with enforcing the Biologics Control Act. In 1930, this laboratory was renamed the National Institutes of Health (NIH). In 1937, the Division of Biologics Control (later renamed as the Bureau of Biologics) was formed within the NIH to regulate biological products. The FDA began in 1927 as the Food, Drug, and Insecticide Administration, a law enforcement agency within the U.S. Department of Agriculture. The name was changed to FDA in 1930. In 1968, the FDA was transferred to the Public Health Services within what was then known as the Department of Health, Education, and Welfare. The authority for biological products was transferred from the NIH to the FDA in 1972. In May 1980, education functions were removed from the department and it became known as the Department of Health and Human Services.[2,6]

Since 1972, the FDA has overseen the safety, purity, and potency of the U.S. blood supply by ensuring that blood and blood component manufacturers conduct their operations and manufacture their products in accordance with applicable laws and regulations, including CGMP. Biological products are regulated in two FDA centers: the Center for Drugs Evaluation and Research (CDER), which regulates therapeutic biological products, and the Center for Biologics Evaluation and Research (CBER), which regulates biological and related products, including blood, vaccines, allergenics, tissues, cellular and gene therapies, and related devices. The Office of Blood Research and Review (OBRR) and the Office of Compliance and Biologics Quality (OCBQ) in CBER are responsible for overseeing the regulation and enforcement of biologics regulations for blood and blood components.

The Office of Regulatory Affairs (ORA) is responsible for performing FDA postmarket inspections of blood and blood component manufacturing facilities and other surveillance activities.

The FDA has identified five overlapping layers of safety that work together to prevent an unsuitable blood component from being transfused to a patient.[7] Blood and blood component manufacturers must ensure they have processes in place to perform and monitor each of these procedures:

1. Donor screening: Donors are informed about potential risks and are required to answer questions about factors that may affect the safety of their blood. For example, donors with a history of intravenous drug abuse are routinely deferred.
2. Blood testing: After donation, each unit of donated blood undergoes a series of tests for infectious diseases.
3. Donor lists: Blood establishments must keep a current list of deferred donors and use it to make sure they do not collect blood from anyone on this list.
4. Quarantine: Donated blood must be quarantined until it is tested and shown to be free of infectious agents.
5. Problems and deficiencies: Blood centers must investigate manufacturing problems, correct all deficiencies, and notify the FDA when product deviations occur in distributed products.

Regulatory Process

Manufacturers, Manufacturing, and Biological Products

Biological product manufacturers are defined as any legal person or entity engaged in the manufacture of biological products subject to licensure under the PHS Act. The term "manufacturer" also includes any legal person or entity who is an applicant for a license where the applicant assumes responsibility for compliance with applicable product and establishment standards (21 CFR 600.3(t)). Manufacturing for blood and blood products means the collection, preparation, processing, or compatibility testing by chemical, physical, biological or other procedures of any blood product that meets the definition of a drug as defined in section 201(k) of the act. It includes the manipulation, sampling, testing, or control procedures applied to the final product or to any part of the process and to the packaging, labeling, repackaging, or otherwise changing the container, wrapper, or labeling of any blood product package in furtherance of the distribution of the blood product from the original place of manufacture to the person who makes final delivery or sale to the ultimate consumer (21 CFR 607.3(d)).

Biological products are defined as "any virus, therapeutic serum, toxin, antitoxin, vaccine, blood, blood component or derivative, allergenic product, protein (except any chemically synthesized polypeptide), or analogous product or arsphenamine or derivative of arsphenamine (or other trivalent organic arsenic compound), applicable to the prevention, treatment, or cure of diseases or condition of human beings" (42 USC 262(i)). Biological products, including blood and blood components, are unique in that they may be considered as biological products under the PHS Act and as drugs or devices (depending on their mode of action) under the FD&C Act. This means that both the CGMP regulations for finished pharmaceuticals (21 CFR 210 and 211) and the CGMP regulations for blood and blood components (21 CFR 606) apply. Table 25–1 provides a comparison of biological products and drugs.

There are a variety of tools used by the FDA to communicate and enforce the regulatory requirements, agency recommendations, and product standards. These include regulations and guidance documents.

Statutes and Laws

Statutes are the acts passed by Congress and signed into law by the President to establish the FDA and to grant the agency authority to fulfill its mission. Statutes such as the PHS Act and the FD&C Act require biological product, drug, and device manufacturers to demonstrate to the FDA that their products are safe and effective (for drug products) or safe, pure, and potent (for biological products) before they are marketed in interstate commerce in the United States. They also require that all biological product, drug, and device manufacturers follow the applicable CGMP regulations and label their products appropriately. The FD&C and PHS Acts grant the FDA the authority to oversee and enforce the requirements described in the Acts, including inspecting the manufacturing facilities and imposing penalties for violations when appropriate. Over the years, there have been several amendments to the Acts to further define the agency's regulatory authority.

Regulations

Agencies promulgate regulations to establish a specific standard or requirement of conduct set by the federal government under the statutory authority granted by Congress (21 CFR 10.90). Regulations are an interpretation of the statutes and are legally binding on both the manufacturing industry and the government agencies charged with enforcing the laws. The regulations define specific minimum standards that manufacturers must meet. They often do not provide specific procedures on how to meet the standards. There may be many acceptable ways to achieve a required objective, and a requirement that is too specific may become outdated.

Proposed and final regulations are published in the *Federal Register* (FR), an official publication of the federal government, under the authority of the Administrative Procedure Act, which usually requires notice and an opportunity for the public to comment on regulations. FDA regulations are codified in Title 21 of the CFR. The regulations applicable to blood and blood components are found in subchapter F, Parts 600 to 680, and subchapter C, Parts 210 to 211, of Title 21 of the CFR. Major regulations pertaining to blood and blood components are listed in Box 25–2.

Guidance Documents

Guidance documents describe the agency's interpretation of or policy on a regulatory issue. The recommendations in the FDA's guidance documents are not legally binding on the manufacturing industry or other government agencies.

Table 25–1	**Comparison of Biological Products and Drugs**	
	BIOLOGICAL PRODUCTS (EXCLUDES MEDICAL DEVICES REGULATED AS BIOLOGICAL PRODUCTS)	**DRUGS**
Definition	Medical products typically derived from living sources that are used to prevent, treat, or cure diseases or conditions of human beings	Finished dosage form (pill, solution, cream, etc.) that contains an active pharmacological ingredient and is used to prevent, treat, or cure diseases or injuries in man
Examples	• Blood and blood components • Tissues, cellular therapies • Vaccines, antitoxins • Plasma derivatives (e.g., albumin, clotting factors, IGIV)	• Over-the-counter medications • Prescription medications • Chemotherapies
Regulatory authority	• Public Health Service Act • Federal Food, Drug, and Cosmetic Act	• Federal Food, Drug, and Cosmetic Act
CGMP regulations	21 CFR Parts 210 and 211 and 606	21 CFR Parts 210 and 211
Regulatory center in FDA	Center for Biologics Evaluation and Research (CBER)	Center for Drugs Evaluation and Research (CDER)

BOX 25–2

Major Regulations Pertaining to Blood and Blood Components[1]

Title 21 CFR, Chapter I, Subchapter C, Parts

210	Current good manufacturing practice in manufacturing drugs: general
211	Current good manufacturing practice for finished pharmaceuticals

Title 21 CFR, Chapter I, Subchapter F, Parts

600	Biological products: general
601	Licensing
606	Current good manufacturing practice for blood and blood components
607	Establishment registration and product listing for manufacturers of blood and blood components
610	General biological product standards
630	General requirements for blood, blood components, and blood derivatives
640	Additional standards for blood and blood products

However, the recommendations in these documents often become the industry standard of practice. In addition, FDA employees generally act consistently with the recommendations set forth in agency guidance documents, although they may depart from them with appropriate justification and supervisory concurrence (21 CFR 10.115(d)(3)).

Guidance documents (called memoranda up to 1996) are issued in order to (21 CFR 10.115):

- Describe the agency's interpretation of a policy or a regulatory issue
- Establish principles, practices, procedures, or standards
- Assist the manufacturing industry and government agencies by clarifying the regulations
- Explain how the manufacturing industry may comply with the regulations
- Provide application review and compliance approaches

Guidance documents are developed and issued under the Good Guidance Practices (GGP) regulations (21 CFR 10.115). GGP regulations allow for two types of guidance documents: Level 1 and Level 2.

Level I Guidance Documents (21 CFR 10.115(c)(1)):

- Set forth initial interpretations of statutory or regulatory requirements
- Set forth changes in interpretation or policy that are of more than a minor nature
- Can include complex scientific issues
- Sometimes cover highly controversial issues
- Are announced in the *Federal Register* through a Notice of Availability
- Are typically issued in draft format for public comment before implementation, although the FDA will issue a final guidance without an initial draft when the agency finds that prior public participation is not feasible or appropriate
- The FDA reviews comments and issues a final guidance

Level 2 Guidance Documents (21 CFR 10.115(c)(2)):

- Set forth existing practices or minor changes in interpretation or policy
- Include all guidance documents that are not classified as Level 1
- Do not require a Notice of Availability in the *Federal Register*
- Are immediately implemented unless the FDA indicates otherwise
- Invite public comment

The public may comment on any guidance document after final issuance and the FDA will determine if a revised guidance document should be issued. Guidance documents and memoranda applicable to blood and blood components can be found on the CBER website at www.fda.gov/BiologicsBloodVaccines/GuidanceComplianceRegulatoryInformation/Guidances/Blood/default.htm and at www.fda.gov/BiologicsBloodVaccines/GuidanceComplianceRegulatoryInformation/OtherRecommendationsforManufacturers/MemorandumtoBloodEstablishments/default.htm.

Center for Biologics Evaluation and Research

Center for Biologics Evaluation and Research (CBER) regulates allergenic products (e.g., allergenic extracts), cellular and gene therapy products, human tissue and tissue products (e.g., bone, skin, corneas), vaccines, (e.g., hepatitis B vaccine, influenza virus vaccine), and blood and blood components.

The Office of Blood Research and Review (OBRR) regulates the following products:

- Blood components for transfusion such as Whole Blood, Red Blood Cells, platelets, Fresh Frozen Plasma, Cryoprecipitated antihemophiliac factor (AHF), and modifications of these products.
- Blood components for further manufacturing such as Source Plasma, Source Leukocytes, recovered plasma
- Medical devices used for blood component collection and manufacturing, including blood bags (with or without anticoagulants and preservative solutions), nondiagnostic blood bank reagents, infectious disease tests for screening blood donors, blood establishment computer systems, blood irradiators, apheresis collection devices, and blood warmers
- Biological products used to treat and prevent diseases, including plasma derivatives such as clotting factors and immune globulins

Questions about the regulation of blood and blood components should be sent to Office of Communications, Outreach and Development, CBER, FDA (HFM-47), 1401 Rockville Pike, Suite 200N, Rockville, MD 20852-1448.

Registration and Licensure

Registration

The FD&C Act requires manufacturers to register their establishments with the FDA and list the products they manufacture. Regulations for blood establishment registration are found in the CFR (21 CFR 607). The following blood establishments are required to register with the FDA (21 CFR 607.20):

- Collection centers
- Community blood banks
- Component preparation facilities
- Hospital blood banks
- Plasmapheresis centers
- Product testing laboratories
- Storage and distribution centers
- Brokers who take possession and manipulate and/or relabel the product

Blood establishments must register within 5 days after beginning their manufacturing operations or within 5 days after the submission of a Biologics License Application (BLA) (21 CFR 607.21). Blood establishments may register by one of two methods: by completing a hard copy of the registration form (Form FDA-2830) and submitting it to the FDA or by completing an electronic registration form found on the CBER website (www.fda.gov/BiologicsBloodVaccines/GuidanceComplianceRegulatoryInformation/EstablishmentRegistration/BloodEstablishmentRegistration/default.htm).

The manufacturer must list all products and manufacturing processes performed at the establishment on the registration form and must complete a form for each manufacturing facility. Registered establishments are required to update their registration each year (21 CFR 607.21). In addition, all registered establishments are responsible for complying with the applicable FDA regulations, including CGMP and applicable product standards, and are routinely inspected by FDA investigators. Registered blood establishments that do not hold an approved BLA may only distribute their products in intrastate commerce.

The regulations exempt some blood establishments from registration (21 CFR 607.65). The exemption applies to:

- Transfusion services that neither collect nor process blood components and that only perform compatibility testing (crossmatching) and transfusion, pool Platelets and Cryoprecipitated AHF units immediately before transfusion, or issue bedside leukocyte-reduction filters with blood components and are either CLIA certified or have met equivalent requirements as determined by CMS
- Carriers that transport blood products
- Brokers who do not take possession, manipulate, or relabel the product

Table 25–2 summarizes the registration of blood establishments. Additional information about registration can be found on the CBER website at www.fda.gov/BiologicsBloodVaccines/GuidanceComplianceRegulatoryInformation/EstablishmentRegistration/BloodEstablishmentRegistration/default.htm.

Licensure

The PHS Act requires a biologics license to be in effect if a manufacturer wants to distribute biological products in interstate commerce. A biologics license will be issued only after the manufacturer demonstrates that the product is safe, pure, and potent and that the facility where the product is manufactured meets applicable requirements to ensure the biological product continues to be safe, pure, and potent (21 CFR 601.2(d)).

Unlike most licensed biological products, which typically have one Biologics License Application (BLA) approval per product, blood establishments manufacture multiple licensed products under one license and one BLA approval.

Table 25–2 Summary of the Registration of Blood Establishments

THE FOLLOWING FACILITIES ARE REQUIRED TO REGISTER:	THE FOLLOWING FACILITIES ARE EXEMPT FROM REGISTRATION:
Collection centers	
Community blood banks	
Component preparation facilities	
Hospital blood banks	Transfusion services that do not collect blood; only perform crossmatching and transfusion, pool Platelets and Cryoprecipitated AHF units immediately before transfusion, and issue bedside leukocyte-reduction filters, and are either CLIA certified or have met equivalent requirements as determined by CMS
Plasmapheresis centers	
Product testing laboratories	
Storage and distribution centers	Carriers (only transport product)
Brokers (take possession and manipulate and/or relabel product)	Brokers (do not take possession, manipulate, or relabel product)

The review of a BLA involves two steps: evaluating the submitted application documents (e.g., standard operating procedures [SOPs], forms, labels, product quality control, etc.) and conducting a pre-license inspection of the manufacturing facility (21 CFR 601.2). The applicant submits the necessary application forms and information about their operations to CBER (21 CFR 601.2).[8] Consumer safety officers (CSOs) in OBRR evaluate the application and supporting documents. The CSOs will inform the applicant if additional information is needed to complete the evaluation of the documents. As part of the application review, CSOs and ORA investigators will conduct a pre-license inspection of the manufacturing facility. The FDA investigators will observe the manufacturing processes to determine if the product is prepared according to the regulations, CGMP, product standards, and the manufacturing description provided in the application.

The applicant should respond to any inspectional observations noted during the inspection. After the applicant has addressed all deficiencies noted during the evaluation of the submitted application documents and the facility inspection, the CSO will make a decision regarding licensure. Once the manufacturer is licensed, the license number must appear on the label of the licensed products in order for the products to be distributed into interstate commerce. Licensed manufacturers are responsible for complying with all applicable FDA regulations, including CGMP and applicable product standards, and are inspected by FDA investigators at least once every 2 years (21 CFR 600.21).

Licensed manufacturers are required to inform the FDA about any intended change in manufacturing from previously approved procedures (21 CFR 601.12). Originally, when a manufacturer submitted a change to the FDA, the manufacturer had to wait for CBER to approve the change before the products could be distributed into interstate commerce. In 1997, CBER issued a new regulation to streamline some FDA activities and reduce the reporting burden by the manufacturing industry.[9] The regulations in the CFR were revised to be consistent with similar requirements in FDAMA. Title 21 CFR 601.12 is the regulation that addresses how licensed applicants report their manufacturing changes to the FDA. Manufacturing changes are now divided into the following three categories as determined by the potential of the change to adversely affect the safety, purity, and potency of the product. CBER has published guidance to help applicants determine the appropriate reporting category:[10]

- Major changes (based on associated risk) are reported as a Prior Approval Supplement (PAS) (21 CFR 601.12(b)). These submissions must be approved before the applicant can distribute the product made using the change into interstate commerce.
- Moderate changes (based on associated risk) are reported as a Changes Being Effected in 30 Days Supplement (CBE30) (21 CFR 601.12(c)). These submissions must be sent to the FDA for review and approval. The applicant may distribute the product made using the change in interstate commerce 30 days after the FDA has received the submission, unless the FDA has informed the applicant

not to distribute because of deficiencies in the submission. The 30-day wait is waived for some moderate changes, which are reported as a Changes Being Effected Supplement (CBE) (21 CFR 601.12(c)(5)). For submissions reporting these moderate changes, the product is distributed before the FDA has approved the change; therefore implementation of the change and distribution of the product made using the change are performed at the manufacturer's own risk. The FDA will review the submission, and if deficiencies are identified, will notify the manufacturer to submit the necessary information. In some cases, the FDA may require the manufacturer to stop distribution until any identified deficiencies have been corrected.

Minor changes are reported to the FDA in an annual report (21 CFR 601.12(d)). Minor changes do not need to be approved by the FDA before the product made using the minor change is distributed into interstate commerce. The FDA will review the annual report to determine if the changes have been reported in the proper category. The FDA will notify the manufacturer if the annual report contains changes that should be submitted as a supplement for FDA approval and may require the manufacturer to stop distribution until the supplement is reviewed and approved.

Unregistered Transfusion Services

The regulations exempt some blood establishments from registering with the FDA because they do not perform the manufacturing steps requiring registration and are either CLIA certified or have met equivalent requirements as determined by CMS (21 CFR 607.65). The majority of unregistered blood establishments operate as transfusion services that only perform compatibility testing (crossmatching) and transfusion, pool Platelets and Cryoprecipitated AHF units immediately before transfusion, and issue bedside leukocyte-reduction filters. Even though they are not registered or licensed, these manufacturers must still comply with the applicable FDA regulations, including CGMP and applicable product standards. There are certain instances when the FDA will inspect these blood establishments; these are typically "for-cause" inspections, such as investigating a transfusion-related fatality.

In 1983, the FDA entered into an agreement with the Health Care Financing Administration (HCFA), now called the Centers for Medicare and Medicaid Services (CMS).[11] The Memorandum of Understanding (MOU) between the FDA and CMS consolidated within CMS the responsibility for inspecting and surveying unregistered transfusion services in order to minimize duplication of effort and to reduce the burden on the affected blood establishments. Transfusion services that engage in the compatibility testing and transfusion of blood and blood components, but that neither routinely collect nor process blood components, are now covered by CMS. CMS, state survey agencies (including those in CLIA-exempt states), and accreditation organizations (such as CAP and AABB) conduct routine biennial surveys of transfusion services on behalf of the FDA. The FDA does not routinely survey transfusion services, although the FDA may inspect any transfusion service at any time.

Table 25–3 summarizes the regulatory oversight of blood and blood component manufacturing facilities.

Overview of the FDA's Inspection Process

Inspection Authorities

The statutory provisions granting the FDA the authority to enter biological product manufacturing facilities for the purposes of conducting inspections are found in both the PHS and FD&C Acts. The FDA conducts pre-license and pre-approval inspections, routine CGMP inspections, and for-cause inspections.

FDA investigators responsible for conducting inspections receive intensive training in the technical and regulatory aspects of the products and manufacturing facilities they inspect. The investigators for blood-related manufacturing are specialized into two teams: (1) Team Biologics, which is responsible for inspecting plasma derivative, reagent, vaccine, and allergenics manufacturers, and (2) the Biologics Cadre, who inspect blood, plasma, and tissue establishments. This reorganization was designed to facilitate inspections with improved consistency and appropriate citations.

Inspection Procedures

As part of the biologics license application process, CBER and ORA investigators conduct prelicense and preapproval inspections of manufacturing facilities that have submitted a BLA or a supplement to an approved BLA. Following approval of the BLA, ORA investigators who are trained as members of the Biologics Cadre will inspect the manufacturing facility at least once every 2 years (21 CFR 600.21). The Biologics Cadre also inspects unlicensed, registered blood establishments that only distribute blood and blood components in intrastate commerce. All FDA inspections are conducted according to the policies and procedures described in the ORA Investigations Operations Manual (IOM) and in written compliance programs and compliance policy guides. The compliance programs provide instructions on how to conduct the inspection and specify the process for recommending appropriate regulatory actions.[12] The compliance policy guides inform investigators and compliance officers about FDA policies and interpretations on specific regulatory issues.[13] These documents can be found on the ORA website at www.fda.gov/AboutFDA/Centers Offices/ORA/default.htm.

Each FDA inspection is conducted using a risk-based systems approach by covering some or all of the following manufacturing systems in a blood establishment operation to ensure compliance with applicable regulations and standards:[12]

- Quality Assurance System: various planned activities that provide confidence that all procedures and processes that influence product manufacture and overall quality are monitored to ensure they are working as expected.
- Donor (Suitability) Eligibility System: the system that protects donor safety, determines a donor's suitability for blood collection (including donor deferral from either history screening or testing), notifies donors of unsuitability for donation and evaluates donors for reentry.
- Product Testing System: the system that tests for communicable diseases, performs blood grouping and typing, and crossmatches blood for transfusion by direct testing or electronically.
- Quarantine/Inventory Management System: the system pertaining to product storage, distribution, and retrieval; quarantine; and distribution (release for use or destruction).
- Production and Processing System: process controls in the manufacture of specific blood and blood components, and equipment quality control, calibration, and maintenance.

FDA investigators discuss their observations with the manufacturer as the inspection progresses. At the end of the inspection, investigators list significant observations on

Table 25–3	Summary of the Regulatory Oversight of Blood and Blood Component Manufacturing Facilities		
	MANUFACTURERS THAT ENGAGE IN INTERSTATE AND INTRASTATE COMMERCE	**MANUFACTURERS THAT ENGAGE IN INTRASTATE COMMERCE ONLY**	**MANUFACTURERS THAT DO NOT PERFORM MANUFACTURING STEPS THAT REQUIRE REGISTRATION**
Requirements for registration	Must be registered	Must be registered	Exempt from registration
Requirements for licensure	Must hold an approved biologics license application	Do not need to be licensed	Do not need to be licensed
Applicable CGMP regulations include:	21 CFR 210, 211, 606	21 CFR 210, 211, 606	21 CFR 210, 211, 606
Inspections	Conducted by FDA: CBER (pre-license and pre-approval) and ORA investigators	Conducted by FDA: ORA investigators	Covered under CMS (CMS, state survey agencies, accredited organizations); FDA may conduct "for- cause" inspections
Regulatory oversight	FDA	FDA	CMS and FDA

the Form FDA-483, Inspectional Observations. Investigators present the Form FDA-483 to the manufacturer and listen to the proposed corrective actions. Investigators may also discuss less serious observations with the manufacturer to point out areas that could potentially cause significant problems. Both significant and less serious observations, as well as any discussions with the manufacturer, are included in the Establishment Inspection Report (EIR) prepared by the FDA investigators.[14] Most inspections result in voluntary compliance by the manufacturer to take corrective action, but inspections with numerous significant observations may trigger advisory, administrative, or legal actions, such as Warning Letters, license suspension, injunction, and prosecutions. Each year, the FDA conducts an average of 1,200 inspections of blood and blood component manufacturers.

Enforcement Actions

When a biological product manufacturer violates any of the laws or regulations the FDA enforces, the manufacturer is often given an opportunity for voluntary correction before the FDA pursues enforcement actions. There are three types of FDA actions: advisory, administrative, and judicial.[15]

Advisory Actions: Warning Letter

Advisory actions alert manufacturers that they have violated FDA regulations and provide an opportunity for corrective action before further compliance action is taken. Warning Letters are one example of an advisory action. The FDA will issue a Warning Letter to a biological product manufacturer for violations of regulatory significance. A Warning Letter is a written communication from the FDA to the manufacturer notifying them that their product, practice, or other activity is in violation of the law. The Warning Letter serves as a prior notice that the FDA may decide to take further action, and it offers the manufacturer an opportunity to correct the deficiencies listed in the letter. The FDA will conduct a follow-up inspection of the manufacturing facility to determine if corrective actions have been implemented. Warning Letters may have significant financial and legal ramifications for a company. These letters are available on the FDA's website at www.fda.gov/BiologicsBloodVaccines/Guidance ComplianceRegulatoryInformation/ucm135850.htm.

Administrative Actions: Suspension, Revocation

Administrative actions of license suspension or license revocation apply only to licensed manufacturers. These actions are more formal than advisory actions, such as issuing Warning Letters, and the agency usually must follow certain procedures, such as providing notice and an opportunity for a hearing. In addition, an affected company can seek a judicial review of the FDA's administrative decisions. The FDA may suspend a manufacturer's license if a danger to health exists (21 CFR 601.6). The FDA can administer this action immediately, and the manufacturer must take appropriate corrective actions and may not engage in interstate commerce of the product while the license is suspended.

A manufacturer's license can be revoked for several reasons: the FDA's inability to gain access to the facility to conduct a meaningful inspection, the discovery of significant CGMP deficiencies, or a determination that the product is not safe or effective for its intended use or is misbranded (21 CFR 601.5). The FDA may also revoke a license when it observes that the deficiencies have been ongoing and have not been corrected after numerous inspections and prior notice. The FDA may revoke a license or call for a voluntary revocation if the manufacturer no longer makes the product and therefore the FDA cannot conduct a meaningful inspection or evaluation. Revocation will prohibit the manufacturer from distributing the product into interstate commerce.

Judicial Actions: Seizure, Injunction, Prosecution

Seizure is an action taken to condemn violative products and remove them from distribution. The FDA and the U.S. Marshals Service take possession of the product typically under a court order. The court usually gives the owner of the seized product 30 days to decide on a course of action. If the owner does not communicate proposed actions, the FDA will dispose of the product. The owner may contest the charges and litigate in court to have the seized products returned. The owner is required to provide a monetary deposit (e.g., a bond) to ensure the court's orders will be carried out.

An injunction is a civil process initiated to stop or prevent violation of the law, such as to halt the flow of violative products in interstate commerce and to give the manufacturer an opportunity to correct the conditions that caused the violation to occur. The FDA may seek to obtain an injunction when a health hazard has been identified or the manufacturer has a history of violations and the evidence suggests that serious violations will continue.

An injunction may be used whether or not the manufacturer holds a biologics license. If there is no license to suspend or revoke, an injunction may be the only way for the FDA to halt the flow of violative products in interstate commerce and to correct the conditions that caused the violation to occur. If a manufacturer violates the terms of the injunction, a court may impose fines or even hold the company or specific corporate officers in contempt and the FDA may take further enforcement actions. As of 2009, only one blood and blood component manufacturer was under injunction.

A prosecution is a criminal action directed against a manufacturer or responsible individual(s) or both. The FDA may consider referring a matter to the Department of Justice for prosecution when fraud, health hazards, or continuing significant violations are encountered. The FD&C Act allows individuals or corporations for whom prosecution is being considered to be offered an opportunity to explain to the agency why the prosecution is not appropriate. Prosecution will proceed without a hearing if the violations are fraudulent or the responsible individuals are likely to flee. Table 25–4 summarizes the enforcement actions.

Table 25–4   Summary of Enforcement Actions[15]

Advisory actions	Warning Letter	• Notifies manufacturer that their product, practice, or other activity is in violation of the law • Serves as prior notice that the FDA may take further action • May be issued to both licensed and unlicensed manufacturers
Administrative actions	Suspension	• Applies to licensed manufacturers only • May occur if reasonable grounds for revocation and a danger to health exist • Provides immediate withdrawal of the authorization to ship a biological product in interstate commerce • Manufacturer cannot engage in interstate commerce until deviations are corrected and suspension is lifted • FDA can take this action quickly
	Revocation	• Applies to licensed manufacturers only • FDA may take this action if agency staff cannot gain access to facility to inspect or product is not safe or effective or is misbranded • Manufacturer cannot engage in interstate commerce after license is revoked
Judicial actions	Seizure	• Court order needed • FDA may seek seizure to condemn violative products and remove from distribution • FDA and U.S. Marshals Service take possession and may dispose of product
	Injunction	• Civil process to stop or prevent violation of the law (e.g., to stop producing a product; to comply with particular regulations) • Manufacturer can contest injunction in court • Court may impose penalties • Applies to both licensed and unlicensed manufacturers
	Prosecution	• FDA will refer cases to Department of Justice for possible prosecution • Applies to both licensed and unlicensed manufacturers • FDA will seek to prosecute for criminal conduct, including fraud or practices that lead to unsafe products or a pattern of violations

Current Good Manufacturing Practice Regulations

Under the FD&C Act, a drug is adulterated if the methods used in, or the facilities or controls used for, its manufacture, processing, packing, or holding do not conform to or are not operated or administered in conformity with current good manufacturing practice. Drugs must meet the requirements of the FD&C Act as to safety and must have the identity and strength and meet the quality and purity characteristics which it purports or is represented to possess.

CGMP regulations for finished pharmaceuticals are found in 21 CFR 210 and 211, and CGMP regulations specific for blood and blood components are found in 21 CFR Part 606. The CGMP regulations describe the minimum current practice and require all manufacturing facilities to implement and follow these requirements. The FD&C Act similarly provides that a medical device is adulterated if the methods used in, or the facilities or controls used for, its manufacture, packaging, storage, or installation are not in conformity with device CGMP regulations, which the FDA has issued in the Quality System Regulations found in 21 CFR 820.

In 1963, the FDA published the first drug CGMP regulations after observing that unsuitable products were being released to the public.[16] The FDA believed that this was due to an increase in number and complexity of the tests being performed and untrained or undertrained personnel deviating from established standards. During inspections, the FDA observed that there were often no controls in place to monitor the whole manufacturing process. The CGMP regulations were published to provide direction for this control and include the elements of quality assurance, quality control, and process validation. The CGMP regulations for blood and blood components were published in 1975.[17] Blood and blood component manufacturers must follow both the CGMP regulations in 21 CFR 210-211 and the more specific CGMP regulations for blood and blood components. The more specific requirements are in 21 CFR Part 606 supplement and do not supersede the more general CGMP requirements set forth in 21 CFR 210 and 211.

Quality Control Unit

The CGMP regulations require each manufacturer to designate a quality control unit that has the responsibility and authority to approve or reject all components, containers, closures, labeling, and drug products. Although the regulations identify this unit as a "quality control unit" (21 CFR 211.22), many manufacturers identify it as a quality assurance unit.

Under 21 CFR 211.22, the quality control unit has the responsibility and authority, at a minimum, to:

• Approve and reject components, containers (e.g., collection bags), supplies, and drug products

- Review production records for accuracy and completeness
- Investigate errors and deviations
- Review and approve standard operating procedures

The responsibilities and procedures applicable to the quality control unit must be in writing. The CGMP regulations do not prescribe how each manufacturer should develop its quality control unit or program but provide minimum requirements that must be adhered to when developing the program. This is to allow flexibility so that each manufacturer can develop a program that will work best in its own manufacturing environment. The FDA has published a guidance document to assist blood and blood component manufacturers in developing a quality assurance program.[18] The FDA generally recommends that the quality control functions be separate from the manufacturing operations because both have their own goals that may sometimes conflict.

Quality Reviews

The CGMP regulations require manufacturers to retain manufacturing and blood collection records, such as donor selection records (21 CFR 211.180 and 606.160). At least annually, the data from written records and quality standards of each product must be reviewed to determine the need for changes in product specifications or manufacturing or control procedures (21 CFR 211.180(e)). The FDA's Guideline for Quality Assurance in Blood Establishments[18] identifies the systems in a blood and blood component manufacturing operation and the critical control points that should be reviewed. The quality control unit or other assigned individuals are responsible for the quality activities, including the annual reviews.

The review should identify trends that could lead to the release of an unsuitable product. The quality control unit must investigate any unexplained discrepancy or the failure of a lot or unit to meet any of its specifications (21 CFR 606.100(c)). The FDA expects the outcome of such investigations will be the development and implementation of corrective and preventive actions. Implementing corrective and preventive actions could result in changes to product specifications or manufacturing and control procedures. The quality control unit must monitor these changes to ensure they adequately address the error and will result in the manufacture of a quality product. The review, investigation, and corrective actions must be documented. The quality control unit should have the authority to stop production if it determines the quality of the product is being adversely affected. The quality control unit should share the results of the review with the management of the manufacturing operations in order to affect the necessary changes to correct and prevent ongoing problems. Records of the reviews may be requested and reviewed during an FDA inspection.[19]

Additional Requirements of Biological Product Manufacturing

All biological product manufacturers must comply with all applicable biologics regulations in the CFR. This section lists some of the additional elements of biologics regulation.

Alternative Procedures ("Variances")

The regulations allow for blood and blood component manufacturers to perform procedures that vary from what is required in some sections of the CFR with the approval of CBER's Director (21 CFR 640.120). Specifically, manufacturers may request from CBER a variance to a regulation in subchapter F of the CFR (Parts 600 to 680). This provision provides flexibility to accommodate changes in technology and unanticipated circumstances that may warrant a departure from regulations. [20]

The procedures addressed by 21 CFR 640.120 are sometimes called "variances" and fall into two categories: an alternative procedure that is incorporated into blood establishment SOPs and an exception that is a singular event related to a specific emergency situation. Manufacturers wishing to implement a procedure that varies from the regulations in these specific sections of the CFR must submit a written request to CBER. A request for exception or alternate procedure from a licensed blood establishment must be submitted as a PAS supplement and contain sufficient information to show that the safety, purity, or potency of the product manufactured at a variance from the regulations will not be adversely affected. Manufacturers cannot implement an alternate procedure or exception until they have received approval from CBER. Examples of alternative procedures and exceptions that the FDA has approved are posted on the CBER website at www.fda.gov/BiologicsBloodVaccines/BloodBloodProducts/ RegulationoftheBloodSupply/ExceptionsandAlternative Procedures/default.htm.

Contract Manufacturing

Under the current regulations, one manufacturer may employ the services of a contract manufacturer to perform some or all of the product manufacturing steps.[21] The contractor is not under the direct control of the original biological product manufacturer, but the original manufacturer should ensure that the manufacturing steps performed by the contractor conform with FDA regulations. Contract manufacturers must be registered with the FDA because they are performing a manufacturing step on a regulated product (21 CFR 607.20(a)). In addition, the contractor must follow CGMP and all applicable regulatory product standards. Contractors should notify the original manufacturer of any changes in their operations, because these changes could affect the safety, purity, or potency of the product. The original manufacturer's quality control unit is responsible for approving or rejecting drug products manufactured, processed, packed, or held under contract by another company (21 CFR 211.22). Examples of contract manufacturing include an outside testing laboratory performing infectious disease testing on donors or products and a blood center irradiating blood components for a hospital transfusion service.

Short Supply Arrangements

A short supply arrangement is an example of a cooperative manufacturing arrangement. Short supply was introduced in

1948, and the provisions governing short supply are found in the CFR (21 CFR 601.22).[21] The short supply regulations allow a licensed biological product manufacturer to arrange for the partial manufacture of a biological product at an unlicensed facility under controlled conditions. Specifically, it allows an unlicensed product, such as recovered plasma, to be shipped in interstate commerce and used to manufacture a licensed final product. Short supply arrangements are most typically established when a blood or blood component manufacturer wants to market recovered plasma. The short supply arrangement must be in writing and is between the blood establishment and the licensed final product manufacturer. The written arrangement specifies the necessary manufacturing procedures and labeling.

Brokers frequently act as intermediaries between suppliers and licensed final product manufacturers. Selling recovered plasma to a broker does not relieve the supplier of the responsibility of obtaining a short supply arrangement. In addition, brokers who take physical possession of plasma must register with the FDA.

Biological Product Deviation Reporting

The regulations require all biological product manufacturers, including licensed and unlicensed manufacturers of blood and blood components and transfusion services, to report to the FDA any event that resulted in the distribution of an unsuitable biological product. Specifically, a manufacturer of blood and blood components must report to the FDA deviations from CGMP or unexpected events in a manufacturing operation that may adversely affect the safety, purity, or potency of the product that was distributed outside the manufacturer's control (21 CFR 606.171).[22] The biological product deviation report (BPDR) must be submitted to CBER as soon as possible but no later than 45 calendar days from the date the event was discovered. Manufacturers may submit a hard copy report or report the BPDR electronically at www.fda.gov/Biologics BloodVaccines/SafetyAvailability/ReportaProblem/Biological ProductDeviations/default.htm. For additional information on BPDRs, contact the Division of Inspections and Surveillance, OCBQ, CBER (HFM-650), 1401 Rockville Pike, Rockville, MD 20852-1448.

In fiscal year (FY) 2008, CBER received 44,125 BPDRs from blood and blood component manufacturers.[23] The majority of the reports (68.3%) involved postdonation information (Table 25–5), which is information received from donors following the collection of the product. In many instances, this information is known by the donor at the time of donation and would have caused the donor to be deferred had he or she given the information to the blood center. On occasion, the products from these donors are still at the blood center, but often they have already been distributed. The manufacturer should take appropriate action after reviewing the impact of the donor's information on product safety. The manufacturer may need to identify each affected product collected from a donor who is subsequently determined to be unsuitable and recall these products.

Table 25–5	Biological Product Deviations Reported to the CBER in FY 2008[23]	
MANUFACTURING SYSTEM		**% OF TOTAL (44,125)**
Postdonation information		68.3
Quality control and distribution		11.2
Labeling		5.2
Donor screening		5.2
Miscellaneous		4.3
Routine testing (ABO, Rh, antibody screen)		2.5
Blood collection		1.8
Component preparation		1.1
Donor deferral		0.3
Infectious disease testing		0.1

Product Recalls

The FDA may order the recall of a biological product that presents an imminent or substantial hazard to the public health or a medical device if there is a reasonable probability that a device intended for human use would cause serious, adverse health consequences or death. However, the FDA rarely has to resort to these authorities and instead relies on the voluntary recall policy contained in 21 CFR Part 7. Voluntary product recalls are the manufacturer's removal or correction of a marketed product that the FDA considers to be in violation of the laws (21 CFR 7.3 and 7.40). Voluntary recalls can be initiated by the manufacturer or requested by the FDA if the product represents a risk of illness or injury or if there is gross consumer deception, the firm has not initiated a recall, and agency action is necessary to protect the public health.

The manufacturer is responsible for developing a recall strategy and conducting the recall. The manufacturer is also responsible for contacting customers with information identifying the affected products and prescribing appropriate actions to take (21 CFR 7.49). The FDA will monitor the recall, including assessing the manufacturer's efforts to notify the appropriate parties. A recall is classified as completed or closed when all reasonable efforts have been made to remove or to correct the product. The FDA may seize the product if it determines that the recall is ineffective.

Recalls of blood and blood components are different from most drug product recalls because the blood or blood component may already have been transfused. In these cases, there can be no physical recall or return of the unit. When blood or a blood component has already been transfused, a recall is really a notification that the product failed to meet standards for safety, purity, and potency.

Recalls are accompanied by a health hazard evaluation of the recalled product by FDA medical staff and scientists to determine if the product caused or could cause harm to a recipient (21 CFR 7.41). The recall will be classified as a class I, II, or III recall based on the potential for a product to cause serious health problems as outlined below:

- Class I: Situation in which there is a reasonable probability that the use of the product will cause serious adverse health consequences or death
- Class II: Situation in which use of the product may cause temporary or medically reversible adverse health consequences or the probability of serious adverse health consequences is remote
- Class III: Situation in which use of the product is not likely to cause adverse health consequences

In FY 2008, CBER classified 2,070 recalls.[24] Most of the recalls involved blood and blood components that were either not likely to cause an adverse reaction or would at most cause only temporary health problems. Additional information about biological product recalls can be found on the CBER website at www.fda.gov/BiologicsBloodVaccines/SafetyAvailability/Recalls/default.htm.

Fatality Reporting

Blood and blood component manufacturers should initially notify CBER of any transfusion-related fatalities or donation-related deaths. The regulations require the blood and blood component manufacturer to formally notify CBER within 7 days after the fatality is confirmed (21 CFR 606.170(b)).[25] The 7-day written report should describe all information related to the fatality. Collection facilities are required to report donation-related deaths, and the facility that performed the compatibility tests must report transfusion-related fatalities. Fatalities are reported to CBER to:

- Ensure that fatalities are thoroughly investigated
- Determine if appropriate corrective actions have been taken to prevent a recurrence
- Determine if there are trends that may warrant FDA action

FDA investigators may visit the reporting facility to follow up on the fatality reports. In FY 2008, CBER received 72 transfusion recipient fatality reports (46 were assessed to be transfusion-related fatalities) and 10 postdonation fatality reports.[26] Transfusion-Related Acute Lung Injury (TRALI) was the most common cause of transfusion-related fatalities (Table 25-6). Additional information on reporting fatalities can be found on the CBER website at

Table 25–6   Transfusion Related Fatalities Reported to the CBER in FY 2008[26]

COMPLICATION	% OF TOTAL (46)
Transfusion-Related Acute Lung Injury (TRALI)	34.8
Hemolytic transfusion reaction (ABO)	21.7
Hemolytic transfusion reaction (non-ABO)	15.2
Microbial infection	15.2
Transfusion Associated Circulatory Overload (TACO)	6.5
Anaphylaxis	6.5

www.fda.gov/BiologicsBloodVaccines/SafetyAvailability/ReportaProblem/TransfusionDonationFatalities/ucm113649.htm.

Medical Devices

CBER regulates medical devices used in the collection, processing, testing, manufacturing, and administration of blood, blood components, human cells, tissues, and cellular- and tissue-based products.[27] Certain products meeting the definition of a medical device and used in blood collection or processing are subject to license under Section 351 of the PHS Act. Other medical devices used in blood collection or processing are regulated under the device authorities in Section 510(k) of the FD&C Act. Licensed biological products that meet the definition of a device are reviewed in the same manner as other licensed biological products. Examples of such licensed biological products are blood grouping reagents and infectious disease tests used for donor screening. Examples of devices used in blood collection or processing regulated by CBER under the FD&C Act are blood irradiators, blood warmers, blood establishment computer systems, blood filters, and apheresis collection instruments. Manufacturers of licensed biological products that are devices must register with the FDA and list their products under 21 CFR 607, and manufacturers of cleared biological devices must register with the FDA and list their products under 21 CFR 807. Both must follow device CGMP, known as the Quality Systems Regulations (21 CFR 820). Additional information about biological devices can be found on the CBER website at www.fda.gov/BiologicsBloodVaccines/DevelopmentApprovalProcess/510kProcess/default.htm. Additional information about the FDA and regulatory issues related to blood and blood components can be found at www.fda.gov/BiologicsBloodVaccines/default.htm.

SUMMARY CHART

✔ The FDA promulgates and enforces regulations to ensure the safety and efficacy of biological products, drugs, and devices, which include blood and blood components, blood collection supplies and instruments, blood grouping reagents, and donor screening tests for infectious diseases.

✔ A drug or device is misbranded if its labeling is false or misleading.

✔ One reason a drug is considered adulterated is if the methods used to manufacture it do not conform with CGMP to ensure the drug is safe and has the identity and strength and meets the quality and purity characteristics which it is represented to possess.

✔ The ORA is responsible for performing routine FDA inspections and other surveillance activities.

✔ The FDA's five overlapping layers of safety of blood and blood components include determining donor eligibility, testing the donation for certain infectious diseases, checking donor deferral registries, quarantining unsuitable products, and investigating and correcting manufacturing problems.

✔ Biological products are defined as any virus, therapeutic serum, toxin, antitoxin, vaccine, blood, blood component or derivative, allergenic product, protein (except any chemically synthesized polypeptide), or analogous product or arsphenamine or derivative of arsphenamine (or other trivalent organic arsenic compound) applicable to the prevention, treatment, or cure of diseases or conditions of human beings.

✔ Statutes are the laws and acts passed by Congress and signed by the President to establish the FDA and to grant the agency authority to fulfill its mission. The Acts enforced by the FDA that are most relevant to blood regulation are the FD&C Act and the PHS Act.

✔ The blood establishments required to register with the FDA under the FD&C Act include collection centers, community blood banks, component preparation facilities, hospital blood banks, plasmapheresis centers, product testing laboratories, storage and distribution centers, and brokers who take possession and manipulate and/or relabel the product.

✔ The PHS Act requires an approved biologics license to be in effect before biological products are distributed in interstate commerce.

✔ The FDA may suspend or revoke a biologics license if there are continued violations that result in harm to a blood or plasma donor or blood or blood component recipient.

✔ CGMP is the minimum current practice for methods to be used in and the facilities or controls to be used for the manufacture, processing, packing, or holding of a drug to ensure that the drug meets the requirements of the FD&C Act as to safety and has the identity and strength and meets the quality and purity characteristics that it purports or is represented to possess.

✔ CBER must approve alternative procedures or exceptions from the regulations before the product made at a variance from the regulations is distributed.

✔ Deviations in biological product manufacturing that affect the safety, purity, or potency of distributed products must be reported to the FDA if the affected product was distributed.

✔ A product recall is the removal or correction of a marketed product that the FDA considers to be in violation of the laws.

✔ Following a confirmed fatality involving blood collection or transfusion, the manufacturer must notify CBER as soon as possible and provide a written report within 7 days of the incident.

Review Questions

1. Which of the following is responsible for overseeing the safety of the nation's blood supply?
   a. Joint Commission on Accreditation of Healthcare Organizations
   b. Food and Drug Administration
   c. College of American Pathologists (CAP)
   d. Occupational Safety and Health Administration

2. Where are the regulations for blood and blood components published?
   a. The AABB Technical Manual
   b. CAP inspection checklist
   c. The Code of Federal Regulations
   d. State Inspectional Guidance Documents

3. What was an important tragedy that prompted Congress to enact the Public Health Service Act?
   a. Three patients contracted hepatitis C following transfusion
   b. A child died following transfusion of hemolyzed red blood cells
   c. A group O patient received group A blood
   d. Thirteen children died after receiving diphtheria antitoxin contaminated with tetanus

4. What is required to ship blood and blood components across state lines (interstate)?
   a. AABB accreditation
   b. State license
   c. CMS certification
   d. Approved Biologics License Application

5. Which of the following government organizations inspect blood and blood component manufacturers?
   a. CBER
   b. ORA
   c. CMS
   d. All of the above

6. Which of the following is true about CGMP?
   a. CGMP is the minimum current practice for methods and facilities used to manufacture a drug to ensure that it is safe, pure, and potent.
   b. The FDA will approve a Biologics License Application if the manufacturer does not have a quality control plan.
   c. The quality control unit must perform all the quality functions.
   d. Blood and blood components do not have to be in compliance with the drug CGMP regulations.

7. A donor calls the blood bank and informs them that within a year prior to his donation, he had intimate contact with a person diagnosed with HIV. Which of the following action is NOT required by the FDA?
   a. Identify and quarantine all blood and blood components produced from the blood supplied by the donor
   b. Report the biological product deviation to CBER if the product has already been distributed
   c. Enter the donor in a record so that he can be identified and his product not be distributed while he is deferred
   d. Notify the AABB

8. A patient dies following transfusion of ABO-incompatible blood. To whom should this event be reported?
   a. The Center for Biologics Evaluation and Research
   b. Center for Medicare and Medicaid Services
   c. The AABB central office
   d. The Occupational Safety and Health Administration

9. Which federal agency has the responsibility to routinely inspect an unregistered transfusion service that does not collect blood?
   a. Food and Drug Administration
   b. Centers for Medicare and Medicaid Services
   c. Occupational Safety and Health Administration
   d. State health department

10. Which of the following is NOT one of the FDA layers of safety?
    a. Donor screening
    b. Biologics License Application
    c. Investigation of manufacturing problems
    d. Infectious disease testing

References

1. Code of Federal Regulations, Title 21, FDA. US Government Printing Office, Washington, DC, April 1, 2010. Available at www.gpoaccess.gov/CFR/.

2. Commemorating 100 Years of Biologics Regulation. Science and the regulation of biological products from a rich history to a challenging future. Center for Biologics Evaluation and Research, FDA, March 2002. Available at www.fda.gov/AboutFDA/WhatWeDo/History/ProductRegulation/100YearsofBiologicsRegulation/default.htm.

3. The Coroner's Verdict in the St. Louis Tetanus Cases. 1901 New York Medical Journal 74; Special Article: Fatal results from diphtheria antitoxin. Minor comments: Tetanus from antidiphtheria serum. JAMA, 1901; 37:1255, 1260.

4. Public Health Service Act. Regulation of Biological Products. Title 42 United States Code, Chapter 6A, Part F, Section 262 (42USC262). Available at www.fda.gov/RegulatoryInformation/Legislation/ucm148717.htm.

5. Federal Food, Drug and Cosmetic Act. Drugs and Devices. Chapter V, Subchapter A. Available at www.fda.gov/RegulatoryInformation/Legislation/FederalFoodDrugandCosmeticActFDCAct/FDCActChapterVDrugsandDevices/default.htm.

6. History of the FDA. Available at www.fda.gov/AboutFDA/WhatWeDo/History/default.htm.

7. Keeping blood transfusion safe: FDA's multi-layered protections for donated blood. Available at www.fda.gov/BiologicsBloodVaccines/SafetyAvailability/BloodSafety/ucm095522.htm.

8. FDA Guidance for Industry: For the Submission of Chemistry, Manufacturing and Controls and Establishment Description Information for Human Blood and Blood Components Intended for Transfusion or For Further Manufacture and for the Completion of the Form FDA 356h "Application to Market a New Drug, Biologic or an Antibiotic Drug for Human Use," May 1999. Available at www.fda.gov/BiologicsBloodVaccines/GuidanceComplianceRegulatoryInformation/Guidances/Blood/ucm077087.htm.

9. Changes to an Approved Application. Federal Register. 62 FR 39901, July 24, 1997.

10. FDA Guidance for Industry: Changes to an Approved Application: Biological Products: Human Blood and Blood Components Intended for Transfusion or For Further Manufacture, July 2001. Available at www.fda.gov/BiologicsBloodVaccines/GuidanceComplianceRegulatoryInformation/Guidances/Blood/ucm076729.htm.

11. Memorandum of Understanding between the Health Care Financing Administration and the Food and Drug Administration. FDA 225-80-4000, June 6, 1983. Available at www.fda.gov/AboutFDA/PartnershipsCollaborations/MemorandaofUnderstandingMOUs/DomesticMOUs/ucm116313.htm.

12. FDA Compliance Program Guidance Manual—7342.001: Inspection of Licensed and Unlicensed Blood Banks, Brokers, Reference Laboratories, and Contractors. FDA Office of Regulatory Affairs, Implementation Date: October 1, 2006. Available at www.fda.gov/BiologicsBloodVaccines/GuidanceComplianceRegulatoryInformation/ComplianceActivities/Enforcement/Complit/ancePrograms/ucm095226.htm.

13. Chapter 2, Biologics, FDA Compliance Policy Guides, FDA Office of Regulatory Affairs. Available at www.fda.gov/ICECI/ComplianceManuals/CompliancePolicyGuidanceManual/ucm116336.htm.

14. Investigations Operations Manual, FDA Office Of Regulatory Affairs, 2009. Available at www.fda.gov/ICECI/Inspections/IOM/default.htm.

15. FDA Regulatory Procedures Manual. FDA Office of Regulatory Affairs, March 2009. Available at www.fda.gov/ICECI/ComplianceManuals/RegulatoryProceduresManual/default.htm.

16. Drugs: current good manufacturing practice in manufacture, processing, packing, or holding. Federal Register. 28 FR 6385, June 20, 1963.

17. Human blood and blood products: collection, processing and storage. Federal Register. 40 FR 53531, November 18, 1975.

18. FDA Guideline for Quality Assurance in Blood Establishments, July 11, 1995. Available at www.fda.gov/BiologicsBlood Vaccines/GuidanceComplianceRegulatoryInformation/ Guidances/Blood/default.htm.

19. FDA Compliance Policy Guide, Sec. 130.300 FDA access to results of quality assurance program audits and inspections. FDA Office of Regulatory Affairs, June 2, 2007. Available at www. fda.gov/ICECI/ComplianceManuals/CompliancePolicy GuidanceManual/ucm073841.htm.

20. Blood and blood products: amendment to allow for alternative procedures; removal of a labeling requirement. Federal Register. 55 FR 10420, March 21, 1990.

21. FDA Guidance for Industry: Cooperative Manufacturing Arrangements for Licensed Biologics, November 2008. Available at www.fda.gov/BiologicsBloodVaccines/GuidanceCompliance RegulatoryInformation/Guidances/General/ucm069883.htm.

22. FDA Guidance for Industry: Biological Product Deviation Reporting for Blood and Plasma Establishments, October 2006. Available at www.fda.gov/BiologicsBloodVaccines/Guidance ComplianceRegulatoryInformation/Guidances/Blood/ ucm073455.htm.

23. Biological product deviation annual summary for fiscal year 2008. October 1, 2007, through September 30, 2008. Available at www.fda.gov/BiologicsBloodVaccines/SafetyAvailability/ ReportaProblem/BiologicalProductDeviations/ucm169990.htm.

24. The Enforcement Story, FDA Office of Regulatory Affairs, March 2009. Available at www.fda.gov/ICECI/Enforcement Actions/EnforcementStory/default.htm.

25. FDA Guidance for Industry: Notifying FDA of Fatalities Related to Blood Collection or Transfusion, September 2003. Available at www.fda.gov/BiologicsBloodVaccines/GuidanceCompliance RegulatoryInformation/Guidances/Blood/ucm074947.htm.

26. Fatalities Reported to FDA Following Blood Collection and Transfusion: Annual Summary for fiscal year 2008. October 1, 2007, through September 30, 2008. Available at www.fda.gov/ BiologicsBloodVaccines/SafetyAvailability/ReportaProblem/ TransfusionDonationFatalities/ucm113649.htm.

27. CBER's Annual Report for Fiscal Year 2008. Available at www.fda.gov/AboutFDA/CentersOffices/CBER/ucm122880.htm.

Chapter 26

Laboratory Information Systems

Ann Tiehen, MT(ASCP)SBB, Gregory Wright, MT(ASCP)SBB, and Melissa Volny, MT(ASCP)SBB

OBJECTIVES

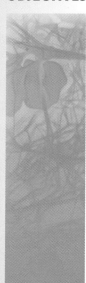

1. Explain the purpose of an information system in a blood bank.
2. Correlate the hardware components of a blood bank information system with their functions.
3. Describe a blood bank information system hardware configuration.
4. Describe the functions of the software components of a blood bank information system.
5. List the responsibilities of operating and maintaining a blood bank information system.
6. Identify regulatory and accrediting agency requirements pertaining to blood bank information systems.
7. Apply the functions of blood bank software applications to blood bank processes.
8. Explain the purpose of a truth table.
9. Construct a truth table for a routine blood bank test.
10. Identify the standard operating procedures (SOPs) needed to manage a blood bank information system.
11. Describe and justify the kinds of testing that should be included in the validation of a blood bank information system.
12. Interpret the results of a software validation test.
13. Identify the times at which validation testing must be performed.
14. Define *control function* and differentiate between process control and decision support.
15. Evaluate a validation test plan and identify its component parts.

Introduction

Information processing plays a vital role in blood banking practice. The proper management of information related to blood donors, blood components, and patients receiving transfusions is crucial to ensuring the safety and traceability of blood products. Blood bank personnel heavily rely on computerized information systems to assist in the handling of this important information.

Regulatory and standard-setting agencies have put increasing pressure on blood banks to store information in a safe manner and retrieve it in a timely fashion. It must be possible to track a blood component from the time of its donation, through all of the processing steps, and to the patient who receives it. It is also essential to be able to perform that trace in reverse order, from the recipient back to the donor.

Before computerized information systems were available, all blood bank data were stored on paper, or "hard copy," records requiring labor-intensive and sometimes error-prone procedures to retrieve it. As blood bank information systems have become more sophisticated, they have made recovering the information much more efficient and have offered the

Table 26–1	**Common Information System Acronyms**
ACRONYM	**DEFINITION**
CPU	Central processing unit
HIS	Hospital information system
LIS	Laboratory information system
PC	Personal computer
RAM	Random access memory
ROM	Read-only memory
SOP	Standard operating procedure

industry a great variety of process controls to reduce errors. Several acronyms unique to the specialty of information systems will be used throughout this chapter and are listed in Table 26–1.

Types of Information Systems

Computerized blood bank **information systems** are available in many different configurations, but they comprise three general categories:

1. A highly complex system like that found in a community blood center
2. A small part of a complete clinical **laboratory information system (LIS)**
3. A stand-alone system, usually found in a hospital blood bank or transfusion service

The functionality of these systems varies from category to category and from vendor to vendor within each category. Some systems may act merely as record keepers, whereas others have the ability to use the information in such a way as to prevent errors in donor acceptance, blood component release, or patient transfusion. For example, a basic system used in a hospital transfusion service may simply allow the entry of an ABO group and Rh type in a patient's record with subsequent generation of a charge for the test. A more complex system in a hospital blood bank can record the donation of an autologous unit in the donor room and then make the transfusion service technologist aware of its presence when the patient is admitted for a type-and-screen test at the time of surgery.

System Components

A computer system includes three major components: hardware, software, and people. **Hardware** components are the physical pieces of equipment. **Software** is a set of instructions written in computer language that tells the computer how to operate and manipulate the data. The people interface with the hardware to enter the data that are manipulated by the software. Just as there are many different kinds of people who enter data, so there are many different kinds of hardware and software.

Hardware

Most of the hardware components of a computer system are readily identifiable because they can be seen and touched, although some are hidden inside a case or a central system unit. Each piece of hardware performs a specific function in the handling of information. The three main functions performed by hardware components are processing, input and output, and storage.

Hardware components include a **central system unit**, sometimes referred to as the *box*, and several different peripheral devices that send or receive information through the system unit. **Peripheral devices** include display terminals, keyboards, bar-code readers, scanners and wands, pointing devices such as mice, printers, and modems. The hardware components and the way in which they are connected to each other is the system configuration. Figure 26–1 illustrates one such configuration.

Processing Hardware

The central hardware component of a computer system is the **central processing unit** (CPU), which is an electric circuit or silicon "chip" that processes information. The CPU, also called a *processor*, is the core of the machine. It controls the interpretation and execution of instructions provided by the software. Other pieces of processing hardware that exist in the system unit are the ROM and RAM chips. **Read-only memory** (ROM) contains the "start-up" instructions for the computer. **Random access memory** (RAM) is an array of chips in which data are temporarily entered while they are being processed. When a computer is turned on, these chips interact with each other and with the operating system software to prepare the computer to accept data and instructions from its users.

Input and Output Devices

Although users can occasionally be seen shouting at their computer systems, most blood bank information systems

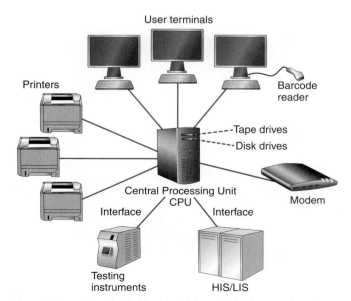

Figure 26–1. Example of a blood bank information hardware configuration.

cannot recognize voice instructions. Commands and data must be entered in a format that the computer can understand. This requires tools that are connected to the system's CPU such as keyboards, pointing devices, bar-code readers, and testing instruments. Keyboards are used to type instructions that tell the computer what to do or to enter data such as donor demographic information or patient test results. Many systems also accept **bar-coded information** from sources such as blood component labels or test tubes. Blood component labels contain many pieces of bar-coded information, including the unit number, blood type, product type, facility identification number, and expiration date. Entry of this information by a bar-code reader is much more accurate than when done by manual entry methods. Figure 26–2 shows a blood component label with this bar-coded information. Scanning the bar codes with an optical or laser device allows efficient entry of the blood component data.

The most common output device is the monitor, which displays information as it is typed on the keyboard. Together, the monitor and the keyboard make up the user terminal. The monitor may also display historical information at the user's request.

Another commonly used output device is the printer, which provides hard-copy output on paper. Printers can produce labels, donor registration records, compatibility tags, management reports, patient chart reports, and donor correspondence. The kind of printer chosen for any of these

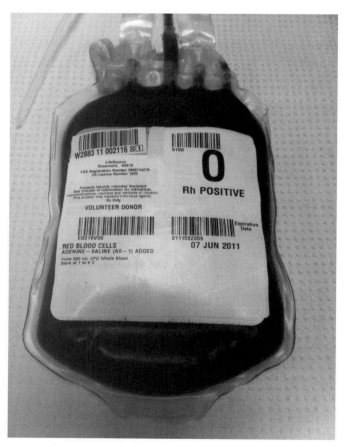

Figure 26–2. Bar codes on unit label.

applications depends on the quality of print desired. For example, a bar-code label requires a high-resolution printing that bar-code readers can accurately interpret. Management reports, which are usually used internally, can be of lower quality print.

An example of a combined input and output device is a modem. Modems allow computer systems to communicate with each other via network or telephone lines. Blood banks can use this mechanism to connect remote facilities to the main computer system so that all sites have access to the system's databases. This configuration is found in blood centers with several collection or testing locations or in a system of hospital affiliates. The technical support staff of software vendors uses modems to investigate and solve system problems and to transfer files to the customer.

Information Storage Hardware

All computer systems have hardware that allows long-term storage of data. This is sometimes referred to as *memory* but should not be confused with RAM, which is only temporary and active when the system is turned on. **Long-term memory** is data saved on a medium from which they can later be retrieved, such as a hard disk. Most systems contain a hard disk controlled by a hard drive. The disk is made of metal coated with a magnetic film and contains software applications (programs) and user-entered data. The hard disk is often contained in the main system unit, but it may also be a peripheral device. The information on the disk is accessed by entering commands, usually with a keyboard connected to a display terminal. Other information storage hardware may be used for archiving old information that has been removed from the hard disk.

Software

Software tells the computer what to do with all of the information it has received. Minimally, every computer system has two kinds of software—operating system software and application software. Some systems may also use interface software, which allows the system to communicate with other computer systems.

Application Software

An application is software that has been designed to perform specific tasks. Personal computers (PCs) can be equipped with application programs such as word processing, spreadsheets, and databases. In a blood bank information system, the **application software** allows users to perform tasks that are specific to blood bank operations. In a donor setting, some of these tasks might include entering donor demographic information and test results, confirming blood component labeling, and generating donor recruitment lists. In a transfusion service, the computer may help with tasks such as searching for a blood component of a particular ABO group, entering blood component modification information, and issuing blood for transfusion. These tasks are distinctly connected to blood banking and would be difficult, if not impossible, to perform in an application not specifically designed for blood bank use.

One of the most important functions performed by blood bank applications is maintaining a database of donors, blood components, and transfusion recipients. A **database** is an organized set of information divided into files and then further subdivided into records. Files exist in one of two ways: they may be static or dynamic. The **dynamic files** contain records related to a specific donor, patient, or blood component. These records are frequently changed as updated information is added to them. For example, the status of a blood component can go from "quarantined" to "transfused," with many intermediate statuses during its shelf life.

The **static files** contain information that is updated infrequently, such as the list of blood products used in the facility. These files, which look different in each blood bank, define the terminology that the blood bank uses. When a new blood bank information system is installed, the static files must be defined before the system can be put into use. One of the most important functions of the static files is to provide a "dictionary" of coded terms that the information system can use to sort and organize the tremendous amount of data entered into it. For example, two static files, one containing codes for physicians and the other codes for blood products, can allow the system to sort information regarding the cross-match-to-transfusion (C:T) ratio of each physician who ordered blood within a particular time period.

Figure 26–3 shows how the parts of a database relate to each other. The database itself can be considered a file cabinet containing folders or files that contain specific records. This illustration is of a dynamic file containing patient records. A static file illustrated in this way—for example, for blood product codes—would list a separate file for each blood product code used in the facility. The associated records would include such information as the official name of the blood component, its maximum allowable shelf life, and whether it contains red blood cells (RBCs) and thus requires crossmatching.

Operating System Software

The tasks performed by the **operating system** are fairly invisible to users because this software works in the background.

It is a set of instructions that controls the computer's hardware, manipulates the application software, and coordinates the flow of data to and from disks and memory. When new data are entered into one of the application programs, it is the operating system that places those data on the disk for storage; when a request for those data is made through the application program, the operating system retrieves them and sends them to the application software for display on a monitor or printed report.

Interface Software

Frequently, different information systems must be allowed to share data with each other to take full advantage of their functionality. Because different systems communicate in different computer languages, they need an interpreter that will allow data to flow between the two systems in a controlled manner. The interpreter is another set of software called an **interface**. Interface software may be used to allow data to flow between a **hospital information system** (HIS) and the blood bank system or between the LIS and the blood bank. For example, an interface between the HIS and the blood bank information system can allow patient demographic information to flow from the HIS to the blood bank system and can allow test results and blood component information to flow from the blood bank system to the HIS, where they can be displayed on terminals in patient care areas.

People

The human components of a blood bank information system are the users and at least one person designated as the system manager. Users have access to the technical applications needed to perform daily blood bank operations. System managers require access to a wider range of applications, including system maintenance functions.

Users

Entry of commands and data into the system is performed by the users. The success with which a blood bank computer

Figure 26–3.   Relationship between database components from general database files to individual patient record items.

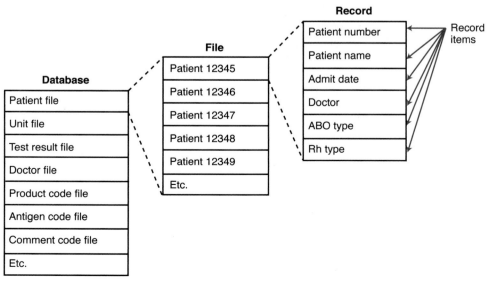

system can be used depends not only on its ease of use but also on the training provided to its users. Most systems are equipped with both a "live" or production database and a "test" database. The static files in both databases are identical, but their dynamic files contain different information. The production database contains real information, whereas the test database consists of fictitious records. The test database offers the user an opportunity to practice the applications of the system (and to make mistakes) without corrupting the database containing actual donor and patient information. Users should be trained in every application they will be expected to use.

System Managers

The configuration and location of the information system will determine the identity and quantity of people performing this task. In a large community blood center, there may be an entire staff dedicated to managing the system. In a hospital blood bank or transfusion service that uses the blood bank module of a complete clinical LIS, the laboratory system manager is likely to have responsibility for the entire system, but there should also be a designated blood bank system manager. In blood banks equipped with a stand-alone blood bank computer, designated system managers may also have other supervisory, technical, or quality assurance duties.

Whatever the duties of the system manager, he or she also oversees the maintenance of the system's hardware and software. Some specific duties include adding or deleting items from the static database files, assigning access codes to new users, and implementing software upgrades from the vendor. In addition, the system manager will be required to investigate problems encountered by the users and to report them to the system vendor.

Blood Bank Software Applications

The kinds of data that must be managed by a particular blood bank information system depend on the types of services provided by the blood bank. Most community blood centers focus on donations and distribution of the donated blood components to customer hospitals. In the hospital transfusion service, the primary concern is the transfusion of patients. However, a community blood center or a hospital blood bank with both a transfusion service laboratory and a donation center must address issues of donor and patient management. Application programs exist for every task, from scheduling donors to assigning a transfused status to a blood component. Many of the typical blood bank information system applications currently available are discussed in this section.

Donation Facility

The applications utilized at a donor center enable the users to manage the flow of donors and blood products from donor recruitment to distribution of the final products to hospital customers.

Donor Management

The system should allow the capture of donor demographic information necessary for definitive donor identification,

telephone contact for recruitment, and notification in the event that abnormal laboratory testing results are obtained. In addition, the system should have a means for preventing a donation from a deferred individual or from one attempting to donate before the required waiting period between donations.

Donor Registration. When a potential donor registers at a donation facility, several pieces of demographic data must be provided, such as name, date of birth, phone number, and mailing address. When this information is entered into the donor database, the system can search for a previous donation record from the same donor. If none is found, a new donor record is created. If there is a record of a previous donation, the system can review the donor's eligibility status. This would include calculating the length of time elapsed since the last donation and examining the record for a deferral because of medical history or disease testing results. If the donor is ineligible because of an inadequate amount of time since the last donation or a previous deferral, the system can alert the registrar and prevent an unsuitable donation from occurring. If the registration is taking place at a location that does not have immediate access to the electronic database, as may happen on a mobile blood drive, the registrars can be equipped with a printed list of eligible and ineligible donors. Alternatively, the database can be downloaded to a portable PC and transported to the mobile site.

Donation Data. Information regarding the donation event can also be entered into the system. This data entry is usually performed after the donation but can include such important information as the unique identification number applied to the collection container, the type of donation made (e.g., whole blood or apheresis), the collection time, and the occurrence of a donor reaction. If the donation is intended for a specific recipient, as in the case of an autologous or designated donation, data regarding the intended recipient can be entered.

Donor Recruitment. The capture of donor demographic information at registration allows the collecting facility to recruit the donor from a system-generated list of eligible donors. Mailing labels, lists of telephone numbers or e-mail addresses can be generated for recruitment efforts. Once laboratory testing is associated with the donor's record, lists of donors meeting special needs can be printed. Such lists may include donors with a specific ABO group, other RBC antigen type, or cytomegalovirus (CMV) seronegativity.

Blood Component Management

Aspects of blood component management include component preparation, laboratory testing, label application and verification, and inventory management and product shipping.

Component Production. After a whole blood unit has been collected, it is usually delivered to a component-processing laboratory where it is separated into different components, including RBCs, fresh frozen plasma, and platelets, and labeled appropriately. Data on the new components created are entered into the system with the unique donation identification number assigned at the time of donation, new blood product codes, time of preparation, and expiration dates.

Laboratory Testing. Samples of the donor's blood that were collected at the time of donation and labeled with the same unique donation identification number are tested for ABO, Rh, atypical antibodies, and markers of transfusion-transmitted diseases such as hepatitis and HIV. The results of all these tests are entered into the system so that they are associated with the unique donation identification number and with the donor. In larger community blood centers, the results of testing performed on automated instruments can be sent directly from the instrument to the system via an instrument interface.

Label Application and Verification. After completion of component production and laboratory testing, the blood products are labeled with the ABO/Rh type. This is a crucial step and must be controlled stringently so that no unsuitable blood products are released into the blood supply. After the label has been applied, the unique donation identification number and ABO/Rh type bar codes on the blood component label can be scanned into the system with a bar-code reader. This allows the system to perform a final check on donor suitability and blood type. If the component "passes" this verification, it can be placed in the available inventory.

Inventory Management and Product Shipping. The collection facility staff members who are responsible for product distribution to customer hospitals must have access to the entire inventory of available blood products. As transfusion services place requests for quantities and ABO/Rh types of blood components, the distribution staff can monitor and control distribution to optimize blood use within the community. For example, blood products nearing their expiration date can be sent to active transfusion services where there is a high probability of transfusion before expiration. As products are shipped to transfusing facilities, their status is updated in the system, along with the identification of the facility to which they were shipped.

Transfusing Facility

The applications utilized at a transfusing facility enable the user to maintain accurate histories of patient and donor unit testing and ensure the release of compatible blood products for transfusion.

Blood Component Management

Aspects of component management unique to the transfusion service include product receipt and entry, inventory management, blood component modification, and component status tracking.

Product Receipt and Entry. When the products are received at the transfusing facility, they are entered into the blood bank information system, where the entire inventory of blood components is maintained. If ABO/Rh confirmation is required, as in the case of components containing RBCs, a status of quarantine will be assigned by the system until confirmation testing is completed. Components not requiring

ABO/Rh confirmation testing may be assigned an "available" status on entry into the system.

Inventory Management. A computerized inventory makes it easy for blood bank staff members to monitor inventory levels so that levels do not drop below predefined minimums. Most systems sort the inventory by product code, ABO/Rh, and expiration date, and output it to a display monitor or printed report. When a selection list of blood components is indexed in this way, the products that are closer to the end of their shelf lives can be chosen for patients with a high likelihood of transfusion.

Blood Component Modification. Many components require modification to meet the special transfusion needs of a particular patient. Modifications include irradiation, leukocyte reduction, aliquoting (dividing), washing, and pooling. As these physical modifications are performed in the blood bank, the steps associated with them are captured by the information system, either by changing the product name or by adding a special attribute to the component data. Some of these steps may also require shortening the component's shelf life, and the system can calculate and apply the new expiration date and time, if needed. Attributes may also be added to components that have undergone special testing, such as tests for antibodies to CMV or specific RBC antigens.

Component Status Tracking. After blood components are received in the transfusion service, they are assigned various statuses, ending with a final disposition of "transfused" or "discarded." Each blood component record in the information system should contain a complete status history. Figure 26–4 illustrates the various statuses that a blood component may be ascribed throughout its shelf life.

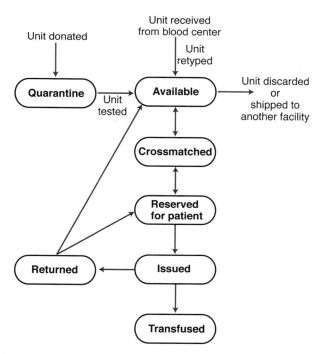

Figure 26–4. Various statuses of a blood component in a blood bank information system.

Patient Management

Blood bank information systems enhance patient safety by providing users with the infrastructure to manage functions such as patient identification, communication of orders and results with a hospital information system (HIS), patient testing, and blood component reservation and issue.

Patient Identification. A blood bank information system used by a facility issuing blood for transfusion should have the capability of capturing patient demographic information such as name and unique facility identification number. Recent developments in technology have made it possible to obtain this information from a bar-coded patient identification wristband at the time of specimen collection. Other essential data that the system should catalog include previous ABO/Rh type, transfusion history, previously identified clinically significant antibodies, and transfusion instructions such as the need for irradiated or leukocyte-reduced cellular components.

Order Entry. On receipt of a specimen for patient testing, the system can retrieve previous test results and alert the technologist to the patient's special transfusion requirements. For example, the record for a patient with a history of a clinically significant antibody can alert the technologist to the need for specific antigen-negative RBC components. Physicians' orders for blood components can also be received from the HIS through an interface or can be entered manually.

Patient Testing. Some systems allow direct entry of test results, thus replacing paper worksheets. If appropriate "truth tables" have been set up in the system, the entered test results can be compared with those of the truth tables for accuracy. Truth tables define the combination of results considered valid for a particular test. This can prevent the release of invalid results such as nonmatching forward and reverse types. Table 26–2 shows an example of a truth table. Each row represents one combination of individual test results and an interpretation, which the system will allow in its ABO test entry function.

In the case of the ABO test, there are only four valid result combinations, and the system warns the user if any other combination is entered. When the results are entered correctly and match one of the valid combinations in the truth table, the results are accepted and verified. Other tests, such as $Rh_0(D)$ and antibody screen, may also have to meet their own truth table requirements. Figure 26–5 illustrates what a user would see on the display monitor when a valid

ABO Truth table
Working behind the Scenes

Anti-A	Anti-B	A_1 cells	B cells	Interpretation
O	O	+	+	O
+	O	O	+	A
O	+	+	O	B
+	+	O	O	AB

ABO Group Test Entry Function

NAME: Doe, Jane   MEDICAL RECORD: 123456789

Anti-A	Anti-B	A_1 cells	B cells	Interpretation	Verification
+	O	O	+	A	YES

Figure 26–5. Display monitor showing entry of a valid ABO group.

ABO group is entered. Invisible to most users is the truth table, which in this figure is highlighted where the valid combination of results has been found to indicate the match with the valid ABO results entered and displayed on the monitor. Truth tables make their presence known when an invalid combination of results is entered.

Figure 26–6 illustrates what a user might see when invalid ABO results are entered. In this example, an incorrect result has been entered for the reaction of the patient's plasma or serum with group B reagent RBCs. When the technologist attempts to verify the results, the computer responds with a warning message, indicating that it was not able to find a match in the truth table for this particular combination of results.

The most critical test performed in the blood bank is the patient ABO/Rh type, and it is required that previous test results be compared with current results. When this comparison, performed by the system, reveals a discrepancy, a warning alerts the technologist to the possibility of a mislabeled specimen or incorrect test results.

Table 26–2   ABO Truth Table

ANTI-A	ANTI-B	A_1 CELLS	B CELLS	INTERPRETATION
0	0	+	+	O
+	0	0	+	A
0	+	+	0	B
+	+	0	0	AB

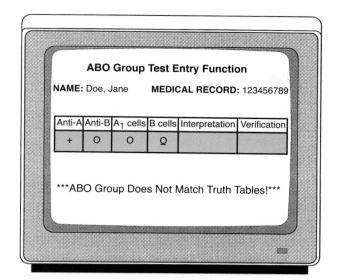

Figure 26–6. Display monitor showing entry of an invalid ABO group.

should be updatable—that is, as the products go from cross-matched or reserved to issued to transfused or returned, the status should be reported.

Blood Component Issue. When blood components are requested for transfusion, the system can assist in issuing them appropriately. For example, if both an autologous RBC and an allogeneic RBC have been reserved for the same patient, it is essential that the autologous unit be issued first. Many systems alert the issuer if he or she attempts to issue the allogeneic unit first. In addition, the system can warn if a special transfusion need is not being met by the product being issued. Verification of unit inspection before issue can also be recorded in the system. When a product is issued, the system updates its status in the inventory.

General System Applications

In addition to the requirements specific to a collection or transfusion facility, there are general applications that are found in all blood bank information systems. These functions assist with system security, quality assurance, and management assistance.

Security

It is critical for only authorized users to have access to the information contained in a blood bank computer system. Access is obtained through the use of assigned user codes and passwords, and it is the users' responsibility to keep their passwords confidential. A second level of security restricts some users to some of the system's functions. This is important for two reasons: donor/patient confidentiality and protection of data from accidental or unauthorized destruction or modification. Sensitive information, such as test results for markers of transfusion-transmitted disease, should be available only to the medical director and selected supervisory personnel. The system manager has access to most or all of the functions, including those that allow modification of the static database files. Technical staff members can access those functions that are specific to their jobs, such as test result entry, labeling, or component production. Clerical staff members may be restricted to inquiry functions that allow them to answer questions from patients or physicians but not to enter or modify patient data. In addition to providing system security, user codes capture the identity of each person performing each step in the information system.

Quality Assurance

Examples of quality assurance activities performed by a blood bank information system include **control functions**, the generation of corrected and amended results, and tools that can be used to monitor blood product utilization.

Control Functions. One of the most useful features that a blood bank information system can offer is assistance to users in ensuring safe transfusion. When blood bank personnel depend on this assistance in making decisions at critical points in

Blood Component Reservation. The system can aid in selecting blood components that will satisfy special transfusion needs and that are compatible with the patient's ABO/Rh. Selections may be made by manual entry or bar-code entry or from an indexed selection list. If autologous or designated blood components are available for a patient, the system can alert the user. As blood components are selected and either crossmatched or reserved for a patient, the system links those products to the patient record and prints compatibility tags.

A fairly recent application available on some systems is the computer crossmatch. It allows electronic verification of recipient and donor compatibility and dispenses with the serologic crossmatch test. A patient is eligible for the computer crossmatch when his or her records indicate that two criteria have been met: (1) there is no current or past history of clinically significant antibodies, and (2) there are at least two concordant ABO grouping test results.

In addition, the system must contain the donation identification number, component name, component ABO group and Rh type, the interpretation of the component ABO confirmatory test, and recipient information, including ABO group and Rh type. The system must process this information to alert the user when there are discrepancies between donor unit labeling and blood group confirmatory test interpretation and when ABO incompatibilities exist between the recipient and donor unit. Finally, the system must require verification of correct entry of data before blood components are released. These stringent requirements for a computer crossmatch must be in place to prevent the issue of ABO-incompatible components.

Result Reporting. Information regarding patient test results and any products linked to the patient should be accessible to the patient's caregivers. This may be in the form of printed reports or monitor displays. The status of linked products the selection of donors and release of blood products for transfusion, the system is said to be exerting "control functions." Control functions can be placed in two general categories: process control and decision support. Process control functions are decisions made by the system without human intervention. Decision support control functions occur when the system displays information to the user, who then decides on the next course of action. Table 26–3 shows some examples of control functions.

Corrected or Amended Results. Sometimes it is necessary to correct or amend incorrect or incomplete information that was entered into the system. This need arises when errors are made in testing or when testing is performed on a mislabeled specimen so that results are associated with the wrong patient. When corrections must be made, both the original erroneous results and the corrected results must be clearly specified as such on monitor displays and printed reports. Figure 26–7 illustrates an example of a corrected result. This method of error correction alerts caregivers who may have made clinical decisions based on the incorrect results. The information system should make it impossible to simply delete the erroneous result and substitute a corrected result.

Blood Product Utilization Review. Transfusion services are required by several accrediting agencies to monitor the utilization of blood products within the facility. This includes both blood ordering and transfusing practices of physicians. An information system can be of tremendous help in sorting and reporting utilization data. C:T ratios can be reported for individual physicians and for services such as surgery and obstetrics.

Management Assistance

Enormous amounts of different kinds of data can be entered into the blood bank information system. When appropriate reporting capabilities are designed into the system, they can provide valuable information to assist in management decisions. Reports of the number of donors drawn and deferred or blood products transfused and expired can help evaluate productivity and future resource needs. In addition, patient or hospital billing can be done more accurately and consistently than with manual systems.

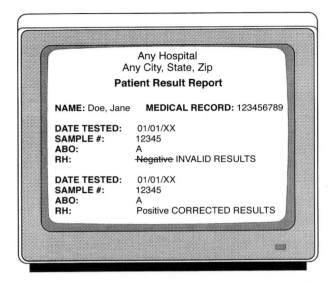

Figure 26–7. Display monitor showing patient report with corrected result.

Regulatory and Accreditation Requirements

As computer systems have assumed greater significance in blood banking, regulatory oversight has also increased. In the late 1980s, the FDA recognized that unsuitable blood components were being released into the blood supply because of inadequately controlled and validated computer systems. In 1988 and 1989, the FDA issued memoranda to registered blood establishments to provide guidance on the use of computer systems. In 1994 and 1995, memoranda were sent to blood establishment computer software manufacturers, advising them that the FDA intended to regulate blood bank software as a medical device under the Safe Medical Devices Act of 1990.

In 2007, the FDA issued an update of a 1993 draft guideline for the validation of blood establishment computer systems, which outlined a validation program in compliance with current good manufacturing practices. These regulatory initiatives have had significant impact on the availability and implementation of blood bank information systems. Both software vendors and users must follow prescribed guidelines in the introduction of new software. Vendors must

Table 26–3 **Examples of Control Functions**		
APPLICATION	**PROCESS CONTROL**	**DECISION SUPPORT**
Donor management	Preventing registration of permanently deferred donor	Warning of current ABO/Rh not matching previous results
Blood component management: collection facility	Preventing unit release if testing unacceptable	Calculation of component expiration date
Blood component management: transfusing facility	Preventing entry of donation identification number that already exists in the system	Warning when entering an expiration date that exceeds the possible shelf life of a blood component
Patient management	Preventing issue of outdated unit	Warning of product not meeting special transfusion needs

perform thorough validation testing before making software available for purchase, and users must document validation procedures on site before using such a system.

Voluntary accreditation agencies, such as the Joint Commission, the American Association of Blood Banks (AABB), and the College of American Pathologists (CAP), also have standards or inspection checklist items that emphasize the responsibilities of operating an information system. A blood bank must have documented evidence of validation of its system as well as written procedures for all aspects of system management so as to comply with regulatory and accreditation requirements.

System Management

Many responsibilities are associated with the operation and maintenance of a computerized blood bank information system. The bulk of these responsibilities occur when a system is first installed as new SOPs are written, the system is validated, and personnel are trained. After a system is established, routine maintenance procedures are performed to ensure the ongoing operation of the system.

Standard Operating Procedures

Written **standard operating procedures** (SOPs) for every blood bank operation are required by all regulatory and accreditation agencies, and computer operations are no exception. The computer-related tasks associated with each of the blood bank's technical operations can be incorporated into each technical procedure or can be addressed in a separate section of the procedures manual. In addition, there are several computer-specific SOPs that must also be available. The subjects of these are included in the following discussions.

Archiving Data

As the system's databases grow in size, the hard disk becomes crowded with this stored information. As a result, the computer's response time slows, and the hard disk is no longer able to store new data. When this happens, additional hard disks may be added to the system, or old data may be removed from the hard disk and placed in archival storage. Removing old data frees up space on the hard disk so that new data can be placed onto it. Old data may be archived to long-term storage media as such as microfiche and flash or external hard drives. A procedure for periodically assessing hard disk space should be instituted so that data can be archived in an orderly fashion before the hard disk becomes full. Procedures for archiving must also be written and should adhere to applicable regulatory and standard-setting agency requirements for data retention. For example, AABB standards require that each donor's ABO group and Rh type be retained for a minimum of 10 years, and patient records of adverse reactions to transfusion must be retained for 5 years. Written procedures for retrieving archived data must ensure that records can be accessed within a reasonable period to maintain patient care.

Backup of Software Programs and Data

Blood banks have come to depend heavily on their information systems, but systems are not infallible. Unexpected, and sometimes inexplicable, failures of software or hardware can occur. Worse, a natural disaster such as a fire or flood can destroy parts or all of an information system. Software and databases should be routinely copied to some storage medium, such as a backup hard drive. The copies can then be used to restore any corrupted or lost information. The frequency with which this backup routine is performed depends on each blood bank's data volume and the recommendations of the software vendor. The copies should be stored in a safe location separate from the information system so that they will not be affected by disastrous events such as a fire or flood. There should also be a procedure to identify and restore any information that was not included in the backup copies. This can be done by manually reentering data that was input between the time of the most recent backup and the disaster.

Computer Downtime

With any computer system, there will be times when the system is not available to users. These disruptions in availability are commonly referred to as **downtime**. Sometimes the downtime is planned, as when the system must undergo maintenance procedures, backup, or software enhancement. Other downtimes are unplanned and usually unpleasant, because the system is experiencing some difficulty such as a power outage. In either case, there must be a written procedure that will allow blood bank operations to continue. The procedure must address the need for retrieving historical patient and donor data and for recording new data obtained during the downtime.

Transfusion service staff must be able to compare current patient test results with previous records before blood components are issued. Donor center staff must have access to permanently deferred donor files. This essential information may be in the form of paper records or may be available to personnel on a PC where the information has been previously downloaded from the blood bank information system. New data generated during downtime—such as test results, blood donations, and distribution or issuance of blood products—can be recorded on hard-copy worksheets or forms and then "backloaded" into the computer when it becomes functional.

Hardware Maintenance

Information system hardware, like all pieces of equipment, requires periodic cleaning, lubrication, and replacement of parts to ensure continued operation. Maintenance procedures usually require that the system be "taken down" or turned off for a period. For that reason, regular maintenance procedures should be scheduled and posted so that blood bank staff members can prepare for downtime. When possible, maintenance should be scheduled to minimize interruption of service, such as during usual periods of low activity.

As the system's databases grow in size, the computer's response time may reach an undesirably slow pace. Procedures should be established for removing the data from the disk. The software will contain programs for purging and archiving older data. Vendors may also offer support services that can examine the system disk(s) to identify potential problems.

Security Maintenance

A procedure for adding users to a system must be established, including the basis on which security levels will be assigned. For example, the list of functions or applications to which a user will have access can be created for each job description. It is also important to have a method for deleting the access codes of users who leave the facility. An additional level of security can be obtained by requiring users to change their passwords periodically; many security applications can be programmed to require this at specified intervals.

Tracking and Correcting Errors

Error management, required by regulatory and accrediting agencies, has become an integral part of blood bank operations. It includes detecting, documenting, and investigating errors; implementing corrective actions; and reporting to appropriate agencies. Errors in the operation of a blood bank information system may be caused by inadequate training, incomplete or cumbersome written procedures, or system problems. In any case, tracking and categorizing errors is essential if corrective actions are to be taken. Identified information system problems should be reported to the software vendor so that other users can be notified and remedies can be included in a future software revision.

Personnel Training

The most elegant and user-friendly information system can be a disaster if staff members are inadequately trained in its use. Training programs should address every function and procedure that each user will be expected to perform. Flowcharts and checklists are useful training tools. Training modules can be designed that present users with the situations that they will encounter in their work. The competence of each staff person must be documented before allowing routine use of the computer. Competence assessment methods can include direct observation, review of system-generated records, and written examinations. Once initial competence has been demonstrated, periodic assessment must be done to document the continued competence of blood bank staff to use the information system appropriately. As previously discussed, it is most beneficial to allow users access to a test database for training purposes. If one is not available, test data can be used in the production database.

Validation of Software

Software validation is the establishment of documented evidence that provides a high degree of assurance that the system will consistently function as expected. It is the responsibility of the software vendor to validate, to the extent possible, the functionality of a software product before it is marketed to blood banks. However, software vendors cannot simulate the conditions in which each system will be used. Differences in environment, hardware, databases,

SOPs, and people require that each blood bank perform on-site validation testing to prove that the system will perform appropriately under those unique conditions.

Validation testing must be performed before a new system can be implemented and whenever new software, databases, or hardware is added to the system. When validation is to be performed on an existing system, the testing should be done in the test database, where it will not affect the production data.

Risk Assessment

Proper validation of the system requires careful planning. Risk assessment is a required analysis tool that focuses validation efforts on system functions or settings that present the greatest potential to harm the patient, donor, or business in the event of a failure. Vendor descriptions of control functions and on-site system configuration settings are reviewed and assigned a risk category (such as high, medium, or low) by the system manager or validation team. A validation test plan is then prepared, ensuring that the highest risk areas receive an appropriate degree of validation.

Test Plan

A **test plan** describes the series of exercises that will be used to validate the blood bank software. Each system function that the blood bank will use must be included in the test plan. A test plan should be created for each function or operation that the computer will perform. Risk analysis will determine the extent of testing required. Test plans should include the following items:

- Control functions
- Data entry methods (keyboard, bar-code reader, instrument interface, LIS, or HIS interface)
- Specific test cases
- Documentation methods
- Acceptance criteria (expected outputs)
- Result review
- Corrective action (if necessary)
- Acceptance

Most of these items will be different in each of the system's applications, so a separate test plan for each application may be necessary. Control functions should be defined by the vendor, but data entry methods will be selected by the user; some applications may have multiple data entry methods. Specific tests cases are discussed below. Screen printouts, written logs, or printed reports can be used to document the testing. After the testing is completed, the results should be compared with acceptance criteria to determine acceptability. If unacceptable results are obtained, they should be investigated, and corrective action should be implemented. When corrective action is necessary, testing should be repeated until it is found acceptable.

Test Cases

Validation test cases include the specific steps to be followed by those performing the testing. **Test cases** should assess the system under normal operating conditions but must also offer challenges to the system. The goal is to make sure that the system repeatedly performs intended functions and does not perform unintended functions. The types of testing that should be performed are:

- Normal testing
- Boundary testing
- Invalid test cases
- Special test cases
- Stress testing

Normal testing uses typical blood bank inputs to produce normal, or routine, outputs. **Boundary testing** involves forcing the system to evaluate data that are slightly below or slightly above valid ranges. This kind of testing might be used for disease test results. **Invalid test cases** assess the system's ability to recognize and reject incorrect inputs. Examples of invalid inputs include entering Q for an ABO interpretation or entering a blood product code that has not been defined in the static database file. **Special test cases** are those that make the system react to unusual inputs. A special case could be designed to see how the system responds when more than one person attempts to add or edit special transfusion instructions in the same patient's record. **Stress testing** involves pushing the system to its physical limits. This might be accomplished by allowing large volumes of data to be entered into the system via all available input devices.

Not every type of test case may be appropriate for each function to be tested. For example, boundary test cases will probably not be applicable in a donor registration function. Another kind of validation testing is parallel testing. This involves running two systems in parallel and comparing the outputs of both. For a blood bank switching from a manual to a computerized system, every procedure would be performed manually and in the computer.

Validating a blood bank information system is a very lengthy and labor-intensive process, but it provides great benefits if undertaken in a thorough manner. Extensive testing will identify potential problems in the way that the blood bank intends to use the system. Sometimes workarounds have to be created, but when it is done as part of validation testing, staff members can be properly trained before going "live" on the new system or software. The creation and performance of comprehensive and detailed validation test cases require allocation of significant resources to the project, but the end result—a well-validated blood bank information system—is worth the resource costs.

SUMMARY CHART

- ✔ Blood bank information systems assist in the management of data and can allow tracing of a blood component through all processing steps from donation through transfusion (final disposition).
- ✔ A computer system is composed of three main components: hardware, software, and people.
- ✔ Hardware components perform functions related to input and output, processing, and storage of data.
- ✔ Software tells the computer what to do with the information it has received.
- ✔ Application software allows users to perform tasks that are specific to blood bank operations.
- ✔ Donor, patient, and blood component information is maintained in databases, which are divided into files and further subdivided into individual records.
- ✔ Static database files define the terminology that the blood bank will use and provide a dictionary of coded terms that the system can use to sort data.
- ✔ Operating system software controls the hardware, manipulates the application software, and coordinates the flow of information between the disks and memory.
- ✔ The system manager oversees the maintenance of the system's hardware and software, including adding or deleting items from the static database files, assigning access codes to new users, implementing software upgrades from the vendor, and investigating and reporting problems encountered by the users.

- ✔ A blood bank information system can have numerous specific applications related to the management of donors, patients, and blood components.
- ✔ User codes and passwords prevent unauthorized use of the system and provide a means for capturing the identity of each person who performs a task on the information system.
- ✔ Control functions assist in making decisions at critical points in the selection of donors and release of blood components for transfusion.
- ✔ When results must be corrected or amended, they must be clearly designated as such on printed reports and monitor displays used by patient caregivers.
- ✔ A blood bank must have documented evidence of validation of its system as well as written procedures for all aspects of system management in order to comply with regulatory and accreditation requirements.
- ✔ Blood bank SOPs must address computer tasks related to blood bank technical duties and must address computer-specific procedures such as computer downtime, backup of software programs and data, system maintenance, security, error management, and personnel training.
- ✔ On-site software validation must provide documented evidence that provides a high degree of assurance that the system will function consistently as expected under the unique combination of hardware, databases, environment, SOPs, and people at the site.

Review Questions

1. Components of an information system consist of all of the following except:
   a. Hardware
   b. Software
   c. Validation
   d. People

2. To be in compliance with regulatory and accreditation agency requirements for blood bank information systems, blood banks must maintain SOPs for all of the following except:
   a. Vendor validation testing
   b. Computer downtime
   c. System maintenance
   d. Personnel training

3. A validation test case that assesses the system's ability to recognize an erroneous input is called:
   a. Normal
   b. Boundary
   c. Stress
   d. Invalid

4. An example of interface software functionality is:
   a. The entry of blood components into the blood bank database
   b. The transmission of patient information from the HIS into the blood bank system
   c. The printing of a workload report
   d. Preventing access to the system by an unauthorized user

5. Backup copies of the information system:
   a. Can be used to restore the information system data and software if the production system is damaged.
   b. Are used to maintain hardware components.
   c. Are performed once a month.
   d. Are created any time changes are made to the system.

6. User passwords should be:
   a. Shared with others.
   b. Kept confidential.
   c. Posted at each terminal.
   d. Never changed.

7. Preventing the issue of an incompatible blood component is an example of:
   a. Inventory management.
   b. Utilization review.
   c. System security.
   d. Control function.

8. Information is stored in a collection of many different files called the:
   a. Database.
   b. Configuration.
   c. Hardware.
   d. Disk drive.

9. Application software communicates with this type of software to retrieve data from the system disks:
   a. Interface
   b. Operating system
   c. Security
   d. Program

10. Validation testing for software should consider all of the following items except:
    a. Data entry methods
    b. Control functions
    c. Performance of testing in production database
    d. Invalid data

11. Complete the truth table below for a negative antibody screen using two screening cells (SCI, SCII) at the immediate spin (IS), 37°C (37), and antihuman globulin (AHG) phases.

Phase	SCI	SCII	Interpretation
IS			
37°C			
AHG			
CC			

12. During validation testing, a computer user entered the following results for an antibody screen test:

SCI	IS	37	AHG	CC	Interpretation
Result	0	0	0	+	Negative

After the user verified the entries, the monitor displayed the following message: "Invalid test results." What caused the error message to display?

a. An invalid entry was made in the check cells (CC) column.
b. The truth table was set up incorrectly.
c. The interpretation does not correlate with the test entries.
d. The interface to the laboratory computer system is down.

13. The following test plan has been created to validate the blood bank computer function used to update the status of blood units that have been transfused. The test plan contains each of the sections, lettered A through H, required for a thorough test plan. Evaluate each section and, using the list below, assign a name to each section.

Section Names

- Acceptance
- Acceptance criteria
- Control functions
- Corrective action
- Data entry methods
- Documentation methods
- Result review
- Test cases

Test Plan Function: Assigning Transfused Status

Section A

Description: This function is used to change the status of issued units to a transfused status. All records pertaining to the unit and patient will be updated:
Name of Section A. _____

Section B

1. Preventing the assignment of transfused status to a quarantined blood unit.
2. Preventing the assignment of transfused status to a blood unit that has already been transfused.
3. Preventing the assignment of transfused status to a blood component that has not been issued.
Name of Section B. _____

Section C

1. The computer will beep and display **Unit Has Not Been Issued** when a blood unit number that has not been issued is entered.
2. The computer will beep and display **Unit Is in Quarantined Status** when a blood component that is in quarantine status is entered.
3. The computer will beep and display **Unit Has Been Transfused** when a blood component that has already been transfused is entered.
4. The Transfusion History screen display will indicate the patient has been transfused and will display the date of the last transfusion.
5. Printed reports will indicate relevant units were assigned transfused status
Name of Section C. _____

Section D

1. Attempt to assign transfused status to the following units:
   a. Quarantined blood component
   b. Selected (but not issued) blood component
   c. Transfused blood component
2. Selection of units from issued inventory list
3. Manual entry of issued blood components
Name of Section D. _____

Section E

1. Operator will input blood component information and select blood components.
2. Operator will input selected patient information.
3. Blood bank computer will update the patient and unit record.
Name of Section E. _____

Section F

The following screen displays and printed reports will be verified for accuracy:

Screen Displays	Printed Reports
Patient Information	Patient History Report
Unit Information	Transfusion Listing
Unit History	
Transfusion History	

Name of Section F. _____

Section G

The acceptability of the results of each test case will be determined by the blood bank manager and documented on the validation documentation form.
Name of Section G. _____

Section H

If the software does not perform as expected, the problem must be recorded on a computer problem report and the supervisor alerted. A remedial action plan will be devised with the assistance of the blood bank computer system vendor.
Name of Section H. _____
Blood bank director signature:_____   Date:_____
Comments: _____

Bibliography

Aller, RD: Pathology's contributions to disease surveillance: Sending our data to public health officials and encouraging our clinical colleagues to do so. Arch Pathol Lab Med 133:926–932, 2009.

Bersch, C, and DiRamio, D: Lab's HIE Solution Connects LIS to EMR and HIS. MLO-Online, 2009.

Bocker, W: ISBT Guidelines for validation and maintaining the validation state of automated systems in blood banking. Vox Sanguinis 85(Suppl. 1): 2003.

Bordowitz, R: Electronic health records: A primer. Lab Med 39(5):301–306, 2008.

Butch, SH: Applying quality improvement tools in the transfusion service. Clin Lab Science 20(2):113–121, 2007.

Butch, SH: Automation in the transfusion service. Immunohematology 24(3):86–92, 2008.

Butch, SH: Computerization in the transfusion service. Vox Sang Sanguinis 83(Suppl 1):105–110, 2002.

Butch, SH: Guidelines for Implementing an Electronic Crossmatch. AABB, Bethesda, 2003.

Butch, SH, and Distler, PB: ISBT 128 blood labeling: Introduction and reference laboratory applications. Immunohematology 22(1):30–36, 2006.

Dzik, WH: Use of a computer assisted system for blood utilization review. Transfusion 47:142, 2007.

Food and Drug Administration: Draft guideline "computer cross-match" (electronic based testing for the compatibility between the donor's cell type and the recipient's serum or plasma type), June 20, 2007.

Food and Drug Administration: "Guidance for industry: Blood establishment computer system validation in the user's facility," October 29, 2007, 72 FR 61171.

Food and Drug Administration: Guidance for Industry: "Computer crossmatch" (computerized analysis of the compatibility between the donor's cell type and the recipient's serum or plasma type), April 28, 2011.

Hicks, BJ: Lean information management: Understanding and eliminating waste. Int J Inform Manage, 27:233–249, 2007.

Levy, R, Pantanowitz, L, Cloutier, D, et al: Development of electronic medical record charting for hospital-based transfusion and apheresis medicine services: Early adoption perspectives. J Pathol Inform 13(1):ii, 2010.

Li, BN, Chao, S, and Dong, MC: Barcode technology in blood bank information systems: Upgrade and its impact. J Med Syst 30(6):449–457, 2006.

Lifshitz, MS, et al: Clinical laboratory informatics. In McPherson, RA: Henry's Clinical Diagnosis and Management by Laboratory Methods, 22nd ed. Elsevier-Mosby-Saunders, Philadelphia, PA, 2012.

Miyata, S: Network computer assisted transfusion-management system for accurate blood component-recipient identification at the bedside. Transfusion 44:364, 2004.

Ohsaka, A, Abe, K, Ohsawa, T, Miyake, N, Sugita, S, and Tojima, I: A computer-assisted transfusion management system and changed transfusion practices contribute to appropriate management of blood components. Transfusion 48(8):1730–1738, 2008.

Overhage, MJ: A comparison of the completeness and timeliness of automated electronic laboratory reporting and spontaneous reporting of notifiable conditions. Am J Public Health 98(2):344–350, 2008.

Ovretveit, J, et al: Implementation of electronic medical records in hospitals: Two case studies. Health Policy 84:181–190, 2007.

Pantanowitz, L, et al: Laboratory reports in the electronic medical record. Lab Med 38(6):339–340, 2007.

Porcella, A, and Walker, K: Patient safety with blood products administration using wireless and bar-code technology. Annual Symposium Proceedings/AMIA Symposium, 614–618, 2005.

Vaquier, C, and Caldani, C: Hospital blood bank: Information system and immuno-hematology. Transfus Clin Biol 17(5–6):345–348, 2010.

Wong, K: Virtual blood bank. J Pathol Inform 2:6, 2011.

Wooster, G: An LIS supports quality initiatives. MLO-Online, 2008.

Chapter 27

Medicolegal and Ethical Aspects of Providing Blood Collection and Transfusion Services

Kathleen Sazama, MD, JD, MS, MT(ASCP)

OBJECTIVES

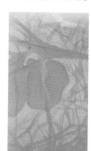

1. Describe the legal and ethical parameters for providing blood collection and transfusion services.
2. Describe the legal bases for liability for providing transfusion medicine services.
3. Explain the necessity of establishing and following standard operating procedures similar to those of other comparable facilities throughout the United States.
4. Identify the evolving legal and ethical concerns that are likely to accompany the increasing complexity of providing blood during the early 21st century.
5. List the two reasons why patients sue for transfusion injury.
6. Describe the steps that blood bank professionals can take to avoid or minimize litigation.

Introduction

Patients who are injured during or as a result of transfusion may seek redress through legal channels, which is usually filed by their families. This has been of particular concern in blood banking and transfusion medicine because of the possibility of disease transmission, especially from previously unknown sources, and because mistakes may mean death. Basing practices on sound ethical principles provides a good foundation to limit liability when these unforeseen events occur. This chapter briefly describes the sources of law and theories of liability, including practical hints for reducing the likelihood of

being found liable, when possible. Emerging concerns for the 21st century are also identified. This chapter is not intended as a substitute for legal advice, which is necessary in particular situations; rather, it is intended to provide the reader with some general principles and definitions so that ethically and legally sound practices continue within transfusion medicine.

Focus of Current Legal Issues

Legal issues for the transfusion medicine professional in the 21st century center around ABO errors, acute lung injury, and patient privacy. There are also concerns about possible transfusion-transmitted diseases, including babesiosis and dengue fever or other exotic diseases that are emerging globally. Concern has also focused on issues regarding transfusion indications, informed consent, and other medically relevant topics. A new concept called patient blood management is gaining prominence in light of the new emphasis on evidence-based medical practice. New studies have been published questioning the safety of blood transfusions, both allogeneic and autologous, with concerns regarding the age of the red blood cells at the time of transfusion and recognition that patient anemia may play a larger role in patient outcomes than previously appreciated.

However, even before transfusion-transmitted acquired immunodeficiency syndrome (TTAIDS) became the basis for numerous lawsuits against blood centers, hospitals, and physicians, there was litigation because of death and serious injury caused by transfusion-transmitted hepatitis B virus (HBV) and a few because of donor injury.[1] (See *Perlmutter v. Beth David Hospital*, 308 NY 100, 123 N.E.2d 792 [1954] in which the court decided that transactions involving blood were not sales but were incidental to the provision of medical services. This decision precludes the application of commercial law, particularly that of warranties, to blood transfusions.)

The HBV cases stimulated nearly every state legislature to enact protection for blood banks through **blood shield statutes**.[2] (California was the first state to enact such protection for blood banks in 1955. Only New Jersey lacks such a law, but it provides similar protection solely through judicial decisions.) Because of these blood shield statutes, most of which extended protection without amendment or modification for TTAIDS and HBV, many TTAIDS lawsuits have been either dismissed or unsuccessful for the person suing (the **plaintiff**).

Recently, however, this premise has come under new challenge in the courts. As most TTAIDS cases have been unsuccessful in compensating plaintiffs (usually patients or their families), new theories of liability are increasingly being raised. When questions of appropriateness of transfusion, availability of blood components, and informed consent arise, the ethical bases of transfusion medicine practice are focused more sharply.

Although blood shield statutes generally protect against application of strict liability, tort liability remains the basis for most lawsuits.

Sources of Law

Laws are created by society through legislation called **statutes** (passed by either the U.S. Congress or by individual state legislatures) or by court decisions, referred to as **case law** (in federal courts, including the U.S. Supreme Court, or in state courts through their own highest state court).

Statutes and Regulations

Federal law (enacted by Congress or by decision in federal courts, including the Supreme Court) may frequently supersede state law, but both federal and state laws can be and often are applied in particular instances. In the absence of federal law, state law can provide precedence for future decisions. However, states may choose to adapt, follow, or ignore decisions made in sister state courts, whereas federal law is applicable to all states. The details of how laws are to be put into action are provided in **regulations**. Regulations, both federal and state, can be applied only if they have been established according to a formal process called the Administrative Procedure Act (APA).[3] Federal regulations that apply specifically to blood banking are found in the Title 21, Code of Federal Regulations, Parts 600–699 and to some extent in Parts 200–299 and 800–899, published annually on April 1.[4] Blood banks and transfusion services are also federally regulated by provisions of the Clinical Laboratories Improvement Act of 1988 (**CLIA 88**) and the Medicare provisions of the Social Security Act. In addition, the 1996 federal law protecting health information (**Health Insurance Portability and Accessibility Act [HIPAA]**), including the 2008 modification (**HITECH**) that extends these protections to electronic records and transmissions and the 2008 federal law protecting persons from discrimination on the basis of genetic information (**GINA**), also apply.

State legislatures also enact laws and publish explanatory regulations about blood banking, clinical laboratories, and transfusion practices, principally covering licensure of facilities and personnel.

Case Law

Case law is established by court decisions, sometimes related to interpretations and applications of statutes and regulations. Patients generally believe that medical treatment administered to them (after obtaining their informed consent) will, on balance, be beneficial. When transfusion causes harm (e.g., through identification error, lung injury, and other causes), patients have understandably reacted by seeking redress in the courts. The legal bases for such suits are generally civil (not criminal) actions for tort. **Tort** is defined as any wrongdoing for which action for damages may be brought.

United States civil law depends on each competent adult in our society behaving reasonably (i.e., not negligently and not aggressively) toward every other person, respecting other people's rights. Civil lawsuits arise because someone disrespects another's rights by:

1. Striking or threatening to strike another person (**battery** and **assault**)
2. Being careless or reckless (**negligence**)
3. Failing to complete an agreement (**breach of contract**)
4. Intruding on another's property or privacy
5. Misbehaving in other similar ways

Civil lawsuits can also arise because of violation of statutes or regulations that require certain types of actions.

Basis of Liability: Torts

Torts arise from improper interactions between individuals. Some of the common torts are described below.

Intentional Tort of Battery

Any touching without consent, including deliberate blows and intentional striking, is the legal definition of *battery*. For transfusion medicine, this concept is used when a donor or a patient claims that he or she never agreed to have the needle placed in his or her arm. If significant harm occurs as a result of the needle, this legal theory may be upheld. Generally, however, the fact that the donor or patient allowed the needle to be placed is sufficient evidence that he or she agreed to the procedure. Informed consent is generally not an issue in battery but is fundamental in the tort of negligence.

Doctrine of Informed Consent

Particularly in the special circumstances of the practice of medicine, the issue of whether a patient (or, in the case of blood collection, a donor) agreed to undergo the procedure actually performed, with full knowledge of the possible benefits, alternatives, and harm that may accompany it, has come to be known as the doctrine of **informed consent**. This doctrine protects the patient (or donor) by requiring that information be provided in a manner understandable to the patient under circumstances that permit the patient to ask questions or express concerns and to receive answers to them (*Canterbury v. Spence*, 464 F.2d 772 [DC Cir 1972]).

For TTAIDS transfusion recipients, this issue first came into sharp focus in the case of *Kozup v. Georgetown University*, 663 F. Supp. 1048 (DC 1987), 851 F.2d 437 (DC Cir 1988), 906 F.2d 783 (DC Cir 1990). In this case, an infant brought by his parents to Georgetown University Hospital for medical care contracted TTAIDS and died. His parents argued that they were insufficiently informed about the harm of the transfusions and did not specifically agree to transfusions as part of the care given their child. The District of Columbia court ruled that their actions in bringing the child to the hospital and not objecting to transfusions that they observed at the time of infusion amounted to tacit consent. The issue of whether specific consent is required for transfusion and who should obtain such consent remains controversial. Generally, physicians have been held responsible (*Ritter v. Delaney*, 790 S.W.2d 29 [Tex. App. San Antonio, 1990] and *Howell v. Spokane*, 785 P.2d 815 [Wash 1990]; *Hoemke v. New York Blood Center*, 90–7182 [2d Cir. 1990] and *Gibson v. Methodist Hospital*, 01-89-00645-CV [Tex. Ct. App. 1991]). However, in 1996, the Joint Commission specifically required hospitals to obtain informed consent for transfusion in some situations.[5]

Another arena in which the informed consent is the key to resolving disputes is that of **donor rights**. With the onset of AIDS, the language of donor histories has been subjected to continuous revising and updating to include information about the disease, how it is acquired, and under what circumstances a person may donate blood. In the United States, unlike other countries, there is no right to donate blood or other tissues. Instead there has been increasing emphasis on educating donors about the restrictions on blood donation. Federal and voluntary requirements for the way in which the history is obtained have emphasized more face-to-face oral questioning, not just self-administration of these questionnaires, until the recent availability of information technology to permit such activities. One part of the donation process has always been for donors to sign a statement of consent or assent to donate.

Until the late 1980s, donors were protected from subpoena in cases of transfusion-transmitted diseases. However, an increasing number of plaintiffs in state courts are insisting that the donor be subject to questioning regarding his or her donation. This questioning may completely or partially protect a donor's identity or may require that donor to appear in open court. Because no one donates blood expecting to have to defend such an altruistic act at some future date, the impact of these decisions on the future availability of blood for transfusion is uncertain.

Negligence

Probably the most common tort is that of negligence. This is the basis for lawsuits when injury occurs.

Elements

Liability for negligence is found when all of the following elements are present:

1. A duty was owed to the injured party.
2. The duty was not met by the injuring party.
3. Because the duty was not met, the injured party was harmed.
4. Failure to meet the duty owed was directly responsible for or could have been predicted to cause the harm suffered by the injured party.
5. Some measurable (compensable) harm (called *damages*) occurred. To be successful in a negligence action, the plaintiff has the responsibility to prove all these factors against the person being sued (the **defendant**).

Standard of Care

There are two standards of care applicable to blood collection and transfusion services: ordinary and professional.

Ordinary Standard of Care. When the alleged negligence involves ordinary things that anyone may encounter in daily life (e.g., injuries caused by traffic accidents, fistfights, etc.), a jury or judge can consider the facts and decide whether the behavior of the defendant was reasonable—that is, did the defendant meet the standard of care required in the situation? For ordinary negligence, this standard of care depends only on what the average person (e.g., a juror) believes is acceptable in our society, or the ordinary standard of care (i.e., the jury decides whether a reasonable person, in the same circumstances as the defendant, would have acted the same way as the defendant did). If the defendant acted reasonably in the circumstances, the plaintiff will be unsuccessful in the lawsuit and vice versa.

In situations in which larger organizations are involved, the question of who is liable for the actions of employees has been resolved under the doctrine of *respondeat superior*. Under this doctrine, the actions of employees are attributable to the employer or person who directs their actions. The person responsible for transfusion services has been defined by federal regulation and general practice to be a physician, a definition that has been reinforced by judicial decision in many states for blood centers as well as for hospitals. The advantage of having a physician as the responsible employer is that the principles and regulations related to medical malpractice usually apply, including the requirement for establishing a professional standard of care.

Professional Standard of Care. When the negligence lawsuit involves professionals such as physicians and scientists, including laboratory professionals, nurses, or other allied health practitioners, the definition of what is reasonable, the "standard of care," depends on expert testimony from other professionals in the same field (e.g., physicians, nurses, or scientists) about what should have been done by other reasonable practitioners (usually of the same specialty). The law makes an extra requirement—in discharging his or her duty to the plaintiff, the defendant must apply the special knowledge and ability he or she possesses by virtue of the profession. This increased professional standard of care is not just what a reasonable person such as the judge or members or the jury would have done but also what other professionals (the expert witnesses) testify should have been done. The judge or jury is not permitted to decide what they would have done but must depend upon testimony by expert witnesses of the same profession as the defendant who define what that reasonable professional standard of care is. For the complex scientific, technical, and medical issues involved in TTAIDS litigation, this distinction has been a key element in protecting blood bankers.

Voluntary and Mandatory Standards

The testimony of experts should generally be supportable by authorities such as statutes, regulations, or other bodies of published knowledge, including published scientific articles and texts. The existence of voluntary standards—particularly those provided by the AABB (formerly known as the American Association of Blood Banks)[6] but also those from the College of American Pathologists (CAP), the American Association of Tissue Banks (AATB), the American Society for Histocompatibility and Immunogenetics (ASHI), the Joint Commission (TJC), and other organizations—are helpful in establishing the professional standard of practice for transfusion medicine. In fact, some state laws and federal regulations cross-reference the AABB standards specifically. Blood bankers and transfusion services that can show that they acted in conformance with these standards are more likely to be found non-negligent than those that do not follow such guidelines.

Blood Banking as a Medical Profession

The question of whether blood banking is a medical profession is being relitigated in courts today, with conflicting results.[7] One possible chilling result is that collecting, processing,

and distributing blood may be considered differently from the crossmatching, issuance, and transfusion of blood to individual patients. Redefining blood banking as *not* medical practice removes the extra protection provided by the requirement for expert medical testimony to establish the standard of care, leaving defendants to be judged by the ordinary negligence standard. There is little dispute that loss of medical professional stature would significantly alter the practice of blood banking. None of the protections of medical malpractice reform would be available, and blood centers may even find themselves subject to strict liability.

Strict Liability

Manufacturers and distributors of goods used in everyday life have been defined by law to have certain responsibilities in their activities to protect consumers. Among other requirements, there are certain warranties that the product purchased—for example, a television set—will actually work and will continue to do so for some fixed period, with small risk of harm from such things as electric shock or blowing up. These warranties, actual or implied, exist for virtually anything a consumer buys and uses. If a product fails to perform as expected or creates harm when none was expected, the consumer has the right to have a replacement or, if the manufacturer denies responsibility, to sue for negligent manufacturing or distribution.

In addition, for some items (such as dynamite), the danger from proper use is so great that manufacturers are legally liable for *all* harm that occurs, which is called **strict liability**. This means that anyone who is harmed when properly using dynamite does not have to prove that the manufacturer or distributor was negligent; he or she has only to show that he or she was injured while properly using it. Imagine how rare and expensive blood transfusions would become if these practices were applied to it. Instead, nearly every state has enacted specific protection—the blood shield statutes described previously—to exclude harm from blood transfusions from suit under these legal theories. It is important that blood bankers avoid implying or stating that blood transfusion is completely safe, because such statements may be construed as creating a warranty, invoking these theories of liability.

Intentional Infliction of Emotional Distress

As the phrase *intentional infliction of emotional distress* suggests, a plaintiff must show that what the defendant did to cause actual and severe emotional distress was intentional, usually some extreme or outrageous conduct that was calculated to deliberately cause harm to the plaintiff. This can take the form the plaintiff's relative claiming wrongful death, particularly in some TTAIDS cases.

Invasion of Privacy Under Civil Case Law

Health-care providers, including blood bankers, are required to respect personal privacy and to maintain patient and donor confidentiality. Plaintiffs may claim remuneration for loss of privacy under four theories:

1. Intruding upon the plaintiff's seclusion or solitude or into his or her private affairs
2. Publicly disclosing embarrassing facts
3. Publicly placing plaintiff in a "false light"
4. Appropriating plaintiff's name or likeness for defendant's benefit

These categories protect a patient or donor from illegal or inadvertent disclosure of his or her personal information, of particular concern with HIV because of the risk of loss of employment, housing, insurance, and other benefits of society. When information is exciting or noteworthy, the media may become aware of and publish private information.

Basis of Liability: HIPAA

In 1996, the U.S. Congress responded to the information age by enacting a law specifically directed toward protecting personal health information (PHI): the Health Information Portability and Accessibility Act (HIPAA). The regulations implementing the provisions of this act occurred in segments beginning in 1996, with the full provision for PHI effective on April 7, 2003. With this new federal requirement, information about donors and patients must be kept in such a manner that inadvertent "use or disclosure" does not occur. Exceptions for health-care providers, insurers, and government scrutiny have been specified, but safeguards should be in place even for these exceptions.

Although few if any cases have been filed, blood banks and transfusion services will be involved in suits under the preexisting civil cases if they are responsible (through negligence or by intention) for releasing confidential data of a donor or patient. Great care should be exercised by blood banking professionals to ensure that private information (whether about donors, patients, or relatives) be kept confidential and not released without written authorization. Procedures to safeguard such release should include proper use of copy and facsimile machines and direct electronic transfer via information systems.

Restrictions on Plaintiff Suits and Recovery

Even when harm or injury occurs, the plaintiff may be unable to pursue legal redress for a number of reasons.

Statutes of Limitations

Some protection for defendants arises because of a statutorily defined limit of time during which a lawsuit can be filed, referred to as the **statute of limitations**. States often have different limits, depending on the legal requirements for initiating suits. Statutes of limitations for medical malpractice are generally shorter (approximately 2 years from the date that the injury should have been discovered in adults) than limitations for other kinds of negligence (2 to 6 years is common).

Doctrine of Charitable Immunity

Historically, courts provided immunity for nonprofit organizations such as hospitals from excess liability because they perform charitable acts. This is referred to as the **doctrine of charitable immunity**. Many state legislatures have enacted and continue to support statutes to provide protection for boards of directors and volunteers using this common law rationale. A 1996 decision in New Jersey redefined this protection in that state (*Snyder v. AABB*, 144 N.J. 269 [1996]). Fortunately for blood bankers, other states have been loathe to accept the Synder decision. Also, many health-care institutions rely less on this doctrine and more on insurance for protection.

Tort Reform

State legislatures, recognizing the need to protect some specialties such as obstetrics, have been active in seeking limits on damages against physicians, protecting them from abusive litigation. For transfusion practices, it is vital that these protections be afforded.

Risk Management

Avoiding liability for TTAIDS and other possible harm from practicing transfusion medicine, whether in hospitals or blood centers, depends on having well-established policies and procedures that are consistent with quality principles and that comply with recognized authorities, regulations, and statutes and that have some measurement of how persons engaged in all activities actually follow those procedures. Complying with accreditation requirements (e.g., AABB, TJC, CAP, and state laws) for **quality systems** will assist in limiting risk. To avoid being negligent, one must behave reasonably. Reasonable behavior for transfusion medicine practice includes continually obtaining and applying new knowledge from all possible sources that will safeguard the donor during collection, the component during handling and delivery, and the patient before and during transfusion.

Specific Donor Issues

Although it is possible to sue another party for many reasons, the most common ones are discussed here.

Screening

What the AIDS epidemic has taught us is that every person who volunteers to donate does not have an unqualified right to do so. In fact, for several years before March 1985 (when a test for HIV antibodies in blood first became available), the best safeguard against TTAIDS was improved donor education and more pertinent questioning regarding behaviors that might put that donor at risk for acquiring HIV. Although numerous lawsuits have been filed against blood collection agencies for improper donor screening, few have been successful when collection facilities could show that they had implemented written procedures and had properly trained employees who followed those procedures and that proper documentation of each screen occurred. Problems occurred when breaches in procedure, typically failures to follow SOPs or to properly document actual practice, were discovered. However, with several state courts demanding release of donor identity or access to donors for questioning, further attention to the process of donor screening is appropriate. Balancing the real threat to patient care that would arise if blood components were not available with the serious nature of litigation will continue to challenge blood banking professionals.

Donations Requested by Patients

Several monetary settlements in the range of hundreds of thousands to millions of dollars have resulted from either failing to offer directed donor services or from improperly characterizing them. With the advent of the HIPAA, patient-requested donations from friends and family require close attention to ensure that inadvertent or overt disclosure of protected health information does not occur.

Untimely Notification

When recipients received notification in years, rather than in weeks or months, after blood centers knew (or should have known) that the recipient had received an HIV-reactive unit, many of them or their families were angry enough to file suit on the basis that they should have been informed sooner. Procedures for look-back and recipient notification were not well established for several years following application of specific testing in most blood collection organizations. It was not until 1996 that the federal government, through the Center for Health Care Financing Administration (now called Centers for Medicaid and Medicare Services, or CMS) and the FDA, issued specific regulations for HIV look-back notification by hospitals. Parallel requirements for HCV are in progress.

Component Collection

Occasionally, lawsuits have occurred from injury that donors received during the collection process. Generally, the injuries are more severe than a simple bruise at the needle site and involve such things as nerve damage, slip-and-fall incidents, and other similar severe reactions. Also, although donor deaths continue to be reported at a rate of approximately two per year, these infrequently result in litigation.

Processing, Labeling, and Distribution

Lack of Standard Protocol for Implementing Testing

Several successful TTAIDS lawsuits awarded millions of dollars against blood-collecting organizations (*Belle Bonfils Memorial Blood Bank v. Denver District Court*, 723 P.2d 1003 [Colo. 1988]) because they had no standard protocol for implementing new testing to ensure that all available components (including those distributed or in active inventory) were test-negative before transfusion once the test kits and equipment were received by the collection facility. The lack of a written plan to implement such testing, including training of personnel, validating instrumentation

and reagents, and establishing the necessary information service support, was seen as negligent by the jury (even *with* expert testimony to the contrary).

Failure to Perform Surrogate Testing

Despite concerted efforts, rarely has a plaintiff prevailed when alleging that blood collection facilities should have performed more or different surrogate tests between 1983 and 1985, when a specific HIV antibody test was first available (*Baker v. JK and Susie Wadley Research Institutes and Blood Bank, aka The Blood Center at Wadley*, 86-2728-C [Tex. Jud. Dist. Ct. 1988] and *Clark v. United Blood Services*, CV 88–6981 [Nev. 2d Jud. Dist. Ct. 1990]).

Failure to Properly Perform Testing

Testing personnel should be constantly alert to proper performance and documentation of all required testing of blood components. There are multiple opportunities for errors to occur during the processes of collecting and transfusing blood components. In addition to mistakes in doing the required testing, failure to document is as damning as failure to perform at all. The FDA has expended considerable effort to inform facilities and to enforce requirements for proper testing for virally transmissible diseases in blood components. Likewise, private accrediting organizations emphasize proper performance and documentation of these activities.

Informed Consent

In TTAIDS cases arising in the early 1980s, it was frequently alleged that patients were insufficiently warned of the hazards of transfusion because transfusion experts failed to warn hospitals and ordering physicians about them. Few cases were successful because the state of scientific knowledge, established by expert testimony relying on published data, was limited. Also, the early HBV cases had established a record that supported the defense position that transfusions were already known by hospitals and other physicians to be unavoidably unsafe, particularly for transfusion-transmitted viral diseases. Some states (e.g., California) enacted specific legislation about informed consent for transfusion.

Medical Malpractice

Several multimillion-dollar lawsuits, decided for the plaintiff, resulted from successful allegations that either the patient did not give adequate informed consent, did not need a transfusion at all, could have waited until test-negative blood was available before receiving a transfusion, or required transfusion solely because of something the physician did. In all these cases, the basis for fault was negligence by the treating physician.

Ethics and Transfusion Medicine

Biomedical ethical principles that must be balanced when considering appropriateness of and informed consent for transfusion include **autonomy**, **beneficence**, and **justice** (see definitions in Box 27–1).

Ethical Principles and Definitions

Autonomy: The right of each person to make decisions based on that person's values and beliefs, having adequate information and an understanding of the choices available to him or her and lacking any compulsion by external forces.

Beneficence: In the health-care setting, professionals seek the well-being of each patient.

Justice: Patients should be treated fairly, with equal, need-based access to beneficial treatment.

In transfusion medicine, autonomy is increasingly important as patients become more aware of the harm, and the benefit, of transfusions and insist on the right to choose the type of therapy and the source of the blood they receive. Although autonomy is not unrestricted, it must form part of the health-care relationship. When transfusions are offered, patients expect that the treatment will benefit them. When the benefit is marginal or even questionable and, in particular, if something harmful occurs, the decision of the health-care professional may be challenged both legally and ethically.

The ethical principle of beneficence will be balanced against autonomy in every instance. Fortunately, the ethical principle of justice is rarely invoked because there are only rare instances in which transfusions are inequitably distributed, generally because of shortage of collections. In times of blood shortages, rationing begins with canceling elective surgical procedures for which transfusion may be indicated and rarely reaches a point at which emergency needs are compromised. An example of balancing ethical principles that has caused legal action is when patients have suffered serious or fatal consequences and were not given the choice of donating for themselves or selecting their own blood donors from among family members, church or social groups, or coworkers.

Emerging Issues

In addition to the concerns listed previously, new issues focused on outcomes related to the concepts of patient blood management challenge the appropriateness of existing transfusion practices that are not fundamentally evidence-based. These include new evidence that raises awareness about the age of red blood cells when transfused, issues surrounding provision of autologous services, use of newer therapies such as recombinant erythropoietin, standards for provision of perioperative blood collection and reinfusion, and control over the use of gene therapy to treat certain transfusion-dependent illnesses. In the TTAIDS area, suits have been filed for false AIDS test results and for fear of AIDS exposure through transfusion or via a health-care worker. There are also ongoing concerns over handling of look-back. New concerns about bacterial contamination, fueled by the still-unexplained upsurge in *Yersinia* growth in RBCs, and newer issues surrounding hepatitis C and other transfusion-transmissible agents (e.g., WNV, babesiosis, and potentially dengue fever and other emerging infections) will surface.

CASE STUDIES

Case 27-1

A 26-year-old woman is critically injured in a two-car collision. She is rushed via helicopter to the nearest trauma center, where 10 units of uncrossmatched O-negative red blood cells (RBCs), 12 units of crossmatch-compatible A-negative RBCs, 4 A-negative apheresis platelet packs, and 8 units of group A fresh frozen plasma are administered within the first 24 hours of her care. Soon after her admission, she is taken to the operating room, where a splenectomy is performed, liver and left kidney lacerations are repaired, numerous fractures of both lower extremities are reset, and a chest tube is placed for a collapsed left lung. She requires only 4 more units of A-negative RBCs during the next several days in the intensive care unit and recovers sufficiently to be discharged home 15 days after the accident to recuperate. Two years later, during her first prenatal visit for a second pregnancy, she tests positive for HIV. Her obstetrician tells her that the blood center reported that one of the units she received came from a donor who was test-positive for HIV a month ago.

1. Was the blood center negligent?
2. Was the physician who transfused the patient negligent?
3. Would using an "ordinary" versus a "professional" standard of care yield a different answer?

Case 27-2

A 43-year-old man received a 1-unit transfusion of RBCs during an emergency coronary artery bypass operation. He experienced sudden unexplained hemolysis, uncontrollable coagulopathy, and renal shutdown, from which he could not be resuscitated despite massive efforts by the cardiac surgeon and anesthesiologist. During the course of the resuscitation, when a new blood sample was sent for additional crossmatch, it was discovered that the patient's blood group was O-positive; the original unit of RBCs was A-positive. His spouse sued his cardiologist for lack of informed consent and negligence and sued the hospital and transfusion service physician for negligence.

1. Which issue is likely to be successful for this plaintiff?
2. Would the result be different if ordinary rather than a professional standard of care were applied?

Case 27-3

A 32-year-old male repeat whole blood donor is found to be positive for HIV through nucleic acid testing, but he has been test-negative for HIV 1/2 antibodies and for HIV p24 antigen on several prior donations. Before all testing is completed, he returns to the blood collection center to donate HLA-matched platelets. At registration, the staff person notices that his prior record indicates his deferral status. She informs the donor that he is not eligible to donate the platelets. The donor is shocked and embarrassed by the news and storms out of the center. Two weeks later, the donor sues the blood center for intentional infliction of emotional distress.

1. Is the donor likely to be successful?
2. Are there other bases on which suit can be brought?
3. Are there established standards for preventing such an occurrence?

Case 27-4

A 59-year-old man was notified in 1999 that he had received a unit of RBCs in 1989 that was negative by first-generation HCV antibody testing, but the donor was found to be positive when subsequently tested by second-generation methods. He was tested by the blood center in late 1999 and found to be HCV-positive. He filed a lawsuit against the treating physician, the hospital, and the blood center in 2002.

1. What legal theory can this man use?
2. What is the likely outcome of this lawsuit?

Case 27-5

A 67-year-old woman, crippled by degenerative arthritis, requests that her own blood and blood from family members be used during her hip replacement surgery. The blood center describes its donation procedures, which do not permit directed donations. Although she is disappointed, she agrees to donate for herself. When her first unit is tested, it is reactive for hepatitis B surface antigen and for antibody to hepatitis B core antigen. The patient-donor is advised that she may no longer donate for herself and that the unit she has already donated will not be available for her surgery. Surgery proceeds. She receives 4 units of volunteer blood and develops TTAIDS 3 years later. She sues the blood-collecting organization.

1. On what legal grounds can this suit be brought?
2. What is the current standard of care regarding patient-directed donations?

3. Can/should health-care organizations deny autologous donor-patients access to their own test-reactive blood?

Case 27-6

On July 5, a Monday afternoon, two trauma victims, both group O-negative, arrive in the same hospital emergency room. Both patients have massive injuries requiring large-volume RBC transfusions. Because of the time of year, the hospital transfusion service is low on O-negative RBCs. As the requests for RBCs rise, units crossmatched for tomorrow's elective surgery are taken to be used for the trauma patients. The transfusion medicine physician (TMP) contacts the department of surgery to cancel elective surgery cases for Tuesday, July 6. The transfusion service manager (TSM) puts in an emergency call to the regional blood center. The blood center informs the TSM that it, too, is short of O-negative RBCs but that it will canvas the neighboring hospitals and put in an emergency request to the blood exchange network.

As several hours pass, during which the trauma surgeons and OR team work diligently to correct the injuries and restore vital organs, it is clear that there will be sufficient RBCs available to adequately support only one patient. The chair of the hospital ethics committee is consulted for assistance in determining how to proceed.

Additional information available includes this: One patient is a 55-year-old bank president who is the sole financial support for his spouse, two college-age children, and widowed mother; the other is a 28-year-old gas service attendant who is unmarried. Both patients are critically injured, but with adequate transfusion support, both are deemed likely to recover by their treating physician.

1. Which ethical principle is being emphasized?
2. How will a decision favoring one patient over the other be viewed ethically? Legally?

SUMMARY CHART

✔ Tort liability is the basis for most lawsuits.

✔ Federal regulations that apply specifically to blood banking are found in Title 21, Code of Federal Regulations.

✔ Claims of the intentional tort of battery is used in transfusion medicine when a donor or a patient claims that he or she never agreed to have the needle placed into his or her arm.

✔ The doctrine of informed consent protects the patient (or donor) by requiring that information be provided in a manner understandable to the patient under circumstances that permit the patient to ask questions and to receive answers to any questions or concerns.

✔ The elements of negligence include:
  • A duty was owed to the injured party.
  • The duty was not met by the injuring party.
  • Because the duty was not met, the injured party was harmed.
  • Failure to meet the duty owed was directly responsible for or could have been predicted to cause the harm suffered by the injured party.
  • Some measurable (compensable) harm occurred (damages).

✔ Under the doctrine of *respondeat superior*, the actions of employees are attributable to the employer or person who directs their actions; for example, in transfusion medicine, this would be a physician.

SUMMARY CHART—cont'd

✔ The concept of product liability implies that a warranty exists for virtually any product a consumer buys, and if the product fails to perform or creates harm when none was expected, the consumer has a right to a replacement or, if denied a replacement, to sue for negligent manufacturing or distribution.

✔ Blood centers may be liable for invasion of privacy lawsuits if confidentiality is breached via public disclosure of embarrassing facts (e.g., HIV-positive results) or for violation of federal law (the HIPAA).

✔ Traditionally, hospitals and other nonprofit organizations are protected under the doctrine of charitable immunity from excess liability because they perform charitable acts.

✔ Biomedical ethical principles that must be balanced when considering appropriateness of and informed consent for transfusion include autonomy, beneficence, and justice.

Review Questions

1. Transfusion-transmitted diseases can result in lawsuits claiming:
   a. Battery.
   b. Invasion of privacy.
   c. Negligence.
   d. A, B, and C

2. Laws applicable to blood banking and transfusion medicine can arise:
   a. In state and federal courts.
   b. In the U.S. Congress, state legislatures, and state and federal courts.
   c. In state legislatures and courts.
   d. In state legislatures and the U.S. Congress.

3. The reasons patients have sued for transfusion injury include:
   a. Failure to perform surrogate testing.
   b. Failure to properly test blood components.
   c. Failure to properly screen donors.
   d. All of the above

4. Blood banking professionals may increase the threat of litigation by:
   a. Following published regulations and guidelines.
   b. Knowing the legal bases for liability.
   c. Disclosing all information about patients and donors.
   d. Practicing good medicine.

5. Issues about transfusion-transmitted diseases:
   a. Are evolving and will continue to result in litigation in the foreseeable future.
   b. Frequently result in plaintiff verdicts.
   c. Have all been litigated.
   d. Are known and avoidable.

References

1. Randall, CH, Jr: Medicolegal Problems in Blood Transfusion. Joint Blood Council, Washington, DC, 1962. Reprinted by Committee on Blood, American Medical Association, Chicago, 1963.
2. Rabkin, B, and Rabkin, MS: Individual and institutional liability for transfusion-acquired disease: An update. JAMA 256:2242, 1986.
3. Administrative Procedure Act, 60 Statutes 237–244, 5 USC Sections 551–559, 1988.
4. Code of Federal Regulations: Food and Drugs, Title 21, Parts 200–299 and 600–699, Title 42, Part 482. U.S. Government Printing Office, Washington, DC, 1997.
5. Sazama, K: Practical issues in informed consent for transfusion. Am J Clin Pathol 107:572, 1997.
6. Klein, HG (ed): Standards for Blood Banks and Transfusion Services, 17th ed. American Association of Blood Banks, Bethesda, MD, 1996.
7. Kelly, C, and Barber, JP: Legal issues in transfusion medicine: Is blood banking a medical profession? Clin Lab Med 12:819, 1992.

Bibliography

Cooper, JS, and Rodrigue, JE: Legal issues in transfusion medicine. Lab Med 23:794, 1992.
Crigger, B-J (ed): Cases in Bioethics, 2nd ed. St. Martin's Press, New York, 1993.
Klein, HG (ed): Standards for Blood Banks and Transfusion Services, 18th ed. American Association of Blood Banks, Bethesda, MD, 1997.
Prosser, WL, Wade, JW, and Schwartz, VE: Torts: Cases and Materials, 7th ed. Foundation Press, Mineola, NY, 1980.
Rabkin, B, and Rabkin, MS: Individual and institutional liability for transfusion-acquired disease: An update. JAMA 256:2242, 1986.
Stowell, C, and Sazama, K (eds): Informed Consent. AABB, Bethesda, MD, 2008.

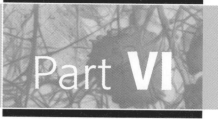

Future Trends | Part VI

Chapter 28

Tissue Banking: A New Role for the Transfusion Service

Holli M. Mason, MD

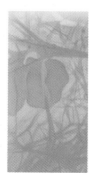

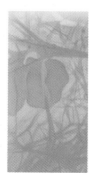

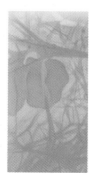

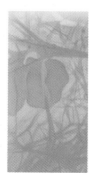

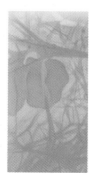

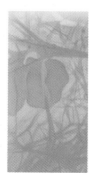

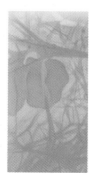

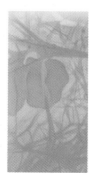

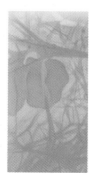

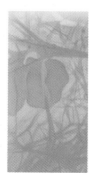

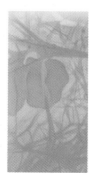

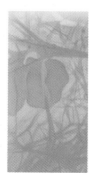

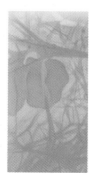

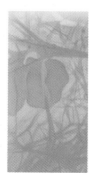

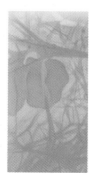

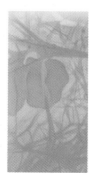

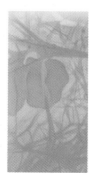

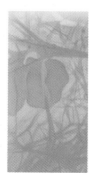

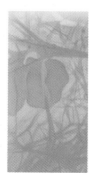

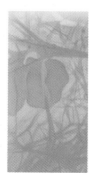

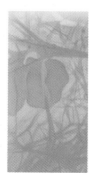

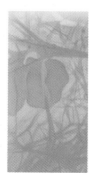

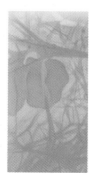

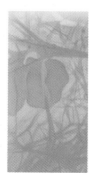

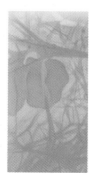

OBJECTIVES

1. Name the principal modern organizations involved in standardization of tissue banks.

2. List examples of tissues contained within the scope of FDA CFR 1270 and 1271, and examples of tissues outside the scope of these regulations.

3. State the minimum requirements for qualifying a tissue supplier and vendor.

4. List the minimum labeling requirements for autologous tissue and the conditions required to utilize autologous tissue without registering with the FDA as a tissue manufacturing establishment.

5. Compare and contrast the similarities and differences between the various regulatory bodies in terms of regulations for tissue banks, and identify voluntary accrediting agencies.

6. Compare the steps taken in an adverse event investigation with those taken in a recall.

Introduction

The function of a **hospital tissue bank** is to consolidate, standardize, and centralize the handling of human-derived tissue. The tissue bank is charged with qualifying tissue vendors, ensuring proper handling and storage of tissues, monitoring of temperature, record keeping, and issuing procedures to ensure traceability. With the advent of the 2005 directive from the Joint Commission to "assign responsibility for overseeing the tissue program throughout the organization including storage and issuance activity" (PC17.10A1), many hospital administrators have begun to look at their hospital structure to determine the best place to assign this responsibility. The blood bank has been a natural fit for many institutions, and many transfusion services have taken on the additional role of tissue bank or **tissue dispensing service**.

The Joint Commission's PC17.10A1 does not require hospitals to locate the tissue bank within the blood bank or require that a specific tissue bank be established; it requires only that there is an assignation of responsibility for oversight.[1] Some hospitals may choose to decentralize and allow surgeons to maintain their own inventories with an administrator who is responsible for ensuring that regulations and standards are followed. Validating vendor qualifications may be handled by the purchasing department and adverse events investigated by the infectious diseases department. This system may be feasible in smaller institutions but becomes unwieldy in large institutions. The AATB Tissue Committee and the AABB Tissue Committee have recommended the centralized model, stating that the ideal location for management and storage of human tissues for transplant is in the hospital blood bank.[2]

The blood bank is a natural fit for a centralized model of tissue banking because tissue is already handled in this field in liquid form. Many of the new standards are quite familiar to blood bankers and can be integrated into those already established for blood and blood products, such as monitored temperature control and record keeping. Storing all tissues under the purview of a single department can simplify standardization and consistent implementation of SOPs. This chapter focuses on the role of transfusion services in storing and issuing tissues. It also touches upon the history of tissue transplantation, the many uses of tissue products, and regulations and standards to give the reader better insight into the requirements for hospital tissue banks. For the purposes of this chapter, the term *hospital tissue bank* refers to tissue management services at the hospital level, generally restricted to receiving, storing, and issuing cells and tissues, and not to FDA-registered tissue establishments.

History and Overview of Tissue Transplantation

Tissue transplantation has had a long and varied history. Early attempts at transplantation were largely experimental and rarely successful. They were also highly controversial from an ethical and religious standpoint. The first bone transplant was recorded as early as 1682.[3] Joints, corneas, and skin were being transplanted by the early 20th century. Organ transplant became feasible with the development of vessel anastomosis through the work of Dr. Alexis Carrel, a French surgeon who worked with cadaver vessels to develop the technique that was introduced in 1911.

In 1949, the U.S. Navy established the first tissue bank. In its 50 years in existence, it created the first model for tissue harvest, processing, storage, and transplant.[4] Many of the principles developed by the U.S. Navy Tissue Bank are standards still followed today. The researchers here affected virtually every aspect of the process, from determining suitable donors, sterilization techniques, **cryopreservation**, and freeze-drying to developing the immunological principles that are so important in modern transplant medicine. The U.S. Navy Tissue Bank was also instrumental in the formation of two major institutions in the tissue transplant field: the National Marrow Donor Program (NMDP) and the American Association of Tissue Banks (AATB).

The AATB was established in 1976. Its mission is to facilitate the provision of high-quality transplantable human tissue in quantities sufficient to meet the national needs. The association publishes standards that cover screening for transmissible disease, donor selection criteria, required testing, record keeping, maintenance of asepsis, labeling, and storage.[5] AATB also carries out accreditation and inspection of tissue banks as well as certification of personnel. Close cooperation is maintained with the FDA.

In 1984, the National Organ Transplant Act (NOTA) was passed (Public Law 98.507).[6] This act established a national, centralized waiting list for organ recipients and outlawed the sale or purchase of organs.

The 1990s saw an increase in the role of the FDA in tissue banking. Beginning in 1993, the FDA required that donors be screened for hepatitis B and HIV and behavioral risk factors. In 1997, the FDA proposed a major overhaul of tissue regulations that eventually led to a more comprehensive approach focusing on three key areas: preventing the unwitting transplant of contaminated tissues that could transmit disease, preventing improper handling that may contaminate or damage tissue, and ensuring the demonstration of safety and effectiveness of tissue products.

In 1998, the FDA proposed a new unified system for the registration and listing of establishments that manufacture human cellular and tissue-based products and the listing of their products. In 2001, the FDA proposed that establishments manufacturing cellular and tissue-based products follow current good manufacturing practices (cGMP), similar to blood collection establishments. These include establishment of standard operating procedures, quality programs, record-keeping standards, and tracking procedures.[7] Additionally, the FDA required that **manufacturing establishments** register with the agency and list their products.[7]

The Joint Commission issued standards in 2005 that included directives to assign a responsible party to oversee tissue programs within institutions for storage and issuing activities. Standards PC17.10, PC17.20, and PC 17.30 also mandate record keeping for traceability and the investigation of adverse events.[1]

The Hospital Tissue Bank

The basic function of the hospital tissue bank is to provide surgeons and their patients with safe, quality tissue products while maintaining detailed records for each tissue handled through final disposition. This includes AABB Hospital Tissue Management:[8]

- Acquisition of safe and effective autografts and allografts
- Oversight of use throughout the organization
- Qualification of suppliers
- Conduction of inspections
- Provision of temperature-controlled, monitored storage
- Record keeping and ensuring traceability
- Quality assurance
- Selection of appropriate allografts
- Investigation of adverse outcomes
- Administration of recalls and look-back investigations
- Compliance with regulations and standards
- Promotion of cost-effective and appropriate tissue use

Common tissues found in tissue banks and used in surgical procedures include bones, ligaments, tendons, heart valves, skin, veins, cartilage, dura mater, hematopoietic stem and progenitor cells, and corneas or eyes. Bone can be sterilized and all living tissue removed. Pieces of bone can be further worked into spacers, wedges, screws of various sizes, and "chips." These have a variety of surgical uses, including decompression of nerves in spinal surgery with donor bone spacers, screws to pin fractured bone together, or chips to aid in the incorporation of hip or knee replacements into the native bone. Once implanted into the patient, bone slowly incorporates into the living native bone and adds strength and structure.

Heart valves are used for valve replacement, most commonly in children and women of childbearing age. The advantage of nonmechanical heart valves for this population is the nonreliance on anticoagulants that are mandatory for recipients of mechanical valves. Drugs such as Coumadin put active children in danger of serious bleeding and are teratogenic in pregnant women, causing birth defects.

Tendons and ligaments are often used in repairs of knee and other orthopedic injuries, particularly in the replacement of the anterior cruciate ligament. Tendons and cartilage are also useful in repair of facial disfigurements.

Skin is widely used for burn victims and often means the difference between life and death. Not only are skin grafts an aesthetic improvement, but they also provide the barrier to the outside world that is essential to protect the body from pathogens. Skin grafts are also used in patients with any large loss of skin, such as pressure sores, nonhealing ulcers, autoimmune disorders, and surgical or traumatic loss of large areas of skin.

Veins are commonly used in coronary artery bypass grafts. They are also used frequently to bypass other vessels that have become blocked by severe atherosclerosis. Such bypasses often make it possible for a patient to avoid limb amputation.

Hematopoietic stem cells and progenitor cells are used to repopulate bone marrow in patients who have undergone chemotherapy and irradiation to destroy tumor cells. This type of therapy destroys the native bone marrow as well, which is fatal without the transplant of donor or autologous stem cells following therapy.

Cornea transplants are used to restore sight in patients with corneas that have been damaged through trauma, disease, or birth defect. Eye tissue, or the sclera, which consists of the "white" part of the eye, is composed of thick fibrous tissue. Sclera can be used as a patch for eyes that have been punctured or torn in a trauma.[9] Sclera is also occasionally used in dental procedures.

The majority of the tissues described here have the advantage of being useful regardless of the donor's or patient's HLA type. No blood type or tissue match is required. Many of the tissues come in standardized shapes and sizes (e.g., bone screws) and can be used by any patient. Other tissues must be ordered in advance specifically for an individual with a specific size, such as heart valves or whole bones. Inventory should take into account not only the "off the shelf" utility of a particular product, but also its frequency of use and expiration date. Tissues that require specific sizes may be ordered in smaller quantities or only ordered in anticipation of specific procedures, depending on the size of the organization and turnover of product. Tissues such as cornea have such a short shelf life that it is best to schedule patient surgeries as the tissue is available and issue the cornea as soon after arrival as possible.[9]

Surgeons should have access to the inventory lists and may even want to look at individual tissue prior to surgery to avoid wasting tissues that do not fit as expected for surgeries requiring tissue of a specific size. At times, surgeons may request a selection of tissues to choose from in the operating room when the patient's situation is better understood. Clear guidelines specifying duration of time out of the tissue bank or regulated temperature ranges in order to reenter the unused tissues into inventory must be made ahead of time.[10] These guidelines should be based upon the tissue manufacturer's recommendations.

In general, the scope of the tissue bank is limited to nonvascularized tissue. Excluded from Parts 1270 and 1271 of the FDA's Code of Federal Regulations (CFR) are vascularized organs such as the liver, kidney, lung, pancreas, and heart.[11] In general, these tissues are immediately transplanted and storage is not necessary or desirable. However, there are exceptions to this general rule. Renal transplants may be stored, if properly packaged, for several days. Because kidneys are vascularized organs, and therefore fall outside the general scope of the hospital tissue bank, it is not necessary to include such tissue in the tissue bank. However, hospital administrators may opt for standardization and for ensuring proper storage and may ask to include organs, such as kidneys, in tissue banks.[1,12]

Other exclusions include autologous tissue, which may also be stored in the tissue bank for convenience and standardization; blood vessels recovered with organs and intended for use in organ transplantation; minimally manipulated bone marrow; tissue intended for education or nonclinical research; **xenografts**; blood components and blood products; and secreted or extracted products such as human milk, collagen, or cell factors.[11,12]

Tissue Bank Oversight

The hospital tissue bank must have a physician-appointed medical director. In keeping with the blood bank model, the AABB requires that the medical director be a medical doctor who investigates adverse outcomes, participates in look-back investigations, approves standard operating procedures with any deviations, and communicates with the physicians using the end product.[10] Hospital tissue banks within the blood bank have the advantage of the presence of a medical director. If the institution chooses to delegate this responsibility to another qualified physician other than the medical director of the blood bank, this individual should participate in the development and review of all policies, procedures, and processes involving the handling of tissue. He or she should also be involved in investigating adverse events, deviations from standard operating procedures, and look-backs. An important part of the Joint Commission requirement from 2005 is that there must be a standard operating procedure that assigns and designates responsibility for the oversight of the organization's tissue-related activities.[1]

Development of a tissue committee is recommended with the intent to ensure and promote best practices based on evidence-based medicine. The tissue committee may be structured similarly to the transfusion committee, including medical staff who are involved in the use of transplantable human tissue. The chair may be the director of the blood bank, but the committee may prefer to choose a chair from the surgery department secondary to that physician's knowledge regarding tissue transplant and use.

Peer review, evidence-based clinical indications, and audits ensuring compliance with standard operating procedures should be major goals of the committee. The committee should review operations, usage trends, shortages, wastages, and errors. All reported adverse outcomes should be brought to the tissue committee and investigated fully. The committee may also be involved in selecting tissue vendors and in educating the hospital staff in the appropriate use of tissue. Often the tissue committee can be successfully incorporated into the transfusion committee with committee members fulfilling both roles.

Additional important roles within the hospital tissue bank are the quality assurance coordinator and the hospital tissue coordinator. The quality assurance coordinator, often known as the compliance officer, is responsible for the quality plan for the transfusion service as mandated by the AABB and CAP.[10] He or she assesses processes, policies, and procedures to make sure they are in compliance with the applicable accrediting agencies. Depending on the size of the organization, the job description may include applying these duties to the entire laboratory or to discrete parts. The quality assurance coordinator should make recommendations to the medical director regarding operations. The hospital tissue coordinator is responsible for all administrative operations of the tissue dispensing service, including handling regulatory issues and hospital policies. He or she defines policies and procedures for the service, ensures competency and training of the staff, manages acquisition and inventory, and prepares reports for the tissue committee, including adverse event reporting. This person is often in the position of supervisor in the blood bank or may be an additional person at the same level.

Acquisition of Allografts and Inventory

The hospital tissue bank serves as the clearing house for all tissues entering the hospital (excluding most or all vascularized organs). It may be necessary or desirable to involve the surgical staff in decisions as to the standard inventory and day-to-day ordering; however, the tissue bank should be responsible for approving tissue vendors and receiving all shipments.

Once a shipment of tissue is received in the tissue bank, it should be inspected for package integrity and correct labeling and reconciled with the packing invoice.[13] Tissue receipt records must contain, at a minimum, name and address of tissue supplier, description of tissue and quantity, date of tissue receipt, condition of tissue upon receipt, and expiration date, if applicable (AATB L4.100).[5] Each tissue specimen must have a **tissue identification number** (TIN). In addition, the name of the person conducting the incoming inspection should be recorded on the tissue receipt record. Joint Commission standards require that the individual receiving the shipment must verify package integrity and ensure that the transport temperature range has been controlled and acceptable, as evidenced by residual dry or wet ice.[1] The vendor should be able to present evidence of validation of transport containers for maintenance of proper temperature range during transport.

Manufacturers' instructions for storage should be rigorously followed and the tissue entered manually or electronically into an inventory list. If necessary, the storage site location should be included in the inventory for ease of locating the tissue upon issue or inspection. Surgeons who transplant tissue should have access to the inventory so they are aware of what tissues are available to them before they begin surgical procedures.

Detailed and accurate inventory management is cost-saving and will reduce wastage of products stored until expiration or will prevent inadvertently reordering when the product is already in inventory. Some products, such as corneas, have a very short shelf life, and careful coordination between the surgical staff and the tissue bank allow for ordering and acquiring the appropriate tissue in time for the surgery, but not so far in advance that the product expires and must be wasted. Duration of storage time will vary greatly between the different types of tissue. Therefore, a system, preferably electronic, must be in place to anticipate replacement of outdated tissues or management of those tissues to avoid outdating.[13]

To avoid waste, some tissue vendors will agree to exchange tissue that is close to outdate with similar tissue that has an expiration date further in the future. This is not true in all cases and must be worked out between individual vendors and hospital tissue banks. Typically vendors who are willing to exchange late-dated products have a network of hospital tissue banks to which they can transfer the product for quick use. Wastage rate for each tissue type should be tracked and examined by the tissue committee for ways to improve the process. Changes in the surgical staff, or focus of the surgical center, may result in unanticipated wastage if the same tissue inventory is kept despite changes in tissue use. Tracking wastage and communicating with other departments using tissue can keep wastage to a minimum.

Storage

Storage conditions vary between the different tissue types. Even the same tissue, such as bone or eye, can have different temperature and duration requirements depending upon its processing and packaging.[14] Therefore it is critical to carefully follow the recommendations and instructions from the tissue vendor or supplier for each specimen. Failure to do so may result in tissue that does not function as intended and may interfere with the tissue's functional and mechanical properties, making it unsuitable for transplant.[14] Special attention should be paid to products stored at "room" or "ambient" temperature. These words may vary in definition between tissue suppliers, and it is advisable to clarify the definition with the vendor. A written response to any such question should be kept on file in the hospital tissue bank.

The Joint Commission and AATB require that tissue storage shall conform to guidelines established by the distributing tissue bank[5] and that organizations use standardized procedures to store tissues.[7] The Joint Commission further requires the hospital to continuously monitor storage refrigerators and freezers with records showing daily storage temperatures.[1] AABB takes a more detailed approach to storage. Standard 3.0 deals with equipment and specifically names tissue that requires the blood bank to identify equipment that is critical to providing blood and tissue services.[13] The blood bank is required to maintain policies, processes, and procedures to ensure that calibration, maintenance, and monitoring of equipment conforms to the blood bank or tissue bank standards.[5]

AABB standard 3.6 states that storage devices must have the capacity and design to ensure proper temperature is maintained.[13] The temperature of refrigerators, freezers, and platelet incubators must be monitored. Storage units using liquid nitrogen must have liquid nitrogen levels checked or the temperature monitored. Tissues that can be stored at room or ambient temperature do not require a monitored storage device, such as a platelet incubator, as long as the definition of room temperature does not include a narrow temperature range.[13] However, many tissue banks will store these products in a monitored device for uniformity and convenience.

Alarm systems have been used in blood banks for decades and are an important assurance that storage temperatures have been consistently maintained, thereby ensuring the integrity of the product being stored. The most important function of the alarm is to allow blood and tissue bank personnel to be aware of an equipment problem before the product is compromised by a temperature that is too high or too low for proper storage. Alarm systems must be set to activate under conditions that will allow action to be taken before products reach unacceptable conditions. Procedures should be in place to instruct the blood and tissue bank personnel on actions to take when the alarm is activated, including corrective action and possible relocation of products to another monitored storage device. An alarm activation must be immediately investigated to find the cause of the malfunction.

Record Keeping and Traceability

Good record keeping is essential in the hospital tissue bank to demonstrate that standard operating procedures are followed (Box 28–1). Also important is the ability to track the tissue bidirectionally, from donor to recipient or disposal and back again. Each change in the status of the product—including receipt into the hospital tissue bank, change in location within the tissue bank, issue, return, transplantation, or disposal—must be documented concurrent with the action. The identity of the person documenting each step and the date should be included. Records must be accurate, legible, written in indelible ink, and as detailed as possible to provide a clear history.

Traceability becomes especially important during recalls. Occasionally a tissue donor is found to have had a disease or disease exposure that was not apparent at the time of donation or may be suspected because one of the tissue recipients became sick following transplant. In cases such as this, all of the tissues that originated from that donor must be investigated and tracked down to prevent transmission of disease to other recipients. Often, transplant has already occurred and the recipient can be tested or treated if necessary. Poor record keeping makes it impossible to track potentially dangerous tissues or to determine who may need

---

BOX 28–1

Standard Operating Procedure (SOP) Checklist

The following SOPs should be written and included in the hospital tissue bank:

- Assignment of responsibility for the oversight of the tissue program
- Validation and qualification of tissue suppliers/vendors
- Tissue ordering
- Tissue receipt
- Tissue storage and temperature control
- Issuance and final inspection of tissue
- Temperature alarms and emergency backup equipment
- Documentation of abnormalities, including instructions on actions such as quarantine
- Quarantine of tissues that are questionable
- Documentation of decisions not to use tissue
- Disposal/disposition of expired tissue

treatment or increased surveillance due to the transplant of a tissue from a donor suspected of transmitting disease. The bidirectional traceability is important so that if a recipient becomes ill after transplant, the tissue bank and supplier can cooperate to trace the source of the tissue in order to initiate a recall.

Records must be maintained for a minimum of 10 years after the expiration of the tissue product.[5] If no expiration date applies to a specific tissue specimen, records must be maintained for 10 years following issue.[5] Each tissue specimen must have a unique TIN, and upon receipt by the hospital tissue bank, must include the name and address of the tissue supplier, a description of the tissue and quantity received, date of receipt, condition upon receipt, and expiration date along with the name of the receiving individual.

When a tissue is **dispensed** to be used for transplant, dispensing records must be created. The dispensing record must include the name, address, and telephone number of the tissue bank; the type and quantity of tissue; the unique TIN; the recipient's name, medical record number, or social security number; transplantation site; date and time of release; name of the ordering physician or other health professional; name of the person dispensing the tissue; and name of the person preparing the tissue if further preparation is necessary prior to transplant.[5] The dispensing records must be maintained in a log format in the hospital tissue bank. It must also be included as part of the recipient's medical record to permit tracing to the appropriate individual. Tracing forms must also be filled out and returned to the tissue supplier or vendor for their records.[5] The records should clearly specify the final disposition of the tissue. The tissue will have been *implanted*, meaning the tissue was implanted in the patient; *discarded*, meaning the tissue was discarded in the operating room and not implanted into the patient; or *explanted*, meaning the tissue came into contact with the patient but was removed either immediately during surgery or at a later date.

Quality Assurance

Quality is the goal of virtually any blood or tissue bank. A quality plan is essential for good tissue practices and excellent patient care. The goals of the quality plan are to maintain safe, functional, and effective products that meet the needs of the patient and the surgeon. Preventing contamination and having an error-free process is critical. To achieve these goals, the quality plan must include written procedures, validation of processes, and investigation of deviations and errors. Errors will occur even in the best-run tissue banks. Well-written standard operating procedures that conform to the regulations and are easy to follow in actual practice decrease errors. However, analysis of deviations and errors, as well as development of corrective action to improve process and prevent future errors, builds quality over time.

The quality plan should also verify supplier qualifications, ensure proper training of personnel, and monitor compliance in the tissue bank. Periodic quality audits should be performed by the tissue service to ensure that standard operating procedures and standards and regulations are being followed.

Qualification of Vendors

Tissue vendors or suppliers must meet a variety of standards. First, the tissue supplied must be safe and effective and of use to the physician who transplants it. The tissue must be readily available in a useful time frame, and its cost must fall within budgetary guidelines and be within the customary price range. The surgeons who will use the tissues should be involved in selecting the tissue vendor based on the tissue's usefulness to them. Most often, a surgeon will request a specific tissue from a specific vendor because of its utility. It is then up to the medical director of the hospital tissue bank to determine whether the vendor qualifies as a supplier of quality, safe, and effective tissues.

Sales representatives must be compelled to seek approval and qualification with the hospital tissue bank prior to demonstrating any new tissue products in the operating room. It is also important to consider other physicians within the organization who may also utilize tissue for patient care in a nonsurgical setting, such as a wound care clinic, and solicit their input as well.

Before the **qualification of a vendor** can commence, the hospital tissue bank must have written guidelines and criteria for the acceptance of a vendor or supplier.[10] Some vendors may be part of a larger entity in which different establishments participated in different parts of the process of supplying a tissue product. For example, one establishment may recover the tissue and pass it on to another that processes and packages the tissue for distribution. The written policy should reflect if each of the **intermediaries** should also be qualified by the hospital tissue bank. Theoretically, qualification of the supplier directly supplying the tissue should be sufficient, as that supplier must have, in turn, qualified its suppliers. However, some medical directors may feel more secure in verifying this for themselves. The medical director may also take into account such things as the transparency and willingness to provide information, method of processing and disinfecting, the involvement of the supplier's medical director, and the ability of the supplier to meet special needs. Table 28–1 outlines the required documentation for tissue vendor and supplier qualification.

The first step in qualifying any vendor is to verify the supplier's FDA registration. On a yearly basis, the tissue bank must verify that its suppliers are registered with the FDA as required by 21 CFR 1271.[15] This can be done by using the FDA's online database: www.fda.gov/cber/tissue/tissregdata.htm. In January 2001, the FDA published a rule requiring establishments that supply human cells, tissues, and cellular and tissue-based products (HCT/Ps) to register with the agency and list their **HCT/Ps**.[15] The final rule, 21 CFR Part 1271, became effective in April 2001 for human tissues intended for transplant that are regulated under section 361 of the Public Health Safety (PHS) Act and 21 CFR 1270.[16] In March 2001, the requirement became effective for all other HCT/Ps except human dura mater and heart valves,

Table 28–1 **Documentation for Tissue Vendor/Supplier Qualification**	
DOCUMENT	**INFORMATION REQUIRED/LOCATION FOUND**
Tissue supplier's FDA registration (Form FDA 3356)*	• Federal registration number • Physical location of the establishment • Reporting official's information • Establishment's function • Product information • Proprietary names (www.fda.gov/cber/tissue/tissregdata.htm)
Tissue supplier's voluntary accreditation	List of accredited suppliers: • www.aatb.org • www.restoresight.org
Tissue supplier's state license and registration	When suppliers are located in states that require licensure by the state.

*Required by the Joint Commission

which became effective when the remaining parts of 21 CFR 1271 were implemented in 2005.[16]

Establishments that meet the requirements for registration with the FDA must do so within 5 days after beginning operations.[15] Registrations must be updated annually in December in conjunction with an update of the HCT/P list unless there is no change. Upon acceptance of the establishment's registration form, the FDA will assign each location a permanent number.[15] This registration number does not imply that the establishment is in compliance with applicable rules and regulations or is approved by the FDA. However, the establishment, once registered, must be available for public inspection by the FDA (CFR 1271).[15] A yearly review of FDA registration of tissue vendors is recommended in the first quarter of each year because of the requirement that the establishments update their registration each December.

A copy of the form used to register with the FDA (Form FDA 3356) should be obtained from the vendor and kept on file in the hospital tissue bank.[15] The registration form contains the following information: **federal registration number**, physical location of the establishment, reporting official's information, the establishment's function (e.g., recovery, packaging, processing, etc.), product information, and proprietary names. Additionally, the hospital tissue bank's medical director may request copies of any observations made during FDA inspection (Form 483), including responses and corrective action.[16] Warning letters to an establishment are available through the Freedom of Information Act and may be found on the FDA website (www.fda.gov).[16]

Some tissue vendors will become voluntarily accredited by a recognized organization. This is not required but may weigh in the medical director's decision to qualify a vendor for his or her tissue bank. This should also be spelled out in the written guidelines. Organizations that accredit tissue establishments are the American Association of Tissue Banks (AATB)[5] and the Eye Bank Association of America (EBAA).[9] Similar to the FDA website, these organizations list their accredited establishments on their websites, which can be found at www.aatb.org and www.restoresight.org, respectively.

Finally, the Joint Commission requires that hospital tissue banks ensure that tissue establishments are licensed by state agencies when required by state law in the physical location of the organization.[1] Not all states require licensure; in fact, most do not. As of this writing, six states require licensure: New York, Florida, New Jersey, California, Georgia, and Maryland (Table 28–2).

Autologous Tissue

The term *autologous tissue* refers to any tissue that is removed from a patient with the intent to reimplant it at a later date and during a different procedure than its removal. Strictly speaking, a bone flap that is elevated and placed in sterile saline during a procedure and then replaced at the end of that same procedure does not qualify as being autologous tissue as defined in this chapter.[17] In order for the regulations and standards pertaining to autologous tissue to apply, that bone flap would require additional processing, storage, and reimplantation at another time within the same facility.[1,17] Ironically, the Joint Commission defines this as the "same procedure," as it is done by the same surgeon in the same facility on the same patient, despite the intervening storage in the tissue bank.[1]

Autologous tissue can be logistically problematic for a hospital tissue bank. First, qualifying the supplier of the tissue is changed in this circumstance. If a tissue is to be used within

Table 28–2	**State Laws Governing Tissue Banking**
STATE	**APPLICABLE LAWS**
California	California Health and Safety Code, Chapter 4.1 and 4.2
Florida	Chapter 893, Florida statutes
Georgia	State law requires tissue banks to be licensed as clinical laboratories.
Maryland	State law requires tissue banks to be licensed as clinical laboratories.
New Jersey	New Jersey Statute 26:2A-1
New York	New York State Public Health Law, Art. 43-B

the same institution and not shipped to an off-site facility under different management for any further processing or storage, there is no requirement to register as a tissue establishment with the FDA. It is important to note that if an autologous tissue is transferred to any other facility, such as a different hospital because the patient was transferred, the hospital tissue bank would be required to register with the FDA as a tissue manufacturing establishment and would be subject to FDA inspection.[16] In order to remain exempt from the requirement to register with the FDA, the hospital tissue bank must retain the tissue until reimplantation at the same facility.

Common autologous tissues include skull bone flaps (most common), ribs, iliac crests, and endocrine tissue such as the pancreas and parathyroid.[18] Occasionally, other tissues such as skin and connective tissue will require storage. The advantage of autologous tissue is the perfect immunological match. Additionally, the size may be ideal, such as is the case for the skull bone flap that is exactly the right size for the hole that must be patched. The risk of infectious disease transmission is diminished. However, one of the main disadvantages to autologous tissue is the possibility of reinfection of bacteria or fungus or the reintroduction of malignant cells.[19] The age and health of the donor-patient may impact the functionality of the tissue as well.

Preparation

The first step in the preparation for harvesting autologous tissue is to define and develop clearly written policies and procedures for both the surgical service and the hospital tissue bank.[18] These policies and standard operating procedures require collaboration between the two services in order to create a seamless operation and to ensure full agreement on all conditions that must apply. The hospital tissue committee may be involved in this process.

The surgical service should include, as part of its procedures, a notification step to alert the tissue bank of a planned procedure that will result in autologous tissue. Clear guidelines should be incorporated to instruct operating room personnel on the steps required both administratively and medically. Informed consent must be obtained from the donor-patient. This is best done by the surgeon treating the patient.

The tissue bank should include a procedure to ascertain whether the donor-patient is being treated for bacteremia or is at high risk for HIV or hepatitis.[20] In general, it is not advisable to use autologous tissue for reimplant if the patient was bacteremic at the time of harvest because of the risk of reinfection. However, this is not true in every case, and procedures for sterilization exist, so each case must be approved individually by the tissue bank medical director and the surgeon jointly. The tissue bank should keep a donor-patient record on file for each autologous tissue. Any **deviations**, test results, **adverse reactions**, and the **disposition** should be documented and retained in this file.

Within the operating room, the preparation of the autologous tissue falls under the regulatory standards of the Joint Commission, the AATB, and the Association of periOperative Registered Nurses (AORN). AORN has developed guidelines and recommendations for autologous tissue recovery that maintain aseptic techniques and prevent contamination.[21] The recommended guidelines include:

1. **Removal of tissue.** The surgeon removes the tissue and hands it off to an assistant in an aseptic manner. The assistant places the tissue in a sterile container. More than one piece of tissue may be placed in the container if removed from the same site at the same time. Otherwise, separate containers should be used.
2. **Culturing of tissue.** If the procedure requires tissue culture, complete written instructions should be available. Culturing should include swabbing the entire tissue surface, including edges. Culture swabs are labeled with at least two unique patient identifiers and sent to the microbiology laboratory. Note: Culture should be done before any antibiotic is used as additive.
3. **Addition of storage solution.** If the tissue requires addition of storage media or antibiotics, it should be added after the culture step. Written protocols for each tissue type must clearly establish which tissues require additives and which additives are required. Because of the possibility of allergic reactions, hospital personnel must confirm that the patient does not have an allergy to an additive antibiotic. The container must be labeled with the name of the antibiotic used.
4. **Containers for storage.** Containers may vary depending on the tissue and the institution. AORN recommends sterile plastic bags or sterile Nalgene jars. The Nalgene jars are useful because they are able to withstand temperatures to −40°C for up to 5 years and can be used with irradiation sterilization procedures.[21]
5. **Wrapping the container.** The sterile container is further protected with at least two sterile outer wraps.
6. **Labeling the container.** The outer wrap of the container must be labeled with two unique patient identifiers, patient age, date of collection, type of tissue, name and address of the facility, physician's name, time of collection and expiration date, if applicable. It may require further biohazard labels according to FDA CFR 1271.90 and must contain a label stating "FOR AUTOLOGOUS USE ONLY" and "NOT EVALUATED FOR INFECTIOUS SUBSTANCES."[16]
7. **Tissue storage.** The tissue must be placed immediately into a temperature-monitored storage unit. If there is a delay, the tissue should be transported on wet ice.
8. **Tissue processing.** Tissue that is to be processed is done in a controlled environment.

The Joint Commission also adds a requirement to "track and identify materials used to prepare or process tissues and instructions used for preparation."[1] (JC Standard TS. 3.2.1) Careful documentation of materials, including name, lot number, expiration date, and amount should be made in the medical record.

Storage

Ideally, the tissue bank will be expecting the arrival of the autologous tissue, having been informed by the surgical staff of the procedure ahead of time. Prior to tissue recovery, the surgical team and the tissue bank should confer on the procedure and verify that written standard operating procedures address any individual issues that may be present for each donor-patient.[1] Once the tissue arrives at the tissue bank, the tissue bank personnel must inspect the label to make sure all elements are present (Box 28–2). The surgical team should be immediately involved to solve any discrepancies or unclear labeling.

As per written standard operating procedure and recommendation on the label, the tissue is placed in the proper storage site to ensure the correct temperature is maintained. A separate area should be reserved for autologous tissues to keep them away from **allogeneic tissue**, as is done with autologous blood. Tissue from donor-patients who are known to have infectious diseases should be stored in a quarantine area.

A common complaint from tissue banks who store autologous tissues is what to do with tissues that never get used. It is surprisingly common for surgeons to decide not to use autologous tissue after it has been harvested. This can be solved with good communication with the surgical staff and agreement of a reasonable expiration date for all tissues. If agreement cannot be reached and an expiration date is assigned by the tissue bank, care should be taken to be sure the container is suitable for the temperature and duration of storage. The surgeon should be informed of the expiration date at the time it is assigned. According to AATB standards, autologous tissues should have the same shelf life as a similar allogeneic tissue under the same storage conditions.[5]

Discard of autologous tissue should require the medical director's approval. As with blood products and allogeneic tissue, proper documentation of discard is required. Documentation must clearly outline the manner and location of disposal according to local, state, and federal regulations for medical waste.[16] Occasionally, a request will be made that the tissue be sent to a funeral home for burial with the deceased donor-patient. This is permissible as long as regulations are followed and documentation is complete.

Sterilization and Testing

Sterilization is not required and not possible with many tissues. A medical director in conjunction with the surgeon may choose a sterilization technique. For skull bone flaps, a common and popular method of sterilization has been high heat by using an autoclave. This has the advantage of killing bacteria and even removing malignant cells; however, the disadvantage is that the high heat denatures proteins and collagen in the bone, making it less suitable for reimplant. Steam has also been utilized but has the same denaturing effect. Many surgeons will opt for irradiation as a method to destroy bacteria. This is useful if there is an irradiator on-site at the hospital and clear guidelines are worked out for exposure times and radiation amount. Note: If the tissue is taken to another facility under different management for sterilization techniques, the hospital tissue bank must register as a tissue manufacturing establishment with the FDA and become subject to FDA inspection.[15]

Testing is optional for autologous tissue, as it is for autologous blood. Culture of autologous tissue is also optional and should be clearly spelled out in the operating procedures as to what tissues, if any, require culture. If the facility opts to culture or test the tissue donor-patient for infectious diseases, the same testing should be performed as for blood donors (HBsAg, anti-HBc, anti-HCV, HCV NAT, anti-HIV-1/2, HIV NAT, anti-HTLV I/II, syphilis, and West Nile virus NAT).[22] If any testing or culture is positive, the tissue should be released only with the medical director's approval. The surgical team should be notified of any positive tests, and the medical director may approve or disapprove based on consultation with the transplanting surgeon. If any test is positive or if donor-patient screening indicates an increased risk for infectious disease, a biohazard label is mandatory for the tissue container. If the facility opts not to test the autologous tissue, a label stating "NOT EVALUATED FOR INFECTIOUS SUBSTANCES" must be affixed to the container.[16]

Implantation

Issuing or dispensing autologous tissue is much the same as for allogeneic tissue. There are a few differences, however, and the tissue bank that is located within the blood bank can utilize familiarity with autologous blood products to construct standard operating procedures that cover all of the necessary requirements. As with autologous blood, the blood bank and tissue bank personnel should be made aware of the expected surgical date for reimplantation. Prior to the surgery date, the tissue bank must perform a thorough record review and all deviations and discrepancies resolved before the tissue is needed for surgery. Suitability should be documented in the donor-patient file. The issuing procedure should be the same as for allogeneic tissue and must include a final visual inspection of the outer wrapping for integrity

---

BOX 28–2

Requirements for Autologous Tissue Labels

- Must read "For Autologous Use Only"
- Name and address of the tissue bank
- Two unique patient identifiers
- Complete description of tissue
- Date of collection
- Name of surgeon
- Date of expiration according to validation of packaging and tissue type
- Disinfection or sterilization steps (if performed)
- Presence and name of any additives
- Biohazard label if testing is positive or screening is positive for risk factors
- "NOT EVALUATED FOR INFECTIOUS SUBSTANCES" unless complete donor testing has been done
- Recommended storage temperatures

and inspection of the label to verify all required elements are present. If any problems or deviations are discovered, the tissue should be placed into quarantine until the medical director resolves the matter in consultation with the transplanting surgeon.

Regulatory Overview

The number of organizations involved in tissue regulations and standards can be daunting to a facility intending to set up a hospital tissue bank. It can be overwhelming to look at the various documents to be sure that all requirements are carried out and satisfied. Table 28–3 is a "crosswalk" that compares each of the major regulatory agencies, matching the categories of regulations for easy cross-reference and comparison.

In taking a broad overview of the regulatory agencies, it is clear that they have evolved in parallel. One may require more than the others in one area but less in another, depending upon the focus of the organization. However, they overlap significantly and it is not difficult to develop an organization that is in compliance with them all. It is important to note that compliance with AABB *Standards* often exceeds requirements from other agencies, another important reason to house the tissue bank within the blood bank.[13] While the author has attempted to summarize the relevant standards and regulations for each of the major organizations listed here, it is recommended that a full review of each regulation is done prior to developing a hospital tissue bank structure or standard operating procedures (SOP) designed for compliance.

Federal Laws

The Code of Federal Regulations, Title 21 was established for food and drugs, and part 1271 deals with human cells,

Table 28–3   "Crosswalk" for HCT/P-Related Standards of the AABB, AATB, EBAA, and the Joint Commission*

AABB[1]	AATB[2]	EBAA[3]	Joint Commission[4]
1.0 Organization	L1.000 L1.100	C1.000–C1.300 C2.000	PC.17.10/QC.5.300 EP1
1.3 Policies, Processes, and Procedures	D1.000 D5.000 E1.000 F1.000 L1.00	C3.400 D1.000 E1.000 F1.000 G1.000 I.1000 J.1000 K1.000 L1.000 L2.000 M1.000	PC.17.10/QC.5.300 EPs 1–10
1.4 Emergency Preparedness	E4.150	C3.200	PC.17.10/QC.5.300 EP 8 EPs 1–10
3.0 Equipment 3.6 Storage Devices for Blood, Components, Reagents, Tissue and Derivatives Alarm Systems	E4.100 E4.140 E4.150 L2.200	C3.200 I1.000	PC.17.10/QC.5.300 EP 8 EPs 6, 7
4.0 Supplier and Customer Issues 4.1 Supplier Qualification 4.3 Incoming Receipt, Inspection, and Testing	F1.200 L4.100	C3.500 C3.510 G1.200 J1.000	PC.17.10/QC.5.300 EPs 2, 5, 10
5.0 Process Control 5.1.6 Identification and Traceability 5.1.6.1 Process or Procedure Steps 5.1.6.2 Traceability 5.1.8 Handling, Storage, and Transportation 5.10 Final Inspection Transfusion Service Related Activities: 5.11 Samples and Requests 5.18 Final Inspection Before Issue	C1.100 D5.300 E1.000 (series) F1.200 (g) K2.220 L1.000 L3.100 L4.200	G1.000 G1.100 E1.000–E1.300 D1.200 J1.000 I1.000 L1.100 L2.000 F1.400 K1.000–K1.200 M1.500	PC.17.10/QC.5.300 EPs 4, 10 PC.17.20/QC.5.310 EPs 1, 2, 3, 4, 6, 7

Table 28–3   "Crosswalk" for HCT/P-Related Standards of the AABB, AATB, EBAA, and the Joint Commission*—cont'd

AABB[1]	AATB[2]	EBAA[3]	Joint Commission[4]
6.0 Documents and Records Reference Standard 6.2D Retention of Tissue Records	C1.300 L4.000 L4.100 L4.200	D1.100–D1.120 K1.100 M1.00-M1.500 C3.400	PC.17.20/QC.5.310 EPs 1–6
10.0 Facilities and Safety 10.3 Discard of Blood, Components, Tissue, and Derivatives	L3.300	C3.600 C.700	PC.17.10/QC.5.3 EP 3 PC.17.20/QC.5.310 EP1

*Horizontal alignment represents only general relationships among standards. This table represents only selected highlights of AABB HCT/OP-related standards. See Chapters 9 through 12 for more detail on the above standards and organizations; see Frizzo[5] for a fuller treatment of all relevant AABB standards and those of the AATB, the College of American Pathologists, and the Joint Commission.
[1]Price, TH (ed): Standards for Blood Banks and Transfusion Services, 25th ed. AABB, Bethesda, MD, 2008.
[2]Pearson, K, Dock, N, and Brubaker S (eds): Standards for Tissue Banking, 12th ed. American Association of Tissue Banks, McLean, VA, 2008.
[3]Eye Bank Association of America: Medical Standards. EBAA, Washington, DC, 2008.
[4]The Joint Commission: Comprehensive Accreditation Manual for Hospitals. PC.17.10–PC.17.30. Joint Commission, Oakbrook Terrace, IL, 2008.
[5]Frizzo, WL: Tissue Management Self-Assessment Tool for Transfusion Services and Hospitals. AABB, Bethesda, MD, 2008.
Key: AABB = American Association of Blood Banks; AATB = American Association of Tissue Banks; EBAA = Eye Bank Association of America; HCT/P = human cells, tissues, and cellular and tissue-based products
Reprinted with permission from Eisenbrey, AB, and Eastlund, T (eds): Hospital Tissue Management: A Practitioner's Handbook, 1st ed. AABB, Bethesda, 2008.

tissues, and cellular and tissue-based products. Part 1271 is subdivided into subparts A through F:[16]

- A: General provisions
- B: Procedures for registration and listing
- C: Donor eligibility
- D: Current good tissue practices
- E and F: Additional requirements, inspection, and enforcement of establishments covered in 1271.10.

Section 361 of the PHS Act refers specifically to regulations to control communicable diseases (42 USC, section 264).[23]

General Provisions

The purpose of part 1271 was to create a system to register and list establishments that manufacture HCT/Ps.[16] Additionally, it is meant to establish guidelines for donor eligibility and incorporate principles of good tissue practice in order to prevent the introduction, transmission, and spread of communicable diseases through tissue transplant. An establishment is defined as a business, which may include any individual, partnership, corporation, or association, under single management, in a single location that engages in the manufacture of HCT/Ps as well as facilities who contract manufacturing services.

Human cells, tissues, or cellular tissue-based products are defined as articles containing or consisting of human cells or tissues intended for transplantation or otherwise transferred into a human recipient. Some examples include bone, ligament, skin, hematopoietic stem cells derived from peripheral and cord blood, manipulated autologous cells, epithelial cells on a synthetic matrix, semen, and other reproductive tissue.[7] This list is by no means exhaustive and represents a small number of examples of HCT/Ps.

HCT/Ps that are regulated under section 361 of the PHS Act meet the following criteria: The tissue is minimally

manipulated; it is intended for and labeled for homologous use only; it is not combined with another vehicle except for water, crystalloids, and sterilizing and preserving agents, unless such additives compromise the clinical safety of the HCT/P; and the HCT/P does not have a systemic effect and is not dependent upon the metabolic activity of living cells for its primary function.[6] Alternatively, the HCT/P may have a systemic effect or may depend on the metabolic activity of living cells for primary function if it is for autologous use, allogeneic use in a first- or second-degree blood relative, or reproductive use.

Tissues that are not considered HCT/Ps include vascularized human organs for transplantation; whole blood or blood components or blood derivative products; secreted or extracted human products (except for semen), such as milk, collagen, and cell factors; minimally manipulated bone marrow for homologous use and not combined with another article, except for additives for preservation and storage; ancillary products used in the manufacture of HCT/P; cells, tissue, and organs derived from animals; in vitro diagnostic products; and blood vessels recovered with an organ intended for transplant and labeled "For use in organ transplant only."[5] Although these items are not HCT/Ps, they may be found as part of a hospital tissue bank at the discretion of the hospital administration and for the sake of uniformity in handling biological items for human transplant, transfer, or infusion.

There are a few exceptions to who must comply with the requirements of part 1271. HCT/Ps used solely for nonclinical or educational purposes are exempt.[16] Entities that merely receive, carry, and deliver HCT/Ps and entities that do not recover, screen, test, process, label, package, or distribute but only receive and store tissues for use on patients only in that facility are also exempt.[16] The latter type of institution is the usual model for hospital tissue banks. Thus, the requirements set forth in 21 CFR 1271 are not regulations that hospital tissue banks that only store and issue HCT/Ps must meet. However, it is important that the tissue banker be aware of the requirements of its suppliers, how the tissues are handled, and what tests are routinely run. Hospital tissue banks that participate in harvesting, processing, packaging, or distribution of tissues must comply with the Code of Federal Regulations (21 CFR 1271) and become registered establishments.[15] *Distribution* is defined as the transfer of HCT/Ps to another facility for use on a patient. It does not include the return of tissue to a supplier.

Procedures for Registration and Listing

Establishments that meet the requirements for registration with the FDA must do so within 5 days after beginning operations using Form FDA 3356.[15] Registrations must be updated annually in December in conjunction with an update of HCT/P list, unless there is no change. If a change in the HCT/P list occurs between December and June, the change must be updated in June.[15]

In addition to the annual renewal and notifications of change in HCT/P list within 6 months, any change in location or ownership of the establishment must be amended on the registration within 5 days of the change.[15] Upon acceptance of the establishment's registration form, the FDA will assign each location a permanent number.[15] This registration number does not imply that the establishment is in compliance with applicable rules and regulations or is approved by the FDA. However, the establishment, once registered, must be available for public inspection by the FDA.[16]

Donor Eligibility

Establishments that manufacture HCT/Ps must develop and maintain procedures for all steps in testing, screening, donor eligibility, and all other requirements.[16] The procedures are subject to review and approval of a responsible individual. Donor eligibility is determined by screening relevant medical records to ensure that the donor is free from risk factors and clinical evidence of relevant communicable diseases, that there are no communicable disease risks associated with xenotransplantation, and that results of donor testing for relevant disease agents are negative or nonreactive. Relevant communicable diseases include HIV, types 1 and 2; hepatitis B virus; hepatitis C virus; human transmissible spongiform encephalopathy; Creutzfeldt-Jakob disease; and *Treponema pallidum*.[24] For leukocyte-rich tissue, there should be additional testing for human T-lymphotropic virus, types 1 and 2. Cells and tissue that are reproductive in nature must also be tested for *Chlamydia trachomatis* and *Neisseria gonorrhea*.[24]

Relevant medical records that must be reviewed include a current donor medical history interview; a current report of the physical assessment of a cadaveric donor or a physical examination of a living donor, if available; laboratory test results in addition to those outlined above; medical records; coroner or autopsy reports; and records from any source pertaining to risk factors for communicable diseases.

Once the donor is deemed eligible, records pertaining to the donor eligibility must accompany the tissue at all times.

The required documentation includes a distinct identification code that links the HCT/P to the donor. Except in the cases of autologous tissues or HCT/Ps donated directly to a first- or second-degree relative, the identification code should not include the donor's name, social security number, or medical record number. A statement that the donor has been determined "eligible" or "ineligible," along with a summary of the records used to make this determination, is required. In addition, a statement that disease testing was performed by a CLIA-certified laboratory or equivalent, a list of tests performed with results, and the name and address of the establishment determining eligibility are required.

Donor eligibility determination is not required in some circumstances. Examples of this include cells and tissues for autologous use, reproductive cells or tissue donated by a sexually intimate partner of the recipient, or cryopreserved cells for reproductive use (when possible, measures should be taken to test the semen and oocyte donors before transfer of an embryo). In these cases, the tissue must be clearly labeled "FOR AUTOLOGOUS USE ONLY" or, for allogeneic tissue, "NOT EVALUATED FOR INFECTIOUS SUBSTANCES" and "WARNING: Advise recipient of communicable disease risks."[16]

Current Good Manufacturing Practice

Subpart D sets forth current good tissue practice (CGTP) requirements.[16] These requirements are intended to prevent the introduction, transmission, or spread of communicable diseases by HTC/Ps by ensuring that they do not contain disease agents, are not contaminated, and do not become contaminated during manufacturing. The CGTP requirements govern all steps in the manufacture of HCT/Ps, specifically donor eligibility, screening, and testing. Core CGTP requirements cover facility control, environment control, equipment, supplies and reagents, recovery, processing, labeling, storage, receipt, distribution, and donor eligibility.[16] Contracts between tissue suppliers are addressed here. Establishments that recover and process tissue must be in compliance with subparts C and D as they apply to the operations performed at that establishment.[16] If another establishment performs some of the operations, such as sterilization, that establishment is also required to conform to the regulations for the operations performed at that facility. Before entering into a contract, the primary establishment is responsible for verifying that the second establishment is in compliance. If at any time the primary establishment becomes aware of noncompliance at the secondary establishment, the contract or agreement must be terminated.

Also part of CGTP is the establishment and maintenance of a quality program. Functions of the quality program must include having appropriate procedures relating to core CGTP requirements and procedures for receiving, evaluating, and documenting core CGTP requirements; ensuring that appropriate corrective actions relating to core CGTP requirements are done, including reaudits of deficiencies and verification that corrective actions are effective; ensuring proper training and education of personnel; establishing appropriate monitoring systems; and investigating and documenting deviations and trends.[16]

State Laws

Only a few states (New York, Florida, California, Maryland, and New Jersey) have enacted laws regarding the transplant and manufacture of human tissue products (see **Table 28–2**). Only three of these states (New York, Florida, and California) have comprehensive laws regarding regulation of tissue banks. Georgia and Maryland only require that tissue banks be licensed as clinical laboratories. New York and Florida have adopted extensive technical regulations. If readers reside in any of these six states, it is recommended they study the laws of that state to ensure compliance with those laws. The Joint Commission requires that tissue banks in states that have additional laws pertaining to tissue must be in compliance.[1]

American Association of Blood Banks

The AABB has been involved in setting standards for tissue banking for almost two decades. In 1993, in its 15th edition of the *Standards for Blood Banks and Transfusion Services* (*Standards*), a section was added to address tissue storage and issue. Since 1947, it has been involved in blood banking, another form of human tissue transplant, which makes AABB-accredited hospital blood banks the recognized and logical leaders in the field of tissue banking. In the 1990s, the AABB revised its quality plan to reflect what the organization considers to be its ten quality system essentials (QSE):

1. Organization
2. Resources
3. Equipment
4. Supplier and customer issues
5. Process control
6. Documents and records
7. Deviations, nonconformances, and adverse events
8. Internal and external assessments
9. Process improvement through corrective and preventative action
10. Facilities and safety

Human tissues for transplantation are treated in an almost identical manner to blood by the AABB *Standards*.[13] In general, hospital tissue banks that operate within hospital blood banks can assume compliance because the same standards apply to blood and tissue equally, unless a standard explicitly excludes tissue. Table 28–4 lists AABB standards that specifically mention tissue.

Table 28–4	AABB Standards Pertaining to Tissue
STANDARD	**PURPOSE**
1.0 Organization	Clearly defined structure
1.3 Policies, Processes, and Procedures	Quality SOPs to ensure the requirements of the *Standards* are satisfied
1.4 Emergency Preparedness	SOPs for internal or external emergencies
3.0 Equipment	Calibration, maintenance, and monitoring of critical equipment
3.6 Storage Devices	Capacity, temperature monitoring
3.7 Alarm Systems	Set to alarm before tissue is compromised, investigate
4.0 Supplier and Customer Issues	Supplier qualification, testing in AABB or equivalent accredited laboratory, registered with FDA
4.3 Incoming Receipt, Inspection, and Testing	Inspection, testing as necessary, label verification
5.0 Process Control	SOPs to ensure quality of tissue, derivatives, and services
5.1 Identification and Traceability	Documentation of each step and identification of person who performed it, traceability, no more than two donation identifications per container, handling, storage, and transportation
6.0 Documents and Records	SOPs for documents to be identified, reviewed, approved, and archived
6.2.3	Record system shall make it possible to trace any tissue from source to final disposition
7.0 Deviations, Nonconformances, and Adverse Events	SOPs to capture, assess, investigate, and monitor deviations, responsibility for review, prevention of issue, quarantine, and notification
7.1.4 Released Nonconforming Tissue	Determination of effect, notification of customer if necessary, records created
7.2 Fatality Reporting	Fatalities related to blood shall be reported to outside agencies as required
7.4.4 Adverse Events Related to Tissue	SOP for investigating and reporting adverse events
10.0 Facilities and Safety	Safe environmental conditions
10.3 Discarded Tissue	Minimize potential for human exposure to infectious agents

(Data from: Price, T, ed: Standards for Blood Banks and Transfusion Services, 26th ed. AABB, Bethesda, 2009.)

American Association of Tissue Banks

The AATB was founded in 1976 by a group of scientists and doctors from the U.S. Navy Tissue Bank.[4] These individuals recognized that the scope of tissue banking should be widened to include the entire nation. It is the only national tissue bank organization and accredits over 100 tissue suppliers nationwide. AATB's *Standards* was first published in 1984. The *Standards*, now in its 12th edition, is a comprehensive and detailed guide to tissue banking.[5] This guide has been used internationally as a framework for other national tissue banking organizations. At least six states (including California, Georgia, and Maryland) require that tissue-manufacturing establishments be accredited by the AATB. In 1988, the organization initiated a certification program, Certified Tissue Banking Specialist (CTBS), for individual workers in the tissue banking industry. It currently certifies over 4,000 people.

In the 1990s, the AATB expanded its scope from tissue manufacturing establishments to include hospital tissue banks. This era also saw the beginnings of a partnership and collaboration between the AABB and the AATB. In 1993, a new section appeared in AATB's *Standards* entitled "Medical Facility Tissue Storage and Issuance." Subsequently, several more sections that apply to the hospital tissue bank were added, including "Records Management," "Release and Transfer of Tissues," "General Operations," and "Quality Assurance and Quality Control Programs." Following AABB's change to the ten QSEs, the AATB *Standards* were reorganized in the same format. In widening its scope to include the hospital

tissue bank, the AATB's intention was to provide greater safety and traceability to final disposition, whether implanted into a patient or disposed.

The section in the AATB *Standards* that is most applicable to the hospital tissue bank is the L1.000 series for tissue dispensing services.[5] Standards that apply to autologous tissue can be found throughout. See Table 28–5 for a list of standards relevant to the hospital tissue bank. A comparison of **Tables 28–4 and 28–5** shows the similarity between the *Standards for Blood Banks and Tissue Services* and the *Standards for Tissue Banking* as they each pertain to tissue banking.

The Joint Commission

The Joint Commission is a nonprofit accrediting agency that accredits and certifies over 17,000 health-care organizations in the United States. Its mission is "to continuously improve health care for the public, in collaboration with other stakeholders, by evaluating health care organizations and inspiring them to excel in providing safe and effective care of the highest quality and value."[25] Its history reaches back to 1910, when Ernest Codman, MD, proposed the "end result system of hospital standardization."[26] He felt that if every hospitalized patient could be tracked long enough to determine effectiveness of treatment, medicine would benefit. The benefit would come primarily in determining for whom treatment was not effective, determining why, and changing practices for future patients. In 1917, a one-page list of minimum standards for hospitals was published, and the following year, the organization began inspections based on

Table 28–5   AATB Standards Pertaining to Hospital Tissue Banks

STANDARD	PURPOSE
L1.000 General, Director	SOPs addressing receipt, storage, final disposition, traceability, supervision by a qualified medical professional
L2.000 Storage	Storage in conformance to guidelines
L2.200 Equipment	Maintenance, calibration, QC
L2.300 Labeling	Tissue shall not be relabeled; labels shall not be altered
L3.100 Dispensing	Physician's order required, all associated written material is to be available to the end user
L3.200 Release to Intermediary	All original written materials, label, and tissue identification number must accompany, documentation of transfer to another facility
L3.300 Tissue Disposal	Minimize hazard to staff or environment, comply with applicable laws and regulations
L3.400 Return of Tissue	Cryopreserved reproductive tissue may not be redistributed for use, except as required by local or state regulations
L4.000 Records	Concurrently record all steps for traceability, maintain records for 10 years after expiration
L4.100 Tissue Receipt Records	Each specimen must have a unique tissue identification number, minimum requirements for receipt records
L4.2 Dispensing Records	Minimum requirements for disposition records, maintained in log format
L5.000 Adverse Outcomes	Potential or suspect adverse outcomes, directly or indirectly related to tissue shall be reported to tissue processor, investigated, and documented
L6.000 Recalls	SOPs for the recall of tissue

(Data from: Pearson, K, Dock, N, and Brubaker, S (eds): Standards for Tissue Banking, 12th ed. American Association of Tissue Banks, McLean, VA, 2008.)

these minimum standards.[26] Of the 692 hospitals surveyed that year, only 89 met the minimum standards.[26]

By 1950, the original document grew significantly, and there were as many as 3,200 accredited hospitals.[26] In 1951, the American College of Physicians (ACP), the American Hospital Association (AHA), the American Medical Association (AMA), and the Canadian Medical Association (CMA) joined with the original American College of Surgeons (ACS) to create the Joint Commission on Accreditation of Hospitals (JCAH).[26]

In 1965, Congress passed the Social Security Amendments with the provision that hospitals accredited by JCAH had **deemed status** with the Medicare Conditions of Participation for Hospitals and could, therefore, participate in Medicare and Medicaid programs.[26] In 1978, JCAH joined forces with the College of American Pathologists (CAP) to further evaluate laboratories. JCAH adopted the name Joint Commission on Accreditation of Healthcare Organizations (JCAHO) in 1987 to reflect its expanding scope of activities.[26]

Effective July 1, 2005, JCAHO adopted the tissue storage and issuance standards for the ambulatory care, office-based surgery, critical access hospitals, and hospital accreditation programs that store and/or issue human tissue. These were in the form of standards PC.17.10, PC.17.20, and PC17.30. In 2007, JCAHO officially shortened its name to "Joint Commission."[26]

Hospital Standard PC.17.10 (Laboratory Standard QC.5.300) addresses the use of standardized procedures to receive, store, and issue tissues. This standard is broken down into ten parts, or elements of performance (EP):[26]

EP 1: Assign responsibility for overseeing the tissue program throughout the hospital.
EP 2: Validate that source facilities are registered with the FDA.
EP 3: Coordinate tissue ordering, receipt, storage, and issuance throughout the hospital.
EP 4: Transport, handle, store, and use tissues according to manufacturer's instructions.
EP 5: Log in all incoming tissue.
EP 6: Maintain continuous temperature monitoring of storage equipment.
EP 7: Maintain daily records of appropriate storage temperature.
EP 8: Make sure there are functional alarms and emergency backup for storage equipment.
EP 9: Comply with state and federal regulations when acting as a source facility.
EP 10: Verify package integrity and transport temperature at receipt.

Hospital Standard PC.17.20 (Laboratory Standard QC.5.310) is concerned with record keeping, particularly in the traceability from donor to final disposition. There are seven parts to this standard:

EP 1: Records must permit tracing of any tissue.
EP 2: Records must track and identify material used to prepare or process tissue.

EP 3: Records must identify who accepted the tissue, who prepared the tissue, and the date and time of preparation.
EP 4: Documentation in the recipient's clinical record of tissue use, including unique identifier of tissue.
EP 5: Maintenance of records for at least 10 years following expiration.
EP 6: Documentation of minimum required elements in records maintained for at least 10 years.
EP 7: Compliance with completion and return of tissue usage information cards requested by the source facility.

Hospital Standard PC.17.30 (Laboratory Standard QC.5.320) concerns the process of investigating adverse reactions to tissue or donor infections. This standard is in five parts:

EP 1: Having SOPs to investigate recipient adverse events related to tissue use.
EP 2: Reporting to the source facility any post-transplant infections and adverse events.
EP 3: Quarantining tissue identified by the source facility as possibly contaminated.
EP 4: Informing and tracking patients whose donors are subsequently found to have a transmissible infectious disease.
EP 5: Following procedures for real or suspected adverse events

A review of the tissue standards from the Joint Commission reveals striking similarity to regulations from AABB, AATB, and FDA. The most notable addition is the requirement for source facilities to comply with applicable state laws for registration and accreditation.

Eye Bank Association of America

The EBAA accredits facilities that provide eye tissue for surgery, education, or research.[9] It is a nonprofit organization that also certifies eye bank technicians. The organization was established in 1961 by the American Academy of Ophthalmology's Committee on Eye Banks.[9] It is the oldest national tissue transplant organization in the United States, and its mission is to "restore sight through the promotion and advancement of eye banking." In addition to accreditation and certification, EBAA also develops uniform medical standards and procedures for its member banks to maintain proficiency in eye tissue recovery, storage, preservation, and transplantation.[9] These medical standards are reviewed and approved semiannually by the American Academy of Ophthalmology.

The EBAA requires facilities providing tissue to be registered with the FDA.[9] The source facility may voluntarily be accredited by EBAA; however, the Joint Commission does not require this as a condition for hospital tissue banks to receive tissue from an establishment. The hospital tissue bank medical director may select suppliers of ocular tissue from EBAA-accredited facilities as an added level of safety and security.[9]

Adverse Events

An **adverse event** is a negative change, unexpected outcome, or reaction to the tissue implant. Adverse events can be due to infectious disease, failure of the allograft to function as expected, or transmission of malignancy. It is important to discover and report adverse events primarily for the protection of other patients who may receive tissue from the same donor.[2,7]

Infection

Transmission of infectious disease through allograft transplantation is relatively rare. Many of the recorded cases of disease transmission occurred in years prior to the current, comprehensive standards and improved donor testing. Infections are most often transmitted by tissues that are fresh or cryopreserved. These methods of storage allow some infectious entities to survive and cause disease in the new host. Fortunately, the most common type of tissue used, freeze-dried bone, has not been seen to transmit disease readily. Often the biggest cause of disease transmission is human error. Inadequate donor screening, inadequate sterilization, and other system failures allow potentially contaminated tissue to remain in the system. For these reasons, the above regulations have been developed.

Similar to blood donation, the first step in ensuring safe tissue is to search the donor population for individuals with low risk of disease. This can be a challenging task for manufacturing facilities. Medical records may be incomplete, and if family of a deceased donor is available for interview, they may not be aware of all the details that may be important. It may also be unclear what caused the donor's death. A misdiagnosis of a fatal infection could result in that infection passing on to a tissue recipient. This was the case for a rural man who died with "chest numbness and back pain" in 1979, reported by Houff and colleagues.[27] His corneas were transplanted into an individual who died six weeks later, following development of headaches, eye pain, and respiratory failure. Studies on both donor and recipient revealed a rabies infection in both individuals. Had the clinical history of the deceased been more accurate, the transplant and subsequent second death could have been avoided. Infections may lie dormant for years. There may be only limited mention in medical records, or none at all for a virus that is dormant with an undetectable antibody titer. Antibody titers may also be unreliable and in the "window period" shortly after initial infection. For these reasons, RNA testing for HIV and Hepatitis C has become standard practice.

Bacterial and fungal infections transmitted by tissue transplant are getting more attention in recent years due to increased awareness and regulatory oversight. It is likely that many adverse events due to fungal and bacterial contamination went undetected, usually with the assumption that the recipient acquired the infection de novo. Investigation into the source of these types of adverse events have shown that the organism was often not part of the premortem condition in the donor but was introduced during the surgical harvest of the tissue or the subsequent processing. Many tissue products undergo minimal processing without sterilization steps. These include heart valves, tendons, ligaments, and cartilage. The tissue bank medical director should be certain to make transplanting surgeons aware of bacterial and fungal risks.

Dura mater has been known to transmit **Creutzfeldt-Jakob disease** (CJD) in more than 100 cases of transplant.[24] CJD is caused by a prion, which is neither virus, bacteria, or fungus but rather is a self-replicating protein known to invade neurological tissue and cause death. Incubation times vary, and patients have shown symptoms as early as 6 months following transplant and as late as 16 years.

Another possibility for introduction of infectious agents is through perimortem blood transfusions. The author is currently investigating several donors whose blood was transfused to a trauma victim who died and subsequently became a tissue donor. A recipient has contracted parvovirus B19. Appropriate investigation of the tissue donor has been unrevealing. Because blood is not routinely tested for parvovirus B19, the donors of the units transfused at death are being investigated. Fortunately, transfusion-transmitted disease is rare.

Malignancy

Malignancy transmitted through tissue transplant is extremely rare. Two cases of carcinoma transmitted through corneal transplant have been recorded.[19] Almost all other known cases of malignancy transmission have been through organ transplant and include a number of adenocarcinomas, melanoma, sarcoma, lymphoma, glioblastoma, and choriocarcinoma.[19] Tissues, such as bone, tendon, and ligament, have few viable cells present at transplant and undergo several sterilization steps. Heart valves and vascular tissue rarely harbor malignancies and are therefore less likely to transmit it. Of note, there has never been a recorded incident of transmission of malignancy through blood transfusion. Both tissue and blood donors are excluded from donation on the basis of malignancy present at time of donation.

Allograft Failure

The allograft may fail to function as expected or intended. In many cases, this may be because of the patient's underlying condition. However, it is important to investigate other causes not related to the patient. Failure of the tissue manufacturer to faithfully adhere to standard operating procedures can cause changes that may affect the stability and durability of the tissue product. Discovering the source of tissue failure, either intrinsic to the donor or because of an irregularity in manufacturing, will lead to recall of other products that may have potential to harm other patients.

Reporting and Investigation

Reporting and investigating suspected adverse outcomes is important for many reasons. This area of medicine has recently received a great deal of attention with efforts to create a national biovigilance network. **Biovigilance**, as a structured, region-wide entity, has been in practice for many years in Europe. The backbone of a quality program is the ability to capture errors and unexpected outcomes and then investigate them to determine, as much as possible, the root cause. This information is of little value if it is not shared with everyone involved in the process so that meaningful change can take place. In the individual case, it is crucial to alert the tissue supplier of a suspected disease transmission or contamination so that the supplier may track down all other tissue harvested from the same donor to prevent other adverse events. Often, tissue tracked from the same donor may have already been transplanted. In that case, it is equally important to know of possible contamination so that the patient may be appropriately tested or treated.

The most basic, and arguably the most important, step in the reporting process is recognizing an adverse event by the clinical staff. Postoperative infections are not uncommon, and a true adverse reaction may be dismissed as a routine postoperative complication. Some adverse reactions may take weeks, months, or even years to express themselves, such as hepatitis C infection or CJD. The medical director of the tissue bank should communicate regularly with the surgeons, especially on this topic. It may be helpful to schedule grand rounds or other educational talks to ensure that all surgical staff are aware of the risks and what to look for. Some clinical staff may be falsely assured by sterile packaging or disinfecting steps in processing. While contamination is rare, it is more common in tissues with viable cells, such as valves and vessels. Disinfection steps may not be effective for every organism. Additionally, steps may be missed due to human error.

Contamination by bacteria or fungus should be suspected based on the type of organism cultured, especially if the infection is deep and not a superficial wound infection. Unusual organisms for the wound or tissue should also be suspect. Although the time frame of onset can be factored into the overall decision to report the infection as a suspected adverse event, it is less reliable, as it may vary greatly depending on the organism. Once the surgeon has sufficient information to suspect that the transplant is the reason for the infection, he or she should immediately report the suspected event to the tissue bank.

Suspicion of viral or prion transmission by tissue should similarly be reported as soon as the physician becomes aware. Obvious other causes of infection should be sought at the time of diagnosis. For example, a patient newly diagnosed with hepatitis C at some point following tissue transplant should be questioned about IV drugs, tattoos, needle sticks, and household contacts as possible sources of infection.

The surgeon may also report the suspected disease transmission to the FDA through the MedWatch program (www.fda.gov/medwatch). However, it is important that the hospital tissue bank is not bypassed in the process, as an important function of the medical director is to report to the tissue supplier and investigate the case.

In the tissue bank, there are several important steps to the investigation process. First, every complaint or suspicion should be taken seriously, even if there is a low chance that the event is related to tissue transplant. A file should be opened on each case, and all documents generated in the investigation should be kept together in the file. Immediately following a complaint, the personnel in the tissue bank should look for and quarantine any tissue from the same donor, pending outcome of the investigation. The medical director must be notified as soon as possible. The tissue supplier must also be notified as soon as possible so that steps may be taken to quickly sequester any other tissue from that donor that may exist at different facilities.

The medical director must then confirm the complaint and begin to determine what other causes may be responsible. He or she should look into the possibility of **nosocomial infection**, other potential routes of infection, and risk factors independent of tissue transplant and should examine patient records for any irregularities associated with tissue transplant procedures. If warranted, corrective action should be implemented depending on the result of the investigation. The tissue bank must cooperate fully with the tissue supplier's investigation.

Other ancillary investigation should include testing of any unused tissue from the same donor and investigation into the postoperative course of other patients who received tissue from the donor. The results of the investigation must be reported to all parties involved, including the transplanting surgeon and the tissue supplier, as well as the hospital risk management department and the tissue committee. Although not required, the tissue bank is encouraged to report the findings to the Joint Commission. If the event is severe or fatal, the Joint Commission recognizes this as a sentinel event requiring root cause analysis and corrective action. Although not required, the event may be reported to the FDA through MedWatch. Reporting to the state is necessary for those cases involving reportable disease. A final report should be placed in the file created for the case, and another copy should be kept in the tissue vendor's qualification file.

It is important to remember to keep the patient informed as well. The Code of Medical Ethics and the Joint Commission are clear that the patient has a right to know when errors or unanticipated outcomes occur, particularly if the adverse event is severe or considered a sentinel event. It is best if the treating surgeon conveys this information because a relationship and level of trust already exists. If another physician must inform the patient, care should be taken not to alienate the patient and treating physician, and the treating physician should be fully informed beforehand. When informing a patient of an error or allograft-related infection, it should be done compassionately, factually, and without blame. Expressions of concern and regret are appropriate, and there should be a plan for how to proceed. An offer of assistance in further treatment as appropriate should be made as well.

Recalls

Recalls are almost always voluntary and may be initiated at virtually any step in the process from the donor to the recipient. The recall is initiated after an error is discovered, even if it is months to years after the tissue has been processed. An irregularity may be discovered in an FDA inspection that initiates the recall, or a problem may be reported by workers or doctors who discover it in the course of using or handling the tissue. When a problem is discovered in the course of an investigation, the FDA may compel the establishment to initiate a recall.

There are three classes of FDA recalls (Box 28–3). Class I is the most severe and serious. These recalls are reserved for products that may cause serious harm, health problems, or death if used. Class II is intermediate and is for products that may cause temporary health problems or less serious injury. Class III is likely the most common type of recall and pertains to products in which a manufacturing irregularity or violation in labeling is discovered, but the product is unlikely to cause harm if used.

Typically, the manufacturing establishment where the tissue was originally processed notifies its customers of recalls. The FDA also disseminates information on recalls of all types. These recalls can be found on the FDA website through MedWatch, the FDA's safety information and adverse event reporting tool. Hospital tissue banks may also subscribe to a national recall reporting service such as the National Recall Alert Center, although that is not required.

Just as there are steps in reporting adverse events, notification of a recall has several important steps. Upon receiving notification of a recall, the hospital tissue bank must verify that the product is or was in inventory, determine the disposition of any and all tissue included in the recall, and quarantine any unused tissue. All tissues that have been transplanted must be tracked to the recipient. If any tissues have been sold, transferred, or returned, the receiving facility must be notified of the recall. Just as in the adverse event investigation, a file should be created for any investigation into the disposition of recalled tissue and maintained for 10 years.

Regulations on notification of the recipient have been addressed by the Joint Commission and AABB. Both require that recipients of tissue from donors who are subsequently found to be positive for HIV, human T-cell lymphotropic virus (HTLV) type I or II, viral hepatitis, or other known infectious agents transmissible by tissue must be notified. This would include making reasonable attempts to notify the implanting physician and request that he or she notify the patient. If the surgeon cannot be reached or does not wish to notify the patient, it becomes the tissue bank's responsibility and reasonable attempts to reach the patient must be made. Reasonable attempts to notify should occur in less than 12 weeks of the recall. The explanation to the patient should include information regarding the reason for the recall, possible effects to him or her, and the opportunity to make a decision regarding further testing or counseling with a list of testing locations.

CASE STUDIES

Case 28-1

A new orthopedic surgeon has just been hired at the hospital. He has a great deal of experience using a particular type of processed bone that can be acquired from only one tissue vendor. He requests that the hospital tissue bank begin ordering this product for his upcoming scheduled surgeries. When the approved vendor list is consulted, the vendor is not on the list.

1. What do you tell the surgeon who is expecting the tissue next week?
2. What is the minimum requirement to qualify the new vendor?

Case 28-2

A neurosurgeon calls the hospital tissue bank in advance of a planned craniotomy. He explains that he will not be able to replace the bone flap at the completion of the surgery planned for the next day, but within 1 to 2 weeks, he would like to close the head wound with the patient's own bone. He further states that it is possible that once stabilized, the patient may be moved to another facility for the second procedure. He requests that the autologous tissue be stored in the tissue bank and inquires as to the procedure for transferring the tissue with the patient.

1. What are the minimum requirements for labeling autologous tissue?
2. Under what condition could the hospital tissue bank transfer the tissue?
3. Give two examples of procedural steps that should be discussed prior to the surgery.

BOX 28-3

FDA Recall Classes

- Class I recall: Potential to cause serious injury or death
- Class II recall: Potential to cause temporary or less serious health problems
- Class III recall: Unlikely to cause harm but violates FDA regulations or labeling

SUMMARY CHART

✔ In 2005, the Joint Commission ruled that hospitals must assign responsibility for overseeing the tissue program throughout the organization, including storage and issuance activity (PC17.10A1).

✔ AABB and AATB recommend a centralized model of tissue banking, and AABB states that the ideal location for the tissue bank is in the hospital blood bank.

✔ The FDA requires that any tissue-manufacturing establishment must register yearly with the FDA and submit to inspection.

✔ Hospital tissue banks that receive, store, and issue tissue do not need to register with the FDA unless their function also involves procurement, processing, or distribution.

✔ Transfer of tissue to another facility is considered distribution.

✔ Vascularized organs, such as liver, kidney, lung, pancreas, and heart are excluded from FDA CFR 1270 and 1271.

✔ The tissue bank should have a physician-appointed medical director in line with the AABB's model for blood bank.

✔ A tissue committee should be established that is similar to, or part of, the transfusion committee.

✔ Tissue delivered to the tissue bank must be inspected for package integrity and labeling and reconciled with packaging invoice, and must receive verification that temperature conditions have been maintained appropriate to the tissue delivered.

✔ The hospital tissue bank must maintain continual monitoring of storage refrigerators and freezers.

✔ Record keeping must detail each step or change in status of the tissue with notation of the person who performed it and the date to allow for bidirectional tracking from donor to final disposition.

✔ Records must be maintained for 10 years following the expiration of a tissue product or 10 years after issue if there is no expiration date.

✔ Each tissue product must have a unique tissue identification number (TIN).

✔ The hospital tissue bank must verify any supplier and vendor's FDA registration on a yearly basis.

✔ The Joint Commission requires that hospital tissue banks ensure that suppliers are licensed by state agencies as the laws apply for the state in which the vendor or tissue bank is located.

✔ Autologous tissue, used within the same facility with no intervening shipments off-site for further processing, may be stored and issued with no requirement to register with the FDA as a tissue manufacturing establishment.

Review Questions

1. Implant records must be kept for what duration?
   a. Ten years after the tissue has been harvested
   b. Indefinitely
   c. For a reasonable time to ensure that the recipient is not still alive when records are destroyed
   d. Ten years following the expiration of the tissue

2. FDA CFR 1270 and 1271 include all of the following tissues EXCEPT:
   a. Cancellous bone chips.
   b. Blood vessels associated with vascular organs for transplant.
   c. Cornea.
   d. Heart valve.

3. Hospital tissue banks must register with the FDA if:
   a. Tissue for transplant is stored.
   b. Autologous tissue is stored and issued.
   c. Tissue is transferred to another facility.
   d. The tissue bank is located outside the blood bank.

4. The Joint Commission requires all of the following EXCEPT:
   a. Hospital tissue banks must ensure that suppliers are complying with applicable state laws.
   b. Tissue manufacturing establishments must register with the FDA.
   c. Hospitals must assign responsibility for overseeing the tissue program throughout the organization.
   d. Hospital tissue banks must verify supplier's registration with the FDA yearly.

5. The American Association of Tissue Banks (AATB) is:
   a. A mandatory accrediting agency for all tissue banks.
   b. A voluntary accrediting agency for tissue-manufacturing establishments.
   c. An historic name for the U.S. Navy Tissue Bank.
   d. A subdivision within the AABB.

6. Transmission of malignancy in tissue:
   a. Is most likely to occur with the use of bone.
   b. Is relatively common (1/10,000 cases)
   c. Is more likely to occur in whole organ transplant.
   d. Has never been reported in cornea transplant.

7. The medical director for the tissue bank can be:

    a. Any individual appointed by the hospital medical director.

    b. The lead supervisor in the blood bank.

    c. The head nurse/transplant coordinator from surgical nursing.

    d. A qualified physician involved in tissue transplant or blood banking.

8. Notification of a recipient of tissue that has been recalled because of possible contamination should be conducted by:

    a. The tissue bank director only.

    b. The patient's transplanting surgeon.

    c. The patient does not need to be told unless he develops an infection.

    d. The informed consent covers this contingency and no further notification is necessary.

9. Tissue receipt records must include all of the following EXCEPT:

    a. Unique tissue identification number.

    b. Name and address of tissue supplier.

    c. Expiration date.

    d. Tissue supplier's FDA registration number.

10. Records that must be reviewed to determine donor eligibility by the tissue manufacturer include:

    a. Donor family history.

    b. Records from any source pertaining to risk factors for communicable diseases.

    c. Interview of next-of-kin.

    d. Consent to harvest tissue.

References

1. Joint Commission: Tissue Storage and Issuance Standards: PC.17.10, PC.17.20, PC.17.30, QC.5.300, QC.5.310, QC.5.320. Joint Commission, Oakbrook Terrace, IL, 2008.
2. Eastlund, T, and Eisenbrey, AB (eds): Guidelines for Managing Tissue Allografts in Hospitals. AABB, Bethesda, 2006.
3. New York Organ Donor Network: Transplantation—the history, 2009. Available at www.donatelifeny.org/all-about-transplantation/tissue-transplant-history/. Accessed November 17, 2011.
4. Strong, DM: The US Navy Tissue Bank: 50 Years on the Cutting Edge. Cell Tissue Bank 1:9–16, 2000.
5. Pearson, K, Dock, N, and Brubaker, S (eds): Standards for Tissue Banking, 12th ed. American Association of Tissue Banks, McLean, VA, 2008.
6. Public Law 98-507. October 19, 1984. The National Organ Transplant Act. Available at www.history.nih.gov/research/downloads/PL98-507.pdf. Accessed November 17, 2011.
7. Food and Drug Administration: Guidance for Industry: MedWatch Form FDA 3500A: Mandatory Reporting of Adverse Reactions Related to Human Cells, Tissues, and Cellular and Tissue-Based Products (HCT/Ps), 2009. Rockville, MD: CBER Office of Communication, Training, and Manufacturers Assistance. Available at www.fda.gov/Safety/MedWatch/HowToReport/ucm085568.htm. Accessed January 25, 2010.
8. Eisenbrey, AB, and Eastlund, T (eds): Hospital Tissue Management: A Practitioner's Handbook, 1st ed. AABB, Bethesda, 2008.
9. Eye Bank Association of America: Medical Standards. Washington, DC: EBAA, 2008. Available at www.restoresight.org/aboutus. Accessed January 25, 2010.
10. Eastlund, T: Tissue and organ transplantation and the hospital transplantation service. In Roback, J, Combs, MR, Grossman, B, and Hillyer, C (eds): Technical Manual, 16th ed. AABB, Bethesda, pp 833–864, 2008.
11. Code of Federal Regulations: Title 21 CFR Part 1270 and 1271. Washington, DC: US Government Printing Office, 2009 (revised annually). Available at www.accessdata.fda.gov/scripts/cdrh/cfdocs/cfCFR/CFRSearch.cfm?CFRPart=1271. Accessed January 25, 2010.
12. Hillyer, CD, and Josephson, CD: Tissue oversight in hospitals: The role of the transfusion services (editorial). Transfusion 47:185–187, 2007.
13. Price, T (ed): Standards for Blood Banks and Transfusion Services, 26th ed. AABB, Bethesda, 2009.
14. Frizzo, W: Tissue Management Self-Assessment Tool for Transfusion Services and Hospitals. AABB, Bethesda, 2008.
15. Code of Federal Regulations: Tissue Establishment Registration. Title 21 CFR Part 1270 and 1271. Available at www.fda.gov/BiologicsBloodVaccines/GuidanceComplianceRegulatoryInformation/EstablishmentRegistration/TissueEstablishmentRegistration/default.htm. Accessed January 25, 2010.
16. Code of Federal Regulations: Current Good Tissue Practice for Human Cell, Tissue, and Cellular and Tissue-Based Product Establishments; Inspection and Enforcement. Title 21 CFR Parts 16, 1270, and 1271; Final Rule. Federal Register 69:68612, 2004.
17. Shulman, IA (forum ed and moderator): Should Blood Banks Store Autologous Bone Flaps in Their Freezers? California Blood Bank Society e-Network Forum. 2001. Available at www.cbbsweb.org/enf/2001/bonestorage.html. Accessed January 25, 2010.
18. Shulman, IA (forum ed and moderator): Management and Ensuring Compliance of "Tissue Banking/Tissue Dispensing Services." California Blood Bank Society e-Network Forum. 2006. Available at www.cbbsweb.org/enf/2006/tissue_mgmt.html. Accessed November 18, 2011.
19. Gandhi, MJ, and Strong, DM (eds): Donor derived malignancy following transplantation: A review. Cell Tissue Bank 8:267–286, 2007.
20. Southeast Tissue Alliance: The Truth About Tissue Donation. 2007. Available at www.donorcare.org/pdfs/ceu_the_truth_about_tissue_donation_web.pdf. Accessed January 25, 2010.
21. Association of periOperative Registered Nurses: Standards, Recommended Practices, and Guidelines. AORN Publications, Denver, CO, 2006.
22. Centers for Disease Control and Prevention: West Nile virus infections in organ transplant recipients—New York and Pennsylvania, August–September, 2005. MMWR Morb Mortal Wkly Rep 54:1021–1023, 2005.
23. United States Code: Regulations to Control Communicable Diseases. Section 361 Public Health Service Act, 42 USC § 264(a). Washington, DC. US Government Printing Office, 2006.
24. Eastlund, T, and Strong, DM: Infectious disease transmission through tissue transplantation. In Phillips, GO (ed): Advances in Tissue Banking. Vol 7. World Scientific Publishing, Singapore, 2003, pp 51–131.
25. Joint Commission: About The Joint Commission. Available at www.jointcommission.org/about_us/about_the_joint_commission_main.aspx. Accessed 2011
26. Joint Commission: History of The Joint Commission. Available at www.jointcommission.org/about_us/history.aspx. Accessed 2011.
27. Houff, SA, Burton, RC, Wilson, RW, et al: Human-to-human transmission of rabies virus by corneal transplant. N Engl J Med 300:603–604, 1979.

Answer Key

Chapter 1

Review Questions

1. c	6. c	11. b	16. a
2. c	7. d	12. d	17. d
3. b	8. d	13. d	18. c
4. c	9. a	14. c	19. c
5. d	10. a	15. c	20. a

Chapter 2

Review Questions

1. b	5. d	9. c	13. a
2. b	6. d	10. a	14. a
3. c	7. b	11. b	15. c
4. d	8. a	12. a	

Chapter 3

Review Questions

1. a	7. b	13. d	19. a
2. c	8. c	14. c	20. b
3. b	9. d	15. a	21. d
4. d	10. c	16. b	
5. d	11. a	17. c	
6. c	12. a	18. d	

Chapter 4

Review Questions

1. a	5. d	9. c	13. c
2. c	6. a	10. b	
3. c	7. d	11. b	
4. b	8. d	12. d	

Chapter 5

Case 5-1

1. No. Adding check cells to all tubes negative at the AHG phase provides a quality-control measure to the test. The expected result is positive agglutination. A negative result deems our test invalid.
2. The blood bank tech is required to repeat the test, starting from step 1.
3. The most likely cause is failure to adequately wash cells after the incubation phase.
4. Failing to add AHG reagent is also common; AHG reagent that has failed QC or is expired should never be used for patient testing.

Case 5-2

1. Yes.
2. The initial antibody screen gel reaction is positive but may be demonstrating a method-dependent antibody. Some antibodies, both specific and nonspecific, have the ability to demonstrate method dependency. The results show reactivity in one method but not others. The negative reactions in the LISS panel confirm the prediction of the method-dependent antibody.
3. The use of PCR technology to genotype the patient might be useful in situations of method-dependent antibodies. It should also be noted in the patient's record that future testing should be conducting using the LISS method.

Review Questions

1. d	5. b	9. b	13. a
2. c	6. b	10. a	14. b
3. a	7. d	11. c	15. c
4. a	8. a	12. c	16. b

Chapter 6

Case 6-1

1. The results indicate an ABO discrepancy in the reverse grouping since there is only a 2+ reaction with the reagent A1 red cells. Normally, ABO forward and reverse testing show strong 3+ to 4+ reactions.
2. Since the antibody screen was negative, the blood bank technologist proceeded to type the patient's RBCs with anti-A_1 lectin, *Dolichos biflorus*. This was decided because, based on the negative antibody screen and patient history, an alloantibody was most likely not causing the ABO discrepancy.
3. The reaction with anti-A1 lectin indicates the patient's cells are not type A1. The additional serum studies show that the antibody is not directed toward a possible alloantibody reacting at room temperature and that the antibody is not anti-A, in that only anti-A would react with A2 cells. If a cold autoantibody or alloantibody was causing the discrepancy, the patient's serum would likely react with the reagent O cells.

    Results indicate the patient is a likely group A2 and has formed an anti-A1.
4. During surgery, the OR ordered 2 units of packed RBCs. Two type O–positive packed RBCs were crossmatched with the patient serum and found to be compatible. Only 1 unit was transfused without episode. The patient was discharged 4 days later.

    In this case, there was an ABO discrepancy caused by anti-A1 in the reverse grouping. Although anti-A1 is considered to be nonreactive at 37°C, it was decided to transfuse type O–positive cells to this patient since there was ample supply.

Review Questions

1. d	4. b	7. a	10. b
2. a.	5. c	8. a	
3. d.	6. b	9. c	

Chapter 7

Case 7-1

1. The patient's ABO, Rh type is O Rh-negative.
2. Both screening cells 1 and 2 show positive reactivity.
3. Given the patient is Rh-negative, elderly, and has six children, it is very likely the positive antibody screen is due to anti-D. In addition, both screening cells are D+.
4. An antibody identification panel should be performed.
5. Anti-D is present in the patient's plasma. All D-positive panel cells are reactive (2+), and all D-negative cells are negative. In addition, all other common alloantibodies are ruled out using at least one double-dose donor cell.

Case 7-2

1. The patient's ABO, Rh type is O Rh-positive. The antibody detection test (screen) is positive. NOTE: In this case study, antibodies are excluded only if the patient's serum does not react with panel cells that possess a double-dose expression of the antigen (from a donor with homozygous expression).
2. Anti-c, anti-E, and anti-K on a double-dose cell (K+k-).
3. Test the patient's serum or plasma against selected cells that are c-E+K- and c-E-K+ and phenotype the patient's RBCs.
4. DCe/DCe (R_1/R_1), DCe/dCe (R_1/r')
5. k
6. Confirm the patient has an anti-c and her red cells lack the c antigen. Now that we know the patient is K+, we do not need to run additional selected cells to rule anti-K out.
7. Anti-E is difficult to rule out in the presence of anti-c because a D+C+c-E+e- (DCE/DCE or RzRz) individual occurs in less than 1% of the population

Case 7-3

1. The patient's ABO, Rh type is interpreted as A Rh-negative, and the antibody detection test (screen) is negative, indicating no unexpected antibodies present in her plasma.
2. DCe/dce (R_1r) or Dce/dCe (R_0r')
3. DCe/dce (R_1r) is most probable; however, if the patient has weakened expression of RhD due to C in *Trans* to *RHD*, she could possess the Dce/dCe (R_0r').

Review Questions

1. a	4. a	7. d	10. c
2. c	5. c	8. c	11. d
3. b	6. c	9. e	12. c

13.

R_1r	DCe/dce	Rh:1,2,-3,4,5
R_2R_0	DcE/Dce	Rh:1,-2,3,4,5
R_zR_1	DCE/DCe	Rh:1,2,3,-4,5
r'r	dCE/dce	RH:-1,2,3,4,5

(see **Table 7–3**)

14. d
15. b
16. d
17. a

Chapter 8

Review Questions

1. d	4. c	7. a	10. c
2. b	5. a	8. d	11. a
3. a	6. d	9. b	12. c

13. d	18. b	23. c	28. b
14. c	19. c	24. d	29. d
15. c	20. d	25. c	30. c
16. b	21. b	26. d	
17. c	22. a	27. b	

Chapter 9

Case 9-1

1. There is inconsistent reactivity (1+ to 3+). The pattern of reactivity appears to fit anti-Fy^b; however, one homozygous cell (cell 2) reacts 3+ while others (cells 8 and 9) react only 2+. This inconsistency is seen in the cells with heterozygous antigen expression as well. Cell 7 reacts 2+, while cells 1, 6, and 11 react only 1+.

2. Anti-C, anti-C^w, anti-K, anti-Kp^a, anti-Js^a, anti-Fy^b, anti-Jk^a, and anti-Lu^a have not been excluded. Fy^b antigens would be destroyed or diminished after treatment with enzymes. C, C^w, Jk^a, and Lu^a would have enhanced antigen expression. K, Kp^a and Js^a would be unaffected by routine enzymes.

3. The specificity of the antibodies was unclear after the initial panel. After repeating the panel using ficin-treated cells, it appears that the antibodies present are anti-K and anti-Fy^b. The enzyme treatment removed the Fy^b antigens, thereby eliminating the anti-Fy^b reactivity, which allows the anti-K to present clearly. Anti-C and anti-Jk^a were also not eliminated by the initial panel. However, one would expect these antibodies to demonstrate enhanced reactivity with the ficin-treated cells. Anti-Jk^a may be excluded using cell 8 of the ficin panel. Whereas anti-C cannot be excluded using a homozygous cell, the pattern of reactivity and lack of response to enzyme treatment suggest it is not present in this sample.

4. Testing a C+, c−, K−, Fy^b− cell would be necessary for exclusion.

Case 9-2

1. The positive reactions on this panel are all the same strength. Cell 10, the only cell that failed to react with the patient's serum, has been identified as being Yt^a negative. As Yt^a is a high-prevalence antigen, one may be suspicious that this is the antibody present in this specimen.

2. For this case, the ideal solution is to test two additional Yt^a-negative cells, which would provide 95% confidence of correct antibody identification and allow for additional exclusions. If antigen-negative cells are not readily available, it may be necessary to consult a reference laboratory that maintains a stock of rare cells. Any other antibodies not excluded following this testing may require patient phenotyping or absorption studies to confirm their presence or absence. The services of a reference laboratory may be required to antigen type the patient for the Yt^a antigen.

3. When working up *any* antibody identification, it is good practice to get the patient's history of transfusions, transplantations, and, if female, pregnancies. A list of medications and the patient's diagnosis may prove helpful. Knowing the patient's ethnicity may give clues as to the identity of the antibody, as antigen frequencies vary among races. One example of a high-prevalence antigen associated with a specific ethnicity is the U antigen, which is present in virtually all whites and all but approximately 1% of blacks. Anti-U is produced mainly in multiparous black females or those patients who have been repeatedly transfused.

Case 9-3

1. A positive reaction was seen with cell 4 only, which is Js^a positive. All other antibody specificities have been eliminated except for anti-Lu^a (an antibody to another other low-prevalence antigen).

2. Testing with additional antigen-positive cells will be required to confirm the specificity. Panel cells that are positive for these rare antigens are normally indicated on the panel profile sheet or listed on the extended typing form. Testing two other cells positive for the Js^a antigen to satisfy the 3 and 3 rule and phenotyping the patient for the Js^a antigen should be done to complete the antibody identification workup. If additional cells are not readily available, consult a reference laboratory.

Case 9-4

1. All cells (except the I-negative cord blood cells) are positive at the immediate spin phase of testing, and the autocontrol is positive. The reactivity does not persist into the AHG phase of testing.

2. The use of cord blood cells, which lack the I antigen, confirms the presence of anti-I in this sample.

3. Many laboratories avoid detection of cold autoantibodies by omitting the immediate spin phase of the antibody screen (and panel) and by using monospecific anti-IgG Coombs' reagent.

   One of the least complex methods used to prevent cold autoantibodies from interfering in antibody detection or identification tests is the **prewarm technique**. In this procedure, the serum being tested and the screen or panel cells are heated to 37°C in separate test tubes. Once at 37°C, a drop of warm RBCs is added to each of the tubes containing serum, and the test proceeds with incubation, washing, and AHG steps. The wash step uses saline that has also been maintained at 37°C so that at no time is the test system allowed to drop below that temperature, thus avoiding the optimal temperature range of the autoantibody. Because this method does not usually have enhancement media in the system, it is possible to fail to detect some weak significant antibodies. Also, the warm saline may result in the dissociation of some significant antibodies from the cells.

A more complex method, discussed previously, is adsorption. The patient's autologous cells may be incubated with the patient's serum at 4°C to remove the autoantibodies before antibody detection steps are performed. This method provides autoantibody-free serum for antibody detection and identification procedures and for compatibility testing. If the autoantibody is particularly strong or if the patient has been recently transfused, RESt may be used to perform the adsorption instead of the patient's RBCs. RESt-adsorbed serum is not suitable for crossmatch, as anti-B may be removed.

Sulfhydryl compounds, such as DTT and 2-mercaptoethanol (2-ME), are known to break the disulfide bonds in IgM. Treating the patient's serum with such a reagent before the antibody detection test will denature the cold autoantibody. IgG antibodies are not affected by these reagents and will remain detectable. A control of saline and serum is tested in parallel with the treated serum to ensure that the autoantibody was truly denatured, not merely diluted.

Case 9-5

1. Warm autoantibody with an underlying alloantibody. The reactivity with all cells, including the autocontrol, at the AHG phase of testing is typical for a warm autoantibody. The increased reactivity on cells 2, 6, and 10 suggests that an additional antibody is present. With the patient's transfusion history, one must consider the possible presence of an alloantibody.

2. Typically with an antibody to a high-prevalence antigen, the autocontrol will be negative. However, if the patient has been recently transfused with RBCs that possess the high-prevalence antigen, the autocontrol may be positive, as the antibody will react with the antigen-positive donor RBCs remaining in circulation.

3. Autoadsorption is the method of choice when the patient has not been recently transfused (transfusion in the past 3 months) and when a sufficient quantity of autologous RBCs is available. The patient's RBCs must first be stripped of autoantibody before they can be used to adsorb autoantibody from the serum. Partial elution using gentle heat or chemical methods is used to produce an antibody-free cell. ZZAP is one chemical that works particularly well for this. It is composed of DTT and papain, resulting in the destruction of enzyme-sensitive antigens and denaturing Kell, LW, Dombrock, Knops, and Cromer antigens. Once the autoantibody has been removed from the cells, the treated cells can be incubated with the patient's serum at 37°C to absorb autoantibody from the serum. Multiple steps are necessary to treat the cells and adsorb the autoantibody, which makes this procedure very time-consuming. Once the autoantibody is removed, the adsorbed serum can be tested for underlying alloantibodies.

When patient cells are limited or when the patient has been recently transfused, allogeneic cells are used for adsorption. The cells used for homologous or differential adsorption are usually treated with enzymes or with ZZAP to enhance expression of certain antigens and facilitate autoantibody removal. These treatment and adsorption steps are time-consuming. There is an alternative method, in which PEG is used to enhance antibody removal, cutting the processing time approximately in half while still providing for adequate autoantibody removal.[50,51]

4. The pattern of reactivity in the "absorbed serum" column of **Figure 9–14** matches that of anti-K. Positive reactions in the autoabsorbed serum were found with cells 2, 6, and 10, which were positive for the K antigen. All other antibody specificities could be ruled out except for C^w, Kp^a, Js^a, and Lu^a. These are low-prevalence antigens and generally do not need to be excluded. Additional phenotyping strategies should be employed to determine if the patient is negative for the K antigen.

5. Transfusion requirements include RBC units negative for the K antigen that appear to be less incompatible with the warm autoantibody than the patient's own cells (least incompatible) when tested with the antiglobulin crossmatch method using unabsorbed serum.

Review Questions

1. d	5. c	9. b	13. a
2. a	6. c	10. c	
3. c	7. d	11. b	
4. b	8. a	12. d	

Chapter 10

Case 10-1

1. Since she has had two previous deliveries at this facility, then our patient's history should also include a previous ABO/Rh and antibody screen determination, which expands the crossmatch options. The first and most common crossmatch option is an immediate spin crossmatch. Of course, an AHG crossmatch option is also available but is not a very good STAT procedure, even though some facilities still have this option as their standard protocol in all situations. The final option, which is the least common, is a computer crossmatch. Since there are two separate determinations of the patient's ABO and no unexpected antibodies are present (both currently and previously), then this option is also available, if the facility's computer system has been validated for computer crossmatching.

2. Playing the odds, the most likely crossmatch selected for this situation is going to be the immediate spin crossmatch, since it is the most widely accepted and used. It is fast and effective in STAT situations. Transfusion service technologists can rapidly perform an immediate spin crossmatch and tag compatible units.

The computer crossmatch is also quite efficient and may even be faster since no serologic testing is required. Just let the computer select the packed cells and print up the tags. The reality is that only about 2% of transfusion services in the United States have computer crossmatching capabilities.

Case 10-2

1. Scenario 1: Patient could have an antibody to a low-incidence antigen that wasn't present on the screening cells of the antibody screening test that was present on the donor red blood cells.

   Scenario 2: Another explanation is that the technologist performing the antibody screening test did not add patient serum to the screen cells but did to the crossmatch test.

2. Scenario 1: Perform an antibody identification using selected panel cells with low-incidence antigens present. Determine specificity of antibody, then antigen-type both the patient and donor cells (all 3 units) for the corresponding antigen. Transfuse antigen-negative, crossmatch (AHG crossmatch) compatible units. Make sure units are labeled with antigen typing results.

   Scenario 2: Repeat all testing, including the antibody screen, this time adding patient serum to all screening cells. If antibody screen is positive, then identify antibody and antigen-type both the patient and donor red cells (all 3 units) for the corresponding antigen. Transfuse antigen-negative, crossmatch (AHG crossmatch) compatible units. Make sure units are labeled with antigen typing results.

Review Questions

1. c	5. b	9. d	13. b
2. d	6. d	10. c	14. a
3. d	7. b	11. b	15. d
4. c	8. b	12. d	

Chapter 11

Review Questions

1. d	3. d	5. a	7. c
2. a	4. c	6. d	8. d

Chapter 12

Review Questions

1. a	4. b	7. c	10. c
2. d	5. c	8. b	
3. d	6. a	9. c	

Chapter 13

Case 13-1

1. Yes, the incubation period for *Babesia microti* is 2 to 8 weeks. The component transfused is red blood cells, which the organism is able to penetrate.

2. Symptoms include malaise, fever, fatigue, anorexia, vomiting, and abdominal pain.

3. Yes, the donor with the high titer should be permanently deferred.

4. No, the donor who was not tested should be indefinitely deferred until he or she can be tested.

Case 13-2

1. After transfusion of 1 unit of leukoreduced RBCs, the hgb should increase approximately 1 g/dl or 11.6; hematocrit should have increased 3% or approximately 35%.

2. One unit of apheresis platelets will usually increase the platelet count of a 70 kg adult by 30,000 to 60,000/uL. This is consistent with the patient platelet count results from 5-23 to 5-24, which increased from 72,000 to 103,000.

3. FFP is frozen within 8 hours of collection and PF24 is frozen within 24 hours of collection. FFP contains all coagulation factors, and PF24 contains all factors contained in FFP with reduced amounts of factors V and VIII. Since this patient had liver abnormalities and not a specific factor deficiency and was taken off Coumadin, standard of practice dictates that FFP and PF24 can be used interchangeably except in hemophilic cases where there is a specific deficiency of factor VIII.

Review Questions

1. c	6. e	11. a	16. d
2. d	7. a	12. e	17. c
3. e	8. b	13. b	18. a
4. a	9. c	14. b	19. c
5. a	10. e	15. a	20. c

Chapter 14

Case 14-1

1. Top five possible diagnoses for this case:
   - Hemolytic uremic syndrome
   - Thrombotic thrombocytopenic purpura (TTP)
   - Disseminated intravascular coagulation (DIC)
   - Malignant hypertension
   - Sepsis

2. Thrombotic thrombocytopenic purpura (TTP). Why? See below + normal coagulation studies and the ADAMTS13 will be significantly decreased.

3. In classic cases, patients present with a pentad of clinical and laboratory findings:
   - Microangiopathic hemolytic anemia (MAHA);
   - Thrombocytopenia
   - Neurological symptoms and signs
   - Renal function abnormalities
   - Fever

4. Plasma exchange with fresh frozen plasma (FFP).

Review Questions

1. d	4. a	7. b	10. d
2. a	5. c	8. a	
3. b	6. d	9. c	

Chapter 15

Case 15-1

1. It is necessary to know the patient's hemoglobin and hematocrit levels, the surgeon's usual blood usage, whether this is the first surgical procedure on this hip (redo surgery uses more blood), and whether the patient has any pretransfusion compatibility problems.
2. Considerations should be the patient's general health, hemoglobin and hematocrit levels, amount of time between request for donation and the time of surgery, and whether the patient has infectious diseases that might interfere (e.g., bacterial infections).
3. Tests should include PT, PTT, and platelet count. If these tests are normal and von Willebrand's disease is suspected, vWF workup should be considered.
4. If the patient has moderate to severe von Willebrand's disease, the patient may need factor VIII concentrate known to contain vWF.

Case 15-2

1. Both answers can be justified. If the answer is yes, her hemoglobin is close to 6 g/dL, which is the criterion for RBC transfusion. She will be less tired and weak if she receives a transfusion. If the answer is no, she is not in any acute distress. She is iron-deficient (from chronic blood loss) and should be treated with iron replacement rather than with transfusion, which has higher risk of complications. The safest, least-expensive, and the most effective long-term strategy is to prescribe iron and not transfuse.
2. For adults, each unit of blood should increase the hemoglobin 1 g/dL and the hematocrit 3 percentage points. For accuracy, this is based on a hypothetical 70-kg man. For smaller men and women, the increase is greater; for larger ones, less.

Case 15-3

1. The platelet count is 5,000/μL; therefore, a platelet transfusion is indicated. Without the platelet transfusion, she would be at increased risk of bleeding from the site of the bone marrow biopsy. Although the hemoglobin and hematocrit levels are lower than normal for a woman of this age, an RBC transfusion is not indicated (hemoglobin greater than 6 g/dL in an otherwise healthy young adult).
2. For an adult, each unit (bag) of platelet concentrate should increase the patient's platelet count by 5,000 to 10,000/μL. The platelet count should be at about 20,000/μL because a bone marrow biopsy is an invasive procedure. Thus, one unit of platelets (plateletpheresis or pool) would be indicated.

3. If it is anticipated that the patient will experience bone marrow recovery soon (after the chemotherapy), no RBC transfusion is indicated. If, however, the bone marrow will be suppressed for several weeks, one or two units are indicated, with a recheck in a couple weeks for another possible transfusion. Each unit of RBCs is expected to increase the hemoglobin level about 1 g/dL.

Case 15-4

1. The blood group for RBC transfusions is O, which is the universal blood group.
2. Group AB should be selected for plasma and platelet transfusion. If AB platelets are not available, any other blood group can be selected.
3. RBCs, plasma, and platelets in the amount specified by your massive transfusion protocol.
4. RBCS, plasma, and platelets should be B. The Rh can be positive because the patient is male. If group B RBCs are in short supply, group O can continue to be used.
5. Workup of the positive antibody screen should start as soon as possible, but without delay of providing products for the massive transfusion. Transfusing RBCs in massive hemorrhage is more important than obtaining "compatible" units. With massive transfusion, the patient's antibody will be removed and diluted by the hemorrhage and the replacement of blood components. The "incompatible" RBCs will be removed more slowly because the mechanism is extravascular hemolysis. When the serologic problem is solved, compatible RBC units can be obtained and transfused.

Review Questions

1. d	4. c	7. a	10. a
2. c	5. a	8. b	
3. c	6. a	9. d	

Chapter 16

Case 16-1

1. A reaction in which signs and symptoms occur during or within 24 hours of transfusion.
2. Hemolysis.
3. Volume of incompatible blood transfused.
4. Look for matching or discrepant information between the information on the labels on the pre- and post-transfusion samples, transfused units, patient transfusion service records.

Case 16-2

1. Communication with other health professionals served as the key to resolving this incident.
2. Chemical or mechanical damage such as improper shipping, storage temperatures, incomplete deglycerolization of frozen red blood cells, inappropriate needle bore size for transfusion rapid infusion, improper use of blood warmers, unapproved fluid infusion.

Case 16-3

1. Laboratory workup for the diagnosis of TAS must rule out hemolysis and perform a gram stain and culture of the implicated component and patient. The culture must be obtained from the container and not the segments attached to the product. Blood cultures from the patient should be drawn from a site other than the site of transfusion.
2. Symptoms implicated with TAS include a fever with greater than 2°C increase in body temperature, rigors, and hypotension.

Review Questions

1. c	5. c	9. d	13. b
2. c	6. b	10. d	14. d
3. b	7. c	11. d	15. d
4. b	8. b	12. a	

Chapter 17

Case 17-1

1. The blood group for RBC transfusion is O, which is the only blood group compatible with both the donor and recipient. If A is chosen, the cells will be hemolyzed or have a shortened life span because of the preexisting anti-A in the patient. If B is chosen, engraftment will be difficult to determine.
2. Group AB should be selected for FFP and platelet transfusion. If group A is selected, the anti-B in the plasma is incompatible with the recipient's RBC and tissue antigens (B). The anti-A in group B products is incompatible with the donor RBCs and, if selected, may contribute to delayed engraftment of RBC precursors.
3. On day 117, the interpretation is B, as B cells and anti-A are present.
4. On day 200, the interpretation is group A, because A cells are present, and B cells and anti-A are absent. On day 156, the forward type is group O (remember that the patient is receiving group O RBC transfusions), but the reverse type still has anti-A; thus, the interpretation is indeterminate. The source of the anti-A may be small amount of plasma in RBC transfusions or anti-A in ABO-incompatible platelet transfusions.

Review Questions

1. a	4. b	7. c	10. a
2. e	5. c	8. c	11. b
3. d	6. d	9. c	12. c

Chapter 18

Review Questions

1. a	8. b	15. a	22. c
2. b	9. d	16. c	23. a
3. d	10. c	17. a	24. d
4. a	11. c	18. d	25. b
5. c	12. d	19. c	
6. b	13. a	20. d	
7. c	14. d	21. b	

Chapter 19

Case 19-1

1. The most probable cause is that the mother received prophylactic Rh immune globulin at 28 weeks gestation. The antibody screen was negative at 28 weeks gestation prior to the administration of Rh immune globulin. The antibody titer of anti-D due to Rh immune globulin is typically less than 1:4.[4]
2. Yes, unless the newborn infant is Rh(D)-negative.

Case 19-2

1. The maternal history, the same father, and the father homozygous for the D antigen suggest that the infant is Rh(D)-positive.
2. The titer should be repeated in 6 weeks (16 weeks' gestation).
3. The infant is only 8 weeks gestational age, so it is too early in the pregnancy to perform any intervention (MCA-PSV, cordocentesis, intrauterine transfusion). The earliest an intervention can take place is 16 weeks.
4. The patient should be scheduled for MCA-PSV at 16 to 18 weeks gestation to determine if the test is positive.

Case 19-3

1. The most probable cause is ABO HDFN. Group O mothers produce IgG anti-A, which can cross the placenta.
2. No. Anti-Le^a does not cause HDFN because Lewis antigens are poorly developed at birth.

Case 19-4

1. The blood types of the cord blood and heel-stick specimens are different—A-negative versus O-negative. The severely anemic infant could have HDFN, although the cord blood results do not indicate severe disease (DAT +/–). On the other hand, a large fetomaternal hemorrhage could have occurred.

2. Cord blood should be collected by needle and syringe from the umbilical cord vein. Collecting the specimen by allowing blood from the placenta or cord to drip into the tube can contaminate the specimen with maternal blood. In this case, the tube marked "cord blood" could be a mislabeled maternal sample. The heel-stick is nearly all adult blood because of the recent intrauterine transfusion. Group O blood is usually used. As discussed in this chapter, transfusion may cause suppression of erythropoiesis and therefore the production of few fetal RBCs. The cells produced are being hemolyzed by the high-titered maternal antibody. This leads to anemia, in this case quite severe, with elevated bilirubin levels indicating that hemolysis is occurring. The eluate of the heel-stick specimen confirms HDFN caused by anti-D.

Review Questions

1. c	4. d	7. d	10. b
2. a	5. d	8. d	11. a
3. b	6. a	9. b	12. c

Chapter 20

Case 20-1

1. There is an ABO serologic discrepancy and a positive albumin control, so ABO/Rh results are invalid.
2. The antibody screen shows a strongly reactive immediate spin (room temperature) reading and weak reactivity at LISS 37°C phase. These preliminary results suggest a cold agglutinin. Because the patient's RBCs are also reactive with his own serum, this appears to be a cold autoantibody, which would also affect the ABO serum typing (tested at room temperature).
3. The patient's RBCs are complement coated.
4. The most likely cause of these atypical results is a cold autoantibody. To obtain valid ABO/Rh typing results, the patient's RBCs should be warmed to 37°C and washed with warm saline. His serum and plasma should be cold autoadsorbed and used for repeating the ABO serum typing and antibody screen.
5. The patient's warm-washed RBCs type group A Rh-positive. The cold autoadsorbed serum confirms that anti-B is present, but not anti-A. This resolves the ABO serologic discrepancy. The antibody screening performed with the cold autoadsorbed serum also confirms that group O RBCs are nonreactive and that there is no alloantibody present.
6. The cold autoadsorbed serum is suitable for crossmatching group A RBCs for transfusion (if still deemed necessary).
7. A cold agglutinin titer and thermal amplitude would be very useful to investigate whether the patient has cold hemagglutinin disease (CHD), as suggested by the preliminary testing and by his symptoms. If a diagnosis of CHD were made, such testing might save him having to endure the bone marrow biopsy.

Case 20-2

1. The patient is group O Rh-positive.
2. Her antibody screening is positive with all three screening cells and with the autologous control at the indirect antiglobulin phase. None of the four units crossmatched are compatible. There is some variability in the strength of the IAT reactivity. Because the patient has no history of recent transfusion (within the last 3 months), the positive auto control by IAT suggests a warm autoantibody is present. The variability of reactivity suggests alloantibody may also be present.
3. A direct antiglobulin test should be done. Warm autoadsorption of the patient's serum should also be done, and an antibody identification panel tested with the adsorbed serum.
4. The DAT shows that the patient's cells are coated with both IgG and complement. The predictive value of the positive DAT in a patient with clinical indications of hemolytic anemia (e.g., decreased hemoglobin and hematocrit, increased reticulocyte count) is high; combined with evidence of a warm autoantibody in the serum, these results support a diagnosis of warm autoimmune hemolytic anemia.
5. Anti-Jk^a is evident in the autoadsorbed serum. Further testing could include typing the patient's RBC for the Jk^a antigen, which might be done using monoclonal anti-Jk^a or using an IgG removal technique to treat her RBCs before typing her RBCs with a conventional anti-Jk^a reagent. Although the patient has a history of prior transfusion when she might have been exposed to Jk(a+) RBCs, it is somewhat unusual to find anti-Jk^a strongly detectable so many years after last exposure.
6. The patient's autoadsorbed serum may be used to crossmatch group O Jk(a–) red blood cells for transfusion.
7. Transfusion to remedy the current anemia is a temporary solution and may stimulate additional alloantibody and increase autoantibody production. Her physician is likely to recommend steroid therapy (e.g., prednisone) to suppress her immune system to try to control the autoimmune hemolytic process.

Case 20-3

1. The patient's RBCs are group B Rh-positive. There is nothing unusual about the blood grouping.
2. The antibody screening is negative, indicating no alloantibodies to RBC antigens are present.
3. Because the antibody screening is negative, crossmatches of the patient's serum with three units of group B Rh-positive units of red cells would be expected to be compatible. The positive autocontrol and the color of the patient's serum are unexpected. Although there is no history of recent transfusion, a DAT could be helpful if the patient is anemic due to an autoimmune process. If the DAT is positive, preparing and testing an eluate of the patient's RBCs could be informative.
4. The DAT shows that the patient's RBCs are coated with IgG and complement. These results could be seen in a

normal individual. (Approximately 1 in 1,000 healthy blood donors have positive DATs.[8]) But since this patient has severe anemia that developed in 1 week and frank hemolysis noted in the sample, there is likely to be more clinical significance to these DAT results.

5. The eluate is nonreactive with the three antibody detection cells but reacts with the patient's own RBCs even after they have been EGA-treated to remove in vivo IgG. The results are consistent with a drug-induced antibody that reacts with the patient's drug-coated RBCs. Typical results seen in cases like this, called the "penicillin-type" drug-induced immune hemolytic anemia, are a negative antibody screen and negative eluate in a patient with a positive DAT and clinical signs of acute hemolysis. In these cases, adsorption of the drug by the patient's RBCs causes them to react selectively with the drug antibody in the patient's serum or eluate.

6. Determining what drug the patient has been receiving is key to knowing what drug antibody to suspect. In this case, the patient was unaware of taking any drugs or antibiotics during or following her hospitalization for labor and delivery by C-section. A careful review of the surgical record revealed that she was given a single dose of Cefotetan during surgery, presumably to prevent postoperative infection.

Review Questions

1. d
2. b
3. a
4. a
5. a
6. d
7. b
8. b
9. c
10. a
11. d
12. b
13. d
14. a
15. c
16. b
17. c
18. d

Chapter 21

Review Questions

1. c
2. c
3. b
4. a
5. d
6. b
7. d
8. a

Chapter 22

Case 22-1

1. b
2. a

Case 22-2

1. c
2. d
3. c

In DNA polymorphisms, the mutation rate can be as high as 2 per 1,000; thus, a single mismatch, when all other systems are consistent with paternity, may represent a mutation. A minimum of two mismatches is necessary before an interpretation of exclusion is rendered.

Review Questions

1. b
2. a
3. b
4. a

Chapter 23

Review Questions

1. b
2. d
3. d
4. b
5. c
6. d
7. c
8. a
9. a
10. c

Chapter 24

Case 24-1

1. A blood utilization management program is intended to ensure blood components are administered appropriately, in accordance with hospital guidelines and evidence-based criteria. Its primary focus is to improve patient safety by ensuring patients are not unnecessarily exposed to the risks of transfusion. If there is a large deviation from standard practice in a facility, reduction in inappropriate ordering may be reflected in reduced expenditure for blood components. However, if this is not the case, a utilization management program may still reduce cost in terms of expenditures for treating transfusion-associated adverse events, impact on length of stay and clinical course, and improved blood component availability.

2. First steps include recruiting a multidisciplinary cross-functional team. This team should define the program's overall goal, then assess the current state and perform a gap analysis. This process will involve using evidence-based criteria and guidelines. Once improvement opportunities are identified, the team may prioritize interventions to promote evidence-based practice.

3. The blood utilization management team should include the blood bank medical director and the blood bank supervisor. Additional members will depend upon the individual facility, but representation from nursing, clinical staff (especially from areas with greater blood use), and quality should be considered. Participation by an information technology associate may be particularly useful in developing tools for queries and to track the metrics the team agrees upon. Administrative support, if not active participation, is critical.

4. Appropriate utilization criteria should be gleaned from evidence-based literature and the recommendations of consensus panels from various subspecialties. Active discussion of proposed guidelines with clinical staff is necessary to gain approval and promote compliance. Where necessary, exceptions for specific clinical populations or diagnoses should be included. The literature upon which

the guidelines are based should be widely disseminated and readily available to clinical staff.

5. Any of the types of review (retrospective, concurrent, targeted, or discontinuous prospective) may be utilized depending on the facility. However, for a medium- or small-sized facility, retrospective review is most likely to be the primary method, due to resource limitations. Large facilities such as academic institutions are more likely to have the available personnel to conduct concurrent and prospective review actions. Targeted or discontinuous prospective review may be appropriate for smaller facilities, since the benefits of "real-time" intervention are balanced by the limited scope.

Case Study 24-2

1. The first step is to determine the gap between the current and desired state. This gap defines the scope of the problem and should be qualified and quantified as succinctly as possible. Review of the value stream will help identify the source of the problem. In this case, review of the nursing units and physician services show that the plasma trend appears to be related to a recent expansion in the hospital's coronary care unit. This is further supported by the observation that the increased usage and waste trends vanish when the data from the coronary unit are excluded from the utilization report. Review of the timing of the blood orders showed that the majority of the increased utilization appeared just prior to the performance of cardiac procedures and surgeries.

2. Further auditing revealed multiple types of waste with plasma usage among patients awaiting cardiac surgery and procedures. In nearly every case, there was an excess of plasma ordered in advance of the procedure that was thawed by the blood bank but was either never dispensed or never transfused. Regarding the dispensed plasma, most of these patients had an average of 2 units of unused thawed plasma. In a few cases, the product was improperly returned and had to be discarded. This overproduction type of waste increased the number of expired plasma components, resulting in increased inventory waste. Further waste was identified through a detailed medical chart audit, which demonstrated that nearly half of the plasma transfused was likely inappropriately administered when compared to the institution's transfusion guidelines.

3. Solutions and improvements arise from the collaborative input of multiple sources such as the medical director of the blood bank, the blood bank supervisor, members of the transfusion committee, and appropriate members from administration. If a specific unit or specialty is identifiable, as in this case, input should also be requested from clinical staff in that area. In this case, after investigation by the medical director, the new coronary unit was employing antiquated order sets copied from another institution. These order sets included template standing plasma orders that were not appropriate for a large institution with readily available thawed plasma. Unfortunately, in spite of discussion with the involved practitioners, many were unwilling to change their practice patterns. Following review by the transfusion committee, the antiquated order sets were removed and a discontinuous prospective review was adopted, focusing on plasma orders for coronary care patients. In addition, educational measures were employed, in the form of several short lectures on current plasma guidelines presented to the coronary unit's physicians and nursing staff.

4. Over the following three quarters, the transfusion safety officer continued the discontinuous prospective review of the coronary care patients in addition to the monthly retrospective reporting. At the end of the third quarter, blood utilization appeared to be at the desired state and the labor-intensive discontinuous prospective review strategy was retired. It is important to always reassess and revaluate the blood utilization management process to determine the effectiveness of corrective strategies and to identify new areas of waste.

Review Questions

1. d	4. c	7. b	10. b
2. a	5. d	8. d	
3. b	6. b	9. a	

Chapter 25

Review Questions

1. b	4. d	7. d	10. b
2. c	5. c	8. a	
3. d	6. a	9. b	

Chapter 26

Review Questions

1. c	4. b	7. d	10. c
2. a	5. a	8. a	
3. d	6. b	9. b	

11.

Phase	SCI	SCII	Interpretation
IS	0	0	Negative
37°C	0	0	
AHG	0	0	
CC	+	+	

12. b

13. A. Control functions
    B. Acceptance Criteria
    C. Test Cases
    D. Data entry methods
    E. Documentation methods
    F. Result review
    G. Corrective action
    H. Acceptance

Chapter 27

Cases 27-1 through 27-6

Editor's Note: Because of the nature of these cases, answers are not provided. Answers to these questions would be decided by a judge or jury.

Review Questions

1. d
2. b
3. d
4. c
5. a

Chapter 28

Case 28-1

1. This tissue manufacturer must be qualified by the medical director of the tissue bank prior to ordering any tissue. The surgeon may consider postponing surgeries until the vendor has been qualified or use tissue from a vendor currently qualified.

2. The supplier's facility and all intermediaries must be registered with the FDA and hold state licenses, if applicable by state.

Case 28-2

1. See **Box 28–2**.
2. The hospital tissue bank must register with the FDA as a tissue distributer.
3. A decision should be made as to whether the tissue should be cultured and if so, with which method. The storage container and appropriate temperature for storage should also be decided. (Any of the AORN recommendations for harvest of autologous tissue are correct answers to this question.)

Review Questions

1. d	4. b	7. d	10. d
2. b	5. b	8. b	
3. c	6. c	9. d	

Glossary

Abruptio placentae Premature detachment of normally situated placenta.

Absorbed anti-A$_1$ If serum from a group B individual that contains anti-A plus anti-A$_1$ is incubated with A$_2$ cells, the anti-A will adsorb onto the cells. Removal of the cells yields a serum containing only anti-A$_1$; thus, it is absorbed anti-A$_1$.

Absorption Removal of an unwanted antibody.

Acid-citrate-dextrose (ACD) An anticoagulant and preservative solution that was once used routinely for blood donor collection but now used only occasionally.

Acid phosphatase (ACP) A red blood cell enzyme used as an identification marker in paternity testing and criminal investigation.

Adenosine deaminase (ADA) A red blood cell enzyme used as an identification marker in paternity testing and criminal investigation.

Adenosine triphosphate (ATP) A compound composed of adenosine (nucleotide containing adenine and ribose) and three phosphoric acid groups, which, when split by enzyme action, produces energy that can be used to support other reactions.

Adenylate kinase (AK) A red blood cell enzyme used as an identification marker in paternity testing and criminal investigation.

Adjuvant One of a variety of substances that, when combined with an antigen, enhance the antibody response to that antigen.

Adsorption Providing an antibody with its corresponding antigen under optimal conditions so that the antibody will attach to the antigen, thereby removing the antibody from the serum; often used interchangeably with *absorption*.

Agammaglobulinemia A rare disorder in which gamma globulin is virtually absent.

Agarose Seaweed extract used to make gels used in electrophoresis. Molten agarose (0.5% to 3.5%, depending on application) is poured into a mold where a plastic comb is suspended. As it cools, the agarose hardens to form a porous gel slab.

Agglutination The clumping together of red blood cells or any particulate matter resulting from interaction of antibody and its corresponding antigen.

Agglutinin An antibody that agglutinates cells.

Agglutinogen A substance that stimulates the production of an agglutinin, thereby acting as an antigen.

Agranulocytosis An acute disease in which the white blood cell count drops to extremely low levels, and neutropenia becomes pronounced.

Albumin Protein found in the highest concentration in human plasma; used as a diluent for blood typing antisera and a potentiator solution in serologic testing to enhance antigen-antibody reactions.

Aldomet *See* Methyldopa.

Alkaline phosphatase (ALP) A red blood cell enzyme used as an identification marker in paternity testing and criminal investigation.

Allele One of two or more different genes that may occupy a specific locus on a chromosome.

Allo- Prefix indicating differences within a species (e.g., an alloantibody is produced in one individual against the red blood cell antigens of another individual).

Allogeneic Transplant donor who is related or unrelated to the recipient.

Allograft A tissue transplant between individuals of the same species.

Allosteric change A change in conformation that exposes a new reactive site on a molecule.

Alpha-adrenergic receptor A site in autonomic nerve pathways wherein excitatory responses occur when adrenergic agents such as norepinephrine and epinephrine are released.

Alum precipitation A method for obtaining an enhanced response when producing an antibody; *see also* Adjuvant.

Aminoacyl-tRNA synthetase An enzyme involved in protein synthesis by attaching a specific amino acid to transfer RNA (tRNA), based on a three-nucleotide sequence present in the loop area of the tRNA called anticodon. Once the amino acid is attached to the tRNA, it may be joined in the ribosome with the growing peptide chain.

Amniocentesis Transabdominal puncture of the amniotic sac, using a needle and syringe, in order to remove amniotic fluid. The material may then be studied to detect genetic disorders or fetomaternal blood incompatibility.

Amniotic fluid Liquid or albuminous fluid contained in the amnion.

Amorph A gene that does not appear to produce a detectable antigen; a silent gene, such as *Jk, Lu, O*.

Amplicon The product of polymerase chain reaction.

Anamnestic response An accentuated antibody response following a secondary exposure to an antigen. Antibody levels from the initial exposure are not detectable in the patient's serum until the secondary exposures, when a rapid rise in antibody titer is observed.

Anaphylaxis An allergic hypersensitivity reaction of the body to a foreign protein or drug.

Anastomosis A connection between two blood vessels, either direct or through connecting channels.

Anemia A condition in which there is reduced oxygen delivery to the tissues; may result from increased destruction of red blood cells, excessive blood loss, or decreased production of red blood cells.

Angina pectoris Severe pain and constriction about the heart caused by an insufficient supply of blood to the heart.

Anion An ion carrying a negative charge.

Annealing Process in which single strands of DNA anneal to each other by formation of hydrogen bonds, under certain temperature conditions, due to complementarity. Annealing, renaturation, and hybridization are chemically the same processes. Two strands of DNA, separated by heat denaturation, will start annealing (renaturation) upon cooling to approximately 5°C (or more) below DNA melting point (Tm). This phenomenon is used in polymerase chain reaction when oligonucleotide primers must anneal to denatured DNA prior to starting DNA synthesis by the enzyme polymerase.

Antecubital In front of the elbow, at the bend of the elbow; usual site for blood collection.

Antenatal Occurring before birth.

Anti-A₁ lectin A reagent anti-A_1 serum produced from the seeds of the plant *Dolichos biflorus*; reacts with A_1 cells but not with A subgroup cells, such as A_2, A_3, and so on; reacts weakly with A_{int} cells.

Anti-B lectin A reagent anti-B serum produced from the seeds of the plant *Bandeiraea simplicifolia*.

Antibody A protein substance secreted by plasma cells that is developed in response to, and interacting specifically with, an antigen. In blood banking, it is found in serum, from either a commercial manufacturer or a patient.

Antibody screen Testing the patient's serum with group O reagent red blood cells in an effort to detect atypical antibodies.

Anticoagulant An agent that prevents or delays blood coagulation.

Anticodon A sequence of three nucleotides in the loop region of the transfer RNA (tRNA), which aligns in the ribosome with the corresponding mRNA codon and attaches the amino acid to the growing peptide chain.

Anti-dl An antibody implicated in warm autoimmune hemolytic anemia, which reacts with all Rh cells, including Rh_{null} and Rh-deleted cells.

Antigen A substance recognized by the body as being foreign, which can cause an immune response. In blood banking, antigens are usually, but not exclusively, found on the red blood cell membrane.

Antihemophilic factor *See* Hemophilia A.

Antihemophilic globulin *See* Hemophilia A.

Antihistamine Drug that opposes the action of histamine.

Anti-H lectin A reagent anti-H produced from the seeds of the plant *Ulex europaeus*.

Antihuman globulin or **antiglobulin serum** *See* Antihuman serum.

Antihuman globulin or **antiglobulin test (AGT)** Test to ascertain the presence or absence of red blood cell coating by immunoglobulin G (IgG) or complement or both; uses a xenoantibody (rabbit antihuman serum) or monoclonal antibody (to IgG or complement) to act as a bridge between sensitized cells, thus yielding agglutination as a positive result. *Direct antihuman globulin test (DAT):* Used to detect in vivo cell sensitization. *Indirect antihuman globulin test (IAT):* Used to detect antigen-antibody reactions that occur in vitro.

Antihuman serum An antibody prepared in rabbits or other suitable animals that is directed against human immunoglobulin or complement or both; used to perform the antihuman globulin or Coombs' test. The serum may be either polyspecific (anti-IgG plus anticomplement) or monospecific (anti-IgG or anticomplement).

Anti-M lectin A reagent anti-M serum produced from the plant *Iberis amara*.

Anti-nl An antibody implicated in warm autoimmune hemolytic anemia, which reacts with all normal Rh cells except Rh_{null} cells and deleted Rh cells.

Anti-N lectin A reagent anti-N serum produced from the plant *Vicia graminea*.

Anti-pdl An antibody implicated in warm autoimmune hemolytic anemia, which reacts with all normal Rh cells and deleted Rh cells but not with Rh_{null} cells.

Antipyretic An agent that reduces fever.

Antiserum A reagent source of antibody, as in a commercial antiserum.

Antithetical Referring to antigens that are the product of allelic genes (e.g., Kell [K] and Cellano [k]).

Apheresis A method of blood collection in which whole blood is withdrawn, a desired component separated and retained, and the remainder of the blood returned to the donor. *See also* Plateletpheresis and Plasmapheresis.

Aplasia Failure of an organ or tissue to develop normally.

Aplastic anemia Anemia caused by aplasia of bone marrow or bone marrow's destruction by chemical agents or physical factors.

Apoptotic Adjective of *apoptosis*, the programmed (non-traumatic) cell death. A natural process occurring in senescent cells.

Arachis hypogaea A peanut lectin used to differentiate T polyagglutination from Tn polyagglutination.

Asphyxia Condition caused by insufficient intake of oxygen.

Asthma Paroxysmal dyspnea accompanied by wheezing caused by a spasm of the bronchial tubes or by swelling of their mucous membrane.

Atypical antibodies Any antibody other than anti-A, anti-B, or anti-A,B.

Australia antigen Old terminology referring to the hepatitis B–associated antigen.

Auto- Prefix indicating *self* (e.g., an autoantibody is reactive against one's own red blood cell antigens); usually associated with a disease state.

Autoabsorption A procedure to remove a patient's antibody, using the patient's own cells.

Autoimmune hemolytic anemia Shortened RBC survival mediated through the immune response of humoral antibody directed at "self" antigenic determinants. Acquired disorder characterized by premature erythrocyte destruction owing to abnormalities in the individual's immune system.

Autologous Donor and recipient are the same person.

Autologous control Testing the patient's serum with his or her own cells in an effort to detect autoantibody activity.

Autologous transfusion blood taken from a patient to be used for the same patient.

Autoradiography An image recorded on a photographic film or plate produced by the radiation emitted from a specimen, such as DNA labeled with radioactive phosphorus isotope.

Autosomal-recessive pattern An inheritance pattern in which a condition or disease determined by a gene located on an autosomal (nonsex) chromosome occurs when both genes on the homologous chromosomes are affected. Individuals with only one gene affected are considered carriers and do not have symptoms due to proper function of the unaffected gene on the other chromosome.

Autosome Any chromosome other than the sex (X and Y) chromosomes.

Bacterial artificial chromosomes (BACs) In recombinant DNA technology, **vectors** capable of carrying DNA fragments (inserts) of up to 350 kb.

Bactericidal Destructive to or destroying bacteria.

Bacteriophage A virus that infects and reproduces in bacterial cells. Often carries genes coding for antibiotic resistance. Basic tools used in molecular biology (vectors) frequently used to introduce and clone (multiply) foreign genes or their fragments inside of a bacterium.

Bandeiraea simplicifolia See Anti-B lectin.

Bar-code reader An optical input device that reads and interprets data from a bar code for entry into a computer system.

Beta globin chain A structural peptide subunit of hemoglobin molecule that consists of two beta globin and two alpha globin chains. Alpha and beta chains are coded for by different genes located on different chromosomes.

Bilirubin The orange-yellow pigment in bile carried to the liver by the blood; produced from hemoglobin of red blood cells by reticuloendothelial cells in bone marrow, spleen, and elsewhere. *Direct bilirubin*: The conjugated water-soluble form of bilirubin. *Indirect bilirubin*: The unconjugated water-insoluble form of bilirubin.

Bilirubinemia Pathological condition in which excessive destruction of red blood cells occurs, increasing the amount of bilirubin found in the blood.

Binding constant The "goodness of fit" in an antigen-antibody complex.

Biphasic Reactivity occurring in two phases.

Blood bank information system Computer system that has been developed specifically to assist blood bank professionals in the management of the patient, donor, and blood component information.

Blood gases Determination of pH, PCO_2, PO_2, and HCO_3; performed on a blood gas analyzer.

Blood group genotyping DNA typing, aimed at genes coding for blood group antigens.

Blood group–specific substances (BGSSs) Soluble antigens present in fluids that can be used to neutralize their corresponding antibodies; systems that demonstrate BGSSs include ABO, Lewis, and P blood group systems.

Blood order sets A means of standardization to clarify indications and enforce guidelines during physician order entry.

Blood utilization management A process incorporating blood utilization review with particular intervention strategies to reduce inappropriate transfusion and improve patient safety.

Blood utilization review A focused audit of a population or subpopulation of transfused patients to determine the appropriateness of transfusion.

Blunt ends The ends of a DNA sequence resulting from restriction enzymes that cut both strands in the middle of the target sequence, leaving no "overhangs." Blunt ends may be rejoined using enzyme ligase.

Bombay Phenotype occurring in individuals who possess normal *A* or *B* genes but are unable to express them because they lack the gene necessary for production of H antigen, the required precursor for A and B. These persons often have a potent anti-H in their serum, which reacts with all cells except other Bombays. Also known as O_h.

Bovine Pertaining to cattle.

Bradykinin A plasma kinin.

Bromelin A proteolytic enzyme obtained from the pineapple.

Bromophenol blue A "tracking" dye mixed with DNA sample and used in electrophoresis to monitor its progress in order to prevent the escape of bands out of the gel. In a 1% gel it runs at around 500 bp.

Buffy coat Light stratum of a blood clot seen when the blood is centrifuged or allowed to stand in a test tube. The red blood cells settle to the bottom, and between the plasma and the red blood cells is a light-colored layer that contains mostly white blood cells.

Burst-forming unit committed to erythropoiesis (BFU-E) A primitive progenitor cell committed to erythropoiesis and believed to be a precursor to the CFU-E.

C3a A biologically active fragment of the complement C3 molecule that demonstrates anaphylactic capabilities upon liberation.

C3b A biologically active fragment of the complement C3 molecule that is an opsonin and promotes immune adherence.

C3d A biologically inactive fragment of the C3b complement component formed by inactivation by the C3b inactivator substance present in serum.

C4 A complement component present in serum that participates in the classic pathway of complement activation.

C5a A biologically active fragment of the C5 molecule, which demonstrates anaphylactic capabilities and chemotactic properties upon liberation. This fragment is also a potent aggregator of platelets.

Cadaveric Source of organs and tissues from a person who has been declared dead.

Capillary electrophoresis The electrophoresis platform consisting of a small capillary filled with some form of separation medium that fractionates a mixture of molecules based upon size or charge.

Capillary gel electrophoresis The process of electrophoresis that occurs in a thin glass capillary filled with polyacrylamide or other synthetic polymer rather than in a slab.

Cardiac output The amount of blood discharged from the left or right ventricle per minute.

Catecholamines Biologically active amines, epinephrine and norepinephrine, derived from the amino acid tyrosine. They have a marked effect on nervous and cardiovascular systems, metabolic rate, temperature, and smooth muscle.

Cathode ray tube (CRT) A display device in an information system.

Cation An ion carrying a positive charge.

CD34 Cell membrane marker of stem cells.

Central dogma A theory developed originally by Francis Crick, claiming that basic information of life flows from DNA through RNA to proteins.

Central processing unit (CPU) The part of a computer that contains the semiconductor chips that process the instructions of the computer programs.

Central venous pressure The pressure within the superior vena cava reflecting the pressure by which the blood is returned to the right atrium.

Chain termination method (Sanger sequencing) The most common method of DNA sequencing, developed by Fred Sanger, which uses DNA synthesis terminating ddNTPs.

Chargaff's rules Established in 1950 by chemist Erwin Chargaff, these rules describe the quantitative ratios of nitrogen-containing bases: adenine, thymine, cytosine, and guanine in DNA. The first rule stated that the amount of adenine in a given molecule was always equal to the amount of thymine and that the amount of cytosine was always equal to the amount of guanine. The second rule stated that the amount of all pyrimidine bases (T and C) in a given DNA molecule was equal to the amount of all purine bases (A and G) in that molecule.

Chemically modified anti-D IgG anti-D reagent antisera in which the immunoglobulin has been chemically modified to react in the saline phase of testing by breaking disulfide bonds at the hinge region of the molecule, converting the Y-shaped antibody structure to a T-shaped form through the use of sulfhydryl-reducing reagents.

Chemotaxis Movement toward a stimulus, particularly that movement displayed by phagocytic cells toward bacteria and sites of cell injury.

Chimera An individual who possesses a mixed cell population.

Chloroquine diphosphate Substance that dissociates IgG antibody from red blood cells with little or no damage to the red blood cell membrane.

Chorionic villus sampling A prenatal procedure of retrieval of tissue from the chorionic villi (the villi in the external membrane surrounding the fetus).

Chromogen Any chemical that may be changed into coloring matter.

Chromosome The structures within a nucleus that contain a linear thread of DNA, which transmits genetic information. Genes are arranged along the strand of DNA and constitute portions of the DNA.

Cis position The location of two or more genes on the same chromosome of a homologous pair.

Citrate Compound of citric acid and a base; used in anticoagulant solutions.

Citrate-phosphate-dextrose (CPD) The anticoagulant preservative solution that replaced ACD in routine donor collection. It has been replaced by CPDA-1 in routine use.

Citrate-phosphate-dextrose-adenine (CPDA-1) The anticoagulant preservative solution in current use. It has extended the shelf life of blood from 21 days (ACD and CPD) to 35 days.

Clone A group of genetically identical cells.

Codominant A pair of genes in which neither is dominant over the other—that is, they are both expressed.

Codon A sequence of three nucleotides (bases) in the strand of DNA that provides the genetic code for specific amino acid. The complementary triplets are found in the messenger RNA (mRNA), which is synthesized based on the DNA template in the nucleus, and then proceeds to the ribosomes for protein synthesis, where the transfer RNA (tRNA), upon alignment with the mRNA, attaches the corresponding amino acid to the growing peptide chain.

Colloid A gluelike substance, such as protein or starch, whose particles, when dispersed in a solvent to the greatest possible degree, remain uniformly distributed and fail to form a true solution.

Colony-forming unit committed to erythropoiesis (CFU-E) A progenitor cell that is committed to forming cells of the red blood cell series.

Colony-forming unit—culture (CFU-C) Generation of stem cells using tissue culture methods. Current synonym is CFU-GM, which is a colony-forming unit committed to the production of myeloid cells (granulocytes and monocytes).

Colostrum Thin yellowish breast fluid secreted 2 to 3 days after birth but before the onset of true lactation; it contains a great quantity of proteins and calories as well as antibodies and lymphocytes.

Compatibility test A series of tests to determine if a particular blood component is appropriate for transfusion to a particular patient. This series of tests usually includes the ABO/Rh of the component and the intended recipient, antibody detection of the recipient, and a crossmatch (serologic or electronic) of the recipient's serum/plasma with the RBCs of the donor unit.

Competent cells Cells (usually various strains of *E. coli*) that possess easily altered cell membrane and readily incorporate foreign DNA (are prone to transformation). Competence may be achieved by exposure to calcium chloride and heat shock.

Complement A series of proteins in the circulation that, when sequentially activated, causes disruption of bacterial and other cell membranes. Activation occurs via one of two pathways; once activated, the components are involved in a great number of immune defense mechanisms, including anaphylaxis, chemotaxis, and phagocytosis. Red blood cell antibodies that activate complement may be capable of causing hemolysis.

Complementarity A phenomenon occurring in nucleic acids, resulting from formation of noncovalent hydrogen bonds between the nitrogen containing bases in the nucleotides on the opposite strands of the double helix. Due to this process, adenine (A) always pairs by two hydrogen bonds with thymine (T) or uracil (U), and guanine (G) always pairs by three hydrogen bonds with cytosine (C).

Complementary DNA (cDNA) An in vitro enzymatically synthesized DNA from an RNA template. A product of reverse transcription.

Complement fixation (CF) An immunologic test.

Component therapy Transfusion of specific components (e.g., red blood cells, platelets, plasma) rather than whole blood to treat a patient. Components are separable by physical means such as centrifugation.

Compound antibody An antibody whose corresponding antigen is an interaction product of two or more antigens.

Compound antigen Two or more antigens that interact and are recognized as a single antigen by an antibody.

Computer crossmatch Comparison of recent serologic results and interpretations on computer file for both the donor and the recipient being matched, establishing compatibility based on the comparison.

Concurrent review A blood utilization review that occurs shortly after transfusion events.

Configuration The physical layout and design of the central processing unit and the peripheral devices of an information system.

Conglutinin A substance present in bovine serum that will agglutinate sensitized cells in the presence of complement.

Constant region The portion of the immunoglobulin chain that shows a relatively constant amino acid sequence within each class of immunoglobulin. Both light and heavy chains have these constant portions, which originate at the carboxyl region of the molecule.

Convulsion Involuntary muscle contraction and relaxation.

Coombs' serum *See* Antihuman serum.

Coombs' test *See* Antihuman globulin test (AGT).

Cord cells Fetal cells obtained from the umbilical cord at birth; may be contaminated with Wharton's jelly.

Cordocentesis Umbilical cord blood sampling performed by ultrasound-guided needle insertion through the uterine wall.

Cosmids Vectors that can accept DNA 28 to 45 kb long. They have a small region of bacteriophage lambda (λ) necessary for packaging viral DNA into λ particles. They are useful for producing large-insert genomic libraries.

Coumarin (Coumadin) A commonly employed anticoagulant that acts as a vitamin K antagonist to prolong prothrombin time.

Counterelectrophoresis (CEP) An immunologic procedure.

Crossmatch The testing of the patient's serum with the donor red blood cells, including an antiglobulin phase or simply an immediate spin phase to confirm ABO compatibility.

Cross-reacting antibody Antibody that reacts with antigens functionally similar to its specific antigen.

Cryoprecipitate A concentrated source of coagulation factor VIII prepared from a single unit of donor blood; it also contains fibrinogen, factor XIII, and von Willebrand's factor.

Cryopreservation Preservation by freezing at very low temperatures.

Cryoprotectant A substance that protects blood cells from damage caused by freezing and thawing. Glycerol and dimethyl sulfoxide are examples.

Cryptantigens Hidden receptors that may be exposed when normal erythrocyte membranes are altered by bacterial or viral enzymes.

Crystalloid A substance capable of crystallization; opposite of colloid.

Cyanosis Slightly bluish or grayish skin discoloration resulting from accumulations of reduced hemoglobin or deoxyhemoglobin in the blood caused by oxygen deficiency or carbon dioxide buildup.

Cycle sequencing A variation of Sanger DNA sequencing conducted in a thermocycler and during the elongation (extension) step of a modified polymerase chain reaction.

Cytapheresis A procedure performed using a machine by which one can selectively remove a particular cell type normally found in peripheral blood of a patient or donor.

Cytokines A family of signaling molecules, such as interferons or interleukins, secreted by certain cell types and triggering various physiological processes by interacting with receptors located either on cell membranes or inside of cells.

Cytomegalovirus (CMV) One of a group of species-specific herpesviruses.

Cytotoxicity Ability to destroy cells.

Cytotoxicity testing Procedure commonly used in HLA typing and crossmatching.

Dane particle Hepatitis B virion.

Database An organized group of files in which information is stored in an information system.

Degenerate In molecular biology, the quality of the genetic code that refers to each amino acid being encoded by more than one nucleotide triplet (codon) in messenger RNA (mRNA) corresponding to a triplet in DNA. Degeneracy is also called *redundancy* of the genetic code. For example, the amino acid leucine is coded by UUA, UUG, CUU, CUC, CUA, or CUG codons.

Deglycerolization Removal of glycerol from a unit of red blood cells after thawing has been performed; required to return the cells to a normal osmolality.

Deletion The loss of a portion of chromosome.

Denaturation In molecular biology, a term that describes separation of two DNA strands upon thermal or chemical treatment, which destroys the noncovalent hydrogen bonds between the complementary nitrogen-containing bases. Thermal denaturation is reversible (*see* renaturation). The temperature at which a given double-stranded DNA denatures is proportional to the number of hydrogen bonds in the molecule and increases with the increase of G-C pair content. In reference to DNA, *denaturation* is a chemical or thermal process of breaking hydrogen bonds between the opposite nucleotides in the double helix, resulting in reversible separation of the two strands. Denaturation is the first step of polymerase chain reaction (PCR).

Deoxyribonucleic acid (DNA) The chemical basis of heredity and the carrier of genetic information for all organisms, except RNA viruses. Structured as a double helix of polymers of nucleotides, each consisting of one of the nitrogen-containing bases (A, T, C, and G), sugar deoxyribose, and a phosphate.

Deoxyribonucleoside triphosphates (dNTPs) Chemical compounds (nucleotides) used during DNA synthesis. They consist of one of the nitrogen-containing bases (A, T, C, and G), sugar deoxyribose, and three phosphates. They become monophosphates once they are built into the DNA molecule.

Dexamethasone A topical steroid with anti-inflammatory, antipruritic, and vasoconstrictive actions.

Dextran A plasma expander that may be used as a substitute for plasma; can be used to treat shock by increasing blood volume. Rouleaux may be observed in the recipient's serum or plasma.

Diagnosis-related group (DRG) Classification system that organizes short-term, general hospital inpatients into statistically stable groups based on age and illness.

Diaphoresis Profuse sweating.

Diastolic pressure The point of least pressure in the arterial vascular system; the lower or bottom value of a blood pressure reading.

Dideoxyribonucleoside triphosphates (ddNTPs) Deoxyribonucleoside triphosphates deprived of an oxygen atom located on the third sugar in the deoxyribose molecule. Lack of this oxygen prevents polymerization of nucleotides during DNA synthesis. Used as terminators of DNA synthesis in the process of DNA sequencing.

Dielectric constant A measure of the electrical conductivity of a suspending medium.

Differential count Counting 100 leukocytes to ascertain the relative percentages of each.

2,3-Diphosphoglycerate (2,3-DPG) An organic phosphate in red blood cells that alters the affinity of hemoglobin for oxygen. Blood cells stored in a blood bank lose 2,3-DPG, but once infused, the substance is resynthesized or reactivated.

Diploid Having two sets of 23 chromosomes, for a total of 46.

Direct antiglobulin test (DAT) Test that detects in vivo coating of an individual's red blood cells with IgG or complement (C3).

Direct transfusion Transfer of blood directly from one person to another.

Discontinuous prospective review A temporary, focused prospective blood utilization review strategy that is performed on a combination of particular product types, DRGs, clinical services, or individual clinicians that can be employed in areas of increased inappropriate blood utilization.

Disk drive A hardware device in an information system that contains a disk on which data are stored; provides for quick access to storing or retrieving data.

Disseminated intravascular coagulation (DIC) Clinical condition of altered blood coagulation secondary to a variety of diseases.

Dithiothreitol (DTT) A sulfhydryl compound used to disrupt the disulfide bonds of immunoglobulin M, yielding monomeric units rather than the typical pentameric molecule.

Diuresis Secretion and passage of large amounts of urine.

Diuretic An agent that increases the secretion of urine, either by increasing glomerular filtration or by decreasing reabsorption from the tubules.

Dizygotic twins Twins who are the product of two fertilized ova (also called *fraternal twins*).

DMSO Dimethyl sulfoxide, a cryoprotectant used for hematopoietic progenitor cells.

DNA *See* Deoxyribonucleic acid.

DNA fingerprinting DNA typing of multiple loci simultaneously in order to establish a genetic profile unique for every individual. A method initially developed by Alex Jeffreys and performed using restriction enzymes and DNA probes complementary to short repetitive sequences. Later, improved by the polymerase chain reaction (PCR).

DNA libraries Collections of clones (cells produced in molecular cloning) that contain all genomic or mRNA sequences of a particular cell type.

DNA polymerase An enzyme that catalyzes the template—dependent on synthesis of DNA. Also known as the HBeAg of the hepatitis B virion.

DNA polymerase III Bacterial enzyme synthesizing a new DNA strand using deoxyribonucleoside triphosphates (dNTPs) as substrates, double-stranded DNA as template, and magnesium as an enzyme cofactor.

DNA typing Also called *genetic profiling*, this is a process in which it is established which polymorphic version or variant of a gene (allele, locus) is present in an individual. Typing of multiple loci is called *DNA fingerprinting*.

Dolichos biflorus *See* Anti-A$_1$ lectin.

Domain Portions along the immunoglobulin chain that show specific biological function.

Dominant A trait or characteristic that will be expressed in the offspring even though it is carried on only one of the homologous chromosomes.

Donath-Landsteiner test A test usually performed in the blood bank to detect the presence of the Donath-Landsteiner antibody, which is a biphasic immunoglobulin G antibody with anti-P specificity found in patients suffering from paroxysmal cold hemoglobinuria.

Donor An individual who donates a pint of blood.

Dopamine A catecholamine synthesized by the adrenal gland, used especially in the treatment of shock.

Dosage A phenomenon whereby an antibody reacts more strongly with a red blood cell carrying a double dose (homozygous inheritance of the appropriate gene) than with a red blood cell carrying a single dose (heterozygous inheritance) of an antigen.

Dot blotting In molecular biology, a technique in which the nucleic acid extracted from specimen is immobilized on a membrane (blot) in a form of a dot. This procedure does not require electrophoresis like other blotting techniques (Southern, Northern, or Western). The membrane is subsequently incubated in a solution with labeled probes, complementary to sequences, expected to be present in the tested specimen. Microarrays are an example of a modified (reversed) dot blotting technique.

Drug-induced immune hemolytic anemia Shortened RBC survival caused by an antibody to a therapeutic agent (e.g., antibiotic) that has become bound to the RBC membrane or that has altered the RBC membrane.

Dyscrasia An old term now used as a synonym for disease.

Ecchymosis A form of macula appearing in large irregularly formed hemorrhagic areas of the skin; first blue-black, then changing to greenish brown or yellow.

Edema A local or generalized condition in which the body tissues contain an excessive amount of tissue fluid.

Electrolyte A substance that in solution conducts an electric current; common electrolytes are acids, bases, and salts.

Electrophoresis The movement of charged particles through a medium (paper, agar gel) in the presence of an electrical field; useful in the separation and analysis of proteins.

Eluate *See* Elution.

Elution A process whereby cells that are coated with antibody are treated in such a manner as to disrupt the bonds between the antigen and antibody. The freed antibody is collected in an inert diluent such as saline or 6% albumin. This antibody serum then can be tested to identify its specificity using routine methods. The mechanism to free the antibody may be physical (heating, shaking) or chemical (ether, acid), and the harvested antibody-containing fluid is called an *eluate*.

Embolism Obstruction of a blood vessel by foreign substances or a blood clot.

Embolus A mass of undissolved matter present in a blood or lymphatic vessel, brought there by the blood or lymph circulation.

Endemic A disease that occurs continuously in a particular population but has a *low* mortality rate; used in contrast to *epidemic*.

Endogenous Produced or arising from within a cell or organism.

Endothelium A form of squamous epithelium consisting of flat cells that line the blood and lymphatic vessels, the heart, and various other body cavities; derived from mesoderm.

Endotoxemia The presence of endotoxin in the blood; endotoxin is present in the cells of certain bacteria (e.g., gram-negative organisms).

Engraftment The successful establishment, proliferation, and differentiation of transplanted hematopoietic stem cells.

Enzyme A substance capable of catalyzing a reaction; proteins that induce chemical changes in other substances without being changed themselves.

Enzyme-linked immunosorbent assay (ELISA) An immunologic test.

Enzyme treatment A procedure in which red blood cells are incubated with an enzyme solution that cleaves some of the membrane's glycoproteins, then washed free of the enzyme and used in serologic testing. Enzyme treatment cleaves some antigens and exposes others.

Epistaxis Hemorrhage from the nose; nosebleed.

Epitope The portion of the antigen molecule that is directly involved in the interaction with the antibody; the antigenic determinant.

Equivalence zone The zone in which antigen and antibody concentrations are optimal and lattice formation is most stable.

Erythroblast A precursor form of nucleated red blood cell that is not normally seen in the circulating blood.

Erythroblastosis fetalis *See* Hemolytic disease of the fetus and newborn (HDFN).

Erythrocyte The blood cell that transports oxygen and carbon dioxide; a mature red blood cell.

Ethidium bromide (EB) A fluorescent dye intercalating between the grooves of the double-stranded DNA. Used for staining of DNA in electrophoretic gels for UV visualization. Mutagenic and carcinogenic is being replaced by safer SYBR green dye.

Ethylenediaminetetraacetic acid (EDTA) An anticoagulant useful in hematologic testing and preferable when direct antihuman globulin testing is indicated.

Euglobulin lysis Coagulation procedure testing for fibrinolysin.

Exchange transfusion Transfusion and withdrawal of small amounts of blood, repeated until blood volume is almost entirely exchanged; used in infants born with hemolytic disease.

Exclusion An exclusion occurs when a child has inherited a genetic marker not detected in an alleged parent. Exclusions can be direct or indirect, which are distinguished in the following way: A direct exclusion refers to the presence of a genetic marker in the child that is not detectable in the alleged parent. An indirect exclusion occurs when the alleged parent has a marker that should be transmitted to all his or her children, but the child in question lacks that genetic marker. Indirect exclusions can result when mutations occur during meiosis or when the gene transmitted to the child is silent or "null."

Exogenous Originating outside an organ or part.

Exon The coding part of a gene in eukaryotes. Only this part of the gene is translated into protein product. In genomic DNA, exons are separated by introns.

Expression library A DNA library generated in a vector that not only replicates itself, but also drives protein synthesis in *E. coli* (an expression vector).

Extracorporeal Outside of the body.

Extravascular Outside of the blood vessel.

Factor assay Coagulation procedure to assay the concentration of specific plasma coagulation factors.

Factor VIII concentrate A commercially prepared source of coagulation factor VIII.

Febrile reaction A transfusion reaction caused by leukoagglutinin that is characterized by fever; usually observed in multiply transfused or multiparous patients.

Fetal and neonatal alloimmune thrombocytopenia (FNAIT) A rare condition that occurs when a mother becomes sensitized to a foreign antigen of paternal origin that is present on fetal thrombocytes (platelets). These platelet antigens provoke production of maternal antibodies that cross the placenta and destroy fetal platelets.

Fibrin A whitish filamentous protein or clot formed by the action of thrombin on fibrinogen, converting it to fibrin.

Fibrinogen A protein produced in the liver that circulates in plasma. In the presence of thrombin, an enzyme produced by the activation of the clotting mechanism, fibrinogen is cleaved into fibrin, which is an insoluble protein that is responsible for clot formation.

Fibrinolysin The substance that has the ability to dissolve fibrin; also called *plasmin*.

Fibrinolysis Dissolution of fibrin by fibrinolysin, caused by the action of a proteolytic enzyme system that is continually active in the body but that is increased greatly by various stress stimuli.

Fibroblast Cells found throughout the body that synthesize connective tissue.

Ficin A proteolytic enzyme derived from the fig.

Ficoll A macromolecular additive that enhances the agglutination of red blood cells.

Ficoll-Hypaque A density-gradient medium used to separate and harvest specific white blood cells, most commonly lymphocytes.

Fluorescent antibody Antibody reaction made visible by incorporating a fluorescent dye into the antigen-antibody reaction and examining the specimen with a fluorescent microscope.

Fluorescent in situ hybridization (FISH) A technique in molecular biology in which fluorescent DNA probes are used to detect homologous DNA or RNA sequences in preserved chromosomes or intact cells.

Fluorescent resonance energy transfer (FRET) probes A type of DNA probe used in real-time PCR. Instead of a quencher, attached to the TaqMan probes or molecular beacons, in the FRET system the fluorescence "donor" and "acceptor" are attached to two separate hybridization probes designed to bind to adjacent DNA sequences within the amplified region. Until there is not any PCR product (amplicon) present in the tube, these probes may not get close, as there is nothing for them to bind to. Once the PCR product starts to accumulate in the tube, the probes bind to the sequences within the product in close proximity and the energy from the donor is transferred to the reporter, which results in emission of light that may now be detected.

Formaldehyde A disinfectant solution.

Forward grouping Testing unknown red blood cells with known reagent antisera to determine which ABO antigens are present.

Frameshift mutation A change in which a message is read incorrectly either because a base is missing or an extra base is added, which results in an entirely new polypeptide because the triplet sequence has been shifted one base.

Fresh frozen plasma (FFP) A frozen plasma product (from a single donor) that contains all clotting factors, especially the labile factors V and VIII; useful for clotting factor deficiencies other than hemophilia A, von Willebrand's disease, and hypofibrinogenemia.

Freund's adjuvant Mixture of killed microorganisms, usually mycobacteria, in an oil-and-water emulsion. The material is administered to induce antibody formation and yields a much greater antibody response.

Furosemide (Lasix) An oral diuretic.

G-CSF Granulocyte-colony stimulating factor, filgrastim.

GM-CSF Granulocyte macrophage–colony stimulating factor, sargramostim.

G6PD (glucose-6-phosphate dehydrogenase) A red cell enzyme involved in the glycolytic pathway.

Gamete A mature male or female reproductive cell.

Gamma globulin A protein found in plasma and known to be involved in immunity.

Gamma marker Allotypic marker on the gamma heavy chain of the IgG immunoglobulin.

Gel test A blood group serology test method that uses a microtube containing gel (with or without antisera or antiglobulin sera) that acts as a reaction vessel for agglutination.

Gene A unit of inheritance within a chromosome.

Gene chips Microarrays.

Gene expression A term generally describing the processes of transcription and translation. A gene that is not transcribed (not expressed) is considered "silent."

Gene therapy An introduction of new genetic material into the cells of an organism for therapeutic purposes.

Genetic code A key according to which a sequence of sets of three DNA nucleotides within a gene is transcribed into a sequence of sets of three nucleotides within mRNA (codon) and then translated into amino acids, the building blocks of a peptide or protein.

Genetic transformation Process of foreign DNA uptake by a cell, usually enforced by use of chemicals, electricity, or liposomes that enable penetration of cell membrane.

Genotype An individual's actual genetic makeup.

Gestation In mammals, the length of time from conception to birth.

Globin A protein constituent of hemoglobin. There are four globin chains in the hemoglobin molecule.

Glomerulonephritis A form of nephritis in which the lesions involve primarily the glomeruli.

Glutamic pyruvate transaminase A liver enzyme used to monitor liver function; also called *serum glutamic pyruvate transaminase* (SGPT) or *alanine transferase* (ALT).

Gluten enteropathy A condition associated with malabsorption of food from the intestinal tract.

Glycerol A cryoprotective agent.

Glycerolization Adding glycerol to a unit of red blood cells for the purpose of freezing.

Glycine soja Soybean extract or lectin used to differentiate different forms of polyagglutination.

Glycophorin A A major glycoprotein of the red blood cell membrane. MN antigen activity is found on it.

Glycophorin B An important red blood cell glycoprotein: SsU antigen activity is found here.

Glycoprotein A protein with linked carbohydrates.

Glycosyl transferase A protein enzyme that promotes the attachment of a specific sugar molecule to a predetermined acceptor molecule. Many blood group genes code for transferases, which reproduce their respective antigens by attaching sugars to designated precursor substances.

Goodpasture's syndrome A disease entity that represents a rapidly progressive glomerulonephritis associated with pulmonary lesions. Usually the patients possess an antibody to the basement membrane of the renal glomeruli.

Graft-versus-host (GVH) disease A disorder in which the grafted tissue attacks the host tissue.

Granulocytopenia Abnormal reduction of granulocytes in the blood.

Griffith's transformation A famous genetic experiment performed in 1928 by Frederick Griffith using two strains of *Streptococcus pneumoniae*. Griffith demonstrated that a heat-resistant "transforming principle" from one strain could change the virulence of another strain. This was the first event that eventually led to discovery of DNA as carrying the genetic information on molecules.

Hageman's factor Synonym for coagulation factor XII.

Half-life The time that is required for the concentration of a substance to be reduced by one half.

Haploid Possessing half the normal number of chromosomes found in somatic or body cells; seen in germ cells (sperm and ova).

Haplotype A term used in HLA testing to denote the five genes (*HLA-A, HLA-B, HLA-C, HLA-D, HLA-DR*) on the same chromosome.

Haptene The portion of an antigen containing the grouping on which the specificity depends.

Haptoglobin A mucoprotein to which hemoglobin released into plasma is bound; it is increased in certain inflammatory conditions and decreased in hemolytic disorders.

Hardware Components of an information computer system that are the tangible, physical pieces of equipment, such as the central processing unit, cathode ray tube, and keyboard.

HBcAg Hepatitis core antigen, referring to the nucleocapsid of the virion.

HBeAg Hepatitis DNA polymerase of the nucleus of the virion.

HBsAg Hepatitis B surface antigen.

Hemangioma A benign tumor of dilated blood vessels.

Hemarthrosis Bloody effusion into the cavity of a joint.

Hematinic Pertaining to blood; an agent that increases the amount of hemoglobin in the blood.

Hematocrit The proportion of red blood cells in whole blood, expressed as a percentage.

Hematoma A swelling or mass of blood confined to an organ, tissue, or space and caused by a break in a blood vessel.

Hematopoietic progenitor cell Stem cells that are committed to produce blood cells.

Hematuria Blood in the urine.

Heme The iron-containing protoporphyrin portion of the hemoglobin wherein the iron is in the ferrous (Fe^{2+}) state.

Hemodialysis Removal of chemical substances from the blood by passing it through tubes made of semipermeable membranes that are continually bathed by solutions that selectively remove unwanted material; used to cleanse the blood of patients in whom one or both kidneys are defective or absent and to remove excess accumulation of drugs or toxic chemicals in the blood.

Hemodilution An increase in the volume of blood plasma, resulting in reduced relative concentration of red blood cells.

Hemoglobin The iron-conjugated protein in the red blood cells whose function is to carry oxygen from the lungs to the tissues. This protein contains heme plus globin.

Hemoglobinemia Presence of hemoglobin in the blood plasma.

Hemoglobin-oxygen dissociation curve The relationship between the percent saturation of the hemoglobin molecule with oxygen and the environmental oxygen tension.

Hemoglobinuria The presence of hemoglobin in the urine freed from lysed red blood cells, which occurs when hemoglobin from disintegrating red blood cells or from rapid hemolysis of red blood cells exceeds the ability of the blood proteins to combine with the hemoglobin.

Hemolysin An antibody that activates complement, leading to cell lysis.

Hemolysis Disruption of the red blood cell membrane and the subsequent release of hemoglobin into the suspending medium or plasma.

Hemolytic anemia Anemia caused by hemolysis of red blood cells, resulting in reduction of normal red blood cell life span.

Hemolytic disease of the fetus and newborn (HDFN) A disease, characterized by anemia, jaundice, enlargement of the liver and spleen, and generalized edema (hydrops fetalis), that is caused by maternal IgG antibodies crossing the placenta and attacking fetal red blood cells when there is a fetomaternal blood group incompatibility (usually ABO or Rh antibodies). Synonym is *erythroblastosis fetalis*.

Hemolytic transfusion reaction (HTR) A reaction from red blood cell destruction caused by patient's antibody(ies) directed to donor red blood cell antigen(s).

Hemophilia A A hereditary disorder characterized by greatly prolonged coagulation time (↑PTT). The blood fails to clot and bleeding occurs; caused by inheritance of a factor VIII deficiency, it occurs almost exclusively in males.

Hemophilia B "Christmas disease," which is a hemophilia-like disease caused by a lack of factor IX.

Hemopoiesis Formation of blood cells. Synonym is *hematopoiesis*.

Hemorrhage Abnormal internal or external bleeding; may be venous, arterial, or capillary; from blood vessels into the tissues or out of the body.

Hemorrhagic diathesis Uncontrolled spontaneous bleeding.

Hemosiderin An iron-containing pigment derived from hemoglobin from disintegration of red blood cells; a method of storing iron until it is needed for making hemoglobin.

Hemostasis Arrest of bleeding; maintaining blood flow within vessels by repairing rapidly any vascular break without compromising the fluidity of the blood.

Hemotherapy Blood transfusion as a therapeutic measure.

Heparin An anticoagulant used for collecting whole blood that is to be filtered for the removal of leukocytes.

Hepatitis Inflammation of the liver.

Hepatitis-associated antigen (HAA) Older terminology currently replaced by HBsAg.

Hepatitis B immunoglobulin (HBIg) An immune serum given to individuals exposed to the hepatitis B virus.

Hereditary spherocytosis An inherited anemia characterized by fragile, spherical RBCs prone to hemolysis. The condition occurs due to mutations within genes coding for cytoskeleton proteins like spectrin, ankyrin, or others.

Heterogenous RNA (hnRNA) *See* pre-mRNA.

Heterozygote An individual with different alleles on a gene for a given characteristic.

Heterozygous Possessing different alleles at a given gene locus.

High-prevalence antigen Also known as *high-incidence antigen*; antigen whose frequency in the population is 98% to 99%.

High protein anti-D Reagent anti-D consisting of human source IgG anti-D with potentiators (bovine albumin and macromolecular additives) to enhance antibody reactivity on direct testing.

Histocompatibility The ability of cells to survive without immunologic interference; especially important in blood transfusion and transplantation.

HLA Human leukocyte antigen.

Homeostasis State of equilibrium of the internal environment of the body that is maintained by dynamic processes of feedback and regulation.

Homozygote An individual developing from gametes with similar alleles and thus possessing like pairs of genes for a given hereditary characteristic.

Homozygous Possessing a pair of identical alleles.

Hormone A substance originating in an organ or gland that is conveyed through the blood to another part of the body, chemically stimulating it to increase functional activity and increase secretion.

Hoshin kanri In Lean, a total quality management principle to prioritize the elimination of waste via policy deployment and control.

Hyaluronidase An enzyme found in the testes; present in semen.

Hybrid gene A gene that results from combining two different genes.

Hybridization Formation of hydrogen bonds between complementary strands of nucleic acids to form either DNA:DNA or DNA:RNA hybrids. Chemically, a process identical with renaturation or annealing. *Nucleic acid hybridization* is a fundamental tool in molecular genetics that takes advantage of the ability of individual single-stranded nucleic acid molecules to form double-stranded molecules—that is, to hybridize to each other. The interacting single-stranded molecules must have a sufficiently high degree of base complementarity. Standard nucleic acid hybridization assays involve using a labeled nucleic acid probe to identify related DNA or RNA molecules—ones with a significantly high degree of sequence similarity—within a complex mixture of unlabeled nucleic acid molecules, the target nucleic acid.

Hybridization protection (HPA) A molecular detection technology, in which ssDNA probes labeled with chemiluminescent molecules are added to form hybrids with the amplified RNA molecules produced during transcription mediated amplification (TMA). Light is emitted upon hybridization of the probes to the RNA and captured by a luminometer.

Hybridoma A hybrid (cross) between a plasmacytoma cell and a spleen (or Ab-producing) cell that produces a monoclonal antibody, resulting in a cell line that can grow indefinitely in culture and can produce high quantities of Ab. This antibody is monoclonal because only one Ab-producing cell combined with the plasmacytoma cell is present.

Hydatid cyst fluid Source of P_1 substance.

Hydrocortisone A corticosteroid with anti-inflammatory properties.

Hydrogen bonds Noncovalent, heat-labile chemical bonds that occur between hydrogen atom and either nitrogen or oxygen atom of the adjacent molecule. In DNA, hydrogen bonding holds together the two strands of double helix by formation of two bonds between adenine and thymine and three bonds between cytosine and guanine.

Hydrops fetalis *See* Hemolytic disease of the fetus and newborn (HDFN).

Hydroxyethyl starch (HES) A red blood cell sedimenting agent used to facilitate leukocyte withdrawal during leukapheresis.

Hypertension Increase in blood pressure.

Hyperventilation Rapid breathing that results in carbon dioxide depletion and that accompanies hypotension, vasoconstriction, and fainting.

Hypogammaglobulinemia Decreased levels of gamma globulins seen in some disease states.

Hypotension Decrease in blood pressure.

Hypothermia Having a body temperature below normal.

Hypovolemia Diminished blood volume.

Hypoxia Deficiency of oxygen.

Iberis amara *See* Anti-M lectin.

Icterus A condition characterized by yellowish skin, whites of the eyes, mucous membranes, and body fluids caused by increased circulating bilirubin resulting from excessive hemolysis or from liver damage due to hepatitis. Synonym is jaundice.

Idiopathic Pertaining to conditions without clear pathogenesis, or disease without recognizable cause, as of spontaneous origin.

Idiopathic thrombocytopenic purpura (ITP) Bleeding owing to a decreased number of platelets; the etiology is unknown, with most evidence pointing to platelet auto-antibodies.

Idiopathic thrombocythemia An increase in blood platelets of unknown etiology.

Idiotype The portion of the immunoglobulin variable region that is the antigen-combining site, which interacts with the antigenic epitope.

Immune response The reactions of the body to substances that are foreign or are interpreted as being foreign. Cell-mediated or cellular immunity pertains to tissue destruction mediated by T cells, such as graft rejection and hypersensitivity reactions. Humoral immunity pertains to cell destruction response during the early period of the reaction.

Immune serum globulin Gamma globulin protein fraction of serum-containing antibodies.

Immunoblast A mitotically active T or B cell.

Immunoblotting A technique for detecting proteins extracted from cells, separated by polyacrylamide gel electrophoresis, transferred from the gel onto a filter membrane and then incubated with a specific labeled antibody.

Immunodeficiency A decrease from the normal concentration of immunoglobulins in serum.

Immunodominant sugar In reference to glycoprotein or glycolipid antigens, the sugar molecule that gives the antigen its specificity (e.g., galactose, which confers B antigen specificity).

Immunogen Any substance capable of stimulating an immune response.

Immunogenicity The ability of an antigen to stimulate an antibody response.

Immunoglobulin (Ig) One of a family of closely related though not identical proteins that are capable of acting as antibodies: IgA, IgD, IgE, IgG, and IgM. IgA is the principal immunoglobulin in exocrine secretions such as saliva and tears. IgD may play a role in antigen recognition and the initiation of antibody synthesis. IgE, produced by the cells lining the intestinal and respiratory tracts, is important in forming reagin. IgG is the main immunoglobulin in human serum. IgM is formed in almost every immune response during the early period of the reaction.

Immunologic memory The development of T and B memory cells that have been sensitized by exposure to an antigen and that respond rapidly under subsequent encounters with the antigen.

Immunologic unresponsiveness Development of a tolerance to certain antigens that would otherwise evoke an immune response.

Immunoprecipitin An antigen-antibody reaction that results in precipitation.

Inclusion The opposite of an exclusion, in which all of the genetic information inherited by the child from the parent whose identity is in question, is present in the alleged parent.

Incubation In vitro combination of antigen and antibody under certain conditions of time and temperature to allow antigen-antibody complexes to occur.

Indirect transfusion Transfusion of blood from a donor to a suitable storage container and then to a patient.

Initiation The deposition of N-formylmethionine on the ribosome, which begins the synthesis of all proteins.

In Lu A rare dominant gene that inhibits the production of all Lutheran antigens as well as i, P_1, and Au^a (Auberger). The quantity of antigen on the red blood cell is markedly reduced in the presence of *In Lu*; it may be virtually undetectable.

Interface Software that allows a computer system to send data to or receive data from another computer system.

Intergenic recombination Recombination of genetic material in noncoding regions of DNA.

Intracellular Occurs within a cell.

Intraoperative salvage A procedure to reclaim a patient's blood loss from an operation by reinfusion.

Intrauterine transfusion Transfusion of blood into a fetus in utero.

Intravascular Within the blood vessel.

Intron A noncoding part of the gene. This fragment of the gene is transcribed into RNA but is excised out during the process of splicing so it is not translated into a protein product.

In utero Within the uterus.

Inversion The breaking of a chromosome during division, with subsequent reattachment occurring in an inverted or upside-down position.

In vitro Outside the living body, as in a laboratory setting.

In vivo Inside the living body.

Ion exchange resin Synthetic organic substances of high molecular weight. They replace certain positive or negative ions, which they encounter in solutions.

Ionic strength Refers to the number of charged particles present in a solution.

Ir genes Immune response genes found within the region of the major histocompatibility complex. *Ir* genes in humans are likely to exist; preliminary evidence shows genes at the D-related locus may be analogous to the *Ir* genes of mice.

Iron-deficiency anemia Anemia resulting from a greater demand on stored iron than can be met.

Irradiation Gamma or electron treatment of a cellular blood product for protection against graft-versus-host disease.

Ischemia Local and temporary deficiency of blood supply caused by obstruction of the circulation to a cell, tissue, or organ.

Isoagglutinins The ABO antibodies anti-A, anti-B, and anti-A,B.

Isoimmune An antibody produced against a foreign antigen in the same species.

Isotype The subclasses of an immunoglobulin molecule.

Jaundice *See* Icterus.

Kaizen In Lean, a continuous improvement process required for long-term success.

Karyotype A photomicrograph of a single cell in the metaphase stage of mitosis that is arranged to show the chromosomes in descending order of size.

kb (or kbp) A measure of DNA length. One thousand ("kilo") nucleotides (or "bases" for simplification) in single-stranded DNA. In double-stranded DNA, this is referred to as one thousand base pairs.

Kernicterus A form of icterus neonatorum occurring in infants, developing at 2 to 8 days of life; prognosis poor if untreated. This condition is due to an increase in unconjugated bilirubin.

Kinin A group of polypeptides that have considerable biological activity (e.g., vasoactivity).

Kleihauer-Betke technique Quantitative procedure used to determine the amount of fetal cells present in the maternal circulation.

Km Light chain marker on the kappa light chains of IgG (formerly known as InV).

Knockout transgenic animal A model to study the consequences of lack of function of a gene that is blocked, or "knocked out" (e.g., by RNA interference) and introduced into the egg using transgenic technology (a microinjection of external/modified genetic material). The egg, upon implantation into a surrogate mother, develops into genetically modified organism missing the desired structural or functional protein.

Labile Capable of deteriorating rapidly upon storage.

Lambda (λ) vectors Vectors that contain the part of the bacterial virus Lambda genome necessary for lytic replication in *E. coli* and one or more restriction sites for insertion of the DNA fragment of interest. They can carry foreign DNA 5 to 14 kb long. The recombinant DNA is "packaged" into viral particles and used to infect *E. coli* in order to produce multiple copies of the fragment.

Lean A systematic approach for identifying actions within a process that create value, then optimizing the alignment of these actions to the customer.

Lectin Proteins present in plants (usually seeds), which bind specifically to carbohydrate determinants and agglutinate erythrocytes through their cell surface of oligosaccharide determinants.

Leukemia Malignant proliferation of leukocytes, which spill into the blood, yielding an elevated leukocyte count.

Leukoagglutinin Antibodies to white blood cells.

Ligases A class of enzymes that catalyze the linkage of two molecules, generally utilizing ATP as the energy donor. In recombinant DNA technology, these are enzymes linking the adjacent nucleotides between two DNA fragments being joined after restriction enzyme digestion.

Ligature Process of binding or tying; a band or bandage; a thread or wire for tying a blood vessel or other structure in order to constrict it.

LightCycler A special type of thermocycler with built-in fluorescence detector, designed for real-time PCR applications.

Linkage The association between distinct genes that occupy closely situated loci on the same chromosome, resulting in an association in the inheritance of these genes.

Linkage disequilibrium Genes associated in a haplotype more often than would be expected on the basis of chance alone.

Locus The site of a gene on a chromosome.

Low ionic-polycation test A compatibility test that incorporates both glycine (low ionic) and protamine (polycation) in an effort to obtain maximal sensitivity and to minimize the need for antibody screening.

Low ionic strength solution (LISS) A type of potentiating medium in use for serologic testing. Reducing the ionic strength of the red blood cell–suspending medium increases the affinity of the antigen for its corresponding antibody such that sensitivity can be increased and incubation time decreased. LISS contains glycine or glucose in addition to saline.

Low melting point agarose Agarose specially formulated to melt in temperatures much lower than normal, which allows for easy dissolving of the gel in order to isolate and purify DNA that was run in it.

Low-prevalence antigen Also known as *low-incidence antigen*; antigen whose frequency in a random population is very low—less than 10%.

Luminometer An instrument that detects and quantifies the amount of light emitted as a result of chemical reaction (chemiluminescence).

Lymphocyte A type of white blood cell involved in the immune response. Lymphocytes normally total 20% to

45% of total white blood cells. T lymphocytes mature during passage through the thymus or after interaction with thymic hormones; these cells function both in cellular and humoral immunity. Subsets include helper T-cells (T_h), which enhance B-cell antibody production, and suppressor T-cells (T_s), which inhibit B-cell antibody production. B-lymphocyte cells are not processed by the thymus. Through morphologic and functional differentiation, they mature into plasma cells that secrete immunoglobulin.

Lymphoma A solid tumor of lymphocyte cells.

Lysosomes Part of an intracellular digestive system that exists as separate particles in the cell. Even though their importance in health and disease is certain, all the precise ways lysosomes effect changes are not understood.

Macroglobulinemia Abnormal presence of high-molecular-weight immunoglobulins (IgM) in the blood.

Macrophages End-stage development for the blood monocyte; these cells can ingest (phagocytose) a variety of substances for subsequent digestion or storage and are located in a number of sites in the body (e.g., spleen, liver, lung), existing as free mobile cells or as fixed cells. Functions include elimination of senescent blood cells and participation in the immune response.

Major ABO incompatibility ABO antibody in the recipient that is incompatible with the donor.

Major histocompatibility complex (MHC) Present in all mammalian and ovarian species; analogous to HLA complex. HLA antigens are within the MHC at a locus on chromosome 6.

Malaria An acute and sometimes chronic infectious disease caused by the presence of a parasite within red blood cells. The parasite is *Plasmodium* (*P. vivax, P. falciparum, P. malariae, P. ovale*), which is introduced through bites of infected female *Anopheles* mosquitoes or through blood transfusion.

Maternal antibody Antibody produced in the mother and transferred to the fetus in utero.

Megaloblastic anemia Anemia in which megaloblasts are found in the blood.

Meiosis Type of cell division of germ cells in which two successive divisions of the nucleus produce cells that contain half the number of chromosomes present in somatic cells.

Melting curve analysis A postamplification analysis of the amplicon produced in the real-time PCR by slowly increasing the temperature and monitoring the decrease of fluorescence as a result of DNA strand separation from the probes used in the reaction. The fluorescent probes detach from the PCR product at lower temperatures if the product has a mutation. This method may be used to distinguish between homo- and heterozygosity underlying certain conditions (the presence of the mutation in one or both homologous chromosomes).

Melting point (Tm) The temperature at which half of all hydrogen bonds in the double-stranded DNA molecule are broken, while the other half are still intact. It determines how much energy is needed to keep the strands of the helix apart. As a general rule, temperatures above the Tm promote the separation of the strands. Knowing the Tm is necessary for calculating temperatures for hybridization-based assays and for annealing primers in the polymerase chain reaction. The primers generally anneal to DNA at about 5°C (or more) below the Tm. If the temperature is decreased more, they will start to anneal to sequences with only partial complementarity, which affects the specificity of the reaction. For short DNA sequences, the simplified formula to calculate the Tm is 2AT + 4GC, where AC is the total number of adenines and thymines, and GC is the total number of guanines and cytosines in the molecule. Based on this formula, it is evident that GC-rich molecules will have higher Tm than AT-rich sequences, because there are always three hydrogen bonds between guanines and cytosines, while there are only two bonds between adenines and thymines.

Mendel's laws The classical principles of inheritance defined by the Moravian monk Gregor Mendel in 1866. The first law of genetics (the law of segregation) stated that the hereditary characteristics are determined by particulate units (presently called genes) that occur in an individual as pairs (diploid), but in the formation of germ cells/gametes they segregate so the gamete contains only one member of the pair (haploid). The second law (the law of independent assortment) stated that the particulate units (genes) that determine different characteristics are inherited independently of other units (now we know that if the genes are close to one another on the chromosome, they will be inherited together).

Menorrhagia Excessive menstrual bleeding, in number of days or amount of blood, or both.

2-Mercaptoethanol (2-ME) A sulfhydryl compound used to disrupt the disulfide bonds of immunoglobulin M, yielding monomeric units rather than the typical pentameric units.

Messenger RNA (mRNA) *See* Ribonucleic acid.

Metastasis Movement of bacteria or body cells, especially cancer cells, from one part of the body to another; change in location of a disease or of its manifestations or transfer from one organ or part of another not directly connected. Spread is by the lymph or blood circulation.

Methemoglobin An abnormal form of hemoglobin wherein the ferrous (Fe^{2+}) iron has been oxidized to ferric (Fe^{3+}) iron.

Methyldopa (Aldomet) Common drug used to treat hypertension; frequently the cause of a positive direct Coombs' test result.

Microaggregates Aggregates of platelets and leukocytes that accumulate in stored blood.

Microarrays (gene chips) Devices consisting of glass slides or membrane filters with fragments of DNA printed by a robot in small spots at high density. These DNA fragments serve as multiple probes that will bind (hybridize with) the complementary regions of DNA (or RNA) present in the analyzed specimen applied to the chip. The chips are scanned with a laser to identify the regions detected by the probes.

Microglobulin (β_2) A protein synthesized by all nucleated cell types; an integral part of the class I MHC antigens.

Microsatellites DNA regions composed of back-back-repeated units of 1-8 nucleotides (also called short tandem repeats; STRs).

Microspherocytes Red blood cells, small and spherical, in certain kinds of anemia (i.e., hereditary spherocytosis).

Miniprep A rapid method for making a small preparation of purified plasmid DNA from 1 to 5 mL of bacterial culture.

Minisatellites DNA regions composed of back-to-back repeated units ranging in size from 9 to 80 bp (also called VNTR; variable number of tandem repeats).

Minor ABO incompatibility ABO antibody in the donor that is incompatible with the recipient.

Mitosis Type of cell division in which each daughter cell contains the same number of chromosomes as the parent cell. All cells except sex cells undergo mitosis.

Mixed-field agglutination A type of agglutination pattern in which numerous small clumps of cells exist amid a sea of free cells. This usually occurs when there is more than one population of RBCs present in the sample (e.g., in a recently transfused individual).

MLC Mixed lymphocyte culture.

MLR Mixed lymphocyte reaction.

Modem Hardware device that provides the ability to attach to a computer system via telephone communication lines.

Molecular beacons Fluorescent DNA probes structured like a hairpin loop with reporter and quencher, used in real-time PCR. The emission of fluorescent light from the reporter, indicating the presence of an amplicon, occurs upon unfolding of the loop structure, which physically separates the quencher.

Molecular cloning Reproduction of recombinant DNA molecules in host cells that, due to universality of the genetic code, replicate the foreign DNA along with its own. The daughter cells of a single cell carrying the recombinant molecule propagate to produce a clone.

Monoclonal Antibody derived from a single ancestral antibody-producing parent cell.

Monocytes *See* Macrophage.

Monospecific antiglobulin reagent Antiserum specific for one type of immunoglobulin (e.g., anti-IgG).

Monozygotic twins Two offspring that develop from a single fertilized ovum.

Mosaic An antigen composed of several subunits, such as the $Rh_0(D)$ antigen. A mixture of characteristics that may result from a genetic crossover or mutation.

Multiparous Having borne more than one child.

Multiple myeloma A neoplastic proliferation of plasma cells, which is characterized by very high immunoglobulin levels of monoclonal origin.

Multiplex assay In molecular biology, refers primarily to multiplex polymerase chain reaction (PCR). Multiplex PCR is a concurrent amplification of several DNA fragments from the same DNA target using several sets of primers that must be carefully designed so that they don't interfere with each other.

Mutation A change in a gene potentially capable of being transmitted to offspring.

Myelofibrosis Replacement of bone marrow by fibrous tissue.

Myeloproliferative An autonomous, purposeless increase in the production of the myeloid cell elements of the bone marrow, which includes granulocytic, erythrocytic, and megakaryocytic cell lines as well as the stromal connective tissue.

N-acetylneuraminic acid (NANA) *See* Sialic acid.

Naturally occurring antibody Antibody present in a patient without known prior exposure to the corresponding red blood cell antigen.

Neonatal alloimmune neutropenia (NAN) A rare condition that occurs when a mother becomes sensitized to a foreign antigen of paternal origin that is present on fetal granulocytes. These fetal granulocyte antigens provoke antibody production. The maternal IgG antibody crosses the placenta and destroys fetal granulocytes. This neutropenia is typically self-limiting and lasts for several weeks but can persist for as long as 6 months. During this period, neonates are at high risk of developing infections.

Neonate A newborn infant up to 4 months of age.

Network Configuration of personal computers linked together with cables; allows all of the personal computers to access common data and software located on a file server.

Neuraminidase An enzyme that cleaves sialic acid from the red blood cell membrane.

Neutralization Inactivating an antibody by reacting it with an antigen against which it is directed.

Neutrophil A leukocyte that ingests bacteria and small particles and plays a role in combating infection.

Nondisjunction Failure of a pair of chromosomes to separate during meiosis.

Nonresponder An individual whose immune system does not respond well in antibody formation to antigenic stimulation.

Normal serum albumin *See* Albumin.

Northern blotting A variation of Southern blotting where, instead of DNA, RNA is run on the electrophoretic gel and transferred onto a blot for detection of specific RNA sequence.

Nucleic acid testing (NAT) General term used to describe diagnostic tests (predominately amplification tests: NAATs) based on detection of nucleic acid sequences unique for the organism (pathogen) in question.

Nucleosides Compounds consisting of one of nitrogen containing bases (A, T or U, C and G) and sugar deoxyribose or ribose. Depending on the base (adenine, thymine, uracil, cytosine, and guanine), the nucleosides are named: adenosine, thymidine, uridine, cytidine, and guanosine. Upon phosphorylation, they become nucleotides and are building blocks of nucleic acids: DNA or RNA.

Nucleotides Compounds consisting of one of nitrogen containing bases (A, T or U, C and G), sugar deoxyribose or ribose, and one, two, or three phosphates. Chemically, they are referred to as *nucleoside phosphates*. Nucleotides are the building blocks of nucleic acids: DNA or RNA.

O_h *See* Bombay.

Oligo-dT primers Universal primers starting cDNA synthesis from messenger RNA (mRNA) in the process of reverse transcription. These primers consist of several thymine nucleotides that are complementary to the poly-A tail of mRNA. These primers will not start cDNA synthesis from rRNA or tRNA because these molecules are missing the poly-A tail.

Oligonucleotide A short synthetic segment of DNA, approximately 20 nucleotides in length, used as a probe.

Oliguria Diminished amount of urine formation.

Opsonin A substance in serum that promotes immune adherence and facilitates phagocytosis by the reticuloendothelial system.

Origin of replication (Ori) In DNA, the sequence that signals the beginning of replication. In plasmids, they drive the replication of the foreign DNA fragments along with their own.

Orthostatic Concerning an erect position.

Osmolality The osmotic concentration of a solution determined by the ionic concentration of dissolved substances per unit of solvent.

Ouchterlony diffusion An immunologic procedure in which antibody and antigen are placed in wells of a gel medium plate and allowed to diffuse in order to visualize the reaction by a precipitin line.

Oxyhemoglobin The combined form of hemoglobin and oxygen.

P_{50} The partial pressure of oxygen or oxygen tension at which the hemoglobin molecule is 50% saturated with oxygen.

PAGE Polyacrylamide gel electrophoresis.

Palindromic sequences Four to 8 nucleotide DNA sequences that read the same in the 5′ to 3′ direction on both strands of the double helix—for example, 5′AAATTT3′ or 5′GAATTC3′.

Pallor Paleness; lack of color.

Panagglutinin An antibody capable of agglutinating all red blood cells tested, including the patient's own cells.

Pancytopenia A reduction in all cellular elements of the blood, including red blood cells, white blood cells, and platelets.

Panel A large number of group O reagent red blood cells that are of known antigenic characterization and are used for antibody identification.

Papain A proteolytic enzyme derived from papaya.

Paragloboside The immediate precursor for the H and P antigens of the red blood cell.

Parentage testing The analysis of one or more genetic markers in a group of individuals thought to be related as parent and child. The group normally consists of a known parent (often a mother), a child, and an alleged parent (often an alleged father). The goal of the testing is to confirm or refute the alleged relatedness of the tested individuals as parents and child.

Paroxysm A sudden, periodic attack or recurrence of symptoms of a disease.

Paroxysmal cold hemoglobinuria (PCH) A type of cold autoimmune hemolytic anemia usually found in children suffering from viral infections in which a biphasic immunoglobulin G antibody can be demonstrated with anti-P specificity. *See also* Donath-Landsteiner test.

Paroxysmal nocturnal hemoglobinuria (PNH) An intrinsic defect in the red blood cell membrane, rendering it more susceptible to hemolysins in an acid environment; characterized by hemoglobin in the urine following periods of sleep.

Partial D Red blood cells that are missing normal RhD epitopes, resulting in a qualitative difference in the RhD protein. Individuals with partial D can make anti-D.

Passenger lymphocytes Donor lymphocytes in the transplanted organ or HPC (hereditary progenitor cell) product.

Paternity index Term that refers to a statement of "weight" concerning the probability a tested individual, who cannot be excluded as the parent of the child, is the true parent. The paternity index represents a likelihood ratio that compares two mutually exclusive hypotheses. The numerator of the ratio reflects the probability the tested alleged parent is the true parent of the child and the denominator reflects the probability someone random and unrelated to the alleged parent is the true parent.

Perfusion Supplying an organ or tissue with nutrients and oxygen by passing blood or another suitable fluid through it.

Perioral paresthesia Tingling around the mouth occasionally experienced by apheresis donors, resulting from the rapid return of citrated plasma, which contains citrate-bound calcium and free citrate.

Peroxidase An enzyme that hastens the transfer of oxygen from peroxide to a tissue that requires oxygen; this process is essential to intracellular respiration.

Phagocytosis Ingestion of microorganisms, other cells, and foreign particles by a phagocyte.

Phenotype The outward expression of genes (e.g., a blood type). On blood cells, serologically demonstrable antigens constitute the phenotype, except those sugar sites that are determined by transferases.

Phenylthiocarbamide (PTC) A chemical used in studying medical genetics to detect the presence of a marker gene. About 70% of the population inherits the ability to taste PTC, which tastes bitter; the remaining 30% finds PTC tasteless. The inheritance of this trait is due to a single dominant gene of a pair.

Phlebotomy The procedure used to draw blood from a person.

Phosphoglyceromutase A red blood cell enzyme.

Phototherapy Exposure to sunlight or artificial light for therapeutic purposes.

Plasma The liquid portion of whole blood, containing water, electrolytes, glucose, fats, proteins, and gases. Plasma contains all the clotting factors necessary for coagulation but in an inactive form. Once coagulation occurs, the fluid is converted to serum.

Plasma cell A B lymphocyte–derived cell that secretes immunoglobulins or antibodies.

Plasmapheresis A procedure using a machine to remove only plasma from a donor or patient.

Plasma protein fraction (PPF) Also known as Plasmanate; sterile pooled plasma stored as a fluid or freeze-dried and used for volume replacement.

Plasmid Bacterial circular genetic element, 2 to 4 kb long, that replicates independently from the chromosome. Used as vectors in recombinant DNA technology to carry up to 15 kb foreign DNA into host cells. A vast selection of plasmids are commercially available that are useful for different purposes, such as DNA sequencing, protein expression in bacteria, and protein expression in mammalian cells.

Plasminogen A protein in many tissues and body fluids important in preventing fibrin clot formation.

Plasmodium *See* Malaria.

Plasmodium knowlesi A parasite that causes malaria in monkeys.

Platelet A round or oval disk, 2 to 4 μm in diameter, that is derived from the cytoplasm of the megakaryocyte, a large cell in the bone marrow. Platelets play an important role in blood coagulation, hemostasis, and blood thrombus formation. When a small vessel is injured, platelets adhere to each other and to the edges of the injury, forming a "plug" that covers the area and initially stops the blood loss.

Platelet concentrate Platelets prepared from a single unit of whole blood or plasma and suspended in a specific volume of the original plasma; also known as *random-donor platelets*.

Plateletpheresis A procedure using a machine to remove only platelets from a donor or patient.

Platelet refractoriness Failure to yield an increase in recipient's platelet count on transfusion of suitably preserved platelets. HLA alloimmunization is a common cause.

Point mutation A change in a base in DNA that can lead to a change in the amino acid incorporated into the polypeptide; identifiable by analysis of the amino acid sequences of the original protein and its mutant offspring.

Polarity (3′ and 5′ ends) Also called DNA "directionality," determines the direction of DNA replication and transcription. Results from the antiparallel way that the two strands of nucleotides ran in opposite directions. The labels 3′ and 5′ refer to the number assigned by convention to the deoxyribose' carbon atom linked to either hydroxyl or phosphate group in DNA molecule.

Polyacrylamide gel A polymer of acrylamide, used as a matrix for gel electrophoresis that provides better resolution than agarose electrophoresis.

Polyagglutination A state in which an individual's red blood cells are agglutinated by all sera, regardless of blood type.

Polyagglutinins Naturally occurring immunoglobulin antibodies that are found in most normal human adult sera.

Poly-A tail A long chain of adenine nucleotides that is added in the reaction of polyadenylation to a messenger RNA (mRNA) molecule during RNA processing to increase the stability of the molecule immediately after a gene in a eukaryotic cell is transcribed.

Polybrene A positively charged polymer that causes normal red blood cells to aggregate spontaneously by neutralizing the negative surface charge contributed by sialic acid.

Polyclonal Antibodies derived from more than one antibody-producing parent cell.

Polycythemia vera A chronic life-shortening myeloproliferative disorder involving all bone marrow elements, characterized by an increase in red blood cell mass and hemoglobin concentration.

Polylinker In plasmid, a region with a series of recognition sequences for different restriction endonucleases that may be used to introduce a foreign DNA fragment cut out of its original source with the corresponding enzymes.

Polymer Combination of two or more molecules of the same substance.

Polymerase chain reaction (PCR) An in vitro method of amplifying a specific fragment of DNA using thermostable DNA polymerase enzyme and short synthetic primers that attach to separated strands of DNA and are extended by the addition of deoxyribonucleotides in numerous cyclic changes of temperature. Each PCR cycle consists of denaturation, annealing, and extension (elongation).

Polymorphism A genetic system that possesses numerous allelic forms, such as a blood group system.

Polyspecific Coombs' sera A reagent that contains antihuman globulin sera against immunoglobulin G and C3d.

Polyvinylpyrrolidone (PVP) A neutral polymeric substance used to increase blood volume in patients with extensive blood loss; also used to enhance antigen-antibody reactions in vitro.

Portal hypertension Increased venous pressure in the portal vein as a result of obstruction of the flow of blood through the liver.

Postpartum Occurring after childbirth.

Potentiator A substance that, when added to a serum and cell mixture, will enhance antigen-antibody interactions.

Precipitation The formation of a visible complex (precipitate) in a medium containing soluble antigen (precipitinogen) and the corresponding antibody (precipitin).

Precipitin An antibody formed in the blood serum of an animal by the presence of a soluble antigen, usually a protein. When added to a solution of the antigen, it brings about precipitation. The injected protein is the antigen; the antibody produced is the precipitin.

Precursor substance A substance that is converted to another substance by the addition of a specific constituent (e.g., a sugar residue).

Pre-mRNA Immature messenger RNA right after synthesis in the nucleus. Also called heterogeneous RNA (hnRNA) because it consists of sequences transcribed from both: exons and introns. The introns (the noncoding fragments) are removed during mRNA processing (maturation) by excision (splicing).

Preseroconversion window A period of time during which a person may be infected with a viral pathogen (HIV, HCV, HBV, etc.) but does not yet produce levels of antibodies detectable by serologic methods.

Pretransfusion compatibility testing Series of testing procedures and processes with the ultimate objective of ensuring the best possible results of a blood transfusion, including recipient and donor identification, ABO testing, clerical checks, and so on.

Primer A short segment of single-stranded DNA, usually 17 to 25 nucleotides long, used to initiate DNA replication in PCR.

Primers (forward and reverse) Short, synthetic segments of single-stranded DNA, usually 15 to 25 nucleotides long, used to initiate DNA replication in PCR. Primers are designed to anneal to complementary DNA sequences at the 3′ end of each strand of the DNA fragment desired to be amplified and extended toward the 5′ end. The forward primer anneals to the antisense strand, and the reverse primer anneals to the sense strand.

Private antigen An antigenic characteristic of the red blood cell membrane that is unique to an individual or a related family of individuals and therefore is not commonly found on all cells (usually less than 1% of the population).

Probability of exclusion (PE) Refers to the strength of the test battery to exclude a falsely accused alleged parent.

Probability of parentage The probability of parentage is produced from the likelihood ratio (paternity index for example) using Bayesian statistical logic and reflects the level of conviction that the included alleged parent is the true parent of the child.

Probe A fragment of DNA that is labeled and hybridized to diagnostic material to locate a complementary strand of DNA.

Prodrome A symptom indicative of an approaching disease.

Propositus The initial individual whose condition led to investigation of a hereditary disorder or to a serologic evaluation of family members. Feminine form is proposita. Synonyms are *proband* and *index case*.

Prospective blood utilization review A blood utilization review that occurs prior to transfusion events and is often used to determine the appropriateness of a transfusion order request.

Prospective validation Validation testing of software; done before implementation of the computer system.

Prosthesis An artificial substitute for a missing part, such as an artificial extremity.

Protamine A polycation with applications similar to those of polybrene.

Protamine sulfate A substance used to neutralize the effects of heparin.

Prothrombin complex A concentrate of coagulation factors II, VII, IX, and X in lyophilized form.

Provirus A DNA form of a retrovirus, upon integration into the genome of the infected (host) cell.

Prozone Incomplete lattice formation caused by an excess of antibody molecules relative to the number of antigen sites, resulting in false-negative reactions.

PRP Platelet-rich plasma.

Public antigen An antigen characteristic of the red blood cell membrane found commonly among individuals, usually more than 98% of the population.

Pulmonary artery wedge pressure Pressure measured in the pulmonary artery at its capillary end.

Pulse pressure The difference between the systolic and the diastolic pressures.

Quality assurance (QA) A set of planned actions to provide confidence that systems and elements that influence the quality of the product or service are working as expected, individually and collectively.

Radioimmunoassay (RIA) A very sensitive method for determining substances present in low concentrations in serum or plasma by using specific antibodies and radioactively labeled or tagged substances.

Random man not excluded (RMNE) Refers to the opposite of probability of exclusion, which is the probability that someone who is falsely accused of being the parent would not be excluded by a particular genetic test. The relationship between PE and RMNE is, PE + RMNE = 1.

Random primers (random hexamers) Six-nucleotide-long sequences used as cDNA (**complementary DNA**) synthesis primers in the process of reverse transcription. Random primers will attach to any RNA molecule present in the reaction tube. The resulting cDNA represents the total RNA isolated from the cell, not just mRNA, which is reverse transcribed using oligo-dT primers.

Rapid passive hemagglutination assay (RPHA) A third-generation procedure used in hepatitis testing.

Rapid passive latex assay (RPLA) A second-generation procedure used in hepatitis testing.

Raynaud's disease A peripheral vascular disorder characterized by abnormal vasoconstriction of the extremities upon exposure to cold or emotional stress. A history of symptoms for at least 2 years is necessary for diagnosis.

Real-time PCR A variation of polymerase chain reaction in which the product formed during each cycle of amplification is detected by fluorescence at the same time that it is produced, instead of being detected after the reaction is finished. In addition to primers, the real-time reaction mixture contains DNA probes complementary to the region between the primers (so called TaqMan or molecular beacons or FRET probes), labeled with fluorophores that emit fluorescent light when binding to the newly synthesized amplicon.

Recessive A type of gene that, in the presence of its dominant allele, does not express itself; expression occurs when it is inherited in the homozygous state.

Recipient A patient who is receiving a transfusion of blood or a blood product.

Recombinant DNA technology A process of recombining two DNA fragments from different species and inserting such recombinant molecule into a host organism in order to produce new genetic combinations that are of value in medicine, science, and industry.

Recombinant proteins Proteins produced by translation of recombinant genes (created by the recombinant DNA technology).

Refractory Obstinate; stubborn; resistant to ordinary treatment; resistant to stimulation (said of a muscle or nerve).

Relationship testing *See* Parentage testing.

Renaturation *See* Annealing.

Replication The process of DNA synthesis based on the existing DNA molecule sequence (template) by enzyme DNA polymerase, which recognizes the 3′ end of the template and starts adding the nucleotides, synthesizing the new strand in the 5′ to 3′ direction (*see* polarity). The place where the two original strands are separating is called a *replication fork*—one strand is synthesized in a continuous manner and is called a *leading strand*, while the other strand's synthesis occurs in short fragments called *Okazaki fragments*, named after a Japanese researcher. This strand is called a *lagging strand* because it is formed slightly slower due to the polymerase constantly jumping toward the fork. DNA replication is said to be semiconservative.

Respiratory distress syndrome (RDS) A condition, formerly known as *hyaline membrane disease*, accounting for more than 25,000 infant deaths per year in the United States. Clinical signs, including delayed onset of respiration and low Apgar score, are usually present at birth.

Restriction endonucleases Bacterial enzymes that cleave DNA at specific sequences and allow scientists to cut DNA in a controlled and predictable way.

Restriction enzyme mapping Finding the sequences in a given DNA recognized by restriction enzymes and establishing the distance between such sites.

Restriction fragment length polymorphism (RFLP) Refers to a specific molecular tool that can be used to demonstrate nucleotide sequence polymorphisms in chromosomal DNA. A single nucleotide polymorphism can alter the spatial arrangement of restriction enzyme recognition sequences in chromosomal DNA that will be revealed following restriction enzyme digestion as an altered pattern of restriction fragments.

Reticulocyte Also known as *neocyte*, the last stage of development before becoming a mature erythrocyte. The reticulocyte has lost its nucleus but retains some residual RNA in its cytoplasm, which is stainable by special techniques. It may be slightly larger than the mature red blood cell.

Reticuloendothelial system (RES) The fixed phagocytic cells of the body, such as the macrophage, having the ability to ingest particulate matter.

Retrospective blood utilization review A blood utilization review that occurs after the transfusion events.

Retrospective validation Validation testing of software, which is done after the computer system has been implemented.

Retrovirus A virus in which the genetic material consists of two identical molecules of RNA that, upon entering the infected cell, are converted into DNA by the enzyme reverse transcriptase to form a "provirus" that may be integrated into the host's own genomic DNA.

Reverse genetics Technology in which genes can be inactivated ("knocked out") in the germ line of a mouse or other animal model in order to study systemic consequences of lack of function of the protein coded by that gene. The resulting model animal is a "knockout transgenic animal."

Reverse grouping Testing a patient's serum with commercial or reagent A and B red blood cells to determine which ABO antibodies are present.

Reverse transcription An enzymatic process, naturally occurring in retroviruses, in which RNA sequence is transcribed into the DNA sequence. In vitro reverse transcription may be performed using isolated or synthetic enzymes (reverse transcriptases) to obtain a complementary DNA (cDNA).

Rh immunoglobulin (RhIg) A concentrated, purified anti-Rh_0(D) prepared from human serum (of immunized donors) that is given to Rh_0(D)-negative mothers after they have given birth to an Rh_0(D)-positive baby or after abortion or miscarriage. It acts to prevent the mother from becoming immunized to any Rh_0(D)-positive fetal cells that may have entered her circulation and thereby prevents formation of anti-Rh_0(D) by the mother.

Rh_{mod} Rare Rh phenotype resulting from mutations in the *RHAG* gene, it can result in missing or significantly altered (reduced) RhD and RhCE antigen expression.

Rh-negative Red blood cells lacking the D antigen.

Rh_{null} Rare Rh phenotype in which no Rh antigens are expressed on the red blood cell; results from a mutation in the *RHAG* gene (regulator-type Rh_{null}) or by a deletion of the RHD gene (the amorphic type) and a mutation in *RHCE* genes.

Rh-positive Red blood cells possessing one particular Rh antigen, the D antigen.

Ribonucleic acid (RNA) A nucleic acid that controls protein synthesis in all living cells. There are three different types, and all are derived from the information encoded in the DNA of the cell. Messenger RNA (mRNA) carries the code for specific amino acid sequences from the DNA to the cytoplasm for protein synthesis. Transfer RNA (tRNA) carries the amino acid groups to the ribosome for protein synthesis. Ribosomal RNA (rRNA), which exists within the ribosomes, is thought to assist in protein synthesis.

Ribosome A cellular organelle that contains ribosomal RNA and protein and functions to synthesize protein. Ribosomes may be single units or clusters called *polyribosomes* or *polysomes*.

Rickettsia Any of the microorganisms belonging to the genus *Rickettsia*.

Ringer's lactated injection An aqueous solution suitable for intravenous use.

RNA interference Gene-regulating enzymatic activity of RNA molecules first discovered in nematode *Caenorhabditis elegans*. Also referred to as *gene silencing*. Interfering RNAs prevent mRNA from being translated into protein.

RNase RNA endonuclease, a ubiquitous enzyme that destroys RNA.

Rouleaux Coinlike stacking of red blood cells in the presence of plasma expanders or abnormal plasma proteins.

Saline anti-D A low-protein (6% to 8% albumin) immunoglobulin M anti-D reagent.

Salvia horminum Plant lectin used in the differentiation of various forms of polyagglutination.

Salvia sclarea Plant lectin with anti-Tn activity, used in the differentiation of various forms of polyagglutination.

Screening cells Group O reagent red blood cells that are used in antibody detection or screening tests.

SD Serologically defined antigens.

SDS-PAGE An electrophoretic technique using a polyacrylamide gel (PAGE), in which proteins are denatured by the negatively charged detergent sodium dodecyl sulfate (SDS), which masks their intrinsic electrical charge so that they are separated according to size, not electrical charge.

Secretor An individual who is capable of secreting soluble, glycoprotein ABH-soluble substances into saliva and other body fluids.

Semiconservative Term referring to the DNA replication model (proved by Meselson and Stahl), in which each double-stranded DNA molecule upon replication contains one parental and one newly synthesized complementary strand.

Sensitization A condition of being made sensitive to a specific substance (e.g., an antigen) after the initial exposure to that substance. This results in the development of immunologic memory that evokes an accentuated immune response with subsequent exposure to the substance.

Sepsis Pathological state, usually febrile, resulting from the presence of microorganisms or their toxins in the bloodstream.

Septicemia Presence of pathogenic bacteria in the blood.

Sequence-specific oligonucleotide probe (SSOP) hybridization A molecular method used in HLA testing, in which the individual's DNA is immobilized on a membrane as a dot-blot and incubated with a labeled complementary DNA probe designed to detect specific HLA sequence.

Sequence-specific PCR (SSP) A polymerase chain reaction method variant in which one of the primers is supposed to align exactly where the anticipated mutation is located (sequence-specific primer).

Sequence-specific primers (1) In reverse transcription: sequences used as cDNA (complementary DNA) synthesis primers when only a specific region of cDNA is desired (not cDNA representing total RNA or messenger (mRNA). (2) In PCR: primers designed to anneal to the specific mutated region of the DNA that is supposed to be amplified. In absence of mutation, the PCR product will either not be produced at all or will have a different length than the product resulting from the mutated DNA.

Sequencing A manual or automated process of deciphering the order of nucleotides in DNA to find various polymorphisms (mutations) relevant in biotechnology or clinical applications.

Serologic test for syphilis (STS) First developed in 1906 by Wassermann, present tests are of three main types based on complement fixation, flocculation, and detection of specific antitreponemal antibodies.

Serotonin A chemical present in platelets that is a potent vasoconstrictor.

Serum The fluid that remains after whole blood has clotted.

Sex chromosome Chromosomes associated with determination of sex.

Sex linkage A genetic characteristic located on the X or Y chromosome.

Shelf life The amount of time blood or blood products may be stored upon collection.

Shock A clinical syndrome in which the peripheral blood flow is inadequate to return sufficient blood to the heart for normal function, particularly transport of oxygen to all organs and tissues. Shock may be caused by a variety of conditions, including hemorrhage, infection, drug reaction, trauma, poisoning, myocardial infarction, or dehydration. Symptoms include paleness of skin (pallor), a bluish gray discoloration (cyanosis), a weak and rapid pulse, rapid and shallow breathing, or blood pressure that is decreased and perhaps immeasurable.

Short tandem repeats (STR) A type of genetic polymorphism demonstrated as back-to back repeats of sets of 1 to 8 nucleotides. The number of times each set is repeated is characteristic for each individual and is useful in kinship and crime investigations and in monitoring of graft success or rejection. *See also* microsatellites.

Sialic acid A group of sugars found on the red blood cell membrane attached to a protein backbone; the major source of the membrane's net negative charge.

Sickle cell anemia Hereditary, chronic hemolytic anemia characterized by large numbers of sickle-shaped red blood cells occurring almost exclusively in black people.

Sickle trait Blood that is heterozygous for the gene coding for the abnormal hemoglobin of sickle cell anemia.

Siderosis Increase of iron in the blood that can lead to organ damage.

Single-donor platelets Platelets collected from a single donor by apheresis.

Single nucleotide polymorphisms (SNP) Single-nucleotide differences between DNA sequences. The vast majority of these polymorphisms have no biological effect and are useful in genetic variation studies relevant to crime or kinship investigations.

Sodium dodecyl sulfate (SDS) An anionic detergent that renders a net negative charge to substances it solubilizes.

Software Written instructions for a computer, which result in information being stored, manipulated, and retrieved.

Solid phase test A blood group serology test method that uses red blood cell adherence on an endpoint instead of agglutination.

Somatic gene therapy Gene therapy in which the cells into which a new genetic material is introduced are the somatic cells (not the gametes) so that the material is not transmitted into the next generation.

Southern blotting Technique, developed by E. M. Southern, in which DNA is cut with one or more restriction endonucleases, the fragments are separated by agarose gel electrophoresis, transferred onto a membrane (blot), and incubated with a labeled detection probe (a short fragment of DNA complementary to the desired region).

Specificity The affinity of an antibody and the antigen against which it is directed.

Spectrin A dimeric structural protein of the red blood cell (RBC) cytoskeleton that maintains the shape of the cell by forming a network with other proteins such as actin and ankyrin. Spectrin defects lead to hereditary elliptocytosis or spherocytosis.

Splenomegaly Enlargement of the spleen.

Splicing The process of excision of introns (noncoding sequences) from the immature, newly synthesized RNA (pre-mRNA) in eukaryotes.

Spontaneous agglutination Direct agglutination of antibody-coated RBCs without the presence of antiserum; this usually occurs when RBCs are heavily coated with IgM or IgG autoantibody. Spontaneous agglutination differs from cold agglutination in that it is not dispersed when the sample is warmed to 37°C.

Steatorrhea Increased secretion of the sebaceous glands.

Stem cell An unspecialized cell, capable of self-renewal, that gives rise to a group of differential cells, such as the hematopoietic cells.

Steroid hormones Hormones of the adrenal cortex and the sex hormones.

Stertorous Pertaining to laborious breathing.

Sticky (cohesive) ends The ends of DNA sequence resulting from restriction enzymes that cut both strands leaving "overhangs" that are complementary to any end cut by the same enzyme. These ends will spontaneously join with complementary ends and do not require DNA ligase.

Storage lesion A loss of viability and function associated with certain biochemical changes that are initiated when blood is stored in vitro.

STR Small tandem repeat, or short tandem repeat. The name describes the molecular nature of the DNA that harbors this type of genetic marker, consisting of tetra- or pentanucleotide sequences that are tandemly repeated a variable number of times in unrelated individuals.

Stroma The red blood cell membrane that is left after hemolysis has occurred.

Subgroup Antigens within the ABO group that react less strongly with their corresponding antisera than do A and B antigens.

Survival studies A measure of the in vivo survival of transfused blood cells; usually performed with radioactive isotopes. Normal red blood cells survive approximately 100 to 120 days in circulation.

SYBR Green Fluorescent stain used in UV visualization of nucleic acids in electrophoretic gels or in real-time PCR to detect the amplified product of the reaction.

Syncytiotrophoblast The outermost fetal component of the placenta that allows for exchange of nutrients between the fetus and the mother.

Syngeneic Possessing identical genotypes, as monozygotic twins.

Synteny Genes that are closely situated on a chromosome but cannot be shown to be linked.

Systemic lupus erythematosus (SLE) A disseminated autoimmune disease characterized by anemia, thrombocytopenia, increased immunoglobulin G levels, and the presence of four immunoglobulin G antibodies: antinuclear antibody, antinucleoprotein antibody, anti-DNA antibody, and antihistone antibody; believed to be caused by suppressor T-cell dysfunction.

System manager A specially trained person who is responsible for the maintenance of an information system.

Systolic pressure Maximum blood pressure that occurs at ventricular contraction; upper value of a blood pressure reading.

Tachycardia Abnormally rapid heart action, usually defined as a heart rate greater than 100 beats per minute.

Tachypnea Abnormally rapid respirations.

TaqMan probes Also called *cleavage* or *hydrolysis* DNA probes used to detect the amplicon produced in real-time PCR. These probes, labeled with reporter and quencher molecules, bind to their complementary area in a single strand of DNA region between the primers and get in the way of the Taq polymerase synthesizing the new strand. The polymerase, in order to continue the synthesis, degrades the probe and the reporter and quencher molecules become separated, which results in emission of light.

Targeted review A type of prospective blood utilization review.

Template bleeding time The elapsed time a uniform incision made by a template and blade stops bleeding, which is a test of platelet function, assuming a normal platelet count.

Tetany A nervous affliction characterized by intermittent spasms of the muscles of the extremities.

Thalassemia major The homozygous form of deficient beta-chain synthesis, which is very severe and presents itself during childhood. Prognosis varies; however, the younger the child at disease onset, the less favorable the outcome.

Thermal amplitude The range of temperature over which an antibody demonstrates serologic and/or in vitro activity.

Thermocycler (or thermal cycler) A programmable heating and cooling machine used to conduct polymerase chain reaction.

Thrombin An enzyme that converts fibrinogen to fibrin so that a soluble clot can be formed.

Thrombocytopenia A reduction in platelet count below the normal level, which is associated with spontaneous hemorrhage.

Thrombotic thrombocytopenic purpura (TTP) A coagulation disorder characterized by (1) increased bleeding owing to a decreased number of platelets, (2) hemolytic anemia, (3) renal failure, and (4) changing neurological signs. The characteristic morphological lesion is thrombotic occlusion of small arteries or capillaries in various organs.

Thymidine An essential ingredient used in DNA synthesis and incorporated by T lymphocytes undergoing blast transformation in response to foreign HLA-D antigens in the mixed lymphocyte culture test.

Titer A measure of the strength of an antibody by testing its reactivity at increasing dilutions against the appropriate antigen. The reciprocal of the highest dilution that shows agglutination is the titer.

Titer score A method used to evaluate more precisely than simple dilution by comparing the titers of an antibody. Agglutination at each higher dilution is graded on a continuous scale; the total is the titer score.

Trait A characteristic that is inherited.

Trans The location of two or more genes on opposite chromosomes of a homologous pair.

Transcription The synthesis of RNA based on the sequence of DNA by the enzyme RNA polymerase. Process based on the principle of complementarity. The first stage of deciphering of the genetic code.

Transcription factor A protein that binds to DNA at a specific nucleotide sequence (a promoter or enhancer sequence) to influence the process of DNA transcription.

Transcription mediated amplification (TMA) Developed initially at Gen-Probe, TMA is a molecular method of detecting an organism by isothermal amplification of its RNA using enzyme reverse transcriptase to produce complementary DNA (cDNA), which is subsequently transcribed into multiple RNA molecules, which then undergo another reverse transcription. This cycle repeats several times, resulting in abundance of RNA to the levels that may be detected by chemiluminescent DNA probes.

Transferase An enzyme that catalyzes the transfer of atoms or groups of atoms from one chemical compound to another.

Transfer RNA (t-RNA) *See* Ribonucleic acid.

Transfuse To perform a transfusion.

Transfusion The injection of blood, a blood component, saline, or other fluids into the bloodstream.

Transfusion guidelines Documentation of indications and thresholds for transfusion that is approved by the hospital or facility and based on evidence-based literature.

Transfusion reaction An adverse response to a transfusion.

Transfusion safety officer A specialized member of the blood utilization management team involved with coordination, audits of transfusion records, quality assurance, and educational functions.

Translation The production of protein, according to the genetic code. An enzymatic process occurring in the ribosomes, during which a codon within messenger RNA (mRNA) is aligned with an anticodon from the transfer RNA (tRNA), which attaches a corresponding amino acid into the growing peptide chain.

Translocation Transfer of a portion of one chromosome to its allele.

Transmembrane protein A protein that crosses the red blood cell membrane and is present on both sides of the membrane.

Transposition The location of two genes on opposite chromosomes of a homologous pair.

Trypsin A proteolytic enzyme formed in the intestine.

Type and screen Testing a patient's blood for ABO, Rh, and unexpected antibodies (antibody screen). If no abnormalities exist in the ABO and Rh and no unexpected antibodies are detected in the antibody screen, then the recipient blood sample is retained in the event that subsequent serologic crossmatching is necessary.

Ulex europaeus *See* Anti-H lectin.

Ultracentrifugation Rapid and prolonged centrifugation, used to separate by density gradient those substances of various specific gravities.

Urticaria A vascular reaction of the skin similar to hives.

Vaccine A suspension of infectious organisms or components of them that is given as a form of passive immunization to establish resistance to the infectious disease caused by that organism.

Validation A systematic process of testing the hardware, software, and user components of an information system to ensure that they are functioning correctly for their intended purpose.

Value stream In Lean, identification of all the steps necessary to bring a finished product to the customer.

Valvular Relating to or having a valve.

Variable number of tandem repeats (VNTR) DNA regions composed of back-to-back repeated units ranging in size from 9 to 80 bp. Like other polymorphisms, the VNTRs are useful in genetic fingerprinting performed in kinship and crime investigations. *See also* minisatellites.

Variable region That portion of the immunoglobulin light and heavy chains where amino acid sequences vary tremendously, thereby permitting the different immunoglobulin molecules to recognize different antigenic determinants. In other words, the variable region determines the antigen against which the antibody will react, thus providing each antibody molecule with its unique specificity. The variable region is located at the amino terminal region of the molecule.

Vasculitis Inflammation of a blood or lymph vessel.

Vasoconstriction Constriction of blood vessels.

Vasodilation Dilation of blood vessels, especially small arteries and arterioles.

Vasovagal syncope Syncope resulting from hypotension caused by emotional stress, pain, acute blood loss, fear, or rapid rising from a recumbent position.

Vector In recombinant DNA technology, a molecule of known nucleotide sequence that is used to carry a foreign DNA fragment into a host organism in order to produce multiple copies using the host's replication. Most common vectors are extrachromosomal, circular DNA plasmids, or bacterial viruses (bacteriophages).

Venesection *See* Phlebotomy.

Venipuncture Puncture of a vein for any purpose.

Veno-occlusive disease Disease involving the veins of the liver associated with GVHD.

Venule A tiny vein continuous with a capillary.

Viability Ability of a cell to live or to survive for a reasonably normal life span.

Vicia graminea *See* Anti-N lectin.

Virion A complete virus particle; a unit of genetic material surrounded by a protective coat that serves as a vehicle for its transmission from one cell to another.

VNTR Variable number of tandem repeats.

von Willebrand's disease A congenital bleeding disorder.

von Willebrand's factor Coagulation factor VIII.

WAIHA Warm autoimmune hemolytic anemia. A hemolytic anemia caused by the patient's autoantibody that reacts at 37°C.

Waste Also called Muda, as used within Lean, an action that does not create value as defined by the customer.

Weak D A general term used to describe individuals with weakened expression of RhD. It represents a specific classification used to describe mutations in the RHD gene that cause changes in amino acids present in the transmembrane or intracellular region of the RhD protein, thus causing quantitative differences in the RhD protein.

Western blotting *See* Immunoblotting.

Wharton's jelly A gelatinous intercellular substance consisting of primitive connective tissue of the umbilical cord.

X chromosome The chromosome that determines female sex characteristics. The normal female has two X chromosomes, and the normal male has an X and a Y chromosome.

Xeno- Prefix indicating differing species. For example, a xenoantibody is an antibody produced in one species against an antigen present in another species. Synonym is *hetero-*.

Xenogeneic Transplantation between species.

Yaws An infectious nonvenereal disease caused by the spirochete *Treponema pertenue* and found mainly in humid equatorial regions.

Zeta potential The difference in charge density between the inner and outer layers of the ionic cloud that surrounds red blood cells in an electrolyte solution.

Zygosity testing The process through which DNA sequences are compared to assess whether individuals born from a multiple gestation (twins, triplets, etc.) are monozygotic (identical) or dizygotic (fraternal); often used to identify a suitable donor for organ transplantation or to estimate disease susceptibility risk if one sibling is affected.

Index

Page numbers followed by f indicate figures; t, tables; and b, boxes.

A

A antigen
    formation of, 123, 125f
    soluble, formation of, 126, 126f
A subgroups, in ABO blood group system, 127–132,
        128f, 128t, 129b, 129f, 129t, 130f, 131b
    weak, 131–132, 131t, 133f
AABB (American Association of Blood Banks),
        290–291
    standards of, pertaining to tissue, 593, 593t
AATB (American Association of Tissue Banks),
        594, 594t
ABH antigens
    in disease, 135–136
    formation of, 123, 124f, 124t, 125f
    on red blood cells, comparison of, with A, B, and
        H soluble substances, 127, 127b, 127t
ABO antibodies, 121–122
ABO blood group system, 119–148
    B subgroups in, weak, 133–134, 134t
    case study on, 145
    ethnic frequency of blood groups in,
        120, 122t
    genes for, interaction of *Hh* genes with, 123–125,
        124f, 125f, 126f
    genotypes and phenotypes of, 123b
    grouping/typing in
        benign cold autoantibodies and,
            442–443
        forward, 120, 120t
            ABO discrepancies between reverse
                grouping and, 141–143, 143–144t
        reverse, 120, 120t
            ABO discrepancies between forward
                grouping and, 141–143, 143–144t
        warm autoantibodies and, 452
    historical perspective on, 120–121, 120b, 120t
    inheritance of, 122–127
    molecular genetics of, 125–126
    in pretransfusion patient sample testing, 245
    routine testing, 120–121
    A subgroups of, 127–132, 128f, 128t, 129b, 129f,
        129t, 130f, 131b
        weak, 131–132, 131t, 133f
    testing for, in donor unit processing, 310
ABO discrepancies, 136–143, 143–144t, 145f
    between forward and reverse groupings, 141–143,
        143–144t
    group I, 136, 138, 138t
    group II, 138–140, 138t, 139t, 140t
    group III, 140–141, 140f, 140t
    group IV, 141–143, 141f, 141t, 142f, 142t
    investigations of, 267
    resolution of, 136, 137f
    simplified summary of, 145f
    from technical errors, 136, 136b

ABO incompatibility
    in hematopoietic progenitor cell transplantation,
        397, 397t
        transfusion therapy and, 399, 400t
    in hemolytic disease of fetus/newborn, 435–436,
        435t
Absorption, selection, in apheresis, 345–346, 346f
Achromatin, 31
Acid citrate-dextrose preservative solution, 8t
Acquired immunity, 47, 48t, 50
Acquired immunodeficiency syndrome, in donor
        history, 299
Acute hemolytic transfusion reaction (AHTR), 370,
        372–374, 372f, 373f
Additive solutions
    in platelet preservation, 19–20, 20b
    in red blood cell preservation, 8–10, 9b, 9t
    improved, 11
Adsorption, in antibody identification, 229–231, 230f,
        231f
Affinity, antibody, 63
Agarose, in gel electrophoresis, 84, 85
Agglutination
    in ABO testing, 120–121
    mixed-field. *See* Mixed-field agglutination.
Agglutination inhibition, in transfusion laboratory
        testing, 65
Agglutination reactions
    antigen-antibody ratio and, 66–67, 66f
    antihuman globulin reagents and, 70
    centrifugation and, 66
    chemical reduction of IgG and IgM molecules and,
        70–71
    enhancement media and, 67, 69t, 70f
    factors influencing, 66–71
    in gel test, 275, 276f
    immunoglobulin type and, 67, 68t
    low ionic strength solution media and,
        68–69
    pH and, 67
    polybrene and, 69
    polyethylene glycol and, 69
    protein media and, 68
    proteolytic enzymes and, 69–70
    temperature and, 67, 67f
Agglutinogen theory, 151
AGT. *See* Antiglobulin test (AGT).
AHG. *See* Antihuman globulin (AHG).
Albumin
    in antiglobulin test, 110
    as potentiator in antibody detection, 219
Aliquots
    platelet, preparation of, 317, 317b
    red blood cell, preparation of, 313–314
Alleles, 31
Allergic transfusion reactions, 375–376

Alloantibodies, 63
    detection and identification of, in warm
        autoimmune hemolytic anemia, 455–456,
        457t, 458t, 459t
Allograft failure, in tissue transplantation, 596
Alloimmune response, definition of, 440
Alloimmunization
    complicating transfusion, 384
    HLA, in hematopoietic progenitor cell
        transplantation, 399
Alloimmunized patients, blood groups typing of
        donors for, 97
Allosteric changes, in hemoglobin, 6
Allotypic variations, in immunoglobulins, 58
Alphanumeric terminology for Rh system, 153, 153t
American Association of Blood Banks (AABB),
        290–291
    standards of, pertaining to tissue, 593, 593t
American Association of Tissue Banks (AATB),
        594, 594t
Amino terminal, of immunoglobulin molecule, 56
Aminoacyl tRNA synthetases, 80
Amniocentesis, in HDFN management, 432
Amorph, 31
    O gene as, 122
Amorphic alleles, 174
Anaphylaxis, 72
Anemia
    hemolytic, autoimmune, 439–473. *See also*
        Autoimmune hemolytic anemia(s).
    in hemolytic disease of fetus/newborn, 429–430
ANG reagents, in tube antiglobulin test, 220
Annealing, in molecular testing, 79
Anti-complement, 103, 106, 106t
Anti-IgG, 103, 105–106
Antibiotics, in bacterial cloning, 85, 85b
Antibody(ies), 55. *See also* Immunoglobulins.
    ABO, 121–122
    blood group, characteristics of, 61–63
    characteristics of, 209t
    detection and identification of, 216–240. *See also*
        Antibody identification; Antibody screen.
        benign cold autoantibodies and, 444–445, 445t
        direct antiglobulin test and elution techniques
            in, 231–232
        to high-prevalence antigen, case study on,
            234, 234f
        immune, 62
        incomplete, 102
        to low-prevalence antigen, case study on,
            234, 235f
        in MNS system, 190–191
        monoclonal, 62, 103
        multiple, case study on, 233–234, 233f
        naturally occurring, 62
        nonagglutinating, 102

Antigen-Antibody Characteristic Chart*

ANTIGENS

Antigen System	Antigen Name	ISBT Name	Antigen Freq. % W	Antigen Freq. % B	RBC Antigen Expression at Birth	Antigen Distrib. Plasma/RBC	Demonstrates Dosage	Antigen Modification Enzyme/Other
Kidd	Jk^a	JK1	77	91	strong	RBC only	yes	Enz. ↑
	Jk^b	JK2	73	43	strong	RBC only	yes	Enz. ↑
		JK3	100	100	strong	RBC	no	Enz. ↑
Lewis	Le^a	LE1	22	23	nil	Plasma/RBC	no	Enz. ↑
	Le^b	LE2	72	55	nil	Plasma/RBC	no	Enz. ↑
†P	P1	P1PK1	79	94	moderate	RBC, platelets, WBC	individual variation	Enz. ↑ AET → ZZAP ↑
	P	GLOB1	100	100	moderate	RBC, platelets, WBC	no	Enz. ↑ AET → ZZAP ↑
	‡P^k	P1PK3	100	100	?	RBC, platelets, fibroblast	no	no
MNS	M	MNS1	78	70	strong	RBC only	yes	Enz. ↓ AET → ZZAP ↓
	N	MNS2	72	74	strong	RBC only	yes	Enz. ↓ AET → ZZAP →
	S	MNS3	55	37	strong	RBC only	yes	Enz. ↓ AET → ZZAP ↓
	s	MNS4	89	97	strong	RBC only	yes	Enz. ↓ AET → ZZAP ↓
	U	MNS5	100	100	strong	RBC only	no	Enz. → AET → ZZAP →
Lutheran	Lu^a	LU1	7.6	5.3	poor	RBC only	yes	Enz. → AET → ZZAP ↓
	Lu^b	LU2 LU3	99.8 >99.8	99.9	poor	RBC only	yes	Enz. → AET → ZZAP ↓

*This chart is to be used for general information only. Please refer to the appropriate chapter for more detailed information.
AET = 2-aminoethylisothiouronium bromide; ↑ = enhanced reactivity; → = no effect; ↓ = depressed reactivity; occ = occasionally; HDN = hemolytic disease of the newborn; HTR = hemolytic transfusion reaction; NRBC = non-red blood cell; RBC = red blood cell; WBC = white blood cell; ZZAP = dithiothreitol plus papain. PCH = paroxysmal cold hemoglobinuria; ↑ = enhanced reactivity;
†In the P system, phenotype P$_1$ contains both P1 P, and P^k antigens; phenotype P$_2$ contains only P antigens; phenotype p lacks both P1 P, and P^k antigens.
‡The P^k antigen is typically converted to P; therefore there is no P^k antigen detectable on adult cells. There are rare individuals (P$_1$^{k}, P$_2$^{k}) where p^k antigen is not converted to P.